RANG AND DALE'S
Pharmacology

Content Strategist: **Meghan Ziegler**
Content Development Specialist: **Alexandra Mortimer**
Content Coordinator: **Sam Crowe, Trinity Hutton**
Project Manager: **Joanna Souch**
Design: **Christian Bilbow**
Illustration Manager: **Brett MacNaughton**
Illustrator: **Peter Lamb, Antbits, Jason McAlexander**
Marketing Manager: **Melissa Darling**

RANG AND DALE'S
Pharmacology
EIGHTH EDITION

H P Rang MB BS MA DPhil Hon FBPharmacolS FMedSci FRS
Emeritus Professor of Pharmacology,
University College London, London, UK

J M Ritter DPhil FRCP FBPharmacolS FMedSci
Emeritus Professor of Clinical Pharmacology,
King's College London, and Medical Research Director, Quintiles,
London, UK

R J Flower PhD DSc FBPharmacolS FMedSci FRS
Professor, Biochemical Pharmacology,
The William Harvey Research Institute,
Barts and the London School of Medicine and Dentistry,
Queen Mary University of London, London, UK

G Henderson BSc PhD FBPharmacolS FSB
Professor of Pharmacology, University of Bristol, Bristol, UK

ELSEVIER
CHURCHILL
LIVINGSTONE

For additional online content visit
studentconsult

Student | CONSULT

ELSEVIER
CHURCHILL
LIVINGSTONE

an imprint of Elsevier Limited

© 2016, Elsevier Ltd. All rights reserved.

First edition 1987
Second edition 1991
Third edition 1995
Fourth edition 1999
Fifth edition 2003
Sixth edition 2007
Seventh edition 2012

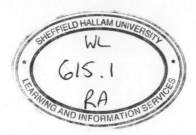

Notices

Knowledge and best practice in this field are constantly changing. As new research and experience broaden our understanding, changes in research methods, professional practices, or medical treatment may become necessary.

Practitioners and researchers must always rely on their own experience and knowledge in evaluating and using any information, methods, compounds, or experiments described herein. In using such information or methods they should be mindful of their own safety and the safety of others, including parties for whom they have a professional responsibility.

With respect to any drug or pharmaceutical products identified, readers are advised to check the most current information provided (i) on procedures featured or (ii) by the manufacturer of each product to be administered, to verify the recommended dose or formula, the method and duration of administration, and contraindications. It is the responsibility of practitioners, relying on their own experience and knowledge of their patients, to make diagnoses, to determine dosages and the best treatment for each individual patient, and to take all appropriate safety precautions.

To the fullest extent of the law, neither the Publisher nor the authors, contributors, or editors, assume any liability for any injury and/or damage to persons or property as a matter of products liability, negligence or otherwise, or from any use or operation of any methods, products, instructions, or ideas contained in the material herein.

ISBN:
Main edition
ISBN-13 978-0-7020-5362-7

International edition
ISBN-13 978-0-7020-5363-4

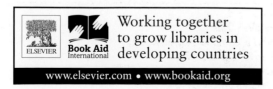

Working together
to grow libraries in
developing countries

www.elsevier.com • www.bookaid.org

Printed in China
Last digit is the print number: 9 8 7 6 5 4 3 2 1

Contents

Section 3: **Drugs affecting major organ systems**

21. The heart **247**

22. The vascular system **265**

23. Atherosclerosis and lipoprotein metabolism **285**

24. Haemostasis and thrombosis **293**

25. Haemopoietic system and treatment of anaemia **308**

26. Anti-inflammatory and immunosuppressant drugs **317**

27. Skin **335**

Section 4: **Nervous system**

Rang and Dale's Pharmacology
Eighth Edition Preface

In this edition, as in its predecessors, we set out not just to describe what drugs do but also to emphasise the mechanisms by which they act. This entails analysis not only at the cellular and molecular level, where knowledge and techniques are advancing rapidly, but also at the level of physiological mechanisms and pathological disturbances. Pharmacology has its roots in therapeutics, where the aim is to ameliorate the effects of disease, so we have attempted to make the link between effects at the molecular and cellular level and the range of beneficial and adverse effects that humans experience when drugs are used for therapeutic or other reasons. Therapeutic agents have a high rate of obsolescence, and more than 100 new ones have been approved since the last edition of this book. An appreciation of the mechanisms of action of the class of drugs to which a new agent belongs provides a good starting point for understanding and using a new compound intelligently.

Pharmacology is a lively scientific discipline in its own right, with an importance beyond that of providing a basis for the use of drugs in therapy, and we aim to provide a good background, not only for future doctors but also for scientists in other disciplines who need to understand how drugs act. We have, therefore, where appropriate, described how drugs are used as probes for elucidating cellular and physiological functions, even when the compounds have no clinical use.

Names of drugs and related chemicals are established through usage and sometimes there is more than one name in common use. For prescribing purposes, it is important to use standard names, and we follow, as far as possible, the World Health Organization's list of recommended international non-proprietary names (rINN). Sometimes these conflict with the familiar names of drugs (e.g. amphetamine becomes amfetamine in the rINN list), and the endogenous mediator prostaglandin I_2 – the standard name in the scientific literature – becomes 'epoprostenol' – a name unfamiliar to most scientists – in the rINN list. In general, we use rINN names as far as possible in the context of therapeutic use, but often use the common name in describing mediators and familiar drugs. Sometimes English and American usage varies (as with adrenaline/epinephrine and noradrenaline/norepinephrine). Adrenaline and noradrenaline are the official names in EU member states and relate clearly to terms such as 'noradrenergic', 'adrenoceptor' and 'adrenal gland' and we prefer them for these reasons.

Drug action can be understood only in the context of what else is happening in the body. So at the beginning of most chapters, we briefly discuss the physiological and biochemical processes relevant to the action of the drugs described in that chapter. We have included the chemical structures of drugs only where this information helps in understanding their pharmacological and pharmacokinetic characteristics, secure in the knowledge that chemical structures are readily available online.

The overall organisation of the book has been retained, with sections covering: (1) the general principles of drug action; (2) the chemical mediators and cellular mechanisms with which drugs interact in producing their therapeutic effects; (3) the action of drugs on specific organ systems; (4) the action of drugs on the nervous system; (5) the action of drugs used to treat infectious diseases and cancer; (6) a range of special topics such as adverse effects, non-medical uses of drugs, etc. This organisation reflects our belief that drug action needs to be understood, not as a mere description of the effects of individual drugs and their uses, but as a chemical intervention that perturbs the network of chemical and cellular signalling that underlies the function of any living organism. In addition to updating all of the chapters, we have covered the receptor-related topics of biased agonism, allosteric modulation and desensitisation in more detail in Chapters 2 and 3, as well as revamping the section on nuclear receptors. A new Chapter 27 on the pharmacology of the skin has been added, and Chapters 17 and 18 on local hormones have been revised. Additional material on cognition-enhancing drugs has been included in Chapter 48.

Despite the fact that pharmacology, like other branches of biomedical science, advances steadily, with the acquisition of new information, the development of new concepts and the introduction of new drugs for clinical use, we have avoided making the 8th edition any longer than its predecessor by cutting out-dated and obsolete material, and have made extensive use of small print text to cover more specialised and speculative information that is not essential to understanding the key message, but will, we hope, be helpful to students seeking to go into greater depth. In selecting new material for inclusion, we have taken into account not only new agents but also recent extensions of basic knowledge that presage further drug development. And where possible, we have given a brief outline of new treatments in the pipeline. Reference lists are largely restricted to guidance on further reading, together with review articles that list key original papers.

ACKNOWLEDGEMENTS

We would like to thank the following for their help and advice in the preparation of this edition: Dr Alistair Corbett, Dr Hannah Gill, Professor Eamonn Kelly, Professor Alastair Poole, Dr Emma Robinson, Dr Maria Usowicz and Professor Federica Marelli-Berg. We would like to put on record our appreciation of the team at Elsevier who worked on this edition: Meghan Ziegler (commissioning editor), Alexandra Mortimer (development editor), Joanna Souch (project manager), Brett MacNaughton (illustration manager), Peter Lamb, Antbits and Jason McAlexander (freelance illustrators), Elaine Leek (freelance copyeditor), Marcela Holmes (freelance proofreader) and Innodata Inc. (freelance indexing services).

London 2014

H. P. Rang
J. M. Ritter
R. J. Flower
G. Henderson

What is pharmacology?

OVERVIEW

In this introductory chapter we explain how pharmacology came into being and evolved as a scientific discipline, and describe the present day structure of the subject and its links to other biomedical sciences. The structure that has emerged forms the basis of the organisation of the rest of the book. Readers in a hurry to get to the here-and-now of pharmacology can safely skip this chapter.

WHAT IS A DRUG?

For the purposes of this book, a drug can be defined as *a chemical substance of known structure, other than a nutrient or an essential dietary ingredient,*[1] *which, when administered to a living organism, produces a biological effect.*

A few points are worth noting. Drugs may be synthetic chemicals, chemicals obtained from plants or animals, or products of genetic engineering. A *medicine* is a chemical preparation, which usually, but not necessarily, contains one or more drugs, administered with the intention of producing a therapeutic effect. Medicines usually contain other substances (excipients, stabilisers, solvents, etc.) besides the active drug, to make them more convenient to use. To count as a drug, the substance must be administered as such, rather than released by physiological mechanisms. Many substances, such as insulin or thyroxine, are endogenous hormones but are also drugs when they are administered intentionally. Many drugs are not used in medicines but are nevertheless useful research tools. In everyday parlance, the word *drug* is often associated with addictive, narcotic or mind-altering substances – an unfortunate negative connotation that tends to bias uninformed opinion against any form of chemical therapy. In this book we focus mainly on drugs used for therapeutic purposes but also describe important examples of drugs used as experimental tools. Although poisons fall strictly within the definition of drugs, they are not covered in this book.

ORIGINS AND ANTECEDENTS

Pharmacology can be defined as the study of the effects of drugs on the function of living systems. As a science, it was born in the mid-19th century, one of a host of new biomedical sciences based on principles of experimentation rather than dogma that came into being in that remarkable period. Long before that – indeed from the dawn of civilisation – herbal remedies were widely used,

pharmacopoeias were written, and the apothecaries' trade flourished. However, nothing resembling scientific principles was applied to therapeutics, which was known at that time as *materia medica*.[2] Even Robert Boyle, who laid the scientific foundations of chemistry in the middle of the 17th century, was content, when dealing with therapeutics (*A Collection of Choice Remedies*, 1692), to recommend concoctions of worms, dung, urine and the moss from a dead man's skull. The impetus for pharmacology came from the need to improve the outcome of therapeutic intervention by doctors, who were at that time skilled at clinical observation and diagnosis but broadly ineffectual when it came to treatment.[3] Until the late 19th century, knowledge of the normal and abnormal functioning of the body was too rudimentary to provide even a rough basis for understanding drug effects; at the same time, disease and death were regarded as semisacred subjects, appropriately dealt with by authoritarian, rather than scientific, doctrines. Clinical practice often displayed an obedience to authority and ignored what appear to be easily ascertainable facts. For example, cinchona bark was recognised as a specific and effective treatment for malaria, and a sound protocol for its use was laid down by Lind in 1765. In 1804, however, Johnson declared it to be unsafe until the fever had subsided, and he recommended instead the use of large doses of calomel (mercurous chloride) in the early stages – a murderous piece of advice that was slavishly followed for the next 40 years.

The motivation for understanding what drugs can and cannot do came from clinical practice, but the science could be built only on the basis of secure foundations in physiology, pathology and chemistry. It was not until 1858 that Virchow proposed the cell theory. The first use of a structural formula to describe a chemical compound was in 1868. Bacteria as a cause of disease were discovered by Pasteur in 1878. Previously, pharmacology hardly had the legs to stand on, and we may wonder at the bold vision of Rudolf Buchheim, who created the first pharmacology institute (in his own house) in Estonia in 1847.

In its beginnings, before the advent of synthetic organic chemistry, pharmacology concerned itself exclusively with understanding the effects of natural substances, mainly plant extracts – and a few (mainly toxic) chemicals such as mercury and arsenic. An early development in chemistry was the purification of active compounds from plants. Friedrich Sertürner, a young German apothecary, purified morphine from opium in 1805. Other substances quickly followed, and, even though their structures were unknown, these compounds showed that chemicals, not magic or vital forces, were responsible for the effects that

---

[1]Like most definitions, this one has its limits. For example, there are a number of essential dietary constituents, such as iron and various vitamins, that are used as medicines. Furthermore, some biological products (e.g. **epoietin**) show batch-to-batch variation in their chemical constitution that significantly affects their properties.

[2]The name persists today in some ancient universities, being attached to chairs of what we would call clinical pharmacology.
[3]Oliver Wendell Holmes, an eminent physician, wrote in 1860: '[I] firmly believe that if the whole materia medica, as now used, could be sunk to the bottom of the sea, it would be all the better for mankind and the worse for the fishes' (see Porter, 1997).

plant extracts produced on living organisms. Early pharmacologists focused most of their attention on such plant-derived drugs as quinine, digitalis, atropine, ephedrine, strychnine and others (many of which are still used today and will have become old friends by the time you have finished reading this book).[4]

PHARMACOLOGY IN THE 20TH AND 21ST CENTURIES

Beginning in the 20th century, the fresh wind of synthetic chemistry began to revolutionise the pharmaceutical industry, and with it the science of pharmacology. New synthetic drugs, such as barbiturates and local anaesthetics, began to appear, and the era of antimicrobial chemotherapy began with the discovery by Paul Ehrlich in 1909 of arsenical compounds for treating syphilis. Further breakthroughs came when the sulfonamides, the first antibacterial drugs, were discovered by Gerhard Domagk in 1935, and with the development of penicillin by Chain and Florey during the Second World War, based on the earlier work of Fleming.

These few well-known examples show how the growth of synthetic chemistry, and the resurgence of natural product chemistry, caused a dramatic revitalisation of therapeutics in the first half of the 20th century. Each new drug class that emerged gave pharmacologists a new challenge, and it was then that pharmacology really established its identity and its status among the biomedical sciences.

In parallel with the exuberant proliferation of therapeutic molecules – driven mainly by chemistry – which gave pharmacologists so much to think about, physiology was also making rapid progress, particularly in relation to chemical mediators, which are discussed in depth elsewhere in this book. Many hormones, neurotransmitters and inflammatory mediators were discovered in this period, and the realisation that chemical communication plays a central role in almost every regulatory mechanism that our bodies possess immediately established a large area of common ground between physiology and pharmacology, for interactions between chemical substances and living systems were exactly what pharmacologists had been preoccupied with from the outset. The concept of 'receptors' for chemical mediators, first proposed by Langley in 1905, was quickly taken up by pharmacologists such as Clark, Gaddum, Schild and others and is a constant theme in present-day pharmacology (as you will soon discover as you plough through the next two chapters). The receptor concept, and the technologies developed from it, have had a massive impact on drug discovery

and therapeutics. Biochemistry also emerged as a distinct science early in the 20th century, and the discovery of enzymes and the delineation of biochemical pathways provided yet another framework for understanding drug effects. The picture of pharmacology that emerges from this brief glance at history (Fig. 1.1) is of a subject evolved from ancient prescientific therapeutics, involved in commerce from the 17th century onwards, and which gained respectability by donning the trappings of science as soon as this became possible in the mid-19th century. Signs of its carpetbagger past still cling to pharmacology, for the pharmaceutical industry has become very big business and much pharmacological research nowadays takes place in a commercial environment, a rougher and more pragmatic place than the glades of academia.[5] No other biomedical 'ology' is so close to Mammon.

ALTERNATIVE THERAPEUTIC PRINCIPLES

Modern medicine relies heavily on drugs as the main tool of therapeutics. Other therapeutic procedures, such as surgery, diet, exercise, psychological treatments etc., are also important, of course, as is deliberate non-intervention, but none is so widely applied as drug-based therapeutics.

Before the advent of science-based approaches, repeated attempts were made to construct systems of therapeutics, many of which produced even worse results than pure empiricism. One of these was *allopathy*, espoused by James Gregory (1735–1821). The favoured remedies included blood letting, emetics and purgatives, which were used until the dominant symptoms of the disease were suppressed. Many patients died from such treatment, and it was in reaction against it that Hahnemann introduced the practice of *homeopathy* in the early 19th century. The implausible guiding principles of homeopathy are:

- like cures like
- activity can be enhanced by dilution.

The system rapidly drifted into absurdity: for example, Hahnemann recommended the use of drugs at dilutions of $1:10^{60}$, equivalent to one molecule in a sphere the size of the orbit of Neptune.

Many other systems of therapeutics have come and gone, and the variety of dogmatic principles that they embodied have tended to hinder rather than advance scientific progress. Currently, therapeutic systems that have a basis that lies outside the domain of science are actually gaining ground under the general banner of 'alternative' or 'complementary' medicine. Mostly, they reject the 'medical model', which attributes disease to an underlying derangement of normal function that can be defined in biochemical or structural terms, detected by objective means, and influenced beneficially by appropriate chemical or physical interventions. They focus instead mainly on subjective malaise, which may be disease-associated or

---

[4]A handful of synthetic substances achieved pharmacological prominence long before the era of synthetic chemistry began. Diethyl ether, first prepared as 'sweet oil of vitriol' in the 16th century, and nitrous oxide, prepared by Humphrey Davy in 1799, were used to liven up parties before being introduced as anaesthetic agents in the mid-19th century (see Ch. 41). Amyl nitrite (see Ch. 21) was made in 1859 and can claim to be the first 'rational' therapeutic drug; its therapeutic effect in angina was predicted on the basis of its physiological effects – a true 'pharmacologist's drug' and the smelly forerunner of the nitrovasodilators that are widely used today. Aspirin (Ch. 26), the most widely used therapeutic drug in history, was first synthesised in 1853, with no therapeutic application in mind. It was rediscovered in 1897 in the laboratories of the German company Bayer, who were seeking a less toxic derivative of salicylic acid. Bayer commercialised aspirin in 1899 and made a fortune.

[5]Some of our most distinguished pharmacological pioneers made their careers in industry: for example, Henry Dale, who laid the foundations of our knowledge of chemical transmission and the autonomic nervous system (Ch. 12); George Hitchings and Gertrude Elion, who described the antimetabolite principle and produced the first effective anticancer drugs (Ch. 56); and James Black, who introduced the first β-adrenoceptor and histamine H_2-receptor antagonists (Chs 13 and 17). It is no accident that in this book, where we focus on the scientific principles of pharmacology, most of our examples are products of industry, not of nature.

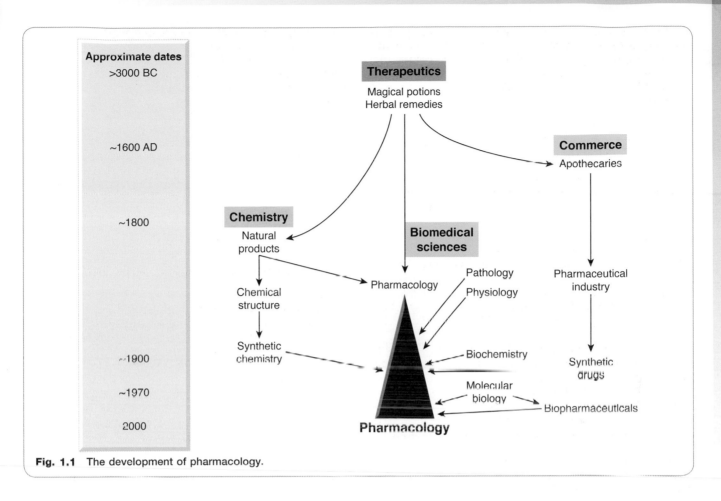

Fig. 1.1 The development of pharmacology.

not. Abandoning objectivity in defining and measuring disease goes along with a similar departure from scientific principles in assessing therapeutic efficacy and risk, with the result that principles and practices can gain acceptance without satisfying any of the criteria of validity that would convince a critical scientist, and that are required by law to be satisfied before a new drug can be introduced into therapy. Demand for 'alternative' therapies by the general public, alas, has little to do with demonstrable efficacy.[6]

THE EMERGENCE OF BIOTECHNOLOGY

Since the 1980s, biotechnology has emerged as a major source of new therapeutic agents in the form of antibodies, enzymes and various regulatory proteins, including hormones, growth factors and cytokines (see Buckel, 1996; Walsh, 2003). Although such products (known as *biopharmaceuticals*) are generally produced by genetic engineering rather than by synthetic chemistry, the pharmacological principles are essentially the same as for conventional drugs. Looking further ahead, gene- and cell-based therapies (Ch. 59), although still in their infancy, will take therapeutics into a new domain. The principles governing the design, delivery and control of functioning artificial genes introduced into cells, or of engineered cells intro-

duced into the body, are very different from those of drug-based therapeutics and will require a different conceptual framework, which texts such as this will increasingly need to embrace if they are to stay abreast of modern medical treatment.

PHARMACOLOGY TODAY

As with other biomedical disciplines, the boundaries of pharmacology are not sharply defined, nor are they constant. Its exponents are, as befits pragmatists, ever ready to poach on the territory and techniques of other disciplines. If it ever had a conceptual and technical core that it could really call its own, this has now dwindled almost to the point of extinction, and the subject is defined by its purpose – to understand what drugs do to living organisms, and more particularly how their effects can be applied to therapeutics – rather than by its scientific coherence.

Figure 1.2 shows the structure of pharmacology as it appears today. Within the main subject fall a number of compartments (neuropharmacology, immunopharmacology, pharmacokinetics, etc.), which are convenient, if not watertight, subdivisions. These topics form the main subject matter of this book. Around the edges are several interface disciplines, not covered in this book, which form important two-way bridges between pharmacology and other fields of biomedicine. Pharmacology tends to have more of these than other disciplines. Recent arrivals on the fringe are subjects such as pharmacogenomics, pharmacoepidemiology and pharmacoeconomics.

---

[6]The UK Medicines and Healthcare Regulatory Agency (MHRA) requires detailed evidence of therapeutic efficacy based on controlled clinical trials before a new drug is registered, but no clinical trials data for homeopathic products or for the many herbal medicines that were on sale before the Medicines Act of 1968.

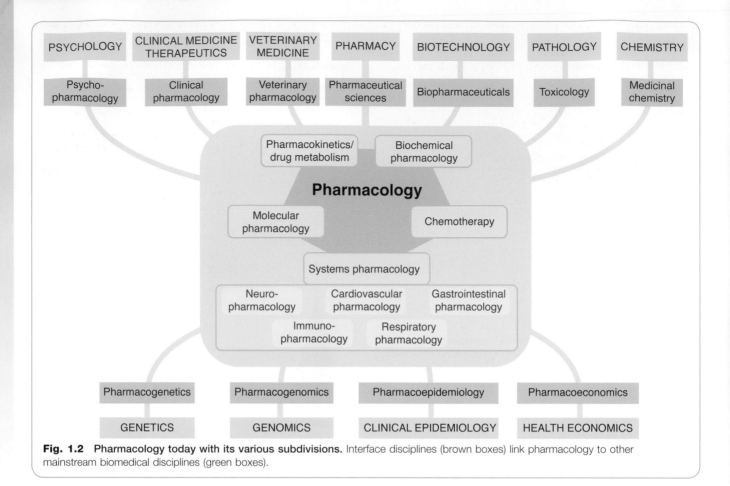

Fig. 1.2 Pharmacology today with its various subdivisions. Interface disciplines (brown boxes) link pharmacology to other mainstream biomedical disciplines (green boxes).

Biotechnology. Originally, this was the production of drugs or other useful products by biological means (e.g. antibiotic production from microorganisms or production of monoclonal antibodies). Currently, in the biomedical sphere biotechnology refers mainly to the use of recombinant DNA technology for a wide variety of purposes, including the manufacture of therapeutic proteins, diagnostics, genotyping, production of transgenic animals, etc. The many non-medical applications include agriculture, forensics, environmental sciences, etc.

Pharmacogenetics. This is the study of genetic influences on responses to drugs, discussed in Chapter 11. Originally, pharmacogenetics focused on familial idiosyncratic drug reactions, where affected individuals show an abnormal – usually adverse – response to a class of drug (see Nebert & Weber, 1990). It now covers broader variations in drug response, where the genetic basis is more complex.

Pharmacogenomics. This recent term overlaps with pharmacogenetics, describing the use of genetic information to guide the choice of drug therapy on an individual basis. The underlying principle is that differences between individuals in their response to therapeutic drugs can be predicted from their genetic make-up. Examples that confirm this are steadily accumulating (see Ch. 11). So far, they mainly involve genetic polymorphism of drug-metabolising enzymes or receptors. Ultimately, linking specific gene variations with variations in therapeutic or unwanted effects of a particular drug should enable the tailoring of therapeutic choices on the basis of an

individual's genotype. Steady improvements in the cost and feasibility of individual genotyping will increase its applicability, potentially with far-reaching consequences for therapeutics (see Ch. 11).

Pharmacoepidemiology. This is the study of drug effects at the population level (see Strom, 2005). It is concerned with the variability of drug effects between individuals in a population, and between populations. It is an increasingly important topic in the eyes of the regulatory authorities who decide whether or not new drugs can be licensed for therapeutic use. Variability between individuals or populations detracts from the utility of a drug, even though its overall effect level may be satisfactory. Pharmacoepidemiological studies also take into account patient compliance and other factors that apply when the drug is used under real-life conditions.

Pharmacoeconomics. This branch of health economics aims to quantify in economic terms the cost and benefit of drugs used therapeutically. It arose from the concern of many governments to provide for healthcare from tax revenues, raising questions of what therapeutic procedures represent the best value for money. This, of course, raises fierce controversy, because it ultimately comes down to putting monetary value on health and longevity. As with pharmacoepidemiology, regulatory authorities are increasingly requiring economic analysis, as well as evidence of individual benefit, when making decisions on licensing. For more information on this complex subject, see Drummond et al. (1997) and Rascati (2009).

REFERENCES AND FURTHER READING

Buckel, P., 1996. Recombinant proteins for therapy. Trends Pharmacol. Sci. 17, 450–456. (*Thoughtful review of the status of, and prospects for, protein-based therapeutics*)

Drummond, M.F., O'Brien, B., Stoddart, G.I., Torrance, G.W., 1997. Methods for the Economic Evaluation of Healthcare Programmes. Oxford University Press, Oxford. (*Coverage of the general principles of evaluating the economic costs and benefits of healthcare, including drug-based therapeutics*)

Nebert, D.W., Weber, W.W., 1990. Pharmacogenetics. In: Pratt, W.B., Taylor, P. (Eds.), Principles of Drug Action, third ed. Churchill Livingstone, New York. (*A detailed account of genetic factors that affect responses to drugs, with many examples from the pregenomic literature*)

Porter, R., 1997. The Greatest Benefit to Mankind. Harper-Collins, London. (*An excellent and readable account of the history of medicine, with good coverage of the early development of pharmacology and the pharmaceutical industry*)

Rascati, K.L., 2009. Essentials of Pharmacoeconomics. Lippincott Williams & Wilkins, Philadelphia.

Strom, B.L. (Ed.), 2005. Pharmacoepidemiology, fourth ed. Wiley, Chichester. (*A multiauthor book covering all aspects of a newly emerged discipline, including aspects of pharmacoeconomics*)

Walsh, G., 2003. Biopharmaceuticals: Biochemistry and Biotechnology. Wiley, Chichester. (*Good introductory textbook covering many aspects of biotechnology-based therapeutics*)

2 How drugs act: general principles

OVERVIEW

The emergence of pharmacology as a science came when the emphasis shifted from describing what drugs do to explaining how they work. In this chapter we set out some general principles underlying the interaction of drugs with living systems (Ch. 3 goes into the molecular aspects in more detail). The interaction between drugs and cells is described, followed by a more detailed examination of different types of drug–receptor interaction. We are still far from the holy grail of being able to predict the pharmacological effects of a novel chemical substance, or to design *ab initio* a chemical to produce a specified therapeutic effect; nevertheless, we can identify some important general principles, which is our purpose in this chapter.

INTRODUCTION

To begin with, we should gratefully acknowledge Paul Ehrlich for insisting that drug action must be explicable in terms of conventional chemical interactions between drugs and tissues, and for dispelling the idea that the remarkable potency and specificity of action of some drugs put them somehow out of reach of chemistry and physics and required the intervention of magical 'vital forces'. Although many drugs produce effects in extraordinarily low doses and concentrations, low concentrations still involve very large numbers of molecules. One drop of a solution of a drug at only 10^{-10} mol/l still contains about 3×10^9 drug molecules, so there is no mystery in the fact that it may produce an obvious pharmacological response. Some bacterial toxins (e.g. diphtheria toxin) act with such precision that a single molecule taken up by a target cell is sufficient to kill it.

One of the basic tenets of pharmacology is that drug molecules must exert some chemical influence on one or more cell constituents in order to produce a pharmacological response. In other words, drug molecules must get so close to these constituent cellular molecules that the two interact chemically in such a way that the function of the latter is altered. Of course, the molecules in the organism vastly outnumber the drug molecules, and if the drug molecules were merely distributed at random, the chance of interaction with any particular class of cellular molecule would be negligible. Pharmacological effects, therefore, require, in general, the non-uniform distribution of the drug molecule within the body or tissue, which is the same as saying that drug molecules must be 'bound' to particular constituents of cells and tissues in order to produce an effect. Ehrlich summed it up thus: '*Corpora non agunt nisi fixata*' (in this context, 'A drug will not work unless it is bound').[1]

These critical binding sites are often referred to as 'drug targets' (an obvious allusion to Ehrlich's famous phrase 'magic bullets', describing the potential of antimicrobial drugs). The mechanisms by which the association of a drug molecule with its target leads to a physiological response constitute the major thrust of pharmacological research. Most drug targets are protein molecules. Even general anaesthetics (see Ch. 41), which were long thought to produce their effects by an interaction with membrane lipid, now appear to interact mainly with membrane proteins (see Franks, 2008).

All rules need exceptions, and many antimicrobial and antitumour drugs (Chs 51 and 56), as well as mutagenic and carcinogenic agents (Ch. 57), interact directly with DNA rather than protein; bisphosphonates, used to treat osteoporosis (Ch. 36), bind to calcium salts in the bone matrix, rendering it toxic to osteoclasts, much like rat poison. There are also exceptions among the new generation of *biopharmaceutical drugs* that include nucleic acids, proteins and antibodies (see Ch. 59).

PROTEIN TARGETS FOR DRUG BINDING

Four main kinds of regulatory protein are commonly involved as primary drug targets, namely:

- receptors
- enzymes
- carrier molecules (transporters)
- ion channels.

Furthermore, many drugs bind (in addition to their primary targets) to plasma proteins (see Ch. 8) and other tissue proteins, without producing any obvious physiological effect. Nevertheless, the generalisation that most drugs act on one or other of the four types of protein listed above serves as a good starting point.

Further discussion of the mechanisms by which such binding leads to cellular responses is given in Chapters 3–4.

DRUG RECEPTORS

WHAT DO WE MEAN BY RECEPTORS?

▼ As emphasised in Chapter 1, the concept of receptors is central to pharmacology, and the term is most often used to describe the target molecules through which soluble physiological mediators – hormones, neurotransmitters, inflammatory mediators, etc.

---

[1]There are, if one looks hard enough, exceptions to Ehrlich's dictum – drugs that act without being bound to any tissue constituent (e.g. osmotic diuretics, osmotic purgatives, antacids and heavy metal chelating agents). Nonetheless, the principle remains true for the great majority.

Targets for drug action

- A drug is a chemical applied to a physiological system that affects its function in a specific way.
- With few exceptions, drugs act on target proteins, namely:
  - receptors
  - enzymes
  - carriers
  - ion channels.
- The term *receptor* is used in different ways. In pharmacology, it describes protein molecules whose function is to recognise and respond to endogenous chemical signals. Other macromolecules with which drugs interact to produce their effects are known as *drug targets*.
- Specificity is reciprocal: individual classes of drug bind only to certain targets, and individual targets recognise only certain classes of drug.
- No drugs are completely specific in their actions. In many cases, increasing the dose of a drug will cause it to affect targets other than the principal one, and this can lead to side effects.

– produce their effects. Examples such as acetylcholine receptors, cytokine receptors, steroid receptors and growth hormone receptors abound in this book, and generally the term *receptor* indicates a recognition molecule for a chemical mediator through which a response is transduced.

'Receptor' is sometimes used to denote *any* target molecule with which a drug molecule (i.e. a foreign compound rather than an endogenous mediator) has to combine in order to elicit its specific effect. For example, the voltage-sensitive sodium channel is sometimes referred to as the 'receptor' for **local anaesthetics** (see Ch. 43), or the enzyme dihydrofolate reductase as the 'receptor' for **methotrexate** (Ch. 50). The term *drug target*, of which receptors are one type, is preferable in this context.

In the more general context of cell biology, the term receptor is used to describe various cell surface molecules (such as *T-cell receptors, integrins, Toll receptors*, etc; see Ch. 6) involved in the cell-to-cell interactions that are important in immunology, cell growth, migration and differentiation, some of which are also emerging as drug targets. These receptors differ from conventional pharmacological receptors in that they respond to proteins attached to cell surfaces or extracellular structures, rather than to soluble mediators.

Various carrier proteins are often referred to as receptors, such as the *low-density lipoprotein receptor* that plays a key role in lipid metabolism (Ch. 23) and the *transferrin receptor* involved in iron absorption (Ch. 25). These entities have little in common with pharmacological receptors. Though quite distinct from pharmacological receptors, these proteins play an important role in the action of drugs such as *statins* (Ch. 23).

RECEPTORS IN PHYSIOLOGICAL SYSTEMS

Receptors form a key part of the system of chemical communication that all multicellular organisms use to coordinate the activities of their cells and organs. Without them, we would be unable to function.

Some fundamental properties of receptors are illustrated by the action of **adrenaline** (epinephrine) on the heart. Adrenaline first binds to a receptor protein (the *β adrenoceptor*, see Ch. 14) that serves as a recognition site for adrenaline and other catecholamines. When it binds to

the receptor, a train of reactions is initiated (see Ch. 3), leading to an increase in force and rate of the heartbeat. In the absence of adrenaline, the receptor is functionally silent. This is true of most receptors for endogenous mediators (hormones, neurotransmitters, cytokines, etc.), although there are examples (see Ch. 3) of receptors that are 'constitutively active' – that is, they exert a controlling influence even when no chemical mediator is present.

There is an important distinction between *agonists*, which 'activate' the receptors, and *antagonists*, which combine at the same site without causing activation, and block the effect of agonists on that receptor. The distinction between agonists and antagonists only exists for pharmacological receptors; we cannot usefully speak of 'agonists' for the other classes of drug target described above.

The characteristics and accepted nomenclature of pharmacological receptors are described by Neubig et al. (2003). The origins of the receptor concept and its pharmacological significance are discussed by Rang (2006).

DRUG SPECIFICITY

For a drug to be useful as either a therapeutic or a scientific tool, it must act selectively on particular cells and tissues. In other words, it must show a high degree of binding site specificity. Conversely, proteins that function as drug targets generally show a high degree of ligand specificity; they bind only molecules of a certain precise type.

These principles of binding site and ligand specificity can be clearly recognised in the actions of a mediator such as **angiotensin** (Ch. 22). This peptide acts strongly on vascular smooth muscle, and on the kidney tubule, but has very little effect on other kinds of smooth muscle or on the intestinal epithelium. Other mediators affect a quite different spectrum of cells and tissues, the pattern in each case reflecting the specific pattern of expression of the protein receptors for the various mediators. A small chemical change, such as conversion of one of the amino acids in angiotensin from L to D form, or removal of one amino acid from the chain, can inactivate the molecule altogether, because the receptor fails to bind the altered form. The complementary specificity of ligands and binding sites, which gives rise to the very exact molecular recognition properties of proteins, is central to explaining many of the phenomena of pharmacology. It is no exaggeration to say that the ability of proteins to interact in a highly selective way with other molecules – including other proteins – is the basis of living machines. Its relevance to the understanding of drug action will be a recurring theme in this book.

Finally, it must be emphasised that no drug acts with complete specificity. Thus tricyclic antidepressant drugs (Ch. 47) act by blocking monoamine transporters but are notorious for producing side effects (e.g. dry mouth) related to their ability to block various other receptors. In general, the lower the potency of a drug and the higher the dose needed, the more likely it is that sites of action other than the primary one will assume significance. In clinical terms, this is often associated with the appearance of unwanted side effects, of which no drug is free.

Since the 1970s, pharmacological research has succeeded in identifying the protein targets of many different types of drug. Drugs such as opioid analgesics (Ch. 42), cannabinoids (Ch. 19) and benzodiazepine tranquillisers (Ch. 44), whose actions had been described in exhaustive detail for many years, are now known to target well-defined receptors, which have been fully characterised by gene-cloning and protein crystallography techniques (see Ch. 3).

RECEPTOR CLASSIFICATION

▼ Where the action of a drug can be associated with a particular receptor, this provides a valuable means for classification and refinement in drug design. For example, pharmacological analysis of the actions of histamine (see Ch. 17) showed that some of its effects (the H_1 effects, such as smooth muscle contraction) were strongly antagonised by the competitive histamine antagonists then known. Black and his colleagues suggested in 1970 that the remaining actions of histamine, which included its stimulant effect on gastric secretion, might represent a second class of histamine receptor (H_2). Testing a number of histamine analogues, they found that some were selective in producing H_2 effects, with little H_1 activity. By analysing which parts of the histamine molecule conferred this type of specificity, they were able to develop selective H_2 antagonists, which proved to be potent in blocking gastric acid secretion, a development of major therapeutic significance (Ch. 30).[2] Two further types of histamine receptor (H_3 and H_4) were recognised later.

Receptor classification based on pharmacological responses continues to be a valuable and widely used approach. Newer experimental approaches have produced other criteria on which to base receptor classification. The direct measurement of ligand binding to receptors (see below) has allowed many new receptor subtypes to be defined that could not easily be distinguished by studies of drug effects. Molecular cloning (see Ch. 3) provided a completely new basis for classification at a much finer level of detail than can be reached through pharmacological analysis. Finally, analysis of the biochemical pathways that are linked to receptor activation (see Ch. 3) provides yet another basis for classification.

The result of this data explosion was that receptor classification suddenly became much more detailed, with a proliferation of receptor subtypes for all the main types of ligand. As alternative molecular and biochemical classifications began to spring up that were incompatible with the accepted pharmacologically defined receptor classes, the International Union of Basic and Clinical Pharmacology (IUPHAR) convened expert working groups to produce agreed receptor classifications for the major types, taking into account the pharmacological, molecular and biochemical information available. These wise people have a hard task; their conclusions will be neither perfect nor final but are essential to ensure a consistent terminology. To the student, this may seem an arcane exercise in taxonomy, generating much detail but little illumination. There is a danger that the tedious lists of drug names, actions and side effects that used to burden the subject will be replaced by exhaustive tables of receptors, ligands and transduction pathways. In this book, we have tried to avoid detail for its own sake and include only such information on receptor classification as seems interesting in its own right or is helpful in explaining the actions of important drugs. A comprehensive database of known receptor classes is available (see www.guidetopharmacology.org/), as well as a regularly updated summary (Alexander et al., 2013).

DRUG–RECEPTOR INTERACTIONS

Occupation of a receptor by a drug molecule may or may not result in *activation* of the receptor. By activation, we mean that the receptor is affected by the bound molecule in such a way as to alter the receptor's behaviour towards the cell and elicit a tissue response. The molecular mechanisms associated with receptor activation are

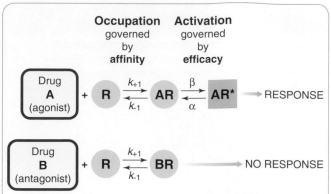

Fig. 2.1   **The distinction between drug binding and receptor activation.** Ligand A is an agonist, because when it is bound, the receptor (R) tends to become activated, whereas ligand B is an antagonist, because binding does not lead to activation. It is important to realise that for most drugs, binding and activation are reversible, dynamic processes. The rate constants k_{+1}, k_{-1}, α and β for the binding, unbinding and activation steps vary between drugs. For an antagonist, which does not activate the receptor, $\beta = 0$.

discussed in Chapter 3. Binding and activation represent two distinct steps in the generation of the receptor-mediated response by an agonist (Fig. 2.1). If a drug binds to the receptor without causing activation and thereby prevents the agonist from binding, it is termed a *receptor antagonist*. The tendency of a drug to bind to the receptors is governed by its *affinity*, whereas the tendency for it, once bound, to activate the receptor is denoted by its *efficacy*. These terms are defined more precisely below (p. 12 and 18). Drugs of high potency generally have a high affinity for the receptors and thus occupy a significant proportion of the receptors even at low concentrations. Agonists also possess significant efficacy, whereas antagonists, in the simplest case, have zero efficacy. Drugs with intermediate levels of efficacy, such that even when 100% of the receptors are occupied the tissue response is submaximal, are known as *partial agonists*, to distinguish them from *full agonists*, the efficacy of which is sufficient that they can elicit a maximal tissue response. These concepts, though clearly an oversimplified description of events at the molecular level (see Ch. 3), provide a useful basis for characterising drug effects.

We now discuss certain aspects in more detail, namely drug binding, agonist concentration–effect curves, competitive antagonism, partial agonists and the nature of efficacy. Understanding these concepts at a qualitative level is sufficient for many purposes, but for more detailed analysis a quantitative formulation is needed (see p. 18-20).

THE BINDING OF DRUGS TO RECEPTORS

▼ The binding of drugs to receptors can often be measured directly by the use of drug molecules (agonists or antagonists) labelled with one or more radioactive atoms (usually ^3H, ^{14}C or ^{125}I). The usual procedure is to incubate samples of the tissue (or membrane fragments) with various concentrations of radioactive drug until equilibrium is reached (i.e. when the rate of association [binding] and dissociation [unbinding] of the radioactive drug are equal). The bound radioactivity is measured after removal of the supernatant. In such experiments, the radiolabelled drug will exhibit both specific binding (i.e. binding to receptors, which is saturable as there are a

---

[2]For this work, and the development of β-adrenoceptor antagonists using a similar experimental approach, Sir James Black was awarded the 1984 Nobel Prize in Physiology or Medicine.

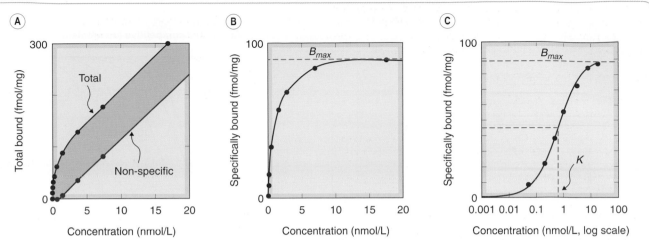

Fig. 2.2 **Measurement of receptor binding (β adrenoceptors in cardiac cell membranes).** The ligand was [³H]-cyanopindolol, a derivative of pindolol (see Ch. 14). **[A]** Measurements of total and non-specific binding at equilibrium. Non-specific binding is measured in the presence of a saturating concentration of a non-radioactive β-adrenoceptor agonist, which prevents the radioactive ligand from binding to β adrenoceptors. The difference between the two lines represents specific binding. **[B]** Specific binding plotted against concentration. The curve is a rectangular hyperbola (equation 2.5). **[C]** Specific binding as in **[B]** plotted against the concentration on a log scale. The sigmoid curve is a *logistic curve* representing the logarithmic scaling of the rectangular hyperbola plotted in panel **[B]** from which the binding parameters K and B_{max} can be determined.

finite number of receptors in the tissue) and a certain amount of 'non-specific binding' (i.e. drug taken up by structures other than receptors, which, at the concentrations used in such studies, is normally non-saturable), which obscures the specific component and needs to be kept to a minimum. The amount of non-specific binding is estimated by measuring the radioactivity taken up in the presence of a saturating concentration of a (non-radioactive) ligand that inhibits completely the binding of the radioactive drug to the receptors, leaving behind the non-specific component. This is then subtracted from the total binding to give an estimate of specific binding (Fig. 2.2). The *binding curve* (Fig. 2.2B, C) defines the relationship between concentration and the amount of drug bound (B), and in most cases it fits well to the relationship predicted theoretically (see Fig. 2.13), allowing the affinity of the drug for the receptors to be estimated, as well as the *binding capacity* (B_{max}), representing the density of receptors in the tissue. When combined with functional studies, binding measurements have proved very valuable. It has, for example, been confirmed that the *spare receptor hypothesis* (p. 10) for muscarinic receptors in smooth muscle is correct; agonists are found to bind, in general, with rather low affinity, and a maximal biological effect occurs at low receptor occupancy. It has also been shown, in skeletal muscle and other tissues, that denervation leads to an increase in the number of receptors in the target cell, a finding that accounts, at least in part, for the phenomenon of *denervation supersensitivity*. More generally, it appears that receptors tend to increase in number, usually over the course of a few days, if the relevant hormone or transmitter is absent or scarce, and to decrease in number if it is in excess, a process of adaptation to drugs or hormones resulting from continued administration (see p. 17).

Non-invasive imaging techniques, such as *positron emission tomography* (PET), can also be used to investigate the distribution of receptors in structures such as the living human brain. This technique has been used, for example, to measure the degree of dopamine-receptor blockade produced by antipsychotic drugs in the brains of schizophrenic patients (see Ch. 46).

Binding curves with agonists often reveal an apparent heterogeneity among receptors. For example, agonist binding to muscarinic receptors (Ch. 13) and also to β adrenoceptors (Ch. 14) suggests at least two populations of binding sites with different affinities. This may be because the receptors can exist either unattached or coupled within the membrane to another macromolecule, the G protein (see Ch. 3), which constitutes part of the transduction system through which the receptor exerts its regulatory effect. Antagonist binding does not show this complexity, probably because antagonists, by their nature, do not lead to the secondary event of G protein coupling. Because agonist binding results in activation, agonist affinity has proved to be a surprisingly elusive concept, about which afficionados love to argue.

THE RELATION BETWEEN DRUG CONCENTRATION AND EFFECT

Although binding can be measured directly, it is usually a biological response, such as a rise in blood pressure, contraction or relaxation of a strip of smooth muscle in an organ bath, the activation of an enzyme, or a behavioural response, that we are interested in, and this is often plotted as a *concentration–effect curve* (*in vitro*) or *dose–response curve* (*in vivo*), as in Figure 2.3. This allows us to estimate the *maximal response* that the drug can produce (E_{max}), and the concentration or dose needed to produce a 50% maximal response (EC_{50} or ED_{50}). A logarithmic concentration or dose scale is often used. This transforms the curve from a rectangular hyperbola to a sigmoidal curve in which the mid portion is essentially linear (the importance of the slope of the linear portion will become apparent later in this chapter when we consider antagonism and partial agonists). The E_{max}, EC_{50} and slope parameters are useful for comparing different drugs that produce qualitatively similar effects (see Fig. 2.7 and Ch. 7). Although they look similar to the binding curve in Figure 2.2C, concentration–effect curves cannot be used to measure the affinity of agonist drugs for their receptors, because the response produced is not, as a rule, directly proportional to receptor occupancy. This often arises because the maximum response of a tissue may be produced by agonists when they are bound to less than 100% of the receptors. Under these circumstances the tissue is said to possess spare receptors (see p. 10).

In interpreting concentration–effect curves, it must be remembered that the concentration of the drug at the

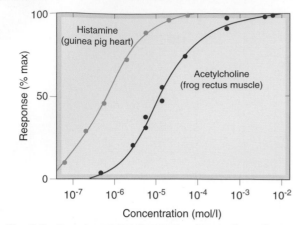

Fig. 2.3 Experimentally observed concentration–effect curves. Although the lines, drawn according to the binding equation 2.5, fit the points well, such curves do not give correct estimates of the affinity of drugs for receptors. This is because the relationship between receptor occupancy and response is usually non-linear.

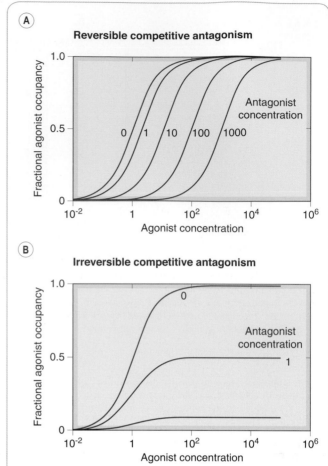

Fig. 2.4 Hypothetical agonist concentration–occupancy curves in the presence of reversible [A] and irreversible [B] competitive antagonists. The concentrations are normalised with respect to the equilibrium constants, K (i.e. 1.0 corresponds to a concentration equal to K and results in 50% occupancy). Note that in [A] increasing the agonist concentration overcomes the effect of a reversible antagonist (i.e. the block is surmountable), so that the maximal response is unchanged, whereas in [B] the effect of an irreversible antagonist is insurmountable and full agonist occupancy cannot be achieved.

receptors may differ from the known concentration in the bathing solution. Agonists may be subject to rapid enzymic degradation or uptake by cells as they diffuse from the surface towards their site of action, and a steady state can be reached in which the agonist concentration at the receptors is very much less than the concentration in the bath. In the case of acetylcholine, for example, which is hydrolysed by cholinesterase present in most tissues (see Ch. 13), the concentration reaching the receptors can be less than 1% of that in the bath, and an even bigger difference has been found with noradrenaline (norepinephrine), which is avidly taken up by sympathetic nerve terminals in many tissues (Ch. 14). The problem is reduced but not entirely eradicated by the use of recombinant receptors expressed in cells in culture. Thus, even if the concentration–effect curve, as in Figure 2.3, looks just like a facsimile of the binding curve (Fig. 2.2C), it cannot be used directly to determine the affinity of the agonist for the receptors.

SPARE RECEPTORS

▼ Stephenson (1956), studying the actions of acetylcholine analogues in isolated tissues, found that many full agonists were capable of eliciting maximal responses at very low occupancies, often less than 1%. This means that the mechanism linking the response to receptor occupancy has a substantial reserve capacity. Such systems may be said to possess *spare receptors*, or a receptor reserve. The existence of spare receptors does not imply any functional subdivision of the receptor pool, but merely that the pool is larger than the number needed to evoke a full response. This surplus of receptors over the number actually needed might seem a wasteful biological arrangement. But in fact it is highly efficient in that a given number of agonist–receptor complexes, corresponding to a given level of biological response, can be reached with a lower concentration of hormone or neurotransmitter than would be the case if fewer receptors were provided. Economy of hormone or transmitter secretion is thus achieved at the expense of providing more receptors.

COMPETITIVE ANTAGONISM

Though one drug can inhibit the response to another in several ways (see p. 15), competition at the receptor level

is particularly important, both in the laboratory and in the clinic, because of the high potency and specificity that can be achieved.

In the presence of a competitive antagonist, the agonist occupancy (i.e. proportion of receptors to which the agonist is bound) at a given agonist concentration is reduced, because the receptor can accommodate only one molecule at a time. However, because the two are in competition, raising the agonist concentration can restore the agonist occupancy (and hence the tissue response). The antagonism is therefore said to be *surmountable*, in contrast to other types of antagonism (see below) where increasing the agonist concentration fails to overcome the blocking effect. A simple theoretical analysis (see p. 19) predicts that in the presence of a fixed concentration of the antagonist, the log concentration–effect curve for the agonist will be shifted to the right, without any change in slope or maximum – the hallmark of competitive antagonism (Fig. 2.4A). The shift is expressed as a *dose ratio*,

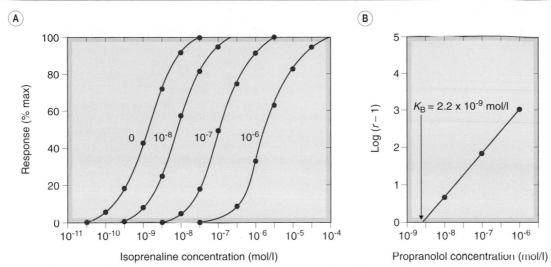

Fig. 2.5 Competitive antagonism of isoprenaline by propranolol measured on isolated guinea pig atria. **[A]** Concentration–effect curves at various propranolol concentrations (indicated on the curves). Note the progressive shift to the right without a change of slope or maximum. **[B]** Schild plot (equation 2.10). The equilibrium dissociation constant (K_B) for propranolol is given by the abscissal intercept, 2.2 × 10^{-9} mol/l. *(Results from Potter LT 1967 Uptake of propranolol by isolated guinea-pig atria. J Pharmacol Exp Ther 55, 91–100.)*

r (the ratio by which the agonist concentration has to be increased in the presence of the antagonist in order to restore a given level of response). Theory predicts that the dose ratio increases linearly with the concentration of the antagonist (see p. 19). These predictions are often borne out in practice (see Fig. 2.5A), providing a relatively simple method for determining the dissociation constant of the antagonist (K_B; Fig. 2.5B). Examples of competitive antagonism are very common in pharmacology. The surmountability of the block by the antagonist may be important in practice, because it allows the functional effect of the agonist to be restored by an increase in concentration. With other types of antagonism (as detailed below), the block is usually insurmountable.

The salient features of competitive antagonism are:

- shift of the agonist log concentration–effect curve to the right, without change of slope or maximum (i.e. antagonism can be overcome by increasing the concentration of the agonist)
- linear relationship between agonist dose ratio and antagonist concentration
- evidence of competition from binding studies.

Competitive antagonism is the most direct mechanism by which one drug can reduce the effect of another (or of an endogenous mediator).

▼ The characteristics of *reversible competitive antagonism* described above reflect the fact that agonist and competitive antagonist molecules do not stay bound to the receptor but bind and rebind continuously. The rate of dissociation of the antagonist molecules is sufficiently high that a new equilibrium is rapidly established on addition of the agonist. In effect, the agonist is able to displace the antagonist molecules from the receptors, although it cannot, of course, evict a bound antagonist molecule. Displacement occurs because, by occupying a proportion of the vacant receptors, the agonist effectively reduces the rate of association of the antagonist molecules; consequently, the rate of dissociation temporarily exceeds that of association, and the overall antagonist occupancy falls.

Competitive antagonism

- Reversible competitive antagonism is the commonest and most important type of antagonism; it has two main characteristics:
  - in the presence of the antagonist, the agonist log concentration–effect curve is shifted to the right without change in slope or maximum, the extent of the shift being a measure of the *dose ratio*
  - the dose ratio increases linearly with antagonist concentration
- Antagonist affinity, measured in this way, is widely used as a basis for receptor classification.

IRREVERSIBLE COMPETITIVE ANTAGONISM

▼ *Irreversible competitive* (or *non-equilibrium*) *antagonism* occurs when the antagonist binds to the same site on the receptor as the agonist but dissociates very slowly, or not at all, from the receptors, with the result that no change in the antagonist occupancy takes place when the agonist is applied.[3]

The predicted effects of reversible and irreversible antagonists are compared in Figure 2.4.

In some cases (Fig. 2.6A), the theoretical effect is accurately reproduced, but the distinction between reversible and irreversible competitive antagonism (or even non-competitive antagonism; see p. 17) is not always so clear. This is because of the phenomenon of spare receptors (see p. 10); if the agonist occupancy required to produce a maximal biological response is very small (say 1% of the total receptor pool), then it is possible to block irreversibly nearly 99% of the receptors without reducing the maximal response. The effect of a lesser degree of antagonist occupancy will be to produce a parallel shift of the log concentration–effect curve that is indistinguishable from reversible competitive antagonism (Fig. 2.6B).

---

[3]This type of antagonism is sometimes called non-competitive, but that term is ambiguous and best avoided in this context.

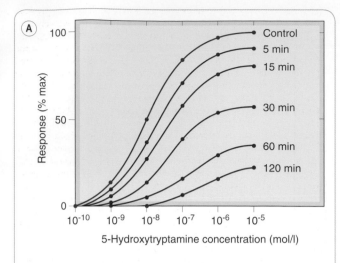

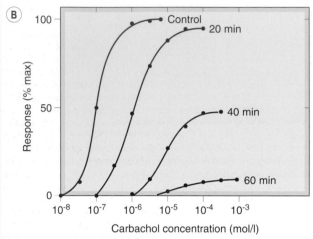

Fig. 2.6 Effects of irreversible competitive antagonists on agonist concentration–effect curves. **[A]** Rat stomach smooth muscle responding to 5-hydroxytryptamine at various times after addition of methysergide (10^{-9} mol/l). **[B]** Rabbit stomach responding to carbachol at various times after addition of dibenamine (10^{-5} mol/l). *(Panel [A] after Frankhuijsen AL, Bonta IL 1974 Eur J Pharmacol 26, 220; panel [B] after Furchgott RF 1965 Adv Drug Res 3, 21.)*

Irreversible competitive antagonism occurs with drugs that possess reactive groups that form covalent bonds with the receptor. These are mainly used as experimental tools for investigating receptor function, and few are used clinically. Irreversible enzyme inhibitors that act similarly are clinically used, however, and include drugs such as **aspirin** (Ch. 26), **omeprazole** (Ch. 30) and monoamine oxidase inhibitors (Ch. 47).

PARTIAL AGONISTS AND THE CONCEPT OF EFFICACY

So far, we have considered drugs either as agonists, which in some way activate the receptor when they occupy it, or as antagonists, which cause no activation. However, the ability of a drug molecule to activate the receptor is actually a graded, rather than an all-or-nothing, property. If a series of chemically related agonist drugs acting on the

same receptors is tested on a given biological system, it is often found that the largest response that can be produced differs from one drug to another. Some compounds (known as *full agonists*) can produce a maximal response (the largest response that the tissue is capable of giving), whereas others (*partial agonists*) can produce only a submaximal response. Figure 2.7A shows concentration–effect curves for several α-adrenoceptor agonists (see Ch. 14), which cause contraction of isolated strips of rabbit aorta. The full agonist **phenylephrine** produced the maximal response of which the tissue was capable; the other compounds could only produce submaximal responses and are partial agonists. The difference between full and partial agonists lies in the relationship between receptor occupancy and response. In the experiment shown in Figure 2.7 it was possible to estimate the affinity of the various drugs for the receptor, and hence (based on the theoretical model described later; p. 18) to calculate the fraction of receptors occupied (known as *occupancy*) as a function of drug concentration. Plots of response as a function of occupancy for the different compounds are shown in Figure 2.7B, showing that for partial agonists the response at a given level of occupancy is less than for full agonists. The weakest partial agonist, **tolazoline**, produces a barely detectable response even at 100% occupancy, and is usually classified as a *competitive antagonist* (see p. 10 and Ch. 14).

These differences can be expressed quantitatively in terms of *efficacy* (*e*), a parameter originally defined by Stephenson (1956) that describes the 'strength' of the agonist–receptor complex in evoking a response of the tissue. In the simple scheme shown in Figure 2.1, efficacy describes the tendency of the drug–receptor complex to adopt the active (AR*), rather than the resting (AR), state. A drug with zero efficacy ($e = 0$) has no tendency to cause receptor activation, and causes no tissue response. A full agonist is a drug whose efficacy[4] is sufficient that it produces a maximal response when less than 100% of receptors are occupied. A partial agonist has lower efficacy, such that 100% occupancy elicits only a submaximal response.

▼ Subsequently, it was appreciated that characteristics of the tissue (e.g. the number of receptors that it possesses and the nature of the coupling between the receptor and the response; see Ch. 3), as well as of the drug itself, were important, and the concept of *intrinsic efficacy* was developed (see Kenakin, 1997), which can account for a number of anomalous findings. For example, depending on tissue characteristics, a given drug may appear as a full agonist in one tissue but a partial agonist in another, and drugs may differ in their relative agonist potencies in different tissues, though the receptor is the same.

It would be nice to be able to explain what efficacy means in physical terms, and to understand why one drug may be an agonist while another, chemically very similar, is an antagonist. We are beginning to understand the molecular events underlying receptor activation (described in Ch. 3) but can still give no clear answer to the question of why some ligands are agonists and some are antagonists, although the simple theoretical two-state model described below provides a useful starting point.

---

[4]In Stephenson's formulation, efficacy is the reciprocal of the occupancy needed to produce a 50% maximal response, thus $e = 25$ implies that a 50% maximal response occurs at 4% occupancy. There is no theoretical upper limit to efficacy.

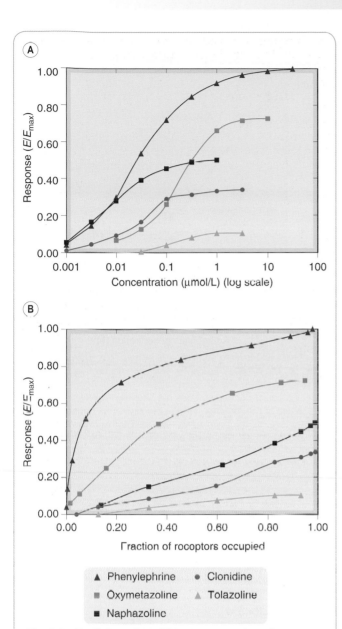

Fig. 2.7 Partial agonists. [A] Log concentration–effect curves for a series of α-adrenoceptor agonists causing contraction of an isolated strip of rabbit aorta. Phenylephrine is a full agonist. The others are partial agonists with different efficacies. The lower the efficacy of the drug the lower the maximum response and slope of the log concentration-response curve. [B] The relationship between response and receptor occupancy for the series. Note that the full agonist, phenylephrine, produces a near-maximal response when only about half the receptors are occupied, whereas partial agonists produce submaximal responses even when occupying all of the receptors. The efficacy of tolazoline is so low that it is classified as an α-adrenoceptor antagonist (see Ch. 14). In these experiments, receptor occupancy was not measured directly, but was calculated from pharmacological estimates of the equilibrium constants of the drugs. *(Data from Ruffolo RR Jr et al. 1979 J Pharmacol Exp Ther 209, 429–436.)*

CONSTITUTIVE RECEPTOR ACTIVATION AND INVERSE AGONISTS

▼ Although we are accustomed to thinking that receptors are activated only when an agonist molecule is bound, there are examples (see De Ligt et al., 2000) where an appreciable level of activation

(*constitutive activation*) may exist even when no ligand is present. These include receptors for benzodiazepines (see Ch. 44), cannabinoids (Ch. 19), serotonin (Ch. 15) and several other mediators. Furthermore, receptor mutations occur – either spontaneously, in some disease states (see Bond & Ijzerman, 2006), or experimentally created (see Ch. 4) – that result in appreciable constitutive activation. Resting activity may be too low to have any effect under normal conditions but become evident if receptors are overexpressed, a phenomenon clearly demonstrated for β adrenoceptors (see Bond et al., 1995), and which may prove to have major pathophysiological implications. Thus if, say, 1% of receptors are active in the absence of any agonist, in a normal cell expressing perhaps 10 000 receptors, only 100 will be active. Increasing the expression level 10-fold will result in 1000 active receptors, producing a significant effect. Under these conditions, it may be possible for a ligand to *reduce* the level of constitutive activation; such drugs are known as *inverse agonists* (Fig. 2.8; see De Ligt et al., 2000) to distinguish them from *neutral antagonists*, which do not by themselves affect the level of activation. Inverse agonists can be regarded as drugs with negative efficacy, to distinguish them from agonists (positive efficacy) and neutral antagonists (zero efficacy). Neutral antagonists, by binding to the agonist binding site, will antagonise both agonists and inverse agonists. Inverse agonism was first observed at the benzodiazepine receptor (Ch. 44) but such drugs are proconvulsive and thus not therapeutically useful! New examples of constitutively active receptors and inverse agonists are emerging with increasing frequency (mainly among G protein-coupled receptors; Seifert & Wenzel-Seifert, 2002). In theory, an inverse agonist, by silencing constitutively active receptors, should be more effective than a neutral antagonist in disease states associated with receptor mutations or with receptor-directed autoantibodies that result in enhanced constitutive activation. These include certain types of hyperthyroidism, precocious puberty and parathyroid diseases (see Bond & Ijzerman, 2006). This remains to be verified, but it turns out that most of the receptor antagonists in clinical use are actually inverse agonists when tested in systems showing constitutive receptor activation. However, most receptors – like cats – show a preference for the inactive state, and for these there is no practical difference between a competitive antagonist and an inverse agonist. It remains to be seen whether the inverse agonist principle will prove to be generally important in therapeutics, but interest is running high. So far, most examples come from the family of G protein-coupled receptors (see Ch. 3 and the review by Costa & Cotecchia, 2005), and it is not clear whether similar phenomena occur with other receptor families.

The following section describes a simple model that explains full, partial and inverse agonism in terms of the relative affinity of different ligands for the resting and activated states of the receptor.

The two-state receptor model

▼ As illustrated in Figure 2.1, agonists and antagonists both bind to receptors, but only agonists activate them. How can we express this difference, and account for constitutive activity, in theoretical terms? The two-state model (Fig. 2.9) provides a simple but useful approach.

As shown in Figure 2.1, we envisage that the occupied receptor can switch from its 'resting' (R) state to an activated (R*) state, R* being favoured by binding of an agonist but not an antagonist molecule.

As described above, receptors may show constitutive activation (i.e. the R* conformation can exist without any ligand being bound), so the added drug encounters an equilibrium mixture of R and R* (Fig. 2.9). If it has a higher affinity for R*than for R, the drug will cause a shift of the equilibrium towards R* (i.e. it will promote activation and be classed as an agonist). If its preference for R* is very large, nearly all the occupied receptors will adopt the R* conformation and the drug will be a full agonist (positive efficacy); if it shows only a modest degree of selectivity for R* (say 5–10-fold), a smaller proportion of occupied receptors will adopt the R* conformation and it will be a partial agonist; if it shows no preference, the prevailing R:R* equilibrium will not be disturbed and the drug will be a neutral antagonist (zero efficacy), whereas if it shows selectivity for R it will

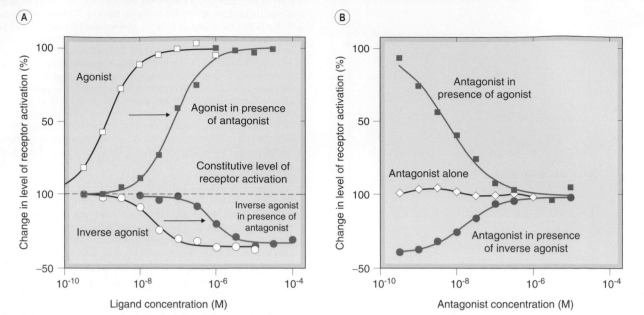

Fig. 2.8 **Inverse agonism.** The interaction of a competitive antagonist with normal and inverse agonists in a system that shows receptor activation in the absence of any added ligands (constitutive activation). **[A]** The degree of receptor activation (vertical scale) increases in the presence of an agonist (open squares) and decreases in the presence of an inverse agonist (open circles). Addition of a competitive antagonist shifts both curves to the right (closed symbols). **[B]** The antagonist on its own does not alter the level of constitutive activity (open symbols), because it has equal affinity for the active and inactive states of the receptor. In the presence of an agonist (closed squares) or an inverse agonist (closed circles), the antagonist restores the system towards the constitutive level of activity. These data (reproduced with permission from Newman-Tancredi A et al. 1997 Br J Pharmacol 120, 737–739) were obtained with cloned human 5-hydroxytryptamine (5-HT) receptors expressed in a cell line. (Agonist, 5-carboxamidotryptamine; inverse agonist, spiperone; antagonist, WAY 100635; ligand concentration [M = mol/l]; see Ch. 15 for information on 5-HT receptor pharmacology.)

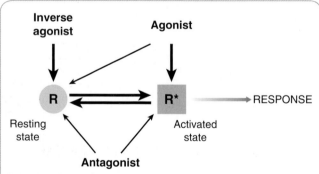

Fig. 2.9 **The two-state model.** The receptor is shown in two conformational states, 'resting' (R) and 'activated' (R*), which exist in equilibrium. Normally, when no ligand is present, the equilibrium lies far to the left, and few receptors are found in the R* state. For constitutively active receptors, an appreciable proportion of receptors adopt the R* conformation in the absence of any ligand. Agonists have higher affinity for R* than for R, so shift the equilibrium towards R*. The greater the relative affinity for R* with respect to R, the greater the efficacy of the agonist. An inverse agonist has higher affinity for R than for R* and so shifts the equilibrium to the left. A 'neutral' antagonist has equal affinity for R and R* so does not by itself affect the conformational equilibrium but reduces by competition the binding of other ligands.

shift the equilibrium towards R and be an inverse agonist (negative efficacy). We can therefore think of efficacy as a property determined by the relative affinity of a ligand for R and R*, a formulation known as the *two-state model*, which is useful in that it puts a physical interpretation on the otherwise mysterious meaning of efficacy, as well as accounting for the existence of inverse agonists.

BIASED AGONISM

A major problem with the two-state model is that, as we now know, receptors are not actually restricted to two distinct states but have much greater conformational flexibility, so that there is more than one inactive and active conformation. The different conformations that they can adopt may be preferentially stabilised by different ligands, and may produce different functional effects by activating different signal transduction pathways (see Ch. 3).

Receptors that couple to second messenger systems (see Ch. 3) can couple to more than one intracellular effector pathway, giving rise to two or more simultaneous responses. One might expect that all agonists that activate the same receptor type would evoke the same array of responses (Fig. 2.10A). However it has become apparent that different agonists can exhibit *bias* for the generation of one response over another even although they are acting through the same receptor (Fig. 2.10B) probably because they stabilise different conformational states of the receptor. Agonist bias has become an important concept in pharmacology recently and might in future have important therapeutic implications (see Kelly, 2013).

Redefining and attempting to measure agonist efficacy for such a multistate model is problematic, however, and

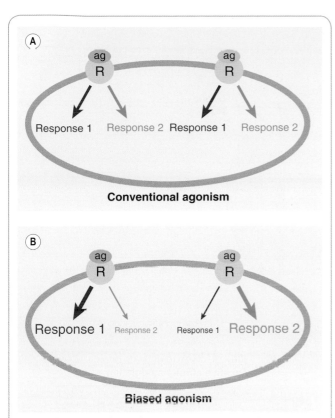

Fig. 2.10 Biased agonism. In the upper panel the receptor R is coupled to two intracellular responses – response 1 and response 2. When different agonists indicated in red and green activate the receptor they evoke both responses in a similar manner. This is what we can consider as being conventional agonism. In the lower panel biased agonism is illustrated in which two agonists bind at the same site on the receptor yet the red agonist is better at evoking response 1 and the green agonist is better at evoking response 2.

proven difficult to develop selective agonists and antagonists for individual subtypes. The hope is that there will be greater variation in the allosteric sites and that receptor-selective allosteric ligands can be developed. Furthermore, positive allosteric modulators will exert their effects only on receptors that are being activated by endogenous ligands and have no effect on those that are not activated. This might provide a degree of selectivity (e.g. in potentiating spinal inhibition mediated by endogenous opioids, see Ch. 42) and a reduction in side effect profile.

Agonists, antagonists and efficacy

- Drugs acting on receptors may be *agonists* or *antagonists*.
- Agonists initiate changes in cell function, producing effects of various types; antagonists bind to receptors without initiating such changes.
- Agonist potency depends on two parameters: *affinity* (i.e. tendency to bind to receptors) and *efficacy* (i.e. ability, once bound, to initiate changes that lead to effects).
- For antagonists, efficacy is zero.
- *Full agonists* (which can produce maximal effects) have high efficacy; *partial agonists* (which can produce only submaximal effects) have intermediate efficacy.
- According to the two-state model, efficacy reflects the relative affinity of the compound for the resting and activated states of the receptor. Agonists show selectivity for the activated state; antagonists show no selectivity. This model, although helpful, fails to account for the complexity of agonist action.
- *Inverse agonists* show selectivity for the resting state of the receptor, this being of significance only in situations where the receptors show *constitutive activity*.
- *Allosteric modulators* bind to sites on the receptor other than the agonist binding site and can modify agonist activity.

requires a more complicated state transition model than the two-state model described above. The errors, pitfalls and a possible way forward have recently been outlined by Kenakin and Christopoulos (2013).

ALLOSTERIC MODULATION

▼ In addition to the agonist binding site (now referred to as the *orthosteric* binding site), to which competitive antagonists also bind, receptor proteins possess many other (*allosteric*) binding sites (see Ch. 3) through which drugs can influence receptor function in various ways, by increasing or decreasing the affinity of agonists for the agonist binding site, by modifying efficacy or by producing a response themselves (Fig. 2.11). Depending on the direction of the effect, the ligands may be allosteric antagonists or allosteric facilitators of the agonist effect, and the effect may be to alter the slope and maximum of the agonist log concentration–effect curve (Fig. 2.11). This type of allosteric modulation of receptor function has attracted much attention recently (see review by May et al., 2007), and may prove to be more widespread than previously envisaged. Well-known examples of allosteric facilitation include glycine at NMDA receptors (Ch. 38), benzodiazepines at GABA$_A$ receptors (Ch. 38), **cinacalcet** at the Ca^{2+} receptor (Ch. 36) and **sulfonylurea** drugs at K$_{ATP}$ channels (Ch. 31). One reason why allosteric modulation may be important to the pharmacologist and future drug development is that across families of receptors such as the muscarinic receptors (see Ch. 13) the orthosteric binding sites are very similar and it has

OTHER FORMS OF DRUG ANTAGONISM

Other mechanisms can also account for inhibitory interactions between drugs.

The most important ones are:

- chemical antagonism
- pharmacokinetic antagonism
- block of receptor–response linkage
- physiological antagonism.

CHEMICAL ANTAGONISM

Chemical antagonism refers to the uncommon situation where the two substances combine in solution; as a result, the effect of the active drug is lost. Examples include the use of chelating agents (e.g. **dimercaprol**) that bind to heavy metals and thus reduce their toxicity, and the use of the neutralising antibody **infliximab**, which has an anti-inflammatory action due to its ability to sequester the inflammatory cytokine tumour necrosis factor (TNF; see Ch. 18).

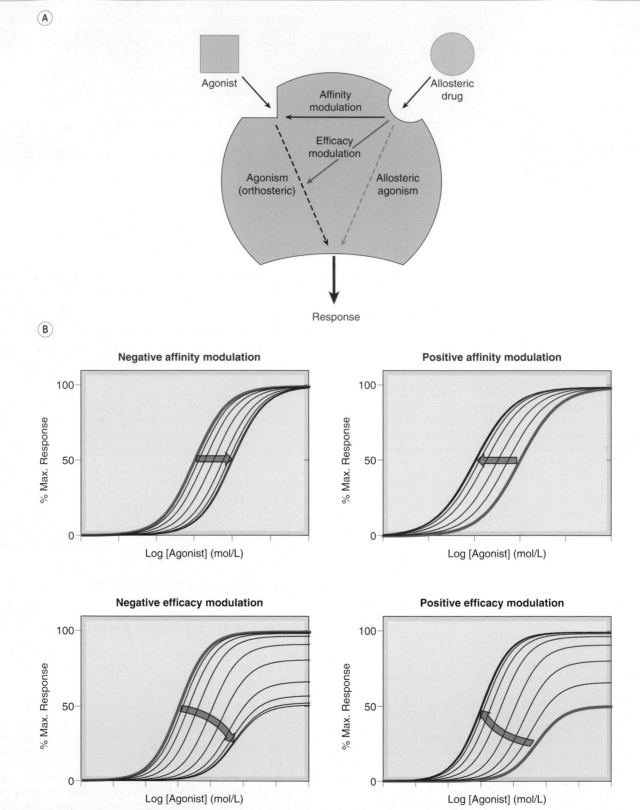

Fig. 2.11 Allosteric modulation. [**A**] Allosteric drugs bind at a separate site on the receptor to 'traditional' agonists (now often referred to as 'orthosteric' agonists). They can modify the activity of the receptor by (i) altering agonist affinity, (ii) altering agonist efficacy or (iii) directly evoking a response themselves. [**B**] Effects of affinity- and efficacy-modifying allosteric modulators on the concentration–effect curve of an agonist (blue line). In the presence of the allosteric modulator the agonist concentration–effect curve (now illustrated in red) is shifted in a manner determined by the type of allosteric modulator until a maximum effect of the modulator is reached. *(Panel [A] adapted with permission from Conn et al., 2009 Nature Rev Drug Discov 8, 41–54; panel [B] courtesy of A Christopoulos.)*

PHARMACOKINETIC ANTAGONISM

Pharmacokinetic antagonism describes the situation in which the 'antagonist' effectively reduces the concentration of the active drug at its site of action. This can happen in various ways. The rate of metabolic degradation of the active drug may be increased (e.g. the reduction of the anticoagulant effect of **warfarin** when an agent that accelerates its hepatic metabolism, such as **phenytoin**, is given; see Chs 9 and 57). Alternatively, the rate of absorption of the active drug from the gastrointestinal tract may be reduced, or the rate of renal excretion may be increased. Interactions of this sort, discussed in more detail in Chapter 57, are common and can be important in clinical practice.

BLOCK OF RECEPTOR–RESPONSE LINKAGE

Non-competitive antagonism describes the situation where the antagonist blocks at some point downstream from the agonist binding site on the receptor, and interrupts the chain of events that leads to the production of a response by the agonist. For example, **ketamine** enters the ion channel pore of the NMDA receptor (see Ch. 38) blocking it and thus preventing ion flux through the channels. Drugs such as **verapamil** and **nifedipine** prevent the influx of Ca^{2+} through the cell membrane (see Ch. 22) and thus block non-selectively the contraction of smooth muscle produced by drugs acting at any receptor that couples to these calcium channels. As a rule, the effect will be to reduce the slope and maximum of the agonist log concentration–response curve, although it is quite possible for some degree of rightward shift to occur as well.

PHYSIOLOGICAL ANTAGONISM

Physiological antagonism is a term used loosely to describe the interaction of two drugs whose opposing actions in the body tend to cancel each other. For example, **histamine** acts on receptors of the parietal cells of the gastric mucosa to stimulate acid secretion, while **omeprazole** blocks this effect by inhibiting the proton pump; the two drugs can be said to act as physiological antagonists.

Types of drug antagonism

Drug antagonism occurs by various mechanisms:
- chemical antagonism (interaction in solution)
- pharmacokinetic antagonism (one drug affecting the absorption, metabolism or excretion of the other)
- competitive antagonism (both drugs binding to the same receptors); the antagonism may be reversible or irreversible
- interruption of receptor–response linkage
- physiological antagonism (two agents producing opposing physiological effects).

DESENSITISATION AND TOLERANCE

Often, the effect of a drug gradually diminishes when it is given continuously or repeatedly. *Desensitisation* and *tachyphylaxis* are synonymous terms used to describe this phenomenon, which often develops in the course of a few minutes. The term *tolerance* is conventionally used to describe a more gradual decrease in responsiveness to a drug, taking hours, days or weeks to develop, but the distinction is not a sharp one. The term *refractoriness* is also sometimes used, mainly in relation to a loss of therapeutic efficacy. *Drug resistance* is a term used to describe the loss of effectiveness of antimicrobial or antitumour drugs (see Chs 50 and 56). Many different mechanisms can give rise to these phenomena. They include:

- change in receptors
- translocation of receptors
- exhaustion of mediators
- increased metabolic degradation of the drug
- physiological adaptation
- active extrusion of drug from cells (mainly relevant in cancer chemotherapy; see Ch. 56).

CHANGE IN RECEPTORS

Among receptors directly coupled to ion channels (see Ch. 3), desensitisation is often rapid and pronounced. At the neuromuscular junction (Fig. 2.12A), the desensitised state is caused by a conformational change in the receptor, resulting in tight binding of the agonist molecule without the opening of the ionic channel. Phosphorylation of intracellular regions of the receptor protein is a second, slower mechanism by which ion channels become desensitised.

Most G protein-coupled receptors (see Ch. 3) also show desensitisation (see Fig. 2.12B). Phosphorylation of the receptor interferes with its ability to activate second messenger cascades, although it can still bind the agonist molecule. The molecular mechanisms of this 'uncoupling' are considered further in Chapter 3. This type of desensitisation usually takes seconds to minutes to develop, and recovers when the agonist is removed.

It will be realised that the two-state model in its simple form, discussed earlier, needs to be further elaborated to incorporate additional 'desensitised' states of the receptor.

TRANSLOCATION OF RECEPTORS

Prolonged exposure to agonists often results in a gradual decrease in the number of receptors expressed on the cell surface, as a result of *internalisation* of the receptors. This is shown for β adrenoceptors in Figure 2.12B and is a slower process than the uncoupling described above. Similar changes have been described for other types of receptor, including those for various peptides. The internalised receptors are taken into the cell by endocytosis of patches of the membrane, a process that normally depends on receptor phosphorylation and the subsequent binding of *arrestin* proteins to the phosphorylated receptor (see Ch. 3, Fig. 3.16). This type of adaptation is common for hormone receptors and has obvious relevance to the effects produced when drugs are given for extended periods. It is generally an unwanted complication when drugs are used clinically.

EXHAUSTION OF MEDIATORS

In some cases, desensitisation is associated with depletion of an essential intermediate substance. Drugs such as **amphetamine**, which acts by releasing amines from nerve

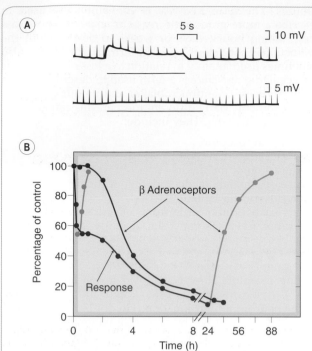

Fig. 2.12 Two kinds of receptor desensitisation.
[**A**] Acetylcholine (ACh) at the frog motor endplate. Brief
depolarisations (upward deflections) are produced by short
pulses of ACh delivered from a micropipette. A long pulse
(horizontal line) causes the response to decline with a time
course of about 20 s, owing to desensitisation, and it recovers
with a similar time course. [**B**] β adrenoceptors of rat glioma
cells in tissue culture. Isoproterenol (1 μmol/l) was added at time
zero, and the adenylyl cyclase response and β-adrenoceptor
density measured at intervals. During the early uncoupling
phase, the response (blue line) declines with no change in
receptor density (red line). Later, the response declines further
concomitantly with disappearance of receptors from the
membrane by internalisation. The green and orange lines show
the recovery of the response and receptor density after the
isoproterenol is washed out during the early or late phase.
*(Panel [A] from Katz B, Thesleff S 1957 J Physiol 138, 63; panel
[B] from Perkins JP 1981 Trends Pharmacol Sci 2, 326.)*

terminals (see Chs 14 and 48), show marked tachyphylaxis
because the amine stores become depleted.

ALTERED DRUG METABOLISM

Tolerance to some drugs, for example **barbiturates** (Ch.
44) and **ethanol** (Ch. 49), occurs partly because repeated
administration of the same dose produces a progressively
lower plasma concentration, because of increased metabolic degradation. The degree of tolerance that results is
generally modest, and in both of these examples other
mechanisms contribute to the substantial tolerance that
actually occurs. On the other hand, the pronounced tolerance to **nitrovasodilators** (see Chs 20 and 22) results
mainly from decreased metabolism, which reduces the
release of the active mediator, nitric oxide.

PHYSIOLOGICAL ADAPTATION

Diminution of a drug's effect may occur because it is nul-
lified by a homeostatic response. For example, the blood

pressure-lowering effect of **thiazide diuretics** is limited
because of a gradual activation of the renin–angiotensin
system (see Ch. 22). Such homeostatic mechanisms are
very common, and if they occur slowly the result will be
a gradually developing tolerance. It is a common experience that many side effects of drugs, such as nausea or
sleepiness, tend to subside even though drug administration is continued. We may assume that some kind of
physiological adaptation is occurring, presumably associated with altered gene expression resulting in changes in
the levels of various regulatory molecules, but little is
known about the mechanisms involved.

QUANTITATIVE ASPECTS OF DRUG–RECEPTOR INTERACTIONS

▼ Here we present some aspects of so-called *receptor theory*, which
is based on applying the Law of Mass Action to the drug–receptor
interaction and which has served well as a framework for
interpreting a large body of quantitative experimental data (see
Colquhoun, 2006).

THE BINDING REACTION

▼ The first step in drug action on specific receptors is the formation
of a reversible drug–receptor complex, the reactions being governed
by the Law of Mass Action. Suppose that a piece of tissue, such as
heart muscle or smooth muscle, contains a total number of receptors,
N_{tot}, for an agonist such as adrenaline. When the tissue is exposed
to adrenaline at concentration x_A and allowed to come to equilibrium, a certain number, N_A, of the receptors will become occupied,
and the number of vacant receptors will be reduced to $N_{tot} - N_A$.
Normally, the number of adrenaline molecules applied to the tissue
in solution greatly exceeds N_{tot}, so that the binding reaction does not
appreciably reduce x_A. The magnitude of the response produced by
the adrenaline will be related (even if we do not know exactly how) to
the number of receptors occupied, so it is useful to consider what
quantitative relationship is predicted between N_A and x_A. The reaction can be represented by:

$$
\begin{array}{ccccc}
A & + & R & \xrightleftharpoons[k_{-1}]{k_{+1}} & AR \\
drug & + & free\ receptor & & complex \\
(x_A) & & (N_{tot} - N_A) & & (N_A)
\end{array}
$$

The Law of Mass Action (which states that the rate of a chemical
reaction is proportional to the product of the concentrations of reac-
tants) can be applied to this reaction.

$$\text{Rate of forward reaction} = k_{+1} x_A (N_{tot} - N_A) \quad (2.1)$$

$$\text{Rate of backward reaction} = k_{-1} N_A \quad (2.2)$$

At equilibrium, the two rates are equal:

$$k_{+1} x_A (N_{tot} - N_A) = k_{-1} N_A \quad (2.3)$$

The *affinity constant* of binding is given by k_{+1}/k_{-1} and from equation
2.3 equals $N_A/x_A(N_{tot} - N_A)$. Unfortunately this has units of reciprocal
concentration (l/mol) which for some of us is a little hard to get our
heads around. Pharmacologists therefore tend to use the reciprocal
of the affinity constant, the *equilibrium dissociation constant* (K_A),
which has units of concentration (mol/l).

$$K_A = k_{-1}/k_{+1} = x_A (N_{tot} - N_A)/N_A \quad (2.4)$$

The proportion of receptors occupied, or occupancy (p_A), is N_A/N_{tot},
which is independent of N_{tot}.

$$p_A = \frac{x_A}{x_A + k_{-1}/k_{+1}} = \frac{x_A}{x_A + K_A} \quad (2.5)$$

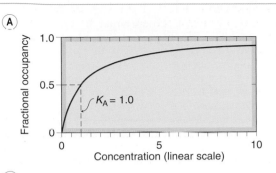

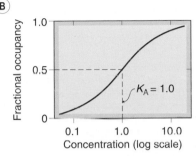

Fig. 2.13 **Theoretical relationship between occupancy and ligand concentration.** The relationship is plotted according to equation 2.5. **[A]** Plotted with a linear concentration scale, this curve is a rectangular hyperbola. **[B]** Plotted with a log concentration scale, it is a symmetrical sigmoid curve.

Thus if the equilibrium dissociation constant of a drug is known we can calculate the proportion of receptors it will occupy at any concentration.

Equation 2.5 can be written:

$$p_A = \frac{x_A / K_A}{x_A / K_A + 1} \qquad (2.6)$$

This important result is known as the Hill–Langmuir equation.[5]

The *equilibrium dissociation constant*, K_A, is a characteristic of the drug and of the receptor; it has the dimensions of concentration and is numerically equal to the concentration of drug required to occupy 50% of the sites at equilibrium. (Verify from equation 2.5 that when $x_A = K_A$, $p_A = 0.5$.) The higher the affinity of the drug for the receptors, the lower will be the value of K_A. Equation 2.6 describes the relationship between occupancy and drug concentration, and it generates a characteristic curve known as a *rectangular hyperbola*, as shown in Figure 2.13A. It is common in pharmacological work to use a logarithmic scale of concentration; this converts the hyperbola to a symmetrical sigmoid curve (Fig. 2.13B).

The same approach is used to analyse data from experiments in which drug binding is measured directly (see p. 9, Fig. 2.2). In this case, the relationship between the amount bound (B) and ligand concentration (x_A) should be:

$$B = B_{max} x_A / (x_A + K_A) \qquad (2.7)$$

where B_{max} is the total number of binding sites in the preparation (often expressed as pmol/mg of protein). To display the results in linear form, equation 2.6 may be rearranged to:

$$B / x_A = B_{max} / (K_A - B / K_A) \qquad (2.8)$$

---

[5]A.V. Hill first published it in 1909, when he was still a medical student. Langmuir, a physical chemist working on gas adsorption, derived it independently in 1916. Both subsequently won Nobel Prizes. Until recently, it was known to pharmacologists as the Langmuir equation, even though Hill deserves the credit.

A plot of B/x_A against B (known as a *Scatchard plot*) gives a straight line from which both B_{max} and K_A can be estimated. Statistically, this procedure is not without problems, and it is now usual to estimate these parameters from the untransformed binding values by an iterative non-linear curve-fitting procedure.

To this point, our analysis has considered the binding of one ligand to a homogeneous population of receptors. To get closer to real-life pharmacology, we must consider (a) what happens when more than one ligand is present, and (b) how the tissue response is related to receptor occupancy.

BINDING WHEN MORE THAN ONE DRUG IS PRESENT

▼ Suppose that two drugs, A and B, which bind to the same receptor with equilibrium dissociation constants K_A and K_B, respectively, are present at concentrations x_A and x_B. If the two drugs compete (i.e. the receptor can accommodate only one at a time), then, by application of the same reasoning as for the one-drug situation described above, the occupancy by drug A is given by:

$$p_A = \frac{x_A / K_A}{x_A / K + x_B / K_B + 1} \qquad (2.9)$$

Comparing this result with equation 2.5 shows that adding drug B, as expected, reduces the occupancy by drug A. Figure 2.4A (p. 10) shows the predicted binding curves for A in the presence of increasing concentrations of B, demonstrating the shift without any change of slope or maximum that characterises the pharmacological effect of a competitive antagonist (see Fig. 2.5). The extent of the rightward shift, on a logarithmic scale, represents the ratio (r_A, given by x_A'/x_A where x_A' is the increased concentration of A) by which the concentration of A must be increased to overcome the competition by B. Rearranging equation 2.9 shows that

$$r_A = (x_B / K_B) + 1 \qquad (2.10)$$

Thus r_A depends only on the concentration and equilibrium dissociation constant of the competing drug B, not on the concentration or equilibrium dissociation constant of A.

If A is an agonist, and B is a competitive antagonist, and we assume that the response of the tissue will be an unknown function of p_A, then the value of r_A determined from the shift of the agonist concentration–effect curve at different antagonist concentrations can be used to estimate the equilibrium constant K_B for the antagonist. Such pharmacological estimates of r_A are commonly termed *agonist dose ratios* (more properly concentration ratios, although most pharmacologists use the older term). This simple and very useful equation (2.10) is known as the *Schild equation*, after the pharmacologist who first used it to analyse drug antagonism.

Equation 2.10 can be expressed logarithmically in the form:

$$\log(r_A - 1) = \log x_B - \log K_B \qquad (2.11)$$

Thus a plot of log (r_A–1) against log x_B, usually called a Schild plot (as in Fig. 2.5 above), should give a straight line with unit slope (i.e. its gradient is equal to 1) and an abscissal intercept equal to log K_B. Following the pH and pK notation, antagonist potency can be expressed as a pA_2 value; under conditions of competitive antagonism, $pA_2 = -\log K_B$. Numerically, pA_2 is defined as the negative logarithm of the molar concentration of antagonist required to produce an agonist dose ratio equal to 2. As with pH notation, its principal advantage is that it produces simple numbers, a pA_2 of 6.5 being equivalent to a K_B of 3.2×10^{-7} mol/l.

For competitive antagonism, r shows the following characteristics:

- It depends only on the concentration and equilibrium dissociation constant of the antagonist, and not on the size of response that is chosen as a reference point for the measurements (so long as it is submaximal).
- It does not depend on the equilibrium dissociation constant of the agonist.

- It increases linearly with x_B, and the slope of a plot of (r_A-1) against x_B is equal to $1/K_B$; this relationship, being independent of the characteristics of the agonist, should be the same for an antagonist against all agonists that act on the same population of receptors.

These predictions have been verified for many examples of competitive antagonism (see Fig. 2.5).

In this section, we have avoided going into great detail and have oversimplified the theory considerably. As we learn more about the actual molecular details of how receptors work to produce their biological effects (see Ch. 3), the shortcomings of this theoretical treatment become more obvious. The two-state model can be incorporated without difficulty, but complications arise when we include the involvement of G proteins (see Ch. 3) in the reaction scheme (as they shift the equilibrium between R and R*), and when we allow for the fact that receptor 'activation' is not a simple on–off switch, as the two-state model assumes, but may take different forms. Despite strenuous efforts by theoreticians to allow for such possibilities, the molecules always seem to remain one step ahead. Nevertheless, this type of basic theory applied to the two-state model remains a useful basis for developing quantitative models of drug action. The book by Kenakin (1997) is recommended as an introduction, and the later review (Kenakin & Christopoulos, 2011) presents a detailed account of the value of quantification in the study of drug action.

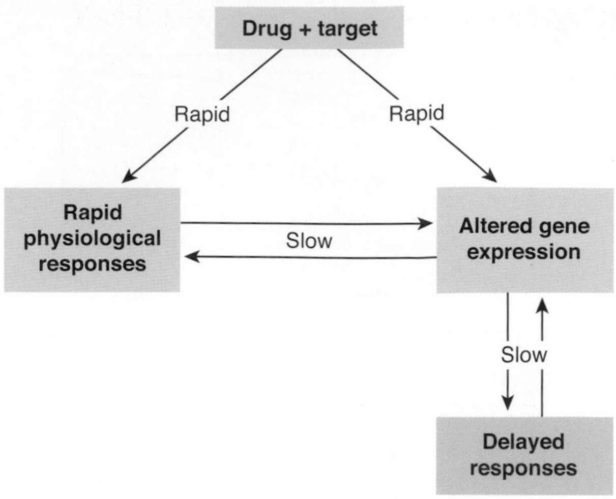

Fig. 2.14 **Early and late responses to drugs.** Many drugs act directly on their targets (left-hand arrow) to produce a rapid physiological response. If this is maintained, it is likely to cause changes in gene expression that give rise to delayed effects. Some drugs (right-hand arrow) have their primary action on gene expression, producing delayed physiological responses. Drugs can also work by both pathways. Note the bidirectional interaction between gene expression and response.

Binding of drugs to receptors

- Binding of drugs to receptors necessarily obeys the *Law of Mass Action*.
- At equilibrium, receptor occupancy is related to drug concentration by the *Hill–Langmuir equation* (2.5).
- The higher the affinity of the drug for the receptor, the lower the concentration at which it produces a given level of occupancy.
- The same principles apply when two or more drugs compete for the same receptors; each has the effect of reducing the apparent affinity for the other.

---

cases long-term addiction. In these and many other examples, the nature of the intervening mechanism is unclear, although as a general rule any long-term phenotypic change necessarily involves alterations of gene expression. Drugs are often used to treat chronic conditions, and understanding long-term as well as acute drug effects is becoming increasingly important. Pharmacologists have traditionally tended to focus on short-term physiological responses, which are much easier to study, rather than on delayed effects. The focus is now clearly shifting.

THE NATURE OF DRUG EFFECTS

In discussing how drugs act in this chapter, we have focused mainly on the consequences of receptor activation. Details of the receptors and their linkage to effects at the cellular level are described in Chapter 3. We now have a fairly good understanding at this level. It is important, however, particularly when considering drugs in a therapeutic context, that their direct effects on cellular function generally lead to secondary, delayed effects, which are often highly relevant in a clinical situation in relation to both therapeutic efficacy and harmful effects (see Fig. 2.14). For example, activation of cardiac β adrenoceptors (see Chs 3 and 21) causes rapid changes in the functioning of the heart muscle, but also slower (minutes to hours) changes in the functional state of the receptors (e.g. desensitisation), and even slower (hours to days) changes in gene expression that produce long-term changes (e.g. hypertrophy) in cardiac structure and function. Opioids (see Ch. 42) produce an immediate analgesic effect but, after a time, tolerance and dependence ensue, and in some

---

Drug effects

- Drugs act mainly on cellular targets, producing effects at different functional levels (e.g. biochemical, cellular, physiological and structural).
- The direct effect of the drug on its target produces acute responses at the biochemical, cellular or physiological levels.
- Acute responses generally lead to *delayed long-term effects*, such as desensitisation or down-regulation of receptors, hypertrophy, atrophy or remodelling of tissues, tolerance, dependence and addiction.
- Long-term delayed responses result from changes in gene expression, although the mechanisms by which the acute effects bring this about are often uncertain.
- Therapeutic effects may be based on acute responses (e.g. the use of bronchodilator drugs to treat asthma; Ch. 28) or delayed responses (e.g. antidepressants; Ch. 47).

REFERENCES AND FURTHER READING

General

Alexander, S.P.H., Benson, H.E., Faccenda, E., et al., 2013. The Concise Guide to Pharmacology 2013/2014. Br. J. Pharmacol. Special Issue 170 (8), 1449–1896. (*Summary data on a vast array of receptors, ion channels, transporters and enzymes and of the drugs that interact with them – valuable for reference*)

Colquhoun, D., 2006. The quantitative analysis of drug–receptor interactions: a short history. Trends Pharmacol. Sci. 27, 149–157. (*An illuminating account for those interested in the origins of one of the central ideas in pharmacology*)

Franks, N.P., 2008. General anaesthesia: from molecular targets to neuronal pathways of sleep and arousal. Nat. Rev. Neurosci. 9, 370–386.

Kenakin, T., 1997. Pharmacologic Analysis of Drug–Receptor Interactions, third ed. Lippincott-Raven, New York. (*Useful and detailed textbook covering most of the material in this chapter in greater depth*)

Kenakin, T., Christopoulos, A., 2013. Signalling bias in new drug discovery: detection, quantification and therapeutic impact. Nat. Rev. Drug Discov. 12, 205–216. (*Detailed discussion of the difficulties in measuring agonist efficacy and bias*)

Neubig, R., Spedding, M., Kenakin, T., Christopoulos, A., 2003. International Union of Pharmacology Committee on receptor nomenclature and drug classification: XXXVIII. Update on terms and symbols in quantitative pharmacology. Pharmacol. Rev. 55, 597–606. (*Summary of IUPHAR-approved terms and symbols relating to pharmacological receptors – useful for reference purposes*)

Rang, H.P., 2006. The receptor concept: pharmacology's big idea. Br. J. Pharmacol. 147 (Suppl. 1), 9–16. (*Short review of the origin and status of the receptor concept*)

Stephenson, R.P., 1956. A modification of receptor theory. Br. J. Pharmacol. 11, 379–393. (*Classic analysis of receptor action introducing the concept of efficacy*)

Receptor mechanisms: agonists and efficacy

Bond, R.A., Ijzerman, A.P., 2006. Recent developments in constitutive receptor activity and inverse agonism, and their potential for GPCR drug discovery. Trends Pharmacol. Sci. 27, 92–96. (*Discussion of pathophysiological consequences of constitutive receptor activation and therapeutic potential of inverse agonists – mainly hypothetical so far, but with important implications*)

Bond, R.A., Leff, P., Johnson, T.D., et al., 1995. Physiological effects of inverse agonists in transgenic mice with myocardial overexpression of the β_2 adrenoceptor. Nature 374, 270–276. (*A study with important clinical implications, showing that overexpression of β adrenoceptors results in constitutive receptor activation*)

Conn, P.J., Christopoulos, A., Lindsley, C.W., 2009. Allosteric modulators of GPCRs: a novel approach for the treatment of CNS disorders. Nat. Rev. Drug Discov. 8, 41–54. (*Outlines how drugs acting at allosteric sites may have therapeutic potential*)

Costa, T., Cotecchia, S., 2005. Historical review: negative efficacy and the constitutive activity of G protein-coupled receptors. Trends Pharmacol. Sci. 26, 618–624. (*A clear and thoughtful review of ideas relating to constitutive receptor activation and inverse agonists*)

De Ligt, R.A.F., Kourounakis, A.P., Ijzerman, A.P., 2000. Inverse agonism at G protein-coupled receptors: (patho)physiological relevance and implications for drug discovery. Br. J. Pharmacol. 130, 1–12. (*Useful review article giving many examples of constitutively active receptors and inverse agonists, and discussing the relevance of these concepts for disease mechanisms and drug discovery*)

Kelly, E., 2013. Efficacy and ligand bias at the μ-opioid receptor. Br. J. Pharmacol. 169, 1430–1446. (*A readable account of the problems of measuring efficacy as well as a discussion of agonist bias at an important brain receptor*)

Kenakin, T., Christopoulos, A., 2011. Analytical pharmacology: the impact of numbers on pharmacology. Trends Pharmacol. Sci. 32, 189–196. (*A theoretical treatment that attempts to take into account recent knowledge of receptor function at the molecular level*)

May, L.T., Leach, K., Sexton, P.M., Christopoulos, A., 2007. Allosteric modulation of G protein-coupled receptors. Annu. Rev. Pharmacol. Toxicol. 47, 1–51. (*Comprehensive review describing the characteristics, mechanisms and pharmacological implications of allosteric interactions at GPCRs*)

Seifert, R., Wenzel-Seifert, K., 2002. Constitutive activity of G protein-coupled receptors: cause of disease and common properties of wild-type receptors. Naunyn-Schmiedeberg's Arch. Pharmacol. 366, 381–416. (*Detailed review article emphasising that constitutively active receptors occur commonly and are associated with several important disease states*)

3 How drugs act: molecular aspects

OVERVIEW

In this chapter, we move from the general principles of drug action outlined in Chapter 2 to the molecules that are involved in recognising chemical signals and translating them into cellular responses. Molecular pharmacology is advancing rapidly, and the new knowledge is changing our understanding of drug action and also opening up many new therapeutic possibilities, further discussed in other chapters.

First, we consider the types of target proteins on which drugs act. Next, we describe the main families of receptors and ion channels that have been revealed by cloning and structural studies. Finally, we discuss the various forms of receptor–effector linkage (signal transduction mechanisms) through which receptors are coupled to the regulation of cell function. The relationship between the molecular structure of a receptor and its functional linkage to a particular type of effector system is a principal theme. In the next two chapters, we see how these molecular events alter important aspects of cell function – a useful basis for understanding the effects of drugs on intact living organisms. We go into more detail than is necessary for understanding today's pharmacology at a basic level, intending that students can, if they wish, skip or skim these chapters without losing the thread; however, we are confident that tomorrow's pharmacology will rest solidly on the advances in cellular and molecular biology that are discussed here.

TARGETS FOR DRUG ACTION

The protein targets for drug action on mammalian cells (Fig. 3.1) that are described in this chapter can be broadly divided into:

- receptors
- ion channels
- enzymes
- transporters (carrier molecules).

The great majority of important drugs act on one or other of these types of protein, but there are exceptions. For example, **colchicine** used to treat arthritic gout attacks (Ch. 26) interacts with the structural protein tubulin, while several immunosuppressive drugs (e.g. **ciclosporin**, Ch. 26) bind to cytosolic proteins known as immunophilins. Therapeutic antibodies that act by sequestering cytokines (protein mediators involved in inflammation; see Ch. 26) are also used. Targets for chemotherapeutic drugs (Chs 50–56), where the aim is to suppress invading microorganisms or cancer cells, include DNA and cell wall constituents as well as other proteins.

RECEPTORS

Receptors (Fig. 3.1A) are the sensing elements in the system of chemical communications that coordinates the function of all the different cells in the body, the chemical messengers being the various hormones, transmitters and other mediators discussed in Section 2 of this book. Many therapeutically useful drugs act, either as agonists or antagonists, on receptors for known endogenous mediators. In most cases, the endogenous mediator was discovered before – often many years before – the receptor was characterised pharmacologically and biochemically, but in recent years, many receptors have been identified initially on the basis of their pharmacological or molecular characteristics. In some cases, such as the cannabinoid and opioid receptors (see Chs 19 and 42), the endogenous mediators were identified later; in others, known as *orphan receptors* (see below) the mediator, if it exists, still remains unknown.

ION CHANNELS

Ion channels[1] are essentially gateways in cell membranes that selectively allow the passage of particular ions, and that are induced to open or close by a variety of mechanisms. Two important types are *ligand-gated channels* and *voltage-gated channels*. The former open only when one or more agonist molecules are bound, and are properly classified as receptors, since agonist binding is needed to activate them. Voltage-gated channels are gated by changes in the transmembrane potential rather than by agonist binding.

In general, drugs can affect ion channel function in several ways:

1. By binding to the channel protein itself, either to the ligand-binding (*orthosteric*) site of ligand-gated channels, or to other (*allosteric*) sites, or, in the simplest case, exemplified by the action of local anaesthetics on the voltage-gated sodium channel (see Ch. 43), the drug molecule plugs the channel physically (Fig. 3.1B), blocking ion permeation. Examples of drugs that bind to allosteric sites on the channel protein and thereby affect channel gating include:
   - **benzodiazepine** tranquillisers (see Ch. 44). These drugs bind to a region of the GABA$_A$ receptor–chloride channel complex (a ligand-gated channel) that is distinct from the GABA binding site and facilitate the opening of the channel by the inhibitory neurotransmitter GABA (see Ch. 38)

---

[1]'Ion channels and the electrical properties they confer on cells are involved in every human characteristic that distinguishes us from the stones in a field' (Armstrong CM 2003 Voltage-gated K channels; http://www.stke.org).

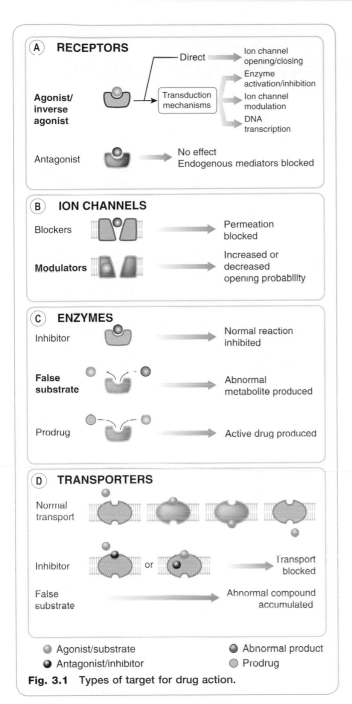

Fig. 3.1 Types of target for drug action.

ENZYMES

Many drugs are targeted on enzymes (Fig. 3.1C). Often, the drug molecule is a substrate analogue that acts as a competitive inhibitor of the enzyme (e.g. **captopril**, acting on angiotensin-converting enzyme; Ch. 22); in other cases, the binding is irreversible and non-competitive (e.g. **aspirin**, acting on cyclo-oxygenase; Ch. 26). Drugs may also act as false substrates, where the drug molecule undergoes chemical transformation to form an abnormal product that subverts the normal metabolic pathway. An example is the anticancer drug **fluorouracil**, which replaces uracil as an intermediate in purine biosynthesis but cannot be converted into thymidylate, thus blocking DNA synthesis and preventing cell division (Ch. 56).

It should also be mentioned that drugs may require enzymic degradation to convert them from an inactive form, the prodrug (see Ch. 9), to an active form (e.g. **enalapril** is converted by esterases to enalaprilat, which inhibits angiotensin converting enzyme). Furthermore, as discussed in Chapter 57, drug toxicity often results from the enzymic conversion of the drug molecule to a reactive metabolite. **Paracetamol** (see Ch. 26) causes liver damage in this way. As far as the primary action of the drug is concerned, this is an unwanted side reaction, but it is of major practical importance.

TRANSPORTERS

The movement of ions and small organic molecules across cell membranes generally occurs either through channels (see above), or through the agency of a transport protein, because the permeating molecules are often too polar (i.e. insufficiently lipid-soluble) to penetrate lipid membranes on their own (Fig. 3.1D). Many such transporters are known; examples of particular pharmacological importance include those responsible for the transport of ions and many organic molecules across the renal tubule, the intestinal epithelium and the blood–brain barrier, the transport of Na^+ and Ca^{2+} out of cells, the uptake of neurotransmitter precursors (such as choline) or of neurotransmitters themselves (such as amines and amino acids) by nerve terminals, and the transport of drug molecules and their metabolites across cell membranes and epithelial barriers. We shall encounter transporters frequently in later chapters.

In many cases, hydrolysis of ATP provides the energy for transport of substances against their electrochemical gradient. Such transport proteins include a distinct ATP binding site, and are termed ABC (ATP-binding cassette) transporters. Important examples include the sodium pump (Na^+-K^+-ATPase; see Ch. 4) and *multi-drug resistance* (MDR) transporters that eject cytotoxic drugs from cancer and microbial cells, conferring resistance to these therapeutic agents (see Ch. 56). In other cases, including the neurotransmitter transporters, the transport of organic molecules is coupled to the transport of ions (usually Na^+), either in the same direction (*symport*) or in the opposite direction (*antiport*), and therefore relies on the electrochemical gradient for Na^+ generated by the ATP-driven sodium pump. The carrier proteins embody a recognition site that makes them specific for a particular permeating species, and these recognition sites can also be targets for drugs whose effect is to block the transport system.

The importance of transporters as a source of individual variation in the pharmacokinetic characteristics of various drugs is becoming increasingly recognised (see Ch. 10).

– vasodilator drugs of the **dihydropyridine** type (see Ch. 22), which inhibit the opening of L-type calcium channels (see Ch. 4)
– **sulfonylureas** (see Ch. 31) used in treating diabetes, which act on ATP-gated potassium channels of pancreatic β-cells and thereby enhance insulin secretion.

2. By an indirect interaction, involving a G protein and other intermediaries (see p. 30).
3. By altering the level of expression of ion channels on the cell surface. For example **gabapentin** reduces the insertion of neuronal calcium channels into the plasma membrane (Ch. 45).

A summary of the different ion channel families and their functions is given below.

RECEPTOR PROTEINS

CLONING OF RECEPTORS

In the 1970s, pharmacology entered a new phase when receptors, which had until then been theoretical entities, began to emerge as biochemical realities following the development of receptor-labelling techniques (see Ch. 2), which made it possible to extract and purify the receptor material.

Once receptor proteins were isolated and purified, it was possible to analyse the amino acid sequence of a short stretch, allowing the corresponding base sequence of the mRNA to be deduced and full-length DNA to be isolated by conventional cloning methods, starting from a cDNA library obtained from a tissue source rich in the receptor of interest. The first receptor clones were obtained in this way, but subsequently expression cloning and, with the sequencing of the entire genome of various species, including human, cloning strategies based on sequence homologies, which do not require prior isolation and purification of the receptor protein, were widely used, and now several hundred receptors of all four structural families (see p. 25) have been cloned. Endogenous ligands for many of these novel receptors identified by gene cloning are so far unknown, and they are described as 'orphan receptors'.[2] Identifying ligands for these presumed receptors is often difficult. However, there are examples (e.g. the cannabinoid receptor; see Ch. 19) where important endogenous ligands have been linked to hitherto orphan receptors, and others, such as PPARs (peroxisome proliferator-activated receptors) that have emerged as the targets of important therapeutic drugs (see Ch. 32) though the endogenous ligand remains unknown. There is optimism that novel therapeutic agents will emerge by targeting this pool of unclaimed receptors.

Much information has been gained by introducing the cloned DNA encoding individual receptors into cell lines, producing cells that express the foreign receptors in a functional form. Such engineered cells allow much more precise control of the expressed receptors than is possible with natural cells or intact tissues, and the technique is widely used to study the binding and pharmacological characteristics of cloned receptors. Expressed human receptors, which often differ in their sequence and pharmacological properties from their animal counterparts, can be studied in this way.

The cloning of receptors revealed many molecular variants (subtypes) of known receptors, which had not been evident from pharmacological studies. This produced some taxonomic confusion, but in the long term molecular characterisation of receptors is essential. Barnard, one of the high priests of receptor cloning, was undaunted by the proliferation of molecular subtypes among receptors that pharmacologists had thought that they understood. He quoted Thomas Aquinas: 'Types and shadows have their ending, for the newer rite is here'. The newer rite, Barnard confidently asserted, was molecular biology. Analysis of the human and other mammalian genomes suggests that many hundreds of receptor-like genes are present, with many still to be fully characterised.

Receptors are proteins normally embedded in membrane lipid and thus have proven very difficult to crystallise. Obtaining crystals of a protein allows its structure to be analysed at very high resolution by X-ray diffraction techniques. Much of our knowledge of ligand-gated ion channel structure comes from work on the nicotinic acetylcholine receptor. Recent years have seen great strides made in crystallising other types of receptors. So far, much of the information obtained relates to how ligands bind to receptors (i.e. the extracellular domains), but we are now beginning to learn more about agonist-induced receptor conformational changes and how signalling is initiated (see Audet & Bouvier, 2012).

Now that the genes have been clearly identified, the emphasis has shifted to characterising the receptors pharmacologically and determining their molecular characteristics and physiological functions.

TYPES OF RECEPTOR

Receptors elicit many different types of cellular effect. Some of them are very rapid, such as those involved in synaptic transmission, operating within milliseconds, whereas other receptor-mediated effects, such as those produced by thyroid hormone or various steroid hormones, occur over hours or days. There are also many examples of intermediate timescales – catecholamines, for example, usually act in a matter of seconds, whereas many peptides take rather longer to produce their effects. Not surprisingly, very different types of linkage between the receptor occupation and the ensuing response are involved. Based on molecular structure and the nature of this linkage (the transduction mechanism), we can distinguish four receptor types, or superfamilies (see Figs 3.2 and 3.3; Table 3.1).

- Type 1: **ligand-gated ion channels** (also known as **ionotropic** receptors).[3] The chain of discoveries culminating in the molecular characterisation of these receptors is described by Halliwell (2007). Typically, these are the receptors on which fast neurotransmitters act (Table 3.1).
- Type 2: **G protein-coupled receptors** (GPCRs). These are also known as **metabotropic receptors** or **7-transmembrane** (7-TM or heptahelical) **receptors**. They are membrane receptors that are coupled to intracellular effector systems primarily via a G protein (see p. 27). They constitute the largest family,[4] and include receptors for many hormones and slow transmitters (Table 3.1).
- Type 3: **kinase-linked and related receptors**. This is a large and heterogeneous group of membrane receptors responding mainly to protein mediators. They comprise an extracellular ligand-binding domain linked to an intracellular domain by a

---

[2]An oddly Dickensian term that seems inappropriately condescending, because we can assume that these receptors play defined roles in physiological signalling, their 'orphanhood' reflects our ignorance, not their status. More information on orphan receptors can be found at www.guidetopharmacology.org/GRAC/FamilyDisplayForward?familyId=115#16.

[3]Here, focusing on receptors, we include ligand-gated ion channels as an example of a receptor family. Other types of ion channels are described later (p. 45); many are also drug targets, although not receptors in the strict sense.

[4]There are 865 human GPCRs comprising 1.6% of the genome (Fredriksson & Schiöth, 2005). Nearly 500 of these are believed to be odorant receptors involved in smell and taste sensations, the remainder being receptors for known or unknown endogenous mediators – enough to keep pharmacologists busy for some time yet.

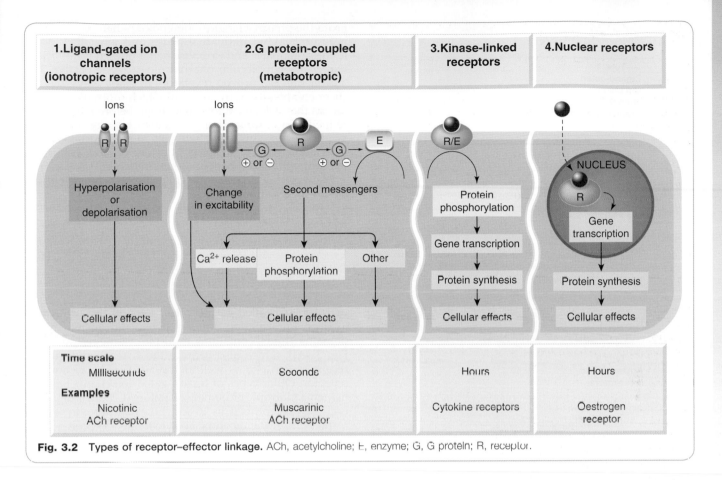

Fig. 3.2 **Types of receptor–effector linkage.** ACh, acetylcholine; E, enzyme; G, G protein; R, receptor.

single transmembrane helix. In many cases, the intracellular domain is enzymic in nature (with protein kinase or guanylyl cyclase activity).

- Type 4: **nuclear receptors.** These are receptors that regulate gene transcription.[5] Receptors of this type also recognise many foreign molecules, inducing the expression of enzymes that metabolise them.

MOLECULAR STRUCTURE OF RECEPTORS

The molecular organisation of typical members of each of these four receptor superfamilies is shown in Figure 3.3. Although individual receptors show considerable sequence variation in particular regions, and the lengths of the main intracellular and extracellular domains also vary from one to another within the same family, the overall structural patterns and associated signal transduction pathways are very consistent. The realisation that just four receptor superfamilies provide a solid framework for interpreting the complex welter of information about the effects of a large proportion of the drugs that have been studied has been one of the most refreshing developments in modern pharmacology.

RECEPTOR HETEROGENEITY AND SUBTYPES

Receptors within a given family generally occur in several molecular varieties, or subtypes, with similar architecture but significant differences in their sequences, and often in

their pharmacological properties.[6] Nicotinic acetylcholine receptors are typical in this respect; distinct subtypes occur in different brain regions (see Table 39.2), and these differ from the muscle receptor. Some of the known pharmacological differences (e.g. sensitivity to blocking agents) between muscle and brain acetylcholine receptors correlate with specific sequence differences; however, as far as we know, all nicotinic acetylcholine receptors respond to the same physiological mediator and produce the same kind of synaptic response, so why many variants should have evolved is still a puzzle.

▼ Much of the sequence variation that accounts for receptor diversity arises at the genomic level, i.e. different genes give rise to distinct receptor subtypes. Additional variation arises from alternative mRNA splicing, which means that a single gene can give rise to more than one receptor isoform. After translation from genomic DNA, the mRNA normally contains non-coding regions (introns) that are excised by mRNA splicing before the message is translated into protein. Depending on the location of the splice sites, splicing can result in inclusion or deletion of one or more of the mRNA coding regions, giving rise to long or short forms of the protein. This is an important source of variation, particularly for GPCRs, which produces receptors with different binding characteristics and different signal transduction mechanisms, although its pharmacological relevance remains to be clarified. Another process that can produce different receptors from the same gene is mRNA editing, which involves the mischievous substitution of one base in the mRNA for another, and hence a small variation in the amino acid sequence of the receptor.

Molecular heterogeneity of this kind is a feature of all kinds of receptors – indeed of functional proteins in

---

[5]The term *nuclear receptor* is something of a misnomer, because some are actually located in the cytosol and migrate to the nuclear compartment when a ligand is present.

[6]Receptors for 5-hydroxytryptamine (see Ch. 15) are currently the champions with respect to diversity, with 14 cloned subtypes.

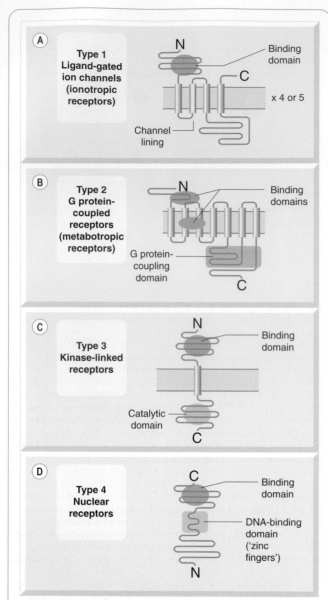

Fig. 3.3   General structure of four receptor families. The rectangular segments represent hydrophobic α-helical regions of the protein comprising approximately 20 amino acids, which form the membrane-spanning domains of the receptors. [**A**] Type 1: ligand-gated ion channels. The example illustrated here shows the subunit structure of the nicotinic acetylcholine receptor. The subunit structure of other ligand-gated ion channels is shown in Fig. 3.20. Many ligand-gated ion channels comprise four or five subunits of the type shown, the whole complex containing 16–20 membrane-spanning segments surrounding a central ion channel. [**B**] Type 2: G protein-coupled receptors. [**C**] Type 3: kinase-linked receptors. Most growth factor receptors incorporate the ligand-binding and enzymatic (kinase) domains in the same molecule, as shown, whereas cytokine receptors lack an intracellular kinase domain but link to cytosolic kinase molecules. Other structural variants also exist. [**D**] Type 4: nuclear receptors that control gene transcription.

general. New receptor subtypes and isoforms continue to be discovered, and regular updates of the catalogue are available (www.guidetopharmacology.org/). The problems of classification, nomenclature and taxonomy resulting from this flood of data have been mentioned earlier.

From the pharmacological viewpoint, where our concern is to understand individual drugs and what they do to living organisms, and to devise better ones, it is important that we keep molecular pharmacology in perspective. The 'newer rite' has proved revelatory in many ways, but the sheer complexity of the ways in which molecules behave means that we have a long way to go before reaching the reductionist Utopia that molecular biology promised. When we do, this book will get much shorter. In the meantime, we try to pick out the general principles without getting too bogged down in detail.

We will now describe the characteristics of each of the four receptor superfamilies.

TYPE 1: LIGAND-GATED ION CHANNELS

In this general description of ligand-gated ion channel structure we will focus primarily on the nicotinic acetylcholine receptor, which we find at the skeletal neuromuscular junction (Ch. 13). It is the one we know most about and is similar in structure and function to other cys-loop receptors (so called because they have in their structure a large intracellular domain between transmembrane domains 3 and 4 containing multiple cystine residues [see Fig. 3.3A]), which also include the $GABA_A$ and glycine receptors (Ch. 38) as well as the $5\text{-}HT_3$ (Chs 15 and 39) receptor. Other types of ligand-gated ion channel exist – namely ionotropic glutamate receptors (Ch. 38) and purinergic P2X receptors (Chs 16 and 39) – that differ in several respects from the nicotinic acetylcholine receptor.

MOLECULAR STRUCTURE

Ligand-gated ion channels have structural features in common with other ion channels, described on p. 45. The nicotinic acetylcholine receptor (Fig. 3.4), the first to be cloned, consists of a pentameric assembly of different subunits, of which there are four types, termed α, β, γ and δ, each of molecular weight (M_r) 40–58 kDa. The subunits show marked sequence homology, and each contains four membrane-spanning α-helices, inserted into the membrane as shown in Figure 3.4B. The pentameric structure (α_2, β, γ, δ) possesses two acetylcholine binding sites, each lying at the interface between one of the two α subunits and its neighbour. Both must bind acetylcholine molecules in order for the receptor to be activated. This receptor is sufficiently large to be seen in electron micrographs, and Figure 3.4B shows its structure, based mainly on a high-resolution electron diffraction study (Miyazawa et al., 2003). Each subunit spans the membrane four times, so the channel comprises no fewer than 20 membrane-spanning helices surrounding a central pore.

▼ The two acetylcholine-binding sites lie on the extracellular N-terminal region of the two α subunits. One of the transmembrane helices (M_2) from each of the five subunits forms the lining of the ion channel (Fig. 3.4). The five M_2 helices that form the pore are sharply kinked inwards halfway through the membrane, forming a constriction. When acetylcholine molecules bind, a conformation change occurs in the extracellular part of the receptor (see review by Gay & Yakel, 2007), which twists the α subunits, causing the kinked M_2 segments to swivel out of the way, thus opening the channel (Miyazawa et al., 2003). The channel lining contains a series of anionic residues, making the channel selectively permeable to cations (primarily Na^+ and K^+, although some types of nicotinic receptor are permeable to Ca^{2+} as well).

The use of site-directed mutagenesis, which enables short regions, or single residues, of the amino acid sequence to be altered, has shown that a mutation of a critical residue in the M_2 helix changes

Table 3.1   The four main types of receptor

	Type 1: Ligand-gated ion channels	Type 2: G protein-coupled receptors	Type 3: Receptor kinases	Type 4: Nuclear receptors
Location	Membrane	Membrane	Membrane	Intracellular
Effector	Ion channel	Channel or enzyme	Protein kinases	Gene transcription
Coupling	Direct	G protein or arrestin	Direct	Via DNA
Examples	Nicotinic acetylcholine receptor, GABA$_A$ receptor	Muscarinic acetylcholine receptor, adrenoceptors	Insulin, growth factors, cytokine receptors	Steroid receptors
Structure	Oligomeric assembly of subunits surrounding central pore	Monomeric or oligomeric assembly of subunits comprising seven transmembrane helices with intracellular G protein-coupling domain	Single transmembrane helix linking extracellular receptor domain to intracellular kinase domain	Monomeric structure with receptor- and DNA-binding domains

the channel from being cation selective (hence excitatory in the context of synaptic function) to being anion selective (typical of receptors for inhibitory transmitters such as GABA and glycine). Other mutations affect properties such as gating and desensitisation of ligand-gated channels.

Other ligand-gated ion channels, such as glutamate receptors (see Ch. 38) and P2X receptors (see Ch. 39), whose structures are shown in Figure 3.5, have a different architecture. Ionotropic glutamate receptors are tetrameric and the pore is built from loops rather than transmembrane helices, in common with many other (non-ligand-gated) ion channels (see p. 29). P2X receptors are trimeric and each subunit has only two transmembrane domains (North, 2002). The nicotinic receptor and other cys-loop receptors are pentamers with two agonist binding sites on each receptor. Binding of one agonist molecule to one site increases the affinity of binding at the other site (positive co-operativity) and both sites need to be bound for the receptor to be activated and the channel to open. Some ionotropic glutamate receptors have as many as four agonist binding sites and P2X receptors have three but they appear to open when two agonist molecules are bound. Once again we realise that the simple model of receptor activation shown in Figure 2.1 is an oversimplification as it only considered one agonist molecule binding to produce a response. For two or more agonist molecules binding, more complex mathematical models are needed (see Colquhoun, 2006).

THE GATING MECHANISM

Receptors of this type control the fastest synaptic events in the nervous system, in which a neurotransmitter acts on the postsynaptic membrane of a nerve or muscle cell and transiently increases its permeability to particular ions. Most excitatory neurotransmitters, such as acetylcholine at the neuromuscular junction (Ch. 13) or glutamate in the central nervous system (Ch. 38), cause an increase in Na^+ and K^+ permeability and in some instances Ca^{2+} permeability. At negative membrane potentials this results in a net inward current carried mainly by Na^+, which depolarises the cell and increases the probability that it will generate an action potential. The action of the transmitter reaches a peak in a fraction of a millisecond, and usually decays within a few milliseconds. The sheer speed of this response implies that the coupling between the receptor and the ion channel is a direct one, and the molecular structure of the receptor–channel complex (see above) agrees with this. In contrast to other receptor families (see below), no intermediate biochemical steps are involved in the transduction process.

▼ The patch clamp recording technique, devised by Neher and Sakmann, allows the very small current flowing through a single ion channel to be measured directly (Fig. 3.6), and the results have fully confirmed the previous interpretation of channel properties based on noise analysis made by Katz and Miledi in 1972. The patch clamp technique provides a view, rare in biology, of the physiological behaviour of individual protein molecules in real time, and has given many new insights into the gating reactions and permeability characteristics of both ligand-gated channels and voltage-gated channels (see p. 30, Fig. 3.6). The magnitude of the single channel conductance confirms that permeation occurs through a physical pore through the membrane, because the ion flow is too large (about 10^7 ions per second) to be compatible with a carrier mechanism. The channel conductance produced by different agonists is the same, whereas the mean channel lifetime varies. The ligand–receptor interaction scheme shown in Chapter 2 is a useful model for ion-channel gating. The conformation R*, representing the open state of the ion channel, is thought to be the same for all agonists, accounting for the finding that the channel conductance does not vary. Kinetically, the mean open time is determined mainly by the closing rate constant, α, and this varies from one drug to another. As explained in Chapter 2, an agonist of high efficacy that activates a large proportion of the receptors that it occupies will be characterised by $\beta/\alpha \gg 1$, whereas for a drug of low efficacy β/α has a lower value.

At some ligand-gated ion channels the situation is more complicated because different agonists may cause individual channels to open to one or more of several distinct conductance levels (Fig. 3.6). This implies that there is more than one R* conformation. Furthermore, desensitisation of ligand-gated ion channels (see Ch. 2) also involves one or more additional agonist-induced conformational states. These findings necessitate some elaboration of the simple scheme in which only a single open state, R*, is represented, and are an example of the way in which the actual behaviour of receptors makes our theoretical models look a little threadbare.

TYPE 2: G PROTEIN-COUPLED RECEPTORS

The abundant GPCR family comprises many of the receptors that are familiar to pharmacologists, such as muscarinic AChRs, adrenoceptors, dopamine receptors, 5-HT receptors, opioid receptors, receptors for many peptides, purine receptors and many others, including the chemoreceptors involved in olfaction and pheromone detection, and also many 'orphans' (see Fredriksson & Schiöth, 2005). For most of these, pharmacological and molecular studies have revealed a variety of subtypes. All have the characteristic heptahelical structure.

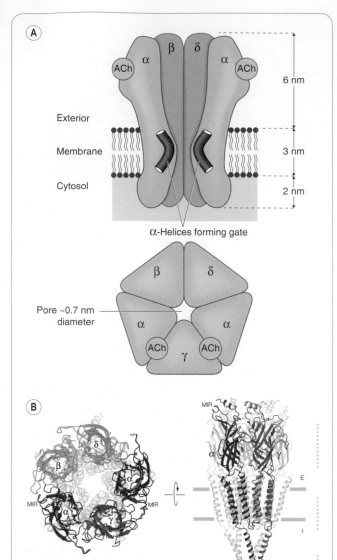

Fig. 3.4 Structure of the nicotinic acetylcholine receptor (a typical ligand-gated ion channel). [**A**] Schematic diagram in side view (upper) and plan view (lower). The five receptor subunits (α_2, β, γ, δ) form a cluster surrounding a central transmembrane pore, the lining of which is formed by the M_2 helical segments of each subunit. These contain a preponderance of negatively charged amino acids, which makes the pore cation selective. There are two acetylcholine binding sites in the extracellular portion of the receptor, at the interface between the α and the adjoining subunits. When acetylcholine binds, the kinked α-helices either straighten out or swing out of the way, thus opening the channel pore. [**B**] High-resolution image showing revised arrangement of intracellular domains. *(Panel [A] based on Unwin N 1993 Nicotinic acetylcholine receptor at 9A resolution. J Mol Biol 229, 1101–1124, and Unwin N 1995 Acetylcholine receptor channel imaged in the open state. Nature 373, 37–43; panel [B] reproduced with permission from Unwin N 2005 Refined structure of the nicotinic acetylcholine receptor at 4A resolution. J Mol Biol 346(4), 967–989.)*

Ligand-gated ion channels

- These are sometimes called ionotropic receptors.
- They are involved mainly in fast synaptic transmission.
- There are several structural families, the commonest being heteromeric assemblies of four or five subunits, with transmembrane helices arranged around a central aqueous channel.
- Ligand binding and channel opening occur on a millisecond timescale.
- Examples include the nicotinic acetylcholine, GABA type A (GABA$_A$), glutamate (NMDA) and ATP (P2X) receptors.

Many neurotransmitters, apart from peptides, can interact with both GPCRs and ligand-gated channels, allowing the same molecule to produce fast (through ligand-gated ion channels) and relatively slow (through GPCRs) effects. Individual peptide hormones, on the other hand, generally act either on GPCRs or on kinase-linked receptors (see below), but rarely on both, and a similar choosiness applies to the many ligands that act on nuclear receptors.[7]

The human genome includes genes encoding about 400 GPCRs (excluding odorant receptors), which constitute the commonest single class of targets for therapeutic drugs, and it is thought that many promising therapeutic drug targets of this type remain to be identified. For a short review, see Hill (2006).

MOLECULAR STRUCTURE

The first GPCR to be fully characterised was the β adrenoceptor (Ch. 14), which was cloned in 1986. Molecular biology caught up very rapidly with pharmacology, and all of the receptors that had been identified by their pharmacological properties have now been cloned. What seemed revolutionary in 1986 is now commonplace. Recently, the difficulties of crystallising GPCRs have been overcome (see Weis & Kobilka, 2008), allowing the use of the powerful technique of X-ray crystallography to study the molecular structure of these receptors in detail (Fig. 3.7). Also, fluorescence methods have been developed to study the kinetics of ligand binding and subsequent conformational changes associated with activation (see Lohse et al., 2008; Bockenhauer et al., 2011). This is starting to provide important information on agonist- and antagonist-bound receptor conformations as well as receptor–G protein interactions. From such studies we are gaining a clearer picture of the mechanism of activation of GPCRs and the factors determining agonist efficacy, as well as having a better basis for designing new GPCR ligands.

G protein-coupled receptors consist of a single polypeptide chain, usually of 350–400 residues, but can in some cases be up to 1100 residues. The general anatomy is shown in Figure 3.3B. Their characteristic structure

---

[7]Examples of promiscuity are increasing, however. Steroid hormones, normally faithful to nuclear receptors, make the occasional pass at ion channels and other targets (see Falkenstein et al., 2000), and some eicosanoids act on nuclear receptors as well as GPCRs. Nature is quite open-minded, although such examples are liable to make pharmacologists frown and students despair.

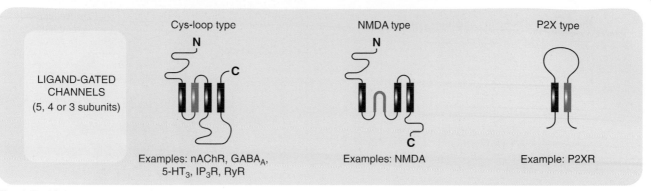

Fig. 3.5 Molecular architecture of ligand-gated ion channels. Red and blue rectangles represent membrane-spanning α-helices and blue hairpins represent the P loop pore-forming regions. Cys-loop receptors are pentameric, NMDA-type receptors are tetrameric and P2X receptors are trimeric. 5-HT$_3$, 5-hydroxytryptamine type 3 receptor; GABA$_A$, GABA type A receptor; IP$_3$R, inositol trisphosphate receptor; nAChR, nicotinic acetylcholine receptor; NMDA, *N*-methyl-D-aspartatic acid receptor; P2XR, purine P2X receptor; RyR, ryanodine receptor.

Table 3.2 G protein-coupled receptor families[a]

Family	Receptors[b]	Structural features
A: rhodopsin family	The largest group. Receptors for most amine neurotransmitters, many neuropeptides, purines, prostanoids, cannabinoids, etc.	Short extracellular (N terminal) tail. Ligand binds to transmembrane helices (amines) or to extracellular loops (peptides)
B: secretin/glucagon receptor family	Receptors for peptide hormones, including secretin, glucagon, calcitonin	Intermediate extracellular tail incorporating ligand-binding domain
C: metabotropic glutamate receptor/calcium sensor family	Small group. Metabotropic glutamate receptors, GABA$_B$ receptors, Ca^{2+}-sensing receptors	Long extracellular tail incorporating ligand-binding domain

[a]A fourth distinct family includes many receptors for pheromones but no pharmacological receptors.
[b]For full lists, see www.guidetopharmacology.org.

comprises seven transmembrane α-helices, similar to those of the ion channels discussed above, with an extracellular N-terminal domain of varying length, and an intracellular C-terminal domain.

GPCRs are divided into three distinct families. There is considerable sequence homology between the members of one family, but little between different families. They share the same seven transmembrane helix (heptahelical) structure, but differ in other respects, principally in the length of the extracellular N-terminus and the location of the agonist binding domain (Table 3.2). Family A is by far the largest, comprising most monoamine, neuropeptide and chemokine receptors. Family B includes receptors for some other peptides, such as calcitonin and glucagon. Family C is the smallest, its main members being the metabotropic glutamate and GABA receptors (Ch. 38) and the Ca^{2+}-sensing receptors[8] (see Ch. 36).

▼ The understanding of the function of receptors of this type owes much to studies of a closely related protein, *rhodopsin*, which is responsible for transduction in retinal rods. This protein is abundant in the retina, and much easier to study than receptor proteins (which are anything but abundant); it is built on an identical plan to that shown in Figure 3.3 and also produces a response in the rod (hyperpolarisation, associated with inhibition of Na$^+$ conductance) through a mechanism involving a G protein (see p. 32, Fig. 3.9). The most obvious difference is that a photon, rather than an agonist molecule, produces the response. In effect, rhodopsin can be regarded as incorporating its own inbuilt agonist molecule, namely *retinal*, which isomerises from the *trans* (inactive) to the *cis* (active) form when it absorbs a photon.

Site-directed mutagenesis experiments show that the third cytoplasmic loop is the region of the molecule that couples to the G protein, because deletion or modification of this section results in receptors that still bind ligands but cannot associate with G proteins or produce responses. Usually, a particular receptor subtype couples selectively with a particular type of G protein, and swapping parts of the cytoplasmic loop between different receptors alters their G protein selectivity. Phosphorylation of serine and threonine residues on the C-terminal tail and other intracellular domains by intracellular kinases can result in receptor desensitisation (see p. 36).

For small molecules, such as noradrenaline (norepinephrine) and acetylcholine, the ligand-binding domain of class A receptors is buried in the cleft between the α-helical segments within the membrane (Figs 3.3B and 3.7), similar to the slot occupied by retinal in the rhodopsin molecule.

[8]The Ca^{2+}-sensing receptor (see Conigrave et al., 2000) is an unusual GPCR that is activated not by conventional mediators, but by extracellular Ca^{2+} in the range of 1–10 mmol/l – an extremely low affinity in comparison with other GPCR agonists. It is expressed by cells of the parathyroid gland, and serves to regulate the extracellular Ca^{2+} concentration by controlling parathyroid hormone secretion (Ch. 36). This homeostatic mechanism is quite distinct from the mechanisms for regulating intracellular Ca^{2+}, discussed in Chapter 4.

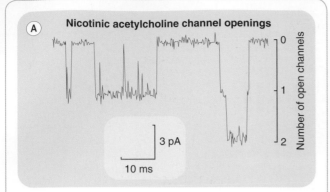

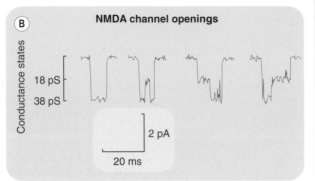

Fig. 3.6 **Single channel openings recorded by the patch clamp technique.** [**A**] Acetylcholine-operated ion channels at the frog motor endplate. The pipette, which was applied tightly to the surface of the membrane, contained 10 μmol/l ACh. The downward deflections show the currents flowing through single ion channels in the small patch of membrane under the pipette tip. Towards the end of the record, two channels can be seen to open with a discrete step from the first to the second. [**B**] Single-channel NMDA receptor currents recorded from cerebellar neurons in the outside-out patch conformation. NMDA was added to the outside of the patch to activate the channel. The channel opens to multiple conductance levels. In [**B**] the openings to the higher conductance level and the subsequent closings are smooth, indicating that one channel is opening (two channels would not be expected to open and close simultaneously) whereas in [**A**] there are discrete steps indicating two channels. *(Panel [A] courtesy of D Colquhoun and DC Ogden; panel [B] reproduced with permission from Cull-Candy SG & Usowicz MM 1987 Nature 325, 525–528.)*

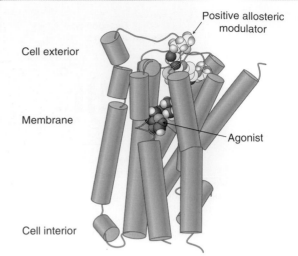

Fig. 3.7 **Structure of the M₄ muscarinic receptor.** High resolution image showing the conformation of the M₄ muscarinic receptor bound with both an agonist (orthosteric) and a positive allosteric modulator. The brown cylinders represent the transmembrane domains. The full extent of the N- and C-terminal domains and the third intracellular loop are not shown. *(Courtesy of A Christopoulos.)*

Peptide ligands, such as substance P (Ch. 18), bind more superficially to the extracellular loops, as shown in Figure 3.3B. From crystal structures and single-site mutagenesis experiments, it is possible to map the ligand-binding domain of these receptors, and the hope is that it may soon be possible to design synthetic ligands based on knowledge of the receptor site structure – an important milestone for the pharmaceutical industry, which has relied up to now mainly on the structure of endogenous mediators (such as histamine) or plant alkaloids (such as morphine) for its chemical inspiration.[9]

---

[9]In the past many lead compounds have come from screening huge chemical libraries (see Ch. 60). No inspiration was required, just robust assays, large computers and efficient robotics. Now with the generation of crystal structures we may be moving to a more sophisticated age in drug discovery.

PROTEASE-ACTIVATED RECEPTORS

▼ Although activation of GPCRs is normally the consequence of a diffusible agonist, it can be the result of protease activation. Four types of protease-activated receptors (PARs) have been identified (see review by Ramachandran & Hollenberg, 2008). Many proteases, such as thrombin (a protease involved in the blood-clotting cascade; see Ch. 24), activate PARs by snipping off the end of the extracellular N-terminal tail of the receptor (Fig. 3.8) to expose five or six N-terminal residues that bind to receptor domains in the extracellular loops, functioning as a 'tethered agonist'. Receptors of this type occur in many tissues (see Ramachandran & Hollenberg, 2008), and they appear to play a role in inflammation and other responses to tissue damage where tissue proteases are released. One of the family of PARs, PAR-2, is activated by a protease released from mast cells, and is expressed on sensory neurons. It is thought to play a role in inflammatory pain (see Ch. 42). A PAR molecule can be activated only once, because the cleavage cannot be reversed, so continuous resynthesis of receptor protein is necessary. Inactivation occurs by a further proteolytic cleavage that frees the tethered ligand, or by desensitisation, involving phosphorylation (Fig. 3.8), after which the receptor is internalised and degraded, to be replaced by newly synthesised protein.

G PROTEINS AND THEIR ROLE

G proteins comprise a family of membrane-resident proteins whose function is to recognise activated GPCRs and pass on the message to the effector systems that generate a cellular response. They represent the level of middle management in the organisational hierarchy, intervening between the receptors – choosy mandarins, alert to the faintest whiff of their preferred chemical – and the effector enzymes or ion channels – the blue-collar brigade that gets the job done without needing to know which hormone authorised the process. They are the go-between proteins, but were actually called G proteins because of their interaction with the guanine nucleotides, GTP and GDP. For more detailed information on the structure and functions of G proteins, see reviews by Milligan & Kostenis (2006) and Oldham & Hamm (2008). G proteins consist of three

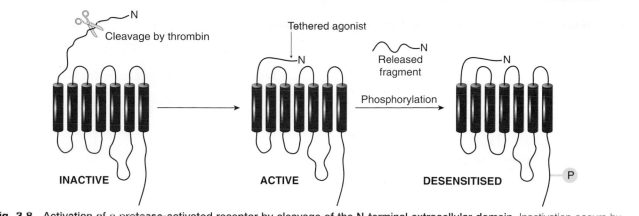

Fig. 3.8 Activation of a protease-activated receptor by cleavage of the N-terminal extracellular domain. Inactivation occurs by phosphorylation. Recovery requires resynthesis of the receptor.

G protein-coupled receptors

- These are sometimes called metabotropic or seven-transmembrane-domain (7-TDM) receptors.
- Structures comprise seven membrane-spanning α-helices, often linked as dimeric structures.
- The third intracellular loop interacts with the G protein.
- The G protein is a membrane protein comprising three subunits (α, β, γ), the α subunit possessing GTPase activity.
- When the trimer binds to an agonist-occupied receptor, the α subunit binds GTP, dissociates and is then free to activate an effector (e.g. a membrane enzyme). In some cases, the βγ subunit is the activator species.
- Activation of the effector is terminated when the bound GTP molecule is hydrolysed, which allows the α subunit to recombine with βγ.
- There are several types of G protein, which interact with different receptors and control different effectors.
- Examples include muscarinic acetylcholine receptors, adrenoceptors, neuropeptide and chemokine receptors, and protease-activated receptors.

subunits: α, β and γ (Fig. 3.9). Guanine nucleotides bind to the α subunit, which has enzymic (GTPase) activity, catalysing the conversion of GTP to GDP. The β and γ subunits remain together as a βγ complex. The 'γ' subunit is anchored to the membrane through a fatty acid chain, coupled to the G protein through a reaction known as *prenylation*. G proteins appear to be freely diffusible in the plane of the membrane, so a single pool of G protein in a cell can interact with several different receptors and effectors in an essentially promiscuous fashion. In the 'resting' state (Fig. 3.9), the G protein exists as an αβγ trimer, which may or may not be precoupled to the receptor, with GDP occupying the site on the α subunit. When a GPCR is activated by an agonist molecule, a conformational change occurs, involving the cytoplasmic domain of the receptor (Fig. 3.3B), inducing a high affinity interaction of αβγ and the receptor. This agonist-induced interaction of αβγ with the receptor occurs within about 50 ms, causing the bound

GDP to dissociate and to be replaced with GTP (GDP-GTP exchange), which in turn causes dissociation of the G protein trimer, releasing α–GTP and βγ subunits; these are the 'active' forms of the G protein, which diffuse in the membrane and can associate with various enzymes and ion channels, causing activation of the target (Fig. 3.9). It was originally thought that only the α subunit had a signalling function, the βγ complex serving merely as a chaperone to keep the flighty α subunits out of range of the various effector proteins that they might otherwise excite. However, the βγ complexes actually make assignations of their own, and control effectors in much the same way as the α subunits. Association of α or βγ subunits with target enzymes or channels can cause either activation or inhibition, depending on which G protein is involved (see Table 3.3). G protein activation results in amplification, because a single agonist–receptor complex can activate several G protein molecules in turn, and each of these can remain associated with the effector enzyme for long enough to produce many molecules of product. The product (see below) is often a 'second messenger', and further amplification occurs before the final cellular response is produced. Signalling is terminated when the hydrolysis of GTP to GDP occurs through the GTPase activity of the α subunit. The resulting α–GDP then dissociates from the effector, and reunites with βγ, completing the cycle.

▼Attachment of the α subunit to an effector molecule actually increases its GTPase activity, the magnitude of this increase being different for different types of effector. Because GTP hydrolysis is the step that terminates the ability of the α subunit to produce its effect, regulation of its GTPase activity by the effector protein means that the activation of the effector tends to be self-limiting. In addition, there is a family of about 20 cellular proteins, regulators of G protein signalling (RGS) proteins (see review by Xie & Palmer, 2007), that possess a conserved sequence that binds specifically to α subunits to increase greatly their GTPase activity, so hastening the hydrolysis of GTP and inactivating the complex. RGS proteins thus exert an inhibitory effect on G protein signalling, a mechanism that is thought to have a regulatory function in many situations.

How is specificity of GPCR function achieved so that each kind of receptor produces a distinct pattern of cellular responses? With a common pool of promiscuous G proteins linking the various receptors and effector systems in a cell, it might seem that all specificity would be lost, but this is clearly not the case. For example, mAChRs and β adrenoceptors, both of which occur in cardiac muscle

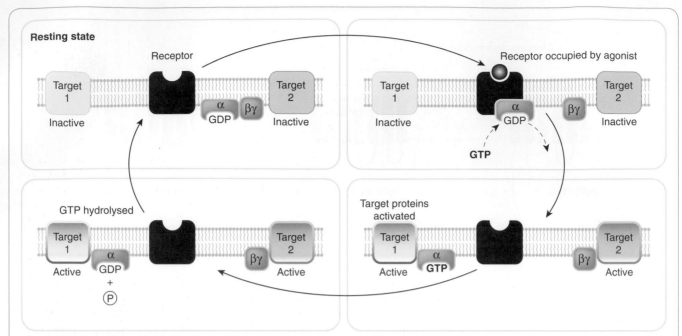

Fig. 3.9 The function of the G protein. The G protein consists of three subunits (α, β, γ), which are anchored to the membrane through attached lipid residues. Coupling of the α subunit to an agonist-occupied receptor causes the bound GDP to exchange with intracellular GTP; the α–GTP complex then dissociates from the receptor and from the βγ complex, and interacts with a target protein (target 1, which may be an enzyme, such as adenylyl cyclase or phospholipase C). The βγ complex also activates a target protein (target 2, which may be an ion channel or a kinase). The GTPase activity of the α subunit is increased when the target protein is bound, leading to hydrolysis of the bound GTP to GDP, whereupon the α subunit reunites with βγ.

Table 3.3 The main G protein subtypes and their functions[a]

Subtypes	Associated receptors	Main effectors	Notes
Gα subunits			
$G\alpha_s$	Many amine and other receptors (e.g. catecholamines, histamine, serotonin)	Stimulates adenylyl cyclase, causing increased cAMP formation	Activated by cholera toxin, which blocks GTPase activity, thus preventing inactivation
$G\alpha_i$	As for $G\alpha_s$, also opioid, cannabinoid receptors	Inhibits adenylyl cyclase, decreasing cAMP formation	Blocked by pertussis toxin, which prevents dissociation of αβγ complex
$G\alpha_o$	As for $G\alpha_s$, also opioid, cannabinoid receptors	? Limited effects of α subunit (effects mainly due to βγ subunits)	Blocked by pertussis toxin. Occurs mainly in nervous system
$G\alpha_q$	Amine, peptide and prostanoid receptors	Activates phospholipase C, increasing production of second messengers inositol trisphosphate and diacylglycerol (see p. 34 and 35)	
Gβγ subunits			
	All GPCRs	Activate potassium channels inhibit voltage-gated calcium channels activate GPCR kinases (GRKs, p. 36) activate mitogen-activated protein kinase cascade Interact with some forms of adenylyl cyclase and with phospholipase Cβ	Many βγ isoforms identified, but specific functions are not yet known

GPCR, G protein-coupled receptor.

[a]This table lists only those isoforms of major pharmacological significance. Many more have been identified, some of which play roles in olfaction, taste, visual transduction and other physiological functions (see Offermanns, 2003).

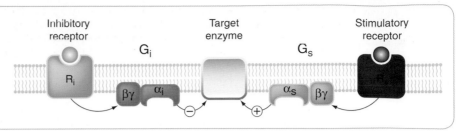

Fig. 3.10 Bidirectional control of a target enzyme, such as adenylyl cyclase by G_s and G_i. Heterogeneity of G proteins allows different receptors to exert opposite effects on a target enzyme.

cells, produce opposite functional effects (Chs 13 and 14). The main reason is molecular variation within the α subunits, of which more than 20 subtypes have been identified[10] (Table 3.3). Four main classes of G protein (G_s, G_i, G_o and G_q) are of pharmacological importance. As summarised in Table 3.3, they show selectivity with respect to both the receptors and the effectors with which they couple, having specific recognition domains in their structure complementary to specific G protein-binding domains in the receptor and effector molecules. G_s and G_i produce, respectively, stimulation and inhibition of the enzyme *adenylyl cyclase* (Fig. 3.10).

The α subunits of these G proteins differ in structure. One functional difference that has been useful as an experimental tool to distinguish which type of G protein is involved in different situations concerns the action of two bacterial toxins, *cholera toxin* and *pertussis toxin* (see Table 3.3). These toxins, which are enzymes, catalyse a conjugation reaction (ADP ribosylation) on the α subunit of G proteins. Cholera toxin acts only on G_s, and it causes persistent activation. Many of the symptoms of cholera, such as the excessive secretion of fluid from the gastrointestinal epithelium, are due to the uncontrolled activation of adenylyl cyclase that occurs. Pertussis toxin specifically blocks G_i and G_o by preventing dissociation of the G protein trimer.

TARGETS FOR G PROTEINS

The main targets for G proteins, through which GPCRs control different aspects of cell function (see Nahorski, 2006; Table 3.3), are:

- *adenylyl cyclase*, the enzyme responsible for cAMP formation
- *phospholipase C*, the enzyme responsible for inositol phosphate and diacylglycerol (DAG) formation
- *ion channels*, particularly calcium and potassium channels
- *Rho A/Rho kinase*, a system that regulates the activity of many signalling pathways controlling cell growth and proliferation, smooth muscle contraction, etc.
- *mitogen-activated protein kinase* (MAP kinase), a system that controls many cell functions, including cell division.

The adenylyl cyclase/cAMP system

The discovery by Sutherland and his colleagues of the role of cAMP (cyclic 3′,5′-adenosine monophosphate) as

an intracellular mediator demolished at a stroke the barriers that existed between biochemistry and pharmacology, and introduced the concept of second messengers in signal transduction. cAMP is a nucleotide synthesised within the cell from ATP by the action of a membrane-bound enzyme, adenylyl cyclase. It is produced continuously and inactivated by hydrolysis to 5′-AMP by the action of a family of enzymes known as phosphodiesterases (PDEs, see below). Many different drugs, hormones and neurotransmitters act on GPCRs and increase or decrease the catalytic activity of adenylyl cyclase, thus raising or lowering the concentration of cAMP within the cell. In mammalian cells there are 10 different molecular isoforms of the enzyme, some of which respond selectively to $G\alpha_s$ or $G\alpha_i$.

Cyclic AMP regulates many aspects of cellular function including, for example, enzymes involved in energy metabolism, cell division and cell differentiation, ion transport, ion channels and the contractile proteins in smooth muscle. These varied effects are, however, all brought about by a common mechanism, namely the activation of *protein kinases* by cAMP – primarily protein kinase A (PKA) in eukaryotic cells. Protein kinases regulate the function of many different cellular proteins by controlling protein phosphorylation. Figure 3.11 shows how increased cAMP production in response to β-adrenoceptor activation affects enzymes involved in glycogen and fat metabolism in liver, fat and muscle cells. The result is a coordinated response in which stored energy in the form of glycogen and fat is made available as glucose to fuel muscle contraction.

Other examples of regulation by cAMP-dependent protein kinases include the increased activity of voltage-gated calcium channels in heart muscle cells (see Ch. 21). Phosphorylation of these channels increases the amount of Ca^{2+} entering the cell during the action potential, and thus increases the force of contraction of the heart.

In smooth muscle, cAMP-dependent protein kinase phosphorylates (thereby inactivating) another enzyme, *myosin light-chain kinase*, which is required for contraction. This accounts for the smooth muscle relaxation produced by many drugs that increase cAMP production in smooth muscle (see Ch. 4).

As mentioned above, receptors linked to G_i rather than G_s inhibit adenylyl cyclase, and thus reduce cAMP formation. Examples include certain types of mAChR (e.g. the M_2 receptor of cardiac muscle; see Ch. 13), α_2 adrenoceptors in smooth muscle (Ch. 14) and opioid receptors (see Ch. 42). Adenylyl cyclase can be activated directly by drugs such as **forskolin**, which is used experimentally to study the role of the cAMP system.

Cyclic AMP is hydrolysed within cells by *phosphodiesterases* (PDEs), an important and ubiquitous family of enzymes. Eleven PDE subtypes exist, of which some (e.g.

---

[10]In humans there are 21 known subtypes of Gα, 6 of Gβ and 12 of Gγ, providing, in theory, about 1500 variants of the trimer. We know little about the role of different α, β and γ subtypes, but it would be rash to assume that the variations are functionally irrelevant. By now, you will be unsurprised (even if somewhat bemused) by such a display of molecular heterogeneity, for it is the way of evolution.

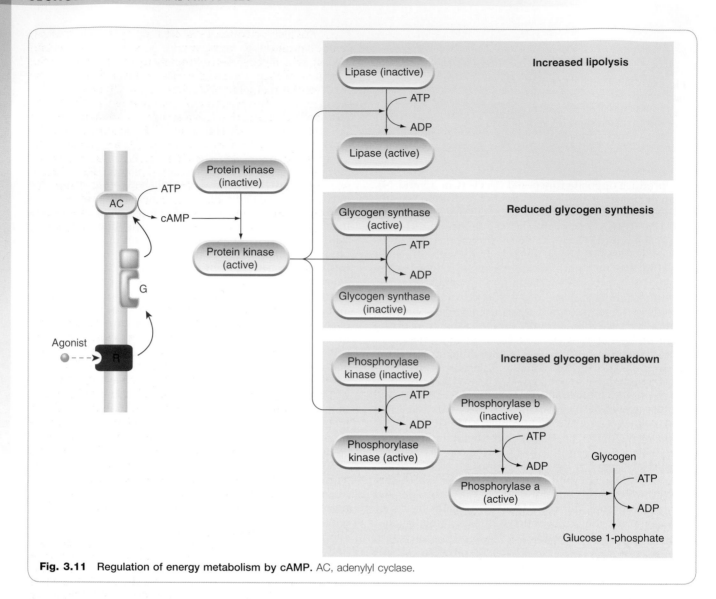

Fig. 3.11 **Regulation of energy metabolism by cAMP.** AC, adenylyl cyclase.

PDE$_3$ and PDE$_4$) are cAMP-selective, while others (e.g. PDE$_5$) are cGMP-selective. Most are weakly inhibited by drugs such as methylxanthines (e.g. **theophylline** and **caffeine**; see Chs 28 and 48). **Rolipram** (used to treat asthma; Ch. 28) is selective for PDE$_4$, expressed in inflammatory cells; **milrinone** (used to treat heart failure; Ch. 21) is selective for PDE$_3$, which is expressed in heart muscle; **sildenafil** (better known as Viagra; Ch. 35) is selective for PDE$_5$, and consequently enhances the vasodilator effects of nitrous oxide (NO) and drugs that release NO, whose effects are mediated by cGMP (see Ch. 20). The similarity of some of the actions of these drugs to those of sympathomimetic amines (Ch. 14) probably reflects their common property of increasing the intracellular concentration of cAMP. Selective inhibitors of the various PDEs are being developed, mainly to treat cardiovascular and respiratory diseases.

The phospholipase C/inositol phosphate system

The *phosphoinositide* system, an important intracellular second messenger system, was first discovered in the 1950s by Hokin and Hokin, whose recondite interests centred on the mechanism of salt secretion by the nasal glands of seabirds. They found that secretion was accompanied by increased turnover of a minor class of membrane phospholipids known as phosphoinositides (collectively known as PIs; Fig. 3.12). Subsequently, Michell and Berridge found that many hormones that produce an increase in free intracellular Ca^{2+} concentration (which include, for example, muscarinic agonists and α-adrenoceptor agonists acting on smooth muscle and salivary glands, and vasopressin acting on liver cells) also increase PI turnover. It was later found that one particular member of the PI family, namely phosphatidylinositol (4,5) bisphosphate (PIP$_2$), which has additional phosphate groups attached to the inositol ring, plays a key role. PIP$_2$ is the substrate for a membrane-bound enzyme, phospholipase Cβ (PLCβ), which splits it into *diacylglycerol* (DAG) and *inositol (1,4,5) trisphosphate* (IP$_3$; Fig. 3.13), both of which function as second messengers as discussed below (p. 35). The activation of PLCβ by various agonists is mediated through a G protein (G$_q$, see Table 3.3). After cleavage of PIP$_2$, the status quo is restored, as shown in Figure 3.13, DAG being phosphorylated to form phosphatidic acid (PA), while the IP$_3$ is dephosphorylated and then recoupled

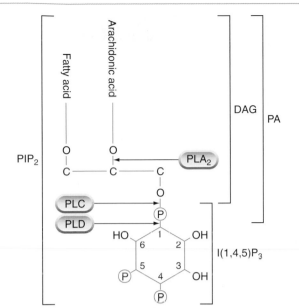

Fig. 3.12 Structure of phosphatidylinositol bisphosphate (PIP$_2$), showing sites of cleavage by different phospholipases to produce active mediators. Cleavage by phospholipase A2 (PLA$_2$) yields arachidonic acid. Cleavage by phospholipase C (PLC) yields inositol trisphosphate (I(1,4,5)P$_3$) and diacylglycerol (DAG). PA, phosphatidic acid; PLD, phospholipase D.

with PA to form PIP$_2$ once again.[11] Lithium, an agent used in psychiatry (see Ch. 47), blocks this recycling pathway (see Fig. 3.13).

Inositol phosphates and intracellular calcium

Inositol (1,4,5) trisphosphate (IP$_3$) is a water-soluble mediator that is released into the cytosol and acts on a specific receptor – the IP$_3$ receptor – which is a ligand-gated calcium channel present on the membrane of the endoplasmic reticulum. The main role of IP, described in more detail in Chapter 4, is to control the release of Ca^{2+} from intracellular stores. Because many drug and hormone effects involve intracellular Ca^{2+}, this pathway is particularly important. IP$_3$ can be converted inside the cell to the (1,3,4,5) tetraphosphate, IP$_4$, by a specific kinase. The exact role of IP$_4$ remains unclear, but some evidence suggests that it, and also higher inositol phosphates, may play a role in controlling gene expression.

Diacylglycerol and protein kinase C

Diacylglycerol is produced as well as IP$_3$ whenever receptor-induced PI hydrolysis occurs. The main effect of DAG is to activate a protein kinase, *protein kinase C* (PKC), which catalyses the phosphorylation of a variety of intracellular proteins. DAG, unlike the inositol phosphates, is highly lipophilic and remains within the membrane. It binds to a specific site on the PKC molecule, causing the enzyme to migrate from the cytosol to the cell membrane, thereby becoming activated. There are at least 10 different mammalian PKC subtypes, which have distinct cellular distributions and phosphorylate different proteins. Several are activated by DAG and raised intracellular Ca^{2+}, both of which are produced by activation of GPCRs.

PKCs are also activated by *phorbol esters* (highly irritant, tumour-promoting compounds produced by certain plants), which have been extremely useful in studying the functions of PKC. One of the subtypes is activated by the lipid mediator arachidonic acid (see Ch. 18) generated by the action of phospholipase A$_2$ on membrane phospholipids, so PKC activation can also occur with agonists that activate this enzyme. The various PKC isoforms, like the tyrosine kinases discussed below (p. 39), act on many different functional proteins, such as ion channels, receptors, enzymes (including other kinases), transcription factors and cytoskeletal proteins. Protein phosphorylation by kinases plays a central role in signal transduction, and controls many different aspects of cell function. The DAG–PKC link provides a mechanism whereby GPCRs can mobilise this army of control freaks.

Ion channels as targets for G proteins

Another major function of G protein-coupled receptors is to control ion channel function directly by mechanisms that do not involve second messengers such as cAMP or inositol phosphates. Direct G protein–channel interaction, through the βγ subunits of G$_i$ and G$_o$ proteins, appears to be a general mechanism for controlling K$^+$ and Ca^{2+} channels. In cardiac muscle, for example, mAChRs enhance K$^+$ permeability in this way (thus hyperpolarising the cells and inhibiting electrical activity; see Ch. 21). Similar mechanisms operate in neurons, where many inhibitory drugs such as opioid analgesics reduce excitability by opening certain K$^+$ channels – known as G protein-activated inwardly rectifying K$^+$ channels (GIRK) – or by inhibiting voltage-activated N and P/Q type Ca^{2+} channels and thus reducing neurotransmitter release (see Chs 4 and 42).

The main postulated roles of GPCRs in controlling enzymes and ion channels are summarised in Figure 3.14.

The Rho/Rho kinase system

▼ This signal transduction pathway (see Bishop & Hall, 2000) is activated by certain GPCRs (and also by non-GPCR mechanisms), which couple to G proteins of the G$_{12/13}$ type. The free G protein α subunit interacts with a *guanosine nucleotide exchange factor*, which facilitates GDP-GTP exchange at another GTPase, Rho. Rho–GDP, the resting form, is inactive, but when GDP–GTP exchange occurs, Rho is activated, and in turn activates Rho kinase. Rho kinase phosphorylates many substrate proteins and controls a wide variety of cellular functions, including smooth muscle contraction and proliferation, angiogenesis and synaptic remodelling. By enhancing hypoxia induced pulmonary artery vasoconstriction, activation of Rho kinase is thought to be important in the pathogenesis of pulmonary hypertension (see Ch. 22). Specific Rho kinase inhibitors (e.g. **fasudil**) are in development for a wide range of clinical indications – an area to watch.

The MAP kinase system

▼ The MAP kinase system involves several signal transduction pathways (Fig. 3.15) that are activated not only by various cytokines and growth factors acting on kinase-linked receptors (see p. 40, Fig. 3.17), but also by ligands activating GPCRs. The coupling of GPCRs to different families of MAP kinases can involve G protein α and βγ subunits as well as Src and arrestins – proteins also involved in GPCR desensitisation (see p. 36) (Pierce & Lefkowitz, 2001). The MAP kinase system controls many processes involved in gene expression, cell division, apoptosis and tissue regeneration

FURTHER DEVELOPMENTS IN GPCR BIOLOGY

▼ By the early 1990s, we thought we had more or less got the measure of GPCR function, as described above. Since then, the plot has thickened, and further developments have necessitated a substantial overhaul of the basic model.

---

[11]Alternative abbreviations for these mediators are PtdIns (PI), PtdIns (4,5)-P$_2$ (PIP$_2$), Ins (1,4,5)-P$_3$ (IP$_3$), and Ins (1,2,4,5)-P4 (IP$_4$).

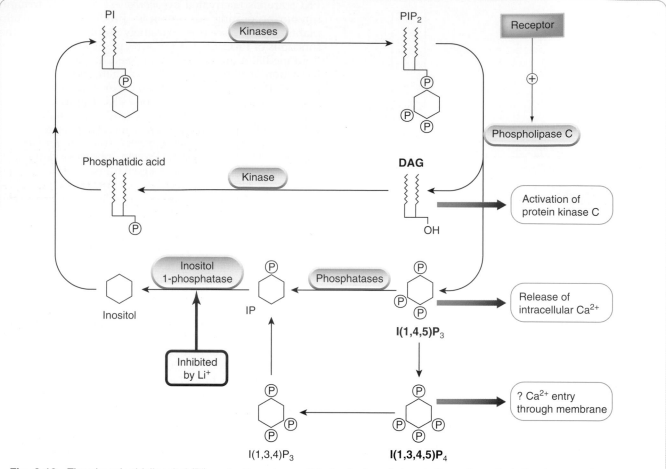

Fig. 3.13 **The phosphatidylinositol (PI) cycle.** Receptor-mediated activation of phospholipase C results in the cleavage of phosphatidylinositol bisphosphate (PIP$_2$), forming diacylglycerol (DAG) (which activates protein kinase C) and inositol trisphosphate (IP$_3$) (which releases intracellular Ca^{2+}). The role of inositol tetraphosphate (IP$_4$), which is formed from IP$_3$ and other inositol phosphates, is unclear, but it may facilitate Ca^{2+} entry through the plasma membrane. IP$_3$ is inactivated by dephosphorylation to inositol. DAG is converted to phosphatidic acid, and these two products are used to regenerate PI and PIP$_2$.

GPCR desensitisation

▼ As described in Chapter 2, desensitisation is a feature of most GPCRs, and the mechanisms underlying it have been extensively studied. *Homologous desensitisation* is restricted to the receptors activated by the desensitising agonist, while *heterologous desensitisation* affects other GPCRs in addition. Two main processes are involved (see Ferguson, 2001; Kelly et al., 2008):

- receptor phosphorylation
- receptor internalisation (endocytosis).

The sequence of GPCRs includes certain residues (serine and threonine), mainly in the C-terminal cytoplasmic tail, which can be phosphorylated by specific membrane-bound GPCR kinases (GRKs) and by kinases such as PKA and PKC.

On receptor activation GRK2 and GRK3 are recruited to the plasma membrane by binding to free G protein βγ subunits. GRKs then phosphorylate the receptors in their activated (i.e. agonist-bound) state. The phosphorylated receptor serves as a binding site for arrestins, intracellular proteins that block the interaction between the receptor and the G proteins producing a selective *homologous desensitisation*. Arrestin binding also targets the receptor for endocytosis in clathrin-coated pits (Fig. 3.16). The internalised receptor can then either be dephosphorylated and reinserted into the plasma membrane (resensitisation) or trafficked to lysosomes for degradation (inactivation). This type of desensitisation seems to occur with most GPCRs but with subtle differences that fascinate the aficionados.

Phosphorylation by PKA and PKC at residues different from those targeted by GRKs generally leads to impaired coupling between the activated receptor and the G protein, so the agonist effect is reduced. This can give rise to either homologous or heterologous desensitisation, depending on whether or not receptors other than that for the desensitising agonist are simultaneously phosphorylated by the kinases, some of which are not very selective. Receptors phosphorylated by second messenger kinases are probably not internalised and are reactivated by dephosphorylation by phosphatases when the agonist is removed.

GPCR oligomerisation

▼ The earlier view that GPCRs exist and function as monomeric proteins (in contrast to ion channels, which generally comprise multimeric complexes; see p. 26) was first overturned by work on the GABA$_B$ receptor. Two subtypes of this GPCR exist, encoded by different genes, and the functional receptor consists of a heterodimer of the two (see Ch. 38). A similar situation arises with G protein-coupled glutamate receptors. Oddly, although such dimers have two potential agonist binding sites, one on each subunit, only one is functional and signalling is transmitted through the dimer to the other receptor in the dimer which couples to the G protein (see Fig 38.9).

Other GPCRs are functional as monomers but it now seems likely that most, if not all, GPCRs can exist as either homomeric or heteromeric oligomers (i.e. dimers or larger oligomers) (Prinster et al., 2005). Within the opioid receptor family (see Ch. 42), the μ receptor

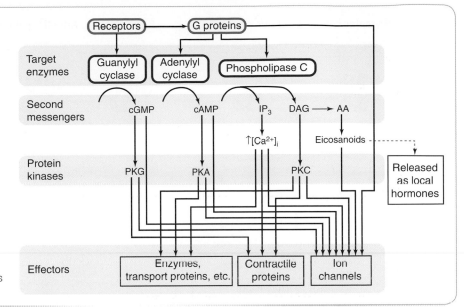

Fig. 3.14 G protein and second messenger control of cellular effector systems. AA, arachidonic acid; DAG, diacylglycerol; IP₃, inositol trisphosphate. Not shown in this diagram are signalling pathways where arrestins, rather than G proteins, link GPCRs to downstream events (see text).

Effectors controlled by G proteins

Two key second messenger pathways are controlled by receptors via G proteins:

- Adenylyl cyclase/cAMP:
  - can be activated or inhibited by pharmacological ligands, depending on the nature of the receptor and G protein
  - adenylyl cyclase catalyses formation of the intracellular messenger cAMP
    cAMP activates various protein kinases that control cell function in many different ways by causing phosphorylation of various enzymes, carriers and other proteins.
- Phospholipase C/inositol trisphosphate (IP₃)/diacylglycerol (DAG):
  - catalyses the formation of two intracellular messengers, IP₃ and DAG, from membrane phospholipid

- IP₃ acts to increase free cytosolic Ca^{2+} by releasing Ca^{2+} from intracellular compartments
- increased free Ca^{2+} initiates many events, including contraction, secretion, enzyme activation and membrane hyperpolarisation
- DAG activates protein kinase C, which controls many cellular functions by phosphorylating a variety of proteins.

Receptor-linked G proteins also control:

- Ion channels:
  - opening potassium channels, resulting in membrane hyperpolarisation
  - inhibiting calcium channels, thus reducing neurotransmitter release.
- Phospholipase A₂ (and thus the formation of arachidonic acid and eicosanoids).

---

was crystallised as a dimer and stable and functional heterodimers of κ and δ receptors, whose pharmacological properties differ from those of either parent, have been created in cell lines. More diverse GPCR combinations have also been found, such as that between dopamine (D₂) and somatostatin receptors, on which both ligands act with increased potency. Roaming even further afield in search of functional assignations, the dopamine receptor D₅ can couple directly with a ligand-gated ion channel, the GABA_A receptor, inhibiting the function of the latter without the intervention of any G protein (Liu et al., 2000). These interactions have so far been studied mainly in engineered cell lines, but they also occur in native cells. Functional dimeric complexes between angiotensin (AT₁) and bradykinin (B₂) receptors occur in human platelets and show greater sensitivity to angiotensin than 'pure' AT₁ receptors (AbdAlla et al., 2001). In pregnant women suffering from hypertension (pre-eclamptic toxaemia), the number of these dimers increases due to increased expression of B₂ receptors, resulting – paradoxically – in increased sensitivity to the vasoconstrictor action of angiotensin. This is the first instance of the role of dimerisation in human disease. It is too early to say what impact this newly discovered versatility of GPCRs in linking up with other receptors to form functional

combinations will have on conventional pharmacology and therapeutics, but it could be considerable.

Constitutively active receptors

▼ G protein-coupled receptors may be constitutively (i.e. spontaneously) active in the absence of any agonist (see Ch. 2 and review by Costa & Cotecchia, 2005). This was first shown for the β adrenoceptor (see Ch. 14), where mutations in the third intracellular loop, or simply overexpression of the receptor, result in constitutive receptor activation. There are now many examples of native GPCRs that show constitutive activity when expressed *in vitro*. The histamine H₃ receptor also shows constitutive activity *in vivo*, and this may prove to be a quite general phenomenon. It means that inverse agonists (see Ch. 2), which suppress this basal activity, may exert effects distinct from those of neutral antagonists, which block agonist effects without affecting basal activity.

Agonist specificity

▼ It was thought that the linkage of a particular GPCR to a particular signal transduction pathway depends mainly on the structure of

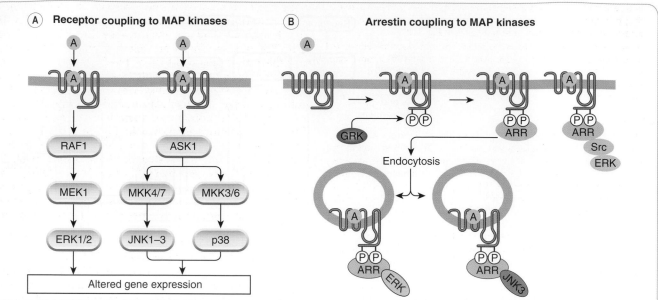

Fig. 3.15 **GPCR activation of MAP kinase cascade.** [A] Sequential activation of the multiple components of the MAP kinase cascade. GPCR activation of MAP kinases can involve Gα and βγ subunits (not shown). [B] Activation of ERK and JNK3 through interaction with arrestins (βARR). Activation of ERK can occur either at the plasma membrane involving Src, or by direct activation after internalisation of the receptor/arrestin complex. ARR, arrestin; GRK, G protein-coupled receptor kinase.

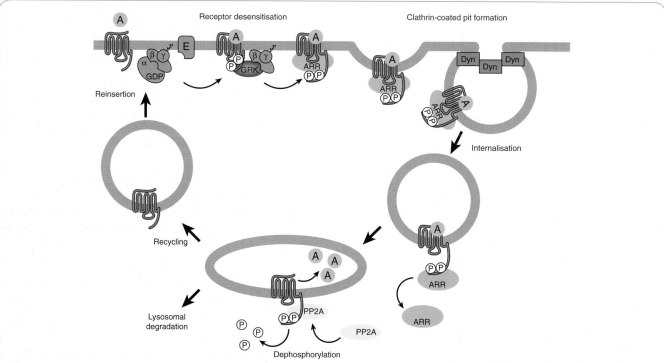

Fig. 3.16 **Desensitisation and trafficking of G protein-coupled receptors (GPCRs).** On prolonged agonist activation of the GPCR selective G protein-coupled receptor kinases (GRKs) are recruited to the plasma membrane and phosphorylate the receptor. Arrestin (ARR) then binds and traffics the GPCR to clathrin-coated pits for subsequent internalisation into endosomes in a dynamin-dependent process. The GPCR is then dephosphorylated by a phosphatase (PP2A) and either recycled back to the plasma membrane or trafficked to lysosomes for degradation. ARR, arrestin; Dyn, dynamin; GRK, G protein-coupled receptor kinase; PP2A, phosphatase 2A.

the receptor, particularly in the region of the third intracellular loop, which confers specificity for a particular G protein, from which the rest of the signal transduction pathway follows. This would imply, in line with the two-state model discussed in Chapter 2, that all agonists acting on a particular receptor stabilise the same activated (R*) state and should activate the same signal transduction pathway, and produce the same type of cellular response. It is now clear that

this is an oversimplification. In many cases, for example with agonists acting on angiotensin receptors, or with inverse agonists on β adrenoceptors, the cellular effects are qualitatively different with different ligands, implying the existence of more than one – probably many – R* states (sometimes referred to as *biased agonism*; see Ch. 2). Binding of arrestins to GPCRs initiates MAP kinase signalling, such that agonists that induce GRK/arrestin 'desensitisation' will terminate some GPCR signalling but may also activate signalling through arrestins that may continue even after the receptor/arrestin complex has been internalised (see Fig. 3.15).

Biased agonism has profound implications – indeed heretical to many pharmacologists, who are accustomed to think of agonists in terms of their affinity and efficacy, and nothing else; it will add a new dimension to the way in which we think about drug efficacy and specificity (see Kelly et al., 2008).

RAMPs

▼ Receptor activity-modifying-proteins (RAMPs) are a family of membrane proteins that associate with some GPCRs and alter their functional characteristics. They were discovered in 1998 when it was found that the functionally active receptor for the neuropeptide **calcitonin gene-related peptide** (CGRP) (see Ch. 18) consisted of a complex of a GPCR – called calcitonin receptor-like receptor (CRLR) – that by itself lacked activity, with another membrane protein (RAMP1). More surprisingly, CRLR when coupled with another RAMP (RAMP2) showed a quite different pharmacology, being activated by an unrelated peptide, **adrenomedulin**. In other words, the agonist specificity is conferred by the associated RAMP as well as by the GPCR itself. More RAMPs have emerged, and so far nearly all the examples involve peptide receptors, the calcium-sensing receptor being an exception. RAMPs are an example of how protein-protein interactions influence the pharmacological behaviour of the receptors in a highly selective way and may be novel targets for drug development (Sexton et al., 2012).

G protein-independent signalling

▼ In using the term *G protein-coupled receptor* to describe the class of receptors characterised by their heptahelical structure, we are following conventional textbook dogma but neglecting the fact that G proteins are not the only link between GPCRs and the various effector systems that they regulate. In this context, signalling mediated through arrestins bound to the receptor (see p. 38), rather than through G proteins, is important (see reviews by Pierce & Lefkowitz; 2001; Delcourt et al., 2007). Arrestins can act as an intermediary for GPCR activation of the MAP kinase cascade (see Fig. 3.15).

There are many examples where the various 'adapter proteins' that link receptors of the tyrosine kinase type to their effectors (see p. 40) can also interact with GPCRs (see Brzostowski & Kimmel, 2001), allowing the same effector systems to be regulated by receptors of either type.

In summary, the simple dogma that underpins much of our current understanding of GPCRs, namely,

> one GPCR gene – one GPCR protein – one functional GPCR – one G protein – one response

is showing distinct signs of wear. In particular:

- one gene, through alternative splicing, RNA editing, etc., can give rise to more than one receptor protein
- one GPCR protein can associate with others, or with other proteins such as RAMPs, to produce more than one type of functional receptor
- different agonists may affect the receptor in different ways and elicit qualitatively different responses
- the signal transduction pathway does not invariably require G proteins, and shows cross-talk with tyrosine kinase-linked receptors.

G protein-coupled receptors are evidently versatile and adventurous molecules around which much modern pharmacology revolves, and nobody imagines that we have reached the end of the story.

TYPE 3: KINASE-LINKED AND RELATED RECEPTORS

These membrane receptors are quite different in structure and function from ligand-gated channels and GPCRs.

They are activated by a wide variety of protein mediators, including growth factors and cytokines (see Ch. 18), and hormones such as insulin (see Ch. 31) and leptin (Ch. 32), whose effects are exerted mainly at the level of gene transcription. Most of these receptors are large proteins consisting of a single chain of up to 1000 residues, with a single membrane-spanning helical region, linking a large extracellular ligand-binding domain to an intracellular domain of variable size and function. The basic structure is shown in Figure 3.3C, but many variants exist (see below). Over 100 such receptors have been cloned, and many structural variations exist. For more detail, see review by Hubbard & Miller (2007). They play a major role in controlling cell division, growth, differentiation, inflammation, tissue repair, apoptosis and immune responses, discussed further in Chapters 5 and 18.

The main types are as follows:

Receptor tyrosine kinases (RTKs). These receptors have the basic structure shown in Figure 3.17A, incorporating a tyrosine kinase moiety in the intracellular region. They include receptors for many growth factors, such as **epidermal growth factor** and **nerve growth factor**, and also the group of *Toll-like receptors* that recognise bacterial lipopolysaccarides and play an important role in the body's reaction to infection (see Ch. 6). The insulin receptor (see Ch. 31) also belongs to the RTK class, although it has a more complex dimeric structure.

Receptor serine/threonine kinases. This smaller class is similar in structure to RTKs but they phosphorylate serine and/or threonine residues rather than tyrosine. The main example is the receptor for **transforming growth factor** (TGF).

Cytokine receptors. These receptors (Fig. 3.17B) lack intrinsic enzyme activity. When occupied, they activate various tyrosine kinases, such as Jak (the Janus kinase). Ligands for these receptors include cytokines such as **interferons** and **colony-stimulating factors** involved in immunological responses.

PROTEIN PHOSPHORYLATION AND KINASE CASCADE MECHANISMS

Protein phosphorylation (see Cohen, 2002) is a key mechanism for controlling the function of proteins (e.g. enzymes, ion channels, receptors, transport proteins) involved in regulating cellular processes. Phosphorylation and dephosphorylation are accomplished by *kinases* and *phosphatases*, respectively – enzymes of which several hundred subtypes are represented in the human genome – which are themselves subject to regulation dependent on their phosphorylation status. Much effort is currently being invested in mapping the complex interactions between signalling molecules that are involved in drug effects and pathophysiological processes such as oncogenesis, neurodegeneration, inflammation and much else. Here we can present only a few pharmacologically relevant aspects of what has become an enormous subject.

In many cases, ligand binding to the receptor leads to dimerisation. The association of the two intracellular kinase domains allows a mutual autophosphorylation of intracellular tyrosine residues to occur. The phosphorylated tyrosine residues then serve as high-affinity docking sites for other intracellular proteins that form the next stage in the signal transduction cascade. One important group of such proteins is known as the *SH2 domain proteins* (standing for Src homology, because they were

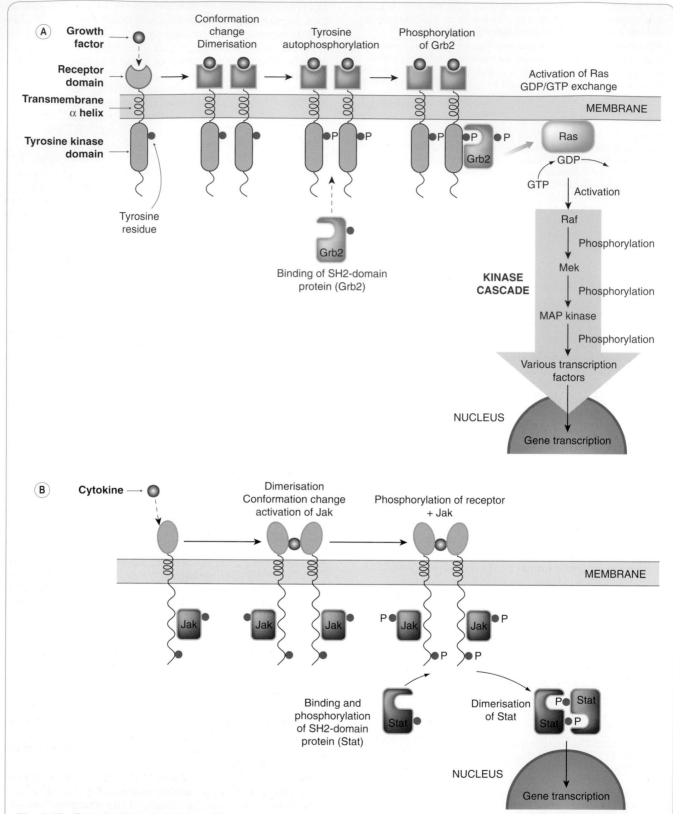

Fig. 3.17 Transduction mechanisms of kinase-linked receptors. The first step following agonist binding is dimerisation, which leads to autophosphorylation of the intracellular domain of each receptor. SH2-domain proteins then bind to the phosphorylated receptor and are themselves phosphorylated. Two well-characterised pathways are shown: [**A**] the growth factor (Ras/Raf/mitogen-activated protein [MAP] kinase) pathway (see also Ch. 5). Grb2 can also be phosphorylated but this negatively regulates its signalling. [**B**] Simplified scheme of the cytokine (Jak/Stat) pathway (see also Ch. 18). Some cytokine receptors may pre-exist as dimers rather than dimerise on cytokine binding. Several other pathways exist, and these phosphorylation cascades interact with components of G protein systems.

Kinase-linked receptors

- Receptors for various growth factors incorporate tyrosine kinase in their intracellular domain.
- Cytokine receptors have an intracellular domain that binds and activates cytosolic kinases when the receptor is occupied.
- The receptors all share a common architecture, with a large extracellular ligand-binding domain connected via a single membrane-spanning helix to the intracellular domain.
- Signal transduction generally involves dimerisation of receptors, followed by autophosphorylation of tyrosine residues. The phosphotyrosine residues act as acceptors for the SH2 domains of a variety of intracellular proteins, thereby allowing control of many cell functions.
- They are involved mainly in events controlling cell growth and differentiation, and act indirectly by regulating gene transcription.
- Two important pathways are:
  - the Ras/Raf/mitogen-activated protein (MAP) kinase pathway, which is important in cell division, growth and differentiation
  - the Jak/Stat pathway activated by many cytokines, which controls the synthesis and release of many inflammatory mediators.
- A few hormone receptors (e.g. atrial natriuretic factor) have a similar architecture and are linked to guanylyl cyclase.

first identified in the Src oncogene product). These possess a highly conserved sequence of about 100 amino acids, forming a recognition site for the phosphotyrosine residues of the receptor. Individual SH2 domain proteins, of which many are now known, bind selectively to particular receptors, so the pattern of events triggered by particular growth factors is highly specific. The mechanism is summarised in Figure 3.17.

What happens when the SH2 domain protein binds to the phosphorylated receptor varies greatly according to the receptor that is involved; many SH2 domain proteins are enzymes, such as protein kinases or phospholipases. Some growth factors activate a specific subtype of phospholipase C (PLCγ), thereby causing phospholipid breakdown, IP_3 formation and Ca^{2+} release (see p. 35). Other SH2-containin-proteins couple phosphotyrosine-containing-proteins with a variety of other functional proteins, including many that are involved in the control of cell division and differentiation. The end result is to activate or inhibit, by phosphorylation, a variety of transcription factors that migrate to the nucleus and suppress or induce the expression of particular genes. For more detail, see Jin and Pawson (2012). *Nuclear factor kappa B* (NFκB) is a transcription factor that plays a key role in multiple disorders including inflammation and cancer (see Chs 17 and 56; Karin et al., 2004). It is normally present in the cytosol complexed with an inhibitor (IκB). Phosphorylation of IκB occurs when a specific kinase (IKK) is activated in response to various inflammatory cytokines and GPCR

agonists. This results in dissociation of IκB from NFκB and migration of NFκB to the nucleus, where it switches on various proinflammatory genes.

▼ Two well-defined signal transduction pathways are summarised in Figure 3.17. The Ras/Raf pathway mediates the effect of many growth factors and mitogens. Ras, which is a proto-oncogene product, functions like a G protein, and conveys the signal (by GDP/GTP exchange) from the SH2-domain protein, Grb. Activation of Ras in turn activates Raf, which is the first of a sequence of three serine/threonine kinases, each of which phosphorylates, and activates, the next in line. The last of these, mitogen-activated protein (MAP) kinase (which is also activated by GPCRs, see above), phosphorylates one or more transcription factors that initiate gene expression, resulting in a variety of cellular responses, including cell division. This three-tiered MAP kinase cascade forms part of many intracellular signalling pathways involved in a wide variety of disease processes, including malignancy, inflammation, neurodegeneration, atherosclerosis and much else. The kinases form a large family, with different subtypes serving specific roles. They are thought to represent an important target for future therapeutic drugs. Many cancers are associated with mutations in the genes coding for proteins involved in this cascade, leading to activation of the cascade in the absence of the growth factor signal (see Chs 5 and 56). For more details, see review by Avruch (2007).

A second pathway, the Jak/Stat pathway (Fig. 3.17B) is involved in responses to many cytokines. Dimerisation of these receptors occurs when the cytokine binds, and this attracts a cytosolic tyrosine kinase unit (Jak) to associate with, and phosphorylate, the receptor dimer. Jaks belong to a family of proteins, different members having specificity for different cytokine receptors. Among the targets for phosphorylation by Jak are a family of transcription factors (Stats). These are SH2-domain proteins that bind to the phosphotyrosine groups on the receptor–Jak complex, and are themselves phosphorylated. Thus activated, Stat migrates to the nucleus and activates gene expression.

Other important mechanisms centre on *phosphatidylinositol-3-kinase* (PI$_3$ kinases, see Vanhaesebroeck et al., 1997), a ubiquitous enzyme family that is activated both by GPCRs and RTKs and attaches a phosphate group to position 3 of PIP$_2$ to form PIP$_3$. Other protein kinases, particularly protein kinase B (PKB, also known as Akt), have recognition sites for PIP$_3$ and are thus activated, controlling a wide variety of cellular functions, including apoptosis, differentiation, proliferation and trafficking. Akt also causes nitric oxide synthase activation in the vascular endothelium (see Ch. 20).

Recent work on signal transduction pathways has produced a bewildering profusion of molecular detail, often couched in a jargon that is apt to deter the faint-hearted. Perseverance will be rewarded, however, for there is no doubt that important new drugs, particularly in the areas of inflammation, immunology and cancer, will come from the targeting of these proteins. A breakthrough in the treatment of chronic myeloid leukaemia was achieved with the introduction of the first specific kinase inhibitor, **imatinib**, a drug that inhibits a specific tyrosine kinase involved in the pathogenesis of the disease (see Ch. 56).

The membrane-bound form of *guanylyl cyclase*, the enzyme responsible for generating the second messenger cGMP in response to the binding of natriuretic peptides (see Chs 18 and 29), resembles the receptor tyrosine kinase family and is activated in a similar way by dimerisation when the agonist is bound.

Figure 3.18 illustrates the central role of protein kinases in signal transduction pathways in a highly simplified and schematic way. Many, if not all, of the proteins involved, including the receptors and the kinases themselves, are substrates for kinases, so there are many mechanisms for feedback and cross-talk between the various signalling pathways. Given that there are over 500 protein kinases, and similarly large numbers of receptors and other signalling molecules, the network of interactions can look bewilderingly complex. Dissecting out the details has become

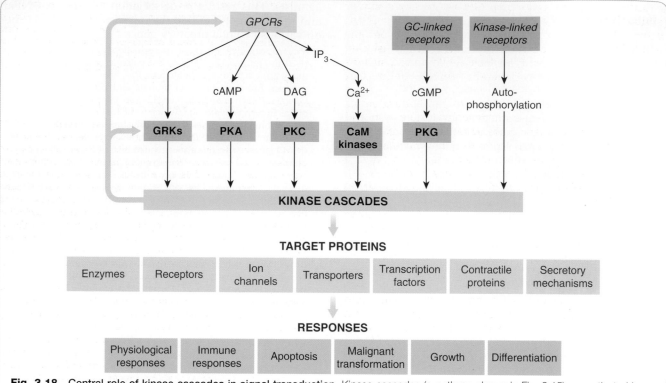

Fig. 3.18 **Central role of kinase cascades in signal transduction.** Kinase cascades (e.g. those shown in Fig. 3.15) are activated by GPCRs, either directly or via different second messengers, by receptors that generate cGMP, or by kinase-linked receptors. The kinase cascades regulate various target proteins, which in turn produce a wide variety of short- and long-term effects. CaM kinase, Ca^{2+}/calmodulin-dependent kinase; DAG, diacylglycerol; GC, guanylyl cyclase; GRK, GPCR kinase; IP_3, inositol trisphosphate; PKA, cAMP-dependent protein kinase; PKC, protein kinase C; PKG, cGMP-dependent protein kinase.

a major theme in cell biology. For pharmacologists, the idea of a simple connection between receptor and response, which guided thinking throughout the 20th century, is undoubtedly crumbling, although it will take some time before the complexities of signalling pathways are assimilated into a new way of thinking about drug action.

Protein phosphorylation in signal transduction

- Many receptor-mediated events involve protein phosphorylation, which controls the functional and binding properties of intracellular proteins.
- Receptor-linked tyrosine kinases, cyclic nucleotide-activated tyrosine kinases and intracellular serine/threonine kinases comprise a 'kinase cascade' mechanism that leads to amplification of receptor-mediated events.
- There are many kinases, with differing substrate specificities, allowing specificity in the pathways activated by different hormones.
- Desensitisation of G protein-coupled receptors occurs as a result of phosphorylation by specific receptor kinases, causing the receptor to become non-functional and to be internalised.
- There is a large family of phosphatases that act to dephosphorylate proteins and thus reverse the effects of kinases.

TYPE 4: NUCLEAR RECEPTORS

By the 1970s, it was clear that receptors for steroid hormones such as oestrogen and the glucocorticoids (Ch. 33) were present in the cytoplasm of cells and translocated into the nucleus after binding with their steroid partner. Other hormones, such as the thyroid hormone T_3 (Ch. 34) and the fat-soluble vitamins D and A (retinoic acid), were found to act in a similar fashion. Comparisons of gene and protein sequence data led to the recognition that these receptors were members of a much larger family of related proteins. We now know these as the *nuclear receptor (NR) family*.

As well as NRs such as the glucocorticoid and retinoic acid receptor, whose ligands are well characterised, this family includes a great many (~40%) *orphan receptors* – receptors with no known well-defined ligands. The first of these to be described, in the 1990s, was the *retinoid X receptor* (RXR), a receptor cloned on the basis of its similarity with the vitamin A receptor, and which was subsequently found to bind the vitamin A derivative 9-*cis*-retinoic acid. Over the intervening years, specific binding partners have been characterised for many NRs ('adopted orphans'; e.g. RXR) but for many others ('true orphans') these have yet to be identified – or perhaps do not exist as such, as one possible function of these receptors is their 'promiscuous' ability to bind to many related compounds (such as dietary factors) with low affinity.

Unlike the other receptors described in this chapter, the NRs can directly interact with DNA. For this reason we should really regard them as *ligand-activated transcription factors* that transduce signals by modifying gene transcription. Another unique property is that NRs are not embedded in membranes like GPCRs or ion channels (although see Ch. 33), but are present in the soluble phase of the cell. Some, such as the steroid receptors, become mobile in the presence of their ligand and can translocate from the cytoplasm to the nucleus, while others, such as the RXR, probably dwell mainly within the nuclear compartment.

The NR superfamily probably evolved from a single distant evolutionary ancestral gene by duplication and other events. In man, there are at least 48 members but more proteins may arise through alternative splicing events. While this represents a rather small proportion of all receptors (less than 10% of the total number of GPCRs), the NRs are very important drug targets (Burris et al., 2013), being responsible for the biological effects of approximately 10–15% of all prescription drugs. They can recognise an extraordinarily diverse group of substances (mostly small hydrophobic molecules), which may exhibit full or partial agonist, antagonist or inverse agonist activity. Some NRs are involved predominantly in endocrine signalling but many act as lipid sensors and are thus crucial links between our dietary and metabolic status and the expression of genes that regulate the metabolism and disposition of lipids. NRs also regulate expression of many drug metabolising enzymes and transporters. Many illnesses are associated with malfunctioning of the NR system, including inflammation, cancer, diabetes, cardiovascular disease, obesity and reproductive disorders (see Kersten et al., 2000; Murphy & Holder, 2000).

STRUCTURE OF NUCLEAR RECEPTORS

▼ All NRs are monomeric proteins that share a broadly similar structural design (see Fig. 3.19 and Bourguet et al., 2000, for further details). The *N-terminal domain* displays the most heterogeneity. It harbours the *AF1* (activation function 1) site that binds to other cell-specific transcription factors in a ligand-independent way and modifies the binding or regulatory capacity of the receptor itself. Alternative splicing of genes may yield several receptor isoforms each with slightly different N-terminal regions. The *core domain* of the receptor is highly conserved and consists of the structure responsible for DNA recognition and binding. At the molecular level, this comprises two *zinc fingers* – cysteine- (or cystine-/histidine-) rich loops in the amino acid chain that are held in a particular conformation by zinc ions. The main function of this portion of the molecule is to recognise and bind to the *hormone response elements* (HREs) located in genes that are regulated by this family of receptors, but it also plays a part in regulating receptor dimerisation.

It is the highly flexible *hinge region* in the molecule that allows it to dimerise with other NRs. This can produce molecular complexes with diverse configurations, able to interact differently with DNA. Finally, the *C-terminal domain* contains the ligand-binding module

and is specific to each class of receptor. The AF2 region is important in ligand-dependent activation and is generally highly conserved although absent in *Rev-erbAα* and *Rev-erbAβ*, NRs that regulate metabolism as part of a circadian molecular clock mechanism. Also located near the C-terminal are motifs that contain nuclear localisation signals and others that may, in the case of some receptors, bind *accessory heat shock* and other proteins.

CONTROL OF GENE TRANSCRIPTION

▼HREs are short (four or five base pairs) sequences of DNA to which the NRs bind to modify gene transcription. They are usually present symmetrically in pairs or *half-sites*, although these may be arranged together in different ways (e.g. simple repeats or inverted repeats). Each NR exhibits a preference for a particular *consensus sequence* but because of the family homology, there is a close similarity between these sequences. Once in the nucleus, the ligand-bound receptor recruits large complexes of other proteins including *co-activators* or *co-repressors* to modify gene expression through its AF1 and AF2 domains. Some of these co-activators are enzymes involved in chromatin remodelling, such as histone acetylase/deacetylase which, together with other enzymes, regulate the unravelling of the DNA to facilitate access by polymerase enzymes and hence gene transcription. Co-repressor complexes are recruited by some receptors and comprise histone deacetylase and other factors that cause the chromatin to become tightly packed, preventing further transcriptional activation. The case of CAR is particularly interesting; like some types of G proteins described earlier in this chapter, CAR can form a constitutively active complex that is terminated when it binds its ligand. The mechanisms of negative gene regulation by NRs are particularly complex (see Santos et al., 2011 for a good account of this phenomenon).

CLASSIFICATION OF NUCLEAR RECEPTORS

NRs are usually classified into subfamilies according to their phylogenetic development. For our purposes, however, it is more useful to make another distinction between them based on their molecular action. Mechanistically then, the NR superfamily consists of two main classes (I and II), and two other minor groups of receptors (III, IV).

Class I consists largely of endocrine steroid receptors, including the glucocorticoid and mineralocorticoid receptors (GR and MR), as well as the oestrogen, progesterone and androgen receptors (ER, PR and AR, respectively). The hormones (e.g. glucocorticoids) recognised by these receptors generally act in a negative feedback fashion to control biological events (see Ch. 33 for more details). In the absence of their ligand, these NRs are predominantly located in the cytoplasm, complexed with heat shock and other proteins and possibly reversibly attached to the cytoskeleton or other structures. Following diffusion (or possibly transportation) into the cell from the blood,

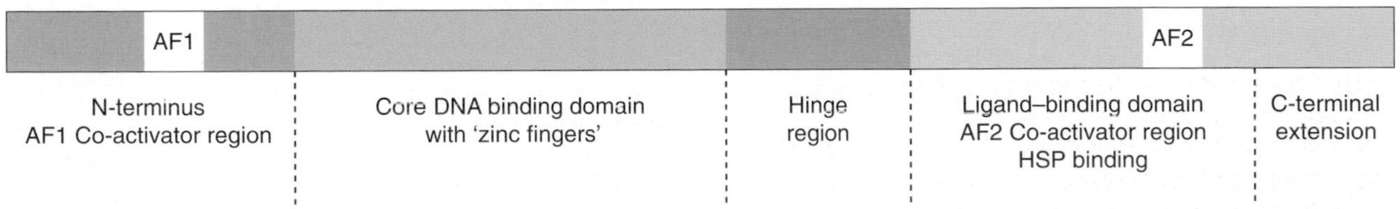

| N-terminus AF1 Co-activator region | Core DNA binding domain with 'zinc fingers' | Hinge region | Ligand–binding domain AF2 Co-activator region HSP binding | C-terminal extension |

Fig. 3.19 **Schematic diagram of a nuclear receptor.** The heterogenous N-terminal domain harbours the AF1 (activation function 1) site. This binds cell-specific transcription factors that modify the properties of the receptor. The highly conserved core domain comprises two 'zinc fingers'; cysteine- (or cystine-/histidine-) rich loops in the amino acid chain that are held in a particular conformation by zinc ions and which are responsible for DNA recognition and binding. The flexible hinge region in the molecule allows the receptor to dimerise with other NRs, and the C-terminal domain, which contains the ligand-binding module, is specific to each class of receptor (see text for more details).

ligands bind their NR partner with high affinity. These liganded receptors generally form homodimers and translocate to the nucleus, where they can *transactivate* or *transrepress* genes by binding to 'positive' or 'negative' HREs. Once bound, the NR recruits other proteins to form complexes that promote transcription of multiple genes. For example, it is estimated that the activated GR itself can regulate transcription of ~1% of the genome either directly or indirectly.

Class II NRs function in a slightly different way. Their ligands are generally lipids already present to some extent within the cell. This group includes the *peroxisome proliferator-activated receptor* (PPAR) that recognises fatty acids; the *liver oxysterol receptor* (LXR) that recognises and acts as a cholesterol sensor, the *farnesoid (bile acid) receptor* (FXR), a *xenobiotic receptor* (SXR; in rodents the PXR) that recognises a great many foreign substances, including therapeutic drugs, and the *constitutive androstane receptor* (CAR), which not only recognises the steroid androstane but also some drugs such as **phenobarbital** (see Ch. 45). Indeed, PXR and CAR are akin to airport security guards who alert the bomb disposal squad when suspicious luggage is found. When they sense foreign molecules (xenobiotics), they induce drug-metabolising enzymes such as CYP3A (which is responsible for metabolising about 60% of all prescription drugs; see Ch. 9 and di Masi et al., 2009). They also bind some prostaglandins and non-steroidal drugs, as well as the antidiabetic **thiazolidinediones** (see Ch. 31) and **fibrates** (see Ch. 23). Unlike the receptors in class I, these NRs almost always operate as heterodimers together with the retinoid X receptor (RXR).

Two types of heterodimer may then be formed: a *non-permissive heterodimer*, which can be activated only by the RXR ligand itself, and the *permissive heterodimer*, which can be activated either by retinoic acid itself or by its partner's ligand. Class II NRs are generally bound to co-repressor proteins. These dissociate when the ligand binds and allows recruitment of co-activator proteins and hence changes in gene transcription. They tend to mediate positive feedback effects (e.g. occupation of the receptor amplifies rather than inhibits a particular biological event).

Class III NRs are very similar to Class I in the sense that they form homodimers, but they can bind to HREs, which do not have an inverted repeat sequence. Class IV NRs may function as monomers or dimers but only bind to one HRE half site. Many of the remaining orphan receptors belong to these latter classes.

The discussion here must be taken only as a broad guide to the action of NRs, as many other types of interaction have also been discovered. For example, some receptors may bring about non-genomic actions by directly interacting with factors in the cytosol, or they may be covalently modified by phosphorylation or by protein-protein interactions with other transcription factors such that their function is altered (see Falkenstein et al., 2000). In addition, there is good evidence for separate membrane and other types of receptor that can bind some steroid hormones such as oestrogen (see Walters & Nemere, 2004).

Table 3.4 summarises the properties of some common NRs of importance to pharmacologists.

Table 3.4 Some common pharmacologically significant nuclear receptors

Receptor name	Abbreviation	Ligand	Drugs	Location	Ligand binding	Mechanism of action
Type I						
Androgen	AR	Tetosterone	All natural and synthetic glucocorticoids (Ch. 33), mineralocorticoids (Ch. 29) and sex steroids (Ch. 35) together with their antagonists (e.g. raloxifine, 4-hydroxy-tamoxifen and mifepristone)	Cytosolic	Homodimers	Translocation to nucleus. Binding to HREs with two half sites with an inverted sequence
Oestrogen	ERα,β	17β-oestradiol				
Glucocorticoid	GRα	Cortisol, corticosterone				
Progesterone	PR	Progesterone				
Mineralocorticoid	MR	Aldosterone				
Type II						
Retinoid X	RXR α,β,γ	9-*cis*-retinoic acid	Retinoid drugs (Ch. 27)	Nuclear	Heterodimers often with RXR	Complexed with co-repressors, which are displaced following ligand binding, allowing the binding of transactivators
Retinoic acid	RAR α,β,γ	Vitamin A				
Thyroid hormone	TR α,β	T3, T4	Thyroid hormone drugs			
Peroxisome proliferator	PPAR α,β,γ,δ	Fatty acids, prostaglandins	Rosiglitazone, pioglitazone			
Constitutive androstane	CAR	Androstane	Stimulation of CYP synthesis and alteration of drug metabolism			
Pregnane X	PXR	Xenobiotics				

Only examples from Classes I and II are included.

Nuclear receptors

- A family of 48 soluble receptors that sense lipid and hormonal signals and modulate gene transcription.
- Their ligands are many and varied, including steroid drugs and hormone, thyroid hormones, vitamins A and D, various lipids and xenobiotics
- There are two main categories:
  - Class I NRs are present in the cytoplasm, form homodimers in the presence of their partner, and migrate to the nucleus. Their ligands are mainly endocrine in nature (e.g. steroid hormones)
  - Class II NRs are generally constitutively present in the nucleus and form heterodimers with the retinoid X receptor. Their ligands are usually lipids (e.g. the fatty acids).
- The liganded receptor complexes initiate changes in gene transcription by binding to hormone response elements in gene promoters and recruiting co-activator or co-repressor factors.
- The receptor family is the target of approximately 10% of prescription drugs, and the enzymes that it regulates affect the pharmacokinetics of some 60% of all prescription drugs.

ION CHANNELS AS DRUG TARGETS

We have discussed ligand gated ion channels as one of the four main types of drug receptor. There are many other types of ion channel that represent important drug targets, even though they are not generally classified as 'receptors' because they are not the immediate targets of fast neurotransmitters, but drugs can act upon them to alter their ability to open and close.[12]

Here we discuss the structure and function of ion channels at the molecular level; their role as regulators of cell function is described in Chapter 4.

Ions are unable to penetrate the lipid bilayer of the cell membrane, and can get across only with the help of membrane-spanning proteins in the form of channels or transporters. The concept of ion channels was developed in the 1950s on the basis of electrophysiological studies on the mechanism of membrane excitation (see Ch. 4). Electrophysiology, particularly the *voltage clamp technique*, remains an essential tool for studying the physiological and pharmacological properties of ion channels. Since the mid-1980s, when the first ion channels were cloned by Numa in Japan, much has been learned about the structure and function of these complex molecules. The use of patch clamp recording, which allows the behaviour of individual channels to be studied in real time, has been particularly valuable in distinguishing channels on the

basis of their conductance and gating characteristics. Accounts by Hille (2001), Ashcroft (2000) and Catterall (2000) give background information.

Ion channels consist of protein molecules designed to form water-filled pores that span the membrane, and can switch between open and closed states. The rate and direction of ion movement through the pore is governed by the electrochemical gradient for the ion in question, which is a function of its concentration on either side of the membrane, and of the membrane potential. Ion channels are characterised by:

- their selectivity for particular ion species, determined by the size of the pore and the nature of its lining
- their gating properties (i.e. the nature of the stimulus that controls the transition between open and closed states of the channel)
- their molecular architecture.

ION SELECTIVITY

Channels are generally either cation selective or anion selective. The main cation-selective channels are selective for Na^+, Ca^{2+} or K^+, or non-selective and permeable to all three. Anion channels are mainly permeable to Cl^-, although other types also occur. The effect of modulation of ion channels on cell function is discussed in Chapter 4.

GATING

VOLTAGE-GATED CHANNELS

In the main these channels open when the cell membrane is depolarised.[13] They form a very important group because they underlie the mechanism of membrane excitability (see Ch. 4). The most important channels in this group are selective sodium, potassium or calcium channels.

Commonly, the channel opening (activation) induced by membrane depolarisation is short lasting, even if the depolarisation is maintained. This is because, with some channels, the initial activation of the channels is followed by a slower process of inactivation.

The role of voltage-gated channels in the generation of action potentials and in controlling other cell functions is described in Chapter 4.

LIGAND-GATED CHANNELS

These (see Fig. 3.5) are activated by binding of a chemical ligand to a site on the channel molecule. Fast neurotransmitters, such as glutamate, acetylcholine, GABA, 5-hydroxytryptamine and ATP (see Chs 13, 16 and 38) act in this way, binding to sites on the outside of the membrane. In addition there are also ligand-gated ion channels that do not respond to neurotransmitters but to changes in their local environment. For example, the TRPV1 channel on sensory nerves that mediates the pain-producing effect of the chilli pepper ingredient capsaicin responds to extracellular protons when tissue pH falls, as occurs in inflamed tissue, as well as to the physical stimulus, heat (see Ch. 42).

---

[12]In truth, the distinction between ligand-gated channels and other ion channels is an arbitrary one. In grouping ligand-gated channels with other types of receptor in this book, we are respecting the historical tradition established by Langley and others, who first defined receptors in the context of the action of acetylcholine at the neuromuscular junction. The advance of molecular biology may force us to reconsider this semantic issue in the future, but for now we make no apology for upholding the pharmacological tradition.

[13]There is always an exception to the rule! The members of the HCN family of potassium channels found in neurons and cardiac muscle cells are activated by hyperpolarisation.

Some ligand-gated channels in the plasma membrane respond to intracellular rather than extracellular signals, the most important being the following:

- Calcium-activated potassium channels, which occur in most cells and open, thus hyperpolarising the cell, when $[Ca^{2+}]_i$ increases.
- Calcium-activated chloride channels, widely expressed in excitable and non-excitable cells where they are involved in diverse functions such as epithelial secretion of electrolytes and water, sensory transduction, regulation of neuronal and cardiac excitability and regulation of vascular tone.
- ATP-sensitive potassium channels, which open when the intracellular ATP concentration falls because the cell is short of nutrients. These channels, which are quite distinct from those mediating the excitatory effects of extracellular ATP, occur in many nerve and muscle cells, and also in insulin-secreting cells (see Ch. 31), where they are part of the mechanism linking insulin secretion to blood glucose concentration.

Other examples of cell membrane channels that respond to intracellular ligands include arachidonic acid-sensitive potassium channels and DAG-sensitive calcium channels, whose functions are not well understood.

CALCIUM RELEASE CHANNELS

The main ones, IP_3 and **ryanodine** receptors (see Ch. 4), are a special class of ligand-gated calcium channels that are present on the endoplasmic or sarcoplasmic reticulum rather than the plasma membrane and control the release of Ca^{2+} from intracellular stores. Ca^{2+} can also be released from lysosomal stores by nicotinic acid adenine dinucleotide phosphate activating two pore domain calcium channels.

STORE-OPERATED CALCIUM CHANNELS

When the intracellular Ca^{2+} stores are depleted, 'store-operated' channels (SOCs) in the plasma membrane open to allow Ca^{2+} entry. The mechanism by which this linkage occurs involves interaction of a Ca^{2+}-sensor protein in the endoplasmic reticulum membrane with a dedicated Ca^{2+} channel in the plasma membrane (see Potier & Trebak, 2008). In response to GPCRs that elicit Ca^{2+} release, the opening of these channels allows the cytosolic free Ca^{2+} concentration, $[Ca^{2+}]_i$, to remain elevated even when the intracellular stores are running low, and also provides a route through which the stores can be replenished (see Ch. 4).

MOLECULAR ARCHITECTURE OF ION CHANNELS

▼Ion channels are large and elaborate molecules. Their characteristic structural motifs have been revealed as knowledge of their sequence and structure has accumulated since the mid-1980s, when the first voltage-gated sodium channel was cloned. The main structural subtypes are shown in Figure 3.20. All consist of several (often four) domains, which are similar or identical to each other,

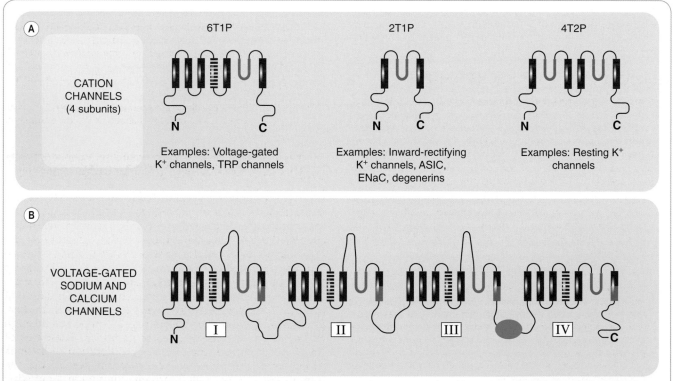

Fig. 3.20 **Molecular architecture of ion channels.** Red and blue rectangles represent membrane-spanning α-helices. Blue hairpins are pore loop (P) domains, present in many channels, blue rectangles being the pore-forming regions of the membrane-spanning α-helices. Cross-shaded rectangles represent the voltage-sensing regions of voltage-gated channels. The green symbol represents the inactivating particle of voltage-gated sodium channels. Potassium channel nomenclature is based on the number of transmembrane helices (T) and pore-forming loops (P) in each subunit. Further information on ion channels is given in Chapter 4. ASIC, acid-sensing ion channel; ENaC, epithelial sodium channel; TRP, transient receptor potential channel.

organised either as an oligomeric array of separate subunits, or as one large protein. Each subunit or domain contains a bundle of two to six membrane-spanning helices.

Voltage-gated channels generally include one transmembrane helix that contains an abundance of basic (i.e. positively charged) amino acids. When the membrane is depolarised, so that the interior of the cell becomes less negative, this region – the voltage sensor – moves slightly towards the outer surface of the membrane, which has the effect of opening the channel (see Bezanilla, 2008). Many voltage-activated channels also show *inactivation*, which happens when an intracellular appendage of the channel protein moves to plug the channel from the inside. Voltage-gated sodium and calcium channels are remarkable in that the whole structure with four six-helix domains consists of a single huge protein molecule, the domains being linked together by intracellular loops of varying length. Potassium channels comprise the most numerous and heterogeneous class.[14] Voltage-gated potassium channels resemble sodium channels, except that they are made up of four subunits rather than a single long chain. The class of potassium channels known as 'inward rectifier channels' because of their biophysical properties has the two-helix structure shown in Figure 3.20A, whereas others are classed as 'two-pore domain' channels, because each subunit contains two P loops.

The various architectural motifs shown in Figure 3.20 only scrape the surface of the molecular diversity of ion channels. In all cases, the individual subunits come in several molecular varieties, and these can unite in different combinations to form functional channels as *hetero-oligomers* (as distinct from *homo-oligomers* built from identical subunits). Furthermore, the channel-forming structures described are usually associated with other membrane proteins, which significantly affect their functional properties. For example, the ATP-gated potassium channel exists in association with the *sulfonylurea receptor* (SUR), and it is through this linkage that various drugs (including antidiabetic drugs of the sulfonylurea class; see Ch. 31) regulate the channel. Good progress is being made in understanding the relation between molecular structure and ion channel function, but we still have only a fragmentary understanding of the physiological role of many of these channels. Many important drugs exert their effects by influencing channel function, either directly or indirectly.

PHARMACOLOGY OF ION CHANNELS

▼ Many drugs and physiological mediators described in this book exert their effects by altering the behaviour of ion channels. Here we outline the general mechanisms as exemplified by the pharmacology of voltage-gated sodium channels (Fig. 3.21). Ion channel pharmacology is likely to be a fertile source of future new drugs.

The gating and permeation of both voltage-gated and ligand-gated ion channels is modulated by many factors, including the following.

- *Ligands that bind directly to various sites on the channel protein.* These include a variety of drugs and toxins that act in different ways, for example by blocking the channel or by affecting the gating process, thereby either facilitating or inhibiting the opening of the channel.
- *Mediators and drugs that act indirectly, mainly by activation of GPCRs.* The latter produce their effects mainly by affecting the state of phosphorylation of individual amino acids located on the intracellular region of the channel protein. As described above, this modulation involves the production of second messengers that activate protein kinases. The opening of the channel may be facilitated or inhibited, depending on which residues are phosphorylated. Drugs such as β-adrenoceptor agonists (Ch. 14) affect calcium and potassium channel function in this way, producing a wide variety of cellular effects.
- *Intracellular signals, particularly Ca^{2+} and nucleotides such as ATP and GTP* (see Ch. 4). Many ion channels possess binding sites for

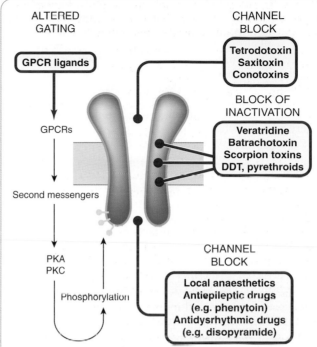

Fig. 3.21 **Drug-binding domains of voltage-gated sodium channels (see Ch. 43).** The multiplicity of different binding sites and effects appears to be typical of many ion channels. DDT, dichlorodiphenyltrichloroethane (dicophane, a well-known insecticide); GPCR, G protein-coupled receptor; PKA, protein kinase A; PKC, protein kinase C.

these intracellular mediators. Increased [Ca^{2+}]$_i$ opens certain types of potassium and chloride channels, and inactivates voltage-gated calcium channels. As described in Chapter 4, [Ca^{2+}]$_i$ is itself affected by the function of ion channels and GPCRs. Drugs of the sulfonylurea class (see Ch. 31) act selectively on ATP-gated potassium channels.

Figure 3.21 summarises the main sites and mechanisms by which drugs affect voltage-gated sodium channels, a typical example of this type of drug target.

CONTROL OF RECEPTOR EXPRESSION

Receptor proteins are synthesised by the cells that express them, and the level of expression is itself controlled, via the pathways discussed above, by receptor-mediated events. We can no longer think of the receptors as the fixed elements in cellular control systems, responding to changes in the concentration of ligands, and initiating effects through the signal transduction pathway – they are themselves subject to regulation. Short-term regulation of receptor function generally occurs through *desensitisation*, as discussed above. Long-term regulation occurs through *an increase or decrease of receptor expression*. Examples of this type of control include the proliferation of various postsynaptic receptors after denervation (see Ch. 12), the upregulation of various G protein-coupled and cytokine receptors in response to inflammation (see Ch. 17), and the induction of growth factor receptors by certain tumour viruses (see Ch. 5). Long-term drug treatment invariably induces adaptive responses, which, particularly with drugs that act on the central nervous system, can limit their effectiveness as in opioid tolerance (see Ch. 42) or

---

[14]The human genome encodes more than 70 distinct potassium channel subtypes – either a nightmare or a golden opportunity for the pharmacologist, depending on one's perspective.

can be the basis for therapeutic efficacy. In the latter instance this may take the form of a very slow onset of the therapeutic effect (e.g. with antidepressant drugs; see Ch. 47). It is likely that changes in receptor expression, secondary to the immediate action of the drug, are involved in delayed effects of this sort – a kind of 'secondary pharmacology' whose importance is only now becoming clearer. The same principles apply to drug targets other than receptors (ion channels, enzymes, transporters, etc.) where adaptive changes in expression and function follow long-term drug administration, resulting, for example, in resistance to certain anticancer drugs (Ch. 56).

RECEPTORS AND DISEASE

Increasing understanding of receptor function in molecular terms has revealed a number of disease states directly linked to receptor malfunction. The principal mechanisms involved are:

- autoantibodies directed against receptor proteins
- mutations in genes encoding receptors, ion channels and proteins involved in signal transduction.

An example of the former is *myasthenia gravis* (see Ch. 13), a disease of the neuromuscular junction due to autoantibodies that inactivate nicotinic acetylcholine receptors. Autoantibodies can also mimic the effects of agonists, as in many cases of thyroid hypersecretion, caused by activation of **thyrotropin** receptors. Activating antibodies have also been discovered in patients with severe hypertension (α adrenoceptors), cardiomyopathy (β adrenoceptors), and certain forms of epilepsy and neurodegenerative disorders (glutamate receptors).

Inherited mutations of genes encoding GPCRs account for various disease states (see Spiegel & Weinstein, 2004; Thompson et al., 2005). Mutated **vasopressin** and **adrenocorticotrophic hormone** receptors (see Chs 29 and 33) can result in resistance to these hormones. Receptor mutations can result in activation of effector mechanisms in the absence of agonists. One of these involves the receptor for thyrotropin, producing continuous oversecretion of thyroid hormone; another involves the receptor for luteinising hormone and results in precocious puberty. Adrenoceptor polymorphisms are common in humans, and recent studies suggest that certain mutations of the β_2 adrenoceptor, although they do not directly cause disease, are associated with a reduced efficacy of β-adrenoceptor agonists in treating asthma (Ch. 28) and a poor prognosis in patients with cardiac failure (Ch. 21). Mutations in G proteins can also cause disease (see Spiegel & Weinstein, 2004). For example, mutations of a particular $G\alpha$ subunit cause one form of *hypoparathyroidism*, while mutations of a $G\beta$ subunit result in hypertension. Many cancers are associated with mutations of the genes encoding growth factor receptors, kinases and other proteins involved in signal transduction (see Ch. 5).

Mutations in ligand-gated ion channels ($GABA_A$ and nicotinic) and other ion channels (Na^+ and K^+) that alter their function give rise to some forms of idiopathic epilepsy (see Ch. 45 and Guerrini et al., 2003).

Research on genetic polymorphisms affecting receptors, signalling molecules, ion channels and effector enzymes is continuing apace, and it is expected that a clearer understanding of the variability between individuals in their disease susceptibility and response to therapeutic drugs (see Ch. 57) will result in the foreseeable future.

REFERENCES AND FURTHER READING

General

IUPHAR/BPS. Guide to Pharmacology. www.guidetopharmacology .org/. (*Comprehensive catalogue of molecular and pharmacological properties of known receptor and ion channels – also transporters and some enzymes involved in signal transduction*)

Nelson, N., 1998. The family of Na^+/Cl^- neurotransmitter transporters. J. Neurochem. 71, 1785–1803. (*Review article describing the molecular characteristics of the different families of neurotransporters*)

Ion channels

Ashcroft, F.M., 2000. Ion Channels and Disease. Academic Press, London. (*A useful textbook covering all aspects of ion channel physiology and its relevance to disease, with a lot of pharmacological information for good measure*)

Bezanilla, F., 2008. How membrane proteins sense voltage. Nat. Rev. Mol. Cell Biol. 9, 323–332. (*Review of recent studies of how membrane proteins respond to changes in transmembrane potential*)

Catterall, W.A., 2000. From ionic currents to molecular mechanisms: the structure and function of voltage-gated sodium channels. Neuron 26, 13–25. (*General review of sodium channel structure, function and pharmacology*)

Colquhoun, D., 2006. Agonist-activated ion channels. Br. J. Pharmacol. 147, S17–S26. (*Review article discussing the relationship between agonist binding and channel opening*)

Gay, E.A., Yakel, J.L., 2007. Gating of nicotinic ACh receptors: new insights into structural transitions triggered by agonist binding that induce channel opening. J. Physiol. 548, 727–733.

Guerrini, R., Casari, G., Marini, C., 2003. The genetic and molecular basis of epilepsy. Trends Mol. Med. 300–306.

Halliwell, R.F., 2007. A short history of the rise of the molecular pharmacology of ionotropic drug receptors. Trends Pharmacol. Sci. 28, 214–219. (*Good account of the main discoveries in this active field*)

Hille, B., 2001. Ionic Channels of Excitable Membranes. Sinauer Associates, Sunderland. (*A clear and detailed account of the basic principles of ion channels, with emphasis on their biophysical properties*)

Miyazawa, A., Fujiyoshi, Y., Unwin, N., 2003. Structure and gating mechanism of the acetylcholine receptor pore. Nature 423, 949–955. (*Description of how the channel is opened by agonists, based on high-resolution crystallography*)

North, R.A., 2002. Molecular physiology of P2X receptors. Physiol. Rev. 82, 1013–1067. (*Encyclopedic review of P2X receptor structure and function*)

Potier, M., Trebak, M., 2008. New developments in the signaling mechanisms of the store-operated calcium entry pathway. Pflugers Arch. 457, 405–415. (*Recent clarification of an old enigma*)

G protein-coupled receptors

AbdAlla, S., Lother, H., El Massiery, A., Quitterer, U., 2001. Increased AT_1 receptor heterodimers in preeclampsia mediate enhanced angiotensin II responsiveness. Nat. Med. 7, 1003–1009. (*The first instance of disturbed GPCR heterodimerisation in relation to human disease*)

Audet, M., Bouvier, M., 2012. Restructuring G protein-coupled receptor activation. Cell 151, 14–23. (*Review of recent developments related to G protein-coupled receptor crystallisation*)

Bockenhauer, S., Yao, X.J., Kobilka, B.K., Moerner, W.E., 2011. Conformational dynamics of single G protein-coupled receptors in solution. J. Phys. Chem. B 115, 13328–13338.

Conigrave, A.D., Quinn, S.J., Brown, E.M., 2000. Cooperative multi-modal sensing and therapeutic implications of the extracellular Ca^{2+}-sensing receptor. Trends Pharmacol. Sci. 21, 401–407. (*Short account of the Ca^{2+}-sensing receptor, an anomalous type of GPCR*)

Costa, T., Cotecchia, S., 2005. Historical review: negative efficacy and the constitutive activity of G protein-coupled receptors. Trends Pharmacol. Sci. 26, 618–624. (*A clear and thoughtful review of ideas relating to constitutive receptor activation and inverse agonists*)

Ferguson, S.S.G., 2001. Evolving concepts in G protein-coupled receptor endocytosis: the role in receptor desensitization and signaling. Pharmacol. Rev. 53, 1–24. (*Detailed account of the role of phosphorylation of receptors in fast and slow desensitisation mechanisms*)

Fredriksson, R., Schiöth, H.B., 2005. The repertoire of G protein-coupled receptors in fully sequenced genomes. Mol. Pharmacol. 67, 1414–1425. (*Estimation of the number of GPCR genes in different species – nearly 500 more in mouse than in human!*)

Hill, S.J., 2006. G protein-coupled receptors: past, present and future. Br. J. Pharmacol. 147 (Suppl.), 27–37. (*Good introductory review*)

Kelly, E., Bailey, C.P., Henderson, G., 2008. Agonist-selective mechanisms of GPCR desensitization. Br. J. Pharmacol. 153 (Suppl. 1), S379–S388. (*Short review of main mechanisms of GPCR desensitisation*)

Liu, F., Wan, Q., Pristupa, Z., et al., 2000. Direct protein–protein coupling enables cross-talk between dopamine D_5 and γ-aminobutyric acid A receptors. Nature 403, 274–280. (*The first demonstration of direct coupling of a GPCR with an ion channel. Look, no G protein!*)

Lohse, M.J., Hein, P., Hoffmann, C., et al., 2008. Kinetics of G protein-coupled receptor signals in intact cells. Br. J. Pharmacol. 153 (Suppl. 1), S125–S132. (*Describes the use of fluorescence methods to measure GPCR signalling events in real time – an important step forward*)

Milligan, G., Kostenis, E., 2006. Heterotrimeric G proteins: a short history. Br. J. Pharmacol. 147 (Suppl.), 46–55.

Offermanns, S., 2003. G proteins as transducers in transmembrane signalling. Prog. Biophys. Mol. Biol. 83, 101–130. (*Detailed review of G protein subtypes and their function in signal transduction*)

Oldham, W.M., Hamm, H.E., 2008. Heterotrimeric G protein activation by G protein-coupled receptors. Nat. Rev. Mol. Cell Biol. 9, 60–71. (*Useful review of the current state of knowledge about the structure and function of G proteins*)

Pierce, K.L., Lefkowitz, R.J., 2001. Classical and new roles of β-arrestins in the regulation of G protein-coupled receptors. Nature Rev. Neurosci. 2, 727–733. (*Good review of non-G protein-mediated signalling of GPCRs through arrestin*)

Prinster, S.C., Hague, C., Hall, R.A., 2005. Heterodimerization of G protein-coupled receptors: specificity and functional significance. Pharmacol. Rev. 57, 289–298. (*Good short review of what the unexpected finding of GPCR dimerisation may signify*)

Ramachandran, R.M.D., Hollenberg, M.D., 2008. Proteinases and signalling: pathophysiological and therapeutic implications via PARs and more. Br. J. Pharmacol. 153 (Suppl. 1), S263–S282. (*Useful short review of PAR mechanisms and relevance to disease states*)

Sexton, P.M., Poyner, D.R., Simms, J., Christopoulos, A., Hay, D.L., 2012. RAMPs as drug targets. Adv. Exp. Med. Biol. 744, 61–74,

Simonds, W.F., 1999. G protein regulation of adenylate cyclase. Trends Pharmacol. Sci. 20, 66–72. (*Review of mechanisms by which G proteins affect adenylyl cyclase at the level of molecular structure*)

Spiegel, A.M., Weinstein, L.S., 2004. Inherited diseases involving G proteins and G protein-coupled receptors. Annu. Rev. Med. 55, 27–39. (*Short review in tick*)

Thompson, M.D., Burnham, W.M., Cole, D.E.C., 2005. The G protein coupled receptors: pharmacogenetics and disease. Crit. Rev. Clin. Lab. Sci. 42, 311–389. (*Extensive review with many examples of GPCR polymorphisms associated with disease*)

Weis, W.I., Kobilka, B.K., 2008. Structural insights into G protein-coupled receptor activation. Curr. Opin. Struct. Biol. 18, 734–740.

Xie, G.-X., Palmer, P.P., 2007. How regulators of G protein signalling achieve selective regulation. J. Mol. Biol. 366, 349–365. (*General review about RGS proteins and how they work*)

Signal transduction

Avruch, J., 2007. MAP kinase pathways: the first twenty years. Biochim. Biophys. Acta. 1773, 1150–1160. (*Short general review. One of a series of articles on MAP kinases in this issue*)

Bishop, A.L., Hall, R.A., 2000. Rho-GTPases and their effector proteins. Biochem. J. 348, 241–255. (*General review article on the Rho/Rho kinase system and the various pathways and functions that it controls*)

Brzostowski, J.A., Kimmel, A.R., 2001. Signaling at zero G: G protein-independent functions for 7TM receptors. Trends Biochem. Sci. 26, 291–297. (*Review of evidence for GPCR signalling that does not involve G proteins, thus conflicting with the orthodox dogma*)

Nahorski, S.R., 2006. Pharmacology of intracellular signalling pathways. Br. J. Pharmacol. 147 (Suppl.), 38–45. (*Useful short review*)

Vanhaesebroeck, B., Leevers, S.J., Panayotou, G., Waterfield, M.D., 1997. Phosphoinositide 3-kinases: a conserved family of signal transducers. Trends Biochem. Sci. 22, 267–272. (*Review by the group that discovered PI-3 kinases, summarising the multiple roles of this signal transduction mechanism – much expanded since 1997*)

Kinase-linked receptors

Cohen, P., 2002. Protein kinases – the major drug targets of the twenty-first century. Nat. Rev. Drug Discov. 1, 309–315. (*General review on pharmacological aspects of protein kinases*)

Cook, D.N., Pisetsky, D.S., Schwartz, D.A., 2004. Toll-like receptors in the pathogenesis of human disease. Nat. Immunol. 5, 975–979. (*Review emphasising the role of this class of receptor tyrosine kinases in many human disease states*)

Delcourt, N., Bockaert, J., Marin, P., 2007. GPCR-jacking: from a new route in RTK signalling to a new concept in GPCR activation. Trends Pharmacol. Sci. 28, 602–607. (*Gives examples of 'cross-talk' between GPCR and RTK signalling pathways*)

Hubbard, S.R., Miller, W.T., 2007. Receptor tyrosine kinases: mechanisms of activation and signaling. Curr. Opin. Cell Biol. 19, 117–123. (*Reviews recent structural results showing mechanism of RTK dimerisation and signalling*)

Ihle, J.N., 1995. Cytokine receptor signalling. Nature 377, 591–594.

Jin, J., Pawson, T., 2012. Modular evolution of phosphorylation-based signalling systems. Philos. Trans. R. Soc. Lond. B. Biol Sci. 367, 2540–2555. (*Informative review on receptor kinase signalling*)

Karin, M., Yamamoto, Y., Wang, M., 2004. The IKK-NFκB system: a treasure trove for drug development. Nat. Rev. Drug Discov. 3, 17–26. (*Describes the transcription factor NFκB, which plays a key role in inflammation, and its control by kinase cascades*)

Nuclear receptors

Bourguet, W., Germain, P., Gronemeyer, H., 2000. Nuclear receptor ligand-binding domains: three-dimensional structures, molecular interactions and pharmacological implications. Trends Pharmacol. Sci. 21, 381–388. (*Accessible review concentrating on distinction between agonist and antagonist effects at the molecular level*)

Burris, T.P., Solt, L.A., Wang, Y., et al., 2012. Nuclear receptors and their selective pharmacologic modulators. Pharmacol. Rev. 65, 710–778. (*A very comprehensive account of the action of drugs at nuclear receptors. Not light reading, but worthwhile if you are interested*)

Falkenstein, E., Tillmann, H.C., Christ, M., Feuring, M., Wehling, M., 2000. Multiple actions of steroid hormones – a focus on rapid non-genomic effects. Pharm. Rev. 52, 513–553. (*Comprehensive review article describing the non-classical effects of steroids*)

Germain, P., Staels, B., Dacquet, C., Spedding, M., Laudet, V., 2006. Overview of nomenclature of nuclear receptors. Pharmacol. Rev. 58, 685–704. (*Comprehensive and authoritative review that deals with receptor biology as well as nomenclature. Recommended*)

Kersten, S., Desvergne, B., Wahli, W., 2000. Roles of PPARs in health and disease. Nature 405, 421–424. (*General review of an important class of nuclear receptors*)

di Masi, A., De Marinis, E., Ascenzi, P., Marino, M., 2009. Nuclear receptors CAR and PXR: molecular, functional, and biomedical aspects. Mol. Aspects Med. 30, 297–343. (*A very comprehensive account of the role played by these nuclear receptors in xenobiotic metabolism but also contains some useful general background information on the receptor family*)

Murphy, G.J., Holder, J.C., 2000. PPAR-γ agonists: therapeutic role in diabetes, inflammation and cancer. Trends Pharmacol. Sci. 21, 469–474. (*Account of the emerging importance of nuclear receptors of the PPAR family as therapeutic targets*)

Santos, G.M., Fairall, L., Schwabe, J.W.R., 2011. Negative regulation by nuclear receptors: a plethora of mechanisms. Trends Endocrinol. Metab. 22, 87–93. (*A very accessible and well written introduction to a very complex subject. Highly recommended*)

Walters, M.R., Nemere, I., 2004. Receptors for steroid hormones: membrane-associated and nuclear forms. Cell. Mol. Life Sci. 61, 2309–2321. (*Good discussion about alternative types of steroid hormone receptors*)

4 How drugs act: cellular aspects – excitation, contraction and secretion

OVERVIEW

The link between a drug interacting with a molecular target and its effect at the pathophysiological level, such as a change in blood glucose concentration or the shrinkage of a tumour, involves events at the cellular level. Whatever their specialised physiological function, cells generally share much the same repertoire of signalling mechanisms. In the next three chapters, we describe the parts of this repertoire that are of particular significance in understanding drug action at the cellular level. In this chapter, we describe mechanisms that operate mainly over a short timescale (milliseconds to hours), particularly excitation, contraction and secretion, which account for many physiological responses; Chapter 5 deals with the slower processes (generally days to months), including cell division, growth, differentiation and cell death, that determine the body's structure and constitution; Chapter 6 describes host defence mechanisms.

The short-term regulation of cell function depends mainly on the following components and mechanisms, which regulate, or are regulated by, the free concentration of Ca^{2+} in the cytosol, $[Ca^{2+}]_i$:

- ion channels and transporters in the plasma membrane
- the storage and release of Ca^{2+} by intracellular organelles
- Ca^{2+}-dependent regulation of a variety of functional proteins, including enzymes, contractile proteins and vesicle proteins.

More detailed coverage of the topics presented in this chapter can be found in Nestler et al. (2008), Berridge (2012) and Kandel et al. (2013).

Because $[Ca^{2+}]_i$ plays such a key role in cell function, a wide variety of drug effects results from interference with one or more of these mechanisms. If love makes the human world go round, $[Ca^{2+}]_i$ does the same for cells. Knowledge of the molecular and cellular details is extensive, and here we focus on the aspects that help to explain drug effects.

REGULATION OF INTRACELLULAR CALCIUM

Ever since the famous accident by Sidney Ringer's technician, which showed that using tap water rather than distilled water to make up the bathing solution for isolated frog hearts would allow them to carry on contracting, the role of Ca^{2+} as a major regulator of cell function has never been in question. Many drugs and physiological mechanisms operate, directly or indirectly, by influencing $[Ca^{2+}]_i$. Here we consider the main ways in which it is regulated, and later we describe some of the ways in which $[Ca^{2+}]_i$ controls cell function. Details of the

molecular components and drug targets are presented in Chapter 3, and descriptions of drug effects on integrated physiological function are given in later chapters.

The study of Ca^{2+} regulation took a big step forward in the 1970s with the development of optical techniques based on the Ca^{2+}-sensitive photoprotein *aequorin*, and fluorescent dyes such as *Fura-2*, which, for the first time, allowed free $[Ca^{2+}]_i$ to be continuously monitored in living cells with a high level of temporal and spatial resolution.

Most of the Ca^{2+} in a resting cell is sequestered in organelles, particularly the *endoplasmic* or *sarcoplasmic reticulum* (ER or SR) and the mitochondria, and the free $[Ca^{2+}]_i$ is kept to a low level, about 100 nmol/l. The Ca^{2+} concentration in extracellular fluid, $[Ca^{2+}]_o$, is about 2.4 mmol/l, so there is a large concentration gradient favouring Ca^{2+} entry. $[Ca^{2+}]_i$ is kept low (a) by the operation of active transport mechanisms that eject cytosolic Ca^{2+} through the plasma membrane and pump it into the ER, and (b) by the normally low Ca^{2+} permeability of the plasma and ER membranes. Regulation of $[Ca^{2+}]_i$ involves three main mechanisms:

- control of Ca^{2+} entry
- control of Ca^{2+} extrusion
- exchange of Ca^{2+} between the cytosol and the intracellular stores.

These mechanisms are described in more detail below and are summarised in Figure 4.1 (see Clapham, 2007; Berridge, 2009).

CALCIUM ENTRY MECHANISMS

There are four main routes by which Ca^{2+} enters cells across the plasma membrane:

- voltage-gated calcium channels
- ligand-gated calcium channels
- store-operated calcium channels (SOCs)
- Na^+–Ca^{2+} exchange (can operate in either direction; see *Calcium extrusion mechanisms*, p. 53).

VOLTAGE-GATED CALCIUM CHANNELS

The pioneering work of Hodgkin and Huxley on the ionic basis of the nerve action potential (see p. 55) identified voltage-dependent Na^+ and K^+ conductances as the main participants. It was later found that some invertebrate nerve and muscle cells could produce action potentials that depended on Ca^{2+} rather than Na^+, and it was then found that vertebrate cells also possess voltage-activated calcium channels capable of allowing substantial amounts of Ca^{2+} to enter the cell when the membrane is depolarised. These voltage-gated channels are highly selective for Ca^{2+} (although they also conduct Ba^{2+} ions, which are often used as a substitute in electrophysiological experiments), and do not conduct Na^+ or K^+; they are ubiquitous in excitable cells

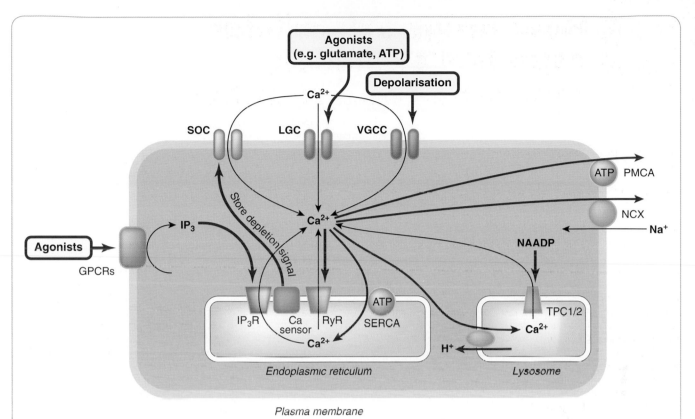

Fig. 4.1 **Regulation of intracellular calcium.** The main routes of transfer of Ca^{2+} into, and out of, the cytosol, endoplasmic reticulum and lysosomal structures are shown for a typical cell (see text for details). Black arrows: routes into the cytosol. Blue arrows: routes out of the cytosol. Red arrows: regulatory mechanisms. The state of the ER store of Ca^{2+} is monitored by the sensor protein Stim1, which interacts directly with the store-operated calcium channel (SOC) to promote Ca^{2+} entry when the ER store is depleted. Normally, $[Ca^{2+}]_i$ is regulated to about 10^{-7} mol/l in a 'resting' cell. Mitochondria (not shown) also function as Ca^{2+} storage organelles but release Ca^{2+} only under pathological conditions, such as ischaemia (see text). There is recent evidence for a lysosomal store of Ca^{2+} activated by the second messenger nicotinic acid adenine dinucleotide phosphate (NAADP) through a two-pore domain calcium channel (TPC). GPCR, G protein-coupled receptor; IP_3, inositol trisphosphate; IP_3R, inositol trisphosphate receptor; LGC, ligand-gated cation channel; NCX, Na^+–Ca^{2+} exchange transporter; PMCA, plasma membrane Ca^{2+}-ATPase; RyR, ryanodine receptor; SERCA, sarcoplasmic/endoplasmic reticulum ATPase; VGCC, voltage-gated calcium channel.

and cause Ca^{2+} to enter the cell whenever the membrane is depolarised, for example by a conducted action potential.

A combination of electrophysiological and pharmacological criteria have revealed five distinct subtypes of voltage-gated calcium channels: L, T, N, P/Q and R.[1] The subtypes vary with respect to their activation and inactivation kinetics, their voltage threshold for activation, their conductance and their sensitivity to blocking agents, as summarised in Table 4.1. The molecular basis for this heterogeneity has been worked out in some detail. The main pore-forming subunits (termed α1, see Fig. 3.4) occur in at least 10 molecular subtypes, and they are associated with other subunits (β, γ and two subunits from the same gene, α2δ, linked by a disulfide bond) that also exist in different forms. Different combinations of these subunits give rise to the different physiological subtypes. In general, L channels are particularly important in regulating

contraction of cardiac and smooth muscle (see p. 60 and 61), and N channels (and also P/Q) are involved in neurotransmitter and hormone release, while T channels mediate Ca^{2+} entry into neurons around the resting membrane potential and can control the rate of repolarisation of neurons and cardiac cells as well as various Ca^{2+}-dependent functions such as regulation of other channels, enzymes, etc. Clinically used drugs that act directly on some forms of calcium channel include the group of 'Ca^{2+} antagonists' consisting of *dihydropyridines* (e.g. **nifedipine**), **verapamil** and **diltiazem** (used for their cardiovascular effects; see Chs 21 and 22), and also **gabapentin** and **pregabalin** (used to treat pain and epilepsy; see Chs 42 and 45). Many drugs affect calcium channels indirectly by acting on G protein-coupled receptors (see Ch. 3). A number of toxins act selectively on one or other type of calcium channel (Table 4.1), and these are used as experimental tools.

LIGAND-GATED CHANNELS

Most ligand-gated cation channels (see Ch. 3) that are activated by excitatory neurotransmitters are relatively non-selective, and conduct Ca^{2+} ions as well as other cations. Most important in this respect is the glutamate

---

[1]P and Q are so similar that they usually get lumped together. The terminology is less than poetic: L stands for *long-lasting*; T stands for *transient*; N stands for *neither long-lasting nor transient*. Although P stands for *Purkinje* – this type of channel was first observed in cerebellar Purkinje cells – it continued the alphabetical sequence (missing out O of course) and so the next discovered were termed Q and R.

Table 4.1 Types and functions of Ca^{2+} channels

Gated by	Main types	Characteristics	Location and function	Drug effects
Voltage	L	High activation threshold Slow inactivation	Plasma membrane of many cells Main Ca^{2+} source for contraction in smooth and cardiac muscle	Blocked by dihydropyridines, verapamil, diltiazem; and calciseptine (peptide from snake venom) Activated by BayK 8644
	N	Low activation threshold Slow inactivation	Main Ca^{2+} source for transmitter release by nerve terminals	Blocked by ω-conotoxin (component of *Conus* snail venom) and ziconotide (marketed preparation of ω-conotoxin used to control pain) (Ch. 42)
	T	Low activation threshold Fast inactivation	Widely distributed Important in cardiac pacemaker and atria (role in dysrhythmias), also neuronal firing patterns	Blocked by mibefradil
	P/Q	Low activation threshold Slow inactivation	Nerve terminals Transmitter release	Blocked by ω-agatoxin-4A (component of funnel-web spider venom)
	R	Low threshold Fast inactivation	Neurons and dendrites Control of firing patterns	Blocked by low concentrations of SNX-482 (a toxin from a member of the tarantula family)
Inositol-trisphosphate	IP$_3$ receptor	Activated by Ca^{2+} and ATP in the presence of IP$_3$	Located in endoplasmic/sarcoplasmic reticulum Mediates Ca^{2+} release produced by GPCR activation	Not directly targeted by drugs Some experimental blocking agents known Responds to GPCR agonists and antagonists in many cells
Ca^{2+}	Ryanodine receptor	Directly activated in skeletal muscle via dihydropyridine receptor of T-tubules. Activated by Ca^{2+} in cardiac muscle	Located in endoplasmic/sarcoplasmic reticulum. Pathway for Ca^{2+} release in striated muscle	Activated by caffeine and ATP in the presence of Ca^{2+} Ryanodine both activates (low concentrations) and closes (high concentrations) the channel. Also closed by Mg^{2+}, K$^+$ channel blockers and dantrolene Mutations may lead to drug-induced malignant hypothermia, sudden cardiac death and central core disease
Store depletion	Store-operated channels	Activated by sensor protein that monitors level of ER Ca^{2+} stores	Located in plasma membrane	Activated indirectly by agents that deplete intracellular stores (e.g. GPCR agonists, thapsigargin) Not directly targeted by drugs

receptor of the NMDA type (Ch. 38), which has a particularly high permeability to Ca^{2+} and is a major contributor to Ca^{2+} uptake by postsynaptic neurons (and also glial cells) in the central nervous system. Activation of this receptor can readily cause so much Ca^{2+} entry that the cell dies, mainly through activation of Ca^{2+}-dependent proteases but also by triggering *apoptosis* (see Ch. 5). This mechanism, termed *excitotoxicity*, probably plays a part in various neurodegenerative disorders (see Ch. 40).

For many years, there was dispute about the existence of 'receptor-operated channels' in smooth muscle, responding directly to mediators such as adrenaline (epinephrine), acetylcholine and histamine. Now it seems (see Berridge, 2009) that the P2X receptor (see Ch. 3), activated by ATP, is the only example of a true ligand-gated channel in smooth muscle, and this constitutes an important route of entry for Ca^{2+}. As mentioned above, many mediators acting on G protein-coupled receptors, affect Ca^{2+} entry indirectly, mainly by regulating voltage-gated calcium channels or potassium channels.

STORE-OPERATED CALCIUM CHANNELS (SOCs)

SOCs are very low-conductance channels that occur in the plasma membrane and open to allow entry when the ER stores are depleted, but are not sensitive to cytosolic [Ca^{2+}]$_i$. The linkage between the ER and the plasma membrane – for long a puzzle – was recently found to involve a Ca^{2+}-sensor protein (*Stim1*) in the ER membrane, which connects directly to the channel protein (*Orai1*) in the plasma membrane (see Clapham, 2007).

Like the ER and SR channels, these channels can serve to amplify the rise in [Ca^{2+}]$_i$ resulting from Ca^{2+} release from the stores. So far, only experimental compounds are known to block these channels, but efforts are being made to develop specific blocking agents for therapeutic use as relaxants of smooth muscle.

CALCIUM EXTRUSION MECHANISMS

Active transport of Ca^{2+} outwards across the plasma membrane, and inwards across the membranes of the ER or SR, depends on the activity of distinct Ca^{2+}-dependent ATPases,[2] similar to the Na^+/K^+-dependent ATPase that pumps Na^+ out of the cell in exchange for K^+. **Thapsigargin** (derived from a Mediterranean plant, *Thapsia garganica*) specifically blocks the ER pump, causing loss of Ca^{2+} from the ER. It is a useful experimental tool but has no therapeutic significance.

Calcium is also extruded from cells in exchange for Na^+, by Na^+–Ca^{2+} exchange. The transporter that does this has been fully characterised and cloned, and (as you would expect) comes in several molecular subtypes whose functions remain to be worked out. The exchanger transfers three Na^+ ions for one Ca^{2+}, and therefore produces a net depolarising current when it is extruding Ca^{2+}. The energy for Ca^{2+} extrusion comes from the electrochemical gradient for Na^+, not directly from ATP hydrolysis. This means that a reduction in the Na^+ concentration gradient resulting from Na^+ entry will reduce Ca^{2+} extrusion by the exchanger, causing a secondary rise in $[Ca^{2+}]_i$, a mechanism that is particularly important in cardiac muscle (see Ch. 21). **Digoxin**, which inhibits Na^+ extrusion, acts on cardiac muscle in this way (Ch. 21), causing $[Ca^{2+}]_i$ to increase.

CALCIUM RELEASE MECHANISMS

There are two main types of calcium channel in the ER and SR membrane, which play an important part in controlling the release of Ca^{2+} from these stores.

- The *inositol trisphosphate receptor* (IP₃R) is activated by inositol trisphosphate (IP₃), a second messenger produced by the action of many ligands on G protein-coupled receptors (see Ch. 3). IP₃R is a ligand-gated ion channel, although its molecular structure differs from that of ligand-gated channels in the plasma membrane (see Mikoshiba, 2007). This is the main mechanism by which activation of G protein-coupled receptors causes an increase in $[Ca^{2+}]_i$.
- *Ryanodine receptors* (RyR) are so called because they were first identified through the specific blocking action of the plant alkaloid **ryanodine**. There are three isoforms – RyR1–3 (Van Petegem, 2012) that are expressed in many different cell types. RyR1 is highly expressed in skeletal muscle, RyR2 in the heart, and RyR3 in brain neurons. In skeletal muscle RyRs on the SR are physically coupled to *dihydropyridine receptors* on the T-tubules (see Fig. 4.9); this coupling results in Ca^{2+} release following the action potential in the muscle fibre. In other muscle types RyRs respond to Ca^{2+} that enters the cell through membrane calcium channels by a mechanism known as *calcium-induced calcium release* (CICR).

The functions of IP₃Rs and RyRs are modulated by a variety of other intracellular signals (see Berridge et al., 2003), which affect the magnitude and spatiotemporal patterning of Ca^{2+} signals. Fluorescence imaging techniques have revealed a remarkable level of complexity of Ca^{2+} signals, and much remains to be discovered about the importance of this patterning in relation to physiological and pharmacological mechanisms. The Ca^{2+} sensitivity of RyRs is increased by caffeine, causing Ca^{2+} release from the SR even at resting levels of $[Ca^{2+}]_i$. This is used experimentally but rarely happens in humans, because the other pharmacological effects of caffeine (see Ch. 48) occur at much lower doses. The blocking effect of **dantrolene**, a compound related to ryanodine, is used therapeutically to relieve muscle spasm in the rare condition of *malignant hyperthermia* (see Ch. 41), which is associated with inherited abnormalities in the RyR protein.

A typical $[Ca^{2+}]_i$ signal resulting from activation of a G protein-coupled receptor is shown in Figure 4.2. The response produced in the absence of extracellular Ca^{2+} represents release of intracellular Ca^{2+}. The larger and more prolonged response when extracellular Ca^{2+} is present shows the contribution of SOC-mediated Ca^{2+} entry. The various positive and negative feedback mechanisms that regulate $[Ca^{2+}]_i$ give rise to a variety of temporal and spatial oscillatory patterns (Fig. 4.2B) that are responsible for spontaneous rhythmic activity in smooth muscle and nerve cells (see Berridge, 2009).

OTHER SECOND MESSENGERS

▼ Two intracellular metabolites, cyclic ADP-ribose (cADPR) and nicotinic acid adenine dinucleotide phosphate (NAADP; see Fliegert et al., 2007), formed from the ubiquitous coenzymes nicotinamide adenine dinucleotide (NAD) and NAD phosphate, also affect Ca^{2+} signalling. cADPR acts by increasing the sensitivity of RyRs to Ca^{2+}, thus increasing the 'gain' of the CICR effect. NAADP releases Ca^{2+} from lysosomes by activating two-pore domain calcium channels.

The levels of these messengers in mammalian cells may be regulated mainly in response to changes in the metabolic status of the cell, although the details are not yet clear. Abnormal Ca^{2+} signalling is involved in many pathophysiological conditions, such as ischaemic cell death, endocrine disorders and cardiac dysrhythmias, where the roles of cADPR and NAADP, and their interaction with other mechanisms that regulate $[Ca^{2+}]_i$, are the subject of much current work (see Morgan et al., 2011).

THE ROLE OF MITOCHONDRIA

▼ Under normal conditions, mitochondria accumulate Ca^{2+} passively as a result of the intramitochondrial potential, which is strongly negative with respect to the cytosol. This negativity is maintained by active extrusion of protons, and is lost – thus releasing Ca^{2+} into the cytosol – if the cell runs short of ATP, for example under conditions of hypoxia. This only happens *in extremis*, and the resulting Ca^{2+} release contributes to the cytotoxicity associated with severe metabolic disturbance. Cell death resulting from brain ischaemia or coronary ischaemia (see Chs 21 and 40) involves this mechanism, along with others that contribute to an excessive rise in $[Ca^{2+}]_i$.

CALMODULIN

Calcium exerts its control over cell functions by virtue of its ability to regulate the activity of many different proteins, including enzymes (particularly kinases and phosphatases), channels, transporters, transcription factors, synaptic vesicle proteins and many others either by binding directly to these proteins or through a Ca^{2+}-binding protein that serves as an intermediate between Ca^{2+} and the regulated functional protein, the best known such binding protein being the ubiquitous *calmodulin* (see Clapham, 2007). This regulates at least 40 different functional

---

[2]Clapham (2007) likens these pumps to Sisyphus, condemned endlessly to push a stone up a hill (also consuming ATP, no doubt), only for it to roll down again.

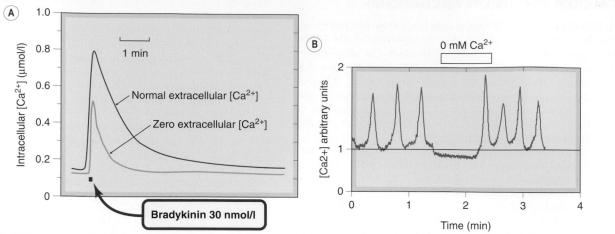

Fig. 4.2 **[A] Increase in intracellular free calcium concentration in response to receptor activation.** The records were obtained from a single rat sensory neuron grown in tissue culture. The cells were loaded with the fluorescent Ca^{2+} indicator Fura-2, and the signal from a single cell monitored with a fluorescence microscope. A brief exposure to the peptide bradykinin, which causes excitation of sensory neurons (see Ch. 42), causes a transient increase in $[Ca^{2+}]_i$ from the resting value of about 150 nmol/l. When Ca^{2+} is removed from the extracellular solution, the bradykinin-induced increase in $[Ca^{2+}]_i$ is still present but is smaller and briefer. The response in the absence of extracellular Ca^{2+} represents the release of stored intracellular Ca^{2+} resulting from the intracellular production of inositol trisphosphate. The difference between this and the larger response when Ca^{2+} is present extracellularly is believed to represent Ca^{2+} entry through store-operated ion channels in the cell membrane. *(Figure kindly provided by GM Burgess and A Forbes.)* **[B] Spontaneous intracellular calcium oscillations in pacemaker cells from the rabbit urethra that regulate the rhythmic contractions of the smooth muscle.** The signals cease when external Ca^{2+} is removed, showing that activation of membrane Ca^{2+} channels is involved in the mechanism. *(From McHale N, Hollywood M, Sargeant G et al. 2006 J Physiol 570, 23–28.)*

Calcium regulation

Intracellular Ca^{2+} concentration, $[Ca^{2+}]_i$, is critically important as a regulator of cell function.
- Intracellular Ca^{2+} is determined by (a) Ca^{2+} entry; (b) Ca^{2+} extrusion; and (c) Ca^{2+} exchange between the cytosol, endoplasmic or sarcoplasmic reticulum (ER, SR), lysosomes and mitochondria.
- Calcium entry occurs by various routes, including voltage- and ligand-gated calcium channels and Na^+–Ca^{2+} exchange.
- Calcium extrusion depends mainly on an ATP-driven Ca^{2+} pump.
- Calcium ions are actively taken up and stored by the ER/SR, from which they are released in response to various stimuli.
- Calcium ions are released from ER/SR stores by (a) the second messenger IP_3 acting on IP_3 receptors; or (b) increased $[Ca^{2+}]_i$ itself acting on ryanodine receptors, a mechanism known as Ca^{2+}-induced Ca^{2+} release.
- Other second messengers, cyclic ADP ribose and nicotinic acid dinucleotide phosphate, also promote the release of Ca^{2+} from Ca^{2+} stores.
- Depletion of ER/SR Ca^{2+} stores promotes Ca^{2+} entry through the plasma membrane, via store-operated channels.
- Calcium ions affect many aspects of cell function by binding to proteins such as calmodulin, which in turn bind other proteins and regulate their function.

proteins – indeed a powerful fixer. Calmodulin is a dimer, with four Ca^{2+} binding sites. When all are occupied, it undergoes a conformational change, exposing a 'sticky' hydrophobic domain that lures many proteins into association, thereby affecting their functional properties.

EXCITATION

Excitability describes the ability of a cell to show a regenerative all-or-nothing electrical response to depolarisation of its membrane, this membrane response being known as an action potential. It is a characteristic of most neurons and muscle cells (including skeletal, cardiac and smooth muscle) and of many endocrine gland cells. In neurons and muscle cells, the ability of the action potential, once initiated, to propagate to all parts of the cell membrane, and often to spread to neighbouring cells, explains the importance of membrane excitation in intra- and intercellular signalling. In the nervous system, and in skeletal muscle, action potential propagation is the mechanism responsible for communication over long distances at high speed, indispensable for large, fast-moving creatures. In cardiac and smooth muscle, as well as in some central neurons, spontaneous rhythmic activity occurs. In gland cells, the action potential, where it occurs, serves to amplify the signal that causes the cell to secrete. In each type of tissue, the properties of the excitation process reflect the special characteristics of the ion channels that underlie the process. The molecular nature of ion channels, and their importance as drug targets, is considered in Chapter 3; here we discuss the cellular processes that depend primarily on ion channel function. For more detail, see Hille (2001).

THE 'RESTING' CELL

The resting cell is not resting at all but very busy controlling the state of its interior, and it requires a continuous supply of energy to do so. In relation to the topics discussed in this chapter, the following characteristics are especially important:

• membrane potential
• permeability of the plasma membrane to different ions
• intracellular ion concentrations, especially $[Ca^{2+}]_i$.

Under resting conditions, all cells maintain a negative internal potential between about −30 mV and −80 mV, depending on the cell type. This arises because (a) the membrane is relatively impermeable to Na^+, and (b) Na^+ ions are actively extruded from the cell in exchange for K^+ ions by an energy-dependent transporter, the Na^+ pump (or Na^+–K^+-ATPase). The result is that the intracellular K^+ concentration, $[K^+]_i$, is higher, and $[Na^+]_i$ is lower, than the respective extracellular concentrations. In many cells, other ions, particularly Cl^-, are also actively transported and unequally distributed across the membrane. In many cases (e.g. in neurons), the membrane permeability to K^+ is relatively high, and the membrane potential settles at a value of −60 to −80 mV, close to the equilibrium potential for K^+ (Fig. 4.3). In other cells (e.g. smooth muscle), anions play a larger part, and the membrane potential is generally lower (−30 to −50 mV) and less dependent on K^+.

ELECTRICAL AND IONIC EVENTS UNDERLYING THE ACTION POTENTIAL

Our present understanding of electrical excitability rests firmly on the work of Hodgkin, Huxley and Katz on squid axons, published in 1949–1952. Their experiments (see Katz, 1966) revealed the existence of voltage-gated ion channels (see p. 57–60) and showed that the action potential is generated by the interplay of two processes:

1. a rapid, transient increase in Na^+ permeability that occurs when the membrane is depolarised beyond about −50 mV
2. a slower, sustained increase in K^+ permeability.

Because of the inequality of Na^+ and K^+ concentrations on the two sides of the membrane, an increase in Na^+ permeability causes an inward (depolarising) current of Na^+ ions, whereas an increase in K^+ permeability causes an outward (repolarising) current. The separability of these two currents can be most clearly demonstrated by the use of drugs blocking sodium and potassium channels, as shown in Figure 4.4. During the physiological initiation or propagation of a nerve impulse, the first event is a small depolarisation of the membrane, produced either by transmitter action or by the approach of an action potential passing along the axon. This opens sodium channels, allowing an inward current of Na^+ ions to flow, which depolarises the membrane still further. The process is thus a regenerative one, and the increase in Na^+ permeability is enough to bring the membrane potential close to E_{Na}. The increased Na^+ conductance is transient, because the channels inactivate rapidly and the membrane returns to its resting state.

In many types of cell, including most nerve cells, repolarisation is assisted by the opening of voltage-dependent

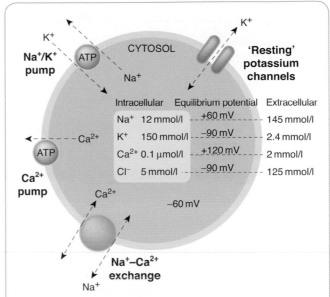

Fig. 4.3 Simplified diagram showing the ionic balance of a typical 'resting' cell. The main transport mechanisms that maintain the ionic gradients across the plasma membrane are the ATP-driven Na^+–K^+ and Ca^{2+} pumps and the Na^+–Ca^{2+} exchange transporter. The membrane is relatively permeable to K^+, because some types of potassium channel are open at rest, but impermeable to other cations. The unequal ion concentrations on either side of the membrane give rise to the 'equilibrium potentials' shown. The resting membrane potential, typically about −60 mV but differing between different cell types, is determined by the equilibrium potentials and the permeabilities of the various ions involved, and by the 'electrogenic' effect of the transporters. For simplicity, anions and other ions, such as protons, are not shown, although these play an important role in many cell types.

The figure shows a cell with the following labels: K+, Na^+/K^+ pump, ATP, CYTOSOL, Na^+, K+, 'Resting' potassium channels, Ca^{2+}, ATP, Ca^{2+} pump, Ca^{2+}, Na^+–Ca^{2+} exchange, Na^+.

	Intracellular	Equilibrium potential	Extracellular
Na^+	12 mmol/l	+60 mV	145 mmol/l
K^+	150 mmol/l	−90 mV	2.4 mmol/l
Ca^{2+}	0.1 μmol/l	+120 mV	2 mmol/l
Cl^-	5 mmol/l	−90 mV	125 mmol/l
		−60 mV	

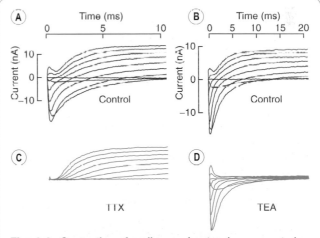

Fig. 4.4 Separation of sodium and potassium currents in the nerve membrane. Voltage clamp records from the node of Ranvier of a single frog nerve fibre. At time 0, the membrane potential was stepped to a depolarised level, ranging from −60 mV (lower trace in each series) to +60 mV (upper trace in each series) in 15-mV steps. **[A] [B]** Control records from two fibres. **[C]** Effect of tetrodotoxin (TTX), which abolishes Na^+ currents. **[D]** Effect of tetraethylammonium (TEA), which abolishes K^+ currents. *(From Hille B 1970. Ionic channels in nerve membranes. Prog Biophys Mol Biol 21, 1–32.)*

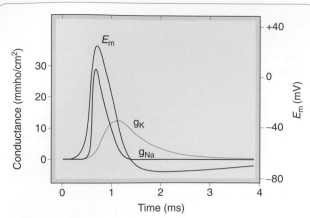

Fig. 4.5 Behaviour of sodium and potassium channels during a conducted action potential. Rapid opening of sodium channels occurs during the action potential upstroke. Delayed opening of potassium channels, and inactivation of sodium channels, causes repolarisation. E_m, membrane potential; g_{Na}, g_K, membrane conductance to Na^+, K^+.

K^+ channels. These function in much the same way as sodium channels, but their activation kinetics are about 10 times slower and they do not inactivate appreciably. This means that the potassium channels open later than the sodium channels, and contribute to the rapid termination of the action potential. The behaviour of the sodium and potassium channels during an action potential is shown in Figure 4.5.

The foregoing account, based on Hodgkin and Huxley's work 60 years ago, involves only Na^+ and K^+ channels. Subsequently (see Hille, 2001), voltage-gated calcium channels (see Fig. 4.1) were discovered. These function in basically the same way as sodium channels if on a slightly slower timescale; they contribute to action potential generation in many cells, particularly cardiac and smooth muscle cells, but also in neurons and secretory cells. Ca^{2+} entry through voltage-gated calcium channels plays a key role in intracellular signalling, as described on p. 50-54.

CHANNEL FUNCTION

The discharge patterns of excitable cells vary greatly. Skeletal muscle fibres are quiescent unless stimulated by the arrival of a nerve impulse at the neuromuscular junction. Cardiac muscle fibres discharge spontaneously at a regular rate (see Ch. 21). Neurons may be normally silent, or they may discharge spontaneously, either regularly or in bursts; smooth muscle cells show a similar variety of firing patterns. The frequency at which different cells normally discharge action potentials also varies greatly, from 100 Hz or more for fast-conducting neurons, down to about 1 Hz for cardiac muscle cells. These very pronounced functional variations reflect the different characteristics of the ion channels expressed in different cell types. Rhythmic fluctuations of $[Ca^{2+}]i$ underlie the distinct firing patterns that occur in different types of cell (see Berridge, 2009).

Drugs that alter channel characteristics, either by interacting directly with the channel itself or indirectly through second messengers, affect the function of many organ systems, including the nervous, cardiovascular, endocrine, respiratory and reproductive systems, and are a frequent theme in this book. Here we describe some of the key mechanisms involved in the regulation of excitable cells.

In general, action potentials are initiated by membrane currents that cause depolarisation of the cell. These currents may be produced by synaptic activity, by an action potential approaching from another part of the cell, by a sensory stimulus or by spontaneous *pacemaker* activity. The tendency of such currents to initiate an action potential is governed by the *excitability* of the cell, which depends mainly on the state of (a) the voltage-gated sodium and/or calcium channels, and (b) the potassium channels of the resting membrane. Anything that increases the number of available sodium or calcium channels, or reduces their activation threshold, will tend to increase excitability, whereas increasing the resting K^+ conductance reduces it. Agents that do the reverse, by blocking channels or interfering with their opening, will have the opposite effect. Some examples are shown in Figures 4.6 and 4.7. Inherited mutations of channel proteins are responsible for a wide variety of (mostly rare) neurological and other genetic disorders (see Ashcroft, 2000, 2006).

USE DEPENDENCE AND VOLTAGE DEPENDENCE

▼ Voltage-gated channels can exist in three functional states (Fig. 4.8): *resting* (the closed state that prevails at the normal resting potential), *activated* (the open state favoured by brief depolarisation) and *inactivated* (the blocked state resulting from a trap door-like occlusion of the open channel by a floppy intracellular appendage of the channel protein). After the action potential has passed, many sodium channels are in the inactivated state; after the membrane potential returns to its resting value, the inactivated channels take time to revert to the resting state and thus become available for activation once more. In the meantime, the membrane is temporarily *refractory*. Each action potential causes the channels to cycle through these states. The duration of the refractory period determines the maximum frequency at which action potentials can occur. Drugs that block sodium channels, such as local anaesthetics (Ch. 43), antidysrhythmic drugs (Ch. 21) and antiepileptic drugs (Ch. 45), commonly show a selective affinity for one or other of these functional states of the channel, and in their presence the proportion of channels in the high-affinity state is increased. Of particular importance are drugs that bind most strongly to the inactivated state of the channel and thus favour the adoption of this state, thus prolonging the refractory period and reducing the maximum frequency at which action potentials can be generated. This type of block is called *use dependent*, because the binding of such drugs increases as a function of the rate of action potential discharge, which governs the rate at which inactivated – and therefore drug-sensitive – channels are generated. This is important for some antidysrhythmic drugs (see Ch. 21) and for antiepileptic drugs (Ch. 45), because high-frequency discharges can be inhibited without affecting excitability at normal frequencies. Drugs that readily block sodium channels in their resting state (e.g. local anaesthetics, Ch. 43) prevent excitation at low as well as high frequencies.

Most sodium channel-blocking drugs are cationic at physiological pH and are therefore affected by the voltage gradient across the cell membrane. They block the channel from the inside, so that their blocking action is favoured by depolarisation. This phenomenon, known as *voltage dependence*, is also of relevance to the action of antidysrhythmic and antiepileptic drugs, because the cells that are the seat of dysrhythmias or seizure activity are generally somewhat depolarised and therefore more strongly blocked than 'healthy' cells. Similar considerations apply also to drugs that block potassium or calcium channels, but we know less about the importance of use and voltage dependence for these than we do for sodium channels.

SODIUM CHANNELS

In most excitable cells, the regenerative inward current that initiates the action potential results from activation of

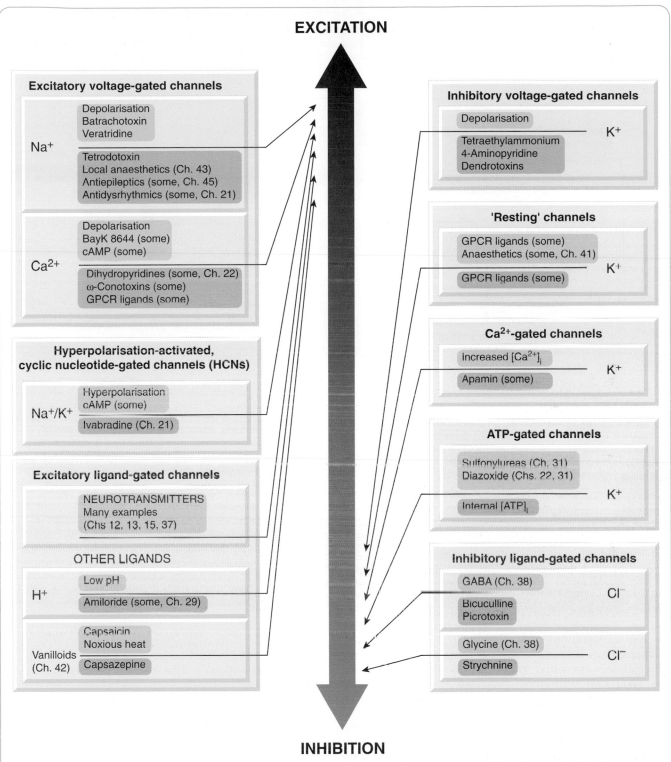

Fig. 4.6 Ion channels associated with excitatory and inhibitory membrane effects, and some of the drugs and other ligands that affect them. Channel openers are shown in green boxes, blocking agents and inhibitors in pink boxes. Hyperpolarisation-activated Na^+/K^+ channels are known as hyperpolarisation-activated, cyclic nucleotide-gated channels (HCNs); H^+ activated channels are known as acid-sensing ion channels (ASICs). GPCR, G protein-coupled receptor.

voltage-gated sodium channels. The early voltage clamp studies by Hodgkin and Huxley on the squid giant axon, described on p. 55, revealed the essential functional properties of these channels. Later, advantage was taken of the potent and highly selective blocking action of **tetrodotoxin** (TTX, see Ch. 43) to label and purify the channel proteins, and subsequently to clone them. Sodium channels consist of a central, pore forming α subunit (shown in Fig. 3.20) and two auxiliary β subunits. Nine α-subunits ($Na_V1.1$ through $Na_V1.9$) and four β subunits have been identified in mammals. The α subunits contain four similar domains each comprising six

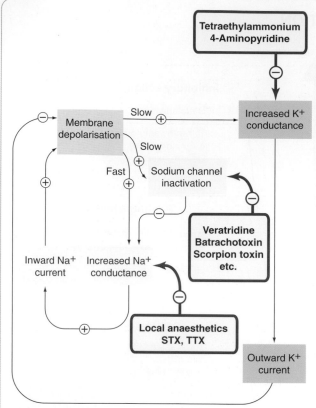

Fig. 4.7 Sites of action of drugs and toxins that affect channels involved in action potential generation. Many other mediators affect these channels indirectly via membrane receptors, through phosphorylation or altered expression. STX, saxitoxin; TTX, tetrodotoxin.

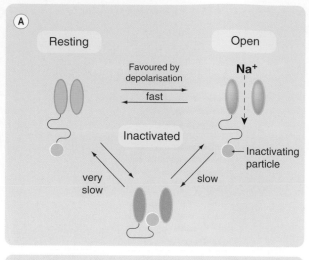
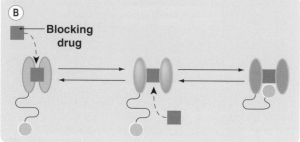

Fig. 4.8 Resting, activated and inactivated states of voltage-gated channels, exemplified by the sodium channel. [**A**] Membrane depolarisation causes a rapid transition from the resting (closed) state to the open state. The inactivating particle (part of the intracellular domain of the channel protein) is then able to block the channel. With prolonged depolarization, below the threshold for opening, channels can go directly from resting to inactivated without opening. [**B**] Some blocking drugs (such as tetrodotoxin) block the channel from the outside, like a plug, whereas others (such as local anaesthetics and antiepileptic drugs) enter from the inside of the cell and often show preference for the open or inactivated states, and thus affect the kinetic behaviour of the channels, with implications for their clinical application.

membrane-spanning helices (reviewed by Catterall, 2000). One of these helices, S4, contains several basic amino acids and forms the voltage sensor, and moves outwards, thus opening the channel, when the membrane is depolarised. One of the intracellular loops is designed to swing across and block the channel when S4 is displaced, thus inactivating the channel.

It was known from physiological studies that the sodium channels of heart and skeletal muscle differ in various ways from those of neurons. In particular, cardiac sodium channels (and also those of some sensory neurons) are relatively insensitive to TTX, and slower in their kinetics, compared with most neuronal sodium channels. This is explained by the relative insensitivity of some α subunits ($Na_v1.5$, $Na_v1.8$ and $Na_v1.9$) to tetrodotoxin. Changes in the level of expression of some sodium channel subunits is thought to underlie the hyperexcitability of sensory neurons in different types of neuropathic pain (see Ch. 42).

In addition to channel-blocking compounds such as tetrodotoxin, other compounds affect sodium channel gating. For example, the plant alkaloid veratridine and the frog skin poison batrachotoxin cause persistent activation, while various scorpion toxins prevent inactivation, mechanisms resulting in enhanced neuronal excitability.

POTASSIUM CHANNELS

In a typical resting cell (see p. 55, Fig. 4.3), the membrane is selectively permeable to K^+, and the membrane potential (about −60 mV) is somewhat positive to the K^+ equilibrium (about −90 mV). This resting permeability comes about because some potassium channels are open. If more potassium channels open, the membrane hyperpolarises and the cell is inhibited, whereas the opposite happens if potassium channels close. As well as affecting excitability in this way, potassium channels also play an important role in regulating the duration of the action potential and the temporal patterning of action potential discharges; altogether, these channels play a central role in regulating cell function. As mentioned in Chapter 3, the number and variety of potassium channel subtypes is extraordinary, implying that evolution has been driven by the scope for biological advantage to be gained from subtle variations in the functional properties of these channels. A recent résumé lists over 60 different pore-forming subunits, plus another 20 or so auxiliary subunits. An impressive evolutionary display, maybe, but hard going for most of us. Here we outline the main types that are known to

Table 4.2 **Types and functions of K+ channels**

Structural class[a]	Functional subtypes[b]	Functions	Drug effects	Notes
Voltage-gated (6T, 1P)	Voltage-gated K+ channels	Action potential repolarisation Limits maximum firing frequency	Blocked by tetraethylammonium, 4-aminopyridine Certain subtypes blocked by dendrotoxins (from mamba snake venom)	Subtypes in the heart include HERG and LQT channels, which are involved in congenital and drug-induced dysrhythmias Other subtypes may be involved in inherited forms of epilepsy
	Ca^{2+}-activated K+ channels	Inhibition following stimuli which increase [Ca^{2+}]$_i$	Certain subtypes blocked by apamin (from bee venom), and charybdotoxin (from scorpion venom)	Important in many excitable tissues to limit repetitive discharges, also in secretory cells
Inward rectifying (2T, 1P)	G protein-activated	Mediate effects of many GPCRs which cause inhibition by increasing K+ conductance	GPCR agonists and antagonists Some are blocked by tertiapin (from honey bee venom)	Other inward rectifying K+ channels important in kidney
	ATP-sensitive	Found in many cells Channels open when [ATP] is low, causing inhibition Important in control of insulin secretion	Association of one subtype with the sulfonylurea receptor (SUR) results in modulation by sulfonylureas (e.g. glibenclamide) which close channel, and by K+ channel openers (e.g. diazoxide, minoxidil) which relax smooth muscle	
Two-pore domain (4T, 2P)	Several subtypes identified (TWIK, TRAAK, TREK, TASK, etc.)	Most are voltage-insensitive; some are normally open and contribute to the 'resting' K+ conductance Modulated by GPCRs	Certain subtypes are activated by volatile anaesthetics (e.g. isoflurane) No selective blocking agents Modulation by GPCR agonists and antagonists	The nomenclature is misleading, especially when they are incorrectly referred to as two-pore channels

GPCR, G protein coupled receptor.

[a]K+ channel structures (see Fig 3.20) are defined according to the number of transmembrane helices (T) and the number of pore-forming loops (P) in each α subunit. Functional channels contain several subunits (often four) which may be identical or different, and they are often associated with accessory (β) subunits.

[b]Within each functional subtype, several molecular variants have been identified, often restricted to particular cells and tissues. The physiological and pharmacological significance of this heterogeneity is not yet understood.

be important pharmacologically. For more details, and information on potassium channels and the various drugs and toxins that affect them, see Shieh et al. (2000), Jenkinson (2006), Alexander et al. (2013).

▼ Potassium channels fall into three main classes (Table 4.2),[3] of which the structures are shown in Figure 3.20.

- *Voltage-gated potassium channels*, which possess six membrane-spanning helices, one of which serves as the voltage sensor, causing the channel to open when the membrane is depolarised. Included in this group are channels of the shaker family, accounting for most of the voltage-gated K+ currents familiar to electrophysiologists, and others such as Ca^{2+}-activated potassium channels and two subtypes that are important in the heart, HERG and LQT channels. Many of these channels are blocked by drugs such as **tetraethylammonium** and **4-aminopyridine**.
- *Inwardly rectifying potassium channels*, so called because they allow K+ to pass inwards much more readily than outwards. These have two membrane-spanning helices and a single pore-forming loop (P loop). These channels are regulated by interaction with G proteins (see Ch. 3) and mediate the inhibitory effects of many agonists acting on G protein-coupled receptors. Certain types are important in the heart, particularly in regulating the duration of the cardiac action potential (Ch. 21); others are the target for the action of **sulfonylureas** (antidiabetic drugs that stimulate insulin

[3]Potassium channel terminology is confusing, to put it mildly. Electrophysiologists have named K+ currents prosaically on the basis of their functional properties (I_{KV}, I_{KCa}, I_{KATP}, I_{KIR}, etc.); geneticists have named genes somewhat fancifully according to the phenotypes associated with mutations (shaker, ether-a-go-go, etc.), while molecular biologists have introduced a rational but unmemorable nomenclature on the basis of sequence data (KCNK, KCNQ, etc., with numerical suffixes). The rest of us have to make what we can of the unlovely jargon of labels such as HERG (which – don't blink – stands for Human Ether-a-go-go Related Gene), TWIK, TREK and TASK.

secretion by blocking them; see Ch. 31) and smooth muscle relaxant drugs, such as **minoxidil** and **diazoxide**, which open them (see Ch. 22).

- *Two-pore domain potassium channels*, with four helices and two P loops (see review by Goldstein et al., 2001). These show outward rectification and therefore exert a strong repolarising influence, opposing any tendency to excitation. They may contribute to the resting K^+ conductance in many cells, and are susceptible to regulation via G proteins; certain subtypes have been implicated in the action of volatile anaesthetics such as **isoflurane** (Ch. 41).

Inherited abnormalities of potassium channels (channelopathies) contribute to a rapidly growing number of cardiac, neurological and other diseases. These include the *long QT syndrome* associated with mutations in cardiac voltage-gated potassium channels, causing episodes of ventricular arrest that can result in sudden death. Drug-induced prolongation of the *QT* interval is an unwanted side effect. Nowadays new drugs are screened for this property at an early stage in the development process (see Ch. 60). Certain familial types of deafness and epilepsy are associated with mutations in voltage-gated potassium channels (Ashcroft, 2000, 2006).

Ion channels and electrical excitability

- Excitable cells generate an all-or-nothing action potential in response to membrane depolarisation. This occurs in most neurons and muscle cells, and also in some gland cells. The ionic basis and time course of the response varies between tissues.
- The regenerative response results from the depolarising current associated with opening of voltage-gated cation channels (mainly Na^+ and Ca^{2+}). It is terminated by inactivation of these channels accompanied by opening of K^+ channels.
- These voltage-gated channels exist in many molecular varieties, with specific functions in different types of cell.
- The membrane of the 'resting' cell is relatively permeable to K^+ but impermeable to Na^+ and Ca^{2+}. Drugs or mediators that open K^+ channels reduce membrane excitability, as do inhibitors of Na^+ or Ca^{2+} channel function. Blocking K^+ channels or activating Na^+ or Ca^{2+} channels increases excitability.
- Cardiac muscle cells, some neurons and some smooth muscle cells generate spontaneous action potentials whose amplitude, rate and rhythm is affected by drugs that affect ion channel function.

MUSCLE CONTRACTION

Effects of drugs on the contractile machinery of smooth muscle are the basis of many therapeutic applications, for smooth muscle is an important component of most physiological systems, including blood vessels and the gastrointestinal, respiratory and urinary tracts. For many decades, smooth muscle pharmacology with its trademark technology – the isolated organ bath – held the

centre of the pharmacological stage, and neither the subject nor the technology shows any sign of flagging, even though the stage has become much more crowded. Cardiac and skeletal muscle contractility are also the targets of important drug effects.

Although in each case the basic molecular basis of contraction is similar, namely an interaction between actin and myosin, fuelled by ATP and initiated by an increase in $[Ca^{2+}]_i$, there are differences between these three kinds of muscle that account for their different responsiveness to drugs and chemical mediators.

These differences (Fig. 4.9) involve (a) the linkage between membrane events and increase in $[Ca^{2+}]_i$, and (b) the mechanism by which $[Ca^{2+}]_i$ regulates contraction.

SKELETAL MUSCLE

Skeletal muscle possesses an array of transverse T-tubules extending into the cell from the plasma membrane. The action potential of the plasma membrane depends on voltage-gated sodium channels, as in most nerve cells, and propagates rapidly from its site of origin, the motor endplate (see Ch. 13), to the rest of the fibre. The T-tubule membrane contains voltage-gated calcium channels termed dihydropyridine receptors (DHPRs),[4] that respond to membrane depolarisation conducted passively along the T-tubule when the plasma membrane is invaded by an action potential. DHPRs are located extremely close to *ryanodine receptors* (RyRs; see Ch. 3) in the adjacent SR membrane, and activation of these RyRs causes release of Ca^{2+} from the SR. Direct coupling between the DHPRs of the T-tubule and the RyRs of the SR (as shown in Fig. 4.9) causes the opening of the RyRs on membrane depolarisation. Through this link, depolarisation rapidly activates the RyRs, releasing a short puff of Ca^{2+} from the SR into the sarcoplasm. The Ca^{2+} binds to troponin, a protein that normally blocks the interaction between actin and myosin. When Ca^{2+} binds, troponin moves out of the way and allows the contractile machinery to operate. Ca^{2+} release is rapid and brief, and the muscle responds with a short-lasting 'twitch' response. This is a relatively fast and direct mechanism compared with the arrangement in cardiac and smooth muscle (see below), and consequently less susceptible to pharmacological modulation.

CARDIAC MUSCLE

Cardiac muscle (see review by Bers, 2002) differs from skeletal muscle in several important respects. The nature of the cardiac action potential, the ionic mechanisms underlying its inherent rhythmicity and the effects of drugs on the rate and rhythm of the heart are described in Chapter 21. The cardiac action potential varies in its configuration in different parts of the heart, but commonly shows a 'plateau' lasting several hundred milliseconds following the initial rapid depolarisation. T-tubules in cardiac muscle contain L-type calcium channels, which open during this plateau and allow Ca^{2+} to enter. This Ca^{2+} entry acts on RyRs (a different molecular type from those of skeletal muscle) to release Ca^{2+} from the SR (Fig. 4.9).

---

[4]Although these are, to all intents and purposes, just a form of L-type calcium channel the term dihydropyridine receptor (DHPR) is used to reflect that they are not identical to the L-type channels in neurons and cardiac muscle.

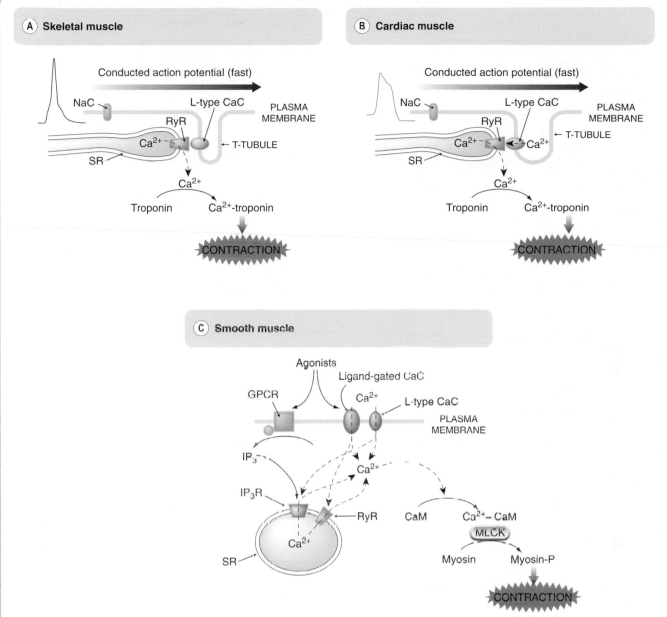

Fig. 4.9 Comparison of excitation–contraction coupling in [A] skeletal muscle, [B] cardiac muscle and [C] smooth muscle. Skeletal and cardiac muscle differ mainly in the mechanism by which membrane depolarisation is coupled to Ca^{2+} release. The calcium channel (CaC) and ryanodine receptor (RyR) are very closely positioned in both types of muscle. In cardiac muscle, Ca^{2+} entry via voltage-gated calcium channels initiates Ca^{2+} release through activation of the Ca^{2+}-sensitive RyRs whereas in skeletal muscle, the sarcolemmal calcium channels activate the ryanodine receptors through a voltage-dependent physical interaction. The control of intracellular Ca^{2+} in smooth muscle cells may vary depending upon the type of smooth muscle. In general terms, smooth muscle contraction is largely dependent upon inositol trisphosphate (IP_3)-induced Ca^{2+} release from SR stores through IP_3 receptors (IP_3R). Smooth muscle contraction can also be produced either by Ca^{2+} entry through voltage- or ligand-gated calcium channels. The mechanism by which Ca^{2+} activates contraction is different, and operates more slowly, in smooth muscle compared with in skeletal or cardiac muscle. CaC, calcium channel; CaM, calmodulin; GPCR, G protein-coupled receptor; MLCK, myosin light-chain kinase; NaC, voltage-gated sodium channel; RyR, ryanodine receptor; SR, sarcoplasmic reticulum.

With minor differences, the subsequent mechanism by which Ca^{2+} activates the contractile machinery is the same as in skeletal muscle. Ca^{2+}-induced Ca^{2+} release via RyRs may play a role in some forms of cardiac arrhythmia. It has been suggested that the antidysrhythmic effects of **flecainide** and β blockers may be due, in part, to their ability to reduce this release. Mutations of RyRs are implicated in various disorders of skeletal and cardiac muscle function (see Priori & Napolitano, 2005).

SMOOTH MUSCLE

The properties of smooth muscle vary considerably in different organs, and the mechanisms linking membrane

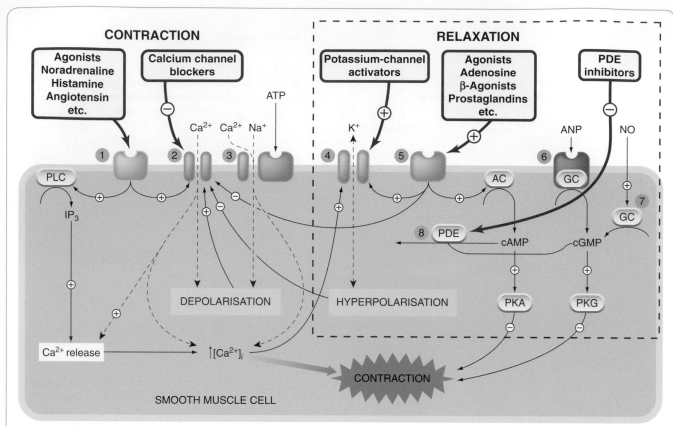

Fig. 4.10 **Mechanisms controlling smooth muscle contraction and relaxation.** 1. G protein-coupled receptors for excitatory agonists, mainly regulating inositol trisphosphate formation and calcium channel function. 2. Voltage-gated calcium channels. 3. P2X receptor for ATP (ligand-gated cation channel). 4. Potassium channels. 5. G protein-coupled receptors for inhibitory agonists, mainly regulating cAMP formation and potassium and calcium channel function. 6. Receptor for atrial natriuretic peptide (ANP), coupled directly to guanylyl cyclase (GC). 7. Soluble guanylyl cyclase, activated by nitric oxide (NO). 8. Phosphodiesterase (PDE), the main route of inactivation of cAMP and cGMP. AC, adenylyl cyclase; PKA, protein kinase A; PKG, protein kinase G; PLC, phospholipase C.

events and contraction are correspondingly variable and more complex than in other kinds of muscle. Spontaneous rhythmic activity occurs in many organs, by mechanisms producing oscillations of $[Ca^{2+}]_i$ (see Berridge, 2009). The action potential of smooth muscle is generally a rather lazy and vague affair compared with the more military behaviour of skeletal and cardiac muscle, and it propagates through the tissue much more slowly and uncertainly. The action potential is, in most cases, generated by L-type calcium channels rather than by voltage-gated sodium channels, and this is one important route of Ca^{2+} entry. In addition, many smooth muscle cells possess P2X receptors, ligand-gated cation channels, which allow Ca^{2+} entry when activated by ATP released from autonomic nerves (see Ch. 12). Smooth muscle cells also store Ca^{2+} in the ER, from which it can be released when the IP_3R is activated (see Ch. 3). IP_3 is generated by activation of many types of G protein-coupled receptor. Thus, in contrast to skeletal and cardiac muscle, Ca^{2+} release and contraction can occur in smooth muscle when such receptors are activated without necessarily involving depolarisation and Ca^{2+} entry through the plasma membrane. RyRs are also present in many smooth muscle cells and calcium-induced Ca^{2+} release via these channels may play a role in generating muscle contraction (Fig. 4.9) or couple to plasma membrane calcium-activated K^+ channels to

regulate membrane potential and thereby Ca^{2+} entry through voltage-gated calcium channels (Fig. 4.10).

The contractile machinery of smooth muscle is activated when the *myosin light chain* undergoes phosphorylation, causing it to become detached from the actin filaments. This phosphorylation is catalysed by a kinase, *myosin light-chain kinase* (MLCK), which is activated when it binds to Ca^{2+}–calmodulin (see p. 61, Fig. 4.9). A second enzyme, *myosin phosphatase*, reverses the phosphorylation and causes relaxation. The activity of MLCK and myosin phosphatase thus exerts a balanced effect, promoting contraction and relaxation, respectively. Both enzymes are regulated by cyclic nucleotides (cAMP and cGMP; see Ch. 3), and many drugs that cause smooth muscle contraction or relaxation mediated through G protein-coupled receptors or through guanylyl cyclase-linked receptors act in this way. Figure 4.10 summarises the main mechanisms by which drugs control smooth muscle contraction. The complexity of these control mechanisms and interactions explains why pharmacologists have been entranced for so long by smooth muscle. Many therapeutic drugs work by contracting or relaxing smooth muscle, particularly those affecting the cardiovascular, respiratory and gastrointestinal systems, as discussed in later chapters, where details of specific drugs and their physiological effects are given.

Muscle contraction

- Muscle contraction occurs in response to a rise in $[Ca^{2+}]_i$.
- In skeletal muscle, depolarisation causes rapid Ca^{2+} release from the sarcoplasmic reticulum (SR); in cardiac muscle, Ca^{2+} enters through voltage-gated channels, and this initial entry triggers further release from the SR; in smooth muscle, the Ca^{2+} signal is due partly to Ca^{2+} entry and partly to IP_3-mediated release from the SR.
- In smooth muscle, contraction can occur without action potentials, for example when agonists at G protein-coupled receptors lead to IP_3 formation.
- Activation of the contractile machinery in smooth muscle involves phosphorylation of the myosin light chain, a mechanism that is regulated by a variety of second messenger systems.

RELEASE OF CHEMICAL MEDIATORS

Much of pharmacology is based on interference with the body's own chemical mediators, particularly neurotransmitters, hormones and inflammatory mediators. Here we discuss some of the common mechanisms involved in the release of such mediators, and it will come as no surprise that Ca^{2+} plays a central role. Drugs and other agents that affect the various control mechanisms that regulate $[Ca^{2+}]_i$ will therefore also affect mediator release, and this accounts for many of the physiological effects that they produce.

Chemical mediators that are released from cells fall into two main groups (Fig. 4.11):

- Mediators that are preformed and packaged in storage vesicles – sometimes called storage granules – from which they are released by *exocytosis*. This large group comprises all the conventional neurotransmitters and neuromodulators (see Chs 12 and 36), and many hormones. It also includes secreted proteins such as cytokines and various growth factors (Ch. 18).
- Mediators that are produced on demand and are released by diffusion or by membrane carriers.[5] This group includes nitric oxide (Ch. 20) and many lipid mediators (e.g. prostanoids, Ch. 17) and endocannabinoids (Ch. 19), which are released from the postsynaptic cell to act retrogradely on nerve terminals.

Calcium ions play a key role in both cases, because a rise in $[Ca^{2+}]_i$ initiates exocytosis and is also the main activator of the enzymes responsible for the synthesis of diffusible mediators.

In addition to mediators that are released from cells, some are formed from precursors in the plasma, two important examples being *kinins* (Ch. 18) and *angiotensin* (Ch. 22), which are peptides produced by protease-mediated cleavage of circulating proteins.

---

[5]Carrier-mediated release can also occur with neurotransmitters that are stored in vesicles but is quantitatively less significant than exocytosis (see Ch. 13).

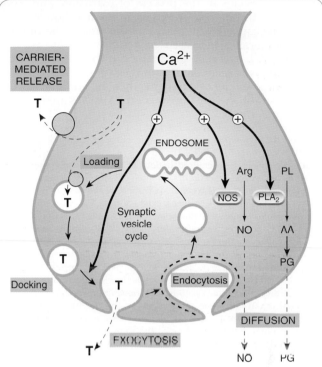

Fig. 4.11 **Role of exocytosis, carrier-mediated transport and diffusion in mediator release.** The main mechanism of release of monoamine and peptide mediators is Ca^{2+}-mediated exocytosis, but carrier-mediated release from the cytosol also occurs. T represents a typical amine transmitter, such as noradrenaline (norepinephrine) or 5-hydroxytryptamine. Nitric oxide (NO) and prostaglandins (PGs) are released by diffusion as soon as they are formed, from arginine (Arg) and arachidonic acid (AA), respectively, through the action of Ca^{2+}-activated enzymes, nitric oxide synthase (NOS) and phospholipase A_2 (PLA_2) (see Chs 17 and 20 for more details).

EXOCYTOSIS

Exocytosis, occurring in response to an increase of $[Ca^{2+}]_i$, is the principal mechanism of transmitter release (see Fig. 4.11) in the peripheral and central nervous systems, as well as in endocrine cells and mast cells. The secretion of enzymes and other proteins by gastrointestinal and exocrine glands and by vascular endothelial cells is also basically similar. Exocytosis (see Burgoyne & Morgan, 2002) involves fusion between the membrane of synaptic vesicles and the inner surface of the plasma membrane. The vesicles are preloaded with stored transmitter, and release occurs in discrete packets, or quanta, each representing the contents of a single vesicle. The first evidence for this came from the work of Katz and his colleagues in the 1950s, who recorded spontaneous 'miniature endplate potentials' at the frog neuromuscular junction, and showed that each resulted from the spontaneous release of a packet of the transmitter, acetylcholine. They also showed that release evoked by nerve stimulation occurred by the synchronous release of several hundred such quanta, and was highly dependent on the presence of Ca^{2+} in the bathing solution. Unequivocal evidence that the quanta represented vesicles releasing their contents by exocytosis came from electron microscopic studies, in which the tissue was rapidly frozen in mid-release, revealing vesicles in the process of extrusion, and from elegant electrophysiological measurements showing that membrane capacitance (reflecting the area of the presynaptic membrane) increased in a stepwise way as each vesicle fused, and then gradually returned as the vesicle membrane was recovered from the surface. There is also biochemical evidence showing that, in addition to the transmitter, other constituents of the vesicles are released at the same time.

▼ In nerve terminals specialised for fast synaptic transmission, Ca^{2+} enters through voltage-gated calcium channels, mainly of the N and P/Q type (see p. 52, Table 4.1), and the synaptic vesicles are 'docked' at active zones – specialised regions of the presynaptic membrane from which exocytosis occurs, situated close to the relevant calcium channels and opposite receptor-rich zones of the postsynaptic membrane. Elsewhere, where speed is less critical, Ca^{2+} may come from intracellular stores, and the spatial organisation of active zones is less clear. It is common for secretory cells, including neurons, to release more than one mediator (for example, a 'fast' transmitter such as glutamate and a 'slow' transmitter such as a neuropeptide) from different vesicle pools (see Ch. 12). The fast transmitter vesicles are located close to active zones, while the slow transmitter vesicles are further away. Release of the fast transmitter, because of the tight spatial organisation, occurs as soon as the neighbouring calcium channels open, before the Ca^{2+} has a chance to diffuse throughout the terminal, whereas release of the slow transmitter requires the Ca^{2+} to diffuse more widely. As a result, release of fast transmitters occurs impulse by impulse, even at low stimulation frequencies, whereas release of slow transmitters builds up only at higher stimulation frequencies. The release rates of the two therefore depend critically on the frequency and patterning of firing of the presynaptic neuron (Fig. 4.12). In non-excitable cells (e.g. most exocrine and endocrine glands), the slow mechanism predominates and is activated mainly by Ca^{2+} release from intracellular stores.

Calcium causes exocytosis by binding to the vesicle-bound protein *synaptotagmin*, and this favours association between a second vesicle-bound protein, *synaptobrevin*, and a related protein, *synaptotaxin*, on the inner surface of the plasma membrane. This association brings the vesicle membrane into close apposition with the plasma membrane, causing membrane fusion. This group of proteins, known collectively as SNAREs, plays a key role in exocytosis.

Having undergone exocytosis, the empty vesicle[6] is recaptured by endocytosis and returns to the interior of the terminal, where it fuses with the larger endosomal membrane. The endosome buds off new vesicles, which take up transmitter from the cytosol by means of specific transport proteins and are again docked on the presynaptic membrane. This sequence, which typically takes several minutes, is controlled by various trafficking proteins associated with the plasma membrane and the vesicles, as well as cytosolic proteins. Further details about exocytosis and vesicle recycling are given by Nestler et al. (2008) and Südhof (2004). So far, there are few examples of drugs that affect transmitter release by interacting with synaptic proteins, although the botulinum neurotoxins (see Ch. 13) produce their effects by proteolytic cleavage of SNARE proteins.

NON-VESICULAR RELEASE MECHANISMS

If this neat and tidy picture of transmitter packets ready and waiting to pop obediently out of the cell in response to a puff of Ca^{2+} seems a little too good to be true, rest assured that the picture is not quite so simple. Acetylcholine, noradrenaline (norepinephrine) and other mediators can leak out of nerve endings from the cytosolic compartment, independently of vesicle fusion, by utilising carriers in the plasma membrane (see Fig. 4.11). Drugs such as **amphetamines**, which release amines from central and peripheral nerve terminals (see Chs 14 and 39), do so by displacing the endogenous amine from storage vesicles into the cytosol, whence it escapes via the monoamine transporter in the plasma membrane, a mechanism that does not depend on Ca^{2+}.

Nitric oxide (see Ch. 20) and arachidonic acid metabolites (e.g. prostaglandins; Ch. 17) are two important examples of mediators that are released from the cytosol by diffusion across the membrane or by carrier-mediated extrusion, rather than by exocytosis. The mediators are not stored but escape from the cell as soon as they are synthesised. In both cases, the synthetic enzyme is activated by Ca^{2+}, and the moment-to-moment control of the rate of synthesis depends on $[Ca^{2+}]_i$. This kind of release is necessarily slower than the classic exocytotic mechanism, but in the case of nitric oxide is fast enough for it to function as a true transmitter (see Fig 12.5 and Ch. 20).

EPITHELIAL ION TRANSPORT

Fluid-secreting epithelia include the renal tubule, salivary glands, gastrointestinal tract and airways epithelia. In each case, epithelial cells are arranged in sheets separating the interior (blood-perfused) compartment from the exterior lumen compartment, into which, or from which, secretion takes place. Fluid secretion involves two main mechanisms, which often coexist in the same cell and indeed interact with each other. Greger (2000) and Ashcroft (2000) give more detailed accounts. The two mechanisms (Fig. 4.13) are concerned, respectively, with Na^+ transport and Cl^- transport.

In the case of Na^+ transport, secretion occurs because Na^+ enters the cell passively at one end and is pumped out actively at the other, with water following passively.

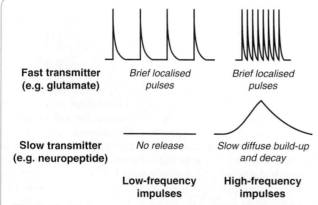

Fast transmitter (e.g. glutamate) — *Brief localised pulses* — *Brief localised pulses*

Slow transmitter (e.g. neuropeptide) — *No release* — *Slow diffuse build-up and decay*

Low-frequency impulses   **High-frequency impulses**

Fig. 4.12 Time course and frequency dependence of the release of 'fast' and 'slow' transmitters. Fast transmitters (e.g. glutamate) are stored in synaptic vesicles that are 'docked' close to voltage-gated calcium channels in the membrane of the nerve terminal, and are released in a short burst when the membrane is depolarised (e.g. by an action potential). Slow transmitters (e.g. neuropeptides) are stored in separate vesicles further from the membrane. Release is slower, because they must first migrate to the membrane, and occurs only when $[Ca^{2+}]_i$ builds up sufficiently.

---

[6]The vesicle contents may not always discharge completely. Instead, vesicles may fuse transiently with the cell membrane and release only part of their contents (see Burgoyne & Morgan, 2002) before becoming disconnected (termed *kiss-and-run exocytosis*).

Mediator release

- Most chemical mediators are packaged into storage vesicles and released by exocytosis. Some are synthesised on demand and released by diffusion or the operation of membrane carriers.
- Exocytosis occurs in response to increased $[Ca^{2+}]_i$ as a result of a Ca^{2+}-mediated interaction between proteins of the synaptic vesicle and the plasma membrane, causing the membranes to fuse.
- After releasing their contents, vesicles are recycled and reloaded with transmitter.
- Many secretory cells contain more than one type of vesicle, loaded with different mediators and secreted independently.
- Stored mediators (e.g. neurotransmitters) may be released directly from the cytosol independently of Ca^{2+} and exocytosis by drugs that interact with membrane transport mechanisms.
- Non-stored mediators, such as prostanoids and nitric oxide, are released by increased $[Ca^{2+}]_i$, which activates the enzymes responsible for their synthesis.

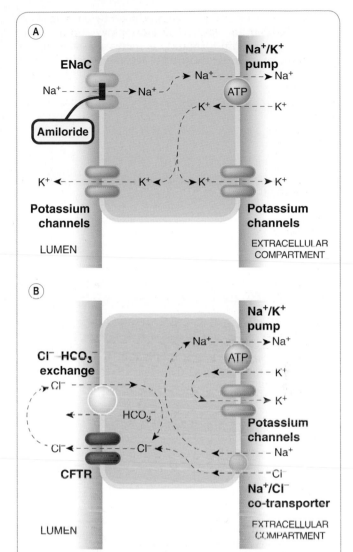

Fig. 4.13 Generalised mechanisms of epithelial ion transport. Such mechanisms are important in renal tubules (see Ch. 29 for more details) and also in many other situations, such as the gastrointestinal and respiratory tracts. The exact mechanism may vary from tissue to tissue depending upon channel and pump expression and location. [**A**] Sodium transport. A special type of epithelial sodium channel (ENaC) controls entry of Na^+ into the cell from the lumenal surface, the Na^+ being actively pumped out at the apical surface by the Na^+–K^+ exchange pump. K^+ moves passively via potassium channels. [**B**] Chloride transport. Cl^- leaves the cell via a special membrane channel, the cystic fibrosis transmembrane conductance regulator (CFTR), after entering the cell either from the apical surface via the Na^+/Cl^- co-transporter, or at the lumenal surface via the Cl^-/HCO_3^- co-transporter.

Critical to this mechanism is a class of highly regulated epithelial sodium channels (ENaCs) that allow Na^+ entry.

Epithelial sodium channels (see De la Rosa et al., 2000) are widely expressed, not only in epithelial cells but also in neurons and other excitable cells, where their function is largely unknown. They are regulated mainly by aldosterone, a hormone produced by the adrenal cortex that enhances Na^+ reabsorption by the kidney (Ch. 29). Aldosterone, like other steroid hormones, exerts its effects by regulating gene expression (see Ch. 3), and causes an increase in ENaC expression, thereby increasing the rate of Na^+ and fluid transport. ENaCs are selectively blocked by certain diuretic drugs, notably amiloride (see Ch. 29), a compound that is widely used to study the functioning of ENaCs in other situations.

Chloride transport is particularly important in the airways and gastrointestinal tract. In the airways it is essential for fluid secretion, whereas in the colon it mediates fluid reabsorption, the difference being due to the different arrangement of various transporters and channels with respect to the polarity of the cells. The simplified diagram in Figure 4.13B represents the situation in the pancreas, where secretion depends on Cl^- transport. The key molecule in Cl^- transport is the *cystic fibrosis transmembrane conductance regulator* (CFTR; see Hwang & Sheppard, 1999), so named because early studies on the inherited disorder cystic fibrosis showed it to be associated with impaired Cl^- conductance in the membrane of secretory epithelial cells, and the CFTR gene, identified through painstaking genetic linkage studies and isolated in 1989, was found to encode a Cl^--conducting ion channel. Severe physiological consequences follow from the impairment of secretion, particularly in the airways but also in many other systems, such as sweat glands and pancreas. Studies on the disease-associated mutations of the CFTR gene have revealed much about the molecular mechanisms involved in Cl^- transport, but as yet no significant therapeutic advance. So far, no therapeutic drugs are known that interact specifically with CFTRs.

Both Na^+ and Cl^- transport are regulated by intracellular messengers, notably by Ca^{2+} and cAMP, the latter exerting its effects by activating protein kinases and thereby causing phosphorylation of channels and transporters. CFTR itself is activated by cAMP. In the gastrointestinal tract, increased cAMP formation causes a large increase in the rate of fluid secretion, an effect that leads to the copious diarrhoea produced by cholera infection (see Ch. 3) and also by inflammatory conditions in which prostaglandin formation is increased (see Ch. 17). Activation of G protein-coupled receptors, which cause release of Ca^{2+}, also stimulates secretion, possibly also by activating CFTR. Many examples of therapeutic drugs that affect epithelial secretion by activating or blocking G protein-coupled receptors appear in later chapters.

Epithelial ion transport

- Many epithelia (e.g. renal tubules, exocrine glands and airways) are specialised to transport specific ions.
- This type of transport depends on a special class of epithelial sodium channels (ENaCs) which allow Na^+ entry into the cell at one surface, coupled to active extrusion of Na^+, or exchange for another ion, from the opposite surface.

- Anion transport depends on a specific chloride channel (the cystic fibrosis transmembrane conductance regulator [CFTR]), mutations of which result in cystic fibrosis.
- The activity of channels, pumps and exchange transporters is regulated by various second messengers and nuclear receptors, which control the transport of ions in specific ways.

REFERENCES AND FURTHER READING

General references

Alexander, S.P.H., Benson, H.E., Faccenda, E., et al., 2013. The Concise Guide to Pharmacology 2013/2014. Br. J. Pharmacol. Special Issue 170 (8), 1449–1896. (*Contains a brief description of a range of ion channels and the drugs that interact with them*)

Berridge, M.J., 2012. Cell Signalling Biology. Portland Press. doi:10.1042/csb0001002 (*Free ebook available on line at www.cellsignallingbiology.org; a regularly updated resource that covers various aspects of cell signalling in a highly readable format*)

Kandel, E.R., Schwartz, J.H., Jessell, T.M., Siegelbaum, S.A., Hudspeth, A.J., 2013. Principles of Neural Science. McGraw-Hill, New York. (*Excellent, well-written textbook of neuroscience*)

Katz, B., 1966. Nerve, Muscle and Synapse. McGraw–Hill, New York. (*A classic account of the ground-breaking electrophysiological experiments that established the basis of nerve and muscle function*)

Nestler, E.J., Hyman, S.E., Malenka, R.C., 2008. Molecular Neuropharmacology, second ed. McGraw–Hill, New York. (*Excellent modern textbook*)

Second messengers and calcium regulation

Berridge, M.J., 2009. Inositol trisphosphate and calcium signalling mechanisms. Biochim. Biophys. Acta. Mol. Cell Res. 1793, 933–940. (*Clear and readable up-to-date account of the mechanisms and versatility of calcium signalling*)

Berridge, M.J., Bootman, M.D., Roderick, H.L., 2003. Calcium signalling: dynamics, homeostasis and remodelling. Nat. Rev. Mol. Cell Biol. 4, 517–529.

Clapham, D.E., 2007. Calcium signalling. Cell 131, 1047–1056. (*Excellent, readable and well-illustrated short review article – recommended*)

Fliegert, R., Gasser, A., Guse, A.H., 2007. Regulation of calcium signalling by adenine-based second messengers. Biochem. Soc. Trans. 35, 109–114. (*Summary of second messenger role of cADPR and NAADP*)

Mikoshiba, K., 2007. IP_3 receptor/Ca^{2+} channel: from discovery to new signaling concepts. J. Neurochem. 102, 1426–1446. (*Interesting account of the discovery of the IP_3 receptor and its functional role*)

Morgan, A.J., Platt, F.M., Lloyd-Evans, E., Galione, A., 2011. Molecular mechanisms of endolysosomal Ca^{2+} signalling in health and disease. Biochem. J. 439, 349–374.

Excitation and ion channels

Ashcroft, F.M., 2000. Ion Channels and Disease. Academic Press, San Diego. (*A very useful textbook that describes the physiology of different kinds of ion channels, and relates it to their molecular structure; the book emphasises the importance of 'channelopathies', genetic channel defects associated with disease states*)

Ashcroft, F.M., 2006. From molecule to malady. Nature 440, 440–447. (*Brief summary and update of the importance of channelopathies*)

Catterall, W.A., 2000. From ionic currents to molecular mechanisms: the structure and function of voltage-gated sodium channels. Neuron 26, 13–25. (*Useful, authoritative review article*)

De la Rosa, D.A., Canessa, C.M., Fyfe, G.K., Zhang, P., 2000. Structure and regulation of amiloride-sensitive sodium channels. Annu. Rev. Physiol. 62, 573–594. (*General review on the nature and function of 'epithelial' sodium channels*)

Goldstein, S.A.N., Bockenhauer, D., Zilberberg, N., 2001. Potassium leak channels and the KCNK family of two-P-domain subunits. Nat. Rev. Neurosci. 2, 175–184. (*Review on this important class of potassium channels*)

Hille, B., 2001. Ionic Channels of Excitable Membranes. Sinauer Associates, Sunderland. (*A clear and detailed account of the basic principles of ion channels, with emphasis on their biophysical properties*)

Jenkinson, D.H., 2006. Potassium channels – multiplicity and challenges. Br. J. Pharmacol. 147 (Suppl.), 63–71. (*Useful short article on the many types of K^+ channel*)

Shieh, C.-C., Coghlan, M., Sullivan, J.P., Gopalakrishnan, M., 2000. Potassium channels: molecular defects, diseases and therapeutic opportunities. Pharmacol. Rev. 52, 557–593. (*Comprehensive review of potassium channel pathophysiology and pharmacology*)

Muscle contraction

Berridge, M.J., 2008. Smooth muscle cell calcium activation mechanisms. J. Physiol. 586, 5047–5061. (*Excellent review article describing the various mechanisms by which calcium signals control activity in different types of smooth muscle – complicated but clear*)

Bers, D.M., 2002. Cardiac excitation–contraction coupling. Nature 415, 198–205. (*Short, well-illustrated review article*)

Priori, S.G., Napolitano, C., 2005. Cardiac and skeletal muscle disorders caused by mutations in the intracellular Ca^{2+} release channels. J. Clin. Invest. 115, 2033–2038. (*Focuses on RyR mutations in various inherited diseases*)

Van Petegem, F., 2012. Ryanodine receptors: structure and function. J. Biol. Chem. 287 (31), 31 624–31 632.

Secretion and exocytosis

Burgoyne, R.D., Morgan, A., 2002. Secretory granule exocytosis. Physiol. Rev. 83, 581–632. (*Comprehensive review of the molecular machinery responsible for secretory exocytosis*)

Greger, R., 2000. The role of CFTR in the colon. Annu. Rev. Physiol. 62, 467–491. (*A useful résumé of information about CFTR and epithelial secretion, more general than its title suggests*)

Hwang, T.-C., Sheppard, D.N., 1999. Molecular pharmacology of the CFTR channel. Trends Pharmacol. Sci. 20, 448–453. (*Description of approaches aimed at finding therapeutic drugs aimed at altering the function of the CFTR channel*)

Südhof, T.C., 2004. The synaptic vesicle cycle. Annu. Rev. Neurosci. 27, 509–547. (*Summarises the mechanism of vesicular release at the molecular level*)

Cell proliferation, apoptosis, repair and regeneration

5

OVERVIEW

About 10 billion new cells are created daily through cell division and this must be counterbalanced by the elimination of a similar number from the body in an ordered manner. This chapter explains how this is managed. We deal with the life and death of the cell – the processes of replication, proliferation, apoptosis, repair and regeneration and how these relate to the actions of drugs. We begin with cell replication. We explain how stimulation by growth factors causes cells to divide and then consider the interaction of these cells with the extracellular matrix which regulates further cell proliferation. We describe the crucial phenomenon of apoptosis (the programmed series of events that lead to cell death), outlining the changes that occur in a cell that is preparing to die and the intracellular pathways that culminate in its demise. We explain how these processes relate to the repair of damaged tissue, to the possibility of its regeneration and whether there is scope for modulating this with novel drugs.

CELL PROLIFERATION

Cell proliferation is, of course, a fundamental biological event. It is integral to many physiological and pathological processes including growth, healing, repair, hypertrophy, hyperplasia and the development of tumours. Because cells need oxygen to survive, *angiogenesis* (the development of new blood vessels) necessarily accompanies many of these processes.

Proliferating cells go through what is termed *the cell cycle*, during which they replicate all their components and then divide into two identical daughter cells. The process is tightly regulated by signalling pathways including receptor tyrosine kinases or receptor-linked kinases and the mitogen-activated protein kinase (MAP kinase) cascade (see Ch. 3). In all cases, the pathways eventually lead to transcription of the genes that control the cell cycle.

THE CELL CYCLE

In the adult, few cells divide repeatedly and most remain in a quiescent phase outside the cycle in the phase termed G_0 (Fig. 5.1). Some cells such as neurons and skeletal muscle cells spend all their lifetime in G_0 whereas others, including bone marrow cells and the epithelium of the gastrointestinal tract, divide daily.

The cell cycle is an ordered sequential series of phases (Fig. 5.1). These are known as:

• G_1: preparation for DNA synthesis
• S: DNA synthesis and chromosome duplication

• G_2: preparation for division
• M: mitosis, division into two daughter cells.

In cells that are dividing continuously, G_1, S and G_2 comprise *interphase* – the phase between one mitosis and the next.

Cell division requires the controlled timing of the critical S phase and M phases. Entry into each of these phases is tightly regulated at *check points* (restriction points) at the start of the S and M phases. DNA damage stops the cycle at one or other of these check points and the integrity of this process is critical for the maintenance of genetic stability. Failure of the check points to stop the cycle when it is appropriate to do so is a hallmark of cancer.

Quiescent cells enter G_1 after exposure to chemical mediators, some of which are associated with damage. For example, a wound can stimulate a quiescent skin cell to divide, thus repairing the lesion. The impetus for a cell to enter the cycle (i.e. to move from G_0 into G_1) may be *growth factors* acting on *growth factor receptors*, though the action of other types of ligands on G protein-coupled receptors (see Ch. 3) can also initiate the process.

Growth factors stimulate the synthesis of both positive regulators of the cell cycle that control the changes necessary for cell division and negative regulators that counterbalance the positive regulators. The maintenance of normal cell numbers in tissues and organs requires a balance between the positive and the negative regulatory signals. *Apoptosis*[1] also controls cell numbers.

POSITIVE REGULATORS OF THE CELL CYCLE

The cycle begins when a growth factor acts on a quiescent cell, provoking it to divide. Growth factors stimulate production of two families of proteins, namely *cyclins* and serine/threonine protein kinases called *cyclin-dependent kinases* (cdks), coded for by the *delayed response* genes. The cdks sequentially phosphorylate various enzymes – activating some and inhibiting others – to coordinate the progression of the cell through the cycle.

Each cdk is inactive and must bind to a cyclin, before it can phosphorylate its target protein(s). After the phosphorylation event the cyclin is degraded (Fig. 5.2) by the *ubiquitin/protease system*. Here, several enzymes sequentially add small molecules of ubiquitin to the cyclin. The resulting ubiquitin polymer acts as an 'address label' that directs the cyclin to the *proteasome* where it is degraded.

There are eight main groups of cyclins. According to the 'classical model' of the cell cycle (see Satayanarayana & Kaldis, 2009), those of principal importance in the control of the cycle are cyclins A, B, D and E. Each cyclin is associated with, and activates, a particular cdk. Cyclin A activates cdks 1 and 2; cyclin B, cdk 1; cyclin D, cdks 4

---

[1]The term is originally a Greek word that describes the falling of leaves or petals from plants.

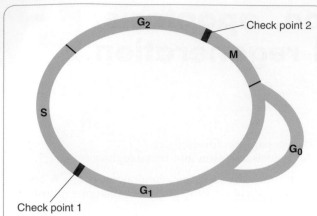

Fig. 5.1 The main phases of the cell cycle of dividing cells.

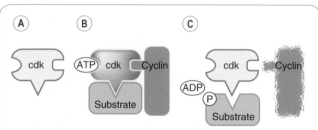

Fig. 5.2 Schematic representation of the activation of a cyclin-dependent kinase (cdk). [**A**] An inactive cdk. [**B**] The inactive cdk binds to a cyclin and is activated; it can now phosphorylate a specific protein substrate (e.g. an enzyme). [**C**] After the phosphorylating event, the cyclin is degraded.

and 6; and cyclin E, cdk 2. Precise timing of each step is essential and many cycle proteins are degraded after they have carried out their functions. The actions of the cyclin/cdk complexes throughout the cell cycle are depicted in Figure 5.3.

The activity of these cyclin/cdk complexes is negatively modulated at one or other of the two check points. In quiescent G_0 cells, cyclin D is present in low concentration, and an important regulatory protein – the *Rb protein*[2] – is hypophosphorylated. This restrains the cell cycle at check point 1 by inhibiting the expression of several proteins critical for further cycle progression. The Rb protein accomplishes this by binding to transcription factors controlling the expression of the genes that code for proteins essential for DNA replication during S phase, such as cyclins E and A, DNA polymerase, thymidine kinase and dihydrofolate reductase.

Growth factor action on a cell in G_0 propels it into G_1, which prepares the cell for S phase. The concentration of cyclin D increases and the cyclin D/cdk complex phosphorylates and activates the proteins required for DNA replication.

In mid-G_1, the cyclin D/cdk complex phosphorylates the Rb protein, releasing a transcription factor that activates the genes for the components essential for the next phase – DNA synthesis. The action of the cyclin E/cdk

complex is necessary for transition from G_1, past check point 1, into S phase.

Once into S phase, the processes that have been set in motion cannot be reversed and the cell is committed to DNA replication and mitosis. Cyclin E/cdk and cyclin A/cdk regulate progress through S phase, phosphorylating and thus activating the proteins/enzymes involved in DNA synthesis.

In G_2 phase, the cell, which now has double the number of chromosomes, produces the messenger RNAs and proteins needed to duplicate all other cellular components for allocation to the two daughter cells.

Cyclin A/cdk and cyclin B/cdk complexes are active during G_2 phase and are necessary for entry into M phase, i.e. for passing check point 2. The presence of cyclin B/cdk complexes in the nucleus is required for mitosis to commence.

Mitosis occurs in four stages:

- *Prophase.* The duplicated chromosomes (which are at this point a tangled mass in the nucleus) condense, each now consisting of two *daughter chromatids* (the original chromosome and a copy). These are released into the cytoplasm as the nuclear membrane disintegrates.
- *Metaphase.* The chromosomes are aligned at the equator of the cell (see Fig. 5.3).
- *Anaphase.* A specialised cytoskeletal device, the mitotic apparatus, captures the chromosomes and draws them to opposite poles of the dividing cell (see Fig. 5.3).
- *Telophase.* A nuclear membrane forms round each set of chromosomes. Finally, the cytoplasm divides between the two forming daughter cells. Each daughter cell will be in G_0 phase and will remain there unless stimulated into G_1 phase as described above.

During metaphase, the cyclin A and B complexes phosphorylate cytoskeletal proteins, nuclear histones and possibly components of the spindle (the microtubules along which the chromatids are pulled during metaphase).

NEGATIVE REGULATORS OF THE CELL CYCLE

One of the main negative regulators is the Rb protein, which restrains the cell cycle while it is hypophosphorylated.

Inhibitors of the cdks also serve as negative regulators, their main action being at check point 1. There are two known families of inhibitors: the *CIP family* (cdk inhibitory proteins, also termed KIP or kinase inhibitory proteins) – proteins p21, p27 and p57; and the *Ink family* (inhibitors of kinases) – proteins p16, p19 and p15.

Protein p21 is a good example of the role of a cyclin/cdk inhibitor. It is under the control of the *p53 gene* – a particularly important negative regulator which is relevant in carcinogenesis – that operates at check point 1.

Inhibition of the cycle at check point 1

The *p53* gene has been called the 'guardian of the genome'. It codes for the p53 protein, a transcription factor found in only low concentrations in normal healthy cells. However, following DNA damage, the protein accumulates and activates the transcription of several genes, one of which codes for p21. Protein p21 inactivates cyclin/cdk complexes, thus preventing Rb phosphorylation, which means that the cycle is arrested at check point 1. This allows for DNA repair. If the repair is successful, the cycle proceeds past check point 1 into S phase. If the repair

[2]So named because mutations of the *Rb* gene are associated with retinoblastoma tumours.

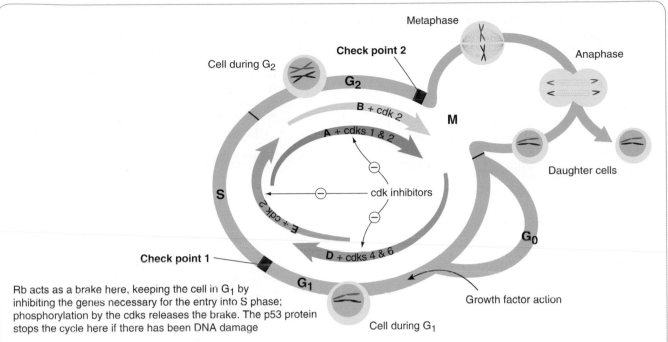

Rb acts as a brake here, keeping the cell in G_1 by inhibiting the genes necessary for the entry into S phase; phosphorylation by the cdks releases the brake. The p53 protein stops the cycle here if there has been DNA damage

Fig. 5.3 Schematic diagram of the cell cycle, showing the role of the cyclin/cyclin-dependent kinase (cdk) complexes. The processes outlined in the cycle occur inside a cell such as the one shown in Figure 5.4. A quiescent cell (in G_0 phase), when stimulated to divide by growth factors, is propelled into G_1 phase and prepares for DNA synthesis. Progress through the cycle is determined by sequential action of the cyclin/cdk complexes – depicted here by coloured arrows, the arrows being given the names of the relevant cyclins: D, E, A and B. The cdks are given next to the relevant cyclins. The thickness of each arrow represents the intensity of the cdk action at that point in the cycle. The activity of the cdks is regulated by cdk inhibitors. If there is DNA damage, the products of the tumour suppressor gene *p53* arrest the cycle at check point 1, allowing for repair. If repair fails, apoptosis (see Fig. 5.5) is initiated. The state of the chromosomes is shown schematically in each G phase – as a single pair in G_1, and each duplicated and forming two daughter chromatids in G_2. Some changes that occur during mitosis (metaphase, anaphase) are shown in a subsidiary circle. After the mitotic division, the daughter cells may enter G_1 or G_0 phase. Rb, retinoblastoma gene.

is unsuccessful, the *p53* gene triggers apoptosis – cell suicide.

Inhibition of the cycle at check point 2

DNA damage can arrest the cycle at check point 2, but the mechanisms involved are poorly understood. Inhibition of the accumulation of cyclin B/cdk complex in the nucleus seems to be a factor. For more detail on the control of the cell cycle, see under MicroRNAs and Swanton (2004).

INTERACTIONS BETWEEN CELLS, GROWTH FACTORS AND THE EXTRACELLULAR MATRIX

Cell proliferation is regulated by the integrated interplay between growth factors, cells, the extracellular matrix (ECM) and the matrix metalloproteinases (MMPs). The ECM is secreted by the cells and provides a supportive framework. It also profoundly influences cell behaviour by signalling through the cell's integrins. Matrix expression by cells is regulated by growth factors and cytokines (see Verrecchia & Mauviel, 2007; Järveläinen et al., 2009). The activity of some growth factors is, in turn, determined by the matrix, because they are sequestered by matrix components and released by proteases (e.g. MMPs) secreted by the cells.

The action of growth factors acting through receptor tyrosine kinases or receptor-coupled kinases (see Ch. 3) is a fundamental part of these processes. Important examples include *fibroblast growth factor* (FGF), *epidermal growth*

The cell cycle

- The term *cell cycle* refers to the sequence of events that take place within a cell as it prepares for division. The quiescent or resting state is called G_0.
- Growth factor action stimulates a cell in G_0 to enter the cycle.
- The phases of the cell cycle are:
  - G_1: preparation for DNA synthesis
  - S: DNA synthesis
  - G_2: preparation for division
  - M, mitosis: division into two daughter cells.
- In G_0 phase, a hypophosphorylated protein, coded for by the *Rb* gene, arrests the cycle by inhibiting expression of critical factors necessary for DNA replication.
- Progress through the cycle is controlled by specific kinases (cyclin-dependent kinases; cdks) that are activated by binding to specific proteins termed cyclins.
- Four main cyclins D, E, A and B, together with their cdk complexes drive the cycle; cyclin D/cdk also releases the Rb protein-mediated inhibition.

  There are protein inhibitors of cdks in the cell. Protein p21 is particularly important; it is expressed when DNA damage triggers transcription of gene *p53* and arrests the cycle at check point 1.

factor (EGF), *platelet-dependent growth factor* (PDGF), *vascular endothelial growth factor* (VEGF) and *transforming growth factor* (TGF)-β.

The main components of the extracellular matrix are:

- Fibre-forming elements, e.g. *collagen species* (the main proteins of the matrix) and *elastin*.
- Non-fibre-forming elements, e.g. proteoglycans, glucoproteins and adhesive proteins such as *fibronectin*. Proteoglycans have a growth-regulating role, in part by functioning as a reservoir of sequestered growth factors. Others are associated with the cell surface, where they bind cells to the matrix. Adhesive proteins link the various elements of the matrix together and also form links between the cells and the matrix through cell surface integrins.

Other proteins in the ECM are *thrombospondin* and *osteopontin*, which are not structural elements but modulate cell–matrix interactions and repair processes. The production of the ECM components is regulated by growth factors, particularly TGF-β.

▼ The ECM is a target for drug action. Both beneficial and adverse effects have been reported. Thus glucocorticoids decrease collagen synthesis in chronic inflammation and cyclo-oxygenase (COX)-2 inhibitors can modify fibrotic processes through a proposed action on TGF-β. Statins can decrease fibrosis by inhibiting angiotensin-induced connective tissue growth factor production (Rupérez et al., 2007) and reduce MMP expression. This may contribute to their effects in cardiovascular diseases (Tousoulis et al., 2010). The adverse actions of some drugs attributable to an effect on the ECM include the osteoporosis and skin thinning caused by glucocortoicoids (discussed in Järveläinen et al., 2009). The ECM is also an important target in the search for new drugs that regulate tissue repair.

THE ROLE OF INTEGRINS

▼ Integrins are transmembrane kinase-linked receptors (see Ch. 3) comprising α and β subunits. Interaction with the ECM elements (e.g. fibronectin) triggers various cell responses, such as cytoskeletal rearrangement (not considered here) and co-regulation of growth factor function.

Intracellular signalling by both growth factor receptors and integrins is important for optimal cell proliferation (Fig. 5.4). Following integrin stimulation an adapter protein and an enzyme (*focal adhesion kinase*), activate the kinase cascade that comprises the growth factor signalling pathway. There is extensive cross-talk between the integrin and growth factor pathways (Streuli & Akhtar, 2009). Autophosphorylation of growth factor receptors (Ch. 3) is enhanced by integrin activation and integrin-mediated adhesion to the extracellular matrix (Fig. 5.4) not only suppresses the concentrations of cdk inhibitors, but is required for the expression of cyclins A and D, and therefore for the progression of the cell cycle. Furthermore, integrin activation inhibits apoptosis (see below), further facilitating growth factor action (see reviews by Gahmberg et al., 2009 and Barczyk et al., 2010). Several monoclonal antibodies are targeted at integrins, including **natalizumab**, used to treat multiple sclerosis and **abciximab**, an antithrombotic (Ch. 24).

THE ROLE OF MATRIX METALLOPROTEINASES

▼ Degradation of the ECM by metalloproteinases is necessary for tissue growth, repair and remodelling. When growth factors stimulate a cell to enter the cell cycle, they also stimulate the secretion of metalloproteinases (as inactive precursors), which then sculpt the matrix, producing the local changes necessary to accommodate the increased cell numbers. Metalloproteinases in turn release growth factors from the ECM and, in some cases (e.g. interleukin [IL]-1β), process them from precursor to active form. The action of these enzymes is regulated by TIMPS (tissue inhibitors of metalloproteinases), which are also secreted by local cells.

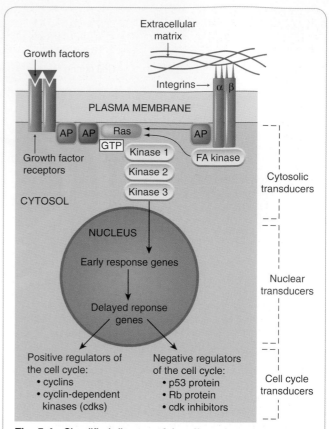

Fig. 5.4 Simplified diagram of the effect of growth factors on a cell in G_0. The overall effect of growth factor action is the generation of the cell cycle transducers. A cell such as the one depicted will then embark on G_1 phase of the cell cycle. Most growth factor receptors have integral tyrosine kinase (see Fig. 3.17). These receptors dimerise, then cross-phosphorylate their tyrosine residues. The early cytosolic transducers include proteins that bind to the phosphorylated tyrosine residues. Optimum effect requires cooperation with integrin action. Integrins (which have α and β subunits) connect the extracellular matrix with intracellular signalling pathways and also with the cell cytoskeleton (not shown here). G protein-coupled receptors can also stimulate cell proliferation, because their intracellular pathways can connect with the Ras/kinase cascade (not shown). AP, adapter protein; FA kinase, focal adhesion kinase; Rb, retinoblastoma protein.

In addition to their physiological function, metalloproteinases are involved in the tissue destruction that accompanies various diseases, such as rheumatoid arthritis, osteoarthritis, periodontitis, macular degeneration and myocardial restenosis. They also have a critical role in the growth, invasion and metastasis of tumours (Skiles et al., 2004; Clark et al., 2008; Marastoni et al., 2008). Because of this, much effort has gone into developing synthetic MMP inhibitors for treating cancers and inflammatory disorders, although clinical trials so far have shown limited efficacy and significant adverse effects (see Fingleton, 2008). **Doxycycline**, an antibiotic, also inhibits MMPs, and is used experimentally for this purpose.

ANGIOGENESIS

Angiogenesis, which normally accompanies cell proliferation, is the formation of new capillaries from existing small blood vessels. Without this, new tissues (including tumours) cannot grow. Angiogenic stimuli include cytokines and various growth factors, in particular *vascular*

Interactions between cells, growth factors and the matrix

- Cells secrete the components of the extracellular matrix (ECM) and become embedded in this tissue.
- The ECM influences the growth and behaviour of the cells. It also acts as a reservoir of growth factors.
- Integrins are transmembrane cellular receptors that can interact with elements of the ECM. They modulate growth factor signalling pathways and also mediate cytoskeletal adjustments within the cell.
- Growth factors cause cells to release metalloproteinases that degrade the local matrix so that it can accommodate the increase in cell numbers.
- Metalloproteinases release growth factors from the ECM and can activate some that are present in precursor form.

endothelial growth factor (VEGF). The sequence of events in angiogenesis is as follows:

1. The basement membrane is degraded locally by proteases.
2. Endothelial cells migrate out, forming a 'sprout'.
3. Following these leading cells, other endothelial cells proliferate under the influence of VEGF.
4. Matrix material is laid down around the new capillary.

A monoclonal antibody, **bevacizumab**, which neutralises VEGF, is used as adjunct treatment for various cancers (see Ch. 56), and following injection into the eye, to treat age-related macular degeneration, a condition in which retinal blood vessels proliferate, causing blindness.

APOPTOSIS AND CELL REMOVAL

Apoptosis is cell suicide. It is regulated by a built-in genetically programmed self-destruct mechanism consisting of specific sequence of biochemical events. It is thus unlike *necrosis*, which is disorganised disintegration of damaged cells that releases substances that trigger the inflammatory response.[3]

Apoptosis plays an essential role in embryogenesis, shaping organs during development by eliminating cells that have become redundant. It is the mechanism that each day unobtrusively removes some 10 billion cells from the human body. It is involved in numerous physiological events, including the shedding of the intestinal lining, the death of time-expired neutrophils and the turnover of tissues as the newborn infant grows to maturity. It is the basis for the development of self-tolerance in the immune system (Ch. 6) and acts as a first-line defence against carcinogenic mutations by purging cells that could become malignant.

Impaired apoptosis is also implicated in the pathophysiology of many conditions, including:

- chronic neurodegenerative diseases such as Alzheimer's, multiple sclerosis and Parkinson's disease (Ch. 40)
- conditions with acute tissue damage or cell loss, such as myocardial infarction (Ch. 21), stroke and spinal cord injury (Ch. 40)
- depletion of T cells in HIV infection (Ch. 52)
- osteoarthritis (Ch. 36)
- haematological disease, such as aplastic anaemia (Ch. 25)
- evasion of the immune response by cancer cells and resistance to cancer chemotherapy (Ch. 56)
- autoimmune/inflammatory diseases such as myasthenia gravis (Ch. 13), rheumatoid arthritis (Ch. 26), and bronchial asthma (Ch. 28)
- viral infections with ineffective eradication of virus-infected cells (Ch. 52).

▼ Apoptosis is particularly important in the regulation of the immune response and in the many conditions in which it is an underlying component. There is evidence that T cells have a negative regulatory pathway controlled by surface *programmed cell death receptors* (e.g. the PD-1 receptor), and that there is normally a balance between the stimulatory pathways triggered by antigens and this negative regulatory apoptosis-inducing pathway. The balance is important in the maintenance of peripheral tolerance. A disturbance of this balance is seen in autoimmune disease, in the 'exhaustion' of T cells in chronic viral diseases such as HIV, and possibly in tumour escape from immune destruction (Zha et al., 2004).

Apoptosis is a *default response*, i.e. continuous active signalling by tissue-specific trophic factors, cytokines and hormones, and cell-to-cell contact factors (adhesion molecules, integrins, etc.) are required for cell survival and viability. The self-destruct mechanism is automatically triggered unless it is actively and continuously inhibited by these antiapoptotic factors. Different cell types require differing sets of survival factors, which function only locally. If a cell strays or is dislodged from the area protected by its paracrine survival signals, it will die.

Withdrawal of these survival factors – which has been termed 'death by neglect' – is not the only pathway to apoptosis (see Fig. 5.5). The death machinery can be activated by ligands that stimulate *death receptors* and by DNA damage. But it is generally accepted that cell proliferation processes and apoptosis are tightly integrated.

MORPHOLOGICAL CHANGES IN APOPTOSIS

As the cell dies it 'rounds up', the chromatin condenses into dense masses, the cytoplasm shrinks and there is blebbing of the plasma membrane. Finally, mediated by a family of proteolytic enzymes known as caspases, the cell is transformed into a cluster of membrane-bound entities. This cellular 'corpse' displays 'eat me' signals, such as phosphatidylserine on its surface, which are recognized by macrophages, which then phagocytose the remains. It is important that these cellular fragments are enclosed by a membrane because otherwise the release of cell constituents could trigger an inflammatory reaction. An additional safeguard against this is that phagocytosing macrophages release anti-inflammatory mediators such as TGF-β, Annexin-1 and IL-10.

THE MAJOR PLAYERS IN APOPTOSIS

The repertoire of reactions in apoptosis is extremely complex and varies between species and cell types. Yet it

---

[3]There are other forms of programmed cell death (PCD) including *autophagy* and (confusingly) *programmed necrosis*. Here we will focus on apoptosis, also known as 'Type I PCD'.

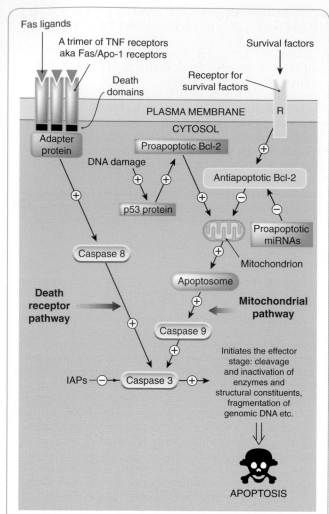

Fig. 5.5 A simplified diagram of the two main signalling pathways in apoptosis. The 'death receptor' pathway is activated when death receptors such as members of the tumour necrosis factor (TNF) family are stimulated by specific death ligands. This recruits adapter proteins that activate initiator caspases (e.g. caspase 8), which in turn activate effector caspases such as caspase 3. The mitochondrial pathway is activated by diverse signals, one being DNA damage. In the presence of DNA damage that cannot be repaired, the p53 protein (see text and Figs 5.3 and 5.4) activates a subpathway that releases cytochrome c from the mitochondrion, with subsequent involvement of the *apoptosome* and activation of an initiator caspase, caspase 9. The apoptosome is a complex of procaspase 9, cytochrome c and apoptotic-activating protease factor-1 (Apaf-1). Both these pathways converge on the effector caspase (e.g. caspase 3), which brings about the demise of the cell. The survival factor subpathway normally restrains apoptosis by inhibiting the mitochondrial pathway through activation of the antiapoptotic factor Bcl-2. The receptor labelled 'R' represents the respective receptors for trophic factors, growth factors, cell-to-cell contact factors (adhesion molecules, integrins), etc. Continuous stimulation of these receptors is necessary for cell survival/ proliferation. If this pathway is non-functional (shown in grey), this antiapoptotic drive is withdrawn. IAP, inhibitor of apoptosis.

could be that the pivotal reaction(s) that lead to either cell survival or cell death are controlled by a single gene or combination of genes. If so, these genes could be desirable targets for drugs used to treat many proliferative diseases.

Only a simple outline of apoptosis can be given here. Portt et al. (2011) have reviewed the whole area in detail. The major players are the *caspases* – a family of cysteine proteases present in the cell in inactive form. These undertake delicate protein surgery, selectively cleaving a specific set of target proteins (enzymes, structural components all of which contain a characteristic motif recognised by the caspases), inactivating some and activating others. A cascade of about nine different caspases are required, some functioning as initiators that transmit the initial apoptotic signals, and others being responsible for the final phase of cell death (Fig. 5.5).

The 'executioner' caspases (e.g. caspase 3) cleave and inactivate cell constituents such as the DNA repair enzymes, protein kinase C, and cytoskeletal components. A DNAase is activated that cuts genomic DNA between the nucleosomes, generating DNA fragments of approximately 180 base pairs.

However, not all caspases are death-mediating enzymes; some have a role in the processing and activating of cytokines (e.g. caspase 8 is active in processing the inflammatory cytokines IL-1 and IL-18).

Besides the caspases, another pathway can be triggered by *apoptotic initiating factor* (AIF), a protein released from the mitochondria that enters the nucleus and triggers cell suicide.

PATHWAYS TO APOPTOSIS

There are two main routes to cell death: stimulation of death receptors by external ligands (the *extrinsic pathway*) and an internal *mitochondrial pathway*. Both routes activate initiator caspases and converge on a final common effector caspase pathway.

THE EXTRINSIC PATHWAY

Lurking in the plasma membrane of most cell types are members of the tumour necrosis factor receptor (TNFR) superfamily (also known as Fas receptors), which function as 'death receptors' (Fig. 5.5). Important family members include TNFR-1 and CD95 (also known as Fas ligands or Apo-1), but there are many others (e.g. PD-1, a death receptor that can be induced on activated T cells, as discussed above).

Each receptor has a 'death domain' in its cytoplasmic tail. Stimulation of the receptors by a ligand such as tumour necrosis factor (TNF) itself or TRAIL[4] causes them to trimerise and recruit an adapter protein that binds to their death domains. The resulting complex activates caspase 8 (and probably caspase 10), which in turn activate the effector caspases (Fig. 5.5).

The mitochondrial pathway

This pathway can be triggered by DNA damage or by withdrawal of cell survival factors or other factors. In

---

[4]TRAIL is tumour necrosis factor-α–related apoptosis-inducing ligand', of course; what else? See Janssen et al. (2005) for discussion of a role of TRAIL. PD-L1, a ligand for the PD-1 receptor, is found on all haemopoietic cells and many other tissues.

some way, the cell can 'audit' such damage and decide whether to initiate the apoptotic pathway. It is possible that *promyelocytic leukaemia bodies*, large complexes of proteins in the nucleus, participate in this task (Wyllie, 2010), although how they do so is not clear.

Regulating the apoptotic event are the members of the Bcl-2 protein family, a group of proteins with homologous domains allowing interactions between individual members. If the cell selects the apoptotic route, the p53 protein activates p21 and proapoptotic members of the Bcl-2 family – Bid, Bax and Bak. In addition to these proapoptotic individuals, this family has antiapoptotic members (e.g. Bcl-2 itself).[5] These factors compete with each other on the surface of the mitochondria and the outcome depends upon the relative concentrations of these molecular players. In the case of a proapoptotic signal, oligomers of Bax and or Bak form pores in the mitochondrial membrane through which proteins such as cytochrome c can leak.

When released, cytochrome c complexes with a protein termed Apaf-1 (apoptotic protease-activating factor-1) and the two then combine with procaspase 9 and activates it. This latter enzyme orchestrates the effector caspase pathway. The triumvirate of cytochrome c, Apaf-1 and procaspase 9 is termed the *apoptosome* (Fig. 5.5; see Riedl & Salvesen, 2007). Nitric oxide (see Ch. 20) is another mediator that can have proapoptotic and antiapoptotic actions.

In normal cells, survival factors (specified above) continuously activate antiapoptotic mechanisms. The withdrawal of survival factors can cause death in several different ways depending on the cell type. A common mechanism is tipping the balance between Bcl-2 family members leading to loss of the antiapoptotic protein action, with the resultant unopposed action of the proapoptotic Bcl-2 proteins (see Fig. 5.5).

The two main cell death pathways are connected to each other, in that caspase 8 in the death receptor pathway can activate the proapoptotic Bcl-2 proteins and thus activate the mitochondrial pathway.

MicroRNAs, the cell cycle and apoptosis

MicroRNAs (miRNAs), discovered only in the past decade, are a family of small non-coding RNAs present in the genomes of plants and animals. They are now known to inhibit the expression of genes coding for cell cycle regulation, apoptosis (Fig 5.5), cell differentiation and development (Carleton et al., 2007; Lynam-Lennon et al., 2009). About 3% of human genes encode for miRNA and some 30% of human genes coding for proteins are regulated by miRNAs.

Altered miRNA expression is now believed to be linked to a variety of diseases, including diabetes, obesity, Alzheimer's, cardiovascular system diseases, inflammatory conditions, neurodegenerative diseases (Barbato et al., 2009), as well as carcinogenesis, metastasis and resistance to cancer therapies (Würdinger & Costa, 2007; Garzon et al., 2009). miRNAs are also believed to function as oncogenes and/or tumour suppressor genes and to regulate T cells (Zhou et al., 2009). Not surprisingly, miRNAs are being heralded as targets for new drug development for a variety of disease states (Liu et al., 2008; Stenvang et al., 2008; Tsai & Yu, 2010).

Apoptosis

- Apoptosis is programmed cell death. It is an essential biological process and critical for (e.g.) embryogenesis and tissue homeostasis.
- Apoptosis depends upon a cascade of proteases called caspases. Two sets of initiator caspases converge on a set of effector caspases, which bring about the apoptotic event.
- Two main pathways activate the effector caspases: the death receptor pathway and the mitochondrial pathway.
  - Stimulation of the tumour necrosis factor receptor family initiates the death receptor pathway. The main initiator is caspase 8.
  - The mitochondrial pathway is activated by internal factors such as DNA damage, which results in transcription of gene *p53*. The p53 protein activates a sub-pathway that releases cytochrome c from the mitochondrion. This, in turn, complexes with protein Apaf-1 and together they activate initiator caspase 9.
- In undamaged cells, survival factors (cytokines, hormones, cell-to-cell contact factors) continuously activate antiapoptotic mechanisms. Withdrawal of survival factors causes cell death through the mitochondrial pathway.
- The effector caspases (e.g. caspase 3) initiate a cascade of proteases that cleave cell constituents, DNA, cytoskeletal components, enzymes, etc. This reduces the cell to a cluster of membrane-bound entities that are eventually phagocytosed by macrophages.

PATHOPHYSIOLOGICAL IMPLICATIONS

As mentioned above, cell proliferation and apoptosis are involved in many physiological and pathological processes. These are:

- the growth of tissues and organs in the embryo and later during childhood
- the replenishment of lost or time-expired cells such as leukocytes, gut epithelium and uterine endometrium
- immunological responses, including development of immunological tolerance to host proteins
- repair and healing after injury or inflammation
- the hyperplasia (increase in cell number and in connective tissue) associated with chronic inflammatory, hypersensitivity and autoimmune diseases (Ch. 6)
- the growth, invasion and metastasis of tumours (Ch. 56)
- regeneration of tissues.

The role of cell proliferation and apoptosis in the first two processes listed is self-evident and needs no further comment. Their involvement in immune tolerance is discussed briefly above but the other processes require further discussion.

---

[5]Another brake on cell death is a family of caspase-inhibiting proteins called IAPs (inhibitors of apoptosis proteins).

REPAIR AND HEALING

Repair occurs when tissues are damaged or lost. It is also implicated in the resolution of the local inflammatory reaction to a pathogen or chemical irritant. In some instances, damage or tissue loss can lead to *regeneration*, which is quite different to repair and is considered separately below.

There is considerable overlap between the mechanisms activated in inflammation and repair. Both entail an ordered series of events including cell migration, angiogenesis, proliferation of connective tissue cells, synthesis of extracellular matrix and finally remodelling – all coordinated by the growth factors and cytokines that are appropriate for the particular tissue involved. TGF-β is a key regulator of several of these processes.

Repair, healing and regeneration

- Repair and healing occurs when tissues are damaged. It is a common sequel to inflammation. Connective tissue cells, white blood cells and blood vessels are commonly involved.
- Regeneration is the replacement of the tissue or organ that has been damaged or lost. It depends upon the presence of a pool of primitive stem cells that have the potential to develop into any cell in the body. Complete regeneration of a tissue or organ is rare in mammals. The more rapid repair processes – often accompanied by scarring – usually make good the damage. This may be an evolutionary trade-off in mammals for the lost power of regeneration.
- However, it might be possible to activate regenerative pathways in mammals – at least to some extent and in some organs.

HYPERPLASIA

Hyperplasia (cell proliferation and matrix expansion) is a hallmark of chronic inflammatory and autoimmune diseases such as rheumatoid arthritis (Chs 6 and 26), psoriasis, chronic ulcers and chronic obstructive lung disease. It also underlies the bronchial hyper-reactivity of chronic asthma (Ch. 28) and glomerular nephritis.

Cell proliferation and apoptotic events are also implicated in atherosclerosis (Ch. 23), restenosis and myocardial repair after infarction (Ch. 21).

THE GROWTH, INVASION AND METASTASIS OF TUMOURS

Growth factor signalling systems, antiapoptotic pathways and cell cycle controllers are of increasing interest as targets for novel approaches to the treatment of cancer. See Chapter 56.

STEM CELLS AND REGENERATION

Regeneration of tissue replaces that lost following damage or disease and allows restoration of function. Many animals (e.g. amphibians) have impressive regenerative powers and can even regrow an entire organ such as a limb or a tail. The essential process is the activation of *stem cells* – a pool of undifferentiated cells that have the potential to develop into any of the more specialised cells in the body ('totipotent' or 'pluripotent' cells). Not only do amphibians have a plentiful supply of these primitive cells but many of their more specialised cells can de-differentiate, becoming stem cells again. These can then multiply and retrace the fetal developmental pathways that generated the organ, proliferating again and again and eventually differentiating into the various cell types needed to replace the missing structure.

However, during evolution, mammals have lost this ability in all but a few tissues. Blood cells, intestinal epithelium and the outer layers of the skin are replaced continuously throughout life but there is a low turnover and replacement of cells in organs such as liver, kidney and bone. This 'physiological renewal' is effected by local tissue-specific stem cells.

Almost alone among mammalian organs, the liver has significant ability to replace itself. It can regenerate to its original size in a remarkably short time, provided that at least 25% has been left intact.[6] The mature parenchymal liver cells participate in this process as well as all the other cellular components of the liver.

It is necessary to distinguish *embryonic stem cells* (ES cells) from *adult stem cells* and *progenitor cells*. ES cells are the true pluripotent cells of the embryo which are able to differentiate into any other cell type. Adult stem cells (AS cells) have a more restricted capability whereas progenitor cells are able to differentiate only into a single cell type. ES cells are absent in the adult mammal, but AS cells are present, although they are few in number. If a mammal is injured or its tissue is removed, repair processes – often with subsequent scarring – usually make good the damage. It seems that rapid closure of the defect after tissue loss (which is much more speedily accomplished by repair mechanisms) takes priority over regeneration.

Until recently, it was assumed that this was (with a few exceptions) an unalterable situation, but recent work has suggested that it might be possible to activate the regenerative pathways in mammals – at least to some extent and in some organs. Replacement of entire limbs is manifestly not possible in humans, but regeneration of limited amounts of tissue or of a small part of an organ may well be feasible. For this to happen, it is necessary to encourage some stem cells to proliferate, develop and differentiate at the relevant sites; or – and this is a rather more remote prospect in humans – to persuade some local specialised cells to de-differentiate. This can occur in some mammals under special circumstances. However, it may be that repair is the Janus face of regeneration, being an evolutionary trade-off in mammals for the lost power of regeneration.

▼ Where are the relevant stem cells that could be coaxed into regenerative service? Various possibilities are being vigorously investigated and in some cases tested clinically. These include:

---

[6]There is an account of liver regeneration in Greek mythology. Prometheus stole the secret of fire from Zeus and gave it to mankind. To punish him, Zeus had him shackled to a crag in the Caucasus and every day an eagle tore at his flesh and devoured much of his liver. During the night, however, it regenerated and in the morning was whole again. The legend doesn't say whether the requisite 25% was left after the eagle had had its fill, and the regeneration described seems unrealistically fast – rat liver takes 2 weeks or more to get back to the original size after 66% hepatectomy.

- embryonic stem cells (limited availability and serious ethical issues)
- bone marrow-derived mesenchymal stem cells (Huang et al., 2009; Stapenbeck & Miyoshi, 2009)
- muscle-derived stem cells (Sinanan et al., 2006)
- human-induced pluripotent stem cells (Nishikawa et al., 2008)
- tissue-resident progenitor cells.

For a tissue such as the liver to regenerate, local tissue-specific stem cells must be stimulated by growth factors to enter the cell cycle and to proliferate. Other essential processes include those already discussed such as angiogenesis, activation of MMPs and interaction between the matrix and fibronectin to link all the new elements together. The concomitant replacement of components of the lost connective tissue (fibroblasts, macrophages, etc.) would also be necessary.

Because most tissues do not regenerate spontaneously, mechanisms that could restore regenerative ability could be of immense therapeutic value. Stem cell therapy has become an attractive prospect for treating all manner of diseases, ranging from erectile dysfunction and urinary incontinence to heart disease and neurodegeneration. Animal studies have confirmed that this is a potentially rewarding area although routine stem cell therapy in humans is still a distant prospect. The literature is daunting but the following examples provide an insight into the obstacles and aspirations of the field: repair of damaged heart muscle (Ch. 21; see Lovell & Mathur, 2011), repair of retinal degeneration (Ong & da Cruz, 2012), stroke (Banerjee et al., 2011) and replacement of insulin-secreting cells to treat type 1 diabetes mellitus (Ch. 31; Voltarelli et al., 2007).

THERAPEUTIC PROSPECTS

Theoretically, all the processes described in this chapter could constitute useful targets for new drug development. Below, we list those approaches that are proving or are likely to prove fruitful.

APOPTOTIC MECHANISMS

Compounds that could modify apoptosis are being intensively investigated (Melnikova & Golden, 2004; MacFarlane, 2009). Here we can only outline some of the more important approaches.

Drugs that promote apoptosis by various mechanisms were heralded as a potential new approach to cancer treatment, and are actively being studied, though none has yet been approved for clinical use. Potential proapoptotic therapeutic approaches need to be targeted precisely to the diseased tissue to avoid the obvious risks of damaging other tissues. Examples include the following:

- An antisense compound against Bcl-2 (**oblimersen**) is being tested for chronic lymphocytic leukaemia.
- **Obatoclax**, a small molecule inhibitor of Bcl-2 action, is being tested for treating haematological malignancies. For details see MacFarlane (2009).
- MicroRNA technology could also be used to promote apoptosis (see Fig. 5.5).
- Monoclonal agonist antibodies to the death receptor ligand TRAIL (e.g. **lexatumumab**) are undergoing clinical trials for treatment of solid tumours and lymphomas (MacFarlane, 2009).

- A new drug, **bortezomib**, which inhibits the proteasome, is available for the treatment of selected cancers. It causes the build-up of Bax, an apoptotic promoter protein of the Bcl-2 family that acts by inhibiting antiapoptotic Bcl-2. Bortezomib acts partly by inhibiting NFκB action (see Ch. 3).
- One of the most cancer-specific genes codes for an endogenous caspase inhibitor, *survivin*. This occurs in high concentrations in certain tumours and a small molecule suppressor of survivin is in clinical trial (Giaccone & Rajan, 2009), the objective being to induce cancer cell suicide.

Inhibiting apoptosis might prevent or treat a wide range of common degenerative disorders. Unfortunately, success in developing such inhibitors for clinical use has so far proved elusive and a number have been found to lack efficacy in clinical trials. Current areas of interest include the following:

- Blocking the PD-1 death receptor with a targeted antibody is a potentially fruitful new avenue to explore for the treatment of HIV, hepatitis B and hepatitis C infections, as well as other chronic infections and some cancers that express the ligand for PD-1 (Williams & Bevan, 2006).
- Several caspase inhibitors are under investigation for treating myocardial infarction, stroke, liver disease, organ transplantation and sepsis. **Emricasan** is one such candidate undergoing trials in patients requiring liver transplants.

ANGIOGENESIS AND METALLOPROTEINASES

The search for clinically useful anti-angiogenic drugs and MMP inhibitors is continuing, but has not so far been successful. At present, only one new drug has been approved for use in cancer treatment: bevacizumab, a monoclonal antibody that neutralises VEGF, which is also used to treat age-related macular degeneration, a disease also associated with excessive proliferation of retinal blood vessels.

CELL CYCLE REGULATION

The main endogenous positive regulators of the cell cycle are the cdks. Several small molecules that inhibit cdks by targeting the ATP-binding sites of these kinases have been developed; an example is **flavopiridol**, currently in clinical trials, which inhibits all the cdks, causing arrest of the cell cycle; it also promotes apoptosis, has anti-angiogenic properties and can induce differentiation (Dickson & Schwartz, 2009).

Some compounds affect upstream pathways for cdk activation and may find a use in cancer treatment. Examples are **perifosine** (although its future is uncertain at the moment) and **lovastatin** (a cholesterol-lowering drug, see Ch. 23, which may also have anticancer properties).

Bortezomib, a boronate compound, covalently binds the proteasome, inhibiting the degradation of proapoptotic proteins. It is used in treating multiple myeloma (see Ch. 56).

Of the various components of the growth factor signalling pathway, receptor tyrosine kinases, the Ras protein and cytoplasmic kinases have been the subjects of most interest. Kinase inhibitors recently introduced for cancer treatment include **imatinib**, **gefitinib** and **erlotinib** (see Ch. 56).

REFERENCES AND FURTHER READING

Cell cycle and apoptosis (general)

Ashkenasi, A., 2002. Targeting death and decoy receptors of the tumour necrosis receptor superfamily. Nat. Rev. Cancer 2, 420–429. (*Exemplary review, comprehensive; good diagrams*)

Aslan, J.E., Thomas, G., 2009. Death by committee: organellar trafficking and communication in apoptosis. Traffic 10, 1390–1404.

Barbato, C., Ruberti, F., Cogoni, C., 2009. Searching for MIND: microRNAs in neurodegenerative diseases. J. Biomed. Biotechnol. 2009, 871313.

Carleton, M., Cleary, M.C., Linsley, P.S., 2007. MicroRNAs and cell cycle regulation. Cell Cycle 6, 2127–2132. (*Describes how specific microRNAs act to control cell cycle check points*)

Cummings, J., Ward, T., Ranson, M., Dive, C., 2004. Apoptosis pathway-targeted drugs – from the bench to the clinic. Biochim. Biophys. Acta 1705, 53–66. (*Good review discussing – in the context of anticancer drug development – Bcl-2 proteins, IAPs, growth factors, tyrosine kinase inhibitors and assays for apoptosis-inducing drugs*)

Danial, N.N., Korsmeyer, S.J., 2004. Cell death: critical control points. Cell 116, 205–219. (*Definitive review of the biology and control of apoptosis; includes evidence from C. elegans, Drosophila and mammals*)

Dickson, M.A., Schwartz, G.K., 2009. Development of cell-cycle inhibitors for cancer therapy. Curr. Oncol. 16, 36–43. (*Discusses drugs that target the cell cycle that have entered clinical trials*)

Elmore, S., 2007. Apoptosis: a review of programmed cell death. Toxicol. Pathol. 35, 495–516. (*A general overview of apoptosis, including structural changes, biochemistry and the role of apoptosis in health and disease*)

Garzon, R., Calin, G.A., Croce, C.M., 2009. MicroRNAs in Cancer. Annu. Rev. Med. 60, 167–179.

Giaccone, G., Rajan, A., 2009. Met amplification and HSP90 inhibitors. Cell Cycle 8, 2682.

Janssen, E.M., Droin, N.M., Lemmens, E.E., 2005. CD4[+] T-cell-help controls CD4[+] T cell memory via TRAIL-mediated activation-induced cell death. Nature 434, 88–92. (*Control of TRAIL expression could explain the role of CD4[+] T cells in CD8[+] T-cell function*)

Liu, Z., Sall, A., Yang, D., 2008. MicroRNA: an emerging therapeutic target and intervention tool. Int. J. Mol. Sci. 9, 978–999.

Lynam-Lennon, N., Maher, S.M., Reynolds, J.V., 2009. The roles of microRNAs in cancer and apoptosis. Biol. Rev. 84, 55–71. (*Detailed review of the role of microRNAs in cell proliferation and cell death and their potential roles as oncogenes and tumour suppressor genes*)

MacFarlane, M., 2009. Cell death pathways – potential therapeutic targets. Xenobiotica 39, 616–624. (*Excellent up-to-date review with table of agents in early clinical trial*)

Melnikova, A., Golden, J., 2004. Apoptosis-targeting therapies. Nat. Rev. Drug Discov. 3, 905–906. (*Crisp overview*)

Ouyang, L., Shi, Z., Zhao, S., et al., 2012. Programmed cell death pathways in cancer: a review of apoptosis, autophagy and programmed necrosis. Cell Prolif. 45, 487–498. (*A wide-ranging review dealing with all types of programmed cell death in cancer cells*)

Portt, L., Norman, G., Clapp, C., Greenwood, M., Greenwood, M.T., 2011. Anti-apoptosis and cell survival: a review. Biochim. Biophys. Acta 1813, 238–259. (*A very detailed review which deals with both pro- and antiapoptotic mechanisms as well as other types of programmed cell death*)

Riedl, S.J., Salvesen, G.S., 2007. The apoptosome: signalling platform of cell death. Nat. Rev. Mol. Cell Biol. 8, 405–413. (*Discusses the formation of the apoptosome and the activation of its effector, caspase 9*)

Riedl, S.J., Shi, Y., 2004. Molecular mechanisms of caspase regulation during apoptosis. Nat. Rev. Mol. Cell Biol. 5, 897–905. (*Systematic review*)

Satyanarayana, A., Kaldis, P., 2009. Mammalian cell-cycle regulation: several Cdks, numerous cyclins and diverse compensatory mechanisms. Oncogene 28, 2925–2939. (*Summarises the results of gene knockout experiments which point to the ability of the cell to compensate for the loss of most cyclins. Interesting review for those who want to delve deeper into the subject*)

Stenvang, J., Lindow, M., Kauppinen, S., 2008. Targeting of microRNAs for therapeutics. Biochem. Soc. Trans. 36, 1197–1200.

Swanton, C., 2004. Cell-cycle targeted therapies. Lancet 5, 27–36. (*Definitive review of the protein families controlling the cell cycle, their alterations in malignancy and their potential as targets for new drugs*)

Tousoulis, D., Andreou, I., Tentolouris, C., et al., 2010. Comparative effects of rosuvastatin and allopurinol on circulating levels of matrix metalloproteinases in patients with chronic heart failure. Int. J. Cardiol. 145, 438–443.

Tsai, L.M., Yu, D., 2010. MicroRNAs in common diseases and potential therapeutic applications. Clin. Exp. Pharmacol. Physiol. 37, 102–107.

Williams, M.A., Bevan, M.J., 2006. Exhausted T cells perk up. Nature 439, 669–670. (*Succinct article assesses the work on reversing T-cell exhaustion*)

Wurdinger, T., Costa, F.F., 2007. Molecular therapy in the microRNA era. Pharmacogenomics J. 7, 297–304.

Wyllie, A.H., 2010. 'Where, O death, is thy sting?' A brief review of apoptosis biology. Mol. Neurobiol. 42, 4–9. (*A short and very accessible review by one of the founders of the field. Highly recommended*)

Yang, B.F., Lu, Y.J., Wang, Z.G., 2009. MicroRNAs and apoptosis: implications in molecular therapy of human disease. Clin. Exp. Pharmacol. Physiol. 36, 951–960. (*Comprehensive review of the apotosis-regulating miRNAs and apoptotic cell death*)

Zha, Y., Blank, C., Gajewski, T.F., 2004. Negative regulation of T-cell function by PD-1. Crit. Rev. Immunol. 24, 229–237. (*Article on the balance between stimulatory and inhibitory signalling and its relevance to self-tolerance and the pathogenesis of autoimmune diseases*)

Zhou, L., Seo, K.H., Wong, H.K., Mi, Q.S., 2009. MicroRNAs and immune regulatory T cells. Int. Immunopharmacol. 9, 524–527.

Integrins, extracellular matrix, metalloproteinases and angiogenesis

Barczyk, M., Carracedo, S., Gullberg, D., 2010. Integrins. Cell Tissue Res. 339, 269–280.

Clark, I.M., Swingler, T.E., Sampieri, C.L., Edwards, D.R., 2008. The regulation of matrix metalloproteinases and their inhibitors. Int. J. Biochem. Cell Biol. 40, 1362–1378.

Fingleton, B., 2008. MMPs as therapeutic targets – still a viable option? Semin. Cell Biol. Dev. 19, 61–68. (*Somewhat discouraging review of clinical trials data with MMP inhibitors*)

Gahmberg, C.G., Fagerholm, S.C., Nurmi, S.M., et al., 2009. Regulation of integrin activity and signalling. Biochim. Biophys. Acta 1790, 431–444. (*Crisp review of the control of cell signalling by integrins*)

Järveläinen, H., Sainio, A., Koulu, M., Wight, T.N., Penttinen, R., 2009. Extracellular matrix molecules: potential targets in pharmacotherapy. Pharmacol. Rev. 61, 198–223. (*Comprehensive review of the role of the extracellular matrix [ECM] in the cellular events involved in proliferation and differentiation with discussion of the ECM as a potential target for new drug development*)

Marastoni, S., Ligresti, G., Lorenzon, E., Colombatti, A., Mongiat, M., 2008. Extracellular matrix: a matter of life and death. Connect. Tissue Res. 49, 203–206. (*Crisp analysis of the ECM and its role in cell survival, growth and proliferation*)

Ruperez, M., Rodrigues-Diez, R., Blanco-Colio, L.M., et al., 2007. HMG-CoA reductase inhibitors decrease angiotensin II-induced vascular fibrosis: role of RhoA/ROCK and MAPK pathways. Hypertension 50, 377–383.

Skiles, J.W., Gonnella, N.C., Jeng, A.Y., 2004. The design, structure and clinical update of small molecular weight matrix metalloproteinase inhibitors. Curr. Med. Chem. 11, 2911–2977. (*Results of trials with early matrix metalloproteinases were disappointing; the authors discuss the proposed usefulness of matrix metalloproteinase inhibitors and review patented drugs*)

Streuli, C.H., Akhtar, N., 2009. Signal co-operation between integrins and other receptor systems. Biochem. J. 418, 491–506. (*Deals with integrin interaction with growth factors to regulate angiogenesis, their interplay with tyrosine kinases and with cytokine receptors*)

Verrecchia, F., Mauviel, A., 2007. Transforming growth factor-beta and fibrosis. World J. Gastroenterol. 13, 3056–3062.

Stem cells, regeneration and repair

Aldhous, P., 2008. How stem cell advances will transform medicine. New Scientist 2654, 40–43. (*Clear, simple article*)

Banerjee, S., Williamson, D., Habib, N., Gordon, M., Chataway, J., 2011. Human stem cell therapy in ischaemic stroke: a review. Age. Ageing 40, 7–13.

Gaetani, R., Barile, L., Forte, E., et al., 2009. New perspectives to repair a broken heart. Cardiovasc. Hematol. Agents Med. Chem. 7, 91–107. (*Discusses sources of cardiomyogenic cells and their potential for diseased or injured myocardium*)

Huang, N.F., Lam, A., Fang, Q., et al., 2009. Bone marrow-derived mesenchymal stem cells in fibrin augment angiogenesis in the chronically infarcted myocardium. Regen. Med. 4, 527–538.

Lovell, M.J., Mathur, A., 2011. Republished review: Cardiac stem cell therapy: progress from the bench to bedside. Postgrad. Med. J. 87,

558–564. (*Useful review on the state of cardiac stem cell therapy highlighting the problems as well as the potential. Easy to read*)

Nature Reviews Drug Discovery, 2006. Vol. 5 (August) has a series of articles on nerve regeneration. (*The articles 'highlight recent progress in knowledge of the molecular, cellular and circuitry level responses to injuries to the adult mammalian CNS, with a view to understanding the underlying mechanism that will enable the development of appropriate therapeutic strategies'*)

Nishikawa, S., Goldstein, R.A., Nierras, C.R., 2008. The promise of human induced pluripotent stem cells for research and therapy. Nat. Rev. Mol. Cell Biol. 9, 725–729. (*Induced pluripotent stem cells [iPS] are human somatic cells that have reprogrammed to be pluripotent*)

Ong, J.M., da Cruz, L., 2012. A review and update on the current status of stem cell therapy and the retina. Br. Med. Bull. 102, 133–146. (*Easy to read review*)

Rosenthal, N., 2003. Prometheus's vulture and the stem-cell promise. N. Engl. J. Med. 349, 267–286. (*Excellent article on the problem of regeneration of tissues and organs*)

Sinanan, A.C., Buxton, P.G., Lewis, M.P., 2006. Muscling in on stem cells. Biol. Cell 98, 203–214.

Stapenbeck, T.S., Miyoshi, H., 2009. The role of stromal cells in tissue regeneration and wound repair. Science 26, 1666–1669. (*Succinct article on the possibility of mammalian stromal cells performing the same function as blastema cells in lower organisms*)

Voltarelli, J.C., Couri, C.E., Stracieri, A.B., et al., 2007. Autologous nonmyeloablative hematopoietic stem cell transplantation in newly diagnosed type 1 diabetes mellitus. JAMA 297, 1568–1576. (*Successful early trial of stem cell transplantation*)

Wilson, C., 2003. The regeneration game. New Scientist 179, 2414–2427. (*Very readable article on the possibility of regeneration of mammalian tissues and organs*)

6 Cellular mechanisms: host defence

OVERVIEW

Everyone has experienced an inflammatory episode at some time or other and will be familiar with the characteristic redness, swelling, heat, pain and loss of function that this generally entails. Inflammatory mediators are considered separately in Chapters 17 and 18; here we list the cellular players involved in the host defence response and explain the bare bones of this crucial and sophisticated mechanism. Understanding these cellular responses and their functions provides an essential basis for understanding the actions of anti-inflammatory and immunosuppressant drugs – a major class of therapeutic agents (see Ch. 26).

INTRODUCTION

All living creatures are born into a universe that poses a constant challenge to their physical well-being and survival. Evolution, which has equipped us with homeostatic systems that maintain a stable internal environment in the face of changing external temperatures and fluctuating supplies of food and water, has also provided us with mechanisms for combating the ever-present threat of infection and for promoting healing and restoration to normal function in the event of injury. In mammals, this function is subserved by the *innate* and *acquired* (or *adaptive*) immune systems, working together with a variety of mediators and mechanisms that collectively give rise to what we term the *inflammatory response*. Generally this acts to protect us, but occasionally it goes awry, leading to a spectrum of inflammatory diseases. It is under these circumstances that we resort to drug therapy to control this overexuberant response.

The main functions of this host inflammatory response then, are *defence* and *repair* – in other words, nothing less than the on-going security of the organism, and crucial to survival. Immunodeficiency due, for example, to genetic causes (e.g. *leukocyte adhesion deficiency*), infection with organisms such as HIV, radiation or immunosuppressant drugs, can be life-threatening.

Like border security systems in the mundane world, the body has the cellular and molecular equivalents of guards, identity checks, alarm systems and a communication network with which to summon back-up when required. It also has access to an astonishing data bank that memorises precise details of previous illegal intruders and prevents them from returning. This host response has two main components, which work hand-in-hand. These are:

- The *innate*, non-adaptive response, which developed early in evolution and is present in some form or other in most multicellular organisms. This is the first line of defence.

The inflammatory response

- The inflammatory response occurs in tissues following injury or exposure to a pathogen or other noxious substance.
- It usually has two components: an *innate* non-adaptive response and an *adaptive* (acquired or specific) immunological response.
- These reactions are generally protective, but if inappropriately deployed they are deleterious.
- The normal outcome of the response is healing with or without scarring; alternatively, if the underlying cause persists, chronic inflammation results.
- Many of the diseases that require drug treatment involve inflammation. Understanding the action and use of anti-inflammatory and immunosuppressive drugs necessitates understanding the inflammatory reaction.

- The *adaptive* immune response. This appeared much later in evolutionary terms and is found only in vertebrates. It provides the physical basis for our immunological 'memory' and is the second, and supremely effective, line of defence.

THE INNATE IMMUNE RESPONSE

Mucosal epithelial tissues constantly secrete antibacterial proteins such as *defensins* together with a type of 'all purpose' immunoglobulin (Ig)A as a sort of pre-emptive defensive strategy, but elsewhere the innate response is activated immediately following infection or injury.[1] It exists in virtually all organisms and some of the mammalian gene families that control it were first identified in plants and insects.

PATTERN RECOGNITION

One of the most important functions of any security system is the ability to establish identity. How does an organism decide whether a cell is a *bona fide* citizen or an invading pathogen? In the case of the innate response this is achieved through a network of pattern recognition receptors (PRRs), found in virtually all organisms. They recognise pathogen-associated molecular patterns (PAMPs), common products produced by bacteria, fungi, viruses and so on that these organisms could not readily

---

[1]One immunologist described the innate response as the organism's 'knee jerk' response to infection; it is an excellent description.

The innate immune response

- The innate response occurs immediately on injury or infection. It comprises vascular and cellular elements. Mediators generated by cells or from plasma modify and regulate the magnitude of the response.
- Utilising Toll and other recognition receptors, sentinel cells in body tissues, such as macrophages, mast and dendritic cells detect specific pathogen-associated molecular patterns. This triggers the release of cytokines, particularly interleukin (IL)-1 and tumour necrosis factor (TNF)-α, as well as various chemokines.
- IL-1 and TNF-α act on local postcapillary venular endothelial cells, causing:
  - vasodilatation and fluid exudation
  - expression of adhesion molecules on the cell surfaces.
- Exudate contains enzyme cascades that generate bradykinin (from kininogen), and C5a and C3a (from complement). Complement activation lyses bacteria.
- C5a and C3a stimulate mast cells to release histamine, which dilates local arterioles.
- Tissue damage and cytokines release prostaglandins PGI$_2$ and PGE$_2$ (vasodilators) and leukotriene (LT)B$_4$ (a chemotaxin).
- Cytokines stimulate synthesis of vasodilator nitric oxide, which increases vascular permeability.
- Using adhesion molecules, leukocytes roll on, adhere to and finally migrate through activated vascular endothelium towards the pathogen (attracted by chemokines, IL-8, C5a, and LTB$_4$), where phagocytosis and killing takes place.

change to evade detection. PRRs include G protein-coupled receptors such as the FPR (formyl peptide receptor) family that recognises N-formylated peptides characteristic of bacterial protein synthesis (and liberated from damaged mitochondria as well) and cytoplasmic receptors such as the *NOD-like receptors* (**N**ucleotide-binding **O**ligomerization **D**omain-like receptors) – a large family of intracellular proteins that can recognise fragments of bacterial proteoglycan.

Among the best-studied of these PRRs are the *Toll-like receptors* (TLRs). The Toll[2] gene was first identified in *Drosophila* in the mid-1990s. Analogous genes were soon found in vertebrates and it was quickly established that as a family, their main job was to detect highly conserved components in pathogens and to signal their presence to both arms of the immune system.

Approximately 10 TLRs occur in mammals. They belong to the class of *receptor tyrosine kinases* (see Ch. 3), and are phylogenetically highly conserved. Unlike the antigen receptors on T and B cells that develop and change through life, endowing each lymphocyte clone with a structurally unique receptor, TLRs are encoded for by discrete genes in the host DNA. Table 6.1 lists these receptors and the pathogenic products they recognise, where these are known. There are two main types of TLR, located respectively on the cell surface and in endosomes. The latter type generally recognises pathogen RNA/DNA (presumably because they appear in phagosomes), while the former recognises other pathogen components such as cell wall material, endotoxin, etc. Some TLRs also recognise ligands released when host cells are damaged (e.g. heat shock proteins). Presumably this provides an additional way of monitoring internal damage.

How a single family of receptors can recognise such a wide spectrum of different chemicals is a molecular mystery. Sometimes recruiting additional 'accessory' binding proteins to the receptors that modulate their binding properties solves the problem. When activated, Toll receptors dimerise and initiate a complex signalling pathway that activates genes coding for proteins and factors crucial to the deployment of the inflammatory response, many of which we will discuss below. Interestingly from the pharmacological viewpoint, TLR 7 also recognises some synthetic antiviral compounds such as *imidazoquinolones*. The ability of these drugs to provoke TLR activation probably underlies their clinical effectiveness (see Ch. 52).

TLRs are strategically located on those 'sentinel' cells which are likely to come into early contact with invaders. These include *macrophages* as well as *mast cells* and *dendritic cells*, are especially abundant in skin and other inside–outside interfaces, as well as some *intestinal epithelial cells* that are exposed to pathogens in the food that we eat. Genetic defects in the TLR system have been observed. These can lead to an inability to mount an effective host defence response or to a low level, constitutively active inflammatory response.

Having outlined how 'non-self' pathogens are detected by the innate immune system, we can now describe the events that follow the 'raising of the alarm'.

RESPONSES TO PATTERN RECOGNITION

Vascular events

Interaction of a PAMP with TLRs triggers the sentinel cells to respond by producing a range of pro-inflammatory polypeptides called *cytokines* including *tumour necrosis factor (TNF)-α* and *interleukin (IL)-1*. The maturation and processing of IL-1 is managed by *inflammasomes*, intracellular multiprotein complexes that vary according to the type of inflammatory stimulus. The inflammasome thus initiates a precisely tailored inflammatory response appropriate to the situation (see Strowig et al., 2012).

Also released, either as a direct consequence of tissue damage or following cytokine stimulation, are lower molecular weight mediators (such as prostaglandins and histamine) that act on the vascular endothelial cells of the postcapillary venules, causing expression of *adhesion molecules* on the intimal surface and an increase in vascular permeability.

Leukocytes adhere to the endothelial cells through interactions between their cell surface *integrins* and adhesion molecules on endothelial cells and this halts their progression through the microcirculation. They are then able to migrate out of the vessels, attracted by *chemotaxins* generated by the microorganisms or as a result of their interaction with the tissues. Polypeptide *chemokines* released during TLR activation play an important

---

[2]The name, which loosely translates from German as 'Great!' or 'Eureka!', has remained firmly attached to the family.

Table 6.1 The TLR family of pattern recognition receptors (PRRs)

PRR	Pathogen recognised	Ligand	Host cell type	Location
TLR 1	Bacteria	Lipoproteins	Monocyte/macrophages Some dendritic cells B lymphocytes	Surface
TLR 2	Bacteria Bacteria (Gm pos) Parasites Yeast Damaged host cells	Lipoproteins Lipoteichoic acid GPI anchors Cell wall carbohydrates Heat shock proteins	Monocyte/macrophages Some dendritic cells Mast cells	Surface
TLR 3	Virus	dsRNA	Dendritic cells B lymphocytes	Intracellular
TLR 4	Bacteria (Gm neg) Virus Damaged host cells	Lipopolysaccharide Some viral proteins Heat shock proteins Fibrinogen Hyaluronic acid	Monocyte/macrophages Some dendritic cells Mast cells Intestinal epithelium	Surface
TLR 5	Bacteria	Flagellin	Monocyte/macrophages Some dendritic cells Intestinal epithelium	Surface
TLR 6	*Mycoplasma* Parasites Yeast	Lipoproteins GPI anchors Cell wall carbohydrates	Monocyte/macrophages Mast cells B lymphocytes	Surface
TLR 7	Virus	ssRNA Some synthetic drugs	Monocyte/macrophages Mast cells B lymphocytes	Intracellular
TLR 8	Virus	ssRNA	Monocyte/macrophages Some dendritic cells Mast cells	Intracellular
TLR 9	Virus/bacteria	CpG containing DNA	Monocyte/macrophages Some dendritic cells B lymphocytes	Intracellular
TLR 10	Unknown	Unknown	Monocyte/macrophages B lymphocytes	Surface
TLR 11[a]	*Toxoplasma*	Profilin	Monocyte/macrophages Liver cells Kidney	Surface

[a]TLR 11 is found in mouse but not human. TLR 12–15 are not included as little is known concerning their function.
CpG DNA, unmethylated CG dinucleotide; dsRNA, double-stranded RNA; Gm neg/pos, Gram-negative/positive (bacteria); GPI, glycosylphosphatidylinositol anchoring proteins; ssRNA, single-stranded RNA.

part in this. (Cytokines and chemokines are considered separately in Ch. 18.)

The initial vascular events also include dilatation of the small arterioles, resulting in increased blood flow. This is followed by a slowing (and sometimes a cessation) of blood flow and an increase in the permeability of the postcapillary venules with exudation of fluid. The vasodilatation is brought about by mediators, including histamine, prostaglandin (PG)E$_2$ and PGI$_2$ (prostacyclin) released from injured cells, some of which act together with cytokines to increase vascular permeability.

The resulting fluid exudate contains the components for four proteolytic enzyme cascades: the *complement system*, the *coagulation system*, the *fibrinolytic system* and the *kinin system* (see Fig. 6.1). The components of these cascades are inactive proteases that are activated by cleavage, each activated component then activating the next. Eventually, the exudate drains through the lymphatics to local lymph nodes or lymphoid tissue, where the products of the invading microorganism trigger the adaptive phase of the response.

▼ The *complement system* comprises nine major components, designated C1 to C9. Activation of the cascade is initiated by substances derived from microorganisms, such as yeast cell walls or endotoxins. This pathway of activation is termed the *alternative pathway* (Fig. 6.1) as opposed to the *classic pathway*, which is dealt with later. One of the main events is the enzymatic splitting of C3, giving rise to various peptides, one of which, *C3a* (termed an *anaphylatoxin*), stimulates mast cells to secrete further chemical mediators and can also directly stimulate smooth muscle, while *C3b* (termed an *opsonin*) attaches to the surface of a microorganism,

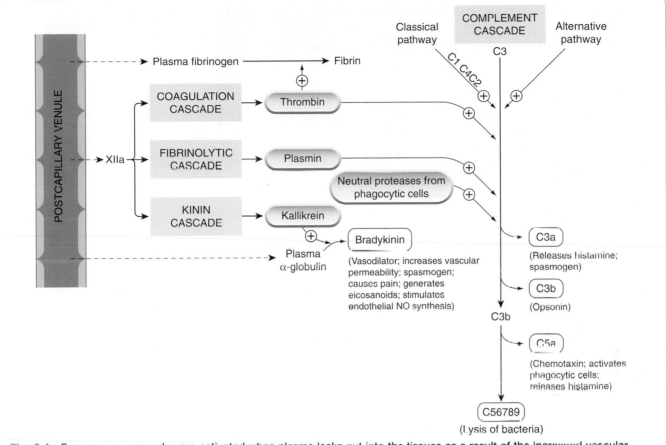

Fig. 6.1 Four enzyme cascades are activated when plasma leaks out into the tissues as a result of the increased vascular permeability of inflammation. Factors causing exudation are depicted in Figure 6.2. Mediators generated are shown in red-bordered boxes. Complement components are indicated by C1, C2, etc. When plasmin is formed, it tends to increase kinin formation and decrease the coagulation cascade. (Adapted from Dale MM, Foreman JC, Fan T-P (eds) 1994 Textbook of Immunopharmacology, third edn. Blackwell Scientific, Oxford.)

facilitating ingestion by phagocytes. *C5a*, generated enzymatically from C5, also releases mediators from mast cells and is a powerful chemotactic attractant and activator of leukocytes.

The final components in the sequence, complement-derived mediators (C5 to C9), coalesce to form a *membrane attack complex* that attaches to certain bacterial membranes, leading to lysis. Complement can therefore mediate the destruction of invading bacteria or damage multicellular parasites; however, it may sometimes cause injury to the host. The principal enzymes of the coagulation and fibrinolytic cascades, thrombin and plasmin, can also activate the cascade by hydrolysing C3, as can enzymes released from leukocytes.

The *coagulation system* and the *fibrinolytic system* are described in Chapter 24. Factor XII is activated to XIIa (e.g. by collagen), and the end product, fibrin, laid down during a host–pathogen interaction, may also serve to limit the extent of the infection. Thrombin is additionally involved in the activation of the kinin (Fig. 6.1) and, indirectly, the fibrinolytic systems (see Ch. 24).

The *kinin system* is another enzyme cascade relevant to inflammation. It yields several mediators, in particular bradykinin (Fig. 6.1).

Cellular events

Of the cells involved in inflammation, some (e.g. vascular endothelial cells, mast cells, dendritic cells and tissue macrophages) are normally present in tissues, while other actively motile cells (e.g. leukocytes) gain access from the circulating blood.

Polymorphonuclear leukocytes

Neutrophil polymorphs are the 'shock troops' of inflammation, and are the first of the blood leukocytes to enter an infected or damaged tissue (Fig. 6.2). The whole process is cleverly choreographed: under direct observation, the neutrophils may be seen first to *roll* along the activated endothelium, then to *adhere* and finally to *migrate* out of the blood vessel and into the extravascular space. This process is regulated by the successive activation of different families of adhesion molecules (*selectins*, *intercellular adhesion molecule* [ICAM] and *integrins*) on the inflamed endothelium that engage corresponding *counter-ligands* on the neutrophil, capturing it as it rolls along the surface, stabilising its interaction with the endothelial cells and enabling it to migrate out of the vessel (using a further adhesion molecule termed *PECAM*, **P**latelet **E**ndothelial **C**ell **A**dhesion **M**olecule). The neutrophil is attracted to the invading pathogen by chemicals termed *chemotaxins*, some of which (such as the tripeptide formyl-Met-Leu-Phe) are released by the microorganism, whereas others, such as C5a, are produced locally or in some cases released (e.g. chemokines such as IL-8), from nearby cells such as macrophages.

Neutrophils can engulf, kill and digest microorganisms. Together with eosinophils, they have surface receptors for C3b, which acts as an *opsonin* that forms a link between

81

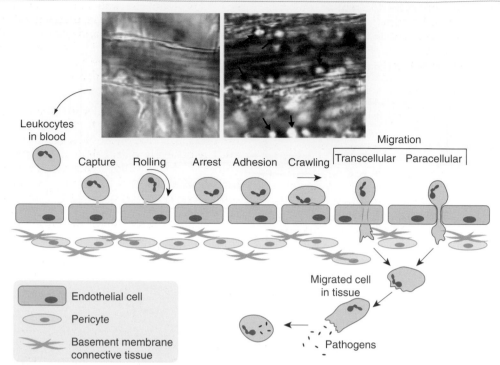

Fig. 6.2 Simplified diagram of the events leading up to polymorphonuclear leukocyte (PMN) migration in a local acute inflammatory reaction. In response to activation of pattern recognition receptors, tissue macrophages release the proinflammatory cytokines interleukin (IL)-1 and tumour necrosis factor (TNF)-α. These act on the endothelial cells of postcapillary venules, causing exudation of fluid and expression of adhesion factors that recognise counter-ligands on blood-borne neutrophils. Free flowing neutrophils in the blood are first 'captured' by *selectins* on activated endothelial cells. These cells then roll along the endothelium before their progress is arrested by the action of *integrins* and they adhere to the vessel wall.

The activated cells then 'crawl' along the endothelium until they find a suitable site for transmigration. This can take two forms: in a minority of cases, cells can actually move through endothelial cells (*transcellular transmigration*) or, in most cases, the neutrophils migrate through the junction between endothelial cells (*paracellular transmigration*). In each case, further adhesion molecules are employed to guide the cell through the gaps.

In addition to traversing this barrier, the migrating cells must now migrate through gaps in the layer of pericytes (contractile cells) that surround the venules as well as the basement membrane (comprised of connective tissue). Chemotactic gradients formed by the release of substances released by or from the pathogen guide the cell to its target where it can kill and or phagocytose the invader. Neutrophils characteristically die after this event, in which case they enter apoptosis and are phagocytosed by macrophages, resolving the inflammatory event.

Photo inset: Photomicrograph of a normal, un-inflamed microcirculation in the mesenteric bed of mouse (left hand panel) and following a period of inflammation (right hand panel). The arrows indicate neutrophils adhering to the endothelium as well as some that have already transmigrated. *(Diagram modified from Nourshargh et al., 2010. Picture courtesy of Drs S. Yazid, G. Leoni and D. Cooper.)*

neutrophil and invading bacterium. (An even more effective link may be made by antibodies.) Neutrophils kill microorganisms by generating toxic oxygen products and other mechanisms, and enzymatic digestion then follows. If the neutrophil is inappropriately activated, these weapons may be turned inadvertently on the host's tissues, causing damage. When neutrophils have released their toxic chemicals, they undergo apoptosis and must be cleared by macrophages. It is this mass of live and apoptotic neutrophils that constitutes 'pus'.

Mast cells

Important 'sentinel' cells that express TLRs, mast cells also have surface receptors both for IgE and for the complement-derived *anaphylotoxins* C3a and C5a. Ligands acting at these receptors trigger mediator release, as does direct physical damage. One of the main substances released is *histamine*; others include *heparin, leukotrienes, PGD₂, platelet-activating factor (PAF), nerve growth factor* and some *interleukins* and proteases. Unusually, mast cells

have preformed packets of cytokines that they can release instantaneously when stimulated. This makes them extremely effective triggers of the inflammatory response.

Monocytes/macrophages

Monocytes follow polymorphs into inflammatory lesions after a delay (sometimes several hours). Adhesion to endothelium and migration into the tissue follow a pattern similar to that of the neutrophils, although monocyte chemotaxis utilises additional chemokines, such as MCP-1[3] (which, reasonably enough, stands for **M**onocyte **C**hemoattractant **P**rotein-1) and RANTES (which very *unreasonably* stands for **R**egulated on **A**ctivation **N**ormal **T** cell **E**xpressed and **S**ecreted; immunological nomenclature has excelled itself here!).

---

[3]Human immunodeficiency virus-1 binds to the surface CD4 glycoprotein on monocytes/macrophages but is able to penetrate the cell only after binding also to MCP-1 and RANTES receptors. This is a case where the innate immune system inadvertently aids the enemy.

Once in tissues, blood monocytes differentiate into *macrophages*.[4] The newly differentiated cell may acquire an *M1* or an *M2 phenotype* depending upon the types of cytokines it secretes. The former is generally regarded as a proinflammatory cell whereas the latter is probably more involved in tissue repair and healing. These cells therefore have a remarkable range of abilities, being not only a jack-of-all-trades but also a master of many.

Activation of monocyte/macrophage TLRs stimulates the generation and release of chemokines and other cytokines that act on vascular endothelial cells, attract other leukocytes to the area and give rise to systemic manifestations of the inflammatory response such as fever. Macrophages engulf tissue debris and dead cells, as well as phagocytosing and killing most (but unfortunately not all) microorganisms. They also play an important part in *antigen presentation*. When stimulated by glucocorticoids, macrophages secrete *annexin-1* (a potent anti-inflammatory polypeptide; see Ch. 33), which controls the development of the local inflammatory reaction limiting any collateral damage.

Dendritic cells

These are present in many tissues, especially those that subserve a barrier function (e.g. the skin, where they are sometimes referred to as *Langerhans cells* after their discoverer). As an important type of 'sentinel cell' they can detect the presence of pathogens and when thus activated they can migrate into lymphoid tissue, where they play an important part in antigen presentation.

Eosinophils

These cells have similar capacities to neutrophils but are also 'armed' with a battery of substances stored in their granules, which, when released, kill multicellular parasites (e.g. helminths). These include *eosinophil cationic protein*, a *peroxidase* enzyme, the *eosinophil major basic protein* and a *neurotoxin*. The eosinophil is considered by many to be of primary importance in the pathogenesis of the late phase of asthma where, it is suggested, secreted granule proteins cause damage to bronchiolar epithelium (see Fig. 28.4).

Basophils

Basophils are very similar in many respects to mast cells. Except in certain inflammatory diseases, such as viral infections and myeloproliferative disorders, the basophil content of the tissues is generally negligible and in health they form only <0.1% of circulating white blood cells.

Vascular endothelial cells

Vascular endothelial cells (see also Chs 22 and 23), originally considered as passive lining cells, are now known to play an active part in inflammation. Small arteriole endothelial cells secrete nitric oxide (NO), causing relaxation of the underlying smooth muscle (see Ch. 20), vasodilatation and increased delivery of plasma and blood cells to the inflamed area. The endothelial cells of the postcapillary venules regulate plasma exudation and thus the delivery of plasma-derived mediators (see Fig. 6.1). Vascular endothelial cells express several adhesion molecules (the ICAM and selectin families; see Fig. 6.2), as well as a variety of receptors, including those for histamine, acetylcholine and IL-1. In addition to NO, the cells can synthesise and release the vasodilator agents PGI_2 and PGE_2, the vasoconstrictor agent endothelin, plasminogen activator, PAF and several cytokines. Endothelial cells also participate in the angiogenesis that occurs during inflammatory resolution, chronic inflammation and cancer (see Chs 5 and 56).

Platelets

Platelets are involved primarily in coagulation and thrombotic phenomena (see Ch. 24) but also play a part in inflammation. They have low-affinity receptors for IgE, and are believed to contribute to the first phase of asthma (Fig. 28.1). In addition to generating thromboxane $(TX)A_2$ and PAF, they can generate free radicals and pro-inflammatory cationic proteins. Platelet-derived growth factor contributes to the repair processes that follow inflammatory responses or damage to blood vessels.

Natural killer cells

Natural killer (NK) cells are a specialised type of lymphocyte. In an unusual twist to the receptor concept, NK cells kill targets (e.g. virus-infected or tumour cells) that lack ligands for inhibitory receptors on the NK cells themselves. The ligands in question are the *major histocompatibility complex* (MHC) molecules, and any cells lacking these become a target for NK-cell attack, a strategy sometimes called the 'mother turkey strategy'.[5] MHC proteins are expressed on the surface of most host cells and, in simple terms, are specific for that individual, enabling the NK cells to avoid damaging host cells. NK cells have other functions: they are equipped with Fc receptors and, in the presence of antibodies directed against a target cell, they can kill the cell by antibody-dependent cellular cytotoxicity.

THE ADAPTIVE IMMUNE RESPONSE

The adaptive response provides the physical basis for an 'immunological memory'. It provides a more powerful defence than the innate response as well as being highly specific for the invading pathogen. Here we will provide only a simplified outline, stressing those aspects relevant for an understanding of drug action; for more detailed coverage, see textbooks in the References and Further Reading section at the end of this chapter.

The key cells are the *lymphocytes*. These are long-lived cells derived from precursor cells within the bone marrow. Following release into the blood and maturation, they dwell in the lymphoid tissues such as the lymph nodes and spleen. Here, they are poised to detect, intercept and identify foreign proteins presented to them by *antigen presenting cells* (APCs) such as the macrophage or the dendritic cells. The three main groups of lymphocytes are:

- *B cells*, which mature in the bone marrow. They are responsible for antibody production, i.e. the *humoral immune response*.
- *T cells*, which mature in the thymus. They are important in the induction phase of the immune response and in *cell-mediated* immune reactions.

---

[4]Literally 'big eaters', compared with neutrophils, originally called microphages or 'little eaters'.

[5]Richard Dawkins in *River out of Eden*, citing the zoologist Schliedt, explains that the 'rule of thumb a mother turkey uses to recognise nest robbers is a dismayingly brusque one; in the vicinity of the nest, attack anything that moves unless it makes a noise like a baby turkey' (quoted by Kärre & Welsh, 1997).

The adaptive response

- The adaptive (specific, acquired) immunological response boosts the effectiveness of the innate responses. It has two phases, the induction phase and the effector phase, the latter consisting of (i) antibody-mediated and (ii) cell-mediated components.
- During the *induction phase*, naive T cells bearing either the CD4 or the CD8 co-receptors are presented with antigen, triggering proliferation:
  - CD8-bearing T cells develop into cytotoxic T cells that can kill virally infected cells
  - CD4-bearing T-helper (Th) cells are stimulated by different cytokines to develop into Th1, Th2, Th17 or Treg cells
  - *Th1* cells develop into cells that release cytokines that activate macrophages; these cells, along with cytotoxic T cells, control cell-mediated responses
  - *Th2* cells control antibody-mediated responses by stimulating B cells to proliferate, giving rise to antibody-secreting plasma cells and memory cells
  - *Th17* cells are similar to Th1 cells and are important in some human diseases such as rheumatoid arthritis
  - *Treg* cells restrain the development of the immune response.
- The effector phase depends on antibody- and cell-mediated responses.
- Antibodies provide:
  - more selective complement activation
  - more effective pathogen phagocytosis
  - more effective attachment to multicellular parasites, facilitating their destruction
  - direct neutralisation of some viruses and of some bacterial toxins.
- Cell-mediated reactions:
  - CD8⁺ cytotoxic T cells that kill virus-infected cells
  - cytokine-releasing CD4⁺ T cells that enable macrophages to kill intracellular pathogens such as the tubercle bacillus
  - memory cells primed to react rapidly to a known antigen
  - provide help for B cell activation.
- Inappropriately deployed immune reactions are termed *hypersensitivity reactions*.
  Anti-inflammatory and immunosuppressive drugs are used when the normally protective inflammatory and/or immune responses escape control.

- *NK (natural killer) cells.* These are really part of the innate system. They are activated by *interferons* and release cytotoxic granules that destroy target cells identified as 'foreign' or abnormal.

T and B lymphocytes express antigen-specific receptors that recognise and react with virtually all foreign proteins and polysaccharides that we are likely to encounter during our lifetime. This receptor repertoire is generated randomly and so would recognise 'self' proteins as well as foreign antigens if it were not that *tolerance* to self-antigens is acquired during fetal life by apoptotic deletion of T-cell

clones in the thymus that recognise the host's own tissues. Dendritic cells and macrophages involved in the innate response also have a role in preventing harmful immune reactions against the host's own cells.

The adaptive immune response occurs in two phases, termed the *induction phase* and the *effector phase*.

THE INDUCTION PHASE

During the induction phase, antigen is 'presented' to T cells in the lymph nodes by macrophages or large dendritic cells. This is followed by complex interactions of those T cells with B cells and other T cells (Fig. 6.3). The antigen may constitute part of an invading pathogen (e.g. the coat of a bacterium) or be released by such an organism (e.g. a bacterial toxin), or it may be a vaccine or a substance introduced experimentally in the laboratory to study the immune response (e.g. the injection of egg albumin into the guinea pig). APCs ingest and proteolytically 'process' the antigen and once they reach local lymph nodes, they 'present' the fragments on their surface to lymphocytes in combination with various *major histocompatibility complex* (MHC) molecules (Fig. 6.4). Two types of lymphocytes 'attend' APCs. They are generally distinguished by the presence, on their surface, of *CD4* or *CD8* receptors. These are *co-receptors* that cooperate with the main antigen-specific receptors in antigen recognition. Macrophages also carry surface CD4 proteins.

The two types of lymphocyte involved in the adaptive response are:

- Uncommitted (naive) CD4⁺ T-helper (Th) lymphocytes, or T-helper precursor (Thp) cells, in association with class II MHC molecules (see Fig. 6.4).
- Naive CD8⁺ T lymphocytes in association with class I MHC molecules.[6]

Activation of a T cell by an APC requires that several signals pass between the two cells at this 'immune synapse' (Fig. 6.4; see Medzhitov & Janeway, 2000). After activation, the T cells both generate IL-2 and acquire IL-2 receptors. Some potent anti-inflammatory drugs block this receptor, thus preventing lymphocyte proliferation (see Ch. 26). IL-2 has an *autocrine*[7] action, stimulating proliferation and giving rise to a clone of T cells termed *Th0* cells, which, depending on the prevailing cytokine milieu, give rise to different subsets of armed helper cells. There are four major types of these 'helper cells', each of which generates a characteristic cytokine profile, possesses a unique surface marker profile and has a different role in disease. These characteristics are summarised in Table 6.2.

Knowledge of the relationship between T-cell subsets, their respective cytokine profiles and pathological conditions can be used to manipulate the immune responses for disease prevention and treatment. There are already many experimental models in which modulation of the Th1/Th2 balance with recombinant cytokines or cytokine antagonists alters the outcome of the disease.

---

[6]The main reason that it is difficult to transplant organs such as kidneys from one person to another is that their respective MHC molecules are different. Lymphocytes in the recipient will react to non-self (*allogeneic*) MHC molecules in the donor tissue, which is then likely to be rejected by a rapid and powerful immunological reaction.

[7]'Autocrine' signalling means that the mediator acts on the cell that released it. 'Paracrine' signalling means that the mediator acts on neighbouring cells.

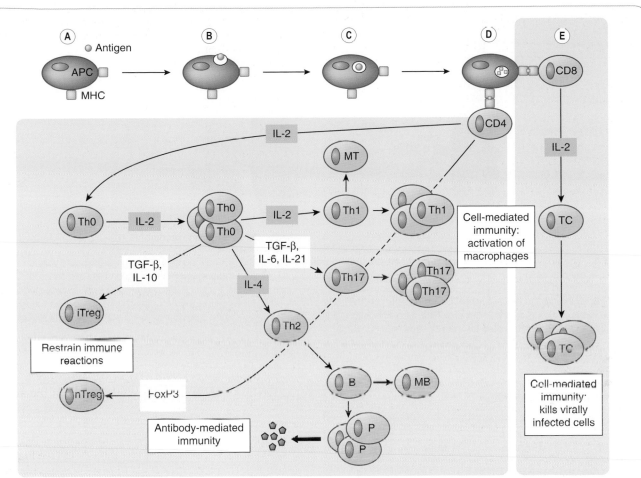

Fig. 6.3 Simplified diagram of the induction and effector phases of lymphocyte activation. Antigen-presenting cells (APCs) ingest and process antigen (A–D) and present fragments to naive, uncommitted CD4 T cells in conjunction with major histocompatibility complex (MHC) class II molecules, or to naive CD8 T cells in conjunction with MHC class I molecules, thus 'arming' them. The armed CD4+ T cells synthesise and express interleukin (IL)-2 receptors and release this cytokine, which stimulates the cells by autocrine action, causing generation and proliferation of T-helper zero (Th0) cells. Autocrine cytokines (e.g. IL-4) cause differentiation of some Th0 cells to give Th2 cells, which are responsible for the development of antibody-mediated immune responses. These Th2 (and sometimes Th1) cells cooperate with and activate B cells to proliferate and give rise eventually to memory B cells (MB) and plasma cells (P), which secrete antibodies. The T cells that aid B cells in this way are referred to as T_{FH} (follicular homing) cells. Other autocrine cytokines (e.g. IL-2) cause proliferation of Th0 cells to give Th1, Th17 or iTreg cells. Th1 and Th17 cells secrete cytokines that activate macrophages (responsible for some cell-mediated immune reactions). iTreg (inducible Treg derived from Th0 precursors) and nTreg (naturally occurring Treg matured in the thymus) cells restrain and inhibit the development of the immune response, thus preventing autoimmunity and excessive immune activation.

The armed CD8+ T cells (F) also synthesise and express IL-2 receptors and release IL-2, which stimulates the cells by autocrine action to proliferate and give rise to cytotoxic T cells (TC). These can kill virally infected cells. IL-2 secreted by CD4+ cells also plays a part in stimulating CD8+ cells to proliferate. Note that the 'effector phase' depicted above relates to the 'protective' action of the immune response. When the response is inappropriately deployed – as in chronic inflammatory conditions such as rheumatoid arthritis – the Th1/Th17 component of the immune response is dominant and the activated macrophages release IL-1 and tumour necrosis factor (TNF)-α, which in turn trigger the release of the chemokines and inflammatory cytokines that play a major role in the pathology of the disease. MT and MB, memory T and B cells, respectively.

THE EFFECTOR PHASE

During the effector phase, the activated B and T lymphocytes differentiate either into *plasma cells* or into *memory cells*. The B plasma cells produce specific antibodies, which are effective in the extracellular fluid, but which cannot neutralise pathogens within cells. T-cell-mediated immune mechanisms overcome this problem by activating macrophages or directly killing virus-infected host cells. Antigen-sensitive *memory cells* are formed when the clone of lymphocytes that are programmed to respond to an antigen is greatly expanded after the first contact with the organism. They allow a greatly accelerated and more effective response to subsequent antigen exposure. In some cases, the response is so rapid and efficient that, after one exposure, the pathogen can never gain a foothold again. Vaccination and immunisation procedures make use of this fact.

THE ANTIBODY-MEDIATED (HUMOURAL) RESPONSE

There are five main classes of antibody – IgG, IgM, IgE, IgA and IgD – which differ from each other in certain structural respects. All are γ-globulins

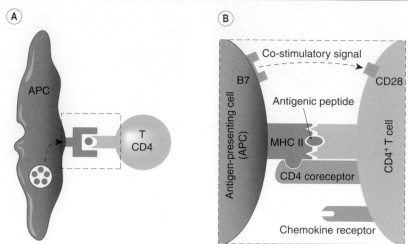

Fig. 6.4 **The activation of a T cell by an antigen-presenting cell (APC).** [A] The APC encounters a foreign protein and this is proteolytically processed into peptide fragments. The activation process then involves three stages: (i) Interaction between the complex of pathogen-derived antigen peptide fragments with major histocompatibility complex (MHC) class II and the antigen-specific receptor on the T cell. [B] (ii) Interaction between the CD4 co-receptor on the T cell and an MHC molecule on the APC. (iii) The B7 protein on the APC cell surface binds to CD28 on the T cell providing a co-stimulatory signal. The CD4 co-receptor, together with a T-cell chemokine receptor, constitute the main binding sites for the HIV virus (see Fig. 52.3).

Table 6.2 Lymphocyte subsets, their role in host defence and relationship to inflammatory disease

Lymphocyte subset	Cytokine stimulus	Main role in adaptive response	Main cytokines produced	Role in disease
Th0	IL-2	To act as a precursor cell type for further differentiation	–	–
Th1	IL-2	'Cell-mediated immunity' Cytokines released from these cells: activate macrophages to phagocytose and kill microorganisms and kill tumour cells; drive proliferation and maturation of the clone into *cytotoxic T cells* that kill virally infected host cells; reciprocally inhibit Th2 cell maturation	IFN-γ, IL-2 and TNF-α	Insulin-dependent diabetes mellitus (Ch. 31), multiple sclerosis, *Helicobacter pylori*-induced peptic ulcer (Ch. 30), aplastic anaemia (Ch. 25) and rheumatoid arthritis (Ch. 26). Allograft rejection
Th2	IL-4	'Humoral immunity' Cytokines released from these cells: stimulate B cells to proliferate and mature into plasma cells producing antibodies; enhance differentiation and activation of eosinophils and reciprocally inhibit Th1/Th17-cell functions. For this reason, they are often thought of as anti-inflammatory	IL-4, IL-5, TGF-β, IL-10 and IL-13	Asthma (Ch. 28) and allergy. AIDS progression is associated with loss of Th1 cells and is facilitated by Th2 responses
Th17	TGF-β, IL-6 and IL-21	A specialised type of Th1 cell	IL-17	The response to infection, organ-specific immune responses and in the pathogenesis of diseases such as rheumatoid arthritis and multiple sclerosis
iTreg	IL-10 and TGF-β	Restraining the immune response, preventing autoimmunity and curtailing potentially damaging inflammatory responses	IL-10 and TGF-β	Failure of this mechanism can provoke excessive inflammation
nTreg	Matured in the thymus			

IFN, interferon; IL, interleukin; iTreg, inducible Treg cells; nTreg, naturally occurring Treg cells; TGF, transforming growth factor; TNF, tumour necrosis factor.

(immunoglobulins), which both recognise and interact specifically with antigens (i.e. proteins or polysaccharides foreign to the host), as well as activating one or more further components of the host's defence systems.

▼ An antibody is a Y-shaped protein molecule (see Ch. 59) in which the arms of the Y (the Fab portion) include the recognition site for specific antigens, and the stem of the Y (the Fc portion) activates host defences. The B cells that are responsible for antibody production recognise foreign molecules by means of surface receptors that are essentially similar to the immunoglobulin that that B-cell clone will eventually produce. Mammals harbour a vast number of B-cell clones that produce different antibodies with recognition sites for different antigens.

The induction of antibody-mediated responses varies with the type of antigen. With most antigens, a cooperative process between Th2 cells and B cells is generally necessary to produce a response. B cells can also present antigen to T cells that then release cytokines that act further on the B cell. The anti-inflammatory glucocorticoids (see Chs 26 and 33) and the immunosuppressive drug **ciclosporin** (see Ch. 26) affect the molecular events at the stage of induction. The cytotoxic immunosuppressive drugs (see Ch. 26) inhibit the proliferation of both B and T cells. Eicosanoids may play a part in controlling these processes as prostaglandins of the E series can inhibit lymphocyte proliferation, probably by inhibiting the release of IL-2.

As you might guess, the ability to make antibodies has huge survival value; children born without this ability[8] suffer repeated infections such as pneumonia, skin infections and tonsillitis. Before the days of antibiotics, they died in early childhood, and even today they require regular replacement therapy with immunoglobulin. Apart from their ability to neutralise pathogens, antibodies can boost the effectiveness and specificity of the host's defence reaction in several ways.

Antibodies and complement
Formation of the antigen–antibody complex exposes a binding site for complement on the Fc domain. This activates the complement sequence and sets in train its attendant biological effects (see Fig. 6.1). This route to C3 activation (the *classic pathway*) provides an especially selective way of activating complement in response to a particular pathogen, because the antigen–antibody reaction that initiates it is not only a highly specific recognition event, but also occurs in close association with the pathogen. The lytic property of complement can be used therapeutically: monoclonal antibodies (mAbs) and complement together can be used to rid bone marrow of cancer cells as an adjunct to chemotherapy or radiotherapy (see Ch. 56).

Antibodies and the phagocytosis of bacteria
When antibodies are attached to their antigens on microorganisms by their Fab portions, the Fc domain is exposed. Phagocytic cells (neutrophils and macrophages) express surface receptors for these projecting Fc portions, which serve as a very specific link between microorganism and phagocyte.

Antibodies and cellular toxicity
In some cases, for example with parasitic worms, the invader may be too large to be ingested by phagocytes.

Antibody molecules can form a link between parasite and the host's white cells (in this case, eosinophils), which are then able to damage or kill the parasite by surface or extracellular actions. NK cells in conjunction with Fc receptors can also kill antibody-coated target cells (an example of *antibody-dependent cell-mediated cytotoxicity*; ADCC).

Antibodies and mast cells or basophils
Mast cells and basophils have receptors for IgE, a particular form of antibody that can attach ('fix') to their cell membranes. When this cell-fixed antibody reacts with an antigen, an entire panoply of pharmacologically active mediators is secreted. This very complex reaction is found widely throughout the animal kingdom and presumably confers clear survival value to the host. Having said that, its precise biological significance is not always entirely clear, although it may be of importance in association with eosinophil activity as a defence against parasitic worms. When inappropriately triggered by substances not inherently damaging to the host, it is implicated in certain types of allergic reaction and seemingly contributes more to illness than to survival in the modern world.

THE CELL-MEDIATED IMMUNE RESPONSE
Cytotoxic T cells (derived from CD8+ cells) and inflammatory (cytokine-releasing) Th1 cells are attracted to inflammatory sites in a similar manner to neutrophils and macrophages, and are involved in cell-mediated responses (see Fig. 6.3).

Cytotoxic T cells
Armed cytotoxic T cells kill intracellular microorganisms such as viruses. When a virus infects a mammalian cell, there are two aspects to the resulting defensive response. The first step is the expression on the cell surface of peptides derived from the pathogen in association with MHC molecules. The second step is the recognition of the peptide–MHC complex by specific receptors on cytotoxic (CD8+) T cells (Fig. 6.4 shows a similar process for a CD4+ T cell). The cytotoxic T cells then destroy virus-infected cells by programming them to undergo apoptosis. Cooperation with macrophages may be required for killing to occur.

Macrophage activating CD4+ Th1 cells
Some pathogens (e.g. *Mycobacteria*, *Listeria*) survive and multiply within macrophages after ingestion. Armed CD4+ Th1 cells release cytokines that activate macrophages to kill these intracellular pathogens. Th1 cells also recruit macrophages by releasing cytokines that act on vascular endothelial cells (e.g. TNF-α) and chemokines (e.g. *macrophage chemotactic factor-1; MCP-1*) that attract the macrophages to the sites of infection.

A complex of microorganism-derived peptides plus MHC molecules is expressed on the macrophage surface and is recognised by cytokine-releasing Th1 cells, which then generate cytokines that enable the macrophage to deploy its killing mechanisms. Activated macrophages (with or without intracellular pathogens) are veritable factories for the production of chemical mediators: they can generate and secrete not only many cytokines but also toxic oxygen metabolites and neutral proteases that kill extracellular organisms (e.g. *Pneumocystis jiroveci* and helminths), complement components, eicosanoids, NO, a fibroblast-stimulating factor, pyrogens and the 'tissue factor' that initiates the extrinsic pathway of the coagulation cascade (Ch. 24), as well as various other coagulation

---

[8]Mainly boys: 'Bruton's agammaglobulinaemia' is caused by a defect in a tyrosine kinase (Btk) coded on the X chromosome (Colonel Bruton was chief of paediatrics at the Walter Reid army hospital).

factors. It is primarily the cell-mediated reaction that is responsible for allograft rejection. Macrophages are also important in coordinating the repair processes that must occur for inflammation to resolve.

The specific cell-mediated or humoral immunological response is superimposed on the innate non-specific vascular and cellular reactions described previously, making them not only markedly more effective but much more selective for particular pathogens.

The general events of the inflammatory and hypersensitivity reactions specified above vary in some tissues. For example, in the airway inflammation of asthma, eosinophils and neuropeptides play a particularly significant role (see Ch. 28). In central nervous system (CNS) inflammation, there is less neutrophil infiltration and monocyte influx is delayed, possibly because of lack of adhesion molecule expression on CNS vascular endothelium and deficient generation of chemokines. It has long been known that some tissues – the CNS parenchyma, the anterior chamber of the eye and the testis – are *immunologically privileged* sites, in that a foreign antigen introduced directly does not provoke an immune reaction (which could be very disadvantageous to the host). However, introduction elsewhere of an antigen already in the CNS parenchyma will trigger the development of immune/inflammatory responses in the CNS.

SYSTEMIC RESPONSES IN INFLAMMATION

In addition to the local changes in an inflammatory site, there are often general systemic manifestations of inflammatory disease, including fever, an increase in blood leukocytes termed *leukocytosis* (or *neutrophilia* if the increase is in the neutrophils only) and the release from the liver of *acute-phase proteins*. These include C-reactive protein, α_2-macroglobulin, fibrinogen, α_1-antitrypsin, serum amyloid A and some complement components. While the function of many of these components is still a matter of conjecture, many seem to have some antimicrobial actions. C-reactive protein, for example, binds to some microorganisms, and the resulting complex activates complement. Other proteins scavenge iron (an essential nutrient for invading organisms) or block proteases, perhaps protecting the host against the worst excesses of the inflammatory response.

THE ROLE OF THE NERVOUS SYSTEM IN INFLAMMATION

It has become clear in recent years that the central, autonomic and peripheral nervous systems all play an important part in the regulation of the inflammatory response. This occurs at various levels:

- *The neuroendocrine system.* Adrenocorticotrophic hormone (ACTH), released from the anterior pituitary gland in response to endogenous circadian rhythm or to stress, releases cortisol from the adrenal glands. This hormone plays a crucial role in regulating immune function at all levels, hence the use of glucocorticoid drugs in the treatment of inflammatory disease. This topic is explored fully in Chs 26 and 33.
- *The central nervous system.* Surprisingly, cytokines such as IL-1 can signal the development of an inflammatory response directly to the brain through receptors on the vagus nerve. This may elicit an 'inflammatory reflex' and trigger activation of a cholinergic anti-inflammatory pathway. See Tracey (2002) and Sternberg (2006) for interesting discussions of this topic.
- *The autonomic nervous system.* Both the sympathetic and parasympathetic systems can influence the development of the inflammatory response. Generally speaking, their influence is anti-inflammatory. Receptors for noradrenaline and acetylcholine are found on macrophages and many other cells involved in the immune response although it is not always entirely clear exactly where their ligands originate.
- *Peripheral sensory neurons.* Some sensory neurons release inflammatory neuropeptides when appropriately stimulated. These neurons are fine afferents (capsaicin-sensitive C and Aδ fibres; see Ch. 42) with specific receptors at their peripheral terminals. Kinins, 5-hydroxytryptamine and other chemical mediators generated during inflammation act on these receptors, stimulating the release of neuropeptides such as the tachykinins (neurokinin A, substance P) and calcitonin gene-related peptide (CGRP), which have proinflammatory or algesic actions. The neuropeptides are considered further in Chapter 18.

UNWANTED INFLAMMATORY AND IMMUNE RESPONSES

The immune response has to strike a delicate balance. According to one school of thought, an infection-proof immune system would be a possibility but would come at a serious cost to the host. With approximately 1 trillion potential antigenic sites in the host, such a 'super-immune' system would be some 1000 times more likely to attack the host itself, triggering *autoimmune disease*. In addition, it is not uncommon to find that ordinarily innocuous substances such as pollen or peanuts sometimes inadvertently activate the immune system. When this happens, the ensuing inflammation itself inflicts damage and may be responsible for the major symptoms of the disease – either acutely as in (for example) anaphylaxis, or chronically in (for example) asthma or rheumatoid arthritis. In either case, anti-inflammatory or immunosuppressive therapy may be required.

▼ Unwanted immune responses, termed *allergic* or *hypersensitivity* reactions, are generally classified into four types.

Type I hypersensitivity

▼ Also called *immediate* or *anaphylactic hypersensitivity* (often known simply as 'allergy'), type I hypersensitivity occurs in individuals who predominantly exhibit a Th2 rather than a Th1 response to antigen. In these individuals, substances that are not inherently noxious (such as grass pollen, house dust mites, certain foodstuffs or drugs, animal fur and so on) provoke the production of antibodies of the IgE type.[9] These fix on mast cells, in the lung, and also to eosinophils. Subsequent contact with the substance causes the release of histamine, PAF, eicosanoids and cytokines. The effects may be localised to the nose (hay fever), the bronchial tree (the initial phase of asthma), the skin (urticaria) or the gastrointestinal tract. In some cases, the reaction is more generalised and produces

---

[9]Such individuals are said to be 'atopic', from a Greek word meaning 'out of place'.

anaphylactic shock, which can be severe and life-threatening. Some important unwanted effects of drugs include anaphylactic hypersensitivity responses (see Ch. 57).

Type II hypersensitivity

▼ Also called *antibody-dependent cytotoxic hypersensitivity*, type II hypersensitivity occurs when the mechanisms outlined above are directed against cells within the host that are (or appear to be) foreign. For example, host cells altered by drugs are sometimes mistaken by the immune system for foreign proteins and evoke antibody formation. The antigen–antibody reaction triggers complement activation (and its sequelae) and may promote attack by NK cells. Examples include alteration by drugs of neutrophils, leading to *agranulocytosis* (see Ch. 56), or of platelets, leading to *thrombocytopenic purpura* (Ch. 24). These type II reactions are also implicated in some types of *autoimmune thyroiditis* (e.g. *Hashimoto's disease*; see Ch. 34).

Type III hypersensitivity

▼ Also called *complex-mediated hypersensitivity*, type III hypersensitivity occurs when antibodies react with *soluble* antigens. The antigen–antibody complexes can activate complement or attach to mast cells and stimulate the release of mediators.

An experimental example of this is the *Arthus reaction* that occurs if a foreign protein is injected subcutaneously into a rabbit or guinea pig with high circulating concentrations of antibody. Within 3–8 hours the area becomes red and swollen because the antigen antibody complexes precipitate in small blood vessels and activate complement. Neutrophils are attracted and activated (by C5a) to generate toxic oxygen species and to secrete enzymes.

Mast cells are also stimulated by C3a to release mediators. Damage caused by this process is involved in *serum sickness*, caused when antigen persists in the blood after sensitisation, causing a severe reaction, as in the response to mouldy hay (known as *farmer's lung*), and in certain types of autoimmune kidney and arterial disease. Type III hypersensitivity is also implicated in *lupus erythematosus* (a chronic, autoimmune inflammatory disease).

Type IV hypersensitivity

▼ The prototype of type IV hypersensitivity (also known as *cell-mediated* or *delayed hypersensitivity*) is the *tuberculin reaction*, a local inflammatory response seen when proteins derived from cultures of the tubercle bacillus are injected into the skin of a person who has been sensitised by a previous infection or immunisation. An 'inappropriate' cell-mediated immune response is stimulated, accompanied by infiltration of mononuclear cells and the release of various cytokines. Cell-mediated hypersensitivity is also the basis of the reaction seen in some other infections (e.g. mumps and measles), as well as with mosquito and tick bites. It is also important in the skin reactions to drugs or industrial chemicals (see Ch. 57), where the

chemical (termed a *hapten*) combines with proteins in the skin to form the 'foreign' substance that evokes the cell-mediated immune response (Fig. 6.3).

In essence, inappropriately deployed T-cell activity underlies all types of hypersensitivity, initiating types I, II and III, and being involved in both the initiation and the effector phase in type IV. These reactions are the basis of the clinically important group of autoimmune diseases. Immunosuppressive drugs (Ch. 26) and/or glucocorticoids (Ch. 33) are routinely employed to treat such disorders.

THE OUTCOME OF THE INFLAMMATORY RESPONSE

It is important not to lose sight of the fact that the inflammatory response is a defence mechanism and not, *ipso facto*, a disease. Its role is to restore normal structure and function to the infected or damaged tissue and, in the vast majority of cases, this is what occurs. The healing and resolution phase of the inflammatory response is an active process and does not simply 'happen' in the absence of further inflammation. This is an area that we are just beginning to understand, but it is clear that it utilises its own unique palette of mediators and cytokines (including various growth factors, annexin-A1, lipoxins, resolvins and IL-10; see Ch. 18) to terminate residual inflammation and to promote remodelling and repair of damaged tissue.

In some cases healing will be complete, but if there has been marked damage, repair is usually necessary and this may result in scarring. If the pathogen persists, the acute inflammatory response is likely to transform into a chronic inflammatory response. This is a slow, smouldering reaction that can continue indefinitely, destroying tissue and promoting local proliferation of cells and connective tissue. The principal cell types found in areas of chronic inflammation are mononuclear cells and abnormal macrophage-derived cells. During healing or chronic inflammation, growth factors trigger angiogenesis and cause fibroblasts to lay down fibrous tissue. Infection by some microorganisms, such as syphilis, tuberculosis and leprosy, bears the characteristic hallmarks of chronic inflammation from the start. The cellular and mediator components of this type of inflammation are also seen in many, if not most, chronic autoimmune and hypersensitivity diseases, and are important targets for drug action.

REFERENCES AND FURTHER READING

The innate and adaptive responses

Abbas, A.K., Murphy, K.M., Sher, A., 1996. Functional diversity of helper lymphocytes. Nature 383, 787–793. (*Excellent review, helpful diagrams; commendable coverage of Th1 and Th2 cells and their respective cytokine subsets*)

Adams, D.H., Lloyd, A.R., 1997. Chemokines: leukocyte recruitment and activation cytokines. Lancet 349, 490–495. (*Commendable review*)

Balamayooran, T., Balamayooran, G., Jeyaseelan, S., 2010. Review: Toll-like receptors and NOD-like receptors in pulmonary antibacterial immunity. Innate Immun. 16, 201–210. (*Although it focuses on the lung, this review is a good introduction to TLRs*)

Delves, P.J., Roitt, I.M., 2000. The immune system. N. Engl. J. Med. 343, 37–49, 108–117. (*A good overview of the immune system – a mini-textbook of major areas in immunology; colourful three-dimensional figures*)

Gabay, C., Kushner, I., 1999. Acute phase proteins and other systemic responses to inflammation. N. Engl. J. Med. 340, 448–454. (*Lists the*

acute-phase proteins and outlines the mechanisms controlling their synthesis and release)

Kärre, K., Welsh, R.M., 1997. Viral decoy vetoes killer cell. Nature 386, 446–447.

Kennedy, M.A., 2010. A brief review of the basics of immunology: the innate and adaptive response. Vet. Clin. North Am. Small Anim. Pract. 40, 369–379. (*Actually written for vets, this little review is an easy-to-read introduction to the subject*)

Kay, A.B., 2001. Allergic diseases and their treatment. N. Engl. J. Med. 344, 30–37, 109–113. (*Covers atopy and Th2 cells, the role of Th2 cytokines in allergies, IgE, the main types of allergy and new therapeutic approaches*)

Mackay, C.R., Lanzavecchia, A., Sallusto, F., 1999. Chemoattractant receptors and immune responses. Immunologist 7, 112–118. (*Masterly short review covering the role of chemoattractants in orchestrating immune responses – both the innate reaction and the Th1 and Th2 responses*)

Medzhitov, R., 2001. Toll-like receptors and innate immunity. Nat. Rev. Immunol. 1, 135–145. (*Excellent review of the role of Toll-like receptors in (a) the detection of microbial infection, and (b) the activation of innate non-adaptive responses, which in turn lead to antigen-specific adaptive responses*)

Medzhitov, R., Janeway, C., 2000. Innate immunity. N. Engl. J. Med. 343, 338–344. (*Outstandingly clear coverage of the mechanisms involved in innate immunity and its significance for the adaptive immune response*)

Mills, K.H., 2008. Induction, function and regulation of IL-17-producing T cells. Eur. J. Immunol. 38, 2636–2649. (*This paper covers the biology of Th17 cells – a relatively recent addition to our understanding of Th biology. Accessible and has good diagrams*)

Murphy, P.M., 2001. Viral exploitation and subversion of the immune system through chemokine mimicry. Nat. Immunol. 2, 116–122. (*Excellent description of viral/immune system interaction*)

Nourshargh, S., Hordijk, P.L., Sixt, M., 2010. Breaching multiple barriers: leukocyte motility through venular walls and the interstitium. Nature Rev. Mol. Cell Biol. 11, 366–378. (*Excellent review of the latest thinking about leukocyte transmigration through blood vessels. Contains excellent diagrams. Recommended*)

Parkin, J., Cohen, B., 2001. An overview of the immune system. Lancet 357, 1777–1789. (*A competent, straightforward review covering the role of the immune system in recognising, repelling and eradicating pathogens and in reacting against molecules foreign to the body*)

Sternberg, E.M., 2006. Neural regulation of innate immunity: a coordinated nonspecific host response to pathogens. Nat. Rev. Immunol. 6, 318–328. (*This paper and the paper by Tracey (below) are both excellent and easy-to-read reviews covering the role of the CNS in inflammation. Some good diagrams*)

Strowig, T., Henao-Mejia, J., Elinav, E., Flavell, R., 2012. Inflammasomes in health and disease. Nature 481, 278–286. (*Excellent, comprehensive review if you want to keep up to date in this area*)

Takeda, K., Akira, S., 2003. Toll receptors and pathogen resistance. Cell. Microbiol. 5, 143–153. (*Useful review and easy to read. Also deals with Toll receptor signalling in some depth*)

Tracey, K.J., 2002. The inflammatory reflex. Nature 420, 853–859.

Vasselon, T., Detmers, P.A., 2002. Toll receptors: a central element in innate immune responses. Infect. Immun. 70, 1033–1041. (*Another comprehensive review on this important topic*)

Wills-Karp, M., Santeliz, J., Karp, C.L., 2001. The germless theory of allergic diseases. Nat. Rev. Immunol. 1, 69–75. (*Discusses the hypothesis that early childhood infections inhibit the tendency to develop allergic disease*)

Books

Dale, M.M., Foreman, J.C., Fan, T.-P. (Eds.), 1994. Textbook of Immunopharmacology, third ed. Blackwell Scientific, Oxford. (*Unfortunately out of print now but if you can get a second hand copy, this excellent textbook contains many sections relevant to this chapter*)

Murphy, K.M., Travers, P., Walport, M., 2011. Janeway's Immunobiology, eighth ed. Taylor & Francis, London. (*A classic textbook now completely updated and available as an e-book also. Excellent diagrams*)

Nijkamp, F.P., Parnham, M. (Eds.), 2011. Principles of Immunopharmacology, third ed. Birkhauser, Basle. (*The latest version of a popular textbook that covers most of the topics in more depth than is possible in this book. Well written and illustrated. Recommended*)

Serhan, C., Ward, P.A., Gilroy, D.W. (Eds.), 2010. Fundamentals of Inflammation. Cambridge University Press, New York. (*A different type of textbook. Individual topics are written by appropriate experts and combined into a single volume. An authoritative and comprehensive volume that provides access to cutting edge thinking in the field. Recommended*)

Method and measurement in pharmacology

7

OVERVIEW

We emphasised in Chapters 2 and 3 that drugs, being molecules, produce their effects by interacting with other molecules. This interaction can lead to effects at all levels of biological organisation, from molecules to human populations.[1]

Gaddum, a pioneering pharmacologist, commented in 1942: 'A branch of science comes of age when it becomes quantitative.' In this chapter, we cover the principles of metrication at the various organisational levels, ranging from laboratory methods to clinical trials. Assessment of drug action at the population level is the concern of pharmaco-epidemiology and pharmacoeconomics (see Ch. 1), disciplines that are beyond the scope of this book.

We consider first the general principles of bioassay, and its extension to studies in human beings; we describe the development of animal models to bridge the predictive gap between animal physiology and human disease; we next discuss aspects of clinical trials used to evaluate therapeutic efficacy in a clinical setting; finally, we consider the principles of balancing benefit and risk. Experimental design and statistical analysis are central to the interpretation of all types of pharmacological data. Kirkwood & Sterne (2003) provide an excellent introduction.

BIOASSAY

Bioassay, defined as the estimation of the concentration or potency of a substance by measurement of the biological response that it produces, has played a key role in the development of pharmacology. Quantitation of drug effects by bioassay is necessary to compare the properties of different substances, or the same substance under different circumstances. It is used:

- to measure the pharmacological activity of new or chemically undefined substances
- to investigate the function of endogenous mediators
- to measure drug toxicity and unwanted effects.

▼ Bioassay plays a key role in the development of new drugs, discussed in Chapter 60.

The use of bioassay to measure the *concentration* of drugs and other active substances in the blood or other body fluids – once an important technology – has now been largely replaced by analytical chemistry techniques.

Many hormones and chemical mediators have been discovered by the biological effects that they produce. For example, the ability of extracts of the posterior lobe of the pituitary to produce a rise in blood pressure and a contraction of the uterus was observed at the beginning of the 20th century. Quantitative assay procedures based on these actions enabled a standard preparation of the extract to be established by international agreement in 1935. By use of these assays, it was shown that two distinct peptides – vasopressin and oxytocin – were responsible, and they were eventually identified and synthesised in 1953. Biological assay had already revealed much about the synthesis, storage and release of the hormones, and was essential for their purification and identification. Nowadays, it does not take 50 years of laborious bioassays to identify new hormones before they are chemically characterised,[2] but bioassay still plays a key role. The recent growth of *biopharmaceuticals* (see Ch. 59) as registered therapeutic agents has relied on bioassay techniques and the establishment of standard preparations. Biopharmaceuticals, whether derived from natural sources (e.g. monoclonal antibodies, vaccines) or by recombinant DNA technology (e.g. erythropoietin), tend to vary from batch to batch, and need to be standardised with respect to their biological activity. Varying glycosylation patterns, for example, which are not detected by immunoassay techniques, may affect biological activity.

BIOLOGICAL TEST SYSTEMS

Nowadays, an important use of bioassay is to provide information that will predict the effect of the drug in the clinical situation (where the aim is to improve function in patients suffering from the effects of disease). The choice of laboratory test systems (*in vitro* and *in vivo* 'models') that provide this predictive link is an important aspect of quantitative pharmacology.

By the 1960s, pharmacologists had become adept at using isolated organs and laboratory animals (usually under anaesthesia) for quantitative experiments, and had developed the principles of bioassay to allow reliable measurements to be made with these sometimes difficult and unpredictable test systems.

Bioassays on different test systems may be run in parallel to reveal the profile of activity of an unknown mediator. Vane and his colleagues studied the generation and destruction of endogenous active substances such as prostanoids (see Ch. 17) in blood by the technique of *cascade superfusion* measuring contraction or relaxation of a series of different smooth muscle test preparations chosen to differentiate between different active constituents of the sample. This technique has been invaluable in studying the production and fate of short-lived mediators such as prostanoids and nitric oxide (Ch. 20).

These 'traditional' assay systems address drug action at the physiological level – roughly, the mid-range of the organisational hierarchy shown in Fig. 7.1. Extension of the range in both directions, towards the molecular and towards the clinical, has taken place since. Binding assays

---

[1]Consider the effect of cocaine on organised crime, of organophosphate 'nerve gases' on the stability of dictatorships or of anaesthetics on the feasibility of surgical procedures for examples of molecular interactions that affect the behaviour of populations and societies.

[2]In 1988, a Japanese group (Yanagisawa et al., 1988) described in a single remarkable paper the bioassay, purification, chemical analysis, synthesis and DNA cloning of a new vascular peptide, *endothelin* (Ch. 22).

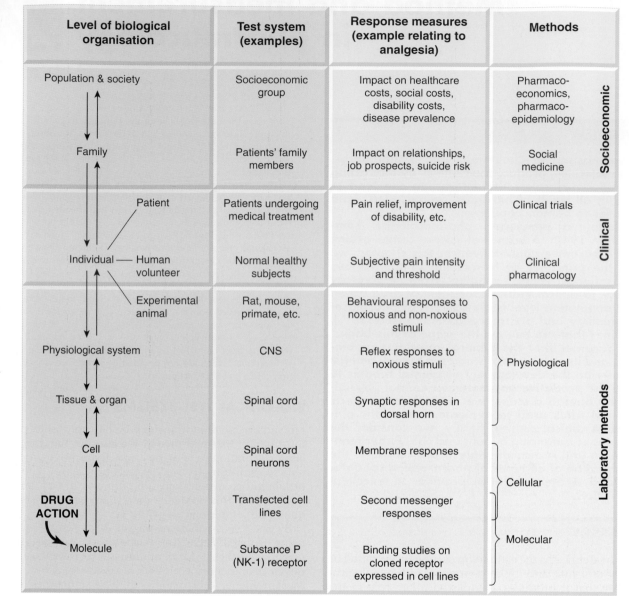

Level of biological organisation	Test system (examples)	Response measures (example relating to analgesia)	Methods	
Population & society	Socioeconomic group	Impact on healthcare costs, social costs, disability costs, disease prevalence	Pharmaco-economics, pharmaco-epidemiology	Socioeconomic
Family	Patients' family members	Impact on relationships, job prospects, suicide risk	Social medicine	
Patient	Patients undergoing medical treatment	Pain relief, improvement of disability, etc.	Clinical trials	Clinical
Individual — Human volunteer	Normal healthy subjects	Subjective pain intensity and threshold	Clinical pharmacology	
Experimental animal	Rat, mouse, primate, etc.	Behavioural responses to noxious and non-noxious stimuli	Physiological	Laboratory methods
Physiological system	CNS	Reflex responses to noxious stimuli		
Tissue & organ	Spinal cord	Synaptic responses in dorsal horn		
Cell	Spinal cord neurons	Membrane responses	Cellular	
DRUG ACTION	Transfected cell lines	Second messenger responses		
Molecule	Substance P (NK-1) receptor	Binding studies on cloned receptor expressed in cell lines	Molecular	

Fig. 7.1 Levels of biological organisation and types of pharmacological measurement.

(Ch. 3) and the use of engineered cell lines expressing normal and mutated receptors and signalling molecules are now widely used. Techniques based on X-ray crystallography, nuclear magnetic resonance spectroscopy and fluorescence signals have thrown much new light on drug action at the molecular level (see reviews by Lohse et al., 2012; Nygaard et al., 2013), and allow for the first time measurement, as well as detection, of the initial molecular events. Indeed, the range of techniques for analysing drug effects at the molecular and cellular levels is now very impressive and expanding rapidly. An example (Fig 7.2) is the use of fluorescence-activated cell sorting (FACS) to measure the effect of a corticosteroid on the expression of a cell surface marker protein by human blood monocytes. Quantitative cellular assays of this kind are now widely used in pharmacology.

These approaches have important implications for basic understanding of drug action, and for drug design, but the need remains for measurement of drug effects at the physiological and clinical level – the focus of this chapter.

Bridging the gap between events at the molecular level and at the physiological and therapeutic levels presents difficulties, because human illness cannot, in many cases, be accurately reproduced in experimental animals. The use of transgenic animals to model human disease is discussed in more detail below.

GENERAL PRINCIPLES OF BIOASSAY

THE USE OF STANDARDS

J.H. Burn wrote in 1950: 'Pharmacologists today strain at the king's arm, but they swallow the frog, rat and mouse, not to mention the guinea pig and the pigeon.' He was referring to the fact that the 'king's arm' had been long since abandoned as a standard measure of length, whereas drug activity continued to be defined in terms of dose

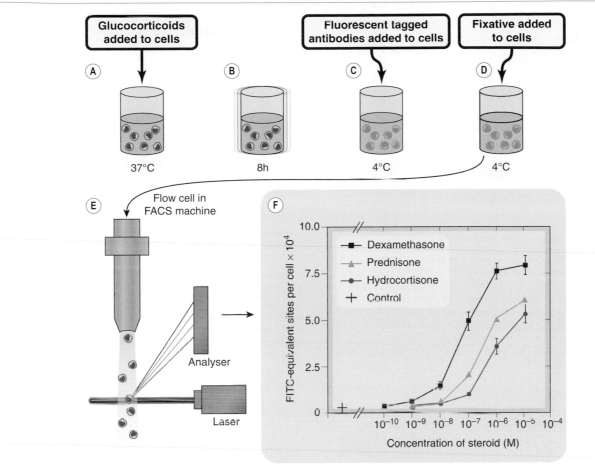

Fig. 7.2 Measuring the effect of glucocorticoid drugs on cell surface receptor expression using FACS (fluorescence activated cell sorting). FACS technology enables the detection and measurement of fluorescent-tagged antibodies attached to structures on individual cells. In this experiment the effect of three glucocorticoids is tested on the expression of a cell-surface haemoglobin scavenger receptor (CD 163). **[A]** Human monocytes were isolated from human venous blood and **[B]** incubated for 8 h alone or with various concentrations of the glucocorticoids dexamethasone, prednisone or hydrocortisone (see Chs 26 and 33). **[C]** The cells were then placed on ice and incubated with fluorescent tagged antibodies to the receptor. **[D]** The cells were then fixed, washed and **[E]** subjected to FACS analysis. In this technique, cells flow through a small tube and are individually scanned by a laser. The reflected light is analysed using a series of filters (so that different coloured fluorescent tags can be used) and the data collected as *fluorescence intensity units*, compared to a standard (FITC) and expressed as 'FITC equivalents' to produce the final results **[F]**, which can be plotted as a conventional log-concentration curve. *(Data courtesy of N Goulding.)*

needed to cause, say, vomiting of a pigeon or cardiac arrest in a mouse. A plethora of 'pigeon units', 'mouse units' and the like, which no two laboratories could agree on, contaminated the literature.[3] Even if two laboratories cannot agree – because their pigeons differ – on the activity in pigeon units of the same sample of an active substance, they should nonetheless be able to agree that preparation X is, say, 3.5 times as active as standard preparation Y on the pigeon test. Biological assays are therefore designed to measure the *relative potency* of two preparations, usually a standard and an unknown. Maintaining stable preparations of various hormones, antisera and other biological

materials, as reference standards, is the task of the UK National Board for Biological Standards Control.

THE DESIGN OF BIOASSAYS

▼ Given the aim of comparing the activity of two preparations, a standard (S) and an unknown (U), on a particular preparation, a bioassay must provide an estimate of the dose or concentration of U that will produce the same biological effect as that of a known dose or concentration of S. As Figure 7.3 shows, provided that the log dose–effect curves for S and U are parallel, the ratio, M, of equiactive doses will not depend on the magnitude of response chosen. Thus M provides an estimate of the potency ratio of the two preparations. A comparison of the magnitude of the effects produced by equal doses of S and U does not provide an estimate of M (see Fig. 7.3).

The main problem with all types of bioassay is that of biological variation, and the design of bioassays is aimed at:

- minimising variation
- avoiding systematic errors resulting from variation
- estimation of the limits of error of the assay result.

---

[3]More picturesque examples of absolute units of the kind that Burn would have frowned on are the PHI and the mHelen. PHI, cited by Colquhoun (1971), stands for 'purity in heart index' and measures the ability of a virgin pure-in-heart to transform, under appropriate conditions, a he-goat into a youth of surpassing beauty. The mHelen is a unit of beauty, 1 mHelen being sufficient to launch one ship.

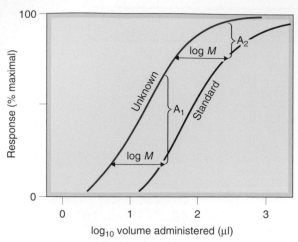

Fig. 7.3 Comparison of the potency of unknown and standard by bioassay. Note that comparing the magnitude of responses produced by the same dose (i.e. volume) of standard and unknown gives no quantitative estimate of their relative potency. (The differences, A_1 and A_2, depend on the dose chosen.) Comparison of equieffective doses of standard and unknown gives a valid measure of their relative potencies. Because the lines are parallel, the magnitude of the effect chosen for the comparison is immaterial; i.e. log M is the same at all points on the curves.

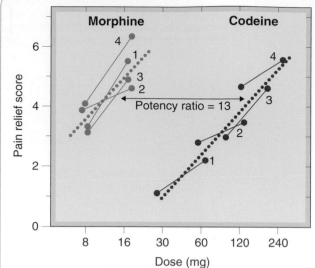

Fig. 7.4 Assay of morphine and codeine as analgesics in humans. Each of four patients (numbered 1–4) was given, on successive occasions in random order, four different treatments (high and low morphine, and high and low codeine) by intramuscular injection, and the subjective pain relief score calculated for each. The calculated regression lines gave a potency ratio estimate of 13 for the two drugs. *(After Houde RW et al. 1965 In: Analgetics. Academic Press, New York.)*

Bioassay

- Bioassay is the measurement of potency of a drug or unknown mediator from the magnitude of the biological effect that it produces.
- Bioassay normally involves comparison of the unknown preparation with a standard. Estimates that are not based on comparison with standards are liable to vary from laboratory to laboratory.
- Comparisons are best made on the basis of dose–response curves, which allow estimates of the equiactive concentrations of unknown and standard to be used as a basis for the potency comparison. Parallel line assays follow this principle.
- The biological response may be *quantal* (the proportion of tests in which a given all-or-nothing effect is produced) or *graded*. Different statistical procedures are appropriate in each case.
- Different approaches to metrication apply according to the level of biological organisation at which the drug effect needs to be measured. Approaches range through molecular and chemical techniques, *in vitro* and *in vivo* animal studies and clinical studies on volunteers and patients, to measurement of effects at the socioeconomic level.

Commonly, comparisons are based on analysis of *dose–response curves*, from which the matching doses of S and U are calculated. The use of a logarithmic dose scale means that the curves for S and U will normally be parallel, and the potency ratio (M) is estimated from the horizontal distance between the two curves (Fig. 7.3).

Assays of this type are known as *parallel line* assays, the minimal design being the 2 + 2 assay, in which two doses of standard (S_1 and S_2) and two of unknown (U_1 and U_2) are used. The doses are chosen to give responses lying on the linear part of the log dose–response curve, and are given repeatedly in randomised order, providing an inherent measure of the variability of the test system, which can be used, by means of straightforward statistical analysis, to estimate the confidence limits of the final result.

A simple example of an experiment to compare two analgesic drugs, morphine and codeine (see Ch. 42) in humans, based on a modified 2 + 2 design is shown in Figure 7.4. Each of the four doses was given on different occasions to each of the four subjects, the order being randomised and both subject and observer being unaware of the dose given. Subjective pain relief was assessed by a trained observer, and the results showed morphine to be 13 times as potent as codeine. This, of course, does not prove its superiority, but merely shows that a smaller dose is needed to produce the same effect. Such a measurement is, however, an essential preliminary to assessing the relative therapeutic merits of the two drugs, for any comparison of other factors, such as side effects, duration of action, tolerance or dependence, needs to be done on the basis of doses that are equiactive as analgesics.

Problems arise if the two log dose–response curves are not parallel, or if the maximal responses differ, which can happen if the mechanism of action of the two drugs differs, or if one is a partial agonist (see Ch. 2). In this case it is not possible to define the relative potencies of S and U unambiguously in terms of a simple ratio and the experimenter must then face up to the fact that the comparison requires measurement of more than a single dimension of potency.

ANIMAL MODELS OF DISEASE

There are many examples where simple intuitive models predict with fair accuracy therapeutic efficacy in humans. Ferrets vomit when placed in swaying cages, and drugs that prevent this are also found to relieve motion sickness and other types of nausea in humans. Irritant chemicals injected into rats' paws cause them to become swollen and tender, and this model predicts very well the efficacy of drugs used for symptomatic relief in inflammatory conditions such as rheumatoid arthritis in humans. As discussed elsewhere in this book, models for many important disorders, such as epilepsy, diabetes, hypertension and gastric ulceration, based on knowledge of the physiology of the condition, are available, and have been used successfully to produce new drugs, even though their success in predicting therapeutic efficacy is far from perfect.[4]

Ideally, an animal model should resemble the human disease in the following ways:

1. similar pathophysiological phenotype (*face validity*)
2. similar causation (*construct validity*)
3. similar response to treatment (*predictive validity*).

In practice, there are many difficulties, and the shortcomings of animal models are one of the main roadblocks on the route from basic medical science to improvements in therapy. The difficulties include the following.

- Many diseases, particularly in psychiatry, are defined by phenomena in humans that are difficult or impossible to observe in animals, which rules out face validity. As far as we know, mania or delusions have no counterpart in rats, nor does anything resembling a migraine attack or autism. Pathophysiological similarity is also inapplicable to conditions such as depression or anxiety disorders, where no clear brain pathology has been defined.
- The 'cause' of many human diseases is complex or unknown. To achieve construct validity for many degenerative diseases (e.g. Alzheimer's disease, osteoarthritis, Parkinson's disease), we need to model the upstream (causative) factors rather than the downstream (symptomatic) features of the disease, although the latter are the basis of most of the simple physiological models used hitherto. The inflammatory pain model mentioned above lacks construct validity for rheumatoid arthritis, which is an autoimmune disease.
- Relying on response to treatment as a test of predictive validity carries the risk that drugs acting by novel mechanisms could be missed, because the model will have been selected on the basis of its responsiveness to known drugs. With schizophrenia (Ch. 46), for example, it is clear that dopamine antagonists are effective, and many of the models used are designed to assess dopamine antagonism in the brain, rather than other potential mechanisms that need to be targeted if drug discovery is to move on to address new targets.

GENETIC AND TRANSGENIC ANIMAL MODELS

Nowadays, genetic approaches are increasingly used as an adjunct to conventional physiological and pharmacological approaches to disease modelling.

Animal models

- Animal models of disease are important for investigating pathogenesis and for the discovery of new therapeutic agents. Animal models generally reproduce imperfectly only certain aspects of human disease states. Models of psychiatric illness are particularly problematic.
- Transgenic animals are produced by introducing mutations into the germ cells of animals (usually mice), which allow new genes to be introduced ('knock-ins') or existing genes to be inactivated ('knockouts') or mutated in a stable strain of animals.
- Transgenic animals are widely used to develop disease models for drug testing. Many such models are now available.
- The induced mutation operates throughout the development and lifetime of the animal, and may be lethal. Techniques of conditional mutagenesis allow the abnormal gene to be switched on or off at a chosen time.

By selective breeding, it is possible to obtain pure animal strains with characteristics closely resembling certain human diseases. Genetic models of this kind include spontaneously hypertensive rats, genetically obese mice, epilepsy-prone dogs and mice, rats with deficient vasopressin secretion, and many other examples. In many cases, the genes responsible have not been identified.

▼ The obese mouse, which arose from a spontaneous mutation in a mouse-breeding facility, is one of the most widely used models for the study of obesity and type 2 diabetes (see Ch. 31). The phenotype results from inactivation of the *leptin* gene, and shows good face validity (high food intake, gross obesity, impaired blood glucose regulation, vascular complications – features characteristic of human obesity) and good predictive validity (responding to pharmacological intervention similarly to humans), but poor construct validity, since obese humans are not leptin deficient.

Genetic manipulation of the germline to generate *transgenic animals* (see Rudolph & Moehler, 1999; Offermanns & Hein, 2004) is of growing importance as a means of generating animal models that replicate human disease and are expected to be predictive of therapeutic drug effects in humans. This versatile technology, first reported in 1980, can be used in many different ways, for example:

- to inactivate individual genes, or mutate them to pathological forms
- to introduce new (e.g. human) genes
- to overexpress genes by inserting additional copies
- to allow gene expression to be controlled by the experimenter.[5]

Currently, most transgenic technologies are applicable in mice but much more difficult in other mammals. Other vertebrates (e.g. zebrafish) and invertebrates (*Drosophila, Caenorhabditis elegans*) are increasingly used for drug screening purposes.

Examples of such models include transgenic mice that overexpress mutated forms of the *amyloid precursor protein* or *presenilins*, which are important in the pathogenesis of Alzheimer's disease (see Ch. 40). When they are a few months old, these mice develop pathological lesions and cognitive changes resembling Alzheimer's disease, and provide very useful models with which to test possible new therapeutic approaches. Another neurodegenerative condition, Parkinson's disease (Ch. 40), has been modelled in transgenic mice that overexpress *synuclein*, a protein found in the brain inclusions that are characteristic of the disease. Transgenic mice with mutations in tumour suppressor genes and oncogenes (see Ch. 5) are widely used as models for human cancers. Mice in which the gene for a particular adenosine receptor subtype has been inactivated show distinct behavioural and cardiovascular abnormalities, such as increased aggression, reduced response to noxious stimuli and raised blood pressure. These findings serve to pinpoint the physiological role of this receptor, whose function was hitherto unknown, and to suggest new ways in which agonists or antagonists for these receptors might be developed for therapeutic use (e.g. to reduce aggressive behaviour or to treat hypertension). Transgenic mice can, however, be misleading in relation to human disease. For example, the gene defect responsible for causing cystic fibrosis (a disease affecting mainly the lungs in humans), when reproduced in mice, causes a disorder that mainly affects the intestine.

PHARMACOLOGICAL STUDIES IN HUMANS

Studies involving human subjects range from experimental pharmacodynamic or pharmacokinetic investigations to formal clinical trials. Non-invasive recording methods, such as *functional magnetic resonance imaging* to measure regional blood flow in the brain (a surrogate for neuronal activity) and *ultrasonography* to measure cardiac performance, have greatly extended the range of what is possible. The scientific principles underlying experimental work in humans, designed, for example, to check whether mechanisms that operate in other species also apply to humans, or to take advantage of the much broader response capabilities of a person compared with a rat, are the same as for animals, but the ethical and safety issues are paramount, and ethical committees associated with all medical research centres tightly control the type of experiment that can be done, weighing up not only safety and ethical issues, but also the scientific importance of the proposed study. At the other end of the spectrum of experimentation on humans are formal *clinical trials*, often involving thousands of patients, aimed at answering specific questions regarding the efficacy and safety of new drugs.

CLINICAL TRIALS

Clinical trials are an important and highly specialised form of biological assay, designed specifically to measure therapeutic efficacy and detect adverse effects. The need to use patients undergoing treatment for experimental purposes raises serious ethical considerations, and imposes many restrictions. Here, we discuss some of the basic principles involved in clinical trials; the role of such trials in the course of drug development is described in Chapter 60.

A clinical trial is a method for comparing objectively, by a prospective study, the results of two or more therapeutic procedures. For new drugs, this is carried out during phases II and III of clinical development (Ch. 60). It is important to realise that, until about 50 years ago, methods of treatment were chosen on the basis of clinical impression and personal experience rather than objective testing.[6] Although many drugs, with undoubted effectiveness, remain in use without ever having been subjected to a controlled clinical trial, any new drug is now required to have been tested in this way before being licensed for clinical use.[7]

On the other hand, **digitalis** (see Ch. 21) was used for 200 years to treat cardiac failure before a controlled trial showed it to be of very limited value except in a particular type of patient.

An introduction to the principles and organisation of clinical trials is given by Hackshaw (2009). A clinical trial aims to compare the response of a test group of patients receiving a new treatment (A) with that of a control group receiving an existing 'standard' treatment (B). Treatment A might be a new drug or a new combination of existing drugs, or any other kind of therapeutic intervention, such as a surgical operation, a diet, physiotherapy and so on. The standard against which it is judged (treatment B) might be a currently used drug treatment or (if there is no currently available effective treatment) a placebo or no treatment at all.

The use of controls is crucial in clinical trials. Claims of therapeutic efficacy based on reports that, for example, 16 out of 20 patients receiving drug X got better within 2 weeks are of no value without a knowledge of how 20 patients receiving no treatment, or a different treatment, would have fared. Usually, the controls are provided by a separate group of patients from those receiving the test treatment, but sometimes a crossover design is possible in which the same patients are switched from test to control treatment or vice versa, and the results compared. Randomisation is essential to avoid bias in assigning individual patients to test or control groups. Hence, the *randomised controlled clinical trial* is now regarded as the essential tool for assessing clinical efficacy of new drugs.

---

[6]Not exclusively. James Lind conducted a controlled trial in 1753 on 12 mariners, which showed that oranges and lemons offered protection against scurvy. However, 40 years passed before the British Navy acted on his advice, and a further century before the US Navy did.

[7]It is fashionable in some quarters to argue that to require evidence of efficacy of therapeutic procedures in the form of a controlled trial runs counter to the doctrines of 'holistic' medicine. This is a fundamentally antiscientific view, for science advances only by generating predictions from hypotheses and by subjecting the predictions to experimental test. 'Alternative' medical procedures, such as homeopathy, aromatherapy, acupuncture or 'detox', have rarely been so tested, and where they have, they generally lack efficacy. Standing up for the scientific approach is the *evidence-based medicine* movement (see Sackett et al., 1996), which sets out strict criteria for assessing therapeutic efficacy, based on randomised, controlled clinical trials, and urges scepticism about therapeutic doctrines whose efficacy has not been so demonstrated.

Concern inevitably arises over the ethics of assigning patients at random to particular treatment groups (or to no treatment). However, the reason for setting up a trial is that doubt exists whether the test treatment offers greater benefit than the control treatment. All would agree on the principle of informed consent,[8] whereby each patient must be told the nature and risks of the trial, and agree to participate on the basis that he or she will be randomly and unknowingly assigned to either the test or the control group. The regularly updated 'Declaration of Helsinki' sets out the widely accepted ground rules governing research on human subjects.

Unlike the kind of bioassay discussed earlier, the clinical trial does not normally give any information about potency or the form of the dose–response curve, but merely compares the response produced by two or more stipulated therapeutic regimens. Survival curves provide one commonly used measure. Figure 7.5 shows rates of disease-free survival in two groups of breast cancer patients treated with conventional chemotherapy with and without the addition of paclitaxel (see Ch. 56). The divergence of the curves shows that paclitaxel significantly improved the clinical response. Additional

questions may be posed, such as the incidence and severity of side effects, or whether the treatment works better or worse in particular classes of patient, but only at the expense of added complexity and numbers of patients. The investigator must decide in advance what dose to use and how often to give it, and the trial will reveal only whether the chosen regimen performed better or worse than the control treatment. Unless different doses are compared, it will not say whether increasing or decreasing the dose would have improved the response. The basic question posed by a clinical trial is thus simpler than that addressed by most conventional bioassays. However, the organisation of clinical trials, with controls against bias, is immeasurably more complicated, time-consuming and expensive than that of any laboratory-based assay. Much of the time and cost of developing a new drug is taken up by clinical trials.

AVOIDANCE OF BIAS

There are two main strategies that aim to minimise bias in clinical trials, namely:

1. randomisation
2. the double-blind technique.

If two treatments, A and B, are being compared on a series of selected patients, the simplest form of randomisation is to allocate each patient to A or B by reference to a series of random numbers. One difficulty, particularly if the groups are small, is that the two groups may turn out to be ill-matched with respect to characteristics such as age, sex or disease severity. *Stratified randomisation* avoids the difficulty by dividing the subjects into age, sex, severity, or other categories, random allocation to A or B being used within each category. It is possible to treat two or more characteristics of the trial population in this way, but the number of strata can quickly become large, and the process is self-defeating when the number of subjects in each becomes too small. As well as avoiding error resulting from imbalance of groups assigned to A and B, stratification can also allow more sophisticated conclusions to be reached. B might, for example, prove to be better than A in a particular group of patients even if it is not significantly better overall.

The double-blind technique, whereby neither subject nor investigator is aware at the time of the assessment which treatment is being used, is intended to minimise subjective bias. It has been repeatedly shown that, with the best will in the world, subjects and investigators both contribute to bias if they know which treatment is which, so the use of a double-blind technique is an important safeguard. It is not always possible, however. A dietary regimen, for example, can seldom be disguised; with drugs, pharmacological effects may reveal to patients what they are taking and predispose them to report accordingly.[9] In general, however, the double-blind

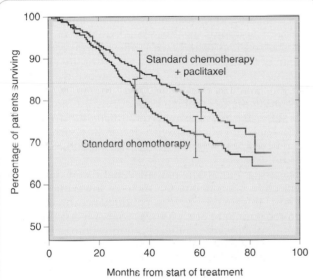

Fig. 7.5 Disease-free survival curves followed for 8 years in matched groups of breast cancer patients treated with a standard chemotherapy regime alone (629 patients), or with addition of paclitaxel (613 patients), showing a highly significant ($P = 0.006$) improvement with paclitaxel. Error bars represent 95% confidence intervals. *(Redrawn from Martin et al. 2008 J Natl Cancer Inst 100, 805–814.)*

---

[8]Even this can be contentious, because patients who are unconscious, demented or mentally ill are unable to give such consent, yet no one would want to preclude trials that might offer improved therapies to these needy patients. Clinical trials in children are particularly problematic but are necessary if the treatment of childhood diseases is to be placed on the same evidence base as is judged appropriate for adults. There are many examples where experience has shown that children respond differently from adults, and there is now increasing pressure on pharmaceutical companies to perform trials in children, despite the difficulties of carrying out such studies. The same concerns apply to trials in elderly patients.

---

[9]The distinction between a true pharmacological response and a beneficial clinical effect produced by the knowledge (based on the pharmacological effects that the drug produces) that an active drug is being administered is not easy to draw, and we should not expect a mere clinical trial to resolve such a tricky semantic issue.

procedure, with precautions if necessary to disguise such clues as the taste or appearance of the two drugs, is used whenever possible.[10]

THE SIZE OF THE SAMPLE

Both ethical and financial considerations dictate that the trial should involve the minimum number of subjects, and much statistical thought has gone into the problem of deciding in advance how many subjects will be required to produce a useful result. The results of a trial cannot be absolutely conclusive, because it is based on a sample of patients, and there is always a chance that the sample was atypical of the population from which it came. Two types of erroneous conclusion are possible, referred to as *type I* and *type II errors*. A type I error occurs if the results show a difference between A and B when none actually exists (false positive). A type II error occurs if no difference is found although A and B do actually differ (false negative). A major factor that determines the size of sample needed is the degree of certainty the investigator seeks in avoiding either type of error. The probability of incurring a type I error is expressed as the *significance* of the result. To say that A and B are different at the $P < 0.05$ level of significance means that the probability of obtaining a false positive result (i.e. incurring a type I error) is less than 1 in 20. For most purposes, this level of significance is considered acceptable as a basis for drawing conclusions.

The probability of avoiding a type II error (i.e. failing to detect a real difference between A and B) is termed the *power* of the trial. We tend to regard type II errors more leniently than type I errors, and trials are often designed with a power of 0.8–0.9. To increase the significance and the power of a trial requires more patients. The second factor that determines the sample size required is the magnitude of difference between A and B that is regarded as clinically significant. For example, to detect that a given treatment reduces the mortality in a certain condition by at least 10 percentage points, say from 50% (in the control group) to 40% (in the treated group), would require 850 subjects, assuming that we wanted to achieve a $P < 0.05$ level of significance and a power of 0.9. If we were content only to reveal a reduction by 20 percentage points (and very likely miss a reduction by 10 points), only 210 subjects would be needed. In this example, missing a real 10-point reduction in mortality could result in abandonment of a treatment that would save 100 lives for every 1000 patients treated – an extremely serious mistake from society's point of view. This simple example emphasises the need to assess clinical benefit (which is often difficult to quantify) in parallel with statistical considerations (which are fairly straightforward) in planning trials.

▼ A trial may give a significant result before the planned number of patients have been enrolled, so it is common for interim analyses to be carried out at intervals (by an independent team so that the trial team remains unaware of the results). If this analysis gives a conclusive result, or if it shows that continuation is unlikely to give a conclusive result, the trial can be terminated, thus reducing the number of subjects tested. In one such large-scale trial (Beta-blocker Heart Attack Trial Research Group, 1982) of the value of long-term treatment with the β-adrenoceptor-blocking drug **propranolol** (Ch. 14) following heart attacks, the interim results showed a significant reduction in mortality, which led to the early termination of the trial. In another, the Cardiac Arrhythmia Suppression Trial (CAST, Echt et al., 1991), the trial was stopped because the treatment group, contrary to expectation, showed increased mortality compared with placebo.

Recently, the tendency has been to perform very large-scale trials, to allow several different treatment protocols, in various different patient groups to be compared. An example is the ALLHAT trial of various antihypertensive and lipid-lowering drugs to improve the outcome in cardiovascular disease (see Ch. 22). This ran from 1994 to 2002, cost US$130 million, and involved more than 42 000 patients in 623 treatment centres, with an army of coordinators and managers to keep it on track. One of its several far-reaching conclusions was that a cheap and familiar diuretic drug in use for more than 50 years was more effective than more recent and expensive antihypertensive drugs.[11]

CLINICAL OUTCOME MEASURES

The measurement of clinical outcome can be a complicated business, and is becoming increasingly so as society becomes more preoccupied with assessing the efficacy of therapeutic procedures in terms of improved length and quality of life, and societal and economic benefit. Various scales for assessing 'health-related quality of life' have been devised and tested (see Walley & Haycocks, 1997); these may be combined with measures of life expectancy to arrive at the measure 'quality-adjusted life years' (QALYs) as an overall measure of therapeutic efficacy, which attempts to combine both survival time and relief from suffering in assessing overall benefit.[12] In planning clinical trials, it is necessary to decide the purpose of the trial in advance, and to define the outcome measures accordingly.

Measuring long-term patient benefit may take years, so objective clinical effects, such as lowering of blood pressure, improved airways conductance or change in white cell count are often used as trial outcome measures. These *surrogate markers* reflect pathophysiological changes of which the patient is most likely unaware. In many cases such changes correlate well with clinical outcome as it affects the patient; not always, though. In the CAST trial (see above), anti-arrhythmic drugs were found to suppress certain ventricular arrhythmias (the surrogate marker), but to *increase* sudden cardiac deaths, So regulatory authorities are rightly cautious about accepting surrogate endpoints as a measure of actual patient benefit.

---

[10]Maintaining the blind can be problematic. In an attempt to determine whether **melatonin** is effective in countering jet lag, a pharmacologist investigator recruited a group of fellow pharmacologists attending a congress in Australia, providing them with unlabelled capsules of melatonin or placebo, with a jet lag questionnaire to fill in when they arrived. Some of them (one of the authors included), with analytical resources easily to hand, opened the capsules and consigned them to the bin on finding that they contained placebo. Pharmacologists are only human.

[11]Though without much impact so far on prescribing habits, owing to the marketing muscle of pharmaceutical companies.

[12]As may be imagined, trading off duration and quality of life raises issues about which many of us feel decidedly squeamish. Not so economists, however. They approach the problem by asking such questions as: 'How many years of life would you be prepared to sacrifice in order to live the rest of your life free of the disability you are currently experiencing?' Or, even more disturbingly: 'If, given your present condition, you could gamble on surviving free of disability for your normal lifespan, or (if you lose the gamble) dying immediately, what odds would you accept?' Imagine being asked this by your doctor. 'But I only wanted something for my sore throat,' you protest weakly.

PLACEBOS

▼ A placebo is a dummy medicine containing no active ingredient (or alternatively, a dummy surgical procedure, diet or other kind of therapeutic intervention), which the patient believes is (or could be, in the context of a controlled trial) the real thing. The 'placebo response' (see review by Enck et al., 2013) is widely believed to be a powerful therapeutic effect,[13] producing a significant beneficial effect in about one-third of patients. While many clinical trials include a placebo group that shows improvement, few have compared this group directly with untreated controls. A survey of these trial results (Hróbjartsson & Gøtzsche, 2001) concluded (controversially) that the placebo effect was often insignificant, except in the case of pain relief, where it was small but significant. They concluded that the popular belief in the strength of the placebo effect is misplaced, and probably reflects in part the tendency of many symptoms to improve spontaneously and in part the reporting bias of patients who want to please their doctors. The ethical case for using placebos as therapy, which has been the subject of much public discussion, may therefore be weaker than has been argued. The risks of placebo therapies should not be underestimated. The use of active medicines may be delayed. The necessary element of deception[14] risks undermining the confidence of patients in the integrity of doctors. A state of 'therapy dependence' may be produced in people who are not ill, because there is no way of assessing whether a patient still 'needs' the placebo.

META-ANALYSIS

▼ It is possible, by the use of statistical techniques, to combine the data obtained in several individual trials (provided each has been conducted according to a randomised design) in order to gain greater power and significance. This procedure, known as meta-analysis or overview analysis, can be very useful in arriving at a conclusion on the basis of several published trials, of which some claimed superiority of the test treatment over the control while others did not. As an objective procedure, it is certainly preferable to the 'take your pick' approach to conclusion-forming adopted by most human beings when confronted with contradictory data. It has several drawbacks, however (see Naylor, 1997), the main one being 'publication bias', because negative studies are less likely to be published than positive studies, partly because they are considered less interesting, or, more seriously, because publication would harm the business of the pharmaceutical company that performed the trial.[15] Double counting, caused by the same data being incorporated into more than one trial report, is another problem.

The published clinical trials literature contains reports of many trials that are poorly designed and unreliable. The Cochrane Collaboration (www.cochrane.org) sifts carefully through the literature and produces *systematic reviews* that collate and combine data only from trials (of drugs and other therapeutic interventions) that meet strict quality criteria. About 5000 such 'gold-standard' summaries are available, and provide the most reliable evaluation of trials data on a wide range of therapeutic drugs.

BALANCING BENEFIT AND RISK

THERAPEUTIC INDEX

▼ The concept of therapeutic index aims to provide a measure of the margin of safety of a drug, by drawing attention to the relationship between the effective and toxic doses:

Clinical trials

- A clinical trial is a special type of bioassay done to compare the clinical efficacy of a new drug or procedure with that of a known drug or procedure (or a placebo).
- At its simplest, the aim is a straight comparison of unknown (A) with standard (B) at a single-dose level. The result may be: 'B better than A', 'B worse than A', or 'No difference detected'. Efficacy, not potency, is compared.
- To avoid bias, clinical trials should be:
  - *controlled* (comparison of A with B, rather than study of A alone)
  - *randomised* (assignment of subjects to A or B on a random basis)
  - *double-blind* (neither subject nor assessor knows whether A or B is being used).
- Type I errors (concluding that A is better than B when the difference is actually due to chance) and type II errors (concluding that A is not different from B because a real difference has escaped detection) can occur; the likelihood of either kind of error decreases as the sample size and number of end-point events is increased.
- Interim analysis of data, carried out by an independent group, may be used as a basis for terminating a trial prematurely if the data are already conclusive, or if a clear result is unlikely to be reached.
- All experiments on human subjects require approval by an independent ethical committee.
- Clinical trials require very careful planning and execution, and are inevitably expensive.
- Clinical outcome measures may comprise:
  - physiological measures (e.g. blood pressure, liver function tests, airways function)
  - subjective assessments (e.g. pain relief, mood)
  - long-term outcome (e.g. survival or freedom from recurrence)
  - overall 'quality of life' measures
  - 'quality-adjusted life years' (QALYs), which combine survival with quality of life.
- Meta-analysis is a statistical technique used to pool the data from several independent trials.

$$\text{Therapeutic index} = LD_{50} / ED_{50}$$

where LD_{50} is the dose that is lethal in 50% of the population, and ED_{50} is the dose that is 'effective' in 50%. Obviously, it can only be measured in animals, and it is not a useful guide to the safety of a drug in clinical use for several reasons:

- LD_{50} does not reflect the incidence of adverse effects in the therapeutic setting.[16]
- ED_{50} depends on what measure of effectiveness is used. For example, the ED_{50} for **aspirin** used for a mild headache is much lower than for aspirin as an antirheumatic drug.

---

[13]Its opposite, the *nocebo effect*, describes the adverse effects reported with dummy medicines.
[14]Surprisingly, deception may not even be necessary. Kaptchuk et al. (2010) found that symptoms of irritable bowel syndrome were improved slightly more in patients given inert sugar pills, described as such by the physician, than in patients given no pills. The effect was, however, small, and the patients were encouraged to think that the pills might engage 'mind-body healing processes'.
[15]Measures are now in place to ensure that all clinical trials are registered and the results published, so this problem should disappear.

---

[16]Ironically, **thalidomide** – probably the most harmful drug ever marketed – was promoted specifically on the basis of its exceptionally high therapeutic index (i.e. it killed rats only when given in extremely large doses).

- Both efficacy and toxicity are subject to individual variation. Individual differences in the effective dose or the toxic dose of a drug makes it inherently less predictable, and therefore less safe, although this is not reflected in the therapeutic index.

OTHER MEASURES OF BENEFIT AND RISK

▼ Alternative ways of quantifying the benefits and risks of drugs in clinical use have received much attention. One useful approach is to estimate from clinical trial data the proportion of test and control patients who will experience (a) a defined level of clinical benefit (e.g. survival beyond 2 years, pain relief to a certain predetermined level, slowing of cognitive decline by a given amount) and (b) adverse effects of defined degree. These estimates of proportions of patients showing beneficial or harmful reactions can be expressed as *number needed to treat* (NNT; i.e. the number of patients who need to be treated in order for one to show the given effect, whether beneficial or adverse). For example, in a recent study of pain relief by antidepressant drugs compared with placebo, the findings were: for benefit (a defined level of pain relief), NNT = 3; for minor unwanted effects, NNT = 3; for major adverse effects, NNT = 22. Thus of 100 patients treated with the drug, on average 33 will experience pain relief, 33 will experience minor unwanted effects, and 4 or 5 will experience major adverse effects, information that is helpful in guiding therapeutic choices. One advantage of this type of analysis is that it can take into account the underlying disease severity in quantifying benefit. Thus if drug A halves the mortality of an often

fatal disease (reducing it from 50% to 25%, say), the NNT to save one life is 4; if drug B halves the mortality of a rarely fatal disease (reducing it from 5% to 2.5%, say), the NNT to save one life is 40. Notwithstanding other considerations, drug A is judged to be more valuable than drug B, even though both reduce mortality by one-half. Furthermore, the clinician must realise that to save one life with drug B, 40 patients must be exposed to a risk of adverse effects, whereas only 4 are exposed for each life saved with drug A.

Determination of risk and benefit

- *Therapeutic index* (lethal dose for 50% of the population divided by effective dose for 50%) is unsatisfactory as a measure of drug safety because:
  - it is based on animal toxicity data, which may not reflect forms of toxicity or adverse reactions that are important clinically
  - it takes no account of idiosyncratic toxic reactions.
- More sophisticated measures of risk–benefit analysis for drugs in clinical use are available, and include the *number needed to treat* (NNT) principle.

REFERENCES AND FURTHER READING

General references

Colquhoun, D., 1971. Lectures on Biostatistics. Oxford University Press, Oxford. (*Standard textbook*)

Kirkwood, B.R., Sterne, J.A.C., 2003. Medical Statistics, second ed. Blackwell, Malden. (*Clear introductory textbook covering statistical principles and methods*)

Walley, T., Haycocks, A., 1997. Pharmacoeconomics: basic concepts and terminology. Br. J. Clin. Pharmacol. 43, 343–348. (*Useful introduction to analytical principles that are becoming increasingly important for therapeutic policy makers*)

Yanagisawa, M., Kurihara, H., Kimura, S., et al., 1988. A novel potent vasoconstrictor peptide produced by vascular endothelial cells. Nature 332, 411–415. (*The first paper describing endothelin – a remarkably full characterisation of an important new mediator*)

Molecular methods

Lohse, M.J., Nuber, S., Hoffmann, C., 2012. Fluorescence/ bioluminescence resonance energy transfer techniques to study G protein-coupled receptor activation and signaling. Pharmacol. Rev. 64, 299–336. (*Review of modern fluorescence-based methods for studying GPCR function*)

Nygaard, R., Zou, Y., Dror, R.O., et al., 2013. The dynamic process of β(2)-adrenergic receptor activation. Cell 152 (3), 532–542. (*Review demonstrating the use of modern spectroscopic techniques to measure the effects of ligands on receptor conformation*)

Animal models

Offermanns, S., Hein, L. (Eds.), 2004. Transgenic models in pharmacology. Handb. Exp. Pharmacol. 159. (*A comprehensive series of review articles describing transgenic mouse models used to study different pharmacological mechanisms and disease states*)

Ristevski, S., 2005. Making better transgenic models: conditional, temporal, and spatial approaches. Mol. Biotechnol. 29, 153–164. (*Description of methods for controlling transgene expression*)

Rudolph, U., Moehler, H., 1999. Genetically modified animals in pharmacological research: future trends. Eur. J. Pharmacol. 375, 327–337. (*Good review of uses of transgenic animals in pharmacological research, including application to disease models*)

Clinical trials

Beta-blocker Heart Attack Trial Research Group, 1982. A randomised trial of propranolol in patients with acute myocardial infarction. 1. Mortality results. JAMA 247, 1707–1714. (*A trial that was terminated early when clear evidence of benefit emerged*)

Echt, D.S., Liebson, P.R., Mitchell, L.B., et al., 1991. Mortality and morbidity in patients receiving encainide, flecainide, or placebo. The Cardiac Arrhythmia Suppression Trial. N. Engl. J. Med. 324, 781–788. (*Important trial showing that antiarrhythmic drugs, which were expected to reduce sudden deaths after a heart attack, have the opposite effect*)

Enck, P., Bigel, U., Schedlowski, M., Rief, W., 2013. The placebo response in medicine: minimize, maximize or personalize? Nat. Rev. Drug Discov. 12, 191–204. (*Comprehensive review of a slippery phenomenon*)

Hackshaw, A., 2009. A Concise Guide to Clinical Trials. Wiley Blackwell. (*Short introductory textbook*)

Hróbjartsson, A., Gøtzsche, P.C., 2001. Is the placebo powerless? An analysis of clinical trials comparing placebo with no treatment. N. Engl. J. Med. 344, 1594–1601. (*An important meta-analysis of clinical trial data, which shows, contrary to common belief, that placebos in general have no significant effect on clinical outcome, except – to a small degree – in pain relief trials. Confirmed in an extended analysis: J. Int. Med. 2004, 256, 91–100*)

Kaptchuk, T.J., Friedlander, E., Kelley, J.M., Sanchez, M.N., Kokkotou, E., et al., 2010. Placebos without deception: A randomized controlled trial in irritable bowel syndrome. PLoS ONE 5 (12), e15591. (*Study showing that placebo pills have a significant effect even if the patient knows that they contain no active ingredient*)

Naylor, C.D., 1997. Meta-analysis and the meta-epidemiology of clinical research. Br. Med. J. 315, 617–619. (*Thoughtful review on the strengths and weaknesses of meta-analysis*)

Sackett, D.L., Rosenburg, W.M.C., Muir-Gray, J.A., et al., 1996. Evidence-based medicine: what it is and what it isn't. Br. Med. J. 312, 71–72. (*Balanced account of the value of evidence-based medicine – an important recent trend in medical thinking*)

Absorption and distribution of drugs

8

OVERVIEW

The physical processes of diffusion, penetration of membranes, binding to plasma protein and partition into fat and other tissues underlie the absorption and distribution of drugs. These processes are described, followed by more specific coverage of the process of drug absorption and related practical issue of routes of drug administration, and of the distribution of drugs into different bodily compartments. Drug interactions caused by one drug altering the absorption or distribution of another are described. There is a short final section on special drug delivery systems designed to deliver drugs efficiently and selectively to their sites of action.

INTRODUCTION

Drug disposition is divided into four stages designated by the acronym 'ADME':

- Absorption from the site of administration
- Distribution within the body
- Metabolism
- Excretion

General aspects of drug absorption and distribution are considered here, together with routes of administration. Absorption and distribution of inhalation general anaesthetics (a special case) are described in Ch. 41. Metabolism and excretion are covered in Chapter 9. We begin with a description of the physical processes that underlie drug disposition.

PHYSICAL PROCESSES UNDERLYING DRUG DISPOSITION

Drug molecules move around the body in two ways:

- bulk flow (i.e. in the bloodstream, lymphatics or cerebrospinal fluid)
- diffusion (i.e. molecule by molecule, over short distances).

The chemical nature of a drug makes no difference to its transfer by bulk flow. The cardiovascular system provides a rapid long-distance distribution system. In contrast, diffusional characteristics differ markedly between different drugs. In particular, ability to cross hydrophobic diffusion barriers is strongly influenced by lipid solubility. Aqueous diffusion is part of the overall mechanism of drug transport, because it is this process that delivers drug molecules to and from the non-aqueous barriers. The rate of diffusion of a substance depends mainly on its molecular size, the *diffusion coefficient* being inversely proportional to the square root of molecular weight. Consequently, while large molecules diffuse more slowly than small ones, the variation with molecular weight is modest. Many drugs fall within the molecular weight range 200–1000 Da, and variations in aqueous diffusion rate have only a small effect on their overall pharmacokinetic behaviour. For most purposes, we can regard the body as a series of interconnected well-stirred compartments within each of which the drug concentration is uniform. It is movement *between* compartments, generally involving penetration of non-aqueous diffusion barriers that determines where, and for how long, a drug will be present in the body after it has been administered. The analysis of drug movements with the help of a simple compartmental model is discussed in Chapter 9.

THE MOVEMENT OF DRUG MOLECULES ACROSS CELL BARRIERS

Cell membranes form the barriers between aqueous compartments in the body. A single layer of membrane separates the intracellular from the extracellular compartments. An epithelial barrier, such as the gastrointestinal mucosa or renal tubule, consists of a layer of cells tightly connected to each other so that molecules must traverse at least two cell membranes (inner and outer) to pass from one side to the other. The anatomical disposition and permeability of vascular endothelium (the cell layer that separates intravascular from extravascular compartments) varies from one tissue to another. Gaps between endothelial cells are packed with a loose matrix of proteins that act as filters, retaining large molecules and letting smaller ones through. The cut-off of molecular size is not exact: water permeates rapidly whereas molecules of 80 000–100 000 Da permeate very slowly. In some organs, especially the central nervous system (CNS) and the placenta, there are tight junctions between the cells, and the endothelium is encased in an impermeable layer of periendothelial cells (*pericytes*). These features prevent potentially harmful molecules from penetrating to brain or fetus and have major consequences for drug distribution and activity.[1]

In other organs (e.g. the liver and spleen), endothelium is discontinuous, allowing free passage between cells. In the liver, hepatocytes form the barrier between intra- and extravascular compartments and take on several

---

[1] This is illustrated by strain and species differences. For example, Collie dogs lack the multidrug resistance gene (*mdr1*) and a P-glycoprotein that contributes importantly to the blood–brain barrier, with consequences for veterinary medicine because **ivermectin** (an anthelminthic drug, Ch. 55) is severely neurotoxic in the many breeds with Collie ancestry.

endothelial cell functions. Fenestrated endothelium occurs in endocrine glands, facilitating transfer to the bloodstream of hormones or other molecules through pores in the endothelium. Formation of fenestrated endothelium is controlled by a specific endocrine gland-derived vascular endothelial growth factor (dubbed EG-VEGF). Endothelial cells lining postcapillary venules have specialised functions relating to leukocyte migration and inflammation and the sophistication of the intercellular junction can be appreciated from the observation that leukocyte migration can occur without any detectable leak of water or small ions (see Ch. 6).

There are four main ways by which small molecules cross cell membranes (Fig. 8.1):

- by diffusing directly through the lipid
- by combination with a *solute carrier* (SLC) or other membrane transporter
- by diffusing through aqueous pores formed by special proteins (*aquaporins*) that traverse the lipid
- by *pinocytosis*.

Of these routes, diffusion through lipid and carrier-mediated transport are particularly important in relation to pharmacokinetic mechanisms.

▼ Diffusion through aquaporins (membrane glycoproteins that can be blocked by mercurial reagents such as *para*-chloromercurobenzene sulfonate) is probably important in the transfer of gases such as carbon dioxide, but the pores are too small in diameter (about 0.4 nm) to allow most drug molecules (which usually exceed 1 nm in diameter) to pass through. Consequently, drug distribution is not notably abnormal in patients with genetic diseases affecting aquaporins. Pinocytosis involves invagination of part of the cell membrane and the trapping within the cell of a small vesicle containing extracellular constituents. The vesicle contents can then be released within the cell, or extruded from its other side. This mechanism is important for the transport of some macromolecules (e.g. **insulin**, which crosses the blood–brain barrier by this process), but not for small molecules.

DIFFUSION THROUGH LIPID

Non-polar molecules (in which electrons are uniformly distributed) dissolve freely in membrane lipids, and consequently diffuse readily across cell membranes. The number of molecules crossing the membrane per unit area

in unit time is determined by the *permeability coefficient, P,* and the concentration difference across the membrane. Permeant molecules must be present within the membrane in sufficient numbers and must be mobile within the membrane if rapid permeation is to occur. Thus, two physicochemical factors contribute to P, namely *solubility* in the membrane (which can be expressed as a partition coefficient for the substance distributed between the membrane phase and the aqueous environment) and *diffusivity*, which is a measure of the mobility of molecules within the lipid and is expressed as a diffusion coefficient. The diffusion coefficient varies only modestly between conventional drugs, as noted above (macromolecular biopharmaceuticals – see Ch. 59 – are an exception), so the most important determinant of membrane permeability for conventional low-molecular-weight drugs is the partition coefficient (Fig. 8.2). Many pharmacokinetic characteristics of a drug – such as rate of absorption from the gut, penetration into different tissues and the extent of renal elimination – can be predicted from knowledge of a drug's lipid solubility.

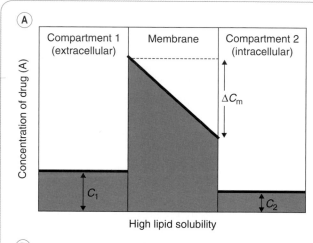

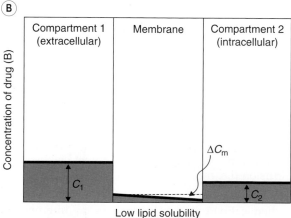

Fig. 8.2 **The importance of lipid solubility in membrane permeation.** [**A**] and [**B**] Figures show the concentration profile in a lipid membrane separating two aqueous compartments. A lipid-soluble drug [**A**] is subject to a much larger transmembrane concentration gradient (ΔC_m) than a lipid-insoluble drug [**B**]. It therefore diffuses more rapidly, even though the aqueous concentration gradient (C_1–C_2) is the same in both cases.

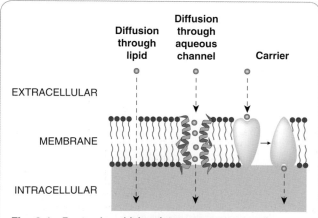

Fig. 8.1 **Routes by which solutes can traverse cell membranes.** (Molecules can also cross cellular barriers by pinocytosis.)

pH and ionisation

One important complicating factor in relation to membrane permeation is that many drugs are weak acids or bases, and therefore exist in both un-ionised and ionised form, the ratio of the two forms varying with pH. For a weak base, B, the ionisation reaction is:

$$BH^+ \underset{K_a}{\rightleftharpoons} B + H^+$$

and the dissociation constant pK_a is given by the Henderson–Hasselbalch equation

$$pK_a = pH + \log_{10} \frac{[BH^+]}{[B]}$$

For a weak acid, AH:

$$AH \underset{K_a}{\rightleftharpoons} A^- + H^+$$

$$pK_a = pH + \log_{10} \frac{[AH]}{[A^-]}$$

In either case, the ionised species, BH^+ or A^-, has very low lipid solubility and is virtually unable to permeate membranes except where a specific transport mechanism exists. The lipid solubility of the uncharged species, B or AH, depends on the chemical nature of the drug; for many drugs, the uncharged species is sufficiently lipid soluble to permit rapid membrane permeation, although there are exceptions (e.g. aminoglycoside antibiotics; see Ch. 51) where even the uncharged molecule is insufficiently lipid-soluble to cross membranes appreciably. This is usually because of the occurrence of hydrogen-bonding groups (such as hydroxyl in sugar moieties in aminoglycosides) that render the uncharged molecule hydrophilic.

pH partition and ion trapping

Ionisation affects not only the rate at which drugs permeate membranes but also the steady-state distribution of drug molecules between aqueous compartments, if a pH difference exists between them. Figure 8.3 shows how a weak acid (e.g. **aspirin**, pK_a 3.5) and a weak base (e.g. **pethidine**, pK_a 8.6) would be distributed at equilibrium between three body compartments, namely plasma

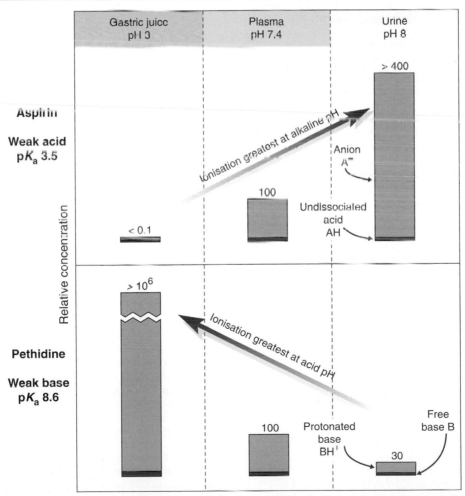

Fig. 8.3 **Theoretical partition of a weak acid (aspirin) and a weak base (pethidine) between aqueous compartments (urine, plasma and gastric juice) according to the pH difference between them.** Numbers represent relative concentrations (total plasma concentration = 100). It is assumed that the uncharged species in each case can permeate the cellular barrier separating the compartments, and therefore reaches the same concentration in all three. Variations in the fractional ionisation as a function of pH give rise to the large total concentration differences with respect to plasma.

(pH 7.4), alkaline urine (pH 8) and gastric juice (pH 3). Within each compartment, the ratio of ionised to un-ionised drug is governed by the pK_a of the drug and the pH of that compartment. It is assumed that the un-ionised species can cross the membrane, and therefore reaches an equal concentration in each compartment. The ionised species is assumed not to cross at all. The result is that, at equilibrium, the total (ionised + un-ionised) concentration of the drug will be different in each compartment, with an acidic drug being concentrated in the compartment with high pH ('ion trapping'), and vice versa. The concentration gradients produced by ion trapping can theoretically be very large if there is a large pH difference between compartments. Thus, aspirin would be concentrated more than four-fold with respect to plasma in an alkaline renal tubule, and about 6000-fold in plasma with respect to the acidic gastric contents. Such large gradients are not achieved in reality for two main reasons. First, assuming total impermeability of the charged species is not realistic, and even a small permeability will attenuate considerably the concentration difference that can be reached. Second, body compartments rarely approach equilibrium. Neither the gastric contents nor the renal tubular fluid stands still, and the resulting bulk flow of drug molecules reduces the concentration gradients well below the theoretical equilibrium conditions. The pH partition mechanism nonetheless correctly explains some of the qualitative effects of pH changes in different body compartments on the pharmacokinetics of weakly acidic or basic drugs, particularly in relation to renal excretion and to penetration of the blood–brain barrier.

pH partition is not the main determinant of the site of absorption of drugs from the gastrointestinal tract. This is because the enormous absorptive surface area of the villi and microvilli in the ileum compared with the much smaller absorptive surface area in the stomach is of overriding importance. Thus, absorption of an acidic drug such as aspirin is promoted by drugs that accelerate gastric emptying (e.g. **metoclopramide**) and retarded by drugs that slow gastric emptying (e.g. **propantheline**), despite the fact that the acidic pH of the stomach contents favours absorption of weak acids. Values of pK_a for some common drugs are shown in Figure 8.4.

There are several important consequences of pH partition:

- Free-base trapping of some antimalarial drugs (e.g. **chloroquine**, see Ch. 54) in the acidic environment in the food vacuole of the malaria parasite contributes to the disruption of the haemoglobin digestion pathway that underlies their toxic effect on the parasite.
- Urinary acidification accelerates excretion of weak bases and retards that of weak acids (see Ch. 9).
- Urinary alkalinisation has the opposite effects: it reduces excretion of weak bases and increases excretion of weak acids.
- Increasing plasma pH (e.g. by administration of sodium bicarbonate) causes weakly acidic drugs to be extracted from the CNS into the plasma. Conversely, reducing plasma pH (e.g. by administration of a carbonic anhydrase inhibitor such as **acetazolamide**) causes weakly acidic drugs to become concentrated in the CNS, increasing their

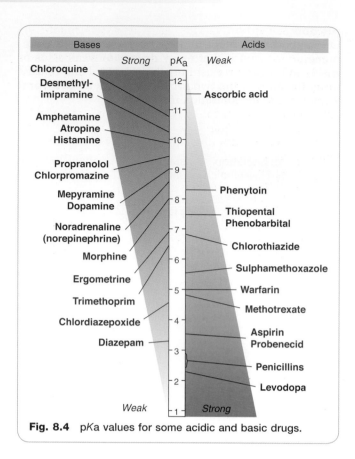

Fig. 8.4 pK_a values for some acidic and basic drugs.

neurotoxicity. This has practical consequences in choosing a means to alkalinise urine in treating aspirin overdose: bicarbonate and acetazolamide each increase urine pH and hence increase salicylate elimination, but bicarbonate reduces whereas acetazolamide increases distribution of salicylate to the CNS.

CARRIER-MEDIATED TRANSPORT

Many cell membranes possess specialised transport mechanisms that regulate entry and exit of physiologically important molecules, such as sugars, amino acids, neurotransmitters and metal ions. They are broadly divided into *solute carrier (SLC) transporters* and *ATP-binding cassette (ABC) transporters*. The former facilitate passive movement of solutes down their electrochemical gradient, while the latter are active pumps fuelled by ATP. Over 300 human genes are believed to code these transporters, most of which act mainly on endogenous substrates, but some also transport foreign chemicals ('xenobiotics') including drugs (see Hediger et al., 2004). The role of such transporters in neurotransmitter function is discussed in Chapters 13, 14 and 37.

Organic cation transporters and organic anion transporters

Two structurally related SLCs of importance in drug distribution are the organic cation transporters (OCTs) and organic anion transporters (OATs). The carrier molecule consists of a transmembrane protein that binds one or more molecules or ions, changes conformation and releases its cargo on the other side of the membrane. Such systems may operate purely passively, without any energy source; in this case, they merely facilitate the process of transmembrane equilibration of a single transported species in the direction of its electrochemical gradient. The OCTs translocate dopamine, choline and various drugs including **vecuronium**, **quinine** and **procainamide**. They are 'uniporters' (i.e. each protein transporter molecule binds one solute molecule at a time and transports it down its gradient). OCT2 (present in proximal renal tubules) concentrates drugs such as **cisplatin** (an important anticancer drug, see Ch. 56) in these cells, resulting in its selective nephrotoxicity; related drugs (e.g. carboplatin, **oxaliplatin**) are not transported by OCT2 and are less nephrotoxic; competition with **cimetidine** for OCT2 offers possible protection against cisplatin nephrotoxicity (Fig. 8.5). Other SLCs are coupled to the electrochemical gradient of Na⁺ or other ions across the membrane, generated by ATP-dependent ion pumps (see Ch. 4); in this case, transport can occur against an electrochemical gradient. It may involve exchange of one molecule for another

('antiport') or transport of two molecules together in the same direction ('symport'). The OATs are responsible for the renal secretion of urate, prostaglandins, several vitamins and *p*-amino hippurate, and for drugs such as **probenecid**, many antibiotics, antiviral, non-steroidal anti-inflammatory and antineoplastic drugs. Uptake is driven by exchange with intracellular dicarboxylic acids (mainly α-ketoglutarate, partly derived from cellular metabolism and partly by co-transport with Na⁺ entering cells down its concentration gradient). Metabolic energy is provided by ATP for Na⁺/K⁺ exchange. Carrier-mediated transport, because it involves a binding step, shows the characteristic of saturation.

Carriers of this type are ubiquitous, and many pharmacological effects are the result of interference with them. Thus nerve terminals have transport mechanisms for accumulating specific neurotransmitters, and there are many examples of drugs that act by inhibiting these transport mechanisms (see Chs 13, 14, 37, 47 and 48). From a

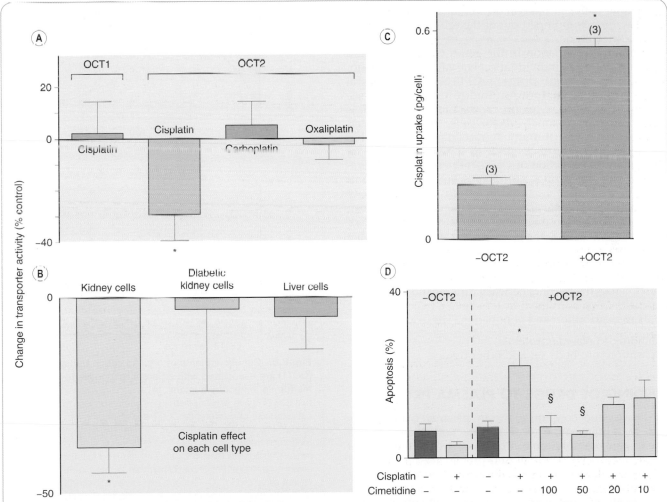

Fig. 8.5 **Human organic cation transporter 2 (OCT2) mediates cisplatin nephrotoxicity.** OCT2 is expressed in kidney whereas OCT1 is expressed in liver. Cisplatin (100 µmol/l) influences the activity of OCT2 but not of OCT1, each expressed in a cultured cell line **[A]**, whereas the less nephrotoxic drugs carboplatin and oxaliplatin do not. Cisplatin similarly influences OCT2 activity in fresh human kidney tubule cells but not in fresh hepatocytes or kidney cells from diabetic patients who are less susceptible to cisplatin nephrotoxicity **[B]**. Cisplatin accumulates in cells that express OCT2 **[C]** and causes cell death **[D]**. Cimetidine competes with cisplatin for OCT2 and concentration dependently protects against cisplatin-induced apoptosis **[D]** – cimetidine concentrations are in µmol/l. *(Data redrawn from Ciarimboli G et al. 2005 Am J Pathol 167, 1477–1484.)*

general pharmacokinetic point of view, however, the main sites where SLCs, including OCTs and OATs, are expressed and carrier-mediated drug transport is important are:

- the blood–brain barrier
- the gastrointestinal tract
- the renal tubule
- the biliary tract
- the placenta.

P-glycoprotein transporters

P-glycoproteins (P-gp; P for 'permeability'), which belong to the ABC transporter superfamily, are the second important class of transporters, and are responsible for multidrug resistance in cancer cells. They are present in renal tubular brush border membranes, in bile canaliculi, in astrocyte foot processes in brain microvessels, and in the gastrointestinal tract. They play an important part in absorption, distribution and elimination of many drugs, and are often co-located with SLC drug carriers, so that a drug that has been concentrated by, for example, an OAT transporter in the basolateral membrane of a renal tubular cell may then be pumped out of the cell by a P-gp in the luminal membrane.

Polymorphic variation in the genes coding SLCs and P-gp contributes to individual genetic variation in responsiveness to different drugs. OCT1 transports several drugs, including **metformin** (used to treat diabetes; see Ch. 31), into hepatocytes (in contrast to OCT2 which is active in renal proximal tubular cells, see above). Metformin acts partly through intracellular effects within hepatocytes. Single nucleotoide polymorphisms (SNPs) that impair the function of OCT1 influence the effectiveness of metformin (Fig. 8.6). This is but one example of many genetic influences on drug effectiveness or toxicity via altered activity of carriers that influence drug disposition. Furthermore, induction or competitive inhibition of transport can occur in the presence of a second ligand that binds the carrier, so there is a potential for drug interaction (see Fig. 8.5 and Ch. 10). In addition to the processes so far described, which govern the transport of drug molecules across the barriers between different aqueous compartments, two additional factors have a major influence on drug distribution and elimination. These are:

- binding to plasma proteins
- partition into body fat and other tissues.

BINDING OF DRUGS TO PLASMA PROTEINS

At therapeutic concentrations in plasma, many drugs exist mainly in bound form. The fraction of drug that is free in aqueous solution can be less than 1%, the remainder being associated with plasma protein. It is the unbound drug that is pharmacologically active. Such seemingly small differences in protein binding (e.g. 99.5% versus 99.0%) can have large effects on free drug concentration and drug effect. Such differences are common between human plasma and plasma from species used in preclinical drug testing, and must be taken into account when estimating a suitable dose for 'first time in human' studies. The most important plasma protein in relation to drug binding is albumin, which binds many acidic drugs (e.g. **warfarin**, non-steroidal anti-inflammatory drugs,

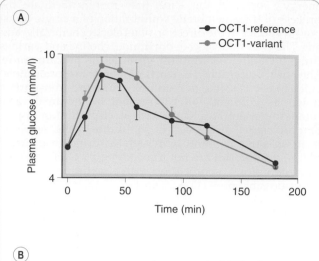

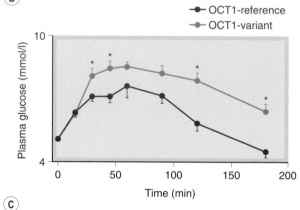

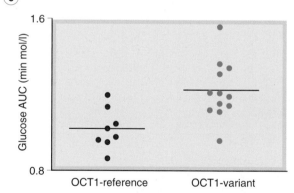

Fig. 8.6 Genetic variants of organic cation transporter 1 (OCT1) are associated with different responses to metformin in healthy humans. **[A]** An oral glucose tolerance test (OGTT) gave similar plasma glucose responses in control subjects with only reference *OCT1* alleles versus subjects with at least one reduced function *OCT1* allele. **[B]** In contrast, after metformin treatment the OGTT response was less in the same reference subjects than in those with reduced function *OCT1* alleles – i.e. the effect of metformin was blunted in the variant-allele group. **[C]** Glucose exposure estimated by area under the glucose time curves (AUC) was significantly lower in subjects with only reference *OCT1* alleles, *P* = 0.004. *(Data redrawn from Yan Shu et al. 2007 J Clin Invest 117, 1422–1431.)*

Movement of drugs across cellular barriers

- To traverse cellular barriers (e.g. gastrointestinal mucosa, renal tubule, blood–brain barrier, placenta), drugs have to cross lipid membranes.
- Drugs cross lipid membranes mainly (a) by passive diffusional transfer and (b) by carrier-mediated transfer.
- The main factor that determines the rate of passive diffusional transfer across membranes is a drug's lipid solubility.
- Many drugs are weak acids or weak bases; their state of ionisation varies with pH according to the Henderson–Hasselbalch equation.
- With weak acids or bases, only the uncharged species (the protonated form for a weak acid, the unprotonated form for a weak base) can diffuse across lipid membranes; this gives rise to pH partition.
- pH partition means that weak acids tend to accumulate in compartments of relatively high pH, whereas weak bases do the reverse.
- Carrier-mediated transport is mediated by solute carriers (SLCs), which include organic cation transporters (OCTs) and organic anion transporters (OATs), and P-gps (ABC transporters) in the renal tubule, blood–brain barrier and gastrointestinal epithelium. These are important in determining the distribution of many drugs, are prone to genetic variation and are targets for drug interactions.

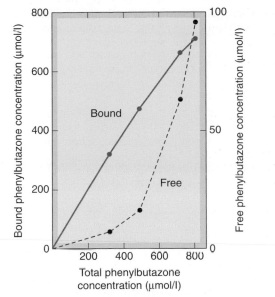

Fig. 8.7 Binding of phenylbutazone to plasma albumin. The graph shows the disproportionate increase in free concentration as the total concentration increases, owing to the binding sites approaching saturation. (Data from Brodie B, Hogben CAM 1957 J Pharm Pharmacol 9, 345.)

sulfonamides) and a smaller number of basic drugs (e.g. tricyclic antidepressants and chlorpromazine). Other plasma proteins, including β-globulin and an acid glycoprotein that increases in inflammatory disease, have also been implicated in the binding of certain basic drugs such as quinine.

The amount of a drug that is bound to protein depends on three factors:

- the concentration of free drug
- its affinity for the binding sites
- the concentration of protein.

As a first approximation, the binding reaction can be regarded as a simple association of the drug molecules with a finite population of binding sites, exactly analogous to drug–receptor binding (see Ch. 2):

$$\begin{array}{ccc} D & + & S & \rightleftharpoons & DS \\ \text{free} & & \text{binding} & & \text{complex} \\ \text{drug} & & \text{site} & & \end{array}$$

The usual concentration of albumin in plasma is about 0.6 mmol/l (4 g/100 ml). With two sites per albumin molecule, the drug-binding capacity of plasma albumin would therefore be about 1.2 mmol/l. For most drugs, the total plasma concentration required for a clinical effect is much less than 1.2 mmol/l, so with usual therapeutic doses the binding sites are far from saturated, and the concentration bound [DS] varies nearly in direct proportion to the free concentration [D]. Under these

conditions, the fraction bound, [DS]/([D] + [DS]), is independent of the drug concentration. However, some drugs, for example **tolbutamide** (Ch. 31), act at plasma concentrations at which its binding to plasma albumin approaches saturation (i.e. on the flat part of the binding curve). This means that increasing the dose increases the free (pharmacologically active) concentration disproportionately. This is illustrated in Figure 8.7.

Plasma albumin binds many different drugs, so competition can occur between them. If two drugs (A and B) compete in this way, administration of drug B can reduce the protein binding, and hence increase the free plasma concentration, of drug A. To do this, drug B needs to occupy an appreciable fraction of the binding sites. Few therapeutic drugs affect the binding of other drugs because they occupy, at therapeutic plasma concentrations, only a tiny fraction of the available sites. *Sulfonamides* (Ch. 51) are an exception, because they occupy about 50% of the binding sites at therapeutic concentrations and so can cause harmful effects by displacing other drugs or, in premature babies, bilirubin (see below). Much has been made of binding interactions of this kind as a source of untoward drug interactions in clinical medicine, but this type of competition is less important than was once thought (see Ch. 57).

PARTITION INTO BODY FAT AND OTHER TISSUES

Fat represents a large, non-polar compartment. In practice, this is important for only a few drugs, mainly because the effective fat:water partition coefficient is relatively low for most drugs. **Morphine**, for example, although lipid-soluble enough to cross the blood–brain barrier, has a lipid:water partition coefficient of only 0.4, so

Binding of drugs to plasma proteins

- Plasma albumin is most important and is a source of species variation; β-globulin and acid glycoprotein also bind some drugs that are bases.
- Plasma albumin binds mainly acidic drugs (approximately two molecules per albumin molecule). Saturable binding sometimes leads to a non-linear relation between dose and free (active) drug concentration.
- Extensive protein binding slows drug elimination (metabolism and/or glomerular filtration).
- Competition between drugs for protein binding can lead to clinically important drug interactions, but this is uncommon.

sequestration of the drug by body fat is of little importance. **Thiopental**, by comparison (fat : water partition coefficient approximately 10), accumulates substantially in body fat. This has important consequences that limit its usefulness as an intravenous anaesthetic to short-term initiation ('induction') of anaesthesia, and it has been replaced by **propofol** even for this indication in many countries (Ch. 41).

The second factor that limits the accumulation of drugs in body fat is its low blood supply – less than 2% of the cardiac output. Consequently, drugs are delivered slowly to body fat, and the theoretical equilibrium distribution between fat and body water is delayed. For practical purposes, therefore, partition into body fat when drugs are given acutely is important only for a few highly lipid-soluble drugs (e.g. general anaesthetics; Ch. 41). When lipid-soluble drugs are given chronically, however, accumulation in body fat is often significant (e.g. benzodiazepines; Ch. 44). Some drugs and environmental contaminants (such as insecticides), if ingested intermittently, accumulate slowly but progressively in body fat.

Body fat is not the only tissue in which drugs can accumulate. **Chloroquine** – an antimalarial drug (Ch. 54) – has a high affinity for melanin and is taken up by the retina, which is rich in melanin granules, accounting for chloroquine's ocular toxicity. Tetracyclines (Ch. 51) accumulate slowly in bones and teeth, because they have a high affinity for calcium, and should not be used in children for this reason. Very high concentrations of **amiodarone** (an antidysrhythmic drug; Ch. 21) accumulate in liver and lung during chronic use, causing hepatitis and interstitial pulmonary fibrosis.

DRUG ABSORPTION AND ROUTES OF ADMINISTRATION

The main routes of drug administration and elimination are shown schematically in Figure 8.8. Absorption is defined as the passage of a drug from its site of administration into the plasma. It is important for all routes of

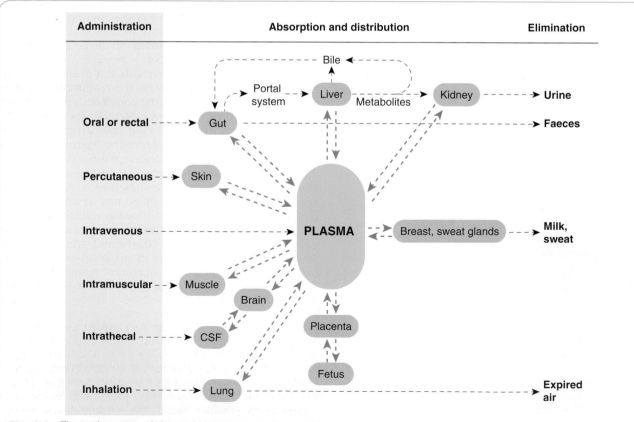

Fig. 8.8 The main routes of drug administration and elimination.

administration except intravenous injection, where it is complete by definition. There are instances, such as topical administration of a steroid cream to skin or inhalation of a bronchodilator aerosol to treat asthma (Ch. 28), where absorption as just defined is not required for the drug to act, but in most cases the drug must enter plasma before reaching its site of action.

The main routes of administration are:

- oral
- sublingual
- rectal
- application to other epithelial surfaces
  (e.g. skin, cornea, vagina and nasal mucosa)
- inhalation
- injection
  - subcutaneous
  - intramuscular
  - intravenous
  - intrathecal
  - intravitreal.

ORAL ADMINISTRATION

Most drugs are taken by mouth and swallowed. Little absorption occurs until the drug enters the small intestine, although a few non-polar drugs applied to the buccal mucosa or under the tongue are absorbed directly from the mouth (e.g. organic nitrates, Ch. 21, and buprenorphine, Ch. 42).

DRUG ABSORPTION FROM THE INTESTINE

For most drugs the mechanism of absorption is the same as for other epithelial barriers, namely passive transfer at a rate determined by the ionisation and lipid solubility of the drug molecules. Figure 8.9 shows the absorption of various weak acids and bases as a function of pK_a. As expected, strong bases of pK_a 10 or higher are poorly absorbed, as are strong acids of pK_a less than 3, because they are fully ionised. The arrow poison curare used by South American Indians contains quaternary ammonium compounds that block neuromuscular transmission

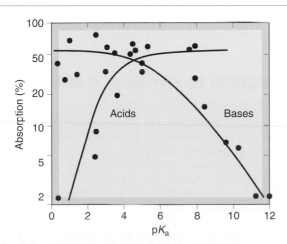

Fig. 8.9 Absorption of drugs from the intestine, as a function of pKa, for acids and bases. Weak acids and bases are well absorbed; strong acids and bases are poorly absorbed. (Redrawn from Schanker LS et al. 1957 J Pharmacol 120, 528.)

(Ch. 13). These strong bases are poorly absorbed from the gastrointestinal tract, so the meat from animals killed in this way was safe to eat.

In a few instances, intestinal drug absorption depends on carrier-mediated transport rather than simple lipid diffusion. Examples include **levodopa**, used in treating Parkinson's disease (see Ch. 40), which is taken up by the carrier that normally transports phenylalanine, and **fluorouracil** (Ch. 56), a cytotoxic drug that is transported by the carrier for pyrimidines (thymine and uracil). Iron is absorbed via specific carriers in the epithelial cell membranes of jejunal mucosa, and calcium is absorbed by a vitamin D-dependent carrier.

FACTORS AFFECTING GASTROINTESTINAL ABSORPTION

Typically, about 75% of a drug given orally is absorbed in 1–3 h, but numerous factors alter this, some physiological and some to do with the formulation of the drug. The main factors are:

- gut content (e.g. fed versus fasted)
- gastrointestinal motility
- splanchnic blood flow
- particle size and formulation
- physicochemical factors, including some drug interactions.

The influence of feeding, which influences both gut content and splanchnic blood flow, is routinely examined in early phase clinical trials and prescribing advice tailored accordingly. Gastrointestinal motility has a large effect. Many disorders (e.g. migraine, diabetic neuropathy) cause gastric stasis and slow drug absorption. Drug treatment can also affect motility, either reducing (e.g. drugs that block muscarinic receptors; see Ch. 13) or increasing it (e.g. **metoclopramide**, an antiemetic used in migraine to facilitate absorption of analgesic). Excessively rapid movement of gut contents (e.g. in some forms of diarrhoea) can impair absorption. Several drugs (e.g. **propranolol**) reach a higher plasma concentration if they are taken after a meal, probably because food increases splanchnic blood flow. Conversely, splanchnic blood flow is greatly reduced by hypovolaemia or heart failure, with a resultant reduction of drug absorption.

Particle size and formulation have major effects on absorption. In 1971, patients in a New York hospital were found to require unusually large maintenance doses of **digoxin** (Ch. 21). In a study on normal volunteers, it was found that standard digoxin tablets from different manufacturers resulted in grossly different plasma concentrations (Fig. 8.10), even though the digoxin content of the tablets was the same, because of differences in particle size. Because digoxin is rather poorly absorbed, small differences in the pharmaceutical formulation can make a large difference to the extent of absorption.

Therapeutic drugs are formulated pharmaceutically to produce desired absorption characteristics. Capsules may be designed to remain intact for some hours after ingestion in order to delay absorption, or tablets may have a resistant coating to give the same effect. In some cases, a mixture of slow- and fast-release particles is included in a capsule to produce rapid but sustained absorption. More elaborate pharmaceutical systems include modified-release preparations that permit less frequent dosing.

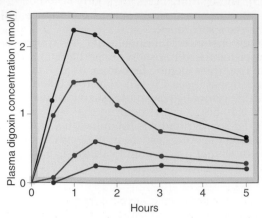

Fig. 8.10 Variation in oral absorption among different formulations of digoxin. The four curves show the mean plasma concentrations attained for the four preparations, each of which was given on separate occasions to four subjects. The large variation has caused the formulation of digoxin tablets to be standardised since this study was published. *(From Lindenbaum J et al. 1971 N Engl J Med 285, 1344.)*

Such preparations not only increase the dose interval but also reduce adverse effects related to high peak plasma concentrations following administration of a conventional formulation.

When drugs are swallowed, the intention is usually that they should be absorbed and cause a systemic effect, but there are exceptions. **Vancomycin** is very poorly absorbed, and is administered orally to eradicate toxin-forming *Clostridium difficile* from the gut lumen in patients with pseudomembranous colitis (an adverse effect of broad-spectrum antibiotics caused by appearance of this organism in the bowel). **Mesalazine** is a formulation of 5-aminosalicylic acid in a pH-dependent acrylic coat that degrades in the terminal ileum and proximal colon, and is used to treat inflammatory bowel disease affecting this part of the gut. **Olsalazine** is a prodrug (see p. 114-115) consisting of a dimer of two molecules of 5-aminosalicylic acid that is cleaved by colonic bacteria in the distal bowel and is used to treat patients with distal colitis.

Bioavailability and bioequivalence

To get into the systemic circulation, for example from the lumen of the small intestine, a drug must not only penetrate local barriers such as the intestinal mucosa, it must also run a gauntlet of inactivating enzymes in the gut wall and liver, referred to as 'presystemic' or 'first-pass' metabolism or clearance. The term *bioavailability* is used to indicate the fraction (F) of an orally administered dose that reaches the systemic circulation as intact drug, taking into account both absorption and local metabolic degradation. F is measured by determining the plasma drug concentration versus time curves in a group of subjects following oral and (on a separate occasion) intravenous administration (the fraction absorbed following an intravenous dose is 1 by definition). The areas under the plasma concentration time curves (AUC) are used to estimate F as $AUC_{oral}/AUC_{intravenous}$. Bioavailability is not a characteristic solely of the drug preparation: variations in enzyme activity of gut wall or liver, in gastric pH or intestinal motility all affect it.

Because of this, one cannot speak strictly of the bioavailability of a particular preparation, but only of that preparation in a given individual on a particular occasion, and F determined in a group of healthy volunteer subjects may differ substantially from the value determined in patients with diseases of gastrointestinal or circulatory systems.

Bioavailability relates only to the total proportion of the drug that reaches the systemic circulation and neglects the rate of absorption. If a drug is completely absorbed in 30 min, it will reach a much higher peak plasma concentration (and have a more dramatic effect) than if it were absorbed over several hours. Regulatory authorities – which have to make decisions about the licensing of products that are 'generic equivalents' of patented products – require evidence of 'bioequivalence' based on the maximum concentration achieved (C_{max}), time between dosing and C_{max} (t_{max}) and $AUC_{(0-\infty)}$. For most drugs, each of these parameters ($AUC_{(0-\infty)}$, C_{max}, t_{max}) must lie between 80% and 125% of a marketed preparation for the new generic product to be accepted as bioequivalent (EMEA, 2009).

SUBLINGUAL ADMINISTRATION

Absorption directly from the oral cavity is sometimes useful (provided the drug does not taste too horrible) when a rapid response is required, particularly when the drug is either unstable at gastric pH or rapidly metabolised by the liver. **Glyceryl trinitrate** and **buprenorphine** are examples of drugs that are often given sublingually (Chs 21 and 41, respectively). Drugs absorbed from the mouth pass directly into the systemic circulation without entering the portal system, and so escape first-pass metabolism by enzymes in the gut wall and liver.

RECTAL ADMINISTRATION

Rectal administration is used for drugs that are required either to produce a local effect (e.g. anti-inflammatory drugs for use in ulcerative colitis) or to produce systemic effects. Absorption following rectal administration is often unreliable, but this route can be useful in patients who are vomiting or are unable to take medication by mouth (e.g. postoperatively). It is sometimes used to administer diazepam to children who are in *status epilepticus* (Ch. 45), in whom it is difficult to establish intravenous access.

APPLICATION TO EPITHELIAL SURFACES

CUTANEOUS ADMINISTRATION

Cutaneous administration is used when a local effect on the skin is required (e.g. topically applied steroids, Ch. 27). Appreciable absorption may nonetheless occur and lead to systemic effects; absorption is sometimes exploited therapeutically, for example in local application of rub-on gels of non-steroidal anti-inflammatory agents such as **ibuprofen** (Ch. 26).

Most drugs are absorbed very poorly through unbroken skin. However, a number of organophosphate insecticides (see Ch. 13), which need to penetrate an insect's cuticle in order to work, are absorbed through skin, and accidental poisoning occurs in farm workers.

▼ A case is recounted of a 35-year-old florist in 1932. 'While engaged in doing a light electrical repair job at a work bench he sat down in a chair on the seat of which some 'Nico-Fume liquid' (a 40% solution of free nicotine) had been spilled. He felt the solution wet through his clothes to the skin over the left buttock, an area about the size of the palm of his hand. He thought nothing further of it and continued at his work for about 15 minutes, when he was suddenly seized with nausea and faintness … and found himself in a drenching sweat. On the way to hospital he lost consciousness.' He survived, just, and then 4 days later: 'On discharge from the hospital he was given the same clothes that he had worn when he was brought in. The clothes had been kept in a paper bag and were still damp where they had been wet with the nicotine solution.' The sequel was predictable. He survived again but felt thereafter 'unable to enter a greenhouse where nicotine was being sprayed'. Transdermal dosage forms of nicotine are now used to reduce the withdrawal symptoms that accompany stopping smoking (Ch. 49).

Transdermal dosage forms, in which the drug is incorporated in a stick-on patch applied to the skin, are used increasingly, and several drugs – for example **oestrogen** and **testosterone** for hormone replacement (Ch. 35) are available in this form. Such patches produce a steady rate of drug delivery and avoid presystemic metabolism. **Fentanyl** is available in a patch to treat intermittent breakthrough pain (Ch. 42). However, the method is suitable only for lipid-soluble drugs and is relatively expensive.

NASAL SPRAYS

Some peptide hormone analogues, for example of **antidiuretic hormone** (Ch. 33) and of **gonadotrophin-releasing hormone** (see Ch. 35), are given as nasal sprays, as is **calcitonin** (Ch. 36). Absorption is believed to take place through mucosa overlying nasal-associated lymphoid tissue. This is similar to mucosa overlying Peyer's patches in the small intestine, which is also unusually permeable.

EYE DROPS

Many drugs are applied as eye drops, relying on absorption through the epithelium of the conjunctival sac to produce their effects. Desirable local effects within the eye can be achieved without causing systemic side effects; for example, **dorzolamide** is a carbonic anhydrase inhibitor that is given as eye drops to lower ocular pressure in patients with glaucoma. It achieves this without affecting the kidney (see Ch. 29), thus avoiding the acidosis that is caused by oral administration of acetazolamide. Some systemic absorption from the eye occurs, however, and can result in unwanted effects (e.g. bronchospasm in asthmatic patients using **timolol** eye drops for glaucoma).

ADMINISTRATION BY INHALATION

Inhalation is the route used for volatile and gaseous anaesthetics, the lung serving as the route of both administration and elimination. The rapid exchange resulting from the large surface area and blood flow makes it possible to achieve rapid adjustments of plasma concentration. The pharmacokinetic behaviour of inhalation anaesthetics is discussed more fully in Chapter 41.

Drugs used for their effects on the lung are also given by inhalation, usually as an aerosol. Glucocorticoids (e.g. **beclometasone dipropionate**) and bronchodilators (e.g. **salbutamol**; Ch. 28) are given in this way to achieve high local concentrations in the lung while minimising systemic side effects. However, drugs given by inhalation in this way are usually partly absorbed into the circulation, and systemic side effects (e.g. tremor following

salbutamol) can occur. Chemical modification of a drug may minimise such absorption. For example, **ipratropium**, a muscarinic-receptor antagonist (Chs 13 and 28), is a quaternary ammonium ion analogue of atropine. It is used as an inhaled bronchodilator because its poor absorption minimises systemic adverse effects.

ADMINISTRATION BY INJECTION

Intravenous injection is the fastest and most certain route of drug administration. Bolus injection rapidly produces a high concentration of drug, first in the right heart and pulmonary vessels and then in the systemic circulation. The peak concentration reaching the tissues depends critically on the rate of injection. Administration by steady intravenous infusion avoids the uncertainties of absorption from other sites, while avoiding high peak plasma concentrations caused by bolus injection.

Subcutaneous or intramuscular injection of drugs usually produces a faster effect than oral administration, but the rate of absorption depends greatly on the site of injection and on local blood flow. The rate-limiting factors in absorption from the injection site are:

• diffusion through the tissue
• removal by local blood flow.

Absorption from a site of injection (sometimes but not always desirable, see below) is increased by increased blood flow. *Hyaluronidase* (an enzyme that breaks down the intercellular matrix, thereby increasing diffusion) also increases drug absorption from the site of injection. Conversely, absorption is reduced in patients with circulatory failure ('shock') in whom tissue perfusion is reduced (Ch. 22).

METHODS FOR DELAYING ABSORPTION

It may be desirable to delay absorption, either to produce a local effect or to prolong systemic action. For example, addition of adrenaline (epinephrine) to a local anaesthetic reduces absorption of the anaesthetic into the general circulation, usefully prolonging the anaesthetic effect (Ch. 43). Formulation of insulin with protamine and zinc produces a long-acting form (see Ch. 31). Procaine penicillin (Ch. 51) is a poorly soluble salt of **penicillin**; when injected as an aqueous suspension, it is slowly absorbed and exerts a prolonged action. Esterification of steroid hormones (e.g. medroxyprogesterone acetate, testosterone propionate; Ch. 35) and antipsychotic drugs (e.g. fluphenazine decanoate; Ch. 46) increases their solubility in oil and slows their rate of absorption when they are injected in an oily solution.

Another method used to achieve slow and continuous absorption of certain steroid hormones (e.g. **oestradiol**; Ch. 35) is the subcutaneous implantation of drug substance, for example formulated as a solid pellet. The rate of absorption is proportional to the surface area of the implant.

INTRATHECAL INJECTION

Injection of a drug into the subarachnoid space via a lumbar puncture needle is used for some specialised purposes. **Methotrexate** (Ch. 56) is administered in this way in the treatment of certain childhood leukaemias to prevent relapse in the CNS. Regional anaesthesia can be produced by intrathecal administration of a local anaesthetic such as **bupivacaine** (see Ch. 43); opioid analgesics can also be used in this way (Ch. 42). **Baclofen** (a GABA analogue; Ch. 38) is used to treat disabling muscle spasms. It has been administered intrathecally to minimise its adverse effects. Some antibiotics (e.g. aminoglycosides) cross the blood–brain barrier very slowly, and in rare clinical situations where they are essential (e.g. nervous system infections with bacteria resistant to other antibiotics) can be given intrathecally or directly into the cerebral ventricles via a reservoir.

INTRAVITREAL INJECTION

Ranibizumab (monoclonal antibody fragment that binds to vascular endothelial growth factor; Ch. 22) is given by intravitreal injection by ophthalmologists treating patients with wet age-related macular degeneration.

Drug absorption and bioavailability

- Drugs of very low lipid solubility, including those that are strong acids or bases, are generally poorly absorbed from the gut.
- A few drugs (e.g. **levodopa**) are absorbed by carrier-mediated transfer.
- Absorption from the gut depends on many factors, including:
  - gastrointestinal motility
  - gastrointestinal pH
  - particle size
  - physicochemical interaction with gut contents (e.g. chemical interaction between calcium and tetracycline antibiotics).
- Bioavailability is the fraction of an ingested dose of a drug that gains access to the systemic circulation. It may be low because absorption is incomplete, or because the drug is metabolised in the gut wall or liver before reaching the systemic circulation.
- Bioequivalence implies that if one formulation of a drug is substituted for another, no clinically untoward consequences will ensue.

DISTRIBUTION OF DRUGS IN THE BODY

BODY FLUID COMPARTMENTS

Body water is distributed into four main compartments (Fig. 8.11). The total body water as a percentage of body weight varies from 50% to 70%, being rather less in women than in men.

Extracellular fluid comprises the blood plasma (about 4.5% of body weight), interstitial fluid (16%) and lymph (1.2%). Intracellular fluid (30–40%) is the sum of the fluid contents of all cells in the body. Transcellular fluid (2.5%) includes the cerebrospinal, intraocular, peritoneal, pleural and synovial fluids, and digestive secretions. The fetus may also be regarded as a special type of transcellular compartment. Within each of these aqueous compartments, drug molecules usually exist both in free solution and in bound form; furthermore, drugs that are weak

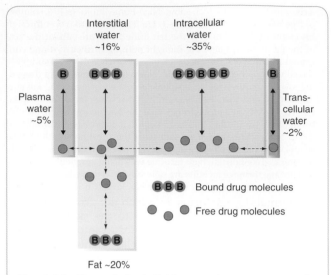

Fig. 8.11 The main body fluid compartments, expressed as a percentage of body weight. Drug molecules exist in bound or free form in each compartment, but only the free drug is able to move between the compartments.

acids or bases will exist as an equilibrium mixture of the charged and uncharged forms, the position of the equilibrium depending on the pH.

The equilibrium pattern of distribution between the various compartments will therefore depend on:

- permeability across tissue barriers
- binding within compartments
- pH partition
- fat : water partition.

To enter the transcellular compartments from the extracellular compartment, a drug must cross a cellular barrier, a particularly important example being the blood–brain barrier.

THE BLOOD–BRAIN BARRIER

The concept of the blood–brain barrier was introduced by Paul Ehrlich to explain his observation that intravenously injected dye stained most tissues but not the brain. The barrier consists of a continuous layer of endothelial cells joined by tight junctions and surrounded by pericytes. The brain is consequently inaccessible to many drugs whose lipid solubility is insufficient to allow penetration of the blood–brain barrier. However, inflammation can disrupt the integrity of the blood–brain barrier, allowing normally impermeant substances to enter the brain (Fig. 8.12); consequently, penicillin (Ch. 51) can be given intravenously (rather than intrathecally) to treat bacterial meningitis (which is accompanied by intense inflammation).

Furthermore, in some parts of the CNS, including the *chemoreceptor trigger zone*, the barrier is leaky. This enables **domperidone**, an antiemetic dopamine-receptor antagonist (Chs 30 and 40) that does not penetrate the blood–brain barrier but does access the chemoreceptor trigger zone, to be used to prevent the nausea caused by dopamine agonists such as **apomorphine** when these are used to treat advanced Parkinson's disease. This is achieved

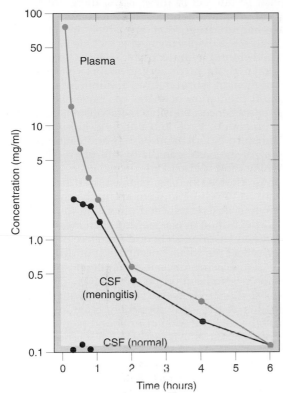

Fig. 8.12 Plasma and cerebrospinal fluid concentrations of an antibiotic (thienamycin) following an intravenous dose (25 mg/kg). In normal rabbits, no drug reaches the cerebrospinal fluid (CSF), but in animals with experimental *Escherichia coli* meningitis the concentration of drug in CSF approaches that in the plasma. *(From Paramasucon P, McCracken Jr GH 1973 Antimicrob Agents Chemother 3, 270.)*

content of the drug (Q) at a concentration equal to that present in the plasma (C_p):

$$V_d = \frac{Q}{C_p}$$

It is important to avoid identifying a given range of V_d too closely with a particular anatomical compartment. Drugs may act at very low concentrations in the key compartment that provides access to their receptors. For example, insulin has a measured V_d similar to the volume of plasma water but exerts its effects on muscle, fat and liver via receptors that are exposed to interstitial fluid but not to plasma (Ch. 31).

DRUGS LARGELY CONFINED TO THE PLASMA COMPARTMENT

The plasma volume is about 0.05 l/kg body weight. A few drugs, such as **heparin** (Ch. 24), are confined to plasma because the molecule is too large to cross the capillary wall easily. More often, retention of a drug in the plasma following a single dose reflects strong binding to plasma protein. It is, nevertheless, the free drug in the interstitial fluid that exerts a pharmacological effect. Following repeated dosing, equilibration occurs and measured V_d increases. Some dyes bind exceptionally strongly to plasma albumin, as with Evans blue, such that its V_d is used experimentally to measure plasma volume.

DRUGS DISTRIBUTED IN THE EXTRACELLULAR COMPARTMENT

The total extracellular volume is about 0.2 l/kg, and this is the approximate V_d for many polar compounds, such as vecuronium (Ch. 13), **gentamicin** and **carbenicillin** (Ch. 51). These drugs cannot easily enter cells because of their low lipid solubility, and they do not traverse the blood–brain or placental barriers freely. Many macromolecular biopharmaceuticals, notably monoclonal antibodies (Ch. 59), distribute in the extracellular space and access receptors on cell surfaces but do not enter cells. Nucleic acid-based biopharmaceuticals which work on intracellular DNA or RNA are often packaged in special delivery systems (see p. 114-115) that facilitate access to the cell interior, often in low amounts that are nevertheless sufficient to exert effects on protein synthesis.

DISTRIBUTION THROUGHOUT THE BODY WATER

Total body water represents about 0.55 l/kg. This approximates the distribution of many drugs that readily cross cell membranes, such as **phenytoin** (Ch. 45) and **ethanol** (Ch. 49). The binding of drugs outside the plasma compartment, or partitioning into body fat, increases V_d beyond total body water. Consequently, there are also many drugs with V_d greater than the total body volume, such as morphine (Ch. 42), tricyclic antidepressants (Ch. 47) and **haloperidol** (Ch. 46). Such drugs are not efficiently removed from the body by haemodialysis, which is therefore unhelpful in managing overdose with such agents.

without loss of efficacy, because dopamine receptors in the basal ganglia are accessible only to drugs that have traversed the blood–brain barrier.

Methylnaltrexone bromide is a peripherally acting μ-opioid-receptor antagonist used in treating opioid-induced constipation in patients requiring opioids as part of palliative care. It has limited gastrointestinal absorption and does not cross the blood–brain barrier, so does not block the desired CNS opioid effects. Several peptides, including bradykinin and enkephalins, increase blood–brain barrier permeability. There is interest in exploiting this to improve penetration of anticancer drugs during treatment of brain tumours. In addition, extreme stress renders the blood–brain barrier permeable to drugs such as **pyridostigmine** (Ch. 13), which normally act peripherally.[2]

VOLUME OF DISTRIBUTION

The apparent volume of distribution, V_d, (see Ch. 10) is defined as the volume that would contain the total body

DRUG INTERACTIONS CAUSED BY ALTERED ABSORPTION

Gastrointestinal absorption is slowed by drugs that inhibit gastric emptying, such as atropine or opiates, or

---

[2]This has been invoked to explain the central symptoms of cholinesterase inhibition experienced by some soldiers during the Gulf War. These soldiers may have been exposed to cholinesterase inhibitors (developed as chemical weapons and also used externally during the conflict to prevent insect infestation) in the context of the stress of warfare.

Drug distribution

- The major compartments are:
  - plasma (5% of body weight)
  - interstitial fluid (16%)
  - intracellular fluid (35%)
  - transcellular fluid (2%)
  - fat (20%).
- Volume of distribution (V_d) is defined as the volume that would contain the total body content of the drug at a concentration equal to that in the plasma.
- Lipid-insoluble drugs are mainly confined to plasma and interstitial fluids; most do not enter the brain following acute dosing.
- Lipid-soluble drugs reach all compartments and may accumulate in fat.
- For drugs that accumulate outside the plasma compartment (e.g. in fat or by being bound to tissues), V_d may exceed total body volume.

accelerated by drugs that hasten gastric emptying (e.g. metoclopramide; see Ch. 30). Alternatively, drug A may interact physically or chemically with drug B in the gut in such a way as to inhibit absorption of B. For example, Ca^{2+} and Fe^{2+} each form insoluble complexes with **tetracycline** that retard their absorption; **colestyramine**, a bile acid-binding resin, binds several drugs (e.g. warfarin, digoxin), preventing their absorption if administered simultaneously. Another example is the addition of **adrenaline** (**epinephrine**) to local anaesthetic injections; the resulting vasoconstriction slows the absorption of the anaesthetic, thus prolonging its local effect (Ch. 43).

DRUG INTERACTIONS CAUSED BY ALTERED DISTRIBUTION

One drug may alter the distribution of another, by competing for a common binding site on plasma albumin or tissue protein, but such interactions are seldom clinically important unless accompanied by a separate effect on drug elimination (see Ch. 9). Displacement of a drug from binding sites in plasma or tissues transiently increases the concentration of free (unbound) drug, but this is followed by increased elimination, so a new steady state results in which total drug concentration in plasma is reduced but the free drug concentration is similar to that before introduction of the second 'displacing' drug. Consequences of potential clinical importance include:

- Toxicity from the transient increase in concentration of free drug before the new steady state is reached.
- If dose is being adjusted according to measurements of total plasma concentration, it must be appreciated that the target therapeutic concentration range will be altered by co-administration of a displacing drug.
- When the displacing drug additionally reduces elimination of the first, so that the free concentration is increased not only acutely but also chronically at the new steady state, severe toxicity may ensue.

Although many drugs have appreciable affinity for plasma albumin, and therefore might potentially be

expected to interact in these ways, there are rather few instances of clinically important interactions of this type. Protein-bound drugs that are given in large enough dosage to act as displacing agents include various *sulfonamides* and **chloral hydrate**; trichloracetic acid, a metabolite of chloral hydrate, binds very strongly to plasma albumin. Displacement of bilirubin from albumin by such drugs in jaundiced premature neonates can have clinically disastrous consequences: bilirubin metabolism is undeveloped in the premature liver, and unbound bilirubin can cross the immature blood–brain barrier and cause kernicterus (staining of the basal ganglia by bilirubin). This causes a distressing and permanent disturbance of movement known as choreoathetosis, characterised by involuntary writhing and twisting movements in the child.

Phenytoin dose is adjusted according to measurement of its concentration in plasma, and such measurements do not routinely distinguish bound from free phenytoin (that is, they reflect the total concentration of drug). Introduction of a displacing drug in an epileptic patient whose condition is stabilised on phenytoin (Ch. 45) reduces the total plasma phenytoin concentration owing to increased elimination of free drug, but there is no loss of efficacy because the concentration of unbound (active) phenytoin at the new steady state is unaltered. If it is not appreciated that the therapeutic range of plasma concentrations has been reduced in this way, an increased dose may be prescribed, resulting in toxicity.

There are several instances where drugs that alter protein binding additionally reduce elimination of the displaced drug, causing clinically important interactions. *Salicylates* displace **methotrexate** from binding sites on albumin and reduce its secretion into the nephron by competition with the organic anion transporter (OAT; Ch. 9). **Quinidine** and several other antidysrhythmic drugs including **verapamil** and **amiodarone** (Ch. 21) displace digoxin from tissue-binding sites while simultaneously reducing its renal excretion; they consequently can cause severe dysrhythmias through digoxin toxicity.

SPECIAL DRUG DELIVERY SYSTEMS

Several approaches are used or in development to improve drug delivery and localise the drug to the target tissue. They include:

- prodrugs
- biologically erodible nanoparticles
- antibody–drug conjugates
- packaging in liposomes
- coated implantable devices.

PRODRUGS

Prodrugs are inactive precursors that are metabolised to active metabolites; they are described in Chapter 9. Some of the examples in clinical use confer no obvious benefits and have been found to be prodrugs only retrospectively, not having been designed with this in mind. However, some do have advantages. For example, the cytotoxic drug **cyclophosphamide** (see Ch. 56) becomes active only after it has been metabolised in the liver; it can therefore be taken orally without causing serious damage to the gastrointestinal epithelium. Levodopa is absorbed from the gastrointestinal tract and crosses the blood–brain barrier via an amino acid transport mechanism before conversion to active dopamine in nerve terminals in the basal ganglia (Ch. 40). **Zidovudine** is phosphorylated to its active triphosphate metabolite only in cells containing the appropriate reverse transcriptase, hence conferring selective toxicity towards cells infected with HIV (Ch. 52). **Valaciclovir** and **famciclovir** are each ester prodrugs, respectively of **aciclovir** and of **penciclovir**. Their bioavailability is greater than that of aciclovir and penciclovir, which are themselves prodrugs that are converted into active metabolites in virally infected cells (Ch. 52). **Diacetyl morphine** ('heroin') is a prodrug that penetrates the blood–brain barrier even faster than its active metabolites morphine and 6-monoacetyl morphine (Ch. 42), accounting for increased 'buzz' and hence abuse potential.

Other problems could theoretically be overcome by the use of suitable prodrugs; for example, instability of drugs at gastric pH, direct gastric irritation (aspirin was synthesised in the 19th century in a deliberate attempt to produce a prodrug of salicylic acid that would be tolerable when taken by mouth), failure of drug to cross the blood–brain barrier and so on. Progress with this approach remains slow, however, and the optimistic prodrug designer 'will have to bear in mind that an organism's normal reaction to a foreign substance is to burn it up for food'.

BIOLOGICALLY ERODIBLE NANOPARTICLES

▼ Microspheres of biologically erodible polymers (see Varde & Pack, 2004) can be engineered to adhere to mucosal epithelium in the gut. Such particles can be loaded with drugs, including high-molecular-weight substances, as a means of improving absorption, which occurs both through mucosal absorptive epithelium and also through epithelium overlying Peyer's patches. Various polymer nanoparticles, that can be loaded with drug molecules and targeted to specific tissues, are in development for many therapeutic applications (see Singh & Lillard, 2008), particularly as a means of delivering cytotoxic drugs specifically to cancer cells (see Ch. 56).

ANTIBODY–DRUG CONJUGATES

▼ One of the aims of cancer chemotherapy is to improve the selectivity of cytotoxic drugs (see Ch. 56). One interesting possibility is to attach the drug to an antibody directed against a tumour-specific antigen, which will bind selectively to tumour cells.

PACKAGING IN LIPOSOMES

▼ Liposomes are vesicles 0.1–1 μm in diameter produced by sonication of an aqueous suspension of phospholipids. They can be filled with non-lipid-soluble drugs, which are retained until the liposome is disrupted. Liposomes are taken up by reticuloendothelial cells, especially in the liver. They are also concentrated in malignant tumours, and there is a possibility of achieving selective delivery of drugs in this way. **Amphotericin**, an antifungal drug used to treat systemic mycoses (Ch. 53), is available in a liposomal formulation that is less nephrotoxic and better tolerated than the conventional form, albeit considerably more expensive. A long acting form of **doxorubicin** encapsulated in liposomes is available for the treatment of malignancies (including ovarian cancer and myeloma), and **paclitaxel** is available in an albumin nanoparticle used to treat breast cancer (Ch. 56). Lipid nanoparticles are being used to deliver small interfering RNA preparations that are in development for a wide range of potential indications (Ch. 59). In the future, it may be possible to direct drugs or genes selectively to a specific target by incorporating antibody molecules into liposomal membrane surfaces.

COATED IMPLANTABLE DEVICES

▼ Impregnated coatings have been developed that permit localised drug delivery from implants. Examples include hormonal delivery to the endometrium from intrauterine devices, and delivery of antithrombotic and antiproliferative agents (drugs or radiopharmaceuticals) to the coronary arteries from *stents* (tubular devices inserted via a catheter after a diseased coronary artery has been dilated with a balloon). Stents reduce the occurrence of re-stenosis, but this can still occur at the margin of the device. Coating stents with drugs such as **sirolimus** (a potent immunosuppressant; see Ch. 26) embedded in a surface polymer prevents this important clinical problem.

REFERENCES AND FURTHER READING

References

EMEA, 2009. Guideline on the investigation of bioequivalence. <www.emea.europa.eu/docs/en_GB/document_library/Scientific_guideline/2009/09/WC500003011.pdf> (accessed 8 April 2014).

Singh, R., Lillard, J.W., 2008. Nanoparticle-based targeted drug delivery. Exp. Mol. Pathol. 86, 215–223.

Varde, N.K., Pack, D.W., 2004. Microspheres for controlled release drug delivery. Exp. Opin. Biol. Ther. 4, 35–51.

Drug absorption

Bailey, D.G., 2010. Fruit juice inhibition of uptake transport: a new type of food–drug interaction. Br. J. Clin. Pharmacol. 70, 645–655.

De Gorter, M.K., Xia, C.Q., Yang, J.J., Kim, R.B., 2012. Drug transporters in drug efficacy and toxicity. Ann. Rev. Pharmacol. Toxicol. 52, 249–273.

Drug distribution (including blood–brain barrier)

Ciarimboli, G., 2008. Organic cation transporters. Xenobiotica 38, 936–971. (*Discusses species- and tissue-specific distribution of different OCT isoforms and polymorphisms in OCTs as a source of variation in drug response*)

Hediger, M.A., Romero, M.F., Peng, J.-B., et al., 2004. The ABCs of solute carriers: physiological, pathological and therapeutic implications of human membrane transport proteins. Pflug. Arch. 447, 465–468.

Miller, D.S., Bauer, B., Hartz, A.M.S., 2008. Modulation of P-glycoprotein at the blood–brain barrier: opportunities to improve central nervous system pharmacotherapy. Pharmacol. Rev. 60, 196–209.

Drug delivery

Huttunen, K.M., Raunio, H., Rautio, J., 2011. Prodrugs – from serendipity to rational design. Pharmacol. Rev. 63, 750–771.

Moghuini, S.M., Hunter, A.C., Andersen, T.L., 2012. Factors controlling nanoparticle pharmacokinetics: an integrated analysis and perspective. Ann. Rev. Pharmacol. Toxicol. 52, 481–503.

9 Drug metabolism and elimination

OVERVIEW

We describe phases 1 and 2 of drug metabolism, emphasising the importance of the cytochrome P450 monooxygenase system. We then cover the processes of biliary excretion and enterohepatic recirculation of drugs, and of drug interactions caused by induction or inhibition of metabolism. Drug and drug metabolite elimination by the kidney are described and drug interactions due to effects on renal elimination considered.

INTRODUCTION

Drug elimination is the irreversible loss of drug from the body. It occurs by two processes: *metabolism* and *excretion*. Metabolism consists of anabolism and catabolism, i.e. respectively the build-up and breakdown of substances by enzymic conversion of one chemical entity to another within the body, whereas excretion consists of elimination from the body of drug or drug metabolites. The main excretory routes are:

- the kidneys
- the hepatobiliary system
- the lungs (important for volatile/gaseous anaesthetics).

Most drugs leave the body in the urine, either unchanged or as polar metabolites. Some drugs are secreted into bile via the liver, but most of these are then reabsorbed from the intestine. There are, however, instances (e.g. **rifampicin**; Ch. 51) where faecal loss accounts for the elimination of a substantial fraction of unchanged drug in healthy individuals, and faecal elimination of drugs such as **digoxin** that are normally excreted in urine (Ch. 21) becomes progressively more important in patients with advancing renal failure. Excretion via the lungs occurs only with highly volatile or gaseous agents (e.g. general anaesthetics; Ch. 41). Small amounts of some drugs are also excreted in secretions such as milk or sweat. Elimination by these routes is quantitatively negligible compared with renal excretion, although excretion into milk can sometimes be important because of effects on the baby (www.fpnotebook.com/ob/Pharm/MdctnsInLctn.htm).

Lipophilic substances are not eliminated efficiently by the kidney. Consequently, most lipophilic drugs are metabolised to more polar products, which are then excreted in urine. Drug metabolism occurs predominantly in the liver, especially by the cytochrome P450 (CYP) system. Some P450 enzymes are extrahepatic and play an important part in the biosynthesis of steroid hormones (Ch. 33) and eicosanoids (Ch. 18), but here we are concerned with catabolism of drugs by the hepatic P450 system.

DRUG METABOLISM

Animals have evolved complex systems that detoxify foreign chemicals ('xenobiotics'), including carcinogens and toxins present in poisonous plants. Drugs are a special case of such xenobiotics and, like plant alkaloids, they often exhibit *chirality* (i.e. there is more than one stereoisomer), which affects their overall metabolism. Drug metabolism involves two kinds of reaction, known as phase 1 and phase 2, which often occur sequentially. Both phases decrease lipid solubility, thus increasing renal elimination.

PHASE 1 REACTIONS

Phase 1 reactions (e.g. oxidation, reduction or hydrolysis) are catabolic, and the products are often more chemically reactive and hence, paradoxically, sometimes more toxic or carcinogenic than the parent drug. Phase 1 reactions often introduce a reactive group, such as hydroxyl, into the molecule, a process known as 'functionalisation'. This group then serves as the point of attack for the conjugating system to attach a substituent such as glucuronide (Fig. 9.1), explaining why phase 1 reactions so often precede phase 2 reactions. The liver is especially important in phase 1 reactions. Many hepatic drug-metabolising enzymes, including CYP enzymes, are embedded in the smooth endoplasmic reticulum. They are often called 'microsomal' enzymes because, on homogenisation and differential centrifugation, the endoplasmic reticulum is broken into very small fragments that sediment only after prolonged high-speed centrifugation in the microsomal fraction. To reach these metabolising enzymes in life, a drug must cross the plasma membrane. Polar molecules do this less readily than non-polar molecules except where there are specific transport mechanisms (Ch. 8), so intracellular metabolism is important for lipid-soluble drugs, while polar drugs are, at least partly, excreted unchanged in the urine.

THE P450 MONOOXYGENASE SYSTEM
Nature, classification and mechanism of P450 enzymes

Cytochrome P450 enzymes are haem proteins, comprising a large family ('superfamily') of related but distinct enzymes, each referred to as CYP followed by a defining set of numbers and a letter. These enzymes differ from one another in amino acid sequence, in sensitivity to inhibitors and inducing agents (see below), and in the specificity of the reactions that they catalyse (see Anzenbacher, 2007 for review). Different members of the family have distinct, but often overlapping, substrate specificities. Purification and cloning of P450 enzymes form the basis of the current classification, which is based on amino acid sequence

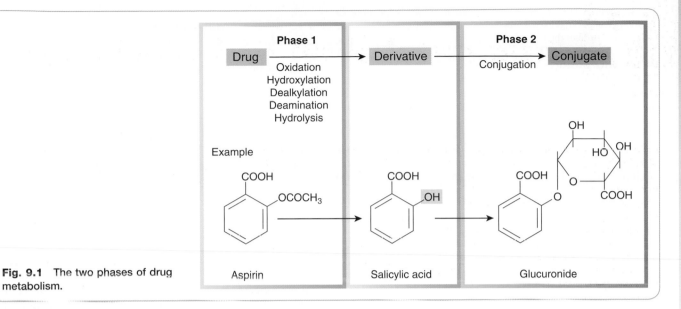

Fig. 9.1 The two phases of drug metabolism.

Table 9.1 Examples of drugs that are substrates of P450 isoenzymes

Isoenzyme P450	Drug(s)
CYP1A2	Caffeine, paracetamol (→NAPQI), tacrine, theophylline
CYP2B6	Cyclophosphamide, methadone
CYP2C8	Paclitaxel, repaglinide
CYP2C19	Omeprazole, phenytoin
CYP2C9	Ibuprofen, tolbutamide, warfarin
CYP2D6	Codeine, debrisoquine, S-metoprolol
CYP2E1	Alcohol, paracetamol
CYP3A4, 5, 7	Ciclosporin, nifedipine, indinavir, simvastatin

Adapted from http://medicine.iupui.edu/flockhart/table.htm

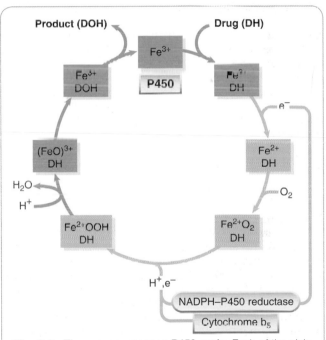

Fig. 9.2 The monooxygenase P450 cycle. Each of the pink or blue rectangles represents one single molecule of cytochrome P450 (P450) undergoing a catalytic cycle. Iron in P450 is in either the ferric (pink rectangles) or ferrous (blue rectangles) state. P450 containing ferric iron (Fe^{3+}) combines with a molecule of drug ('DH'); receives an electron from NADPH–P450 reductase, which reduces the iron to Fe^{2+}; combines with molecular oxygen, a proton and a second electron (either from NADPH–P450 reductase or from cytochrome b_5) to form an $Fe^{2+}OOH$–DH complex. This combines with another proton to yield water and a ferric oxene $(FeO)^{3+}$–DH complex. $(FeO)^{3+}$ extracts a hydrogen atom from DH, with the formation of a pair of short-lived free radicals (see text), liberation from the complex of oxidised drug ('DOH'), and regeneration of P450 enzyme.

similarities. Seventy-four CYP gene families have been described, of which three main ones (CYP1, CYP2 and CYP3) are involved in drug metabolism in human liver. Examples of therapeutic drugs that are substrates for some important P450 isoenzymes are shown in Table 9.1. Drug oxidation by the monooxygenase P450 system requires drug (substrate, 'DH'), P450 enzyme, molecular oxygen, NADPH and NADPH–P450 reductase (a flavoprotein). The mechanism involves a complex cycle (Fig. 9.2), but the outcome of the reaction is quite simple, namely the addition of one atom of oxygen (from molecular oxygen) to the drug to form a hydroxylated product (DOH), the other atom of oxygen being converted to water.

▼ P450 enzymes have unique spectral properties, and the reduced forms combine with carbon monoxide to form a pink compound (hence 'P') with absorption peaks near 450 nm (range 447–452 nm). The first clue that there is more than one form of CYP came from the observation that treatment of rats with 3-methylcholanthrene (3-MC), an inducing agent (see below), causes a shift in the absorption maximum from 450 to 448 nm – the 3-MC-induced isoform of the enzyme absorbs light maximally at a slightly shorter wavelength than the un-induced enzyme.

P450 and biological variation

There are important variations in the expression and regulation of P450 enzymes between species. For instance, the pathways by which certain dietary heterocyclic amines (formed when meat is cooked) generate genotoxic products involves one member of the P450 superfamily (CYP1A2) that is constitutively present in humans and rats (which develop colon tumours after treatment with such amines) but not in cynomolgus monkeys (which do not). Such species differences have crucial implications for the choice of species to be used for toxicity and carcinogenicity testing during the development of new drugs for use in humans.

Within human populations, there are major sources of inter-individual variation in P450 enzymes that are of great importance in therapeutics. These include genetic polymorphisms (alternative sequences at a locus within the DNA strand – alleles – that persist in a population through several generations; Ch. 11). Environmental factors are also important, since enzyme inhibitors and inducers are present in the diet and environment. For example, a component of grapefruit juice inhibits drug metabolism (leading to potentially disastrous consequences, including cardiac dysrhythmias), whereas Brussels sprouts and cigarette smoke induce P450 enzymes. Components of the herbal medicine St John's wort (Ch. 47) induce CYP450 isoenzymes as well as P-glycoprotein (P-gp) (see Ch. 8). Drug interactions based on one drug altering the metabolism of another are common and clinically important (see Ch. 11).

Not all drug oxidation reactions involve the P450 system. Some drugs are metabolised in plasma (e.g. hydrolysis of **suxamethonium** by plasma cholinesterase; Ch. 13), lung (e.g. various prostanoids; Ch. 17) or gut (e.g. **tyramine**, **salbutamol**; Chs 14 and 28). **Ethanol** (Ch. 49) is metabolised by a soluble cytoplasmic enzyme, alcohol dehydrogenase, in addition to CYP2E1. Other P450-independent enzymes involved in drug oxidation include xanthine oxidase, which inactivates **6-mercaptopurine** (Ch. 56), and monoamine oxidase, which inactivates many biologically active amines (e.g. **noradrenaline** [norepinephrine], tyramine, 5-hydroxytryptamine; Chs 14 and 15).

HYDROLYTIC REACTIONS

Hydrolysis (e.g. of **aspirin**; Fig. 9.1) occurs in plasma and in many tissues. Both ester and (less readily) amide bonds are susceptible to hydrolytic cleavage. Reduction is less common in phase 1 metabolism than oxidation, but **warfarin** (Ch. 24) is inactivated by reduction of a ketone to a hydroxyl group by CYP2A6.

PHASE 2 REACTIONS

Phase 2 reactions are synthetic ('anabolic') and involve conjugation (i.e. attachment of a substituent group), which usually results in inactive products, although there are exceptions (e.g. the active sulfate metabolite of **minoxidil**, a potassium channel activator used to treat severe hypertension (Ch. 22) and to promote hair growth. Phase 2 reactions take place mainly in the liver. If a drug molecule or Phase 1 product has a suitable 'handle' (e.g. a hydroxyl, thiol or amino group), it is susceptible to conjugation. The chemical group inserted may

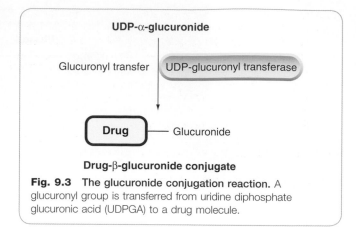

Fig. 9.3 The glucuronide conjugation reaction. A glucuronyl group is transferred from uridine diphosphate glucuronic acid (UDPGA) to a drug molecule.

be glucuronyl (Fig. 9.3), sulfate, methyl or acetyl. The tripeptide glutathione conjugates drugs or their phase 1 metabolites via its sulfhydryl group, as in the detoxification of **paracetamol** (see Fig. 57.1). Glucuronidation involves the formation of a high-energy phosphate ('donor') compound, uridine diphosphate glucuronic acid (UDPGA), from which glucuronic acid is transferred to an electron-rich atom (N, O or S) on the substrate, forming an amide, ester or thiol bond. UDP-glucuronyl transferase, which catalyses these reactions, has very broad substrate specificity embracing many drugs and other foreign molecules. Several important endogenous substances, including bilirubin and adrenal corticosteroids, are conjugated by the same pathway.

Acetylation and methylation reactions occur with acetyl-CoA and S-adenosyl methionine, respectively, acting as the donor compounds. Many conjugation reactions occur in the liver, but other tissues, such as lung and kidney, are also involved.

STEREOSELECTIVITY

Many clinically important drugs, such as **sotalol** (Ch. 21), **warfarin** (Ch. 24) and **cyclophosphamide** (Ch. 56), are mixtures of stereoisomers, the components of which differ not only in their pharmacological effects but also in their metabolism, which may follow completely distinct pathways (Campo et al., 2009). Several clinically important drug interactions involve stereospecific inhibition of metabolism of one drug by another (see Table 9.6, p. 121). In some cases, drug toxicity is mainly linked to one of the stereoisomers, not necessarily the pharmacologically active one. Where practicable, regulatory authorities urge that new drugs should consist of single isomers to lessen these complications.[1]

INHIBITION OF P450

Inhibitors of P450 differ in their selectivity towards different isoforms of the enzyme, and are classified by their mechanism of action. Some drugs compete for the active site but are not themselves substrates (e.g. **quinidine** is a potent competitive inhibitor of CYP2D6 but is not a

---

[1]Well-intentioned – though the usefulness of expensive 'novel' entities that are actually just the pure active isomer of well-established and safe racemates has been questioned, and enzymic interconversion of stereoisomers may subvert such chemical sophistication.

substrate for it). Non-competitive inhibitors include drugs such as **ketoconazole**, which forms a tight complex with the Fe^{3+} form of the haem iron of CYP3A4, causing reversible non-competitive inhibition. So-called mechanism-based inhibitors require oxidation by a P450 enzyme. Examples include the oral contraceptive **gestodene** (CYP3A4) and the anthelmintic drug **diethylcarbamazine** (CYP2E1). An oxidation product (e.g. a postulated epoxide intermediate of gestodene) binds covalently to the enzyme, which then destroys itself ('suicide inhibition'; see Pelkonen et al., 2008).

INDUCTION OF MICROSOMAL ENZYMES

A number of drugs, such as **rifampicin** (Ch. 51), **ethanol** (Ch. 49) and **carbamazepine** (Ch. 45), increase the activity of microsomal oxidase and conjugating systems when administered repeatedly. Many carcinogenic chemicals (e.g. benzpyrene, 3-MC) also have this effect, which can be substantial; Figure 9.4 shows a nearly 10-fold increase in the rate of benzpyrene metabolism 2 days after a single dose. The effect is referred to as *induction*, and is the result of increased synthesis and/or reduced breakdown of microsomal enzymes (Pelkonen et al., 2008).

Enzyme induction can increase drug toxicity and carcinogenicity, because several phase 1 metabolites are toxic or carcinogenic: paracetamol is an important example of a drug with a highly toxic metabolite (see Ch. 57). Enzyme induction is exploited therapeutically by administering **phenobarbital** to premature babies to induce glucuronyltransferase, thereby increasing bilirubin conjugation and reducing the risk of kernicterus (staining and neurological damage of the basal ganglia by bilirubin, Ch. 8).

▼ The mechanism of induction is incompletely understood but is similar to that involved in the action of steroid and other hormones that bind to nuclear receptors (see Ch. 3). The most thoroughly studied inducing agents are polycyclic aromatic hydrocarbons (e.g. 3-MC). These bind to the ligand-binding domain of a soluble protein, termed the aromatic hydrocarbon (Ah) receptor. This complex is transported to the nucleus by an Ah receptor nuclear translocator and binds Ah receptor response elements in the DNA, thereby promoting transcription of the gene CYP1A1. In addition to enhanced transcription, some inducing agents (e.g. ethanol, which induces CYP2E1 in humans) also stabilise mRNA or P450 protein.

FIRST-PASS (PRESYSTEMIC ['FIRST-PASS'] METABOLISM)

Some drugs are extracted so efficiently by the liver or gut wall that the amount reaching the systemic circulation is considerably less than the amount absorbed. This is known as presystemic (or first-pass) metabolism and reduces bioavailability (Ch. 8), even when a drug is well absorbed. Presystemic metabolism is important for many therapeutic drugs (Table 9.2 shows some examples), and is a problem because:

- a much larger dose of the drug is needed when it is taken by mouth than when it is given parenterally
- marked individual variations occur in the extent of first-pass metabolism, both in the activities of drug metabolising enzymes and also as a result of variation in hepatic blood flow. This can be reduced in disease (e.g. heart failure) or by drugs, such as β adrenoceptor antagonists, which impair the clearance of unrelated drugs, such as lidocaine, that are subject to presystemic metabolism due to a high hepatic extraction ratio.

PHARMACOLOGICALLY ACTIVE DRUG METABOLITES

In some cases (see Table 9.3) a drug becomes pharmacologically active only after it has been metabolised. For example, **azathioprine**, an immunosuppressant drug (Ch. 26), is metabolised to **mercaptopurine**; and **enalapril**, an angiotensin-converting enzyme inhibitor (Ch. 22), is hydrolysed to its active form **enalaprilat**. Such drugs, in which the parent compound lacks activity of its own, are known as *prodrugs*. These are sometimes designed deliberately to overcome problems of drug delivery (Ch. 8). Metabolism can alter the pharmacological actions of a drug qualitatively. **Aspirin** inhibits platelet function and has anti-inflammatory activity (Chs 24 and 26). It is hydrolysed to salicylic acid (see Fig. 9.1), which has anti-inflammatory but not antiplatelet activity. In other instances, metabolites have pharmacological actions similar to those of the parent compound (e.g. benzodiazepines, many of which form long-lived active metabolites that cause sedation to persist after the parent drug has disappeared; Ch. 44). There are also cases in which metabolites are responsible for toxicity. Bladder toxicity of **cyclophosphamide**, which is caused by its toxic metabolite acrolein (Ch. 56), is an example. Methanol and ethylene

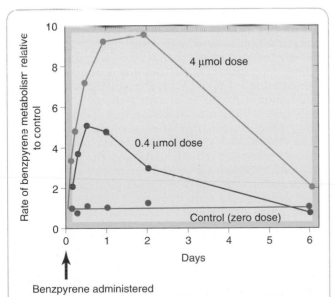

Fig. 9.4 **Stimulation of hepatic metabolism of benzpyrene.** Young rats were given benzpyrene (intraperitoneally) in the doses shown, and the benzpyrene-metabolising activity of liver homogenates was measured at times up to 6 days. (From Conney AH et al. 1957 J Biol Chem 228, 753.)

Table 9.2 Examples of drugs that undergo substantial first-pass elimination

Aspirin	Metoprolol
Glyceryl trinitrate	Morphine
Isosorbide dinitrate	Propranolol
Levodopa	Salbutamol
Lidocaine	Verapamil

Table 9.3 Some drugs that produce active or toxic metabolites

Inactive (prodrugs)	Active drug	Active metabolite	Toxic metabolite	See Chapter
Azathioprine ─────────────────────→		Mercaptopurine		26
Cortisone ─────────────────────→		Hydrocortisone		33
Prednisone ─────────────────────→		Prednisolone		33
Enalapril ─────────────────────→		Enalaprilat		22
Zidovudine ─────────────────────→		Zidovudine trisphosphate		52
Cyclophosphamide ─────────────────────→		Phosphoramide mustard ──────→	Acrolein	56
	Diazepam ──────→	Nordiazepam ──────────→	Oxazepam	44
	Morphine ──────→	Morphine 6-glucuronide		42
	Halothane ─────────────────────→		Trifluoroacetic acid	41
	Methoxyflurane ─────────────────→		Fluoride	41
	Paracetamol ─────────────────────→		N-Acetyl-p-benzoquinone imine	26, 57

glycol both exert their toxic effects via metabolites formed by alcohol dehydrogenase. Poisoning with these agents is treated with ethanol (or with a more potent inhibitor), which competes for the active site of the enzyme.

Drug metabolism

- Phase 1 reactions involve oxidation, reduction and hydrolysis. They:
  - usually form more chemically reactive products, which can be pharmacologically active, toxic or carcinogenic
  - often involve a monooxygenase system in which cytochrome P450 plays a key role.
- Phase 2 reactions involve conjugation (e.g. glucuronidation) of a reactive group (often inserted during phase 1 reaction) and usually lead to inactive and polar products that are readily excreted in urine.
- Some conjugated products are excreted via bile, are reactivated in the intestine and then reabsorbed ('enterohepatic circulation').
- Induction of P450 enzymes can greatly accelerate hepatic drug metabolism. It can increase the toxicity of drugs with toxic metabolites, and is an important cause of drug–drug interaction as in enzyme inhibition.
- Presystemic metabolism in liver or gut wall reduces the bioavailability of several drugs when they are administered by mouth.

DRUG INTERACTIONS DUE TO ENZYME INDUCTION OR INHIBITION

INTERACTIONS CAUSED BY ENZYME INDUCTION

Enzyme induction is an important cause of drug interaction. The slow onset of induction and slow recovery after

withdrawal of the inducing agent together with the potential for selective induction of one or more CYP isoenzymes contributes to the insidious nature of the clinical problems that induction presents. Adverse clinical outcomes from such interactions are very diverse, including graft rejection as a result of loss of effectiveness of immunosuppressive treatment, seizures due to loss of anticonvulsant effectiveness, unwanted pregnancy from loss of oral contraceptive action and thrombosis (from loss of effectiveness of warfarin) or bleeding (from failure to recognise the need to reduce warfarin dose when induction wanes). Over 200 drugs cause enzyme induction and thereby decrease the pharmacological activity of a range of other drugs. Some examples are given in Table 9.4. Because the inducing agent is often itself a substrate for the induced enzymes, the process can result in slowly developing tolerance. This pharmacokinetic kind of tolerance is generally less marked than pharmacodynamic tolerance, for example to opioids (Ch. 42), but it is clinically important when starting treatment with the antiepileptic drug **carbamazepine** (Ch. 45). Treatment starts at a low dose to avoid toxicity (because liver enzymes are not induced initially) and is gradually increased over a period of a few weeks, during which it induces its own metabolism.

Figure 9.5 shows how the antibiotic **rifampicin**, given for 3 days, reduces the effectiveness of **warfarin** as an anticoagulant. Conversely, enzyme induction can increase toxicity of a second drug if the toxic effects are mediated via an active metabolite. **Paracetamol (acetaminophen)** toxicity is a case in point (see Fig. 57.1): this is caused by its CYP metabolite N-acetyl-p-benzoquinone imine. Consequently, the risk of serious hepatic injury following paracetamol overdose is increased in patients in whom CYP has been induced, for example by chronic alcohol consumption.

INTERACTIONS CAUSED BY ENZYME INHIBITION

Enzyme inhibition, particularly of CYP enzymes, slows the metabolism and hence increases the action of other

Table 9.4 Examples of drugs that induce drug-metabolising enzymes

Drugs inducing enzyme action	Drugs with metabolism affected
Phenobarbital	Warfarin
Rifampicin	Oral contraceptives
Griseofulvin	Corticosteroids
Phenytoin	Ciclosporin
Ethanol Carbamazepine	Drugs listed in left-hand column will also be affected

Table 9.5 Examples of drugs that inhibit drug-metabolising enzymes

Drugs inhibiting enzyme action	Drugs with metabolism affected
Allopurinol	Mercaptopurine, azathioprine
Chloramphenicol	Phenytoin
Cimetidine	Amiodarone, phenytoin, pethidine
Ciprofloxacin	Theophylline
Corticosteroids	Tricyclic antidepressants, cyclophosphamide
Disulfiram	Warfarin
Erythromycin	Ciclosporin, theophylline
Monoamine oxidase inhibitors	Pethidine
Ritonavir	Saquinavir

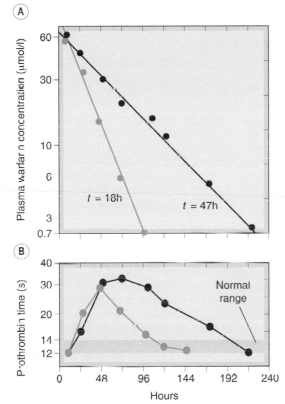

Fig. 9.5 Effect of rifampicin on the metabolism and anticoagulant action of warfarin. **[A]** Plasma concentration of warfarin (log scale) as a function of time following a single oral dose of 5 μmol/kg body weight. After the subject was given rifampicin (600 mg daily for a few days), the plasma half-life of warfarin decreased from 47 h (red curve) to 18 h (green curve). **[B]** The effect of a single dose of warfarin on prothrombin time under normal conditions (red curve) and after rifampicin administration (green curve). *(Redrawn from O'Reilly 1974 Ann Intern Med 81, 337.)*

Table 9.6 Stereoselective and non-stereoselective inhibition of warfarin metabolism

Inhibition of metabolism	Drug(s)
Stereoselective for (S) isomer	Phenylbutazone Metronidazole Sulfinpyrazone Trimethoprim– sulfamethoxazole Disulfiram
Stereoselective for (R) isomer	Cimetidine[a] Omeprazole[a]
Non-stereoselective effect on both isomers	Amiodarone

[a]Minor effect only on prothrombin time.
From Hirsh 1991 N Engl J Med 324, 1865–1875

drugs inactivated by the enzyme. Such effects can be clinically important and are major considerations in the treatment of patients with HIV infection with triple and quadruple therapy, because several protease inhibitors are potent CYP inhibitors (Ch. 52). Other examples of drugs that are enzyme inhibitors are shown in Table 9.5.

To make life even more difficult, several inhibitors of drug metabolism influence the metabolism of different stereo-isomers selectively. Examples of drugs that inhibit the metabolism of the active (S) and less active (R) isomers of warfarin in this way are shown in Table 9.6.

The therapeutic effects of some drugs are a direct conse-quence of enzyme inhibition (e.g. the xanthine oxidase inhibitor **allopurinol**, used to prevent gout; Ch. 26). Xan-thine oxidase metabolises several cytotoxic and immuno-suppressant drugs, including **mercaptopurine** (the active metabolite of **azathioprine**), the action of which is thus potentiated and prolonged by allopurinol. **Disulfiram**, an inhibitor of aldehyde dehydrogenase used to produce an aversive reaction to ethanol (see Ch. 49), also inhibits metabolism of other drugs, including **warfarin**, which it potentiates. **Metronidazole**, an antimicrobial used to treat anaerobic bacterial infections and several protozoal dis-eases (Chs 51 and 54), also inhibits this enzyme, and patients prescribed it are advised to avoid alcohol for this reason.

There are also examples of drugs that inhibit the metabolism of other drugs, even though enzyme inhibition is not the main mechanism of action of the offending agents. Thus, *glucocorticosteroids* and **cimetidine** enhance the actions of a range of drugs, including some antidepressant and cytotoxic drugs.

When a drug works through an active metabolite, inhibition of its metabolism can result in *loss* of activity. Proton pump inhibitors (such as **omeprazole**, Ch. 30) and the antiplatelet drug **clopidogrel** (Ch. 24) have been widely co-prescribed (because clopidogrel is often used with other antithrombotic drugs so there is a high risk of bleeding from the stomach – omeprazole reduces this). Clopidogrel works through an active metabolite formed by CYP2C19 which is inhibited by omeprazole which might thereby reduce the antiplatelet effect. It is unclear how clinically important this may be, but the Food and Drug Administration has warned against concomitant use of these drugs for this reason.

As with induction, interactions caused by enzyme inhibition are hard to anticipate from first principles. If in doubt about the possibility of an interaction, it is best to look it up (e.g. in the *British National Formulary*, which has an invaluable appendix on drug interactions indicating which are of known clinical importance).

DRUG AND METABOLITE EXCRETION

BILIARY EXCRETION AND ENTEROHEPATIC CIRCULATION

Liver cells transfer various substances, including drugs, from plasma to bile by means of transport systems similar to those of the renal tubule; these include organic cation transporters (OCTs), organic anion transporters (OATs) and P-glycoproteins (P-gp) (see Ch. 8). Various hydrophilic drug conjugates (particularly glucuronides) are concentrated in bile and delivered to the intestine, where the glucuronide can be hydrolysed, regenerating active drug; free drug can then be reabsorbed and the cycle repeated, a process referred to as *enterohepatic circulation*. The result is a 'reservoir' of recirculating drug that can amount to about 20% of total drug in the body, prolonging drug action. Examples where this is important include **morphine** (Ch. 42) and **ethinylestradiol** (Ch. 35). Several drugs are excreted to an appreciable extent in bile. **Vecuronium** (a non-depolarising muscle relaxant; Ch. 13) is an example of a drug that is excreted mainly unchanged in bile. **Rifampicin** (Ch. 51) is absorbed from the gut and slowly deacetylated, retaining its biological activity. Both forms are secreted in the bile, but the deacetylated form is not reabsorbed, so eventually most of the drug leaves the body in this form in the faeces.

RENAL EXCRETION OF DRUGS AND METABOLITES

RENAL CLEARANCE

Elimination of drugs by the kidneys is best quantified by the renal clearance (CL_{ren}, see Ch. 10). This is defined as the volume of plasma containing the amount of substance that is removed from the body by the kidneys in unit time. It is calculated from the plasma concentration, C_p, the urinary concentration, C_u, and the rate of flow of urine, V_u, by the equation:

$$CL_{ren} = (C_u \times V_u) / C_p.$$

CL_{ren} varies greatly for different drugs, from less than 1 ml/min to the theoretical maximum set by the renal plasma flow, which is approximately 700 ml/min, measured by *p*-aminohippuric acid (PAH) clearance (renal extraction of PAH approaches 100%).

Drugs differ greatly in the rate at which they are excreted by the kidney, ranging from **penicillin** (Ch. 51), which is (like PAH) cleared from the blood almost completely on a single transit through the kidney, to **amiodarone** (Ch. 21) and **risedronate** (Ch. 36), which are cleared extremely slowly. Most drugs fall between these extremes. Three fundamental processes account for renal drug excretion:

1. glomerular filtration
2. active tubular secretion
3. passive reabsorption (diffusion from the concentrated tubular fluid back across tubular epithelium).

GLOMERULAR FILTRATION

Glomerular capillaries allow drug molecules of molecular weight below about 20 kDa to pass into the glomerular filtrate. Plasma albumin (molecular weight approximately 68 kDa) is almost completely impermeant, but most drugs – with the exception of macromolecules such as **heparin** (Ch. 24) or biological products (Ch. 59) – cross the barrier freely. If a drug binds to plasma albumin, only free drug is filtered. If, like **warfarin** (Ch. 24), a drug is approximately 98% bound to albumin, the concentration in the filtrate is only 2% of that in plasma, and clearance by filtration is correspondingly reduced.

TUBULAR SECRETION

Up to 20% of renal plasma flow is filtered through the glomerulus, leaving at least 80% of delivered drug to pass on to the peritubular capillaries of the proximal tubule. Here, drug molecules are transferred to the tubular lumen by two independent and relatively non-selective carrier systems (see Ch. 8). One of these, the OAT, transports acidic drugs in their negatively charged anionic form (as well as various endogenous acids, such as uric acid), while an OCT handles organic bases in their protonated cationic form. Some important drugs that are transported

Table 9.7 Important drugs and related substances secreted into the proximal renal tubule by OAT or OCT transporters

OAT	OCT
p-Aminohippuric acid	Amiloride
Furosemide	Dopamine
Glucuronic acid conjugates	Histamine
Glycine conjugates	Mepacrine
Indometacin	Morphine
Methotrexate	Pethidine
Penicillin	Quaternary ammonium
Probenecid	compounds
Sulfate conjugates	Quinine
Thiazide diuretics	5-Hydroxytryptamine
Uric acid	(serotonin)
	Triamterene

by these two carrier systems are shown in Table 9.7. The OAT carrier can transport drug molecules against an electrochemical gradient, and can therefore reduce the plasma concentration nearly to zero, whereas OCT facilitates transport down an electrochemical gradient. Because at least 80% of the drug delivered to the kidney is presented to the carrier, tubular secretion is potentially the most effective mechanism of renal drug elimination. Unlike glomerular filtration, carrier-mediated transport can achieve maximal drug clearance even when most of the drug is bound to plasma protein.[2] **Penicillin** (Ch. 51), for example, although about 80% protein-bound and therefore cleared only slowly by filtration, is almost completely removed by proximal tubular secretion, and is therefore rapidly eliminated.

Many drugs compete for the same transport systems (Table 9.7), leading to drug interactions. For example, **probenecid** was developed originally to prolong the action of penicillin by retarding its tubular secretion.

DIFFUSION ACROSS THE RENAL TUBULE

Water is reabsorbed as fluid traverses the tubule, the volume of urine emerging being only about 1% of that of the glomerular filtrate. Consequently, if the tubule is freely permeable to drug molecules, some 99% of the filtered drug will be reabsorbed passively down the resulting concentration gradient. Lipid soluble drugs are therefore excreted poorly, whereas polar drugs of low tubular permeability remain in the lumen and become progressively concentrated as water is reabsorbed. Polar drugs handled in this way include **digoxin** and aminoglycoside antibiotics. These exemplify a relatively small but important group of drugs (Table 9.8) that are not inactivated by metabolism, the rate of renal elimination being the main factor that determines their duration of action. These drugs have to be used with special care in individuals whose renal function may be impaired, including the elderly and patients with renal disease or any severe acute illness.

Table 9.8 Examples of drugs that are excreted largely unchanged in the urine

Percentage	Drugs excreted
100–75	Furosemide, gentamicin, methotrexate, atenolol, digoxin
75–50	Benzylpenicillin, cimetidine, oxytetracycline, neostigmine
~50	Propantheline, tubocurarine

[2]Because filtration involves isosmotic movement of both water and solutes, it does not affect the free concentration of drug in the plasma. Thus the equilibrium between free and bound drug is not disturbed, and there is no tendency for bound drug to dissociate as blood traverses the glomerular capillary. The rate of clearance of a drug by filtration is therefore reduced directly in proportion to the fraction that is bound. In the case of active tubular secretion, this is not so because the carrier transports drug molecules unaccompanied by water. As free drug molecules are taken from the plasma, therefore, the free plasma concentration falls, causing dissociation of bound drug from plasma albumin. Secretion is only retarded slightly, even though the drug is mostly bound, because effectively 100% of the drug, both bound and free, is available to the carrier.

The degree of ionisation of many drugs – weak acids or weak bases – is pH-dependent, and this markedly influences their renal excretion. The ion-trapping effect (see Ch. 8) means that a basic drug is more rapidly excreted in an acid urine that favours the charged form and thus inhibits reabsorption. Conversely, acidic drugs are most rapidly excreted if the urine is alkaline (Fig. 9.6).

DRUG INTERACTIONS DUE TO ALTERED DRUG EXCRETION

The main mechanisms by which one drug can affect the rate of renal excretion of another are by:

- altering protein binding, and hence filtration
- inhibiting tubular secretion
- altering urine flow and/or urine pH.

INHIBITION OF TUBULAR SECRETION

Probenecid (Ch. 26) was developed to inhibit secretion of **penicillin** and thus prolong its action. It also inhibits the excretion of other drugs, including **zidovudine** (see Ch. 52). Other drugs have an incidental probenecid-like effect and can enhance the actions of substances that rely on tubular secretion for their elimination. Table 9.9 gives some examples. Because diuretics act from within the tubular lumen, drugs that inhibit their secretion into the tubular fluid, such as non-steroidal anti-inflammatory drugs, reduce their effect.

ALTERATION OF URINE FLOW AND PH

Diuretics tend to increase the urinary excretion of other drugs and their metabolites, but this is seldom immediately clinically important. Conversely, loop and thiazide diuretics indirectly increase the proximal tubular reabsorption of **lithium** (which is handled in a similar way to Na[+]), and this can cause lithium toxicity in patients treated with lithium carbonate for mood disorders (Ch. 47). The effect of urinary pH on the excretion of weak acids and bases is put to use in the treatment of poisoning with *salicylate* (see Ch. 26), but is not a cause of accidental interactions.

Table 9.9 Examples of drugs that inhibit renal tubular secretion

Drug(s) causing inhibition	Drug(s) affected
Probenecid Sulfinpyrazone Phenylbutazone Sulfonamides Aspirin Thiazide diuretics Indometacin	Penicillin Azidothymidine Indometacin
Verapamil Amiodarone Quinidine	Digoxin
Indometacin	Furosemide (frusemide)
Aspirin Non-steroidal anti-inflammatory drugs	Methotrexate

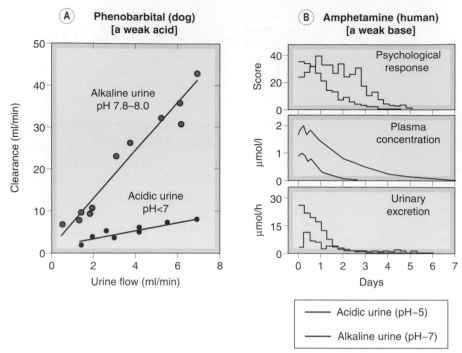

Fig. 9.6 **The effect of urinary pH on drug excretion.** [**A**] Phenobarbital clearance in the dog as a function of urine flow. Because phenobarbital is acidic, alkalinising the urine increases clearance about five-fold. [**B**] Amphetamine excretion in humans. Acidifying the urine increases the rate of renal elimination of amphetamine, reducing its plasma concentration and its effect on the subject's mental state. *(Data from Gunne & Anggard 1974. In: Torrell T et al. (eds) Pharmacology and Pharmacokinetics. Plenum, New York.)*

Elimination of drugs by the kidney

- Most drugs, unless highly bound to plasma protein, cross the glomerular filter freely.
- Many drugs, especially weak acids and weak bases, are actively secreted into the renal tubule and thus more rapidly excreted.
- Lipid-soluble drugs are passively reabsorbed by diffusion across the tubule, so are not efficiently excreted in the urine.
- Because of pH partition, weak acids are more rapidly excreted in alkaline urine, and vice versa.

- Several important drugs are removed predominantly by renal excretion, and are liable to cause toxicity in elderly persons and patients with renal disease.
- There are instances of clinically important drug–drug interactions due to one drug reducing the renal cleance of another (examples include diuretics/lithium, and indometacin/methotrexate), but these are less common than interactions due to altered drug metabolism.

REFERENCES AND FURTHER READING

General further reading

Coon, M.J., 2005. Cytochrome P450: nature's most versatile biological catalyst. Annu. Rev. Pharmacol. Toxicol. 45, 1–25. (*Summarises the individual steps in the P450 and reductase reaction cycles*)

Nassar, A.F., 2009. Drug Metabolism Handbook: Concepts and Applications. Wiley-Blackwell, Hoboken, NJ. (*Multi-authored handbook aimed at bench scientists; will be invaluable for pharmaceutical industry scientists*)

Testa, B., Krämer, S.D., 2009. The biochemistry of drug metabolism. Wiley-VCH, Weinheim. (*Two-volume reference work*)

Drug metabolism

Anzenbach, P., (Ed.), 2007. Special issue: cytochrome P450. BBA General Subjects 1770 (3), 313–494.

Campo, V.L., Bernardes, L.S.C., Carvalho, I., 2009. Stereoselectivity in drug metabolism: molecular mechansims and analytical methods. Curr. Drug Metab. 10, 188–205.

P450 enzyme induction and inhibition

Henderson, L., Yue, Q.Y., Bergquist, C., et al., 2002. St John's wort (*Hypericum perforatum*): drug interactions and clinical outcomes. Br. J. Clin. Pharmacol. 54, 349–356. (*Reviews the induction of CYP450 isoenzymes and of P-glycoprotein by constituents in this herbal remedy*)

Pelkonen, O., Turpeinen, M., Hakkola, J., et al., 2008. Inhibition and induction of human cytochrome P450 enzymes: current status. Arch. Toxicol. 82, 667–715. (*Review*)

Drug elimination

Kusuhara, H., Sugiyama, Y., 2009. In vitro–in vivo extrapolation of transporter-mediated clearance in the liver and kidney. Drug Metab. Pharmacokinet. 24, 37–52. (*Review*)

Pharmacokinetics

OVERVIEW

We explain the importance of pharmacokinetic analysis and present a simple approach to this. We explain how drug clearance determines the steady-state plasma concentration during constant-rate drug administration and how the characteristics of absorption and distribution (considered in Ch. 8) plus metabolism and excretion (considered in Ch. 9) determine the time course of drug concentration in blood plasma during and following drug administration. The effect of different dosing regimens on the time course of drug concentration in plasma is explained. Population pharmacokinetics is mentioned briefly, and a final section considers limitations to the pharmacokinetic approach.

INTRODUCTION: DEFINITION AND USES OF PHARMACOKINETICS

Pharmacokinetics may be defined as the measurement and formal interpretation of changes with time of drug concentrations in one or more different regions of the body in relation to dosing ('what the body does to the drug'). This distinguishes it from pharmacodynamics ('what the drug does to the body', i.e. events consequent on interaction of the drug with its receptor or other primary site of action). The distinction is useful, although the words cause dismay to etymological purists. 'Pharmacodynamic' received an entry in a dictionary of 1890 ('relating to the powers or effects of drugs') whereas pharmacokinetic studies only became possible in the latter part of the 20th century with the development of sensitive, specific and accurate physicochemical analytical techniques, especially high-performance chromatography and mass spectrometry, for measuring drug concentrations in biological fluids. The time course of drug concentration following dosing depends on the processes of absorption, distribution, metabolism and excretion that we have considered qualitatively in Chapters 8 and 9.

In practice, pharmacokinetics usually focuses on concentrations of drug in *blood plasma*, which is easily sampled via venepuncture, since plasma concentrations are assumed usually to bear a clear relation to the concentration of drug in extracellular fluid surrounding cells that express the receptors or other targets with which drug molecules combine. This underpins what is termed the *target concentration strategy*. Individual variation in *response* to a given dose of a drug is often greater than variability in the *plasma concentration* at that dose. Plasma concentrations (C_p) are therefore useful in the early stages of drug development (see below), and in the case of a few drugs plasma drug concentrations are also used in routine clinical practice to individualise dosage so as to achieve the desired therapeutic effect while minimising adverse effects in each individual patient, an approach known as

therapeutic drug monitoring (often abbreviated TDM – see Table 10.1 for examples of some drugs where a therapeutic range of plasma concentrations has been established). Concentrations of drug in other body fluids (e.g. urine,[1] saliva, cerebrospinal fluid, milk) may add useful information.

Formal interpretation of pharmacokinetic data consists of fitting concentration-versus-time data to a model (whether abstract or, more usefully, physiologically based) and determining parameters that describe the observed behaviour. The parameters can then be used to adjust the dose regimen to achieve a desired target plasma concentration estimated initially from pharmacological experiments on cells, tissues or laboratory animals, and modified in light of empirical human pharmacology. Some descriptive pharmacokinetic characteristics can be observed directly by inspecting the time course of drug concentration in plasma following dosing – important examples,[2] illustrated more fully below, are the *maximum plasma concentration* following a given dose of a drug administered in a defined dosing form (C_{max}) and the *time* (T_{max}) between drug administration and achieving C_{max}. Other pharmacokinetic parameters are estimated mathematically from experimental data; examples include *volume of distribution* (V_d) and *clearance* (CL), concepts that have been introduced in Chapters 8 and 9 respectively and to which we return below.

USES OF PHARMACOKINETICS

Knowledge of the pharmacokinetic behaviour of drugs in animals and man is crucial in drug development, both to make sense of preclinical toxicological and pharmacological data[3] and to decide on an appropriate dosing regimen for clinical studies of efficacy (see Ch. 60). Drug regulators need detailed pharmacokinetic information for the same reasons, and have developed concepts such as *bioavailability* and *bioequivalence* (Ch. 8) to assist decisions about licensing generic versions of drugs as originator products lose patent protection. Understanding the general principles of pharmacokinetics is important for clinicians when considering dosage recommendations in the product information provided with licensed drugs. Clinicians also need to understand principles of pharmacokinetics if they are to identify and evaluate possible drug interactions (see Chs 8, 9), to interpret drug concentrations for TDM and to adjust dose regimens rationally. In particular, intensive care specialists and

---

[1] *Clinical* pharmacology became at one time so associated with the measurement of drugs in urine that the canard had it that clinical pharmacologists were the new alchemists – they turned urine into airline tickets.

[2] Important because dose-related adverse effects often occur around C_{max}.

[3] For example, doses used in experimental animals often need to be much greater than those in humans (on a 'per unit body weight' basis), because drug metabolism is commonly much more rapid in rodents – **methadone** (Ch. 42) is one of many such examples.

Table 10.1 Examples of drugs where therapeutic drug monitoring (TDM) of plasma concentrations is used clinically

Category	Example(s)	See Chapter
Immunosuppressants	Ciclosporine, tacrolimus	26
Cardiovascular	Digoxin	21
Respiratory	Theophylline	16, 28
CNS	Lithium, phenytoin	47, 45
Antibacterials	Aminoglycosides	51
Anticancer drugs	Methotrexate	56

anaesthetists dealing with a severely ill patient often need to individualise the dose regimen depending on the urgency of achieving a therapeutic plasma concentration, and whether the pharmacokinetic behaviour of the drug is likely to be affected by the condition of the patient.

SCOPE OF THIS CHAPTER

We aim to familiarise the reader with the meanings of important pharmacokinetic parameters by explaining how:

- total drug clearance determines its steady-state plasma concentration during continuous administration;
- drug concentration versus time can be described by a simple model in which the body is represented as a single well-stirred compartment, of volume V_d. This describes the situation before steady state is reached (or after drug is discontinued) in terms of elimination half-life ($t_{1/2}$);
- to approach situations where this simple model is inadequate, by introducing a two-compartment model and describing situations where clearance varies with drug concentration ('non-linear kinetics');
- situations (such as paediatric pharmacokinetics) where only a few samples may be available, can be addressed by population kinetics.

Finally, we consider some of the limitations inherent in the pharmacokinetic approach. More detailed accounts are provided by Atkinson et al. (2001), Birkett (2002), Jambhekar & Breen (2009) and Rowland & Tozer (2010).

DRUG ELIMINATION EXPRESSED AS CLEARANCE

The overall clearance of a drug by all routes (CL_{tot}) is the fundamental pharmacokinetic parameter describing drug elimination. It is defined as the volume of plasma which contains the total amount of drug that is removed from the body in unit time. It is thus expressed as volume per unit time, e.g. ml/min or l/h. The application of this concept to renal clearance (CL_{ren}) was described in Ch 9.

The overall clearance of a drug (CL_{tot}) is the sum of clearance rates for each mechanism involved in eliminating the drug, usually renal clearance (CL_{ren}) and metabolic clearance (CL_{met}) plus any additional appreciable routes of elimination (faeces, breath, etc.). It relates the rate of elimination of a drug (in units of mass/unit time) to C_p:

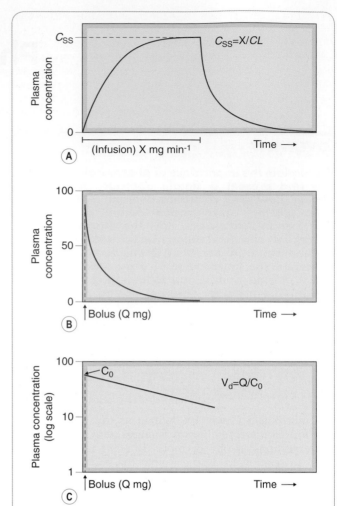

Fig. 10.1 Plasma drug concentration–time curves.
[A] During a constant intravenous infusion at rate X mg/min, indicated by the horizontal bar, the plasma concentration (C) increases from zero to a steady-state value (C_{SS}); when the infusion is stopped, C declines to zero. **[B]** Following an intravenous bolus dose (Q mg), the plasma concentration rises abruptly and then declines towards zero. **[C]** Data from panel **[B]** plotted with plasma concentrations on a logarithmic scale. The straight line shows that concentration declines exponentially. Extrapolation back to the ordinate at zero time gives an estimate of C_0, the concentration at zero time, and hence of V_d, the volume of distribution.

$$\text{Rate of drug elimination} = C_p \times CL_{tot} \qquad (10.1)$$

Drug clearance can be determined in an individual subject by measuring the plasma concentration of the drug (in units of, say, mg/l at intervals during a constant-rate intravenous infusion (delivering, say, X mg of drug per h), until a steady state is approximated (Fig. 10.1A). At steady state, the rate of input to the body is equal to the rate of elimination, so:

$$X = C_{ss} \times CL_{tot} \qquad (10.2)$$

Rearranging this,

$$CL_{tot} = \frac{X}{C_{ss}} \qquad (10.3)$$

where C_{ss} is the plasma concentration at steady state, and CL_{tot} is in units of volume/time (l/h in the example given).

For many drugs, clearance in an individual subject is the same at different doses (at least within the range of doses used therapeutically – but see the section on saturation kinetics below for exceptions), so knowing the clearance enables one to calculate the dose rate needed to achieve a desired steady-state ('target') plasma concentration from equation 10.2.

CL_{tot} can also be estimated by measuring plasma concentrations at intervals following a single intravenous bolus dose of, say, Q mg (Fig. 10.1B):

$$CL_{tot} = \frac{Q}{AUC_{0-\infty}} \qquad (10.4)$$

where $AUC_{0-\infty}$ is the area under the full curve[4] relating C_p to time following a bolus dose given at time $t = 0$. (See Ch. 8, and Birkett, 2002, for a fuller account.)

Note that these estimates of CL_{tot}, unlike estimates based on the rate constant or half-life (see below), do not depend on any particular compartmental model.

SINGLE-COMPARTMENT MODEL

Consider a highly simplified model of a human being, which consists of a single well-stirred compartment, of volume V_d (distribution volume), into which a quantity of drug Q is introduced rapidly by intravenous injection, and from which it can escape either by being metabolised or by being excreted (Fig. 10.2). For most drugs, V_d is an apparent volume rather than the volume of an anatomical compartment. It links the total amount of drug in the body to its concentration in plasma (see Ch. 8). The quantity of drug in the body when it is administered as a single bolus is equal to the administered dose Q. The initial concentration, C_0, will therefore be given by:

$$C_0 = \frac{Q}{V_d} \qquad (10.5)$$

In practice, C_0 is estimated by extrapolating the linear portion of a semilogarithmic plot of C_p against time back to its intercept at time 0 (Fig. 10.1C). C_p at any time depends on the rate of elimination of the drug (i.e. on its total clearance, CL_{tot}) as well as on the dose and V_d. Many drugs exhibit *first-order kinetics* where the rate of elimination is directly proportional to drug concentration. (An analogy is letting your bath drain down the plug hole where the water, analogous to drug, initially rushes out whereas the last bit always takes an age to drain away. Contrast this with so-called zero-order kinetics where the water is pumped out of the bath at a constant rate.) With first-order kinetics drug concentration decays exponentially (Fig. 10.3), being described by the equation:

$$C_{(t)} = C_{(0)} \exp \frac{-CL_{tot}}{V_d} t \qquad (10.6)$$

(Note that exp is another way of writing 'e to the power of', so this has the same form as $C_{(t)} = C_{(0)}.e^{-kt}$.)

Taking logarithms to the base e (written as ln):

$$\ln C_{(t)} = \ln C_{(0)} - \frac{CL_{tot}}{V_d} t \qquad (10.7)$$

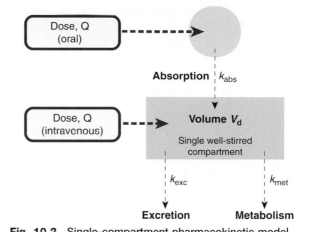

Fig. 10.2 Single-compartment pharmacokinetic model. This model is applicable if the plasma concentration falls exponentially after drug administration (as in Fig. 10.1).

Plotting C_t on a logarithmic scale against t (on a linear scale) yields a straight line with slope $-CL_{tot}/V_d$. The constant CL_{tot}/V_d is the *elimination rate constant* k_{el}, which has units of (time)$^{-1}$. It represents the *fraction* of drug in the body eliminated per unit of time. For example, if the rate constant is 0.1 h^{-1} this implies that one-tenth of the drug remaining in the body is eliminated each hour.

The *elimination half-life*, $t_{1/2}$, is the time taken for C_p to decrease by half, and is equal to $\ln2/k_{el}$ (= $0.693/k_{el}$). The plasma half-life is therefore determined by V_d as well as by CL_{tot}. It enables one to predict the time-course of C_p after bolus of drug is given or after the start or end of an infusion, when C_p is rising to its steady-state level or declining to zero.

When the single-compartment model is applicable, the drug concentration in plasma approaches the steady-state value approximately exponentially during a constant infusion (Fig. 10.1A). When the infusion is discontinued, the concentration falls exponentially towards zero with the same half-life: after one half-life, the concentration will have fallen to half the initial concentration; after two half-lives, it will have fallen to one-quarter the initial concentration; after three half-lives, to one-eighth; and so on. It is intuitively obvious that the longer the half-life, the longer the drug will persist in the body after dosing is discontinued. It is less obvious, but nonetheless true, that during chronic drug administration, the longer the half-life, the longer it will take for the drug to accumulate to its steady-state level: one half-life to reach 50% of the steady-state value, two to reach 75%, three to reach 87.5% and so on. This is extremely helpful to a clinician deciding how to start treatment. If the drug in question has a half-life of approximately 24 h, for example, it will take 3–5 days to approximate the steady-state concentration during a constant-rate infusion. If this is too slow in the face of the prevailing clinical situation, a *loading dose* may be used in order to achieve a therapeutic concentration of drug in the plasma more rapidly (see below). The size of such a dose is determined by the volume of distribution (equation 10.5).

EFFECT OF REPEATED DOSING

Drugs are usually given as repeated doses rather than single injections or a constant infusion. Repeated

---

[4]The area is obtained by integrating from time = 0 to time = ∞, and is designated $AUC_{0-\infty}$. The area under the curve has units of time – on the abscissa – multiplied by concentration (mass/volume) – on the ordinate; so $CL = Q/AUC_{0-\infty}$ has units of volume/time as it should.

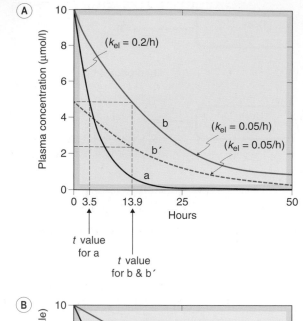

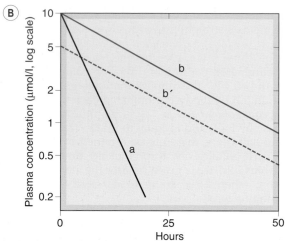

Fig. 10.3 Predicted behaviour of single-compartment model following intravenous drug administration at time 0. Drugs a and b differ only in their elimination rate constant, k_{el}. Curve b' shows the plasma concentration time course for a smaller dose of b. Note that the half-life ($t_{1/2}$) (indicated by broken lines) does not depend on the dose. **[A]** Linear concentration scale. **[B]** Logarithmic concentration scale.

injections (each of dose Q) give a more complicated pattern than the smooth exponential rise during intravenous infusion, but the principle is the same (Fig. 10.4). The concentration will rise to a mean steady-state concentration with an approximately exponential time course, but will oscillate (through a range Q/V_d). The smaller and more frequent the doses, the more closely the situation approaches that of a continuous infusion, and the smaller the swings in concentration. The exact dosage schedule, however, does not affect the mean steady-state concentration, or the rate at which it is approached. In practice, a steady state is effectively achieved after three to five half-lives. Speedier attainment of the steady state can be achieved by starting with a larger dose, as mentioned above. Such a loading dose is sometimes used when starting treatment with a drug with a half-life that is long in the context of the urgency of the clinical situation, as may

be the case when treating cardiac dysrhythmias with drugs such as **amiodarone** or **digoxin** (Ch. 21) or initiating anticoagulation with **heparin** (Ch. 24).

EFFECT OF VARIATION IN RATE OF ABSORPTION

If a drug is absorbed slowly from the gut or from an injection site into the plasma, it is (in terms of a compartmental model) as though it were being slowly infused at a variable rate into the bloodstream. For the purpose of kinetic modelling, the transfer of drug from the site of administration to the central compartment can be represented approximately by a rate constant, k_{abs} (see Fig. 10.2). This assumes that the rate of absorption is directly proportional, at any moment, to the amount of drug still unabsorbed, which is at best a rough approximation to reality. The effect of slow absorption on the time course of the rise and fall of the plasma concentration is shown in Figure 10.5. The curves show the effect of spreading out the absorption of the same total amount of drug over different times. In each case, the drug is absorbed completely, but the peak concentration appears later and is lower and less sharp if absorption is slow. In the limiting case, a dosage form that releases drug at a constant rate as it traverses the ileum (Ch. 8) approximates a constant-rate infusion. Once absorption is complete, the plasma concentration declines with the same half-time, irrespective of the rate of absorption.

▼ For the kind of pharmacokinetic model discussed here, the area under the plasma concentration–time curve (AUC) is directly proportional to the total amount of drug introduced into the plasma compartment, irrespective of the rate at which it enters. Incomplete absorption, or destruction by first-pass metabolism before the drug reaches the plasma compartment, reduces AUC after oral administration (see Ch. 8). Changes in the rate of absorption, however, do not affect AUC. Again, it is worth noting that provided absorption is complete, the relation between the rate of administration and the steady-state plasma concentration (equation 10.3) is unaffected by k_{abs}, although the size of the oscillation of plasma concentration with each dose is reduced if absorption is slowed.

MORE COMPLICATED KINETIC MODELS

So far, we have considered a single-compartment pharmacokinetic model in which the rates of absorption, metabolism and excretion are all assumed to be directly proportional to the concentration of drug in the compartment from which transfer is occurring. This is a useful way to illustrate some basic principles but is clearly a physiological oversimplification. The characteristics of different parts of the body, such as brain, body fat and muscle, are quite different in terms of their blood supply, partition coefficient for drugs and the permeability of their capillaries to drugs. These differences, which the single-compartment model ignores, can markedly affect the time courses of drug distribution and action, and much theoretical work has gone into the mathematical analysis of more complex models (see Atkinson et al., 2001; Rowland & Tozer, 2010). They are beyond the scope of this book, and perhaps also beyond the limit of what is actually useful, for the experimental data on pharmacokinetic properties of drugs are seldom accurate or reproducible enough to enable complex models to be tested critically.

The two-compartment model, which introduces a separate 'peripheral' compartment to represent the tissues, in communication with the 'central' plasma compartment,

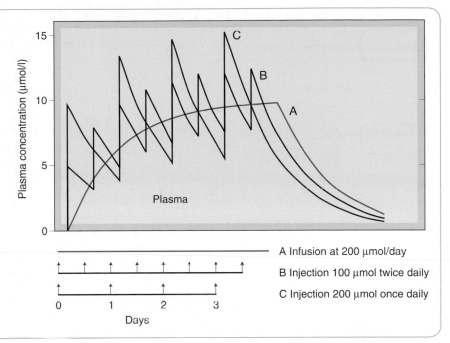

Fig. 10.4 Predicted behaviour of single-compartment model with continuous or intermittent drug administration. Smooth curve A shows the effect of continuous infusion for 4 days; curve B the same total amount of drug given in eight equal doses; and curve C the same total amount of drug given in four equal doses. The drug has a half-life of 17 h and a volume of distribution of 20 l. Note that in each case a steady state is effectively reached after about 2 days (about three half-lives), and that the mean concentration reached in the steady state is the same for all three schedules.

A Infusion at 200 μmol/day

B Injection 100 μmol twice daily

C Injection 200 μmol once daily

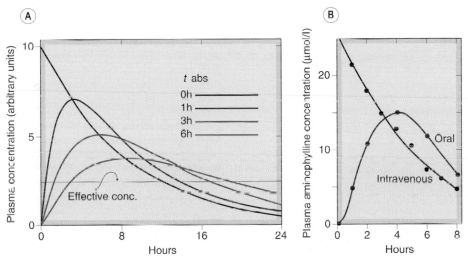

Fig. 10.5 The effect of slow drug absorption on plasma drug concentration. **[A]** Predicted behaviour of single-compartment model with drug absorbed at different rates from the gut or an injection site. The elimination half-time is 6 h. The absorption half-times ($t_{1/2}$ abs) are marked on the diagram. (Zero indicates instantaneous absorption, corresponding to intravenous administration.) Note that the peak plasma concentration is reduced and delayed by slow absorption, and the duration of action is somewhat increased. **[B]** Measurements of plasma aminophylline concentration in humans following equal oral and intravenous doses. *(Data from Swintowsky JV 1956 J Am Pharm Assoc 49, 395.)*

more closely resembles the real situation without involving excessive complications.

TWO-COMPARTMENT MODEL

The two-compartment model is a widely used approximation in which the tissues are lumped together as a peripheral compartment. Drug molecules can enter and leave the peripheral compartment only via the central compartment (Fig. 10.6), which usually represents the plasma (or plasma plus some extravascular space in the case of a few drugs that distribute especially rapidly). The effect of adding a second compartment to the model is to introduce a second exponential component into the predicted time course of the plasma concentration, so that it comprises a fast and a slow phase. This pattern is often found experimentally, and is most clearly revealed when the concentration data are plotted semilogarithmically (Fig. 10.7). If, as is often the case, the transfer of drug between the central and peripheral compartments is relatively fast compared with the rate of elimination, then the fast phase (often called the α *phase*) can be taken to represent the redistribution of the drug (i.e. drug molecules passing from plasma to tissues, thereby rapidly lowering the plasma concentration). The plasma concentration reached when the fast phase is complete, but before appreciable elimination has occurred, allows a measure of the combined distribution volumes of the two compartments; the half-time for the slow

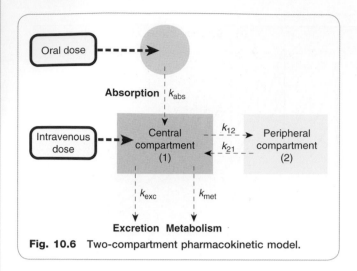

Fig. 10.6   Two-compartment pharmacokinetic model.

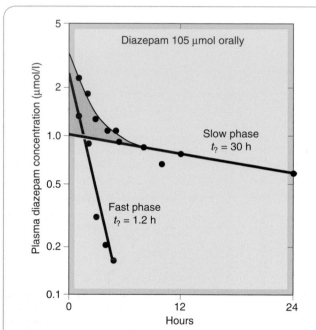

Fig. 10.7   Kinetics of diazepam elimination in humans following a single oral dose. The graph shows a semilogarithmic plot of plasma concentration versus time. The experimental data (black symbols) follow a curve that becomes linear after about 8 h (slow phase). Plotting the deviation of the early points (pink shaded area) from this line on the same coordinates (red symbols) reveals the fast phase. This type of two-component decay is consistent with the two-compartment model (Fig. 10.6) and is obtained with many drugs. *(Data from Curry SH 1980 Drug Disposition and Pharmacokinetics. Blackwell, Oxford.)*

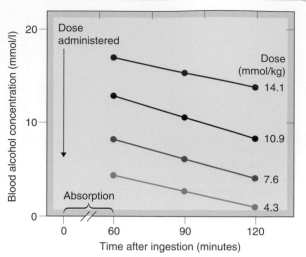

Fig. 10.8   Saturating kinetics of alcohol elimination in humans. The blood alcohol concentration falls linearly rather than exponentially, and the rate of fall does not vary with dose. *(From Drew GC et al. 1958 Br Med J 2, 5103.)*

phase (the β *phase*) provides an estimate of k_{el}. If a drug is rapidly metabolised or excreted, the α and β phases are not well separated, and the calculation of separate V_d and k_{el} values for each phase is not straightforward. Problems also arise with drugs (e.g. very fat-soluble drugs) for which it is unrealistic to lump all the peripheral tissues together.

SATURATION KINETICS

In the case of some drugs, including **ethanol**, **phenytoin** and **salicylate**, the time course of disappearance of drug from the plasma does not follow the exponential or biexponential patterns shown in Figures 10.3 and 10.7 but is

initially linear (i.e. drug is removed at a constant rate that is independent of plasma concentration). This is often called *zero-order kinetics* to distinguish it from the usual first-order kinetics that we have considered so far (these terms have their origin in chemical kinetic theory). *Saturation kinetics* is a better term, because it conveys the underlying mechanism, namely that a carrier or enzyme saturates and so as the concentration of drug substrate increases the rate of elimination approaches a constant value. Figure 10.8 shows the example of ethanol. It can be seen that the rate of disappearance of ethanol from the plasma is constant at approximately 4 mmol/l per h, irrespective of dose or of the plasma concentration of ethanol. The explanation for this is that the rate of oxidation by the enzyme alcohol dehydrogenase reaches a maximum at low ethanol concentrations, because of limited availability of the cofactor NAD^+ (see Ch. 49, Fig. 49.6).

Saturation kinetics has several important consequences (see Fig. 10.9). One is that the duration of action is more strongly dependent on dose than is the case with drugs that do not show metabolic saturation. Another consequence is that the relationship between dose and steady-state plasma concentration is steep and unpredictable, and it does not obey the proportionality rule implicit in equation 10.3 for non-saturating drugs (see Fig. 49.7 for another example related to ethanol). The maximum rate of metabolism sets a limit to the rate at which the drug can be administered; if this rate is exceeded, the amount of drug in the body will, in principle, increase indefinitely and never reach a steady state (Fig. 10.9). This does not actually happen, because there is always some dependence of the rate of elimination on the plasma concentration (usually because other, non-saturating metabolic pathways or renal excretion contribute significantly at high concentrations). Nevertheless, steady-state plasma concentrations of drugs of this kind vary widely and unpredictably with dose. Similarly, variations in the rate of metabolism (e.g. through enzyme induction) cause disproportionately large changes in the plasma concentration. These problems are well recognised for drugs such as phenytoin, an anticonvulsant for which plasma

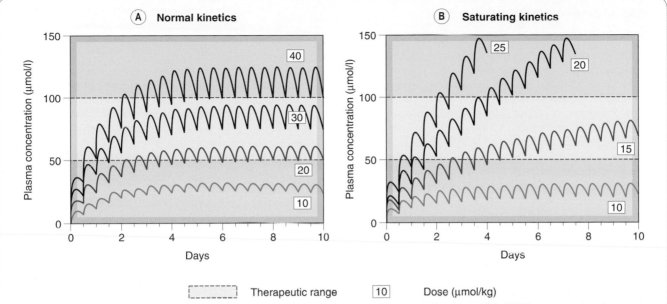

Fig. 10.9 Comparison of non-saturating and saturating kinetics for drugs given orally every 12 h. **[A]** The curves showing an imaginary drug, similar to the antiepileptic drug phenytoin at the lowest dose, but with linear kinetics. The steady-state plasma concentration is reached within a few days, and is directly proportional to dose. **[B]** Curves for saturating kinetics calculated from the known pharmacokinetic parameters of phenytoin (see Ch. 45). Note that no steady state is reached with higher doses of phenytoin, and that a small increment in dose results after a time in a disproportionately large effect on plasma concentration. (Curves were calculated with the Sympak pharmacokinetic modelling program written by Dr JG Blackman, University of Otago.)

concentration needs to be closely controlled to achieve an optimal clinical effect (see Ch. 45, Fig. 45.4). Drugs showing saturation kinetics are less predictable in clinical use than ones with linear kinetics, so may be rejected during drug development if a pharmacologically similar candidate with linear kinetics is available (Ch. 60).

Clinical applications of pharmacokinetics are summarised in the clinical box (see p. 132).

POPULATION PHARMACOKINETICS

▼ In some situations, for example when a drug is intended for use in chronically ill children, it is desirable to obtain pharmacokinetic data in a patient population rather than in healthy adult volunteers. Such studies are inevitably limited and samples for drug analysis are often obtained opportunistically during clinical care, with limitations as to quality of the data and on the number of samples collected from each patient. Population pharmacokinetics addresses how best to analyse such data. Fitting data from all subjects as if there were no kinetic differences between individuals, and fitting each individual's data separately and then combining the individual parameter estimates, have each obvious shortcomings. A better method is to use non-linear mixed effects modelling (NONMEM). The statistical technicalities are considerable and beyond the scope of this chapter: the interested reader is referred to Sheiner et al. (1997).

LIMITATIONS OF PHARMACOKINETICS

Some limitations of the pharmacokinetic approach will be obvious from the above account, such as the proliferation of parameters in even quite conceptually simple models. Here we comment on limitations in its usefulness as an approach to controlling individual variability. Two main assumptions underpin the expectation that by relating response to a drug to its plasma concentration we can reduce variability of response by accounting for

pharmacokinetic variation – that is, variation in absorption, distribution, metabolism and excretion. They are:

1. That plasma concentration of a drug bears a precise relation to the concentration of drug in the immediate environment of its target (receptor, enzyme, etc.).
2. That drug response depends only on the concentration of the drug in the immediate environment of its target.

While the first of these assumptions is very plausible in the few cases of drugs that work through a target in the circulating blood (e.g. a fibrinolytic drug working on fibrinogen) and reasonably plausible for a drug working on an enzyme, ion channel or G protein-coupled or kinase-linked receptor located in the cell membrane, it is less likely in the case of a nuclear receptor or when the target cells are protected by the blood–brain barrier. In the latter case it is not perhaps surprising that, despite considerable efforts, it has never proved clinically useful to measure plasma concentrations of antidepressant or antipsychotic drugs, where there are, in addition, complex metabolic pathways with numerous active metabolites. It is, if anything, surprising that the approach does as well as it does in the case of some other centrally acting drugs, notably antiepileptics and **lithium**.

The second assumption is untrue in the case of drugs that form a stable covalent attachment with their target, and so produce an effect that outlives their presence in solution. Examples include the antiplatelet effects of **aspirin** and **clopidogrel** (Ch. 24) and the effect of some monoamine oxidase inhibitors (Ch. 47). In other cases, drugs in therapeutic use act only after delay (e.g. antidepressants, Ch. 47), or gradually induce tolerance (e.g. opioids, Ch. 42) or physiological adaptations (e.g. corticosteroids, Ch. 33) that alter the relation between concentration and drug effect in a time-dependent manner.

Uses of pharmacokinetics

- Pharmacokinetic studies performed during drug development underpin the standard dose regimens approved by regulatory agencies.
- Clinicians sometimes need to individualise dose regimens to account for individual variation in a particular patient (e.g. a neonate, a patient with impaired and changing renal function, or a patient taking drugs that interfere with drug metabolism; see Ch. 9).
- Drug effect (pharmacodynamics) is often used for such individualisation, but there are drugs (including some anticonvulsants, immunosuppressants and antineoplastics) where a therapeutic range of plasma concentrations has been defined, and for which it is useful to adjust the dose to achieve a concentration in this range.
- Knowledge of kinetics enables rational dose adjustment. For example:
  - the frequency of dosing of a drug such as **gentamicin** eliminated by renal excretion may need to be markedly reduced in a patient with renal impairment (Ch. 51)
  - the dose increment needed to achieve a target plasma concentration range of a drug such as **phenytoin** with saturation kinetics (Ch. 45, Fig. 45.4) is much less than for a drug with linear kinetics.
- Knowing the approximate $t_{1/2}$ of a drug can be very useful, even if a therapeutic concentration is not known:
  - in correctly interpreting adverse events that occur some considerable time after starting regular treatment (e.g. benzodiazepines; see Ch. 44)
  - in deciding on the need or otherwise for an initial loading dose when starting treatment with drugs such as **digoxin** and **amiodarone** (Ch. 21).
- The volume of distribution (V_d) of a drug determines the size of loading dose needed. If V_d is large (as for many tricyclic antidepressants), haemodialysis will not be an effective way of increasing the rate of elimination in treating overdose.

Pharmacokinetics

- Total clearance (CL_{tot}) of a drug is the fundamental parameter describing its elimination: the rate of elimination equals CL_{tot} multiplied by plasma concentration.
- CL_{tot} determines steady-state plasma concentration (C_{ss}): C_{ss} = rate of drug administration/CL_{tot}.
- For many drugs, disappearance from the plasma follows an approximately exponential time course. Such drugs can be described by a model where the body is treated as a single well-stirred compartment of volume V_d. V_d is an apparent volume linking the amount of drug in the body at any time to the plasma concentration.
- Elimination half-life ($t_{1/2}$) is directly proportional to V_d and inversely proportional to CL_{tot}.
- With repeated dosage or sustained delivery of a drug, the plasma concentration approaches a steady value within three to five plasma half-lives.
- In urgent situations, a loading dose may be needed to achieve therapeutic concentration rapidly.
- The loading dose (L) needed to achieve a desired initial plasma concentration C_{target} is determined by V_d: $L = C_{target} \times V_d$.
- A two-compartment model is often needed. In this case, the kinetics are biexponential. The two components roughly represent the processes of transfer between plasma and tissues (α phase) and elimination from the plasma (β phase).
- Some drugs show non-exponential 'saturation' kinetics, with important clinical consequences, especially a disproportionate increase in steady-state plasma concentration when daily dose is increased.

REFERENCES AND FURTHER READING

Atkinson, A.J., Daniels, C.E., Dedrick, R.L., et al. (Eds.), 2001. Principles of Clinical Pharmacology. Academic Press, London. (*Section on pharmacokinetics includes the application of Laplace transformations, effects of disease, compartmental versus non-compartmental approaches, population pharmacokinetics, drug metabolism and transport*)

Birkett, D.J., 2002. Pharmacokinetics Made Easy (revised), second ed. McGraw–Hill Australia, Sydney. (*Excellent slim volume that lives up to the promise of its title*)

Jambhekar, S.S., Breen, P.J., 2009. Basic Pharmacokinetics. Pharmaceutical Press, London. (*Basic textbook*)

Rowland, M., Tozer, T.N., 2010. Clinical Pharmacokinetics and Pharmacodynamics. Concepts and Applications. Wolters Kluwer/ Lippincott Williams & Wilkins, Baltimore. Online simulations by H. Derendorf and G. Hochhaus. (*Excellent text; emphasises clinical applications*)

Population pharmacokinetics

Sheiner, L.B., Rosenberg, B., Marethe, V.V., 1997. Estimation of population characteristics of pharmacokinetic parameters from routine clinical data. J. Pharmacokinet. Biopharm. 5, 445–479.

Individual variation, pharmacogenomics and personalised medicine

11

OVERVIEW

This chapter addresses sources of variation between individuals (inter-individual variation) in their responses to drugs. Important factors including ethnicity, age, pregnancy, disease and drug interaction (i.e. modification of the action of one drug by another) are described. The concept of individualising drug therapy in light of genomic information ('personalised medicine') – a rapidly developing area of clinical pharmacology – is introduced. We explain relevant elementary genetic concepts and describe briefly several single-gene pharmacogenetic disorders that affect drug responses. We then cover pharmacogenomic tests, including tests for variations in human leukocyte antigen (HLA) genes, in genes influencing drug metabolism, and encoding drug targets.

INTRODUCTION

Therapeutics would be a great deal easier if the same dose of drug always produced the same response. In reality, inter- and even intra-individual variation is often substantial. Physicians need to be aware of the sources of such variation to prescribe drugs safely and effectively. Variation can be caused by different concentrations at sites of drug action or by different responses to the same drug concentration. The first kind is called pharmacokinetic variation and can occur because of differences in absorption, distribution, metabolism or excretion (Chs 8 and 9). The second kind is called pharmacodynamic variation. Responses to some therapeutic agents, for example most vaccines and oral contraceptives (Ch. 35), are sufficiently predictable to permit a standard dose regimen, whereas treatment with **lithium** (Ch. 47), antihypertensive drugs (Ch. 22), anticoagulants (Ch. 24) and many other drugs is individualised, doses being adjusted on the basis of monitoring the drug concentration in the plasma or a response such as change in blood pressure, together with any adverse effects.

Inter-individual variation in response to some drugs is a serious problem; if not taken into account, it can result in lack of efficacy or unexpected adverse effects. Variation is partly caused by environmental factors but studies comparing identical with non-identical twins suggest that much of the variation in response to some drugs is genetically determined; for example, elimination half-lives of antipyrine, a probe of hepatic drug oxidation, and of **warfarin**, an oral anticoagulant (Ch. 24), differ much less between identical than between fraternal twins. However, even for drugs with a known genetic component such as **warfarin** (see p. 141 and Ch. 24) addition of pharmacogenetic information to a dosing algorithm incorporating other clinical sources of variation (age, sex and so on) does

not improve outcome significantly, although when compared with a standardised (i.e. trial and error) loading dose strategy a genetically guided dose-initiation strategy does result in a greater fraction of time in the therapeutic range during the first weeks of treatment (see Zineh et al., 2013 for a discussion of recent randomised controlled trials of pharmacogenetics and warfarin dosing).

Genes influence pharmacokinetics by altering the expression of proteins involved in drug absorption, distribution, metabolism or excretion (ADME); pharmacodynamic variation reflects differences in drug targets, G proteins or other downstream pathways; and individual susceptibility to uncommon qualitatively distinct adverse reactions (Ch. 57) can result from genetically determined differences in enzymes or immune mechanisms. It is hoped that as our understanding of the human genome improves, together with the introduction of simpler methods to identify genetic differences between individuals, it will become possible to use genetic information specific to an individual patient to preselect a drug that will be effective and not cause toxicity, rather than relying on trial and error supported by physiological clues as at present – an aspiration referred to as '*personalised medicine*'. Thus far, this approach, which was initially overhyped, has yielded relatively little in the way of clinical benefit. Progress is being made, however, and the US Food and Drug Administration (FDA) has approved over 100 pharmacogenomic additions to drug labelling information – a doubling since the last edition of this book. The use of pharmacogenomic tests is not consistently supported by evidence of improved outcomes from clinical trials (Zineh et al., 2013) and indeed the FDA approach to pharmacogenetic labelling has been criticised (Shah & Shah, 2012). Nevertheless, pharmacogenetic testing seems likely ultimately to make an important contribution to therapeutics, though at a cost.

In this chapter we first describe the most important epidemiological sources of variation in drug responsiveness, before revisiting some elementary genetics as a basis for understanding genetic disorders characterised by abnormal responses to drugs, and conclude with a brief account of currently available pharmacogenomic tests and how these are beginning to be applied to individualise drug therapy (*pharmacogenomics*).

Variation is usually quantitative in the sense that the drug produces a larger or smaller effect, or acts for a longer or shorter time, while still exerting qualitatively the same effect. But importantly, the effect may be qualitatively different in susceptible individuals, often because of genetic or immunological differences. Examples include **primaquine**-induced haemolysis in individuals with glucose 6-phosphate dehydrogenase deficiency whose red blood cells are thereby more susceptible to the effect of oxidative stress (Ch. 57) or immune-mediated haemolytic anaemia caused by **methyldopa** – a

133

drug that commonly causes antidrug antibodies whereas only a few individuals expressing such antibodies develop haemolysis (Ch. 14).

> ### Individual variation
>
> - Variability is a serious problem; if not taken into account, it can result in:
>   - lack of efficacy
>   - unexpected harmful effects.
> - Types of variability may be classified as:
>   - pharmacokinetic
>   - pharmacodynamic.
> - The main causes of variability are:
>   - age
>   - genetic factors
>   - immunological factors (Ch. 57)
>   - disease (especially when this influences drug elimination or metabolism, e.g. kidney or liver disease)
>   - drug interactions.

EPIDEMIOLOGICAL FACTORS AND INTER-INDIVIDUAL VARIATION OF DRUG RESPONSE

ETHNICITY

Ethnic means 'pertaining to race', and many anthropologists are sceptical as to the value of this concept (see, for example, Cooper et al., 2003). Citizens of several modern societies are asked to select their race or ethnicity from a list of options for census purposes (e.g. the UK 2011 National Census). Members of such self-defined groups share some characteristics on the basis of common genetic and cultural heritage, but there is obviously also enormous diversity within each group.

Despite the crudeness of such categorisation, it can give some pointers to drug responsiveness (Wood, 2001). One example is the evidence discussed in Chapter 22 that the life expectancy of African-Americans with heart failure is increased by treatment with a combination of **hydralazine** plus a nitrate, whereas that of white Americans may not be.

Some adverse effects may also be predicted on the basis of race; for example, many Chinese subjects differ from Europeans in the way that they metabolise ethanol, producing a higher plasma concentration of acetaldehyde, which can cause flushing and palpitations (Ch. 49). Chinese subjects are considerably more sensitive to the cardiovascular effects of **propranolol** (Ch. 14) than white Europeans, whereas Afro-Caribbean individuals are less sensitive. Despite their increased sensitivity to β-adrenoceptor antagonists, Chinese subjects metabolise propranolol faster than white people, implying that the difference relates to pharmacodynamic differences at or beyond the β adrenoceptors.

Overall effectiveness of **gefitinib** (Ch. 56) in treating patients with advanced lung tumours has been disappointing, but in about 10% of patients lung tumours shrink rapidly in response to this drug. Japanese patients are three times as likely as whites to respond in this way. The underlying difference is that patients who respond well have specific mutations in the receptor for epidermal growth factor (see Wadman, 2005). It is probable that many such ethnic differences are genetic in origin, but environmental factors, for example relating to distinctive dietary habits, may also contribute. It is important not to abandon the much more sophisticated search for ways to individualise medicine on the basis of pharmacogenomics (see p. 139-141) just because the much simpler and cheaper process of asking patients to define their ethnic group has had some success: this should rather act as a spur. If such a crude and imperfect approach has had some success, we ought surely to be able to do better with genomic testing!

AGE

The main reason that age affects drug action is that drug elimination is less efficient in newborn babies and in old people, so that drugs commonly produce greater and more prolonged effects at the extremes of life. Other age-related factors, such as variations in pharmacodynamic sensitivity, are also important with some drugs. Body composition changes with age, fat contributing a greater proportion to body mass in the elderly, with consequent changes in distribution volume of drugs. Elderly people consume more drugs than do younger adults, so the potential for drug interactions is also increased. For fuller accounts of drug therapy in paediatrics and in the elderly, see the chapters on renal and hepatic disease in Atkinson et al. (2006).

EFFECT OF AGE ON RENAL EXCRETION OF DRUGS

Glomerular filtration rate (GFR) in the newborn, normalised to body surface area, is only about 20% of the adult value. Accordingly, plasma elimination half-lives of renally eliminated drugs are longer in neonates than in adults (Table 11.1). In babies born at term, renal function increases to values similar to those in young adults in less than a week, and continues to increase to a maximum of approximately twice the adult value at 6 months of age. Improvement in renal function occurs more slowly in premature infants. Renal immaturity in premature infants can have a substantial effect on drug elimination. For example, in premature newborn babies, the antibiotic **gentamicin** (see Ch. 51) has a plasma half-life of ≥ 18 h, compared with 1–4 h for adults and approximately 10 h for babies born at term. It is therefore necessary to reduce and/or space out doses to avoid toxicity in premature babies.

Glomerular filtration rate declines slowly from about 20 years of age, falling by about 25% at 50 years and by 50% at 75 years. Figure 11.1 shows that the renal clearance of **digoxin** in young and old subjects is closely correlated with creatinine clearance, a measure of GFR. Consequently, chronic administration over the years of the same daily dose of digoxin to an individual as he or she ages leads to a progressive increase in plasma concentration, and this is a common cause of glycoside toxicity in elderly people (see Ch. 21).

▼ The age-related decline in GFR is not reflected by an increase in plasma creatinine concentration, as distinct from creatinine clearance. Plasma creatinine typically remains within the normal adult range in elderly persons despite substantially diminished GFR. This is because creatinine synthesis is reduced in elderly persons because of their reduced muscle mass. Consequently, a 'normal' plasma creatinine in an elderly person does not indicate that they have a normal GFR. Failure to recognise this and reduce the dose of drugs that are eliminated by renal excretion can lead to drug toxicity.

Table 11.1   Effect of age on plasma elimination half-lives of various drugs

Drug	Mean or range of half-life (h)		
	Term neonate[a]	Adult	Elderly person
Drugs that are mainly excreted unchanged in the urine			
Gentamicin	10	2	4
Lithium	120	24	48
Digoxin	200	40	80
Drugs that are mainly metabolised			
Diazepam	25–100	15–25	50–150
Phenytoin	10–30	10–30	10–30
Sulfamethoxypyridazine	140	60	100

[a]Even greater differences from mean adult values occur in premature babies.

Data from Reidenberg MM 1971 Renal Function and Drug Action. Saunders, Philadelphia; and Dollery CT 1991 Therapeutic Drugs. Churchill Livingstone, Edinburgh.

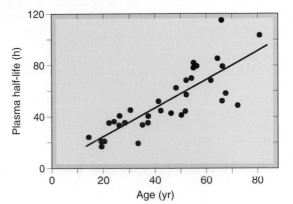

Fig. 11.2 Increasing plasma half-life for diazepam with age in 33 normal subjects. Note the increased variability as well as increased half-life with ageing. *(From Klotz U et al. 1975 J Clin Invest 55, 347.)*

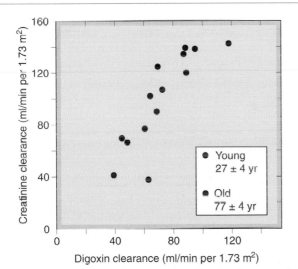

Fig. 11.1 Relationship between renal function (measured as creatinine clearance) and digoxin clearance in young and old subjects. *(From Ewy GA et al. 1969 Circulation 34, 452.)*

EFFECT OF AGE ON DRUG METABOLISM

Several important enzymes, including hepatic microsomal oxidase, glucuronyltransferase, acetyltransferase and plasma esterases, have low activity in neonates, especially if premature. These enzymes take 8 weeks or longer to reach the adult level of activity. The relative lack of conjugating activity in the newborn can have serious consequences, as in *kernicterus* caused by drug displacement of bilirubin from its binding sites on albumin (Ch. 8) and in the 'grey baby' syndrome caused by the antibiotic **chloramphenicol** (see Ch. 51). This sometimes fatal condition, at first thought to be a specific biochemical sensitivity to the drug in young babies, actually results simply from accumulation of very high tissue concentrations of chloramphenicol because of slow hepatic conjugation. Chloramphenicol is no more toxic to babies than to adults provided the dose is reduced to make allowance for this. Slow conjugation is also one reason why **morphine** (which is excreted mainly as the glucuronide, see Ch. 42) is not used as an analgesic in labour, because drug transferred via the placenta has a long half-life in the newborn baby and can cause prolonged respiratory depression.

The activity of hepatic microsomal enzymes declines slowly (and very variably) with age, and the distribution volume of lipid-soluble drugs increases, because the proportion of the body that is fat increases with advancing age. The increasing half-life of the anxiolytic drug **diazepam** with advancing age (Fig. 11.2) is one consequence of this. Some other benzodiazepines and their active metabolites show even greater age-related increases in half-life. Because half-life determines the time course of drug accumulation during repeated dosing (Ch. 10), insidious effects, developing over days or weeks, can occur in elderly people and may be misattributed to age-related memory impairment rather than to drug accumulation. Even if the mean half-life of a drug is little affected, there is often a striking increase in the *variability* of half-life between individuals with increasing age (as in Fig. 11.2). This is important, because a population of old people will contain some individuals with grossly reduced rates of drug metabolism, whereas such extremes do not occur so commonly in young adult populations. Drug regulatory authorities therefore usually require studies in elderly persons as part of the evaluation of drugs likely to be used in older people.

AGE-RELATED VARIATION IN SENSITIVITY TO DRUGS

The same plasma concentration of a drug can cause different effects in young and old subjects. Benzodiazepines (Ch. 44) exemplify this, producing more confusion and less sedation in elderly than in young subjects; similarly, hypotensive drugs (Ch. 22) cause postural hypotension more commonly in elderly than in younger adult patients.

PREGNANCY

Pregnancy causes physiological changes that influence drug disposition (Ch. 8) in mother and fetus. Maternal plasma albumin concentration is reduced, influencing drug protein binding. Cardiac output is increased, leading to increased renal blood flow and GFR, and increased renal elimination of drugs. Lipophilic molecules rapidly traverse the placental barrier, whereas transfer of hydrophobic drugs is slow, limiting fetal drug exposure following a single maternal dose. The placental barrier excludes some drugs (e.g. low-molecular-weight heparins; Ch. 24) so effectively that they can be administered chronically to the mother without causing effects in the fetus. However, drugs that are transferred to the fetus are eliminated more slowly than from the mother. The activity of most drug-metabolising enzymes in fetal liver is much less than in the adult. Furthermore, the fetal kidney is not an efficient route of elimination because excreted drug enters the amniotic fluid, which is swallowed by the fetus. For a fuller account see Atkinson et al. (2006).

DISEASE

Therapeutic drugs are prescribed to patients, so effects of disease on drug response are very important, especially disease of the major organs responsible for drug metabolism and drug (and drug metabolite) excretion. Detailed consideration is beyond the scope of this book, and interested readers should refer to a clinical text such as the chapters on renal and hepatic disease in Atkinson et al. (2006). Disease can cause pharmacokinetic or pharmacodynamic variation. Common disorders such as impaired renal or hepatic function predispose to toxicity by causing unexpectedly intense or prolonged drug effects as a result of increased drug concentration following a 'standard' dose. Drug absorption is slowed in conditions causing gastric stasis (e.g. *migraine, diabetic neuropathy*) and may be incomplete in patients with malabsorption owing to ileal or pancreatic disease or to oedema of the ileal mucosa caused by heart failure or nephrotic syndrome. *Nephrotic syndrome* (characterised by heavy proteinuria, oedema and a reduced concentration of albumin in plasma) alters drug absorption because of oedema of intestinal mucosa; alters drug disposition through changes in binding to plasma albumin; and causes insensitivity to diuretics such as **furosemide** that act on ion transport mechanisms in the lumenal surface of tubular epithelium (Ch. 29), through drug binding to albumin in tubular fluid. *Hypothyroidism* is associated with increased sensitivity to several drugs (e.g. **pethidine**), for reasons that are poorly understood. *Hypothermia* (to which elderly persons, in particular, are predisposed) markedly reduces the clearance of many drugs.

Other disorders affect drug sensitivity by altering receptor or signal-transduction mechanisms (see Ch. 3). Examples include the following:

- Diseases that influence receptors:
  - *myasthenia gravis*, an autoimmune disease characterised by antibodies to nicotinic acetylcholine receptors (Ch. 13) and increased sensitivity to neuromuscular blocking agents (e.g. **vecuronium**) and other drugs that may influence neuromuscular transmission (e.g. *aminoglycoside antibiotics*, Ch. 51)
  - *X-linked nephrogenic diabetes insipidus*, characterised by abnormal antidiuretic hormone (ADH, vasopressin) receptors (Ch. 29) and insensitivity to ADH
  - *familial hypercholesterolaemia*, an inherited disease of low-density-lipoprotein receptors (Ch. 23); the

homozygous form is relatively resistant to treatment with statins (which work mainly by increasing expression of these receptors), whereas the much commoner heterozygous form responds well to statins.
- Diseases that influence signal transduction mechanisms:
  - *pseudohypoparathyroidism*, which stems from impaired coupling of receptors with adenylyl cyclase
  - *familial precocious puberty* and *hyperthyroidism* caused by functioning thyroid adenomas, which are each caused by mutations in G protein-coupled receptors that result in the receptors remaining 'turned on' even in the absence of the hormones that are their natural agonists.

DRUG INTERACTIONS

Many patients, especially elderly ones, are treated continuously with one or more drugs for chronic diseases such as hypertension, heart failure, osteoarthritis and so on. Acute events (e.g. infections, myocardial infarction) are treated with additional drugs. The potential for drug interactions is therefore substantial, and drug interactions account for 5–20% of adverse drug reactions. These may be serious (approximately 30% of fatal adverse drug reactions are estimated to be the consequence of drug interaction). Drugs can also interact with chemical entities in other dietary constituents (e.g. grapefruit juice, which down-regulates expression of CYP3A4 in the gut) and herbal remedies (such as St John's wort; Ch. 47). The administration of one chemical entity (A) can alter the action of another (B) by one of two general mechanisms:[1]

1. Modifying the pharmacological effect of B without altering its concentration in the tissue fluid (pharmacodynamic interaction).
2. Altering the concentration of B at its site of action (pharmacokinetic interaction), as described in Chs 8 and 9.

PHARMACODYNAMIC INTERACTION

Pharmacodynamic interaction can occur in many different ways (including those discussed under *Drug antagonism* in Ch. 2). There are many mechanisms, and some examples of practical importance are probably more useful than attempts at classification.

- β-Adrenoceptor antagonists diminish the effectiveness of β-adrenoceptor agonists such as **salbutamol** (Ch. 14).
- Many diuretics lower plasma K^+ concentration (see Ch. 29), and thereby predispose to **digoxin** toxicity and to toxicity with *type III antidysrhythmic drugs* (Ch. 21).
- **Sildenafil** inhibits the isoform of phosphodiesterase (type V) that inactivates cGMP (Chs 20 and 35); consequently, it potentiates organic nitrates, which activate guanylyl cyclase, and can cause severe hypotension in patients taking these drugs.

---

[1]A third category of pharmaceutical interactions should be mentioned, in which drugs interact *in vitro* so that one or both are inactivated. No pharmacological principles are involved, just chemistry. An example is the formation of a complex between **thiopental** and **suxamethonium**, which must not be mixed in the same syringe. **Heparin** is highly charged and interacts in this way with many basic drugs; it is sometimes used to keep intravenous lines or cannulae open and can inactivate basic drugs if they are injected without first clearing the line with saline.

- *Monoamine oxidase inhibitors* increase the amount of noradrenaline stored in noradrenergic nerve terminals and interact dangerously with drugs, such as **ephedrine** or **tyramine**, that release stored noradrenaline. This can also occur with tyramine-rich foods – particularly fermented cheeses such as Camembert (see Ch. 47).
- **Warfarin** competes with vitamin K, preventing hepatic synthesis of various coagulation factors (see Ch. 24). If vitamin K production in the intestine is inhibited (e.g. by antibiotics), the anticoagulant action of warfarin is increased.
- The risk of bleeding, especially from the stomach, caused by warfarin is increased by drugs that cause bleeding by different mechanisms (e.g. **aspirin**, which inhibits platelet thromboxane A_2 biosynthesis and which can damage the stomach; Ch. 26).
- *Sulfonamides* prevent the synthesis of folic acid by bacteria and other microorganisms; **trimethoprim** inhibits its reduction to its active tetrahydrofolate form. Given together, the drugs have a synergistic action of value in treating *Pneumocystis* infection (Chs 53 and 54).
- *Non-steroidal anti-inflammatory drugs* (NSAIDs; Ch. 26), such as **ibuprofen** or **indometacin**, inhibit biosynthesis of prostaglandins, including renal vasodilator/natriuretic prostaglandins (prostaglandin E_2, prostaglandin I_2). If administered to patients receiving treatment for hypertension, they increase the blood pressure. If given to patients being treated with diuretics for chronic heart failure, they cause salt and water retention and hence cardiac decompensation.[2]
- Histamine H_1-receptor antagonists, such as **promethazine**, commonly cause drowsiness as an unwanted effect. This is more troublesome if such drugs are taken with alcohol, leading to accidents at work or on the road.

Pharmacokinetic interaction

All the four major processes that determine pharmacokinetics – absorption, distribution, metabolism and excretion – can be affected by drugs. Such interactions are covered in Chapters 8 and 9.

Drug interactions

- These are many and varied: if in doubt, look it up.
- Interactions may be pharmacodynamic or pharmacokinetic.
- Pharmacodynamic interactions are often predictable from the actions of the interacting drugs.
- Pharmacokinetic interactions can involve effects on:
  - absorption (Ch. 8)
  - distribution (e.g. competition for protein binding, Ch. 8)
  - hepatic metabolism (induction or inhibition, Ch. 9)
  - renal excretion (Ch. 9).

GENETIC VARIATION IN DRUG RESPONSIVENESS

RELEVANT ELEMENTARY GENETICS

Genes are the fundamental units of heredity; they consist of ordered sequences of nucleotides (adenine, guanine, thymidine and cytosine – A, G, T, C) located in particular positions in a particular DNA strand. Genes are conventionally abbreviated as for the protein they code for, but are written in italics – for example 'CYP2D6' represents a protein while '*CYP2D6*' is the gene that encodes it. Most cellular DNA is located in the chromosomes in cell nuclei, but a small amount is present in mitochondria and is inherited from the mother (since the ovum contributes mitochondria to the gamete). DNA is *transcribed* to complementary messenger RNA (mRNA) which is *translated* in rough endoplasmic reticulum into a sequence of amino acids. The resulting peptide undergoes folding and often post-translational modification to form the final protein product. The DNA sequence of a gene that codes protein is known as the *exon*. Introns are DNA sequences that interrupt the exon; an intron is transcribed into mRNA but this sequence is excised from the message and not translated into protein. The rate of transcription is controlled by promoter regions in the DNA to which RNA polymerase binds to initiate transcription.

Mutations are heritable changes in the base sequence of DNA. This may, or may not,[3] result in a change in the amino acid sequence of the protein for which the gene codes. Most changes in protein structure are deleterious, and so the altered gene dies out in succeeding generations as a result of natural selection. A few changes may confer an advantage, however, at least under some environmental circumstances. A pharmacogenetically relevant example is the X linked gene for *glucose 6 phosphate dehydrogenase* (G6PD); deficiency of this enzyme confers partial resistance to malaria (a considerable selective advantage in parts of the world where this disease is common) at the expense of susceptibility to haemolysis in response to oxidative stress in the form of exposure to various dietary constituents, including several drugs (e.g. the antimalarial drug **primaquine**; see Ch. 54). This ambiguity gives rise to the abnormal gene being preserved in future generations, at a frequency that depends on the balance of selective pressures in the environment. Thus the distribution of G6PD deficiency is similar to the geographical distribution of malaria. The situation where several functionally distinct forms of a gene are common in a population is called a 'balanced' polymorphism (balanced because a disadvantage, for example in a homozygote, is balanced by an advantage, for example in a heterozygote).

Polymorphisms are alternative sequences at a locus within the DNA strand (alleles) that persist in a population through several generations. They arise initially because of a mutation, and are stable if they are non-functional, or die out during subsequent generations if (as

---

[2]The interaction with diuretics may involve a pharmacokinetic interaction in addition to the pharmacodynamic effect described here, because NSAIDs compete with weak acids, including diuretics, for renal tubular secretion; see Ch. 9.

[3]The genetic code is 'redundant', i.e. more than one set of nucleotide base triplets code for each amino acid. If a mutation results in a base change that leads to a triplet that codes for the same amino acid as the original, there is no change in the protein and consequently no change in function – a 'silent' mutation. Such mutations are neither advantageous nor disadvantageous, so they will neither be eliminated by natural selection nor accumulate in the population at the expense of the wild-type gene.

is usually the case) they are disadvantageous. However, if the prevailing selective pressures in the environment are favourable, leading to a selective advantage, a polymorphism may increase in frequency over successive generations. Now that genes can be sequenced readily, it has become apparent that *single nucleotide polymorphisms* (SNPs, DNA sequence variations that occur when a single nucleotide in the genome sequence is altered) are very common. They may entail substitution of one nucleotide for another (usually substitution of C for T), or deletion or insertion of a nucleotide. Insertions and deletions result in a 'frame shift' in translation – for example, after an insertion, the first element of the next triplet in the code becomes the second and all subsequent bases are shifted one 'to the right'. The result can be loss of protein synthesis, abnormal protein synthesis or an abnormal rate of protein synthesis.

SNPs occur every 100–300 bases along the 3 billion base human genome. Approximately two-thirds of SNPs involve C for T substitution. SNPs can occur in coding (gene) and non-coding regions of the genome. A single SNP can be an important determinant of disease – for example, a common genetic variant due to an SNP in one of the coagulation factors, known as factor V Leiden, is the commonest form of inherited thrombophilia (Ch. 24). This confers an increased risk of venous thrombosis in response to environmental factors such as prolonged immobility, but might perhaps have been an advantage to ancestors more at risk of haemorrhage than of thrombosis. Alternatively, predisposition to disease may depend on a combination of several SNPs in or near a gene. Such combinations are known as *haplotypes* and are inherited from each parent.

SINGLE-GENE PHARMACOKINETIC DISORDERS

Where a mutation disrupts gene function profoundly this may result in a 'single-gene disorder', which is inherited in Mendelian fashion. This was recognised for albinism (albinos lack an enzyme that is needed to synthesise the brown pigment melanin) and other 'inborn errors of metabolism' in the early part of the 20th century by Archibald Garrod, a British physician who initiated the study of biochemical genetics. Investigation of this large group of individually rare diseases has contributed disproportionately to our understanding of molecular pathology – familial hypercholesterolaemia and the mechanism of action of statins (Ch. 23) is one example.

PLASMA CHOLINESTERASE DEFICIENCY

In the 1950s Walter Kalow discovered that **suxamethonium** sensitivity is due to genetic variation in the rate of drug metabolism as a result of a Mendelian autosomal recessive trait. This short-acting neuromuscular-blocking drug is widely used in anaesthesia and is normally rapidly hydrolysed by plasma cholinesterase (Ch. 13). About 1 in 3000 individuals fail to inactivate suxamethonium rapidly and experience prolonged neuromuscular block if treated with it; this is because a recessive gene gives rise to an abnormal type of plasma cholinesterase. The abnormal enzyme has a modified pattern of substrate and inhibitor specificity. It is detected by a blood test that measures the effect of **dibucaine**, which inhibits the abnormal enzyme less than the normal enzyme. Heterozygotes

hydrolyse suxamethonium at a more or less normal rate, but their plasma cholinesterase has reduced sensitivity to dibucaine, intermediate between normal subjects and homozygotes. Only homozygotes express the disease: they appear completely healthy unless exposed to suxamethonium (or, presumably, closely related chemicals) but experience prolonged paralysis if exposed to a dose that would cause neuromuscular block for only a few minutes in a healthy person.[4] There are other reasons why responses to suxamethonium may be abnormal in an individual patient, notably *malignant hyperpyrexia* (Ch. 13), a genetically determined idiosyncratic adverse drug reaction involving the ryanodine receptor (Ch. 4). It is important to test family members who may be affected, but the disorder is so rare that it is currently impractical to screen for it routinely before therapeutic use of suxamethonium.

ACUTE INTERMITTENT PORPHYRIA

The hepatic *porphyrias* are prototypic pharmacogenetic disorders in which patients may be symptomatic even if they are not exposed to a drug, but where many drugs can provoke very severe worsening of the course of the disease. They are inherited disorders involving the biochemical pathway of porphyrin haem biosynthesis. *Acute intermittent porphyria* is the least uncommon and most severe form. It is autosomal dominant and is due to one of many different mutations in the gene coding *porphobilinogen deaminase* (PBGD), a key enzyme in haem biosynthesis in red cell precursors, hepatocytes and other cells. All of these mutations reduce activity of this enzyme, and clinical features are caused by the resulting build-up of haem precursors including porphyrins. There is a strong interplay with the environment through exposure to drugs, hormones and other chemicals. The use of sedative, anticonvulsant or other drugs in patients with undiagnosed porphyria can be lethal, though with appropriate supportive management most patients recover completely.[5] Many drugs, especially but not exclusively those that induce CYP enzymes (e.g. barbiturates, **griseofulvin**, **carbamazepine**, oestrogens – see Ch. 9), can precipitate acute attacks in susceptible individuals. Porphyrins are synthesised from δ-amino laevulinic acid (ALA) which is formed by ALA synthase in the liver. This enzyme is induced by drugs such as barbiturates, resulting in increased ALA production and, hence, increased porphyrin accumulation. As mentioned above, the genetic trait is inherited as an autosomal dominant, but frank disease is approximately five times more common in women than in men, because hormonal fluctuations precipitate acute attacks.

---

[4]An apparently healthy middle-aged man saw one of the authors over several months because of hypertension; he also saw a psychiatrist because of depression. This failed to improve with other treatment and he underwent electroconvulsive therapy (ECT). Suxamethonium was used to prevent injury caused by convulsions; this usually results in short-lived paralysis but this poor man recovered consciousness some 2 days later to find himself being weaned from artificial ventilation in an intensive care unit. Subsequent analysis showed him to be homozygous for an ineffective form of plasma cholinesterase.
[5]Life expectancy, obtained from parish records, of patients with porphyria diagnosed retrospectively within large kindreds in Scandinavia was normal until the advent and widespread use of barbiturates and other sedative and anticonvulsant drugs in the 20th century, when it plummeted. There is a long and useful list of drugs to avoid in the *British National Formulary*, together with the warning that drugs not on the list may not necessarily be safe in such patients!

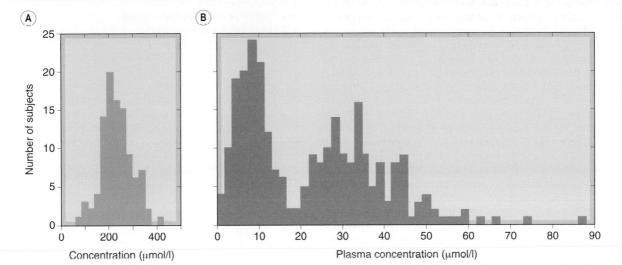

Fig. 11.3 Distribution of individual plasma concentrations for two drugs in humans. [**A**] Plasma salicylate concentration 3 h after oral dosage with sodium salicylate. [**B**] Plasma isoniazid concentration 6 h after oral dosage. Note the normally distributed values for salicylate, compared with the bimodal distribution of isoniazid. *(Panel [A] from Evans DA, Clarke CA 1961 Br Med Bull 17, 234–280; panel [B] from Price-Evans DA 1963 Am J Med 3, 639.)*

DRUG ACETYLATION DEFICIENCY

Both examples considered so far are uncommon diseases. However, in the 1960s Price-Evans demonstrated that the rate of drug acetylation varied in different populations as a result of balanced polymorphism. Figure 11.3 contrasts the approximately Gaussian distribution of plasma concentrations achieved 3 h after administration of a dose of **salicylate** with the bimodal distribution of plasma concentrations after a dose of **isoniazid**. The isoniazid concentration was <20 μmol/l in about half the population, and in this group the mode was approximately 9 μmol/l. In the other half of the population (plasma concentration >20 μmol/l), the mode was approximately 30 μmol/l. Elimination of isoniazid depends mainly on acetylation, catalysed by an acetyltransferase enzyme (Ch. 9). White populations contain roughly equal numbers of 'fast acetylators' and 'slow acetylators'. The characteristic of fast or slow acetylation is controlled by a single recessive gene associated with low hepatic acetyltransferase activity. Other ethnic groups have different proportions of fast and slow acetylators. Isoniazid causes two distinct forms of toxicity. One is peripheral neuropathy, which is produced by isoniazid itself and is commoner in slow acetylators. The other is hepatotoxicity, caused by the acetylated metabolite and is commoner in fast acetylators, at least in some populations. This genetic variation thus produces a qualitative change in the pattern of toxicity caused by the drug in different populations.

Acetyltransferase is also important in the metabolism of other drugs, including **hydralazine** (Ch. 22), **procainamide** (Ch. 21), **dapsone** and various other sulfonamides (Ch. 51) and acetylator status influences drug-induced *lupus* (an autoimmune disorder affecting many organs including skin, joints and kidneys) caused by several of these agents. However, neither phenotyping (by measuring kinetics of drug transformation) nor genotyping for acetyltransferase has found a way into routine clinical practice, probably because these drugs are relatively little

used and there are several alternative treatments available that are usually preferred.

AMINOGLYCOSIDE OTOTOXICITY

In the examples above, variations in chromosomal genes cause variations in drug response. Increased susceptibility to hearing loss caused by aminoglycoside antibiotics (see Ch. 51) is, in some families, inherited quite differently, namely exclusively through the mother to all her children. This is the pattern expected of a mitochondrial gene, and indeed the most common predisposing mutation is *m.1555A>G*, a mitochondrial DNA mutation. This mutation accounts for 30–60% of aminoglycoside ototoxicity in China, where aminoglycoside use is common. Aminoglycosides work by binding to bacterial ribosomes (Ch. 51), which share properties with human mitochondrial ribosomes (mitochondria are believed to have evolved from symbiotic bacteria); aminoglycosides cause ototoxity in all individuals exposed to too high a dose. The *m.1555A>G* mutation makes mitochondrial ribosomes even more similar to their bacterial counterpart, increasing the affinity of the drug which remains bound to ribosomes in the hair cells in the ear for several months following a single dose in susceptible individuals. Screening for this variant may be appropriate in children who are likely to require treatment with aminoglycosides (Bitner-Glindzicz & Rahman, 2007).

THERAPEUTIC DRUGS AND CLINICALLY AVAILABLE PHARMACOGENOMIC TESTS

Clinical tests to predict drug responsiveness were anticipated to be one of the first applications of sequencing the human genome, but their development has been slowed by various scientific, commercial, political and educational barriers (Flockhart et al., 2009). Reimbursement for expensive drugs, whether provided by the state or by insurance schemes, depends increasingly on evidence of cost-effectiveness. New tests need to improve demonstrably on our current ability to prescribe optimally, and must lead to a clear-cut change in prescribing, such as using a different drug or a different dosing regimen. So far the evidence in support of any pharmacogenetic test is less convincing than the ideal of a randomised controlled trial of a pharmacogenomics-informed prescribing strategy versus current best practice, but several of the tests mentioned below are increasingly used in clinical practice. They include tests for (a) variants of different human leukocyte antigens (HLAs) that have been strongly linked to susceptibilities to several severe qualitatively distinct off-target harmful drug reactions; (b) genes controlling aspects of drug metabolism; and (c) genes encoding drug targets. For one drug (**warfarin**), a test combines genetic information about metabolism with information about its target. The genetic susceptibility of Collie dogs to neurotoxic effects of **ivermectin** mentioned in Chapter 8 is of importance in veterinary medicine. It results from a variant of P-glycoprotein that alters the properties of the blood–brain barrier of dogs with Collie ancestry, and in future genes coding for proteins influencing drug distribution in man may also be fertile territory for new tests.

Methodology: Mutations in the germline are passed to the next generation where they are present in all cells; in practice, tests for such germline mutations are usually made on venous blood samples that contain chromosomal and mitochondrial DNA in white blood cells. Somatic cell mutations underlie the pathogenesis of some tumours (Ch. 5), and the presence or absence of such somatic cell mutations guides drug selection. The genomic tests are performed on DNA from samples of the tumour obtained surgically. The tests themselves involve amplification of the relevant sequence(s) and molecular biological methods, often utilising chip technology, to identify the various polymorphisms.

HLA GENE TESTS

ABACAVIR AND *HLAB*5701*

▼ **Abacavir** (Ch. 52) is a reverse transcriptase inhibitor that is highly effective in treating HIV infection. Its use has been limited by severe rashes. Susceptibility to this adverse effect is closely linked to the human leukocyte antigen (HLA) variant *HLAB*5701*, and testing for this variant is used widely and supported by prospective trials; see Figure 11.4 (Lai-Goldman & Faruki, 2008).

ANTICONVULSANTS AND *HLAB*1502*

▼ **Carbamazepine** (Ch. 45) can also cause severe (life-threatening) rashes including *Stevens–Johnson syndrome* (in which a multiform rash with blistering and other lesions extends into the gastrointestinal tract) and *toxic epidermal necrolysis* (in which the outer layer of the skin peels away from the dermis as though it has been scalded). These are associated with a particular HLA allele, *HLAB*1502*, which occurs almost exclusively in people with Asian ancestry (Man et al., 2007); the FDA recommends that Chinese patients should be screened for this allele before starting treatment. People who develop such a reaction to carbamazepine may develop a similar problem if treated with **phenytoin**, and the same allele has been associated with hypersensitivity reactions to this drug too.

CLOZAPINE AND *HLA-DQB1*0201*

▼ **Clozapine** is a uniquely effective antipsychotic drug with a different pattern of adverse effects from classical antipsychotic drugs (Ch. 46); its use is limited by agranulocytosis which occurs in approximately 1% of treated patients. This has been associated with *HLA-DQB1*0201*, but so far studies have been small and the specificity and sensitivity of the test remain to be established.

Pharmacogenetics and pharmacogenomics

- Several inherited disorders influence responses to drugs, including:
  - glucose-6-phosphatase deficiency, a sex-linked disorder in which affected men (or rare homozygous women) experience haemolysis if exposed to various chemicals including the antimalarial drug **primaquine**
  - plasma cholinesterase deficiency, an autosomal recessive disorder that confers sensitivity to the neuromuscular blocker suxamethonium
  - acute intermittent porphyria, an autosomal dominant disease more severe in women and in which severe attacks are precipitated by drugs or endogenous sex hormones that induce CYP enzymes
  - drug acetylator deficiency, a balanced polymorphism
  - increased susceptibility to ototoxicity from aminoglycosides, which is conferred by a mutation in mitochondrial DNA.
- These pharmacogenetic disorders prove that drug responses can be genetically determined in individuals.
- Single nucleotide polymorphisms (SNPs) and combinations of SNPs (haplotypes) in genes coding for proteins involved in drug disposition or drug action are common and may predict drug response. Pharmacogenomic tests in blood or tissue removed surgically have established associations between several such variants and individual drug response, and several such tests are available for clinical use although their status in individualising drug treatment is still being established.
- Such tests are available for:
  - several HLA variants that predict toxicity of **abacavir**, **carbamazepine** and **clozapine**
  - genes for several enzymes in drug metabolism including CYP2D6 and CYP2C9, and thiopurine-*S*-methyltransferase (TPMT)
  - germline and somatic mutations in growth-factor receptors that predict responsiveness to cancer treatments including **imatinib** and **trastuzumab**.

DRUG METABOLISM-RELATED GENE TESTS

THIOPURINES AND TPMT

▼ Thiopurine drugs (**tioguanine**, **mercaptopurine** and its prodrug **azathioprine**; Ch. 56) have been used for the past 50 years to treat leukaemias, including acute lymphoblastic leukaemia (ALL, which accounts for approximately one-fifth of all childhood malignancies), and more recently to cause immunosuppression, e.g. in treating inflammatory bowel disease. All of these drugs cause bone marrow and liver toxicity, and are detoxified by thiopurine-*S*-methyltransferase (TPMT), which is present in blood cells, as well as by xanthine oxidase. There are large inherited variations in TPMT activity with a trimodal frequency distribution (Weinshilboum & Sladek, 1980); low TPMT activity in blood is associated with high concentrations of active 6-thioguanine nucleotides (TGN) in blood and with bone marrow toxicity whereas high TPMT activity is associated with lower concentrations of TGN and reduced efficacy. Before starting treatment, phenotyping (by a blood test for TPMT activity) or genotyping of *TMPT* alleles *TPMT*3A*, *TPMT*3C*, *TPMT*2*, is

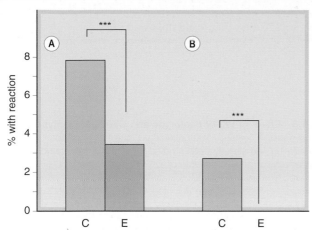

Fig. 11.4 **Incidence of abacavir hypersensitivity is reduced by pharmacogenetic screening.** In the PREDICT-1 study (Mallal et al., 2008), patients were randomised to standard care (control group, C) or prospective pharmacogenetic screening (experimental group, E). All the control subjects were treated with abacavir, but only those experimental subjects who were *HLA-B*5701* negative were treated with abacavir. There were two prespecified end points: clinically suspected hypersensitivity reactions [**A**] and clinically suspected reactions that were immunologically confirmed by a positive patch test [**B**]. Both end points favoured the experimental group (*P* < 0.0001). *(Figure redrawn from Hughes AR et al. 2008 Pharmacogenet J 8, 365–374.)*

recommended. Even with such testing, careful monitoring of the white blood cell count is needed because of environmental susceptibility factors (e.g. drug interaction with **allopurinol** via inhibition of xanthine oxidase).

5-FLUOROURACIL (5-FU) AND DPYD

▼ **5-FU** (Ch. 56, Fig. 56.6) is used extensively to treat solid tumours, but has variable efficacy and unpredictable mucocutaneous toxicity. It is detoxified by dihydropyrimidine dehydrogenase (DPYD), which has multiple clinically identifiable functional genetic variants. Currently available genetic information is neither highly sensitive nor specific, but the FDA recommends that the drug not be given to patients with DPYD deficiency.

TAMOXIFEN AND CYP2D6

▼ **Tamoxifen** (Chs 35 and 56) is metabolised to an oestrogen antagonist endoxifen by CYP2D6, an enzyme that is subject to marked polymorphic variation; several small association studies have suggested a link between *CYP2D6* genotype and efficacy. Genotyping tests for *CYP2D6* are available, but genetic results from larger comparative trials of tamoxifen versus aromatase inhibitors are awaited. Treatment with other CYP2D6 substrates, for example **tetrabenazine**, used to treat Huntington's disease (Ch. 40) may also be influenced by knowledge of *CYP2D6* genotype: the FDA recommends that patients who are CYP2D6 poor metabolisers should not be prescribed more than 50 mg daily because of the risk of severe depression.

IRINOTECAN AND UGT1A1*28

▼ **Irinotecan**, a topoisomerase I inhibitor (Ch. 56) has marked activity against colorectal and lung cancers in a minority of patients, but toxicity (diarrhoea and bone marrow suppression) can be severe. It works through an active metabolite (SN-38) which is detoxified by glucuronidation by UDP-glucuronyltransferase (UGT; Ch. 9, Fig. 9.3). Reduced activity of this enzyme is common and gives rise to the inherited benign condition of hyperbilirubinaemia known as *Gilbert's syndrome* in which unconjugated bilirubin accumulates in plasma. UGT1A1 genetic testing is clinically available and predicts irinotecan pharmacokinetics and clinical outcomes. The best way to use information from the test is still uncertain, however.

DRUG TARGET-RELATED GENE TESTS

TRASTUZUMAB AND HER2

▼ **Trastuzumab** ('Herceptin'; Ch. 56) is a monoclonal antibody that antagonises epidermal growth factor (EGF) by binding to one of its receptors (human epidermal growth factor receptor 2 – HER2) which can occur in tumour tissue as a result of somatic mutation. It is used in patients with breast cancer whose tumour tissue overexpresses this receptor. Other patients do not benefit from it.

DASATINIB, IMATINIB AND BCR-ABL1

▼ **Dasatinib** is a tyrosine kinase inhibitor used in haematological malignancies characterised by the presence of a Philadelphia chromosome, namely chronic myeloid leukaemia (CML) and some adults with acute lymphoblastic leukaemia (ALL). The Philadelphia chromosome results from a translocation defect when parts of two chromosomes (9 and 22) swap places; part of a 'breakpoint cluster region' (BCR) in chromosome 22 links to the 'Abelson-1' (ABL) region of chromosome 9. A mutation (T315I) in BCR/ABL confers resistance to the inhibitory effect of dasatinib and patients with this variant do not benefit from this drug. Pharmacogenetic testing is also being evaluated for **imatinib** (Ch. 56), another tyrosine kinase inhibitor used in patients with CML and other myelodysplastic disorders associated with rearrangements in the gene for platelet-derived growth factor receptor or for BCR-ABL.

COMBINED (METABOLISM AND TARGET) GENE TESTS

WARFARIN AND CYP2C9 + VKORC1 GENOTYPING

▼ **Warfarin** is *par excellence* a drug where dosing must be individualised. This is done by measuring the *international normalised ratio* (INR), a measure of its effect on blood coagulability (Ch. 24), but thrombotic events despite treatment (lack of efficacy) and serious adverse effects (usually bleeding) remain all too common. Warfarin is the most widely used drug for which pharmacogenetic testing has been proposed, based on a study showing that polymorphisms in its key target, vitamin K epoxide reductase (VKOR; see Fig. 24.5) and in CYP2C9, involved in its metabolism, are associated with outcomes. Figure 11.5 shows the effects of VKOR haplotype and of CYP2C9 genotype on the mean dose of warfarin needed to achieve therapeutic INR. Dosing algorithms have been proposed based on the results of testing for polymorphisms of these genes (Schwarz et al., 2008). A randomised trial favoured this strategy for initiating treatment versus a standard loading dose approach, but genetic testing did not improve on an individualised algorithm for dose initiation based on other clinical variables (Zineh et al., 2013).

CONCLUSIONS

Twin studies as well as several well-documented single-gene disorders (including Mendelian chromosomal – autosomal recessive, autosomal dominant and X-linked – and maternally inherited mitochondrial disorders) prove the concept that susceptibility to adverse drug effects can be genetically determined. Pharmacogenomic testing offers the possibility of more precise 'personalised' therapeutics for several drugs and disorders. This is a field of intense research activity, rapid progress and high expectations, but proving that these tests add to present best practice and improve outcomes remains a challenge.

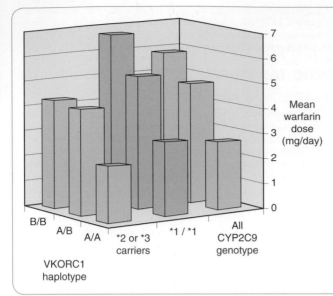

Fig. 11.5 Effect of *VKOR* haplotype and *CYP2C9* genotype on warfarin dose. A series of 186 patients on long-term warfarin treatment who had already been studied for *CYP2C9* were studied retrospectively for genetic variants of *VKOR* (Rieder et al., 2005). *VKOR* haplotype as well as *CYP2C9* genotype influenced the mean warfarin dose (which had been adjusted to achieve therapeutic INR). A, Haplotypes 1 and 2; B, haplotypes 7, 8 and 9. A/A, A/B and B/B represent haplotype combinations. *1/*1 represents CYP2C9 wild-type homozygotes; *2 and *3 represent CYP2C9 variants. *(Figure redrawn from Beitelshees AL, McLeod HL 2006 Applying pharmacogenomics to enhance the use of biomarkers for drug effect and drug safety. TIPS 27, 498–502.)*

REFERENCES AND FURTHER READING

Further reading

Carmichael, D.J.S., 2005. Handling of drugs in kidney disease. In: Davison, A.M., Cameron, J.S., Grunfeld, J.P., et al. (Eds.), Oxford Textbook of Clinical Nephrology, third ed. Oxford University Press, Oxford, pp. 2599–2618. (*Principles and practice of dose adjustment in patients with renal failure*)

Davis, J.C., Furstenthal, L., Desai, A.A., et al., 2009. The microeconomics of personalized medicine: today's challenge and tomorrow's promise. Nat. Rev. Drug Discov. 8, 279–286. (*Argues that major barriers to genomic testing, previously scientific, are now increasingly related to economics*)

Flockhart, D.A., Skaar, T., Berlin, D.S., et al., 2009. Clinically available pharmacogenomics tests. Clin. Pharmacol. Ther. 86, 109–113.

Hertz, D.L., McLeod, H.L., Irvin, W.J., 2012. Tamoxifen and CYP2D6: a contradiction of data. The Oncologist May 1, 620–630.

Pavlos, R., Mallal, S., Phillips, E., 2012. HLA and pharmacogenetics of drug hypersensitivity. Pharmacogenomics 13, 1285–1306.

Phillips, E.J., Mallal, S.A., 2011. HLA-B*1502 Screening and toxic effects of carbamazepine. N. Engl. J. Med. 365, 672.

Wang, L., McLeod, H.L., Weinshilboum, R.M., 2011. Genomics and drug response. N. Engl. J. Med. 364, 1144–1153.

Weng, L.M., Zhang, L., Peng, Y., Huang, R.S., 2013. Pharmacogenetics and pharmacogenomics: a bridge to individualized cancer therapy. Pharmacogenomics 14, 315–324.

Zineh, I., Huang, S.-M., 2011. Biomarkers in drug development and regulation: a paradigm for clinical implementation of personalized medicine. Biomark. Med. 5, 705–713.

References

Atkinson, A.J., Jr., Abernethie, D.R., Daniels, C.E., et al., 2006. Principles of Clinical Pharmacology, second ed. Academic Press, San Diego. (*Includes detailed accounts of clinical aspects including effects of renal and liver disease on pharmacokinetics, of effects of age and on drug therapy in pregnant and nursing women*)

Bitner-Glindzicz, M., Rahman, S., 2007. Ototoxicity caused by aminoglycosides is severe and permanent in genetically susceptible people. BMJ 335, 784–785.

Cooper, R.S., Kaufman, J.S., Ward, R., 2003. Race and genomics. N. Engl. J. Med. 348, 1166–1170. (*Scholarly and appropriately sceptical analysis*)

Lai-Goldman, M., Faruki, H., 2008. Abacavir hypersensitivity: a model system for pharmacogenetic test adoption. Genet. Med. 10, 874–878.

Maitland, M.L., Vasisht, K., Ratain, M.J., 2006. TPMT, UGT1A1 and DPYD: genotyping to ensure safer cancer therapy? TIPS 27, 432–437. (*Reviews gene/drug–phenotype relationships of 6-MP, irinotecan and 5-FU*)

Mallal, S., Phillips, E., Carosi, G., et al., 2008. HLA-B*5701 screening for hypersensitivity to abacavir. N. Engl. J. Med. 358, 568–579.

Man, C.B., Kwan, P., Baum, L., et al., 2007. Association between HLA-B*1502 allele and anti-epileptic drug-induced cutaneous reactions in Han Chinese. Epilepsia 48, 1015–1018.

Rieder, M.J., Reiner, A.P., Gage, B.F., et al., 2005. Effect of VKORC1 haplotype on transcriptional regulation and warfarin dose. N. Engl. J. Med. 352, 2285–2293.

Schwarz, U.I., Ritchie, M.D., Bradford, Y., et al., 2008. Genetic determinants of response to warfarin during initial anticoagulation. N. Engl. J. Med. 358, 999–1008.

Shah, R.R., Shah, D.R., 2012. Personalized medicine: is it a pharmacogenetic mirage? Br. J. Clin. Pharmacol. 74, SI 698–SI 721.

Teml, A., Schaeffeler, E., Schwab, M., 2009. Pretreatment determination of TPMT – state of the art in clinical practice. Eur. J. Clin. Pharmacol. 65, 219–221. and related articles, (*Introduces an issue devoted to the impact of TPMT polymorphisms on thiopurine use in clinical practice*)

Wadman, M., 2005. Drug targeting: is race enough? Nature 435, 1008–1009. (*No!*)

Weinshilboum, R.M., Sladek, S.L., 1980. Mercaptopurine pharmacogenetics: monogenic inheritance of erythrocyte thiopurine methyltransferase activity. Am. J. Hum. Genet. 32, 651–662.

Wood, A.J.J., 2001. Racial differences in response to drugs – pointers to genetic differences. N. Engl. J. Med. 344, 1393–1396.

Zineh, I., Pacanowski, M., Woodcock, J., 2013. Pharmacogenetics and coumarins dosing – recalibrating expectations. N. Engl. J. Med. 369, 2273–2275. (*Discuss the results of three randomised controlled trials published in the same issue which addressed related questions with different outcomes*)

Chemical mediators and the autonomic nervous system

OVERVIEW

The network of chemical signals and associated receptors by which cells in the body communicate with one another provides many targets for drug action, and has always been a focus of attention for pharmacologists. Chemical transmission in the peripheral autonomic nervous system, and the various ways in which the process can be pharmacologically subverted, is the main focus of this chapter, but the mechanisms described operate also in the central nervous system. In addition to neurotransmission, we also consider briefly the less clearly defined processes, collectively termed neuromodulation, by which many mediators and drugs exert control over the function of the nervous system. The relative anatomical and physiological simplicity of the peripheral nervous system has made it the proving ground for many important discoveries about chemical transmission, and the same general principles apply to the central nervous system (see Ch. 37). For more detail than is given here, see Robertson (2004), Burnstock (2009) and Iversen et al. (2009).

HISTORICAL ASPECTS

▼ Studies initiated on the peripheral nervous system have been central to the understanding and classification of many major types of drug action, so it is worth recounting a little history. Excellent accounts are given by Bacq (1975) and Valenstein (2005).

Experimental physiology became established as an approach to the understanding of the function of living organisms in the middle of the 19th century. The peripheral nervous system, and particularly the autonomic nervous system, received a great deal of attention. The fact that electrical stimulation of nerves could elicit a whole variety of physiological effects – from blanching of the skin to arrest of the heart – presented a real challenge to comprehension, particularly of the way in which the signal was passed from the nerve to the effector tissue. In 1877, Du Bois-Reymond was the first to put the alternatives clearly: 'Of known natural processes that might pass on excitation, only two are, in my opinion, worth talking about – either there exists at the boundary of the contractile substance a stimulatory secretion … or the phenomenon is electrical in nature.' The latter view was generally favoured. In 1869, it had been shown that an exogenous substance, **muscarine**, could mimic the effects of stimulating the vagus nerve, and that **atropine** could inhibit the actions both of muscarine and of nerve stimulation. In 1905, Langley showed the same for **nicotine** and **curare** acting at the neuromuscular junction. Most physiologists interpreted these phenomena as stimulation and inhibition of the nerve endings, respectively, rather than as evidence for chemical transmission. Hence the suggestion of T.R. Elliott, in 1904, that **adrenaline (epinephrine)** might act as a chemical transmitter mediating the actions of the sympathetic nervous system was coolly received, until Langley, the Professor of Physiology at Cambridge and a powerful figure at that time, suggested, a year later, that transmission to skeletal muscle involved the secretion by the nerve terminals of a substance related to nicotine.

One of the key observations for Elliott was that degeneration of sympathetic nerve terminals did not abolish the sensitivity of smooth muscle preparations to adrenaline (which the electrical theory predicted) but actually enhanced it. The hypothesis of chemical transmission was put to direct test in 1907 by Dixon, who tried to show that vagus nerve stimulation released from a dog's heart into the blood a substance capable of inhibiting another heart. The experiment failed, and the atmosphere of scepticism prevailed.

It was not until 1921, in Germany, that Loewi showed that stimulation of the vagosympathetic trunk connected to an isolated and cannulated frog's heart could cause the release into the cannula of a substance ('*Vagusstoff*') that, if the cannula fluid was transferred from the first heart to a second, would inhibit the second heart. This is a classic and much-quoted experiment that proved extremely difficult for even Loewi to perform reproducibly. In an autobiographical sketch, Loewi tells us that the idea of chemical transmission arose in a discussion that he had in 1903, but no way of testing it experimentally occurred to him until he dreamed of the appropriate experiment one night in 1920. He wrote some notes of this very important dream in the middle of the night, but in the morning could not read them. The dream obligingly returned the next night and, taking no chances, he went to the laboratory at 3 a.m. and carried out the experiment successfully. Loewi's experiment may be, and was, criticised on numerous grounds (it could, for example, have been potassium rather than a neurotransmitter that was acting on the recipient heart), but a series of further experiments proved him to be right. His findings can be summarised as follows:

- Stimulation of the vagus caused the appearance in the perfusate of the frog heart of a substance capable of producing, in a second heart, an inhibitory effect resembling vagus stimulation.
- Stimulation of the sympathetic nervous system caused the appearance of a substance capable of accelerating a second heart. By fluorescence measurements, Loewi concluded later that this substance was adrenaline.
- Atropine prevented the inhibitory action of the vagus on the heart but did not prevent release of Vagusstoff. Atropine thus prevented the effects, rather than the release, of the transmitter.
- When Vagusstoff was incubated with ground-up heart muscle, it became inactivated. This effect is now known to be due to enzymatic destruction of acetylcholine by cholinesterase.
- **Physostigmine**, which potentiated the effect of vagus stimulation on the heart, prevented destruction of Vagusstoff by heart muscle, providing evidence that the potentiation is due to inhibition of cholinesterase, which normally destroys the transmitter substance acetylcholine.

A few years later, in the early 1930s, Dale showed convincingly that acetylcholine was also the transmitter substance at the neuromuscular junction of striated muscle and at autonomic ganglia. One of the keys to Dale's success lay in the use of highly sensitive bioassays, especially the leech dorsal muscle, for measuring acetylcholine release. Chemical transmission at sympathetic nerve terminals was demonstrated at about the same time as cholinergic transmission and by very similar methods. Cannon and his colleagues at Harvard first showed unequivocally the phenomenon of chemical transmission at sympathetic nerve endings, by experiments *in vivo* in which tissues made supersensitive to adrenaline by prior sympathetic denervation were shown to respond, after a delay, to the transmitter released by stimulation of the sympathetic nerves to other parts of the body. The chemical identity of the transmitter, tantalisingly like adrenaline but not identical to it, caused confusion for many years, until in 1946 von Euler showed it to be the non-methylated derivative **noradrenaline (norepinephrine)**.

THE AUTONOMIC NERVOUS SYSTEM

The autonomic nervous system for a long time occupied centre stage in the pharmacology of chemical transmission.

BASIC ANATOMY AND PHYSIOLOGY

The autonomic nervous system (see Robertson, 2004) consists of three main anatomical divisions: *sympathetic, parasympathetic* and *enteric* nervous systems. The sympathetic and parasympathetic systems (Fig. 12.1) provide a link between the central nervous system and peripheral organs. The enteric nervous system comprises the intrinsic nerve plexuses of the gastrointestinal tract, which are closely interconnected with the sympathetic and parasympathetic systems.

The autonomic nervous system conveys all the outputs from the central nervous system to the rest of the body, except for the motor innervation of skeletal muscle. The enteric nervous system has sufficient integrative capabilities to allow it to function independently of the central nervous system, but the sympathetic and parasympathetic systems are agents of the central nervous system and cannot function without it. The autonomic nervous system is largely outside the influence of voluntary control. The main processes that it regulates, to a greater or lesser extent, are:

- contraction and relaxation of vascular and visceral smooth muscle

- all exocrine and certain endocrine secretions
- the heartbeat
- energy metabolism, particularly in liver and skeletal muscle.

A degree of autonomic control also affects many other systems, including the kidney, immune system and somatosensory system. The autonomic efferent pathway consists of two neurons arranged in series, whereas in the somatic motor system a single motor neuron connects the central nervous system to the skeletal muscle fibre (see Fig. 12.2). The two neurons in the autonomic pathway are known, respectively, as *preganglionic* and *postganglionic*. In the sympathetic nervous system, the intervening synapses lie in *autonomic* ganglia, which are outside the central nervous system, and contain the nerve endings of preganglionic fibres and the cell bodies of postganglionic neurons. In parasympathetic pathways, the postganglionic cells are mainly found in the target organs, discrete parasympathetic ganglia (e.g. the ciliary ganglion) being found only in the head and neck.

The cell bodies of the sympathetic preganglionic neurons lie in the *lateral horn* of the grey matter of the thoracic and lumbar segments of the spinal cord, and the fibres leave the spinal cord in the spinal nerves as the *thoracolumbar sympathetic outflow*. The preganglionic fibres synapse in the *paravertebral chains* of sympathetic ganglia, lying on either side of the spinal column. These ganglia contain the cell bodies of the postganglionic sympathetic

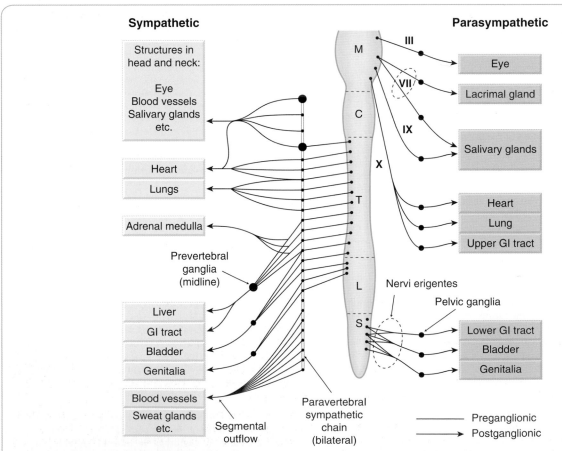

Fig. 12.1 **Basic plan of the mammalian autonomic nervous system.** C, cervical; GI, gastrointestinal; L, lumbar; M, medullary; S, sacral; T, thoracic.

neurons, the axons of which rejoin the spinal nerve. Many of the postganglionic sympathetic fibres reach their peripheral destinations via the branches of the spinal nerves. Others, destined for abdominal and pelvic viscera, have their cell bodies in a group of unpaired *prevertebral ganglia* in the abdominal cavity. The only exception to the two-neuron arrangement is the innervation of the adrenal medulla. The catecholamine-secreting cells of the adrenal medulla are, in effect, modified postganglionic sympathetic neurons, and the nerves supplying the gland are equivalent to preganglionic fibres.

The parasympathetic nerves emerge from two separate regions of the central nervous system. The *cranial outflow* consists of preganglionic fibres in certain cranial nerves, namely the *oculomotor nerve* (carrying parasympathetic fibres destined for the eye), the *facial* and *glossopharyngeal nerves* (carrying fibres to the salivary glands and the nasopharynx), and the *vagus nerve* (carrying fibres to the thoracic and abdominal viscera). The ganglia lie scattered in close relation to the target organs; the postganglionic neurons are very short compared with those of the sympathetic system. Parasympathetic fibres destined for the pelvic and abdominal viscera emerge as the *sacral outflow* from the spinal cord in a bundle of nerves known as the *nervi erigentes* (because stimulation of these nerves evokes genital erection – a fact of some importance to those responsible for artificial insemination of livestock). These fibres synapse in a group of scattered *pelvic ganglia*, whence the short postganglionic fibres run to target tissues such as the bladder, rectum and genitalia. The pelvic ganglia carry both sympathetic and parasympathetic fibres, and the two divisions are not anatomically distinct in this region.

The enteric nervous system (reviewed by Goyal & Hirano, 1996) consists of the neurons whose cell bodies lie in the intramural plexuses in the wall of the intestine. It is estimated that there are more cells in this system than in the spinal cord, and functionally they do not fit simply into the sympathetic/parasympathetic classification. Incoming nerves from both the sympathetic and the parasympathetic systems terminate on enteric neurons, as well as running directly to smooth muscle, glands and blood vessels. Some enteric neurons function as mechanoreceptors or chemoreceptors, providing local reflex pathways that can control gastrointestinal function without external inputs. The enteric nervous system is pharmacologically more complex than the sympathetic or parasympathetic systems, involving many neuropeptide and other transmitters (such as 5-hydroxytryptamine, nitric oxide and ATP; see Ch. 30).

In some places (e.g. in the visceral smooth muscle of the gut and bladder, and in the heart), the sympathetic and the parasympathetic systems produce opposite effects, but there are others where only one division of the autonomic system operates. The *sweat glands* and most *blood vessels*, for example, have only a sympathetic innervation, whereas the *ciliary muscle* of the eye has only a parasympathetic innervation. *Bronchial smooth muscle* has only a parasympathetic (constrictor) innervation (although its tone is highly sensitive to circulating adrenaline – acting probably to inhibit the constrictor innervation rather than on the smooth muscle directly). *Resistance arteries* (see Ch. 22) have a sympathetic vasoconstrictor innervation but no parasympathetic innervation; instead, the constrictor tone is opposed by a background release of nitric oxide from the endothelial cells (see Ch. 20). There are other examples, such as the *salivary glands*, where the two systems produce similar, rather than opposing, effects.

It is therefore a mistake to think of the sympathetic and parasympathetic systems simply as physiological opponents. Each serves its own physiological function and can be more or less active in a particular organ or tissue according to the need of the moment. Cannon rightly emphasised the general role of the sympathetic system in evoking 'fight or flight' reactions in an emergency, but emergencies are rare for most animals. In everyday life, the autonomic nervous system functions continuously to control specific local functions, such as adjustments to postural changes, exercise or ambient temperature (see Jänig & McLachlan, 1992). The popular concept of a continuum from the extreme 'rest and digest' state (parasympathetic active, sympathetic quiescent) to the extreme emergency fight or flight state (sympathetic active, parasympathetic quiescent) is an oversimplification, albeit one that provides the student with a generally reliable *aide memoire*.

Table 12.1 lists some of the more important autonomic responses in humans.

TRANSMITTERS IN THE AUTONOMIC NERVOUS SYSTEM

The two main neurotransmitters that operate in the autonomic system are **acetylcholine** and **noradrenaline**, whose sites of action are shown diagrammatically in Figure 12.2. This diagram also shows the type of postsynaptic receptor with which the transmitters interact at the different sites (discussed more fully in Chs 13 and 14). Some general rules apply:

- All autonomic nerve fibres leaving the central nervous system release acetylcholine, which acts on *nicotinic receptors* (although in autonomic ganglia a minor component of excitation is due to activation of *muscarinic receptors*; see Ch. 13).

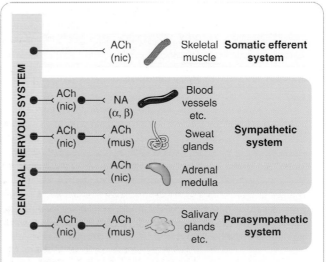

Fig. 12.2 **Acetylcholine and noradrenaline as transmitters in the peripheral nervous system.** The two main types of acetylcholine (ACh) receptor, nicotinic (nic) and muscarinic (mus) (see Ch. 13) and two types of adrenoceptor, α and β (Ch. 14), are indicated. NA, noradrenaline (norepinephrine).

Table 12.1 The main effects of the autonomic nervous system

Organ	Sympathetic effect	Adrenoceptor type[a]	Parasympathetic effect	Cholinoceptor type[a]
Heart				
Sinoatrial node	Rate ↑	β_1	Rate ↓	M_2
Atrial muscle	Force ↑	β_1	Force ↓	M_2
Atrioventricular node	Automaticity ↑	β_1	Conduction velocity ↓	M_2
			Atrioventricular block	M_2
Ventricular muscle	Automaticity ↑	β_1	No effect	M_2
	Force ↑			
Blood vessels				
ARTERIOLES				
Coronary	Constriction	α	No effect	–
Muscle	Dilatation	β_2	No effect	–
Viscera, skin, brain	Constriction	α	No effect	–
Erectile tissue	Constriction	α	Dilatation	M_3[b]
Salivary gland	Constriction	α	Dilatation	M_3[b]
VEINS	Constriction	α	No effect	–
	Dilatation	β_2	No effect	–
Viscera				
BRONCHI				
Smooth muscle	No sympathetic innervation, but dilated by circulating adrenaline (epinephrine)	β_2	Constriction	M_3
Glands	No effect	–	Secretion	M_3
GASTROINTESTINAL TRACT				
Smooth muscle	Motility ↓	$\alpha_1, \alpha_2, \beta_2$	Motility ↑	M_3
Sphincters	Constriction	$\alpha_1, \alpha_2, \beta_2$	Dilatation	M_3
Glands	No effect	–	Secretion	M_3
			Gastric acid secretion	M_1
BLADDER	Relaxation	β_2	Contraction	M_3
	Sphincter contraction	α_1	Sphincter relaxation	M_3
UTERUS				
Pregnant	Contraction	α	Variable	–
Non-pregnant	Relaxation	β_2		
MALE SEX ORGANS	Ejaculation	α	Erection	M_3[b]
Eye				
Pupil	Dilatation	α	Constriction	M_3
Ciliary muscle	Relaxation (slight)	β	Contraction	M_3
Skin				
Sweat glands	Secretion (mainly cholinergic via M_3 receptors)	–	No effect	–
Pilomotor	Piloerection	α	No effect	–
Salivary glands	Secretion	α, β	Secretion	M_3
Lacrimal glands	No effect	—	Secretion	M_3
Kidney	Renin secretion	β_1	No effect	–
Liver	Glycogenolysis	α, β_2	No effect	–
	Gluconeogenesis			
Adipose tissue[c]	Lipolysis	β_3	No effect	–
	Thermogenesis			
Pancreatic islets[c]	Insulin secretion ↓	α_2	No effect	–

[a]The adrenoceptor and cholinoceptor types shown are described more fully in Chapters 13 and 14. Transmitters other than acetylcholine and noradrenaline contribute to many of these responses (see Table 12.2).
[b]Vasodilator effects of M_3 receptors are due to nitric oxide release from endothelial cells (see Ch. 20).
[c]No direct innervation. Effect mediated by circulating adrenaline released from the adrenal medulla.

Basic anatomy and physiology of the autonomic nervous system

Anatomy

- The autonomic nervous system comprises three divisions: *sympathetic*, *parasympathetic* and *enteric*.
- The basic (two-neuron) pattern of the sympathetic and parasympathetic systems consists of a *preganglionic* neuron with a cell body in the central nervous system (CNS) and a *postganglionic* neuron with a cell body in an autonomic ganglion.
- The parasympathetic system is connected to the CNS via:
  – cranial nerve outflow (III, VII, IX, X)
  – sacral outflow.
- Parasympathetic ganglia usually lie close to or within the target organ.
- Sympathetic outflow leaves the CNS in thoracic and lumbar spinal roots. Sympathetic ganglia form two paravertebral chains, plus some midline ganglia.
- The enteric nervous system consists of neurons lying in the intramural plexuses of the gastrointestinal tract. It receives inputs from sympathetic and parasympathetic systems, but can act on its own to control the motor and secretory functions of the intestine.

Physiology

- The autonomic system controls smooth muscle (visceral and vascular), exocrine (and some endocrine) secretions, rate and force of contraction of the heart, and certain metabolic processes (e.g. glucose utilisation).
- Sympathetic and parasympathetic systems have opposing actions in some situations (e.g. control of heart rate, gastrointestinal smooth muscle), but not in others (e.g. salivary glands, ciliary muscle).
- Sympathetic activity increases in stress ('fight or flight' response), whereas parasympathetic activity predominates during satiation and repose. Both systems exert a continuous physiological control of specific organs under normal conditions, when the body is at neither extreme.

- All postganglionic parasympathetic fibres release acetylcholine, which acts on muscarinic receptors.
- All postganglionic sympathetic fibres (with one important exception) release noradrenaline, which may act on either *α* or *β adrenoceptors* (see Ch. 14). The exception is the sympathetic innervation of sweat glands, where transmission is due to acetylcholine acting on muscarinic receptors. In some species, but not humans, vasodilatation in skeletal muscle is produced by cholinergic sympathetic nerve fibres.

Acetylcholine and noradrenaline are the grandees among autonomic transmitters, and are central to understanding autonomic pharmacology. However, many other chemical mediators are also released by autonomic neurons (see p. 149-151), and their functional significance is gradually becoming clearer.

SOME GENERAL PRINCIPLES OF CHEMICAL TRANSMISSION

The essential processes in chemical transmission – the release of mediators, and their interaction with receptors on target cells – are described in Chapters 4 and 3, respectively. Here we consider some general characteristics of chemical transmission of particular relevance to pharmacology. Many of these principles apply also to the central nervous system and are taken up again in Chapter 37.

DALE'S PRINCIPLE

▼ Dale's principle, advanced in 1934, states, in its modern form: 'A mature neuron releases the same transmitter (or transmitters) at all of its synapses.' Dale considered it unlikely that a single neuron could store and release different transmitters at different nerve terminals, and his view was supported by physiological and neurochemical evidence. It is now known, however, that there are situations where different transmitters are released from different terminals of the same neuron. Further, most neurons release more

Transmitters of the autonomic nervous system

- The principal transmitters are **acetylcholine** (ACh) and **noradrenaline**.
- Preganglionic neurons are cholinergic, and ganglionic transmission occurs via nicotinic ACh receptors (although excitatory muscarinic ACh receptors are also present on postganglionic cells).
- Postganglionic parasympathetic neurons are cholinergic, acting on muscarinic receptors in target organs.
- Postganglionic sympathetic neurons are mainly noradrenergic, although a few are cholinergic (e.g. sweat glands).
- Transmitters other than noradrenaline and acetylcholine (NANC transmitters) are also abundant in the autonomic nervous system. The main ones are nitric oxide and vasoactive intestinal peptide (parasympathetic), ATP and neuropeptide Y (sympathetic). Others, such as 5-hydroxytryptamine, GABA and dopamine, also play a role.
- Co-transmission is a general phenomenon.

---

than one transmitter (see co-transmission, p. 149) and may change their transmitter repertoire, for example during development or in response to injury. Moreover (see Fig. 4.12), the balance of the cocktail of mediators released by a nerve terminal can vary with stimulus conditions, and in response to presynaptic modulators. Dale's principle was, of course, framed long before these complexities were discovered, and it has probably now outlived its usefulness, although purists seem curiously reluctant to let it go.

DENERVATION SUPERSENSITIVITY

It is known, mainly from the work of Cannon on the sympathetic system, that if a nerve is cut and its terminals allowed to degenerate, the structure supplied by it becomes supersensitive to the transmitter substance released by the terminals. Thus skeletal muscle, which normally responds to injected acetylcholine only if a large dose is given directly into the arterial blood supply, will, after denervation, respond by contracture to much smaller amounts. Other organs, such as salivary glands and blood vessels, show similar supersensitivity to acetylcholine and noradrenaline when the postganglionic nerves degenerate, and there is evidence that pathways in the central nervous system show the same phenomenon.

▼ Several mechanisms contribute to denervation supersensitivity, and the extent and mechanism of the phenomenon varies from organ to organ. Reported mechanisms include the following (see Luis & Noel, 2009).

- *Proliferation of receptors.* This is particularly marked in skeletal muscle, in which the number of acetylcholine receptors increases 20-fold or more after denervation; the receptors, normally localised to the endplate region of the fibres (Ch. 13), spread over the whole surface. Elsewhere, increases in receptor number are much smaller, or absent altogether.
- *Loss of mechanisms for transmitter removal.* At noradrenergic synapses, the loss of neuronal uptake of noradrenaline (see Ch. 14) contributes substantially to denervation supersensitivity. At cholinergic synapses, a partial loss of cholinesterase occurs (see Ch. 13).
- *Increased postjunctional responsiveness.* Smooth muscle cells become partly depolarised and hyperexcitable after denervation (due in part to reduced Na^+-K^+-ATPase activity; see Ch. 4) and this phenomenon contributes appreciably to their supersensitivity. Increased Ca^{2+} signalling, resulting in enhanced excitation–contraction coupling, may also occur.

Supersensitivity can occur, but is less marked, when transmission is interrupted by processes other than nerve section. Pharmacological block of ganglionic transmission, for example, if sustained for a few days, causes some degree of supersensitivity of the target organs, and long-term blockade of postsynaptic receptors also causes receptors to proliferate, leaving the cell supersensitive when the blocking agent is removed. Phenomena such as this are of importance in the central nervous system, where such supersensitivity can cause 'rebound' effects when drugs that impair synaptic transmission are given for some time and then discontinued.

PRESYNAPTIC MODULATION

The presynaptic terminals that synthesise and release transmitter in response to electrical activity in the nerve fibre are often themselves sensitive to transmitter substances and to other substances that may be produced locally in tissues (for review see Boehm & Kubista, 2002). Such presynaptic effects most commonly act to inhibit transmitter release, but may enhance it. Figure 12.3A shows the inhibitory effect of adrenaline on the release of acetylcholine (evoked by electrical stimulation) from the postganglionic parasympathetic nerve terminals of the intestine. The release of noradrenaline from nearby sympathetic nerve terminals can also inhibit release of acetylcholine. Noradrenergic and cholinergic nerve terminals often lie close together in the myenteric plexus, so the opposing effects of the sympathetic and parasympathetic systems result not only from the opposite effects of the two transmitters on the smooth muscle cells, but also from the inhibition of acetylcholine release by noradrenaline acting on the parasympathetic nerve terminals. A similar situation of mutual presynaptic inhibition exists in the heart, where noradrenaline inhibits acetylcholine release, as in the myenteric plexus, and acetylcholine also inhibits noradrenaline release. These are examples of *heterotropic interactions*, where one neurotransmitter affects the release of another. *Homotropic interactions* also occur, where the transmitter, by

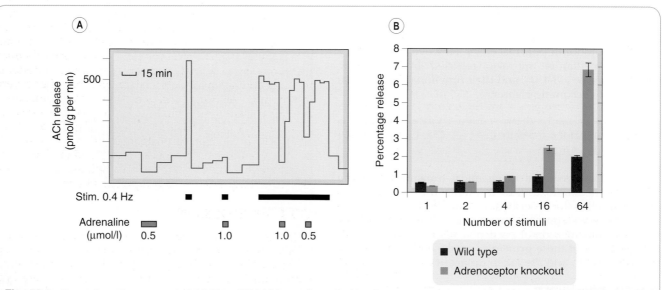

Fig. 12.3 **Examples of presynaptic inhibition.** [A] Inhibitory effect of adrenaline on acetylcholine (ACh) release from postganglionic parasympathetic nerves in the guinea pig ileum. The intramural nerves were stimulated electrically where indicated, and the ACh released into the bathing fluid determined by bioassay. Adrenaline strongly inhibits ACh release. [B] Noradrenaline release from mouse hippocampal slices in response to trains of electrical stimuli. Blue bars show normal (wild type) mice. Red bars show α_2-adrenoceptor knockout mice. The lack of presynaptic autoinhibition in the knockout mice results in a large increase in release with a long stimulus train, but does not affect release by fewer than four stimuli, because the autoinhibition takes a few seconds to develop. This example is taken from a study of brain noradrenergic nerves, but similar findings have been made on sympathetic nerves. (Panel [A] from Vizi ES 1979 Prog Neurobiol 12, 181; panel [B] redrawn from Trendelenburg et al. 2001 Naunyn Schmiedeberg's Arch Pharmacol 364, 117–130.)

binding to presynaptic autoreceptors, affects the nerve terminals from which it is being released. This type of *autoinhibitory feedback* acts powerfully at noradrenergic nerve terminals (see Starke et al., 1989). Figure 12.3B shows that in normal mice, noradrenaline release increases only slightly as the number of stimulus trains increases from 1 to 64. In transgenic mice lacking a specific type of presynaptic α_2 adrenoceptor (see Ch. 14), the amount released by the longer stimulus train is greatly increased, though the amount released by a single stimulus is unaffected. This is because with one or a few stimuli, there is no opportunity for autoinhibitory feedback to develop, whereas with longer trains the inhibition operates powerfully. A similar autoinhibitory feedback occurs with many transmitters, including acetylcholine and 5-hydroxytryptamine.

In both the noradrenergic and cholinergic systems, the presynaptic autoreceptors are pharmacologically distinct from the postsynaptic receptors (see Fig. 12.4 and Chs 13 and 14), and there are drugs that act selectively, as agonists or antagonists, on the pre- or postsynaptic receptors.

Cholinergic and noradrenergic nerve terminals respond not only to acetylcholine and noradrenaline, as described above, but also to other substances that are released as co-transmitters, such as ATP and neuropeptide Y (NPY), or derived from other sources, including nitric oxide, prostaglandins, adenosine, dopamine, 5-hydroxytryptamine, GABA, opioid peptides, endocannabinoids and many other substances. The physiological role and pharmacological significance of these various interactions is still unclear (see review by Vizi, 2001), but the description of the autonomic nervous system represented in Figure 12.2 is undoubtedly oversimplified. Figure 12.4 shows some of the main presynaptic interactions between autonomic neurons, and summarises the many chemical influences that regulate transmitter release from noradrenergic neurons.

Presynaptic receptors regulate transmitter release mainly by affecting Ca^{2+} entry into the nerve terminal (see Ch. 4), but also by other mechanisms (see Kubista & Boehm, 2006). Most presynaptic receptors are of the G protein-coupled type (see Ch. 3), which control the function of calcium channels and potassium channels either through second messengers that regulate the state of phosphorylation of the channel proteins, or by a direct interaction of G proteins with the channels. Transmitter release is inhibited when calcium channel opening is inhibited, or when potassium channel opening is increased (see Ch. 4); in many cases, both mechanisms operate simultaneously. Presynaptic regulation by receptors linked directly to ion channels (ionotropic receptors; see Ch. 3) rather than to G proteins also occurs (see Kubista & Boehm, 2006). Nicotinic acetylcholine receptors (nAChRs) are particularly important in this respect. They can either facilitate or inhibit the release of other transmitters, such as glutamate (see Ch. 38), and most of the nAChRs expressed in the central nervous system are located presynaptically. Another example is the $GABA_A$ receptor, whose action is to inhibit transmitter release (see Chs 4 and 37). Other ionotropic receptors, such as those activated by ATP and 5-hydroxytryptamine (Chs 15, 16 and 38), may have similar effects on transmitter release.

POSTSYNAPTIC MODULATION

Chemical mediators often act on postsynaptic structures, including neurons, smooth muscle cells, cardiac muscle

cells, etc., in such a way that their excitability or spontaneous firing pattern is altered. In many cases, as with presynaptic modulation, this is caused by changes in calcium and/or potassium channel function mediated by a second messenger. We give only a few examples here.

- The slow excitatory effect produced by various mediators, including acetylcholine and peptides such as **substance P** (see Ch. 17), results mainly from a decrease in K^+ permeability. Conversely, the inhibitory effect of various opioids in the gut is mainly due to increased K^+ permeability.
- **Neuropeptide Y** (**NPY**), which is released as a co-transmitter with noradrenaline at many sympathetic nerve endings and acts on smooth muscle cells to enhance the vasoconstrictor effect of noradrenaline, thus greatly facilitating transmission.

The pre- and postsynaptic effects described above are often described as *neuromodulation*, because the mediator acts to increase or decrease the efficacy of synaptic transmission without participating directly as a transmitter. Many neuropeptides, for example, affect membrane ion channels in such a way as to increase or decrease excitability and thus control the firing pattern of the cell. Neuromodulation[1] is loosely defined but, in general, involves slower processes (taking seconds to days) than neurotransmission (which occurs in milliseconds), and operates through cascades of intracellular messengers (Ch. 3) rather than directly on ligand-gated ion channels.

TRANSMITTERS OTHER THAN ACETYLCHOLINE AND NORADRENALINE

As mentioned above, acetylcholine or noradrenaline are not the only autonomic transmitters. The rather grudging realisation that this was so dawned many years ago when it was noticed that autonomic transmission in many organs could not be completely blocked by drugs that abolish responses to these transmitters. The dismal but tenacious term *non-adrenergic non-cholinergic* (NANC) transmission was coined. Later, fluorescence and immunocytochemical methods showed that neurons, including autonomic neurons, contain many potential transmitters, often several in the same cell. Compounds now known to function as NANC transmitters include ATP, vasoactive intestinal peptide (VIP), NPY and nitric oxide (see Fig. 12.5 and Table 12.2), which function at postganglionic nerve terminals, as well as substance P, 5-hydroxytryptamine, GABA and dopamine, which play a role in ganglionic transmission (see Lundberg, 1996, for a comprehensive review).

CO-TRANSMISSION

It is the rule rather than the exception that neurons release more than one transmitter or modulator (see Kupfermann, 1991; Lundberg, 1996), each of which interacts with specific receptors and produces effects, often both pre- and postsynaptically. The example of noradrenaline/ATP co-transmission at sympathetic nerve endings is shown in Figure 12.5, and the best-studied examples and

---

[1]Confusingly, the same term has been used to embrace a range of experimental therapeutic approaches based on nerve stimulation techniques, which have been claimed to be effective in a variety of neurological disorders such as bladder dysfunction, epilepsy and depression.

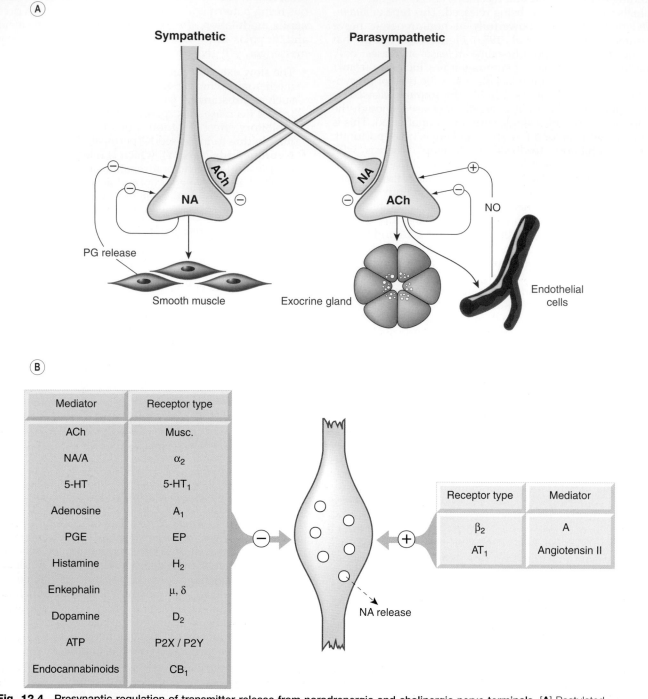

Fig. 12.4 **Presynaptic regulation of transmitter release from noradrenergic and cholinergic nerve terminals. [A]** Postulated homotropic and heterotropic interactions between sympathetic and parasympathetic nerves. **[B]** Some of the known inhibitory and facilitatory influences on noradrenaline release from sympathetic nerve endings. 5-HT, 5-hydroxytryptamine; A, adrenaline; ACh, acetylcholine; NA, noradrenaline; NO, nitric oxide; PG, prostaglandin; PGE, prostaglandin E.

mechanisms are summarised in Table 12.2 and Figures 12.6 and 12.7.

What, one might well ask, could be the functional advantage of co-transmission, compared with a single transmitter acting on various different receptors? The possible advantages include the following.

• One constituent of the cocktail (e.g. a peptide) may be removed or inactivated more slowly than the other

(e.g. a monoamine), and therefore reach targets further from the site of release and produce longer-lasting effects. This appears to be the case, for example, with acetylcholine and gonadotrophin-releasing hormone in sympathetic ganglia (Jan & Jan, 1983).

• The balance of the transmitters released may vary under different conditions. At sympathetic nerve terminals, for example, where noradrenaline and NPY are stored in separate vesicles, NPY is

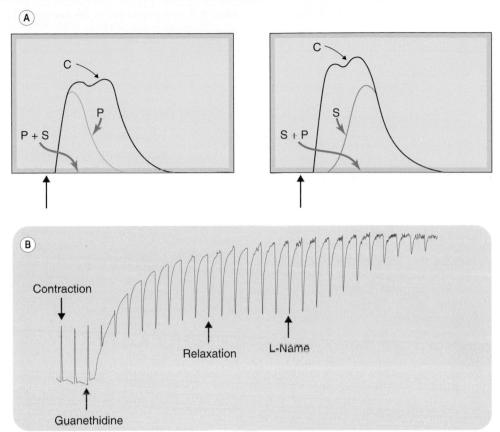

Fig. 12.5 ATP and nitric oxide as neurotransmitters. [A] Noradrenaline and ATP are co-transmitters released from the same nerves in the guinea pig vas deferens. Contractions of the tissue are shown in response to a single electrical stimulus causing excitation of sympathetic nerve endings. With no blocking drugs present, a twin-peaked response is produced (C). The early peak is selectively abolished by the ATP antagonist suramin (S), while the late peak is blocked by the α1-adrenoceptor antagonist prazosin (P). The response is completely eliminated when both drugs are present. **[B]** Noradrenaline and nitric oxide are neurotransmitters in the rat anococcygeus muscle but are probably released from different nerves. The nerves innervating the muscle were stimulated with brief trains of pulses. Initially nerve stimulation evoked rapid contractions by releasing noradrenaline. Application of guanethidine blocked stimulus-evoked noradrenaline release and raised the tone of the preparation revealing nerve-evoked relaxations that were blocked by L-NAME an inhibitor of nitric oxide synthesis. *(Panel [A] reproduced with permission from von Kugelgen I, Starke K 1991 Trends Pharmacol Sci 12, 319–324; data in panel [B] are from a student practical class at Glasgow Caledonian University, courtesy of A Corbett.)*

preferentially released at high stimulation frequencies, so that differential release of one or other mediator may result from varying impulse patterns. Differential effects of presynaptic modulators are also possible; for example, activation of β adrenoceptors inhibits ATP release while enhancing noradrenaline release from sympathetic nerve terminals (Gonçalves et al., 1996).

TERMINATION OF TRANSMITTER ACTION

Chemically transmitting synapses other than the peptidergic variety (Ch. 17) invariably incorporate a mechanism for disposing rapidly of the released transmitter, so that its action remains brief and localised. At cholinergic synapses (Ch. 13), the released acetylcholine is inactivated very rapidly in the synaptic cleft by *acetylcholinesterase*. In most other cases (see Fig. 12.8), transmitter action is terminated by active reuptake into the presynaptic nerve, or into supporting cells such as glia. Such reuptake depends on transporter proteins (see Ch. 4), each being specific for a particular transmitter. The major class

(Na^+/Cl^- co-transporters), whose molecular structure and function are well understood (see Nelson, 1998; Torres et al., 2003; Gether et al., 2006), consists of a family of membrane proteins, each possessing 12 transmembrane helices. Different members of the family show selectivity for each of the main monoamine transmitters (e.g. the noradrenaline [norepinephrine] transporter, NET, the serotonin transporter, SERT, which transports 5-hydroxytryptamine and the dopamine transporter, DAT). These transporters are important targets for psychoactive drugs, particularly antidepressants (Ch. 47), anxiolytic drugs (Ch. 44) and stimulants (Ch. 48). Transporters for glycine and GABA belong to the same family.

Vesicular transporters (Ch. 4), which load synaptic vesicles with transmitter molecules, are closely related to the membrane transporters. Membrane transporters usually act as co-transporters of Na^+, Cl^- and transmitter molecules, and it is the inwardly directed 'downhill' gradient for Na^+ that provides the energy for the inward 'uphill' movement of the transmitter. The simultaneous transport of ions along with the transmitter means that the process generates a net current across the membrane, which can

Table 12.2 Examples of non-adrenergic non-cholinergic transmitters and co-transmitters in the peripheral nervous system

Transmitter	Location	Function
Non-peptides		
ATP	Postganglionic sympathetic neurons	Fast depolarisation/contraction of smooth muscle cells (e.g. blood vessels, vas deferens)
GABA, 5-HT	Enteric neurons	Peristaltic reflex
Dopamine	Some sympathetic neurons (e.g. kidney)	Vasodilatation
Nitric oxide	Pelvic nerves Gastric nerves	Erection Gastric emptying
Peptides		
Neuropeptide Y	Postganglionic sympathetic neurons	Facilitates constrictor action of noradrenaline; inhibits noradrenaline release (e.g. blood vessels)
Vasoactive intestinal peptide (VIP)	Parasympathetic nerves to salivary glands NANC innervation of airways smooth muscle	Vasodilatation; co-transmitter with acetylcholine Bronchodilatation
Gonadotrophin-releasing hormone	Sympathetic ganglia	Slow depolarisation; co-transmitter with acetylcholine
Substance P	Sympathetic ganglia, enteric neurons	Slow depolarisation; co-transmitter with acetylcholine
Calcitonin gene-related peptide	Non-myelinated sensory neurons	Vasodilatation; vascular leakage; neurogenic inflammation

5-HT, 5-hydroxytryptamine; ATP, adenosine triphosphate; GABA, gamma-aminobutyric acid; NANC, non-adrenergic non-cholinergic.

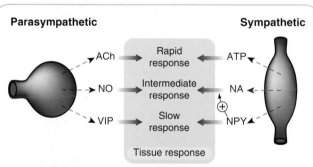

Fig. 12.6 The main co-transmitters at postganglionic parasympathetic and sympathetic neurons. The different mediators generally give rise to fast, intermediate and slow responses of the target organ. ACh, acetylcholine; ATP, adenosine triphosphate; NA, noradrenaline; NO, nitric oxide; NPY, neuropeptide Y; VIP, vasoactive intestinal peptide.

Neuromodulation and presynaptic interactions

- As well as functioning directly as neurotransmitters, chemical mediators may regulate:
  - presynaptic transmitter release
  - neuronal excitability.
- Both are examples of *neuromodulation* and generally involve second messenger regulation of membrane ion channels.
- Presynaptic receptors may inhibit or increase transmitter release, the former being more important.
- Inhibitory *presynaptic autoreceptors* occur on noradrenergic and cholinergic neurons, causing each transmitter to inhibit its own release (*autoinhibitory feedback*).
- Many endogenous mediators (e.g. GABA, prostaglandins, opioid and other peptides), as well as the transmitters themselves, exert presynaptic control (mainly inhibitory) over autonomic transmitter release.

be measured directly and used to monitor the transport process. Very similar mechanisms are responsible for other physiological transport processes, such as glucose uptake (Ch. 31) and renal tubular transport of amino acids. Because it is the electrochemical gradient for sodium that drives the inward transport of transmitter molecules, a reduction of this gradient can reduce or even reverse the flow of transmitter. This is probably not important under normal conditions, but when the nerve terminals are depolarised or abnormally loaded with sodium (e.g. in ischaemic conditions), the resulting non-vesicular release of transmitter (and inhibition of the normal synaptic reuptake mechanism) may play a significant role in the effects of ischaemia on tissues such as heart and brain (see Chs 21 and 40). Studies with transgenic 'knockout' mice

(see Torres et al., 2003) show that the store of releasable transmitter is substantially depleted in animals lacking the membrane transporter, showing that synthesis is unable to maintain the store if the recapture mechanism is disabled. As with receptors (see Ch. 3), many genetic polymorphisms of transporter genes occur in humans, which raised hopes of finding associations with various neurological, cardiovascular and psychiatric disorders. But despite intensive research efforts, the links remain elusive (see Lin & Madras, 2006).

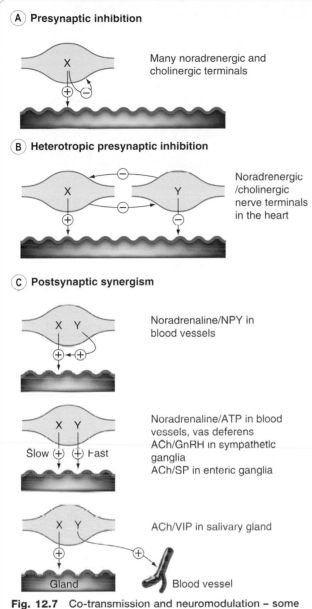

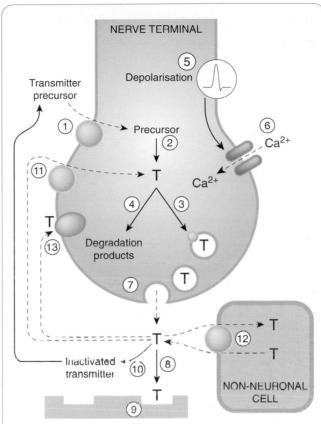

Fig. 12.7 Co-transmission and neuromodulation – some examples. [**A**] Presynaptic inhibition. [**B**] Heterotropic presynaptic inhibition. [**C**] Postsynaptic synergism. ACh, acetylcholine; ATP, adenosine triphosphate; GnRH, gonadotrophin-releasing hormone (luteinising hormone-releasing hormone); NPY, neuropeptide Y; SP, substance P; VIP, vasoactive intestinal peptide.

Fig. 12.8 The main processes involved in synthesis, storage and release of amine and amino acid transmitters. 1, Uptake of precursors; 2, synthesis of transmitter; 3, uptake/ transport of transmitter into vesicles; 4, degradation of surplus transmitter; 5, depolarisation by propagated action potential; 6, influx of Ca^{2+} in response to depolarisation; 7, release of transmitter by exocytosis; 8, diffusion to postsynaptic membrane; 9, interaction with postsynaptic receptors; 10, inactivation of transmitter; 11, reuptake of transmitter or degradation products by nerve terminals; 12, uptake and release of transmitter by non-neuronal cells; and 13, interaction with presynaptic receptors. The transporters (11 and 12) can release transmitter under certain conditions by working in reverse. These processes are well characterised for many transmitters (e.g. acetylcholine, monoamines, amino acids, ATP). Peptide mediators (see Ch. 17) differ in that they may be synthesised and packaged in the cell body rather than the terminals.

As we shall see in subsequent chapters, both membrane and vesicular transporters are targets for various drug effects, and defining the physiological role and pharmacological properties of these molecules is the focus of much current research.

BASIC STEPS IN NEUROCHEMICAL TRANSMISSION: SITES OF DRUG ACTION

Figure 12.8 summarises the main processes that occur in a classical chemically transmitting synapse, and provides a useful basis for understanding the actions of the many different classes of drug, discussed in later chapters, that act by facilitating or blocking neurochemical transmission.

All the steps shown in Figure 12.8 (except for transmitter diffusion, step 8) can be influenced by drugs. For example, the enzymes involved in synthesis or inactivation of the transmitter can be inhibited, as can the transport systems responsible for the neuronal and vesicular uptake of the transmitter or its precursor. The actions of the great majority of drugs that act on the peripheral nervous system (Chs 13 and 14) and the central nervous system fit into this general scheme.

REFERENCES AND FURTHER READING

General references

Bacq, Z.M., 1975. Chemical Transmission of Nerve Impulses: A Historical Sketch. Pergamon Press, Oxford. (*Lively account of the history of the discovery of chemical transmission*)

Burnstock, G., 2009. Autonomic neurotransmission: 60 years since Sir Henry Dale. Ann. Rev. Pharmacol. 49, 1–30. (*Elegant and well-illustrated account of many of the topics discussed in this chapter. Recommended*)

Goyal, R.K., Hirano, I., 1996. The enteric nervous system. N. Engl. J. Med. 334, 1106–1115. (*Excellent review article*)

Iversen, L.L., Iversen, S.D., Bloom, F.E., Roth, R.H., 2009. Introduction to Neuropsychopharmacology. Oxford University Press, New York. (*Excellent general account covering many aspects of neuropharmacology*)

Jänig, W., McLachlan, E.M., 1992. Characteristics of function-specific pathways in the sympathetic nervous system. Trends Neurosci. 15, 475–481. (*Short article emphasising that the sympathetic system is far from being an all-or-none alarm system*)

Luis, E.M.Q., Noel, F., 2009. Mechanisms of adaptive supersensitivity in vas deferens. Auton. Neurosci. 146, 38–46. (*Summarises mechanisms contributing to denervation supersensitivity in a typical organ supplied by the sympathetic nervous system*)

Robertson, D.W. (Ed.), 2004. Primer on the Autonomic Nervous System. Academic Press, New York. (*An excellent comprehensive textbook on all aspects, including pharmacology, of the autonomic nervous system. By no means elementary despite its title*)

Valenstein, E.S., 2005. The War of the Soups and the Sparks. Columbia University Press, New York. (*Readable and informative account of origins of the theory of chemical transmission*)

Presynaptic modulation

Boehm, S., Kubista, H., 2002. Fine tuning of sympathetic transmitter release via ionotropic and metabotropic receptors. Pharm. Rev. 54, 43–99. (*Comprehensive review of presynaptic modulation, focusing on sympathetic neurons though mechanisms are widespread*)

Gonçalves, J., Bueltmann, R., Driessen, B., 1996. Opposite modulation of cotransmitter release in guinea-pig vas deferens: increase of noradrenaline and decrease of ATP release by activation of prejunctional β-receptors. Naunyn-Schmiedeberg's Arch. Pharmacol 353, 184–192. (*Shows that presynaptic regulation can affect specific transmitters in different ways*)

Kubista, H., Boehm, S., 2006. Molecular mechanisms underlying the modulation of exocytotic noradrenaline release via presynaptic receptors. Pharm. Ther. 112, 213–242. (*Describes the wide variety of mechanisms by which presynaptic receptors affect transmitter release*)

Starke, K., Gothert, M., Kilbinger, H., 1989. Modulation of neurotransmitter release by presynaptic autoreceptors. Physiol. Rev. 69, 864–989. (*Comprehensive review article*)

Co-transmission

Jan, Y.N., Jan, L.Y., 1983. A LHRH-like peptidergic neurotransmitter capable of 'action at a distance' in autonomic ganglia. Trends Neurosci. 6, 320–325. (*Electrophysiological analysis of co-transmission*)

Kupfermann, I., 1991. Functional studies of cotransmission. Physiol. Rev. 71, 683–732. (*Good review article*)

Lundberg, J.M., 1996. Pharmacology of co-transmission in the autonomic nervous system: integrative aspects on amines, neuropeptides, adenosine triphosphate, amino acids and nitric oxide. Pharmacol. Rev. 48, 114–192. (*Detailed and informative review article*)

Transporters

Gether, U., Andersen, P.H., Larsson, O.M., et al., 2006. Neurotransmitter transporters: molecular function of important drug targets. Trends Pharmacol. Sci. 27, 375–383. (*Useful short review article*)

Lin, Z., Madras, B.K., 2006. Human genetics and pharmacology of monoamine transporters. In: Sitte, H.H., Freissmuth, M. (Eds.), Neurotransmitter transporters. Handb. Exp. Pharmacol. 175, 327–371. (*Summarises evidence of linkage between transporter polymorphisms and human disease – complex and unclear so far*)

Nelson, N., 1998. The family of Na^+/Cl^- neurotransmitter transporters. J. Neurochem. 71, 1785–1803. (*Review article describing the molecular characteristics of the different families of neurotransporters*)

Torres, G.E., Gainetdinov, R.R., Caron, M.G., 2003. Plasma membrane monoamine transporters: structure, regulation and function. Nat. Rev. Neurosci. 4, 13–25. (*Describes molecular, physiological and pharmacological aspects of transporters*)

Vizi, E.S., 2001. Role of high-affinity receptors and membrane transporters in non-synaptic communication and drug action in the central nervous system. Pharmacol. Rev. 52, 63–89. (*Comprehensive review on pharmacological relevance of presynaptic receptors and transporters; useful for reference*)

Cholinergic transmission

OVERVIEW

This chapter is concerned mainly with cholinergic transmission in the periphery, and the ways in which drugs affect it. Here we describe the different types of acetylcholine (ACh) receptors and their functions, as well as the synthesis and release of ACh. Drugs that act on ACh receptors, many of which have clinical uses, are described in this chapter. Cholinergic mechanisms in the central nervous system (CNS) and their relevance to dementia are discussed in Chapters 39 and 40.

MUSCARINIC AND NICOTINIC ACTIONS OF ACETYLCHOLINE

▼ The discovery of the pharmacological action of ACh came, paradoxically, from work on adrenal glands, extracts of which were known to produce a rise in blood pressure owing to their content of adrenaline (epinephrine) In 1900, Reid Hunt found that after adrenaline had been removed from such extracts, they produced a fall in blood pressure instead of a rise. He attributed the fall to the presence of choline, but later concluded that a more potent derivative of choline must be responsible. With Taveau, he tested a number of choline derivatives and discovered that ACh was some 100 000 times more active than choline in lowering the rabbit's blood pressure. The physiological role of ACh was not apparent at that time, and it remained a pharmacological curiosity until Loewi and Dale and their colleagues discovered its transmitter role in the 1930s.

Analysing the pharmacological actions of ACh in 1914, Dale distinguished two types of activity, which he designated as *muscarinic* and *nicotinic* because they mimicked, respectively, the effects of injecting **muscarine**, the active principle of the poisonous mushroom *Amanita muscaria*, and of injecting **nicotine**. Muscarinic actions closely resemble the effects of parasympathetic stimulation, as shown in Table 12.1. After the muscarinic effects have been blocked by **atropine**, larger doses of ACh produce nicotine-like effects, which include:

- stimulation of all autonomic ganglia
- stimulation of voluntary muscle
- secretion of adrenaline from the adrenal medulla.

The muscarinic and nicotinic actions of ACh are demonstrated in Figure 13.1. Small and medium doses of ACh produce a transient fall in blood pressure due to arteriolar vasodilatation and slowing of the heart – muscarinic effects that are abolished by atropine. A large dose of ACh given after atropine produces nicotinic effects: an initial rise in blood pressure due to a stimulation of sympathetic ganglia and consequent vasoconstriction, and a secondary rise resulting from secretion of adrenaline.

Dale's pharmacological classification corresponds closely to the main physiological functions of ACh in the body. The muscarinic actions correspond to those of ACh released at postganglionic parasympathetic nerve endings, with two significant exceptions:

1. Acetylcholine causes generalised vasodilatation, even though most blood vessels have no parasympathetic innervation. This is an indirect effect: ACh (like many other mediators) acts on vascular endothelial cells to release **nitric oxide** (see Ch. 20), which relaxes smooth muscle. The physiological function of this is uncertain, because ACh is not normally present in circulating blood.
2. Acetylcholine evokes secretion from sweat glands, which are innervated by cholinergic fibres of the sympathetic nervous system (see Table 12.1).

The nicotinic actions correspond to those of ACh acting on autonomic ganglia of the sympathetic and parasympathetic systems, the motor endplate of voluntary muscle and the secretory cells of the adrenal medulla.

ACETYLCHOLINE RECEPTORS

Although Dale himself dismissed the concept of receptors as sophistry rather than science, his functional classification provided the basis for distinguishing the two major classes of ACh receptor (see Ch. 3).

NICOTINIC RECEPTORS

Nicotinic ACh receptors (nAChRs) fall into three main classes – the muscle, ganglionic and CNS types – whose subunit compositions are summarised in Table 13.1. Muscle receptors are confined to the skeletal neuromuscular junction; ganglionic receptors are responsible for transmission at sympathetic and parasympathetic ganglia; and CNS-type receptors are widespread in the brain, and are heterogeneous with respect to their molecular composition and location (see Ch. 39). Most of the CNS-type nAChRs are located presynaptically and serve to facilitate or inhibit the release of other mediators, such as glutamate and dopamine.

▼ All nAChRs are pentameric structures that function as ligand-gated ion channels (see Ch. 3). The five subunits that form the receptor–channel complex are similar in structure, and so far 17 different members of the family have been identified and cloned, designated α (10 types), β (four types), γ, δ and ε (one of each). The five subunits each possess four membrane-spanning helical domains, and one of these helices (M_2) from each subunit defines the central pore (see Ch. 3). nAChR subtypes generally contain both α and β subunits, the exception being the homomeric $(\alpha7)_5$ subtype found mainly in the brain (Ch. 39). The adult muscle receptor has the composition $(\alpha1)_2/\beta1\epsilon\delta$, while the main ganglionic subtype is $(\alpha3)_2(\beta2)_3$. The two binding sites for ACh (both of which need to be occupied to cause the channel to open) reside at the interface between the extracellular domain of each of the α subunits and its neighbour. The diversity of the nAChR family (for details see Kalamida et al., 2007), which emerged from cloning studies in the

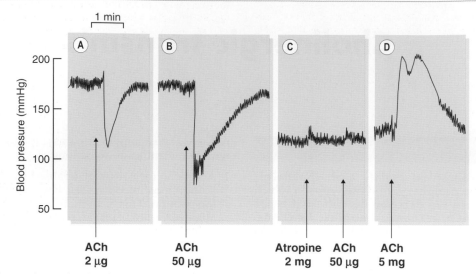

Fig. 13.1 Dale's experiment showing that acetylcholine (ACh) produces two kinds of effect on the cat's blood pressure. Arterial pressure was recorded with a mercury manometer from a spinal cat. **[A]** ACh causes a fall in blood pressure due to vasodilatation. **[B]** A larger dose also produces bradycardia. Both **[A]** and **[B]** are muscarinic effects. **[C]** After atropine (muscarinic antagonist), the same dose of ACh has no effect. **[D]** Still under the influence of atropine, a much larger dose of ACh causes a rise in blood pressure (due to stimulation of sympathetic ganglia), accompanied by tachycardia, followed by a secondary rise (due to release of adrenaline from the adrenal gland). These effects result from its action on nicotinic receptors. *(From Burn JH 1963 Autonomic Pharmacology. Blackwell, Oxford.)*

Table 13.1 Nicotinic receptor subtypes[a]

	Muscle type	Ganglion type	CNS types		Notes
Main molecular form	$(\alpha 1)_2 \beta 1 \delta \varepsilon$ (adult form)	$(\alpha 3)_2 (\beta 2)_3$	$(\alpha 4)_2 (\beta 2)_3$	$(\alpha 7)_5$	–
Main synaptic location	Skeletal neuromuscular junction: mainly postsynaptic	Autonomic ganglia: mainly postsynaptic	Many brain regions: pre- and postsynaptic	Many brain regions: pre- and postsynaptic	–
Membrane response	Excitatory Increased cation permeability (mainly Na^+, K^+)	Excitatory Increased cation permeability (mainly Na^+, K^+)	Pre- and postsynaptic excitation Increased cation permeability (mainly Na^+, K^+)	Pre- and postsynaptic excitation Increased cation permeability	$(\alpha 7)_5$ receptor produces large Ca^{2+} entry, evoking transmitter release
Agonists	Acetylcholine Carbachol Succinylcholine	Acetylcholine Carbachol Nicotine Epibatidine Dimethylphenyl-piperazinium	Nicotine Epibatidine Acetylcholine Cytosine Varenicline[b]	Epibatidine Dimethylphenyl-piperazinium Varenicline[b]	$(\alpha 4)_2 (\beta 2)_3$ is main brain 'nicotine receptor'. See Ch. 39
Antagonists	Tubocurarine Pancuronium Atracurium Vecuronium α-Bungarotoxin α-Conotoxin	Mecamylamine Trimetaphan Hexamethonium α-Conotoxin	Mecamylamine Methylaconitine	α-Bungarotoxin α-Conotoxin Methylaconitine	

[a]This table shows only the main subtypes expressed in mammalian tissues. Several other subtypes are expressed in selected brain regions, and also in the peripheral nervous system and in non-neuronal tissues. For further details, see Ch. 39 and review by Kalamida et al. (2007).
[b]Varenicline is a recently introduced drug for smoking cessation. It acts as a partial agonist on $(\alpha 4)_2 (\beta 2)_3$ receptors and a full agonist on $(\alpha 7)_5$ receptors (see Ch. 49).

1980s, took pharmacologists somewhat by surprise. Although they knew that the neuromuscular and ganglionic synapses differed pharmacologically, and suspected that cholinergic synapses in the CNS might be different again, the molecular diversity goes far beyond this, and its functional significance is only slowly emerging.

The different action of agonists and antagonists on neuromuscular, ganglionic and brain synapses is of practical importance and mainly reflects the differences between the muscle and neuronal nAChRs (Table 13.1).

MUSCARINIC RECEPTORS

Muscarinic receptors (mAChRs) are typical G protein-coupled receptors (see Ch. 3), and five molecular subtypes (M_1–M_5) are known. The odd-numbered members of the group (M_1, M_3, M_5) couple with G_q to activate the inositol phosphate pathway (Ch. 3), while the even-numbered receptors (M_2, M_4) open potassium (K_{ATP}) channels causing

membrane hyperpolarisation as well as acting through G_i to inhibit adenylyl cyclase and thus reduce intracellular cAMP. Both groups activate the MAP kinase pathway. The location and pharmacology of these subtypes are summarised in Table 13.2.

M_1 receptors ('neural') are found mainly on CNS and peripheral neurons and on gastric parietal cells. They mediate excitatory effects, for example the slow muscarinic excitation mediated by ACh in sympathetic ganglia (Ch. 12) and central neurons. This excitation is produced by a decrease in K^+ conductance, which causes membrane depolarisation. Deficiency of this kind of ACh-mediated effect in the brain is possibly associated with dementia (see Ch. 40), although transgenic M_1-receptor knockout mice show only slight cognitive impairment (see Wess et al., 2007). M_1 receptors are also involved in the increase of gastric acid secretion following vagal stimulation (see Ch. 30).

Table 13.2 Muscarinic receptor subtypes[a]

	M_1 ('neural')	M_2 ('cardiac')	M_3 ('glandular/ smooth muscle')	M_4	M_5
Main locations	Autonomic ganglia (including intramural ganglia in stomach) Glands: salivary, lacrimal, etc. Cerebral cortex	Heart: atria CNS: widely distributed	Exocrine glands: gastric (acid-secreting parietal cells), salivary, etc. Smooth muscle: gastrointestinal tract, eye, airways, bladder Blood vessels: endothelium	CNS	CNS: very localised expression in substantia nigra Salivary glands Iris/ciliary muscle
Cellular response	↑ IP_3, DAG Depolarisation Excitation (slow epsp) ↓ K^+ conductance	↓ cAMP Inhibition ↓ Ca^{2+} conductance ↑ K^+ conductance	↑ IP_3 Stimulation ↑ $[Ca^{2+}]_i$	↓ cAMP Inhibition	↑ IP_3 Excitation
Functional response	CNS excitation (? improved cognition) Gastric secretion	Cardiac inhibition Neural inhibition Central muscarinic effects (e.g. tremor, hypothermia)	Gastric, salivary secretion Gastrointestinal smooth muscle contraction Ocular accommodation Vasodilatation	Enhanced locomotion	Not known
Non-selective agonists (see also Table 13.3)	Acetylcholine Carbachol Oxotremorine Pilocarpine **Bethanechol**				
Selective agonists	McNA343		**Cevimeline**		
Non-selective antagonists (see also Table 13.5)	**Atropine** **Dicycloverine** **Tolterodine** **Oxybutynin** **Ipratropium**				
Selective antagonists	**Pirenzepine** Mamba toxin MT7	Gallamine (see p. 158)	**Darifenacin**		Mamba toxin MT3

[a]This table shows only the predominant subtypes expressed in mammalian tissues. For further details, see Ch. 39 and review by and Kalamida et al. (2007).

CNS, central nervous system; DAG, diacylglycerol; epsp, excitatory postsynaptic potential; IP_3, inositol trisphosphate.

Drugs in clinical use are shown in **bold**.

M_2 *receptors* ('*cardiac*') occur in the heart, and also on the presynaptic terminals of peripheral and central neurons. They exert inhibitory effects, mainly by increasing K^+ conductance and by inhibiting calcium channels (see Ch. 4). M_2-receptor activation is responsible for cholinergic inhibition of the heart, as well as presynaptic inhibition in the CNS and periphery (Ch. 12). They are also co-expressed with M_3 receptors in visceral smooth muscle, and contribute to the smooth-muscle-stimulating effect of muscarinic agonists in several organs.

M_3 *receptors* ('*glandular/smooth muscle*') produce mainly excitatory effects, i.e. stimulation of glandular secretions (salivary, bronchial, sweat, etc.) and contraction of visceral smooth muscle. M_3 receptors also mediate relaxation of smooth muscle (mainly vascular), which results from the release of nitric oxide from neighbouring endothelial cells (Ch. 20). M_3 receptors occur also in specific locations in the CNS (see Ch. 39).

M_4 *and* M_5 *receptors* are largely confined to the CNS, and their functional role is not well understood, although mice lacking these receptors do show behavioural changes (Wess et al., 2007). Recently it has been discovered that cytokine secretion from lymphocytes and other cells is regulated by M_1 and M_3 receptors, while M_2 and M_4 receptors affect cell proliferation in various situations, opening up the possibility of new therapeutic roles for muscarinic receptor ligands (see Wessler & Kirkpatrick, 2008).

The agonist binding region is highly conserved between the different subtypes, so attempts to develop selective agonists and antagonists have had limited success. Most known agonists are non-selective, though two experimental compounds, **McNA343** and **oxotremorine**, are selective for M_1 receptors, on which **carbachol** is relatively inactive. **Cevimeline,** a selective M_3-receptor agonist, is used to improve salivary and lacrimal secretion in Sjögren's syndrome, an autoimmune disorder characterised by dryness of mouth and eyes. It is possible that new allosteric mAChR ligands, targeted at sites outside the agonist binding domain (see Ch. 3, Fig. 3.7), will allow better subtype selectivity for drugs acting on this important class of receptors (see Conn et al., 2009).

There is more selectivity among antagonists. Although most of the classic muscarinic antagonists (e.g. **atropine**, **hyoscine**) are non-selective, **pirenzepine** (previously used for peptic ulcer disease) is selective for M_1 receptors, and **darifenacin** (used for urinary incontinence in adults with detrusor muscle instability, known as 'overactive bladder') is selective for M_3 receptors. **Gallamine**, once used as a neuromuscular-blocking drug, is also a selective, although weak, M_2 receptor antagonist.[1] Toxins from the venom of the green mamba have been discovered to be highly selective mAChR antagonists (see Table 13.2).

PHYSIOLOGY OF CHOLINERGIC TRANSMISSION

The physiology of cholinergic neurotransmission is described in detail by Nicholls et al. (2012). The main ways in which drugs can affect cholinergic transmission are shown in Figure 13.2.

[1]Unlike most other antagonists, gallamine acts *allosterically* (i.e. at a site distinct from the ACh binding site).

Acetylcholine receptors

- Main subdivision is into nicotinic (nAChR) and muscarinic (mAChR) subtypes.
- nAChRs are directly coupled to cation channels, and mediate fast excitatory synaptic transmission at the neuromuscular junction, autonomic ganglia and various sites in the central nervous system (CNS). Muscle and neuronal nAChRs differ in their molecular structure and pharmacology.
- mAChRs and nAChRs occur presynaptically as well as postsynaptically, and function to regulate transmitter release.
- mAChRs are G protein-coupled receptors causing:
  - activation of phospholipase C (hence formation of inositol trisphosphate and diacylglycerol as second messengers)
  - inhibition of adenylyl cyclase
  - activation of potassium channels or inhibition of calcium channels.
- mAChRs mediate acetylcholine effects at postganglionic parasympathetic synapses (mainly heart, smooth muscle and glands), and contribute to ganglionic excitation. They occur in many parts of the CNS.
- Three main types of mAChR occur:
  - M_1 receptors ('neural') producing slow excitation of ganglia. They are selectively blocked by **pirenzepine**.
  - M_2 receptors ('cardiac') causing decrease in cardiac rate and force of contraction (mainly of atria). They are selectively blocked by **gallamine**. M_2 receptors also mediate presynaptic inhibition.
  - M_3 receptors ('glandular') causing secretion, contraction of visceral smooth muscle, vascular relaxation. **Cevimeline** is a selective M_3 agonist.
- Two further molecular mAChR subtypes, M_4 and M_5, occur mainly in the CNS.
- All mAChRs are activated by acetylcholine and blocked by **atropine**. There are also subtype-selective agonists and antagonists.

ACETYLCHOLINE SYNTHESIS AND RELEASE

ACh is synthesised within the nerve terminal from choline, which is taken up into the nerve terminal by a specific transporter (Ch. 12), similar to those that operate for many transmitters. The difference is that it transports the precursor, choline, not ACh, so it is not important in terminating the action of the transmitter. The concentration of choline in the blood and body fluids is normally about $10\ \mu mol/l$, but in the immediate vicinity of cholinergic nerve terminals it increases, probably to about $1\ mmol/l$, when the released ACh is hydrolysed, and more than 50% of this choline is normally recaptured by the nerve terminals. Free choline within the nerve terminal is acetylated by a cytosolic enzyme, *choline acetyltransferase* (CAT), which transfers the acetyl group from acetyl coenzyme A. The rate-limiting process in ACh synthesis appears to be choline transport, which is determined by the extracellular choline concentration and hence is linked to the rate at which ACh is being released (Fig. 13.2). *Cholinesterase*

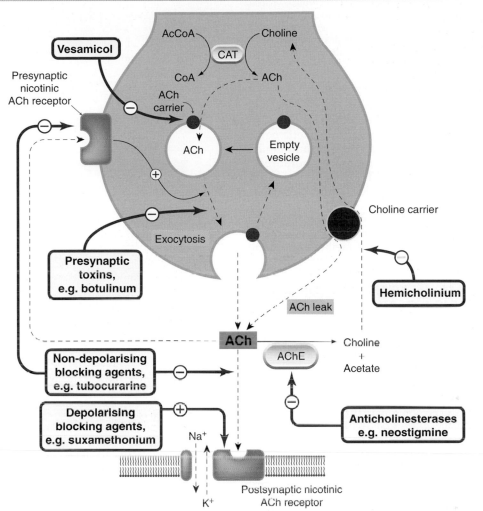

Fig. 13.2 Events and sites of drug action at a nicotinic cholinergic synapse. Acetylcholine (ACh) is shown acting postsynaptically on a nicotinic receptor controlling a cation channel (e.g. at the neuromuscular or ganglionic synapse), and also on a presynaptic nicotinic receptor that acts to facilitate ACh release during sustained synaptic activity. The nerve terminal also contains acetylcholinesterase (not shown); when this is inhibited, the amount of free ACh, and the rate of leakage of ACh via the choline carrier, is increased. Under normal conditions, this leakage of ACh is insignificant. At muscarinic cholinergic junctions (e.g. heart, smooth muscle and exocrine glands), both postsynaptic and presynaptic (inhibitory) receptors are of the muscarinic type. AcCoA, acetyl coenzyme A; AChE, acetylcholinesterase; CAT, choline acetyltransferase; CoA, coenzyme A.

is present in the presynaptic nerve terminals, and ACh is continually being hydrolysed and resynthesised. Inhibition of the nerve terminal cholinesterase causes the accumulation of 'surplus' ACh in the cytosol, which is not available for release by nerve impulses (although it is able to leak out via the choline carrier). Most of the ACh synthesised, however, is packaged into synaptic vesicles, in which its concentration is extraordinarily high (about 100 mmol/l), and from which release occurs by exocytosis triggered by Ca^{2+} entry into the nerve terminal (see Ch. 4).

Cholinergic vesicles accumulate ACh actively, by means of a specific transporter belonging to the family of amine transporters described in Chapter 12. Accumulation of ACh is coupled to the large electrochemical gradient for protons that exists between acidic intracellular organelles and the cytosol; it is blocked selectively by the experimental drug **vesamicol**. Following its release, ACh diffuses across the synaptic cleft to combine with receptors on the postsynaptic cell. Some of it succumbs on the way to hydrolysis by *acetylcholinesterase* (AChE), an enzyme that

is bound to the basement membrane that lies between the pre- and postsynaptic membranes. At fast cholinergic synapses (e.g. the neuromuscular and ganglionic synapses), but not at slow ones (smooth muscle, gland cells, heart, etc.), the released ACh is hydrolysed very rapidly (within 1 ms), so that it acts only very briefly.

▼ At the neuromuscular junction, which is a highly specialised synapse, a single nerve impulse releases about 300 synaptic vesicles (altogether about 3 million ACh molecules) from the nerve terminals supplying a single muscle fibre, which contain altogether about 3 million synaptic vesicles. Approximately two million ACh molecules combine with receptors, of which there are about 30 million on each muscle fibre, the rest being hydrolysed without reaching a receptor. The ACh molecules remain bound to receptors for, on average, about 2 ms, and are quickly hydrolysed after dissociating, so that they cannot combine with a second receptor. The result is that transmitter action is very rapid and very brief, which is important for a synapse that has to initiate speedy muscular responses, and that may have to transmit signals faithfully at high frequency. Muscle cells are much larger than neurons and require much more synaptic current to generate an action potential. Thus all the chemical events happen on a larger scale than at a neuronal synapse; the number of transmitter molecules in a quantum, the number of quanta released, and the number of receptors activated by each quantum are all 10–100 times greater. Our brains would be huge, but not very clever, if their synapses were built on the industrial scale of the neuromuscular junction.

PRESYNAPTIC MODULATION

Acetylcholine release is regulated by mediators, including ACh itself, acting on presynaptic receptors, as discussed in Chapter 12. At postganglionic parasympathetic nerve endings, inhibitory M_2 receptors participate in autoinhibition of ACh release; other mediators, such as noradrenaline, also inhibit the release of ACh (see Ch. 12). At the neuromuscular junction, on the other hand, presynaptic nAChRs facilitate ACh release, a mechanism that may allow the synapse to function reliably during prolonged high-frequency activity whereas, as mentioned above, presynaptic CNS-type nAChRs either facilitate or inhibit the release of other mediators.

ELECTRICAL EVENTS IN TRANSMISSION AT FAST CHOLINERGIC SYNAPSES

Acetylcholine, acting on the postsynaptic membrane of a nicotinic (neuromuscular or ganglionic) synapse, causes a large increase in its permeability to cations, particularly to Na^+ and K^+, and to a lesser extent Ca^{2+}. The resulting inflow of Na^+ depolarises the postsynaptic membrane. This transmitter-mediated depolarisation is called an *endplate potential (epp)* in a skeletal muscle fibre, or a *fast excitatory postsynaptic potential (fast epsp)* at the ganglionic synapse. In a muscle fibre, the localised epp spreads to adjacent, electrically excitable parts of the muscle fibre; if its amplitude reaches the threshold for excitation, an action potential is initiated, which propagates to the rest of the fibre and evokes a contraction (Ch. 4).

In a nerve cell, depolarisation of the soma or a dendrite by the fast epsp causes a local current to flow. This depolarises the axon hillock region of the cell, where, if the epsp is large enough, an action potential is initiated. Figure 13.3 shows that **tubocurarine**, a drug that blocks postsynaptic ACh receptors, reduces the amplitude of the fast epsp until it no longer initiates an action potential, although the cell is still capable of responding when it is stimulated electrically. Most ganglion cells are supplied by several presynaptic axons, and it requires simultaneous activity in more than one to make the postganglionic cell fire (integrative action). At the neuromuscular junction, only one nerve fibre supplies each muscle fibre – like a relay station in a telegraph line the synapse ensures faithful 1:1 transmission despite the impedance mismatch between the fine nerve fibre and the much larger muscle fibre. The amplitude of the epp is normally more than enough to initiate an action potential – indeed, transmission still occurs when the epp is reduced by 70–80%, showing a large margin of safety so that fluctuations in transmitter release (e.g. during repetitive stimulation) do not affect transmission.

▼ Transmission at the ganglionic synapse is more complex than at the neuromuscular junction. Although the primary event at both is the epp or fast epsp produced by ACh acting on nAChRs, this is followed in the ganglion by a succession of much slower postsynaptic responses:

• A *slow inhibitory (hyperpolarising) postsynaptic potential (slow ipsp)*, lasting 2–5 s. This mainly reflects a muscarinic (M_2)-

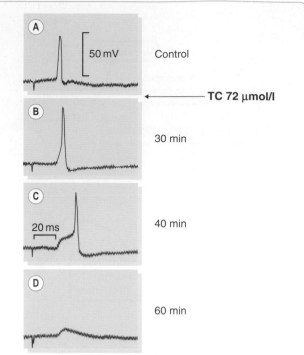

Fig. 13.3 Cholinergic transmission in an autonomic ganglion cell. Records were obtained with an intracellular microelectrode from a guinea pig parasympathetic ganglion cell. The artefact at the beginning of each trace shows the moment of stimulation of the preganglionic nerve. Tubocurarine (TC), an acetylcholine antagonist, causes the epsp to become smaller. In record [**C**], it only just succeeds in triggering the action potential, and in [**D**] it has fallen below the threshold. Following complete block, antidromic stimulation (not shown) will still produce an action potential (cf. depolarisation block, Fig. 13.4). *(From Blackman JG et al. 1969 J Physiol 201, 723.)*

receptor-mediated increase in K^+ conductance, but other transmitters, such as dopamine and adenosine, also contribute.
• A *slow epsp*, which lasts for about 10 s. This is produced by ACh acting on M_1 receptors, which close K^+ channels.
• A *late slow epsp*, lasting for 1–2 min. This is thought to be mediated by a peptide co-transmitter, which may be substance P in some ganglia, and a gonadotrophin-releasing hormone-like peptide in others (see Ch. 12). Like the slow epsp, it is produced by a decrease in K^+ conductance.

DEPOLARISATION BLOCK

▼ Depolarisation block occurs at cholinergic synapses when the excitatory nAChRs are persistently activated, and it results from a decrease in the electrical excitability of the postsynaptic cell. This is shown in Figure 13.4. Application of nicotine to a sympathetic ganglion activates nAChRs, causing a depolarisation of the cell, which at first initiates action potential discharge. After a few seconds, this discharge ceases and transmission is blocked. The loss of electrical excitability at this time is shown by the fact that electrical stimuli also fail to produce an action potential. The main reason for the loss of electrical excitability during a period of maintained depolarisation is that the voltage-sensitive sodium channels (see Ch. 4) become inactivated (i.e. refractory) and no longer able to open in response to a brief depolarising stimulus.

A second type of effect is also seen in the experiment shown in Figure 13.4. After nicotine has acted for several minutes, the cell partially repolarises and its electrical excitability returns but, despite this, transmission remains blocked. This type of secondary, *non-depolarising block* occurs also at the neuromuscular junction if

Cholinergic transmission

- Acetylcholine (ACh) synthesis:
  - requires choline, which enters the neuron via carrier-mediated transport
  - choline is acetylated to form ACh by choline acetyl transferase, a cytosolic enzyme found only in cholinergic neurons. Acetyl coenzyme A is the source of acetyl groups.
- ACh is packaged into synaptic vesicles at high concentration by carrier-mediated transport.
- ACh release occurs by Ca^{2+}-mediated exocytosis. At the neuromuscular junction, one presynaptic nerve impulse releases 100–500 vesicles.
- At the neuromuscular junction, ACh acts on nicotinic receptors to open cation channels, producing a rapid depolarisation (endplate potential), which normally initiates an action potential in the muscle fibre. Transmission at other 'fast' cholinergic synapses (e.g. ganglionic) is similar.
- At 'fast' cholinergic synapses, ACh is hydrolysed within about 1 ms by acetylcholinesterase, so a presynaptic action potential produces only one postsynaptic action potential.
- Transmission mediated by muscarinic receptors is much slower in its time course, and synaptic structures are less clearly defined. In many situations, ACh functions as a modulator rather than as a direct transmitter.
- Main mechanisms of pharmacological block: inhibition of choline uptake, inhibition of ACh release, block of postsynaptic receptors or ion channels, persistent postsynaptic depolarisation.

repeated doses of the depolarising drug **suxamethonium**[2] (see below) are used. The main factor responsible for the secondary block (known clinically as *phase II block*) appears to be receptor desensitisation (see Ch. 2). This causes the depolarising action of the blocking drug to subside, but transmission remains blocked because the receptors are desensitised to ACh.

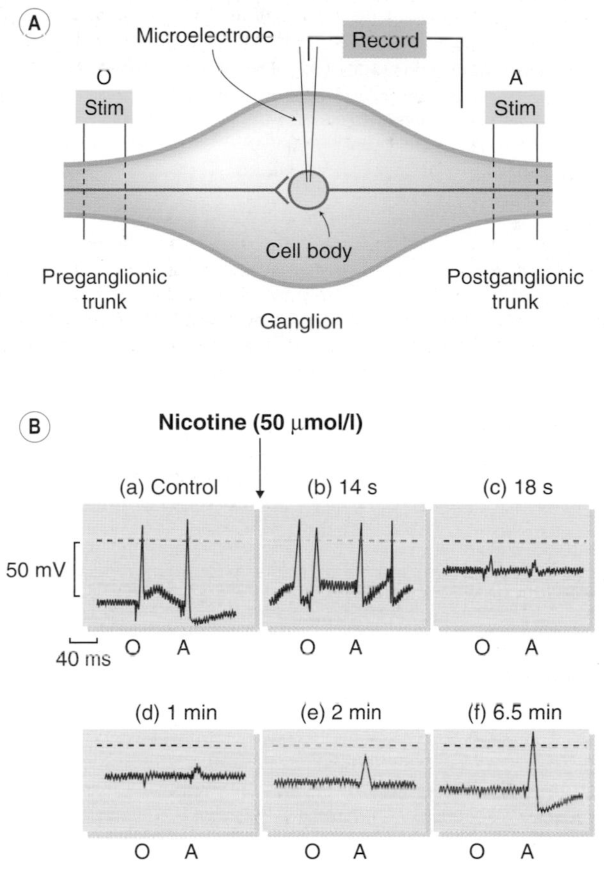

EFFECTS OF DRUGS ON CHOLINERGIC TRANSMISSION

As shown in Figure 13.2, drugs can influence cholinergic transmission either by acting on postsynaptic ACh receptors as agonists or antagonists (Tables 13.1 and 13.2), or by affecting the release or destruction of endogenous ACh.

In the rest of this chapter, we describe the following groups of drugs, subdivided according to their site of action:

- muscarinic agonists
- muscarinic antagonists
- ganglion-stimulating drugs
- ganglion-blocking drugs
- neuromuscular-blocking drugs
- anticholinesterases and other drugs that enhance cholinergic transmission.

[2]Known in the USA as **succinylcholine**.

Fig. 13.4 **Depolarisation block of ganglionic transmission by nicotine.** **[A]** System used for intracellular recording from sympathetic ganglion cells of the frog, showing the location of orthodromic (O) and antidromic (A) stimulating (stim) electrodes. Stimulation at O excites the cell via the cholinergic synapse, whereas stimulation at A excites it by electrical propagation of the action potential. **[B]** The effect of nicotine. (a) Control records. The membrane potential is −55 mV (dotted line = 0 mV), and the cell responds to both O and A. (b) Shortly after adding nicotine, the cell is slightly depolarised and spontaneously active, but still responsive to O and A (c and d). The cell is further depolarised, to −25 mV, and produces only a vestigial action potential. The fact that it does not respond to A shows that it is electrically inexcitable (e and f). In the continued presence of nicotine, the cell repolarises and regains its responsiveness to A, but it is still unresponsive to O because the ACh receptors are desensitised by nicotine. *(From Ginsborg BL, Guerrero S 1964 J Physiol 172, 189.)*

DRUGS AFFECTING MUSCARINIC RECEPTORS

MUSCARINIC AGONISTS

Structure–activity relationships

Muscarinic agonists, as a group, are often referred to as *parasympathomimetic*, because the main effects that they produce in the whole animal resemble those of parasympathetic stimulation. The structures of acetylcholine and related choline esters are given in Table 13.3. They are agonists at both mAChRs and nAChRs, but act more potently on mAChRs (see Fig. 13.1). **Bethanechol, pilocarpine** and **cevimeline** are the only ones used clinically.

The key features of the ACh molecule that are important for its activity are the quaternary ammonium group, which

Table 13.3 Muscarinic agonists

Compound	Structure	Receptor specificity		Hydrolysis by cholinesterase	Clinical uses
		Muscarinic	*Nicotinic*		
Acetylcholine		+++	+++	+++	None
Carbachol		++	+++	–	None
Methacholine		+++	+	++	None
Bethanechol		+++	–	–	Treatment of bladder and gastrointestinal hypotonia[a]
Muscarine		+++	–	–	None[b]
Pilocarpine		++	–	–	Glaucoma
Oxotremorine		++	–	–	None
Cevimeline		++[c]	–	–	Sjögren's syndrome (to increase salivary and lacrimal secretion)

[a]Essential to check that bladder neck is not obstructed.
[b]Cause of one type of mushroom poisoning.
[c]Selective for M_3 receptors.

bears a positive charge, and the ester group, which bears a partial negative charge and is susceptible to rapid hydrolysis by cholinesterase. Variants of the choline ester structure (Table 13.3) have the effect of reducing the susceptibility of the compound to hydrolysis by cholinesterase, and altering the relative activity on mAChRs and nAChRs.

Carbachol and **methacholine** are used as experimental tools. Bethanechol, which is a hybrid of these two molecules, is stable to hydrolysis and selective for mAChRs, and is occasionally used clinically (see clinical box, p. 164). Pilocarpine is a partial agonist and shows some selectivity in stimulating secretion from sweat, salivary, lacrimal and bronchial glands, and contracting iris smooth muscle (see below), with weak effects on gastrointestinal smooth muscle and the heart.

Effects of muscarinic agonists

The main actions of muscarinic agonists are readily understood in terms of the parasympathetic nervous system.

Cardiovascular effects. These include cardiac slowing and a decrease in cardiac output due both to the reduced heart rate and to a decreased force of contraction of the atria (the ventricles have only a sparse parasympathetic innervation and a low sensitivity to muscarinic agonists). Generalised vasodilatation also occurs (mediated by nitric oxide, NO; see Ch. 20) and, combined with the reduced cardiac output, produces a sharp fall in arterial pressure (Fig. 13.1). The mechanism of action of muscarinic agonists on the heart is discussed in Chapter 21 (see Fig. 21.7).

Smooth muscle. Smooth muscle generally *contracts* in direct response to muscarinic agonists, in contrast to the indirect effect via NO on vascular smooth muscle. Peristaltic activity of the gastrointestinal tract is increased, which can cause colicky pain, and the bladder and bronchial smooth muscle also contract.

Sweating, lacrimation, salivation and bronchial secretion. These result from stimulation of exocrine glands. The combined effect of bronchial secretion and constriction can interfere with breathing.

Effects on the eye. These effects are clinically important. The parasympathetic nerves to the eye supply the constrictor pupillae muscle, which runs circumferentially in the iris, and the ciliary muscle, which adjusts the curvature of the lens (Fig. 13.5). Contraction of the ciliary muscle in response to activation of mAChRs pulls the ciliary body forward and inward, thus relaxing the tension on the suspensory ligament of the lens, allowing the lens to bulge more and reducing its focal length. This parasympathetic reflex is thus necessary to accommodate the eye for near vision. The constrictor pupillae is important not only for adjusting the pupil in response to changes in light intensity, but also in regulating the intraocular pressure. Aqueous humour is secreted slowly and continuously by the cells of the epithelium covering the ciliary body, and it drains into the *canal of Schlemm* (Fig. 13.5), which runs around the eye close to the outer margin of the iris. The intraocular pressure is normally 10–15 mmHg above atmospheric, which keeps the eye slightly distended. Abnormally raised intraocular pressure (which leads to

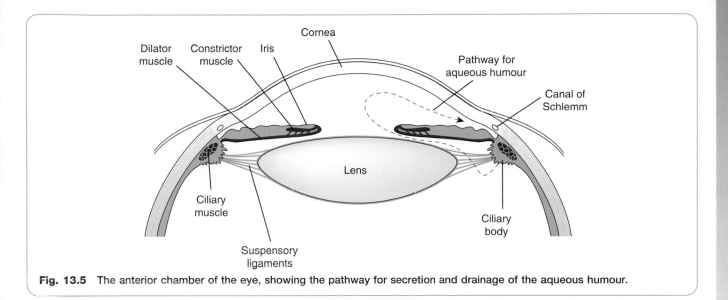

Fig. 13.5 The anterior chamber of the eye, showing the pathway for secretion and drainage of the aqueous humour.

Table 13.4 Drugs that lower intraocular pressure

Drug[a]	Mechanism	Notes	See Chapter
Timolol, carteolol	β-adrenoceptor antagonist	Given as eye drops but may still cause systemic side effects: bradycardia, bronchoconstriction	14
Acetazolamide, dorzolamide	Carbonic anhydrase inhibitor	Acetazolamide is given systemically Side effects include diuresis, loss of appetite, tingling, neutropenia Dorzolamide is used as eye drops Side effects include bitter taste and burning sensation	29
Clonidine, apraclonidine	α₂-adrenoceptor agonist	Used as eye drops	14
Latanoprost	Prostaglandin analogue	Can alter iris pigmentation	17
Pilocarpine	Muscarinic agonist	Used as eye drops	This chapter
Ecothiophate	Anticholinesterase	Used as eye drops Can cause muscle spasm and systemic effects	This chapter

[a]The most important drugs are shown in **bold**.

the pathological condition of *glaucoma*) damages the eye and is one of the commonest preventable causes of blindness. In acute glaucoma, drainage of aqueous humour becomes impeded when the pupil is dilated, because folding of the iris tissue occludes the drainage angle, causing the intraocular pressure to rise. Activation of the constrictor pupillae muscle by muscarinic agonists in these circumstances lowers the intraocular pressure, although in a normal individual it has little effect. The increased tension in the ciliary muscle produced by these drugs may also play a part in improving drainage by realigning the connective tissue trabeculae through which the canal of Schlemm passes. Drugs used in the treatment of glaucoma are summarised in Table 13.4.

In addition to these peripheral effects, muscarinic agonists that are able to penetrate the blood–brain barrier produce marked central effects due to activation mainly of M_1 receptors in the brain. These include tremor,

hypothermia and increased locomotor activity, as well as improved cognition (see Ch. 40).

Clinical use
Currently there are few important uses for muscarinic agonists (though there are still hopes that new, more selective agents may prove useful in various CNS disorders). Current clinical uses are summarised in the clinical box (p. 164).

MUSCARINIC ANTAGONISTS

Muscarinic receptor antagonists (*parasympatholytic drugs*; Table 13.5) are competitive antagonists whose chemical structures usually contain ester and basic groups in the same relationship as ACh, but they have a bulky aromatic group in place of the acetyl group. The two naturally occurring compounds, **atropine** and **hyoscine** (also known as **scopolamine**), are alkaloids found in

Table 13.5   Muscarinic antagonists[a]

Compound	Pharmacological properties		Notes
Atropine	Non-selective antagonist Well absorbed orally CNS stimulant		Belladonna alkaloid Main side effects: urinary retention, dry mouth, blurred vision Dicycloverine (dicyclomine) is similar and used mainly as an antispasmodic agent
Hyoscine	Similar to atropine CNS depressant		Belladonna alkaloid (also known as scopolamine) Causes sedation; other side effects as atropine
Hyoscine butylbromide	Similar to atropine but poorly absorbed and lacks CNS effects Significant ganglion-blocking activity		Quaternary ammonium derivative Similar drugs include atropine methonitrate, propantheline
Tiotropium	Similar to atropine methonitrate Does not inhibit mucociliary clearance from bronchi		Quaternary ammonium compound Ipratropium similar
Tropicamide	Similar to atropine May raise intraocular pressure		–
Cyclopentolate	Similar to tropicamide		–
Darifenacin	Selective for M_3 receptors	Urinary incontinence	Few side effects

Other non-selective muscarinic antagonists in clinical use, with very similar actions and side effects, include oxybutynin, tolterodine, fesoterodine, solifenacin and trospium – an example of me-too development by pharmaceutical companies.

[a]For chemical structures, see Brunton L et al. 2006. Goodman and Gilman's Pharmacological Basis of Therapeutics, 11th edn. McGraw–Hill, New York.

Clinical uses of muscarinic agonists and related drugs

- **Pilocarpine** eye drops cause constriction of the pupils (miosis) and have been used to treat glaucoma (raised pressure within the eye).
- **Pilocarpine** or **cevimeline**, a selective M_3 agonist, can be used to increase salivation and lacrimal secretion in patients with dry mouth or dry eyes (e.g. following irradiation, or in patients with autoimmune damage to the salivary or lacrimal glands as in Sjögren's syndrome).
- **Bethanechol** or **distigmine** (a cholinesterase inhibitor) are now seldom used as stimulant laxatives or to stimulate bladder emptying.

solanaceous plants. The deadly nightshade (*Atropa belladonna*) contains mainly atropine, whereas the thorn apple (*Datura stramonium*) contains mainly hyoscine. These are tertiary ammonium compounds that are sufficiently lipid-soluble to be readily absorbed from the gut or conjunctival sac and, importantly, to penetrate the blood–brain barrier. Quaternary ammonium compounds, which have peripheral actions very similar to those of atropine but, because of their exclusion from the brain, lack central actions, include **hyoscine butylbromide** and **propantheline**. **Ipratropium**, another quaternary ammonium compound, is used by inhalation as a bronchodilator. **Cyclopentolate**

and **tropicamide** are tertiary amines developed for ophthalmic use and administered as eye drops. **Oxybutynin**, **tolterodine** and **darifenacin** (M_3-selective) are drugs that act on the bladder to inhibit micturition, and are used for treating urinary incontinence. They produce unwanted effects typical of muscarinic antagonists, such as dry mouth, constipation and blurred vision, but these are less severe than with earlier drugs.

Effects of muscarinic antagonists

All the muscarinic antagonists produce basically similar peripheral effects, although some show a degree of selectivity, for example for the heart or bladder, reflecting heterogeneity among mAChRs.

The main effects of atropine are:

Inhibition of secretions. Salivary, lacrimal, bronchial and sweat glands are inhibited by very low doses of atropine, producing an uncomfortably dry mouth and skin. Gastric secretion is only slightly reduced. Mucociliary clearance in the bronchi is inhibited, so that residual secretions tend to accumulate in the lungs. Ipratropium lacks this effect.

Effects on heart rate. Atropine causes tachycardia through block of cardiac mAChRs. The tachycardia is modest, up to 80–90 beats/min in humans. This is because there is no effect on the sympathetic system, but only inhibition of tonic parasympathetic tone. Tachycardia is most pronounced in young people, in whom vagal tone at rest is highest; it is often absent in the elderly. At very low doses, atropine causes a paradoxical bradycardia, possibly due to a central action. Arterial blood pressure and the response of the heart to exercise are unaffected.

Effects on the eye. The pupil is dilated (*mydriasis*) by atropine administration, and becomes unresponsive to light. Relaxation of the ciliary muscle causes paralysis of accommodation (*cycloplegia*), so that near vision is impaired. Intraocular pressure may rise; although this is unimportant in normal individuals, it can be dangerous in patients suffering from narrow-angle glaucoma.

Effects on the gastrointestinal tract. Gastrointestinal motility is inhibited by atropine, although this requires larger doses than the other effects listed, and is not complete since excitatory transmitters other than ACh are important in normal function of the myenteric plexus (see Ch. 12). Atropine is used in pathological conditions in which there is increased gastrointestinal motility. Pirenzepine, owing to its selectivity for M_1 receptors, inhibits gastric acid secretion in doses that do not affect other systems.

Effects on other smooth muscle. Bronchial, biliary and urinary tract smooth muscle are all relaxed by atropine. Reflex bronchoconstriction (e.g. during anaesthesia) is prevented by atropine, whereas bronchoconstriction caused by local mediators, such as histamine and leukotrienes (e.g. in asthma; Ch. 28) is unaffected. Biliary and urinary tract smooth muscle are only slightly affected in normal individuals, probably because transmitters other than ACh (see Ch. 12) are important in these organs; nevertheless, atropine and similar drugs commonly precipitate urinary retention in elderly men with prostatic enlargement. Incontinence due to bladder overactivity is reduced by muscarinic antagonists.

Effects on the CNS. Atropine produces mainly excitatory effects on the CNS. At low doses, this causes mild restlessness; higher doses cause agitation and disorientation. In atropine poisoning, which occurs mainly in young children who eat deadly nightshade berries, marked excitement and irritability result in hyperactivity and a considerable rise in body temperature, which is accentuated by the loss of sweating. These central effects are the result of blocking mAChRs in the brain, and they are opposed by anticholinesterase drugs such as **physostigmine**, which have been used to treat atropine poisoning. Hyoscine in low doses causes marked sedation, but has similar effects in high dosage. Hyoscine also has a useful antiemetic effect and is used to prevent motion sickness. Muscarinic antagonists also affect the extrapyramidal system, reducing the involuntary movement and rigidity of patients with Parkinson's disease (Ch. 40) and counteracting the extrapyramidal side effects of many antipsychotic drugs (Ch. 46).

Clinical use

The main uses of muscarinic antagonists are summarised in the clinical box (p. 166).

DRUGS AFFECTING AUTONOMIC GANGLIA

GANGLION STIMULANTS

Most nAChR agonists act on either neuronal (ganglionic and CNS) nACh receptors or on striated muscle (motor endplate) receptors but not, apart from nicotine and ACh, on both (Table 13.6).

Nicotine and **lobeline** are tertiary amines found in the leaves of tobacco and lobelia plants, respectively. Nicotine belongs in pharmacological folklore, as it was the substance on the tip of Langley's paintbrush causing

> ### Drugs acting on muscarinic receptors
>
> #### Muscarinic agonists
> - Important compounds include **acetylcholine**, **carbachol**, **methacholine**, **muscarine** and **pilocarpine**. They vary in muscarinic/nicotinic selectivity, and in susceptibility to cholinesterase.
> - Main effects are bradycardia and vasodilatation (endothelium-dependent), leading to fall in blood pressure; contraction of visceral smooth muscle (gut, bladder, bronchi, etc.); exocrine secretions, pupillary constriction and ciliary muscle contraction, leading to decrease of intraocular pressure.
> - Main use is in treatment of glaucoma (especially **pilocarpine**).
> - Most agonists show little receptor subtype selectivity, but more selective compounds are in development.
>
> #### Muscarinic antagonists
> - Most important compounds are **atropine**, **hyoscine**, **ipratropium** and **pirenzepine**.
> - Main effects are inhibition of secretions; tachycardia; pupillary dilatation and paralysis of accommodation; relaxation of smooth muscle (gut, bronchi, biliary tract, bladder); inhibition of gastric acid secretion (especially **pirenzepine**); central nervous system effects (mainly excitatory with **atropine**; depressant, including amnesia, with **hyoscine**), including antiemetic effect and antiparkinsonian effect.

stimulation of muscle fibres when applied to the endplate region, leading him to postulate in 1905 the existence of a 'receptive substance' on the surface of the fibres (Ch. 12). **Epibatidine**, found in the skin of poisonous frogs, is a highly potent nicotinic agonist selective for ganglionic and CNS receptors. It was found, unexpectedly, to be a powerful analgesic (see Ch. 42), though its autonomic side effects ruled out its clinical use. **Varenicline**, a synthetic agonist relatively selective for CNS receptors, is used (as is nicotine itself) to treat nicotine addiction (Ch. 49). Otherwise these drugs are used only as experimental tools.

They cause complex peripheral responses associated with generalised stimulation of autonomic ganglia. The effects of nicotine on the gastrointestinal tract and sweat glands are familiar to neophyte smokers (see Ch. 49), although usually insufficient to act as an effective deterrent.

GANGLION-BLOCKING DRUGS

Ganglion blocking drugs are used experimentally to study autonomic function, but their clinical use is obsolete. Ganglion block can occur by several mechanisms:

- By interference with ACh release, as at the neuromuscular junction (Ch. 12).
- By prolonged depolarisation. Nicotine (see Fig. 13.4) can block ganglia, after initial stimulation, in this way, as can ACh itself if cholinesterase is inhibited so that it can exert a continuing action on the postsynaptic membrane.
- By interference with the postsynaptic action of ACh. The few ganglion-blocking drugs of practical

Table 13.6 Nicotinic receptor agonists and antagonists

Drug	Main site	Type of action	Notes
Agonists			
Nicotine	Autonomic ganglia CNS	Stimulation then block Stimulation	See Ch. 49
Lobeline	Autonomic ganglia Sensory nerve terminals	Stimulation Stimulation	–
Epibatidine	Autonomic ganglia, CNS	Stimulation	Isolated from frog skin Highly potent No clinical use
Varenicline	CNS, autonomic ganglia	Stimulation	Used for nicotine addiction (see Ch. 49)
Suxamethonium	Neuromuscular junction	Depolarisation block	Used clinically as muscle relaxant
Decamethonium	Neuromuscular junction	Depolarisation block	No clinical use
Antagonists			
Hexamethonium	Autonomic ganglia	Transmission block	No clinical use
Trimetaphan	Autonomic ganglia	Transmission block	Blood pressure-lowering in surgery (rarely used)
Tubocurarine	Neuromuscular junction	Transmission block	Now rarely used
Pancuronium Atracurium Vecuronium	Neuromuscular junction	Transmission block	Widely used as muscle relaxants in anaesthesia

Clinical uses of muscarinic antagonists

Cardiovascular

- Treatment of sinus bradycardia (e.g. after myocardial infarction; see Ch. 21): for example **atropine**.

Ophthalmic

- To dilate the pupil: for example **tropicamide** or **cyclopentolate** eye drops.

Neurological

- Prevention of motion sickness: for example **hyoscine** (orally or transdermally).
- Parkinsonism (see Ch. 40), especially to counteract movement disorders caused by antipsychotic drugs (see Ch. 46): for example, **benzhexol**, **benztropine**.

Respiratory

- Asthma and chronic obstructive pulmonary disease (see Ch. 28): **ipratropium** or **tiotropium** by inhalation.

Anaesthetic premedication

- To dry secretions: for example **atropine**, **hyoscine**. (Current anaesthetics are relatively non-irritant, see Ch. 41, so this use is now less important.)

Gastrointestinal

- To facilitate endoscopy and gastrointestinal radiology by relaxing gastrointestinal smooth muscle (antispasmodic action; see Ch. 30): for example, **hyoscine**.
- As an antispasmodic in irritable bowel syndrome or colonic diverticular disease: for example **dicycloverine** (**dicyclomine**).

importance act by blocking neuronal nAChRs or the associated ion channels.

▼ Sixty-five years ago, Paton and Zaimis investigated a series of linear bisquaternary compounds. Compounds with five or six carbon atoms (**hexamethonium**, no longer used clinically but famous as the first effective antihypertensive agent) in the methylene chain linking the two quaternary groups produced ganglionic block.[3]

Effects of ganglion-blocking drugs

The effects of ganglion-blocking drugs are numerous and complex, as would be expected, because both divisions of the autonomic nervous system are blocked indiscriminately. The description by Paton of 'hexamethonium man' cannot be bettered:

▼ He is a pink-complexioned person, except when he has stood in a queue for a long time, when he may get pale and faint. His hand-shake is warm and dry. He is a placid and relaxed companion; for instance he may laugh but he can't cry because the tears cannot come. Your rudest story will not make him blush, and the most unpleasant circumstances will fail to make him turn pale. His collars and socks stay very clean and sweet. He wears corsets and may, if you meet him out, be rather fidgety (corsets to compress his splanchnic vascular pool, fidgety to keep the venous return going from his legs). He dislikes speaking much unless helped with something to moisten his dry mouth and throat. He is long-sighted and easily blinded by bright light. The redness of his eyeballs may suggest irregular habits and in fact his head is rather weak. But he always behaves like a gentleman and never belches or hiccups. He tends to get cold and keeps well wrapped up. But his health is good; he does not have chilblains and those diseases of modern civilisation, hypertension and peptic ulcer, pass him by. He gets thin because his appetite is modest; he never feels hunger pains and his stomach never rumbles.

---

[3]Based on their structural similarity to ACh, these compounds were originally assumed to compete with ACh for its binding site. However, they are now known to act mainly by blocking the ion channel rather than the receptor itself.

He gets rather constipated so that his intake of liquid paraffin is high. As old age comes on, he will suffer from retention of urine and impotence, but frequency, precipitancy and strangury (i.e. an intensely painful sensation of needing to pass urine coupled with an inability to do so) will not worry him. One is uncertain how he will end, but perhaps if he is not careful, by eating less and less and getting colder and colder, he will sink into a symptomless, hypoglycaemic coma and die, as was proposed for the universe, a sort of entropy death.

(From Paton WDM 1954 The principles of ganglion block. Lectures on the scientific basis of medicine, vol. 2.)

In practice, the main effect is a marked fall in arterial blood pressure resulting mainly from block of sympathetic ganglia, which causes arteriolar vasodilatation, and the block of cardiovascular reflexes. In particular, the venoconstriction, which occurs normally when a subject stands up and which is necessary to prevent the central venous pressure (and hence cardiac output) from falling sharply, is reduced. Standing thus causes a sudden fall in arterial pressure (*postural hypotension*) that can cause fainting. Similarly, the vasodilatation of skeletal muscle during exercise is normally accompanied by vasoconstriction elsewhere (e.g. splanchnic area) produced by sympathetic activity. If this adjustment is prevented, the overall peripheral resistance falls and the blood pressure also falls (*post-exercise hypotension*).

Drugs acting on autonomic ganglia

Ganglion-stimulating drugs

- Compounds include **nicotine**, **dimethylphenylpiperazinium** (**DMPP**)
- Both sympathetic and parasympathetic ganglia are stimulated, so effects are complex, including tachycardia and increase of blood pressure; variable effects on gastrointestinal motility and secretions; increased bronchial, salivary and sweat secretions. Additional effects result from stimulation of other neuronal structures, including sensory and noradrenergic nerve terminals.
- Ganglion stimulation may be followed by depolarisation block.
- **Nicotine** also has important central nervous system effects.
- No therapeutic uses, except for **nicotine** to assist giving up smoking.

Ganglion-blocking drugs

- Compounds include **hexamethonium**, **tubocurarine** (also **nicotine**; see p. 160).
- Block all autonomic ganglia and enteric ganglia. Main effects: hypotension and loss of cardiovascular reflexes, inhibition of secretions, gastrointestinal paralysis, impaired micturition.
- Clinically obsolete.

NEUROMUSCULAR-BLOCKING DRUGS

Drugs can block neuromuscular transmission either by acting presynaptically to inhibit ACh synthesis or release, or by acting postsynaptically.

Neuromuscular block is an important adjunct to anaesthesia (Ch. 40), when artificial ventilation is available. The drugs used for this purpose all work postsynaptically, either (a) by blocking ACh receptors (or in some cases the ion channel) or (b) by activating ACh receptors and thus causing persistent depolarisation of the motor endplate. Apart from **suxamethonium** (see p. 169-170) all of the drugs used clinically are *non-depolarising agents*.

NON-DEPOLARISING BLOCKING AGENTS

In 1856, Claude Bernard, in a famous experiment, showed that 'curare' causes paralysis by blocking neuromuscular transmission, rather than by abolishing nerve conduction or muscle contractility. Curare is a mixture of naturally occurring alkaloids found in various South American plants and used as arrow poisons by South American Indians. The most important component is **tubocurarine**, itself now rarely used in clinical medicine, being superseded by synthetic drugs with improved properties. The most important are **pancuronium**, **vecuronium**, **cisatracurium** and **mivacurium** (Table 13.7), which differ mainly in their duration of action. These substances are all quaternary ammonium compounds, so are poorly absorbed (they are administered intravenously) and generally are efficiently excreted by the kidneys. They do not cross the placenta, which is important in relation to their use in obstetric anaesthesia.

Mechanism of action

Non-depolarising blocking agents act as competitive antagonists (see Ch. 2) at the ACh receptors of the endplate.

▼ The amount of ACh released by a nerve impulse normally exceeds by several-fold what is needed to elicit an action potential in the muscle fibre. It is therefore necessary to block 70–80% of the receptor sites before transmission actually fails. In any individual muscle fibre, transmission is all or nothing, so graded degrees of block represent a varying proportion of muscle fibres failing to respond. In this situation, where the amplitude of the epp in all the fibres is close to threshold (just above in some, just below in others), small variations in the amount of transmitter released, or in the rate at which it is destroyed, will have a large effect on the proportion of fibres contracting, so the degree of block is liable to vary according to various physiological circumstances (e.g. stimulation frequency, temperature and cholinesterase inhibition), which normally have relatively little effect on the efficiency of transmission.

Non-depolarising blocking agents also block facilitatory presynaptic autoreceptors, and thus inhibit the release of ACh during repetitive stimulation of the motor nerve, resulting in the phenomenon of 'tetanic fade', which is often used by anaesthetists to monitor postoperative recovery of neuromuscular transmission.

Effects of non-depolarising blocking drugs

The effects of non-depolarising neuromuscular-blocking agents are mainly due to motor paralysis, although some of the drugs also produce clinically significant autonomic effects.

▼ The first muscles to be affected are the extrinsic eye muscles (causing double vision), reminiscent of the disease myasthenia gravis, which is caused by autoantibodies directed against nAChR (see p. 175-176), and the small muscles of the face, limbs and pharynx (causing difficulty in swallowing). Respiratory muscles are the last to be affected and the first to recover. An experiment in 1947 in which a heroic volunteer was fully curarised while conscious under artificial ventilation established this orderly paralytic march, and showed that consciousness and awareness of pain were quite normal even when paralysis was complete.[4]

---

[4]The risk of patients waking up paralysed during surgery is a serious worry for anaesthetists.

Table 13.7 Characteristics of neuromuscular-blocking drugs[a]

Drug	Speed of onset	Duration of action	Main side effects	Notes
Tubocurarine	Slow (>5 min)	Long (1–2 h)	Hypotension (ganglion block plus histamine release) Bronchoconstriction (histamine release)	Plant alkaloid, now rarely used Alcuronium is a semisynthetic derivative with similar properties but fewer side effects
Pancuronium	Intermediate (2–3 min)	Long (1–2 h)	Slight tachycardia Hypertension	The first steroid-based compound Better side effect profile than tubocurarine Widely used Pipecuronium is similar
Vecuronium	Intermediate	Intermediate (30–40 min)	Few side effects	Widely used Occasionally causes prolonged paralysis, probably owing to active metabolite Rocuronium is similar, with faster onset
Atracurium	Intermediate	Intermediate (<30 min)	Transient hypotension (histamine release)	Unusual mechanism of elimination (spontaneous non-enzymic chemical degradation in plasma); degradation slowed by acidosis Widely used Doxacurium is chemically similar but stable in plasma, giving it long duration of action Cisatracurium is the pure active isomeric constituent of atracurium, more potent but with less histamine release
Mivacurium	Fast (~2 min)	Short (~15 min)	Transient hypotension (histamine release)	Chemically similar to atracurium but rapidly inactivated by plasma cholinesterase (therefore longer acting in patients with liver disease or with genetic cholinesterase deficiency [see p. 172 and Ch. 11])
Suxamethonium	Fast	Short (~10 min)	Bradycardia (muscarinic agonist effect) Cardiac dysrhythmias (increased plasma K^+ concentration – avoid in patients with burns or severe trauma) Raised intraocular pressure (nicotinic agonist effect on extraocular muscles) Postoperative muscle pain	Acts by depolarisation of endplate (nicotinic agonist effect) – the only drug of this type still in use Paralysis is preceded by transient muscle fasciculations Short duration of action owing to hydrolysis by plasma cholinesterase (prolonged action in patients with liver disease or genetic deficiency of plasma cholinesterase) Used for brief procedures (e.g. tracheal intubation, electroconvulsive shock therapy) Rocuronium has similar speed of onset and recovery, with fewer unwanted effects

[a]For chemical structures, see Hardman JG, Limbird LE, Gilman AG, Goodman-Gilman A et al. 2001 Goodman and Gilman's Pharmacological Basis of Therapeutics, tenth ed. McGraw–Hill, New York.

Unwanted effects
The main side effect of tubocurarine is a fall in arterial pressure, due to (a) ganglion block and (b) histamine release from mast cells (see Ch. 17), which can also give rise to bronchospasm in sensitive individuals. This is unrelated to nAChRs but also occurs with **atracurium** and **mivacurium** (as well as with some unrelated drugs such as morphine; see Ch. 42). The other non-depolarising blocking drugs lack these side effects, and hence cause less hypotension. **Pancuronium** also blocks mAChRs, particularly in the heart, which results in tachycardia.

Pharmacokinetic aspects
Neuromuscular-blocking agents are used mainly in anaesthesia to produce muscle relaxation. They are given intravenously but differ in their rates of onset and recovery (Fig. 13.6 and Table 13.7).

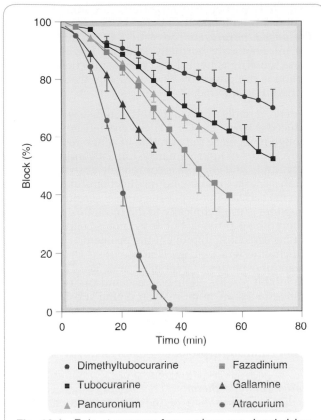

Fig. 13.6 Rate of recovery from various non-depolarising neuromuscular-blocking drugs in humans. Drugs were given intravenously to patients undergoing surgery, in doses just sufficient to cause 100% block of the tetanic tension of the indirectly stimulated adductor pollicis muscle. Recovery of tension was then followed as a function of time. *(From Payne JP, Hughes R 1981 Br J Anaesth 53, 45.)*

Legend:
- Dimethyltubocurarine
- Tubocurarine
- Pancuronium
- Fazadinium
- Gallamine
- Atracurium

Most of the non-depolarising blocking agents are metabolised by the liver or excreted unchanged in the urine, exceptions being **atracurium**, which hydrolyses spontaneously in plasma, and **mivacurium**, which, like **suxamethonium** (see below), is hydrolysed by plasma cholinesterase. Their duration of action varies between about 15 min and 1–2 h (Table 13.7), by which time the patient regains enough strength to cough and breathe properly. The route of elimination is important, because many patients undergoing anaesthesia have impaired renal or hepatic function, which, depending on the drug used, can enhance or prolong the paralysis to an important degree.

Atracurium was designed to be chemically unstable at physiological pH (splitting into two inactive fragments by cleavage at one of the quaternary nitrogen atoms), although indefinitely stable when stored at an acid pH. It has a short duration of action, which is unaffected by renal or hepatic function. Because of the marked pH dependence of its degradation, however, its action becomes considerably briefer during respiratory alkalosis caused by hyperventilation.

Rapid postoperative recovery of muscle strength is needed to reduce the risk of complications. The cholinesterase inhibitor, **neostigmine** (see Table 13.8) is often used to reverse the action of non-depolarising drugs postoperatively. Co-administration of atropine is necessary to prevent unwanted parasympathomimetic effects. An alternative approach (recently licensed for reversal of neuromuscular blockade induced by **rocuronium** or **vecuronium**) is the use of a synthetic cyclodextrin, **sugammadex**, a macromolecule that selectively binds steroidal neuromuscular blocking drugs as an inactive complex in the plasma. The complex is excreted unchanged in the urine. Sugammadex is claimed to produce more rapid reversal of block with fewer unwanted effects than neostigmine.

DEPOLARISING BLOCKING AGENTS

▼ This class of neuromuscular-blocking drugs was discovered by Paton and Zaimis in their study of the effects of symmetrical bis-quaternary ammonium compounds. One of these, **decamethonium**, was found to cause paralysis without appreciable ganglion-blocking activity. Several features of its action showed it to be different from competitive blocking drugs. In particular, it was found to produce a transient twitching of skeletal muscle (fasciculation) before causing block, and when it was injected into chicks it caused a powerful extensor spasm,[5] rather than flaccid paralysis. In 1951, B.D. Burns and Paton showed that it acted as an agonist, causing a maintained depolarisation at the endplate region of the muscle fibre, which led to a loss of electrical excitability, and they coined the term 'depolarisation block'. Fasciculation occurs because the developing endplate depolarisation initially causes a discharge of action potentials in the muscle fibre. This subsides after a few seconds as the electrical excitability of the endplate region of the fibre is lost. Decamethonium itself was used clinically but has the disadvantage of too long a duration of action.

Suxamethonium (Table 13.7) – the only depolarising blocking drug currently used – is closely related in structure to both decamethonium and ACh (consisting of two ACh molecules linked by their acetyl groups) and acts similarly, but its action lasts only a few minutes, because it is quickly hydrolysed by plasma cholinesterase. When given intravenously, however, its depolarising action lasts for long enough to cause the endplate region of the muscle fibres to become inexcitable. ACh, in contrast, when released from the nerve, reaches the endplate in very brief spurts and is rapidly hydrolysed *in situ*, so it never causes sufficiently prolonged depolarisation (10 to 100 milliseconds) to result in block. If cholinesterase is inhibited, however, it is possible for the circulating ACh concentration to reach a level sufficient to cause depolarisation block.

Comparison of non-depolarising and depolarising blocking drugs

▼ There are several differences in the pattern of neuromuscular block produced by depolarising and non-depolarising mechanisms:

- Anticholinesterase drugs are very effective in overcoming the blocking action of competitive, non-depolarising agents. This is because the released ACh, protected from hydrolysis, can diffuse further within the synaptic cleft, and so gains access to a wider area of postsynaptic membrane. The chances of an ACh molecule finding an unoccupied receptor before being hydrolysed are thus increased. This diffusional effect seems to be of more importance than a truly competitive interaction, for it is unlikely that appreciable dissociation of the antagonist can occur in the

---

[5]Birds (and frogs) possess a special type of skeletal muscle, rare in mammals, that has many endplates scattered over the surface of each muscle fibre. Agonists cause a diffuse depolarisation in such muscles, resulting in a graded and maintained contracture. In normal skeletal muscle, with only one endplate per fibre, endplate depolarisation is too localised to cause contracture on its own.

short time for which the ACh is present. In contrast, depolarisation block is unaffected, or even increased (via potentiation of the depolarising action of ACh), by anticholinesterase drugs.

- The fasciculations seen with suxamethonium (see Table 13.7) as a prelude to paralysis do not occur with competitive drugs. There appears to be a correlation between the amount of fasciculation and the severity of the postoperative muscle pain reported after suxamethonium.
- *Tetanic fade* (a term used to describe the failure of muscle tension to be maintained during a brief period of nerve stimulation at a frequency high enough to produce a fused tetanus) is increased by non-depolarising blocking drugs, compared with normal muscle. This is due mainly to the block of presynaptic nAChRs, which normally serve to sustain transmitter release during a tetanus, and it does not occur with depolarisation block.

Unwanted effects and dangers of suxamethonium

Suxamethonium has several adverse effects (see Table 13.7), but remains in use because of the rapid recovery that follows its withdrawal – significantly more rapid than the recovery from non-depolarising agents.

Bradycardia. This is preventable by atropine and is due to a direct muscarinic action.

Potassium release. The increase in cation permeability of the motor endplates causes a net loss of K^+ from muscle, and thus a small rise in plasma K^+ concentration. In normal individuals, this is not important, but in cases of trauma, especially burns or injuries causing muscle denervation, it may be (Fig. 13.7). This is because denervation causes ACh receptors to spread to regions of the muscle fibre away from the endplates (see Ch. 12), so that a much larger area of membrane is sensitive to suxamethonium. The resulting hyperkalaemia can be enough to cause ventricular dysrhythmia or even cardiac arrest.

Increased intraocular pressure. This results from contracture of extraocular muscles applying pressure to the eyeball. It is particularly important to avoid this if the eyeball has been injured.

Prolonged paralysis. The action of suxamethonium given intravenously normally lasts for less than 5 min, because the drug is hydrolysed by plasma cholinesterase. Its action is prolonged by various factors that reduce the activity of this enzyme:

- Genetic variants of plasma cholinesterase with reduced activity (see Ch. 11). Severe deficiency, enough to increase the duration of action to 2 h or more, occurs in approximately 1 in 3500 individuals. Very rarely, the enzyme is completely absent and paralysis lasts for many hours. Biochemical testing of enzyme activity in the plasma and its sensitivity to inhibitors is used clinically to diagnose this problem; genotyping is possible but as yet not practicable for routine screening to prevent the problem.
- Anticholinesterase drugs. The use of organophosphates to treat glaucoma (see Table 13.4) can inhibit plasma cholinesterase and prolong the action of suxamethonium. Competing substrates for plasma cholinesterase (e.g. **procaine**, **propanidid**) can also have this effect.
- Neonates may have low plasma cholinesterase activity and show prolonged paralysis with suxamethonium.

Malignant hyperthermia. This is a rare inherited condition, due to a mutation of the Ca^{2+} release channel of the sarcoplasmic reticulum (the ryanodine receptor, see Ch. 4), which results in intense muscle spasm and a dramatic rise in body temperature when certain drugs are given (see Ch. 11). Suxamethonium is now the commonest culprit, although it can be precipitated by a variety of other drugs. The condition carries a very high mortality (about 65%) and is treated by administration of **dantrolene**, a drug that inhibits muscle contraction by preventing Ca^{2+} release from the sarcoplasmic reticulum.

DRUGS THAT ACT PRESYNAPTICALLY

DRUGS THAT INHIBIT ACETYLCHOLINE SYNTHESIS

The steps in the synthesis of ACh in the presynaptic nerve terminals are shown in Figure 13.2. The rate-limiting process appears to be the transport of choline into the nerve terminal. **Hemicholinium** blocks this transport and thereby inhibits ACh synthesis. It is useful as an experimental tool but has no clinical applications. Its blocking effect on transmission develops slowly, as the existing stores of ACh become depleted. **Vesamicol**, which acts by blocking ACh transport into synaptic vesicles, has a similar effect.

DRUGS THAT INHIBIT ACETYLCHOLINE RELEASE

Acetylcholine release by a nerve impulse involves the entry of Ca^{2+} into the nerve terminal; the increase in $[Ca^{2+}]_i$ stimulates exocytosis and increases the rate of quantal release (Fig. 13.2). Agents that inhibit Ca^{2+} entry include Mg^{2+} and various aminoglycoside antibiotics (e.g. **streptomycin** and **neomycin**; see Ch. 51), which can unpredictably prolong muscle paralysis when used clinically in patients treated with neuromuscular blocking agents as an adjunct to general anaesthesia.

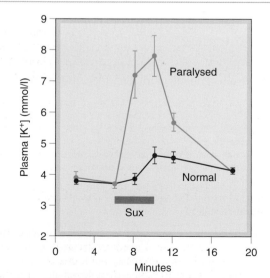

Fig. 13.7 **Effect of suxamethonium (Sux) on plasma potassium concentration in humans.** Blood was collected from veins draining paralysed and non-paralysed limbs of seven injured patients undergoing surgery. The injuries had resulted in motor nerve degeneration, and hence denervation supersensitivity of the affected muscles. *(From Tobey RE et al. 1972 Anaesthesiology 37, 322.)*

Neuromuscular-blocking drugs

- Substances that block choline uptake: for example **hemicholinium** (not used clinically).
- Substances that block acetylcholine release: **aminoglycoside antibiotics**, **botulinum toxin**.
- Drugs used to cause paralysis during anaesthesia are as follows:
  - Depolarising neuromuscular-blocking agents: **suxamethonium**, short acting and used during induction of anaesthesia and intubation of the airway.
  - Non-depolarising neuromuscular-blocking agents: **tubocurarine, pancuronium, atracurium, vecuronium, mivacuronium**. These act as competitive antagonists at nicotinic acetylcholine receptors and differ mainly in duration of action; used to maintain neuromuscular relaxation throughout an operation which may be of several hours duration or when unconscious in an intensive care unit.
- Important characteristics of non-depolarising and depolarising blocking drugs:
  - Non-depolarising block is reversible by anticholinesterase drugs, depolarising block is not.
  - Steroidal ('curonium') drugs (**rocuronium, vecuronium**) are reversed by **sugammadex**.
  - Depolarising block produces initial fasciculations and often postoperative muscle pain.
  - **Suxamethonium** is hydrolysed by plasma cholinesterase and is normally very short-acting, but may cause long-lasting paralysis in a small group of congenitally cholinesterase-deficient individuals.
- Main side effects: early curare derivatives caused ganglion block, histamine release, hence hypotension, bronchoconstriction; newer non-depolarising blocking drugs have fewer side effects; **suxamethonium** may cause bradycardia, cardiac dysrhythmias due to K^+ release (especially in burned or injured patients), increased intraocular pressure, malignant hyperthermia (rare).

Two potent neurotoxins, namely **botulinum toxin** and **β-bungarotoxin**, act specifically to inhibit ACh release. Botulinum toxin is a protein produced by the anaerobic bacillus *Clostridium botulinum*, an organism that can multiply in preserved food and can cause botulism, an extremely serious type of food poisoning.[6]

▼ The potency of botulinum toxin is extraordinary, the minimum lethal dose in a mouse being less than 10^{-12} g – only a few million molecules. It belongs to the group of potent bacterial exotoxins that includes tetanus and diphtheria toxins. They possess two subunits, one of which binds to a membrane receptor and is responsible for cellular specificity. By this means, the toxin enters the cell, where

the other subunit produces the toxic effect. Botulinum toxin contains several components (A–G, see Chen et al., 2012). They are peptidases that cleave specific proteins involved in exocytosis (*synaptobrevins, syntaxins*, etc.; see Ch. 4), thereby producing a long-lasting block of synaptic function. Each toxin component inactivates a different functional protein – a remarkably coordinated attack by a humble bacterium on a vital component of mammalian physiology.

Botulinum poisoning causes progressive parasympathetic and motor paralysis, with dry mouth, blurred vision and difficulty in swallowing, followed by progressive respiratory paralysis. Treatment with antitoxin is effective only if given before symptoms appear, for once the toxin is bound its action cannot be reversed. Mortality is high, and recovery takes several weeks. Anticholinesterases and drugs that increase transmitter release are ineffective in restoring transmission. **Botulinum toxin**, given by local injection, has a number of clinical and cosmetic uses (a testament to Paracelsus' dictum that all drugs are poisons, the distinction lying in the dose), including:

- *blepharospasm* (persistent and disabling eyelid spasm) and other forms of unwanted movement disorder including *torsion dystonia* and *spasmodic torticollis* (twisting movements of, respectively, limbs or neck)
- *spasticity* (excessive extensor muscle tone, associated with developmental brain abnormalities or birth injury)
- *urinary incontinence* associated with bladder overactivity (given by intravesical injection)
- *squint* (given by injection into extraocular muscles)
- *hyperhidrosis* (injected intradermally into axillary skin), for excessive sweating resistant to other treatment
- *sialorrhoea* (excessive salivary secretion)
- *headache prophylaxis* (in adults with chronic migraine and frequent headaches)
- *forehead wrinkles* (injected intradermally it removes frown lines by paralysing the superficial muscles that pucker the skin).

Injections need to be repeated every few months. Botulinum toxin is antigenic, and may lose its effectiveness due to its immunogenicity. There is a risk of more general muscle paralysis if the toxin spreads beyond the injected region.

▼ β-Bungarotoxin is a protein contained in the venom of various snakes of the cobra family, and has a similar action to botulinum toxin, although its active component is a phospholipase rather than a peptidase. The same venoms also contain α-bungarotoxin (Ch. 3), which blocks postsynaptic ACh receptors. These snakes evidently cover all eventualities as far as causing paralysis of their victims is concerned.

DRUGS THAT ENHANCE CHOLINERGIC TRANSMISSION

Drugs that enhance cholinergic transmission act either by inhibiting cholinesterase (the main group) or by increasing ACh release. In this chapter, we focus on the peripheral actions of such drugs; drugs affecting cholinergic transmission in the CNS, used to treat senile dementia, are discussed in Chapter 40.

DISTRIBUTION AND FUNCTION OF CHOLINESTERASE

There are two distinct types of cholinesterase, namely *acetylcholinesterase* (AChE) and *butyrylcholinesterase* (BuChE, sometimes called pseudocholinesterase), closely related in

[6]Among the more spectacular outbreaks of botulinum poisoning was an incident on Loch Maree in Scotland in 1922, when all eight members of a fishing party died after eating duck pâté for their lunch. Their ghillies, consuming humbler fare no doubt, survived. The innkeeper committed suicide.

molecular structure but differing in their distribution, substrate specificity and functions. Both consist of globular catalytic subunits, which constitute the soluble forms found in plasma (BuChE) and cerebrospinal fluid (AChE). Elsewhere, the catalytic units are linked to accessory proteins, which tether them like a bunch of balloons to the basement membrane (at the neuromuscular junction) or to the neuronal membrane at neuronal synapses (and also, oddly, the erythrocyte membrane, where the function of the enzyme is unknown).

The bound AChE at cholinergic synapses serves to hydrolyse the released transmitter and terminate its action rapidly. Soluble AChE is also present in cholinergic nerve terminals, where it has a role in regulating the free ACh concentration, and from which it may be secreted; the function of the secreted enzyme is so far unclear. AChE is quite specific for ACh and closely related esters such as methacholine. Certain neuropeptides, such as substance P (Ch. 17) are inactivated by AChE, but it is not known whether this is of physiological significance. Overall, there is poor correspondence between the distribution of cholinergic synapses and that of AChE, both in the brain and in the periphery, and AChE most probably has synaptic functions other than disposal of ACh, although the details remain unclear (see review by Silman & Sussman, 2005; Zimmerman & Soreq, 2006).

Butyrylcholinesterase (BuChE) has a widespread distribution, being found in tissues such as liver, skin, brain and gastrointestinal smooth muscle, as well as in soluble form in the plasma. It is not particularly associated with cholinergic synapses, and its physiological function is unclear. It has a broader substrate specificity than AChE. It hydrolyses the synthetic substrate butyrylcholine more rapidly than ACh, as well as other esters, such as **procaine**, **suxamethonium** and **propanidid** (a short-acting anaesthetic agent; see Ch. 41). The plasma enzyme is important in relation to the inactivation of the drugs listed above. Genetic variants of BuChE causing significantly reduced enzymic activity occur rarely (see Ch. 11), and these partly account for the variability in the duration of action of these drugs. The very short duration of action of ACh given intravenously (see Fig. 13.1) results from its rapid hydrolysis in the plasma. Normally, AChE and BuChE between them keep the plasma ACh at an undetectably low level, so ACh is strictly a neurotransmitter and not a hormone.

▼ Both AChE and BuChE belong to the class of serine hydrolases, which includes many proteases such as trypsin. The active site of AChE comprises two distinct regions (Fig. 13.8): an *anionic site* (glutamate residue), which binds the basic (choline) moiety of ACh; and an *esteratic (catalytic) site* (histidine + serine). As with other serine hydrolases, the acidic (acetyl) group of the substrate is transferred to the serine hydroxyl group, leaving (transiently) an acetylated enzyme molecule and a molecule of free choline. Spontaneous hydrolysis of the serine acetyl group occurs rapidly, and the overall turnover number of AChE is extremely high (over 10 000 molecules of ACh hydrolysed per second by a single active site).

DRUGS THAT INHIBIT CHOLINESTERASE

Peripherally acting anticholinesterase drugs, summarised in Table 13.8, fall into three main groups according to the nature of their interaction with the active site, which determines their duration of action. Most of them inhibit AChE and BuChE about equally. Centrally acting anticholinesterases, developed for the treatment of dementia, are discussed in Chapter 40.

Short-acting anticholinesterases

The only important drug of this type is **edrophonium**, a quaternary ammonium compound that binds to the anionic site of the enzyme only. The ionic bond formed is readily reversible, and the action of the drug is very brief. It is used mainly for diagnostic purposes, because improvement of muscle strength by an anticholinesterase is characteristic of myasthenia gravis (see p. 175-176) but does not occur when muscle weakness is due to other causes.

Medium-duration anticholinesterases

These include **neostigmine** and **pyridostigmine**, which are quaternary ammonium compounds of clinical importance, and **physostigmine** (eserine), a tertiary amine, which occurs naturally in the Calabar bean.[7]

These drugs are all carbamyl, as opposed to acetyl, esters and all possess basic groups that bind to the anionic site. Transfer of the carbamyl group to the serine hydroxyl group of the esteratic site occurs as with ACh, but the carbamylated enzyme is very much slower to hydrolyse (Fig. 13.8), taking minutes rather than microseconds. The anticholinesterase drug is therefore hydrolysed, but at a negligible rate compared with ACh, and the slow recovery of the carbamylated enzyme means that the action of these drugs is quite long-lasting.

Irreversible anticholinesterases

Irreversible anticholinesterases (Table 13.8) are pentavalent phosphorus compounds containing a labile group such as fluoride (in **dyflos**) or an organic group (in **parathion** and **ecothiophate**). This group is released, leaving the serine hydroxyl group of the enzyme phosphorylated (Fig. 13.8). Most of these organophosphate compounds, of which there are many, were developed as war gases, such as **sarin**, and pesticides as well as for clinical use; they interact only with the esteratic site of the enzyme and have no cationic group. **Ecothiophate** is an exception in having a quaternary nitrogen group designed to bind also to the anionic site.

The inactive phosphorylated enzyme is usually very stable. With drugs such as dyflos, no appreciable hydrolysis occurs, and recovery of enzymic activity depends on the synthesis of new enzyme molecules, a process that may take weeks. With other drugs, such as ecothiophate, slow hydrolysis occurs over the course of a few days, so that their action is not strictly irreversible. Dyflos and parathion are volatile non-polar substances of very high lipid solubility, and are rapidly absorbed through mucous membranes and even through unbroken skin and insect cuticles; the use of these agents as war gases or insecticides relies on this property. The lack of a specificity-conferring quaternary group means that most of these drugs block other serine hydrolases (e.g. trypsin, thrombin), although their pharmacological effects result mainly from cholinesterase inhibition.

Effects of anticholinesterase drugs

Cholinesterase inhibitors affect peripheral as well as central cholinergic synapses.

Some organophosphate compounds can produce, in addition, a severe form of neurotoxicity.

---

[7]Otherwise known as the ordeal bean. In the Middle Ages, extracts of these beans were used to determine the guilt or innocence of those accused of crime or heresy. Death implied guilt.

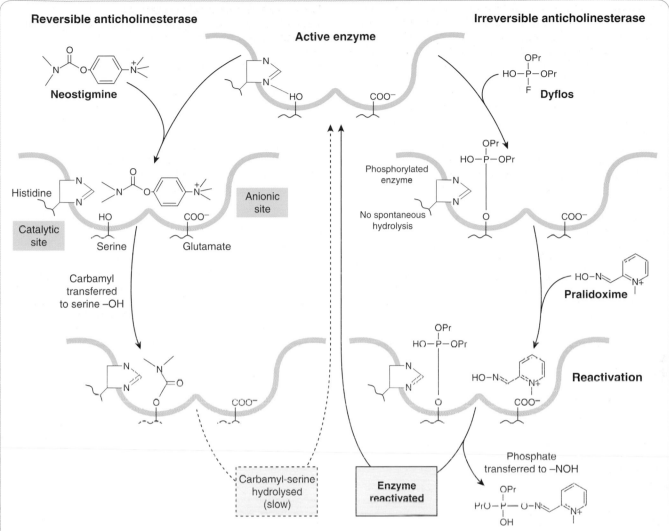

Fig. 13.8 Action of anticholinesterase drugs. Reversible anticholinesterase (neostigmine): recovery of activity by hydrolysis of the carbamylated enzyme takes many minutes. Irreversible anticholinesterase (dyflos): reactivation of phosphorylated enzyme by pralidoxime. The representation of the active site is purely diagrammatic and by no means representative of the actual molecular structure.

Effects on autonomic cholinergic synapses. These mainly reflect enhancement of ACh activity at parasympathetic postganglionic synapses (i.e. increased secretions from salivary, lacrimal, bronchial and gastrointestinal glands; increased peristaltic activity; bronchoconstriction; bradycardia and hypotension; pupillary constriction; fixation of accommodation for near vision; fall in intraocular pressure). Large doses can stimulate, and later block, autonomic ganglia, producing complex autonomic effects. The block, if it occurs, is a depolarisation block and is associated with a build-up of ACh in the plasma and body fluids. Neostigmine and pyridostigmine tend to affect neuromuscular transmission more than the autonomic system, whereas physostigmine and organophosphates show the reverse pattern. The reason is not clear, but therapeutic usage takes advantage of this partial selectivity.

Acute anticholinesterase poisoning (e.g. from contact with insecticides or war gases) causes severe bradycardia, hypotension and difficulty in breathing. Combined with a depolarising neuromuscular block and central effects (see p. 174), the result may be fatal.

Effects on the neuromuscular junction. The twitch tension of a muscle stimulated via its motor nerve is increased by anticholinesterases, owing to repetitive firing in the muscle fibre associated with prolongation of the epp. Normally, the ACh is hydrolysed so quickly that each stimulus initiates only one action potential in the muscle fibre, but when AChE is inhibited this is converted to a short train of action potentials in the muscle fibre, and hence greater tension. Much more important is the effect produced when transmission has been blocked by a nondepolarising blocking agent such as pancuronium. In this case, addition of an anticholinesterase can dramatically restore transmission. If a large proportion of the receptors is blocked, the majority of ACh molecules will normally encounter, and be destroyed by, an AChE molecule before reaching a vacant receptor; inhibiting AChE gives the ACh molecules a greater chance of finding a vacant receptor before being destroyed, and thus increase the epp so that it reaches threshold. In myasthenia gravis (see p. 175-176), transmission fails because there are too few ACh receptors, and cholinesterase inhibition improves transmission just as it does in curarised muscle.

Table 13.8 Anticholinesterase drugs

Drug	Structure	Duration of action	Main site of action	Notes
Edrophonium		Short	NMJ	Used mainly in diagnosis of myasthenia gravis Too short-acting for therapeutic use
Neostigmine		Medium	NMJ	Used intravenously to reverse competitive neuromuscular block Used orally in treatment of myasthenia gravis Visceral side effects
Physostigmine		Medium	P	Used as eye drops in treatment of glaucoma
Pyridostigmine		Medium	NMJ	Used orally in treatment of myasthenia gravis Better absorbed than neostigmine and has longer duration of action
Dyflos		Long	P	Highly toxic organophosphate, with very prolonged action Has been used as eye drops for glaucoma
Ecothiophate		Long	P	Used as eye drops in treatment of glaucoma Prolonged action; may cause systemic effects
Parathion		Long	–	Converted to active metabolite by replacement of sulfur by oxygen Used as insecticide but also causes poisoning in humans

Other anticholinesterase drugs developed for the treatment of dementia are described in Chapter 40.

NMJ, neuromuscular junction; P, postganglionic parasympathetic junction.

In large doses, such as can occur in poisoning, anticholinesterases initially cause twitching of muscles. This is because spontaneous ACh release can give rise to epps that reach the firing threshold. Later, paralysis may occur due to depolarisation block, which is associated with the build-up of ACh in the plasma and tissue fluids.

Effects on the CNS. Tertiary compounds, such as physostigmine, and the non-polar organophosphates penetrate the blood–brain barrier freely and affect the brain. The result is an initial excitation, which can result in convulsions, followed by depression, which can cause unconsciousness and respiratory failure. These central effects result mainly from the activation of mAChRs, and are antagonised by atropine. The use of anticholinesterases to treat senile dementia is discussed in Chapter 40.

Neurotoxicity of organophosphates. Many organophosphates can cause a severe type of delayed peripheral nerve degeneration, leading to progressive weakness and sensory loss. This is not a problem with clinically used anticholinesterases but occasionally results from poisoning with insecticides or nerve gases. In 1931, an estimated 20 000 Americans were affected, some fatally, by contamination of fruit juice with an organophosphate insecticide,

and other similar outbreaks have been recorded. The mechanism of this reaction is only partly understood, but it seems to result from inhibition of a *neuropathy target esterase* distinct from cholinesterase. Chronic low level exposure of agricultural and other workers to organophosphorous pesticides has been associated with neurobehavioural disorders (Jamal et al., 2002).

The main uses of anticholinesterases are summarised in the clinical box (p. 175).

CHOLINESTERASE REACTIVATION

Spontaneous hydrolysis of phosphorylated cholinesterase is extremely slow, so poisoning with organophosphates necessitates prolonged supportive care. **Pralidoxime** (Fig. 13.8) reactivates the enzyme by bringing an oxime group into close proximity with the phosphorylated esteratic site. This group is a strong nucleophile and lures the phosphate group away from the serine hydroxyl group of the enzyme. The effectiveness of pralidoxime in reactivating plasma cholinesterase activity in a poisoned subject is shown in Figure 13.9. The main limitation to its use as an antidote to organophosphate poisoning is that, within a few hours, the phosphorylated enzyme undergoes a

Cholinesterase and anticholinesterase drugs

- There are two main forms of cholinesterase: *acetylcholinesterase* (AChE), which is mainly membrane-bound, relatively specific for acetylcholine, and responsible for rapid acetylcholine hydrolysis at cholinergic synapses; and *butyrylcholinesterase* (BuChE) or pseudocholinesterase, which is relatively non-selective and occurs in plasma and many tissues. Both enzymes belong to the family of serine hydrolases.
- Anticholinesterase drugs are of three main types: short-acting (**edrophonium**); medium-acting (**neostigmine, physostigmine**); irreversible (organophosphates, **dyflos, ecothiophate**). They differ in the nature of their chemical interaction with the active site of cholinesterase.
- Effects of anticholinesterase drugs are due mainly to enhancement of cholinergic transmission at cholinergic autonomic synapses and at the neuromuscular junction. Anticholinesterases that cross the blood–brain barrier (e.g. **physostigmine**, organophosphates) also have marked central nervous system effects. Autonomic effects include bradycardia, hypotension, excessive secretions, bronchoconstriction, gastrointestinal hypermotility and decrease of intraocular pressure. Neuromuscular action causes muscle fasciculation and increased twitch tension, and can produce depolarisation block.
- Anticholinesterase poisoning may occur from exposure to insecticides or nerve gases.

Clinical uses of anticholinesterase drugs

- To reverse the action of non-depolarising neuromuscular-blocking drugs at the end of an operation (**neostigmine**). **Atropine** must be given to limit parasympathomimetic effects.
- To treat myasthenia gravis (**neostigmine** or **pyridostigmine**).
- As a test for myasthenia gravis and to distinguish weakness caused by anticholinesterase overdosage ('cholinergic crisis') from the weakness of myasthenia itself ('myasthenic crisis'): **edrophonium**, a short-acting drug given intravenously.
- Alzheimer's disease (e.g. **donepezil**; see Ch. 40).
- Glaucoma (**ecothiophate** eye drops).

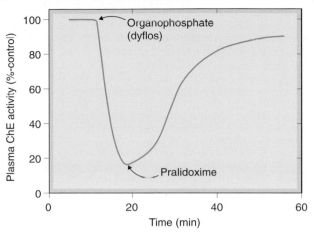

Fig. 13.9 Reactivation of plasma cholinesterase (ChE) in a volunteer subject by intravenous injection of pralidoxime.

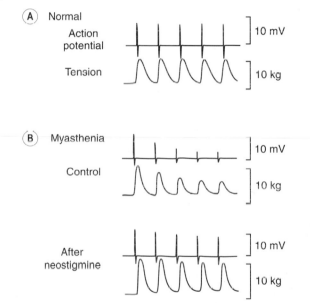

Fig. 13.10 Neuromuscular transmission in a normal and a myasthenic human subject. Electrical activity was recorded with a needle electrode in the adductor pollicis muscle, in response to ulnar nerve stimulation (3 Hz) at the wrist. In a normal subject, electrical and mechanical response is well sustained. In a myasthenic patient, transmission fails rapidly when the nerve is stimulated. Treatment with neostigmine improves transmission. *(From Desmedt JE 1962 Bull Acad R Med Belg VII 2, 213.)*

Myasthenia gravis

▼ The neuromuscular junction is a robust structure that very rarely fails, myasthenia gravis and the Lambert–Eaton myasthenic syndrome (see p. 176) being two of the few disorders that specifically affects it. Myasthenia gravis affects about 1 in 2000 individuals, who show muscle weakness and increased fatiguability resulting from a failure of neuromuscular transmission. The tendency for transmission to fail during repetitive activity can be seen in Figure 13.10. Functionally, it results in the inability of muscles to produce

chemical change ('ageing') that renders it no longer susceptible to reactivation, so that pralidoxime must be given early in order to work. Pralidoxime does not enter the brain, but related compounds have been developed to treat the central effects of organophosphate poisoning.

sustained contractions, of which the characteristic drooping eyelids of myasthenic patients are a sign. The effectiveness of anticholinesterase drugs in improving muscle strength in myasthenia was discovered in 1931, long before the cause of the disease was known.

The cause of the transmission failure is an autoimmune response that causes a loss of nAChRs from the neuromuscular junction, first revealed in studies showing that the number of bungarotoxin-binding sites at the endplates of myasthenic patients was reduced by about 70% compared with normal. It had been suspected that myasthenia had an immunological basis, because removal of the thymus gland is frequently of benefit. Immunisation of rabbits with purified ACh receptor causes, after a delay, symptoms very similar to those of human myasthenia gravis. The presence of antibody directed against the ACh receptor protein can be detected in the serum of myasthenic patients, but the reason for the development of the autoimmune response in humans is unknown (Vrolix et al., 2010).

The improvement of neuromuscular function by anticholinesterase treatment (shown in Fig. 13.10) can be dramatic, but if the disease progresses too far, the number of receptors remaining may be insufficient to produce an adequate epp, and anticholinesterase drugs will then cease to be effective.

Alternative approaches to the treatment of myasthenia are to remove circulating antibody by plasma exchange, which is transiently effective, or, for a more prolonged effect, to inhibit antibody production with immunosuppressant drugs (e.g. **prednisolone**, **azathioprine**; see Ch. 26) or thymectomy.

OTHER DRUGS THAT ENHANCE CHOLINERGIC TRANSMISSION

It was observed many years ago that **tetraethylammonium**, a potassium-channel blocker and ganglion-blocking drug, could reverse the neuromuscular-blocking action of tubocurarine by prolonging the action potential in the nerve terminal and hence increasing the release of transmitter evoked by nerve stimulation. Subsequently, aminopyridines such as **amifampridine**, which also block potassium channels (see Ch. 4) were found to act similarly and to be considerably more potent and selective in their actions than tetraethylammonium. These drugs are not selective for cholinergic nerves but increase the evoked release of many different transmitters. Amifampridine (licensed in 2010) is used to treat the muscle weakness associated with Lambert–Eaton myasthenic syndrome (Maddison & Newsom-Davis, 2003), a complication of certain neoplastic diseases in which acetylcholine release is inhibited because antitumour antibodies cross react with Ca^{2+} channels on the prejunctional membrane.

▼ A related drug, **fampridine**, improves walking in patients whose walking is impaired by the demyelinating disease multiple sclerosis. It works by blocking axonal K^+ channels, thereby facilitating impulse conduction along demyelinated axons.

REFERENCES AND FURTHER READING

General reference

Nicholls, J.G., Martin, A.R., Fuchs, P.A., Brown, D.A., Diamond, M.E., Weisblat, D., 2012. From neuron to brain, fifth ed. Sinauer, Sunderland. (*Excellent general textbook*)

Acetylcholine receptors

Alexander S.P.H., Benson, H.E., Faccenda, E., et al., 2013. Concise Guide to Pharmacology [Acetylcholine receptors (muscarinic), p. 1474 Nicotininc acetylcholine receptors, p. 1597]. Br. J. Pharmacol. 170, 1449–1896.

Conn, P.J., Jones, C.K., Lindsley, C.W., 2009. Subtype-selective allosteric modulators of muscarinic receptors for the treatment of CNS disorders. Trends Pharmacol. Sci. 30 (3), 148–155. (*Describes development of novel allosteric mAChR modulators as potential therapeutic agents*)

Kalamida, D., Poulas, K., Avramopoulou, V., et al., 2007. Muscle and neuronal nicotinic acetylcholine receptors: structure, function and pathogenicity. FEBS J. 274, 3799–3845. (*Excellent comprehensive review*)

Wess, J., Eglen, R.M., Gautam, D., 2007. Muscarinic acetylcholine receptors: mutant mice provide new insights for drug development. Nat. Rev. Drug Discov. 6, 721–733. (*Describes the subtle functional deficits in mice lacking particular receptor subtypes*)

Wessler, I., Kirkpatrick, C.J., 2008. Acetylcholine beyond neurons: the non-neuronal cholinergic system in humans. Br. J. Pharmacol. 154, 1558–1571. (*Summarises recent findings that reveal surprisingly diverse roles for acetylcholine*)

Cholinergic transmission

Fagerlund, M.J., Eriksson, L.I., 2009. Current concepts in neuromuscular transmission. Br. J. Anaesth. 103, 108–114. (*Concentrates on recent findings of potential clinical importance*)

Vrolix, K., Fraussen, J., Molenaar, P.C., et al., 2010. The auto-antigen repertoire in myasthenia gravis. Autoimmunity 43, 380–400. (*Reviews the reported auto-antibodies and their roles in myasthenia gravis*)

Drugs affecting the neuromuscular junction

Chen, Z.X.P., Morris, J.G., Rodriguez, R.L., Shukla, A.W., Tapia-Nunez, J., Okun, M.S., 2012. Emerging opportunities for serotypes of botulinum neurotoxins. Toxins 4, 1196–1222. (*Reviews current research on botulinum serotypes A-G*)

Maddison, P., Newsom-Davis, J., 2003. Treatment for Lambert–Eaton myasthenic syndrome. Cochrane Database Syst. Rev. CD003279, doi:10.1002/14651858.CD003279.

Nicholson, W.T., Sprung, J., Jankowski, C.J., 2007. Sugammadex: a novel agent for the reversal of neuromuscular blockade. Pharmacotherapy 27, 1181–1188. (*An alternative to neostigmine*)

Cholinesterase

Jamal, G.A., Hansen, S., Julu, P.O., 2002. Low level exposures to organophosphorus esters may cause neurotoxicity. Toxicology 181/182, 23–33.

Silman, I., Sussman, J.L., 2005. Acetylcholinesterase: 'classical' and 'non-classical' functions and pharmacology. Curr. Opin. Pharmacol. 5, 293–302. (*Review, covering molecular structure, as well as functions of cholinesterase*)

Zimmerman, G., Soreq, H., 2006. Termination and beyond: acetylcholinesterase as a modulator of synaptic transmission. Cell Tissue Res. 326, 655–669. (*Speculative review of evidence suggesting functions for AChE other than ACh hydrolysis*)

14

Noradrenergic transmission

OVERVIEW

The peripheral noradrenergic neuron and the structures that it innervates are important targets for drug action, both as objects for investigation in their own right and as points of attack for many clinically useful drugs. In this chapter, we describe the physiology and function of noradrenergic neurons and the properties of adrenoceptors (the receptors on which noradrenaline and adrenaline act), and discuss the various classes of drugs that affect them. For convenience, much of the pharmacological information is summarised in tables later in the chapter.

CATECHOLAMINES

Catecholamines are compounds containing a catechol moiety (a benzene ring with two adjacent hydroxyl groups) and an amine side chain (Fig. 14.1). Pharmacologically, the most important ones are:

- **noradrenaline (norepinephrine)**, a transmitter released by sympathetic nerve terminals
- **adrenaline (epinephrine)**, a hormone secreted by the adrenal medulla
- **dopamine**, the metabolic precursor of noradrenaline and adrenaline, also a transmitter/neuromodulator in the central nervous system
- **isoprenaline (isoproterenol)**, a synthetic derivative of noradrenaline, not present in the body.

CLASSIFICATION OF ADRENOCEPTORS

In 1896, Oliver and Schafer discovered that injection of extracts of adrenal gland caused a rise in arterial pressure. Following the subsequent isolation of adrenaline as the active principle, it was shown by Dale in 1913 that adrenaline causes two distinct kinds of effect, namely vasoconstriction in certain vascular beds (which normally predominates and, together with its actions on the heart – see p. 184 – causes the rise in arterial pressure) and vasodilatation in others. Dale showed that the vasoconstrictor component disappeared if the animal was first injected with an ergot derivative[1] (see Ch. 15), and noticed that adrenaline then caused a fall, instead of a rise, in arterial pressure. This result paralleled Dale's demonstration of the

separate muscarinic and nicotinic components of the action of acetylcholine (see Ch. 13). He avoided interpreting it in terms of different types of receptor, but later pharmacological work, beginning with that of Ahlquist, showed clearly the existence of several subclasses of adrenoceptor with distinct tissue distributions and actions (Table 14.1).

Ahlquist found in 1948 that the rank order of the potencies of various catecholamines, including adrenaline, noradrenaline and isoprenaline, fell into two distinct patterns, depending on what response was being measured. He postulated the existence of two kinds of receptor, α and β, defined in terms of agonist potencies as follows:

α: noradrenaline > adrenaline > isoprenaline
β: isoprenaline > adrenaline > noradrenaline

It was then recognised that certain ergot alkaloids, which Dale had studied, act as selective α-receptor antagonists, and that Dale's adrenaline reversal experiment reflected the unmasking of the β effects of adrenaline by α-receptor blockade. Selective β-receptor antagonists were not developed until 1955, when their effects fully confirmed Ahlquist's original classification and also suggested the existence of further subdivisions of both α and β receptors. Subsequently it has emerged that there are two α-receptor subtypes (α_1 and α_2), each comprising three further subclasses (α_{1A}, α_{1B}, α_{1D} and α_{2A}, α_{2B}, α_{2C}) and three β-receptor subtypes (β_1, β_2 and β_3) – altogether nine distinct subtypes – all of which are typical G protein-coupled receptors (Table 14.2). Evidence from specific agonists and antagonists, as well as studies on receptor knockout mice (Philipp & Hein, 2004), has shown that α_1 receptors are particularly important in the cardiovascular system and lower urinary tract, while α_2 receptors are predominantly neuronal, acting to inhibit transmitter release both in the brain and at autonomic nerve terminals in the periphery. The distinct functions of the different subclasses of α_1 and α_2 adrenoceptors remain for the most part unclear; they are frequently co-expressed in the same tissues, and may form heterodimers, making pharmacological analysis difficult.

Each of the three main receptor subtypes is associated with a specific second messenger system (Table 14.2). Thus α_1 receptors are coupled to phospholipase C and produce their effects mainly by the release of intracellular Ca^{2+}; α_2 receptors are negatively coupled to adenylyl cyclase, and reduce cAMP formation as well as inhibiting Ca^{2+} channels and activating K^+ channels; and all three types of β receptor act by stimulation of adenylyl cyclase. The major effects that are produced by these receptors, and the main drugs that act on them, are shown in Tables 14.1 and 14.2; more detailed summaries of adrenoceptor agonists and antagonists are given later in Tables 14.4 and 14.5 respectively.

The distinction between β_1 and β_2 receptors is an important one, for β_1 receptors are found mainly in the heart, where they are responsible for the positive inotropic and chronotropic effects of catecholamines (see Ch. 21). β_2 receptors, on the other hand, are responsible for causing

---

[1] Dale was a new recruit in the laboratories of the Wellcome pharmaceutical company, given the job of checking the potency of batches of adrenaline coming from the factory. He tested one batch at the end of a day's experimentation on a cat that he had earlier injected with an ergot preparation. Because it produced a fall in blood pressure rather than the expected rise, he advised that the whole expensive consignment should be rejected. Unknown to him, he was given the same sample to test a few days later, and reported it to be normal. How he explained this to Wellcome's management is not recorded.

177

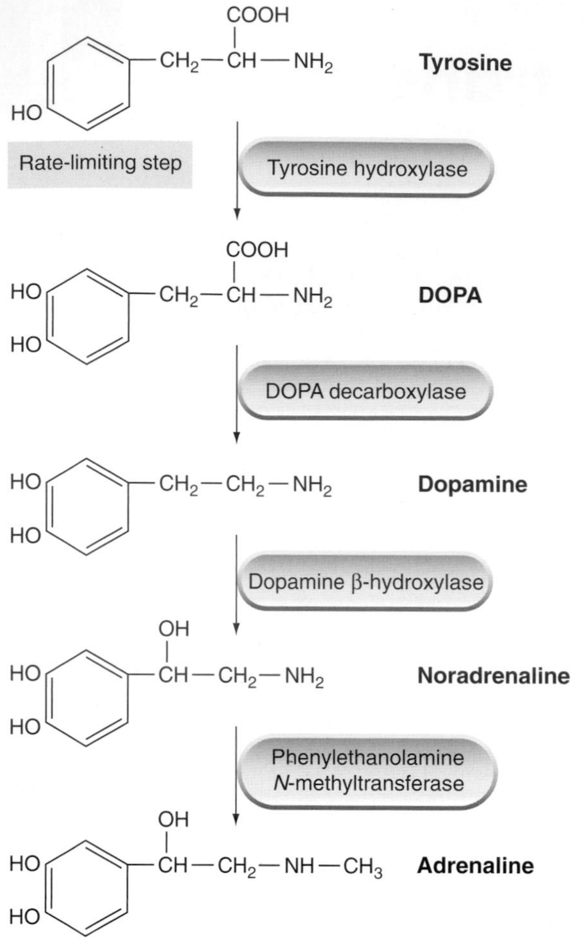

Fig. 14.1 Structures of the major catecholamines.

Tyrosine

Rate-limiting step — Tyrosine hydroxylase

DOPA

DOPA decarboxylase

Dopamine

Dopamine β-hydroxylase

Noradrenaline

Phenylethanolamine N-methyltransferase

Adrenaline

Classification of adrenoceptors

- Main pharmacological classification into α and β subtypes, based originally on order of potency among agonists, later on selective antagonists.
- Adrenoceptor subtypes:
  – two main α-adrenoceptor subtypes, α_1 and α_2, each divided into three further subtypes (1-/2- A,B,C)
  – three β-adrenoceptor subtypes (β_1, β_2, β_3)
  – all belong to the superfamily of G protein-coupled receptors (see Ch. 3).
- Second messengers:
  – α_1 receptors activate phospholipase C, producing inositol trisphosphate and diacylglycerol as second messengers
  – α_2 receptors inhibit adenylyl cyclase, decreasing cAMP formation
  – all types of β receptor stimulate adenylyl cyclase.
- The main effects of receptor activation are as follows:
  – α_1 receptors: vasoconstriction, relaxation of gastrointestinal smooth muscle, salivary secretion and hepatic glycogenolysis
  – α_2 receptors: *inhibition* of: transmitter release (including noradrenaline and acetylcholine release from autonomic nerves); platelet aggregation; vascular smooth muscle contraction; insulin release
  – β_1 receptors: increased cardiac rate and force
  – β_2 receptors: bronchodilatation; vasodilatation; relaxation of visceral smooth muscle; hepatic glycogenolysis; muscle tremor
  – β_3 receptors: lipolysis and thermogenesis; bladder detrusor muscle relaxation.

smooth muscle relaxation in many organs. The latter is often a useful therapeutic effect, while the former is more often harmful; consequently, considerable efforts have been made to find selective β_2 agonists, which would relax smooth muscle without affecting the heart, and selective β_1 antagonists, which would exert a useful blocking effect on the heart without at the same time blocking β_2 receptors in, for example, bronchial smooth muscle (see Table 14.1). It is important to realise that the available drugs are not completely selective, and that compounds used as selective β_1 antagonists invariably have some action on β_2 receptors as well, which can cause unwanted effects such as bronchoconstriction.

In relation to vascular control, it is important to note that both α and β receptor subtypes are expressed in smooth muscle cells, nerve terminals and endothelial cells, and their role in physiological regulation and pharmacological responses of the cardiovascular system is only partly understood (see Guimaraes & Moura, 2001).

PHYSIOLOGY OF NORADRENERGIC TRANSMISSION

THE NORADRENERGIC NEURON

Noradrenergic neurons in the periphery are postganglionic sympathetic neurons whose cell bodies are situated in sympathetic ganglia. They generally have long[2] axons that end in a series of varicosities strung along the branching terminal network. These varicosities contain numerous synaptic vesicles, which are the sites of synthesis and release of noradrenaline and of co-released mediators such as ATP and neuropeptide Y (see Ch. 12), which are stored in vesicles and released by exocytosis (Ch. 4). In most peripheral tissues, the tissue content of noradrenaline closely parallels the density of the sympathetic innervation. With the exception of the adrenal medulla, sympathetic nerve terminals account for all the noradrenaline content of peripheral tissues. Organs such as the heart, spleen, vas deferens and some blood vessels are particularly rich in noradrenaline (5–50 nmol/g of tissue) and have been widely used for studies of noradrenergic transmission. For detailed information on noradrenergic neurons, see Robertson (2004) and Cooper et al. (2002).

NORADRENALINE SYNTHESIS

The biosynthetic pathway for noradrenaline synthesis is shown in Fig. 14.1 and drugs that affect noradrenaline

---

[2]Just how long may be appreciated by scaling up the diameter of a neuronal cell body (4–100 μm) to that of a golf ball (≥42 670 μm diameter, a scaling factor of say 400–10 000); proportionately the axon (length from sympathetic chain ganglion to, say, a blood vessel in the calf, approximately 1 metre) will now reach some 0.4–10 km – some challenge in terms of command and control!

Table 14.1 Distribution and actions of adrenoceptors

Tissues and effects	α_1	α_2	β_1	β_2	β_3
SMOOTH MUSCLE					
Blood vessels	Constrict	Constrict/dilate	–	Dilate	–
Bronchi	Constrict	–	–	Dilate	–
Gastrointestinal tract	Relax	Relax (presynaptic effect)	–	Relax	–
Gastrointestinal sphincters	Contract	–	–	–	–
Uterus	Contract	–	–	Relax	–
Bladder detrusor	–	–	–	Relax	Relax
Bladder sphincter	Contract	–	–	–	–
Seminal tract	Contract	–	–	Relax	–
Iris (radial muscle)	Contract	–	–	–	–
Ciliary muscle	–	–	–	Relax	–
HEART					
Rate	–	–	Increase	Increase[a]	–
Force of contraction	–	–	Increase	Increase[a]	–
OTHER TISSUES/CELLS					
Skeletal muscle	–	–	–	Tremor Increased muscle mass and speed of contraction Glycogenolysis	Thermogenesis
Liver (hepatocytes)	Glycogenolysis	–	–	Glycogenolysis	–
Fat (adipocytes)	–	–	–	–	Lipolysis Thermogenesis
Pancreatic islets (B cells)	–	Decrease insulin secretion	–	–	–
Salivary gland	K⁺ release	–	Amylase secretion	–	–
Platelets	–	Aggregation	–	–	–
Mast cells	–	–	–	Inhibition of histamine release	–
Brain stem	–	Inhibits sympathetic outflow	–	–	–
NERVE TERMINALS					
Adrenergic	–	Decrease release	–	Increase release	–
Cholinergic	–	Decrease release	–	–	–

[a]Minor component normally but may become significant in heart failure.

Table 14.2 Characteristics of adrenoceptors

	α_1	α_2	β_1	β_2	β_3
Second messengers and effectors	Phospholipase C activation $\uparrow$ Inositol trisphosphate $\uparrow$ Diacylglycerol $\uparrow$ Ca²⁺	$\downarrow$ cAMP $\downarrow$ Calcium channels $\uparrow$ Potassium channels	$\uparrow$ cAMP	$\uparrow$ cAMP	$\uparrow$ cAMP
Agonist potency order	NA > A >> ISO	A > NA >> ISO	ISO > NA > A	ISO > A > NA	ISO > NA = A
Selective agonists	Phenylephrine Methoxamine	Clonidine	Dobutamine Xamoterol	Salbutamol Terbutaline Salmeterol Formoterol Clenbuterol	Mirabegron
Selective antagonists	Prazosin Doxazocin	Yohimbine Idazoxan	Atenolol Metoprolol	Butoxamine	–

A, adrenaline; ISO, isoprenaline, NA, noradrenaline.

synthesis are summarised in Table 14.6 (p. 193). The metabolic precursor for noradrenaline is *L-tyrosine*, an aromatic amino acid that is present in the body fluids and is taken up by adrenergic neurons. *Tyrosine hydroxylase*, a cytosolic enzyme that catalyses the conversion of tyrosine to *dihydroxyphenylalanine* (dopa), is found only in catecholamine-containing cells. It is a rather selective enzyme; unlike other enzymes involved in catecholamine metabolism, it does not accept indole derivatives as substrates, and so is not involved in 5-hydroxytryptamine (5-HT) metabolism. This first hydroxylation step is the main control point for noradrenaline synthesis. Tyrosine hydroxylase is inhibited by the end product of the biosynthetic pathway, noradrenaline, and this provides the mechanism for the moment-to-moment regulation of the rate of synthesis; much slower regulation, taking hours or days, occurs by changes in the rate of production of the enzyme.

The tyrosine analogue **α-methyltyrosine** strongly inhibits tyrosine hydroxylase and has been used experimentally to block noradrenaline synthesis.

The next step, conversion of dopa to dopamine, is catalysed by *dopa decarboxylase*, a cytosolic enzyme that is by no means confined to catecholamine-synthesising cells. It is a relatively non-specific enzyme, and catalyses the decarboxylation of various other L-aromatic amino acids, such as *L-histidine* and *L-tryptophan*, which are precursors in the synthesis of histamine (Ch. 17) and 5-HT (Ch. 15), respectively. Dopa decarboxylase activity is not rate-limiting for noradrenaline synthesis. Although various factors, including certain drugs, affect the enzyme, it is not an effective means of regulating noradrenaline synthesis.

Dopamine-β-hydroxylase (DBH) is also a relatively non-specific enzyme, but is restricted to catecholamine-synthesising cells. It is located in synaptic vesicles, mainly in membrane-bound form. A small amount of the enzyme is released from adrenergic nerve terminals in company with noradrenaline, representing the small proportion in a soluble form within the vesicle. Unlike noradrenaline, the released DBH is not subject to rapid degradation or uptake, so its concentration in plasma and body fluids can be used as an index of overall sympathetic nerve activity.

Many drugs inhibit DBH, including copper-chelating agents and **disulfiram** (a drug used mainly for its effect on ethanol metabolism; see Ch. 49). Such drugs can cause a partial depletion of noradrenaline stores and interference with sympathetic transmission. A rare genetic disorder, DBH deficiency, causes failure of noradrenaline synthesis resulting in severe orthostatic hypotension (see Ch. 22).

Phenylethanolamine N-methyl transferase (PNMT) catalyses the *N*-methylation of noradrenaline to adrenaline. The main location of this enzyme is in the adrenal medulla, which contains a population of adrenaline-releasing (A) cells separate from the smaller proportion of noradrenaline-releasing (N) cells. The A cells, which appear only after birth, lie adjacent to the adrenal cortex, and the production of PNMT is induced by an action of the steroid hormones secreted by the adrenal cortex (see Ch. 33). PNMT is also found in certain parts of the brain, where adrenaline may function as a transmitter, but little is known about its role in the central nervous system (CNS).

Noradrenaline turnover can be measured under steady-state conditions by measuring the rate at which labelled noradrenaline accumulates when a labelled precursor, such as tyrosine or dopa, is administered. The turnover time is defined as the time taken for an amount of noradrenaline equal to the total tissue content to be degraded and resynthesised. In peripheral tissues, the turnover time is generally about 5–15 h, but it becomes much shorter if sympathetic nerve activity is increased. Under normal circumstances, the rate of synthesis closely matches the rate of release, so that the noradrenaline content of tissues is constant regardless of how fast it is being released.

NORADRENALINE STORAGE

Most of the noradrenaline in nerve terminals or chromaffin cells is contained in vesicles; only a little is free in the cytoplasm under normal circumstances. The concentration in the vesicles is very high (0.3–1.0 mol/l) and is maintained by the *vesicular monoamine transporter* (VMAT), which is similar to the amine transporter responsible for noradrenaline uptake into the nerve terminal (see Ch. 12), but uses the transvesicular proton gradient as its driving force. Certain drugs, such as **reserpine** (see p. 181; Table 14.3) block this transport and cause nerve terminals to become depleted of their vesicular noradrenaline stores. The vesicles contain two major constituents besides noradrenaline, namely ATP (about four molecules per molecule of noradrenaline) and a protein called *chromogranin A*. These substances are released along with noradrenaline, and it is generally assumed that a reversible complex, depending partly on the opposite charges on the molecules of noradrenaline and ATP, is formed within the vesicle. This would serve both to reduce the osmolarity of the vesicle contents and also to reduce the tendency of noradrenaline to leak out of the vesicles within the nerve terminal.

ATP itself has a transmitter function at noradrenergic synapses (see Fig. 12.5; Ch. 16), being responsible for the fast excitatory synaptic potential and the rapid phase of contraction produced by sympathetic nerve activity in many smooth muscle tissues.

NORADRENALINE RELEASE

The processes linking the arrival of a nerve impulse at a nerve terminal to Ca^{2+} entry and the release of transmitter are described in Chapter 4. Drugs that affect noradrenaline release are summarised in Table 14.6 (p. 193).

An unusual feature of the release mechanism at the varicosities of noradrenergic nerves is that the probability of release, even of a single vesicle, when a nerve impulse arrives at a varicosity is very low (less than 1 in 50). A single neuron possesses many thousand varicosities, so one impulse leads to the discharge of a few hundred vesicles, scattered over a wide area. This contrasts sharply with the neuromuscular junction (Ch. 13), where the release probability at a single terminal is high, and release of acetylcholine is sharply localised.

Regulation of noradrenaline release

Noradrenaline release is affected by a variety of substances that act on presynaptic receptors (see Ch. 12). Many different types of nerve terminal (cholinergic, noradrenergic, dopaminergic, 5-HT-ergic, etc.) are subject to this type of control, and many different mediators (acetylcholine acting through muscarinic receptors, catecholamines acting through α and β receptors, angiotensin II, prostaglandins, purine nucleotides, neuropeptides, etc.) can act on presynaptic terminals. Presynaptic modulation represents an important physiological control mechanism throughout the nervous system.

Table 14.3 Characteristics of noradrenaline (norepinephrine) transport systems

	Neuronal (NET)	Extraneuronal (EMT)	Vesicular (VMAT)
Transport of NA (rat heart) V_{max} (nmol g^{-1} min^{-1})	1.2	100	–
K_m (μmol/l)	0.3	250	~0.2
Specificity	NA > A > ISO	A > NA > ISO	NA = A = ISO
Location	Neuronal membrane	Non-neuronal cell membrane (smooth muscle, cardiac muscle, endothelium)	Synaptic vesicle membrane
Other substrates	Tyramine Methylnoradrenaline Adrenergic neuron-blocking drugs (e.g. guanethidine) Amphetamine[a]	(+)-Noradrenaline Dopamine 5-Hydroxytryptamine Histamine	Dopamine 5-Hydroxytryptamine Guanethidine MPP$^+$ (see Ch. 40)
Inhibitors	Cocaine Tricyclic antidepressants (e.g. desipramine) Phenoxybenzamine Amphetamine[a]	Normetanephrine Steroid hormones (e.g. corticosterone) Phenoxybenzamine	Reserpine Tetrabenazine

[a]Amphetamine is transported slowly, so acts both as a substrate and as an inhibitor of noradrenaline uptake. For details, see Gainetdinov & Caron, 2003.
A, adrenaline; ISO, isoprenaline; NA, noradrenaline.

Furthermore, noradrenaline, by acting on presynaptic β_2 receptors, can regulate its own release, and also that of co-released ATP (see Ch. 12). This is believed to occur physiologically, so that released noradrenaline exerts a local inhibitory effect on the terminals from which it came – the so-called *autoinhibitory feedback* mechanism (Fig. 14.2; see Gilsbach & Hein, 2012). Agonists or antagonists affecting these presynaptic receptors can have large effects on sympathetic transmission. However, the physiological significance of presynaptic autoinhibition in the sympathetic nervous system is still somewhat contentious, and there is evidence that, in most tissues, it is less influential than biochemical measurements of transmitter overflow would seem to imply. Thus, although blocking autoreceptors causes large changes in noradrenaline *overflow* – the amount of noradrenaline released into the bathing solution or the bloodstream when sympathetic nerves are stimulated – the associated changes in the tissue response are often rather small. This suggests that what is measured in overflow experiments may not be the physiologically important component of transmitter release.

The inhibitory feedback mechanism operates through α_2 receptors, which inhibit adenylyl cyclase and prevent the opening of calcium channels. Sympathetic nerve terminals also possess β_2 receptors, coupled to activation of adenylyl cyclase, which *increase* noradrenaline release. Whether they have any physiological function is not yet clear.

UPTAKE AND DEGRADATION OF CATECHOLAMINES

The action of released noradrenaline is terminated mainly by reuptake of the transmitter into noradrenergic nerve terminals. Some is also sequestered by other cells in the vicinity. Circulating adrenaline and noradrenaline are degraded enzymatically, but much more slowly than acetylcholine (see Ch. 13), where synaptically located

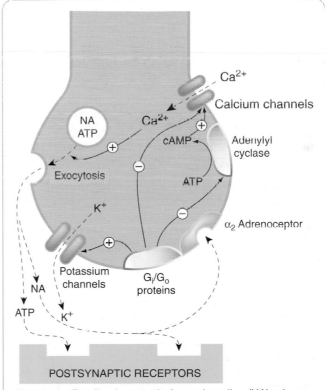

Fig. 14.2 Feedback control of noradrenaline (NA) release. The presynaptic α_2 receptor inhibits Ca^{2+} influx in response to membrane depolarisation via an action of the $\beta\gamma$ subunits of the associated G protein on the voltage-dependent Ca^{2+} channels (Ch. 3).

acetylcholinesterase inactivates the transmitter in milliseconds. The two main catecholamine-metabolising enzymes are located intracellularly, so uptake into cells necessarily precedes metabolic degradation.

UPTAKE OF CATECHOLAMINES

About 75% of the noradrenaline released by sympathetic neurons is recaptured and repackaged into vesicles. This serves to cut short the action of the released noradrenaline, as well as recycling it. The remaining 25% is captured by non-neuronal cells in the vicinity, limiting its local spread. These two uptake mechanisms depend on distinct transporter molecules. Neuronal uptake is performed by the plasma membrane noradrenaline transporter (generally known as NET, the *norepinephrine transporter*), which belongs to the family of neurotransmitter transporter proteins (NET, DAT, SERT, etc.) specific for different amine transmitters, described in Chapter 12; these act as co-transporters of Na^+, Cl^- and the amine in question, using the electrochemical gradient for Na^+ as a driving force. Packaging into vesicles occurs through the *vesicular monoamine transporter* (VMAT), driven by the proton gradient between the cytosol and the vesicle contents. Extraneuronal uptake is performed by the *extraneuronal monoamine transporter* (EMT), which belongs to a large and widely distributed family of organic cation transporters (OCTs, see Ch. 8). NET is relatively selective for noradrenaline, with high affinity and a low maximum rate of uptake, and it is important in maintaining releasable stores of noradrenaline. EMT has lower affinity and higher transport capacity than NET, and transports adrenaline and isoprenaline as well as noradrenaline. The effects of several important drugs that act on noradrenergic neurons depend on their ability either to inhibit NET or to enter the nerve terminal with its help. Table 14.3 summarises the properties of neuronal and extraneuronal uptake.

METABOLIC DEGRADATION OF CATECHOLAMINES

Endogenous and exogenous catecholamines are metabolised mainly by two intracellular enzymes: *monoamine oxidase* (MAO) and *catechol-O-methyl transferase* (COMT). MAO (of which there are two distinct isoforms, MAO-A and MAO-B; see Chs 39 and 47) is bound to the surface membrane of mitochondria. It is abundant in noradrenergic nerve terminals but is also present in liver, intestinal epithelium and other tissues. MAO converts catecholamines to their corresponding aldehydes,[3] which, in the periphery, are rapidly metabolised by *aldehyde dehydrogenase* to the corresponding carboxylic acid (3,4-dihydroxyphenylglycol being formed from noradrenaline; Fig. 14.3). MAO can also oxidise other monoamines, including dopamine and 5-HT. It is inhibited by various drugs which are used mainly for their effects on the central nervous system, where these three amines all have transmitter functions (see Ch. 39). These drugs have important side effects that are related to disturbances of peripheral noradrenergic transmission. Within sympathetic neurons, MAO controls the content of dopamine and noradrenaline, and the releasable store of noradrenaline increases if the enzyme is inhibited. MAO and its inhibitors are discussed in more detail in Chapter 47.

The second major pathway for catecholamine metabolism involves methylation of one of the catechol hydroxyl groups by COMT to give a methoxy derivative. COMT is absent from noradrenergic neurons but present in the adrenal medulla and many other cells and tissues. The final product formed by the sequential action of MAO and COMT is *3-methoxy-4-hydroxyphenylglycol* (MHPG; see Fig. 14.3). This is partly conjugated to sulfate or glucuronide derivatives, which are excreted in the urine, but most of it is converted to *vanillylmandelic acid* (VMA; Fig. 14.3) and excreted in the urine in this form. In patients with tumours of chromaffin tissue that secrete these amines (a rare cause of high blood pressure), the urinary excretion of VMA is markedly increased, this being used as a diagnostic test for this condition.

In the periphery, neither MAO nor COMT is primarily responsible for the termination of transmitter action, most of the released noradrenaline being quickly recaptured by NET. Circulating catecholamines are sequestered and inactivated by a combination of NET, EMT and COMT, the relative importance of these processes varying according to the agent concerned. Thus circulating noradrenaline is removed mainly by NET, whereas adrenaline is more dependent on EMT. Isoprenaline, on the other hand, is not a substrate for NET, and is removed by a combination of EMT and COMT.

In the central nervous system (see Ch. 39), MAO is more important as a means of terminating transmitter action than it is in the periphery, and MAO knockout mice show a greater enhancement of noradrenergic transmission in the brain than do NET knockouts, in which neuronal stores of noradrenaline are much depleted (see Gainetdinov & Caron, 2003). The main excretory product of noradrenaline released in the brain is MHPG.

DRUGS ACTING ON NORADRENERGIC TRANSMISSION

Many clinically important drugs, particularly those used to treat cardiovascular, respiratory and psychiatric disorders (see Chs 21, 22, 28 and 47), act by affecting noradrenergic neuron function, acting on adrenoceptors, transporters or catecholamine-metabolising enzymes. The properties of the most important drugs in this category are summarised in Tables 14.4–4.6.

DRUGS ACTING ON ADRENOCEPTORS

The overall activity of these drugs is governed by their affinity, efficacy and selectivity with respect to different types of adrenoceptor, and intensive research has been devoted to developing drugs with the right properties for specific clinical indications. As a result, the pharmacopoeia is awash with adrenoceptor ligands. Many clinical needs are met, it turns out, by drugs that relax smooth muscle in different organs of the body[4] and those that block the cardiac stimulant effects of the sympathetic nervous system; on the other hand, cardiac stimulation is generally undesirable in chronic disease.

---

[3]Aldehyde metabolites are potentially neurotoxic, and are thought to play a role in certain degenerative CNS disorders (see Ch. 40).

[4]And conversely, contracting smooth muscle is often bad news. This bald statement must not be pressed too far, but the exceptions (such as nasal decongestants and drugs acting on the eye) are surprisingly few. Even adrenaline (potentially life-saving in cardiac arrest) dilates some vessels while constricting others to less immediately essential tissues such as skin).

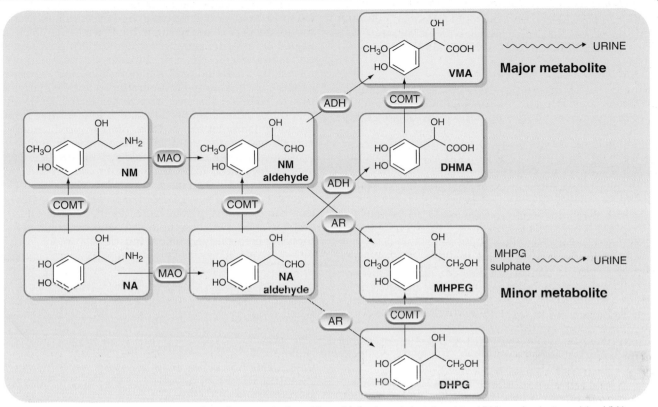

Fig. 14.3 The main pathways of noradrenaline metabolism. The oxidative branch (catalysed by ADH) predominates, giving VMA as the main urinary metabolite. The reductive branch (catalysed by AR) produces the less abundant metabolite, MHPG, which is conjugated to MHPG sulfate before being excreted. ADH, aldehyde dehydrogenase; AR, aldehyde reductase; COMT, catechol-O-methyl transferase; DHMA, 3,4-dihydroxymandelic acid; DHPG, 3,4-dihydroxyphenylglycol; MAO, monoamine oxidase; MHPG, 3-methoxy-4-hydroxyphenylglycol; NA, noradrenaline; NM, normetanephrine; VMA, vanillylmandelic acid.

Noradrenergic transmission

- Transmitter synthesis involves the following:
  - L-tyrosine is converted to dihydroxyphenylalanine (dopa) by tyrosine hydroxylase (rate-limiting step). Tyrosine hydroxylase occurs only in catecholaminergic neurons.
  - Dopa is converted to dopamine by dopa decarboxylase.
  - Dopamine is converted to noradrenaline by dopamine β-hydroxylase (DBH), located in synaptic vesicles.
  - In the adrenal medulla, noradrenaline is converted to adrenaline by phenylethanolamine N-methyltransferase.
- Transmitter storage: noradrenaline is stored at high concentration in synaptic vesicles, together with ATP, chromogranin and DBH, all of which are released by exocytosis. Transport of noradrenaline into vesicles occurs by a reserpine-sensitive transporter (VMAT). Noradrenaline content of cytosol is normally low due to monoamine oxidase in nerve terminals.
- Transmitter release occurs normally by Ca²⁺-mediated exocytosis from varicosities on the terminal network. Non-exocytotic release occurs in response to indirectly acting sympathomimetic drugs (e.g. **amphetamine**), which displace noradrenaline from vesicles. Noradrenaline escapes via the NET transporter (reverse transport).
- Transmitter action is terminated mainly by reuptake of noradrenaline into nerve terminals via the NET transporter. NET is blocked by tricyclic antidepressant drugs and **cocaine**.
- Noradrenaline release is controlled by autoinhibitory feedback mediated by α₂ receptors.
- Co-transmission occurs at many noradrenergic nerve terminals, ATP and neuropeptide Y being frequently co-released with NA. ATP mediates the early phase of smooth muscle contraction in response to sympathetic nerve activity.

Broadly speaking, β-adrenoceptor agonists are useful as smooth muscle relaxants (especially in the airways), while β-adrenoceptor antagonists (often called β blockers) are used mainly for their cardiodepressant effects. α-Adrenoceptor antagonists are used mainly for their vasodilator effects in cardiovascular indications and also for the treatment of prostatic hyperplasia. Adrenaline, with its mixture of cardiac stimulant, vasodilator and vasoconstrictor actions is uniquely important in cardiac arrest (Ch. 21). Selective α-adrenoceptor agonists have relatively few clinical uses.

ADRENOCEPTOR AGONISTS

Examples of adrenoceptor agonists (also known as *directly-acting sympathomimetic* drugs) are given in Table 14.2, and the characteristics of individual drugs are summarised in Table 14.4.

Actions

The major physiological effects mediated by different types of adrenoceptor are summarised in Table 14.1.

Smooth muscle

All types of smooth muscle, except that of the gastrointestinal tract, contract in response to stimulation of α_1-adrenoceptors, through activation of the signal transduction mechanism, leading to intracellular Ca^{2+} release described in Chapter 4.

When α agonists are given systemically to experimental animals or humans, the most important action is on vascular smooth muscle, particularly in the skin and splanchnic vascular beds, which are strongly constricted. Large arteries and veins, as well as arterioles, are also constricted, resulting in decreased vascular compliance, increased central venous pressure and increased peripheral resistance, all of which contribute to an increase in systolic and diastolic arterial pressure and increased cardiac work. Some vascular beds (e.g. cerebral, coronary and pulmonary) are relatively little affected.

In the whole animal, baroreceptor reflexes are activated by the rise in arterial pressure produced by α agonists, causing reflex bradycardia and inhibition of respiration.

Smooth muscle in the vas deferens, spleen capsule and eyelid retractor muscles (or nictitating membrane, in some species) is also stimulated by α agonists, and these organs were once widely used for pharmacological studies.

The α receptors involved in smooth muscle contraction are mainly α_1 in type, although vascular smooth muscle possesses both α_1 and α_2 receptors. It appears that α_1 receptors lie close to the sites of release (and are mainly responsible for neurally mediated vasoconstriction), while α_2 receptors lie elsewhere on the muscle fibre surface and are activated by circulating catecholamines.

Stimulation of β receptors causes relaxation of most kinds of smooth muscle by increasing cAMP formation (see Ch. 4). Additionally, β-receptor activation enhances Ca^{2+} extrusion and intracellular Ca^{2+} binding, both effects acting to reduce intracellular Ca^{2+} concentration.

Relaxation is usually produced by β_2 receptors, although the receptor that is responsible for this effect in gastrointestinal smooth muscle is not clearly β_1 or β_2. In the vascular system, β_2-mediated vasodilatation is (particularly in humans) mainly endothelium dependent and mediated by nitric oxide release (see Ch. 20). It occurs in many vascular beds and is especially marked in skeletal muscle.

The powerful inhibitory effect of the sympathetic system on gastrointestinal smooth muscle is produced by both α and β receptors, this tissue being unusual in that α receptors cause relaxation in most regions. Part of the effect is due to stimulation of presynaptic α_2 receptors (see below), which inhibit the release of excitatory transmitters (e.g. acetylcholine) from intramural nerves, but there are also α receptors on the muscle cells, stimulation of which hyperpolarises the cell (by increasing the membrane permeability to K^+) and inhibits action potential discharge. The sphincters of the gastrointestinal tract are contracted by α-receptor activation.

Bronchial smooth muscle is relaxed by activation of β_2 adrenoceptors, and selective β_2 agonists are important in the treatment of asthma (see Ch. 28). Uterine smooth muscle responds similarly, and these drugs are also used to delay premature labour (Ch. 35). Bladder detrusor muscle is relaxed by activation of β_3 adrenoceptors, and selective β_3 agonists have recently been introduced to treat symptoms of overactive bladder (see Sacco & Bientinesi, 2012).

Also, α_1 adrenoceptors mediate a long-lasting trophic response, stimulating smooth muscle proliferation in various tissues, for example in blood vessels and in the prostate gland, which is of pathological importance. *Benign prostatic hyperplasia* (see Ch. 35) is commonly treated with α-adrenoceptor antagonists. 'Cross-talk' between the α_1 adrenoceptor and the growth factor signalling pathways (see Ch. 3) probably contributes to the clinical effect, in addition to immediate symptomatic improvement which is probably mediated by smooth muscle relaxation.

Nerve terminals

Presynaptic adrenoceptors are present on both cholinergic and noradrenergic nerve terminals (see Chs 4 and 12). The main effect (α_2-mediated) is inhibitory, but a weaker facilitatory action of β receptors on noradrenergic nerve terminals has also been described.

Heart

Catecholamines, acting on β_1 receptors, exert a powerful stimulant effect on the heart (see Ch. 21). Both the heart rate (*chronotropic effect*) and the force of contraction (*inotropic effect*) are increased, resulting in a markedly increased cardiac output and cardiac oxygen consumption. The cardiac efficiency (see Ch. 21) is reduced. Catecholamines can also cause disturbance of the cardiac rhythm, culminating in ventricular fibrillation. (Paradoxically, but importantly, adrenaline is also used to treat ventricular fibrillation arrest as well as other forms of cardiac arrest; Ch. 21). Figure 14.4 shows the overall pattern of cardiovascular responses to catecholamine infusions in humans, reflecting their actions on both the heart and vascular system.

Cardiac hypertrophy occurs in response to activation of both β_1 and α_1 receptors, probably by a mechanism similar to the hypertrophy of vascular and prostatic smooth muscle. This may be important in the pathophysiology of hypertension and of cardiac failure (which is associated with sympathetic overactivity); see Chapter 21.

Metabolism

Catecholamines encourage the conversion of energy stores (glycogen and fat) to freely available fuels (glucose and free fatty acids), and cause an increase in the plasma concentration of the latter substances. The detailed biochemical mechanisms (see review by Nonogaki, 2000) vary from species to species, but in most cases the effects on carbohydrate metabolism of liver and muscle (Fig. 14.5) are mediated through β_1 receptors and the stimulation of lipolysis and thermogenesis is produced by β_3 receptors (see Table 14.1). Activation of α_2 receptors inhibits insulin secretion, an effect that further contributes to the hyperglycaemia. The production of *leptin* by adipose tissue (see Ch. 32) is also inhibited. Adrenaline-induced hyperglycaemia in humans is blocked completely by a combination of α and β antagonists but not by either on its own.

Other effects

Skeletal muscle is affected by adrenaline, acting on β_2 receptors, although the effect is far less dramatic than that

Table 14.4 Mixed (α- and β-) adrenoceptor agonists

Drug	Main action	Uses/function	Unwanted effects	Pharmacokinetic aspects	Notes
Noradrenaline (Norepinephrine)	α/β agonist	Sometimes used for hypotension in intensive care Transmitter at postganglionic sympathetic neurons, and in CNS	Hypertension, vasoconstriction, tachycardia (or reflex bradycardia), ventricular dysrhythmias	Poorly absorbed by mouth Rapid removal by tissues Metabolised by MAO and COMT Plasma $t_{1/2}$ ~2 min	–
Adrenaline (Epinephrine)	α/β agonist	Asthma (emergency treatment), anaphylactic shock, cardiac arrest Added to local anaesthetic solutions Main hormone of adrenal medulla	As norepinephrine	As norepinephrine Given i.m. or s.c. (i.v. infusion in intensive care settings)	See Ch. 28
Isoprenaline	β agonist (non-selective)	Asthma (obsolete)	Tachycardia, dysrhythmias	Some tissue uptake, followed by inactivation (COMT) Plasma $t_{1/2}$ ~2 h	Now replaced by salbutamol in treatment of asthma (see Ch. 28)
Dobutamine	$β_1$ agonist (non-selective)	Cardiogenic shock	Dysrhythmias	Plasma $t_{1/2}$ ~2 min Given i.v.	See Ch. 21
Salbutamol	$β_2$ agonist	Asthma, premature labour	Tachycardia, dysrhythmias, tremor, peripheral vasodilatation	Given orally or by aerosol Mainly excreted unchanged Plasma $t_{1/2}$ ~4 h	See Ch. 28
Salmeterol	$β_2$ agonist	Asthma	As salbutamol	Given by aerosol Long acting	Formoterol is similar
Terbutaline	$β_2$ agonist	Asthma Delay of parturition	As salbutamol	Poorly absorbed orally Given by aerosol Mainly excreted unchanged Plasma $t_{1/2}$ ~4 h	See Ch. 28
Clenbuterol	$β_2$ agonist	'Anabolic' action to increase muscle strength	As salbutamol	Active orally Long acting	Illicit use in sport
Mirabegron	$β_3$ agonist	Symptoms of overactive bladder	Tachycardia	Active orally, given once daily	See Ch. 29
Phenylephrine	$α_1$ agonist	Nasal decongestion	Hypertension, reflex bradycardia	Given intranasally Metabolised by MAO Short plasma $t_{1/2}$	–
Methoxamine	α agonist (non-selective)	Nasal decongestion	As phenylephrine	Given intranasally Plasma $t_{1/2}$ ~1 h	–
Clonidine	$α_2$ partial agonist	Hypertension, migraine	Drowsiness, orthostatic hypotension, oedema and weight gain, rebound hypertension	Well absorbed orally Excreted unchanged and as conjugate Plasma $t_{1/2}$ ~12 h	See Ch. 21

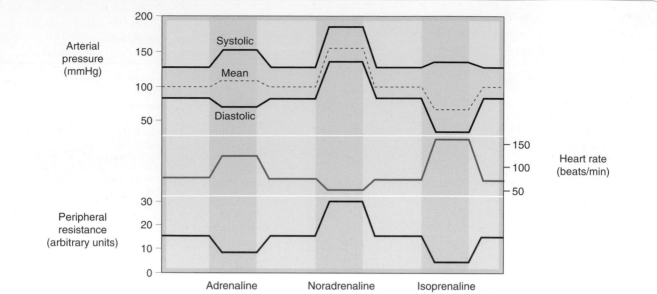

Fig. 14.4 **Schematic representation of the cardiovascular effects of intravenous infusions of adrenaline, noradrenaline and isoprenaline in humans.** Noradrenaline (predominantly α agonist) causes vasoconstriction and increased systolic and diastolic pressure, with a reflex bradycardia. Isoprenaline (β agonist) is a vasodilator, but strongly increases cardiac force and rate. Mean arterial pressure falls. Adrenaline combines both actions.

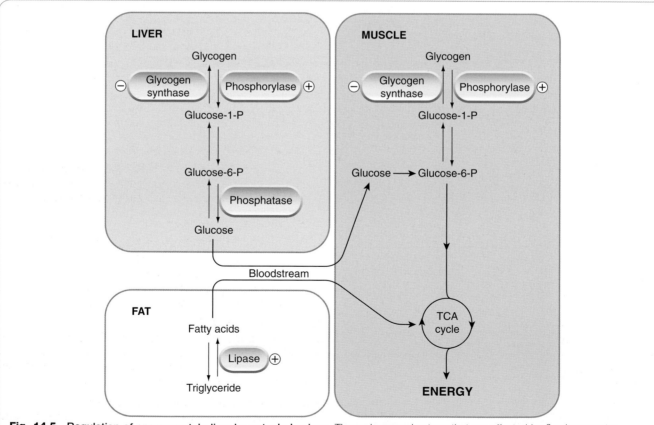

Fig. 14.5 **Regulation of energy metabolism by catecholamines.** The main enzymic steps that are affected by β-adrenoceptor activation are indicated by + and − signs, denoting stimulation and inhibition, respectively. The overall effect is to mobilise glycogen and fat stores to meet energy demands.

on the heart. The twitch tension of fast-contracting fibres (white muscle) is increased by adrenaline, particularly if the muscle is fatigued, whereas the twitch of slow (red) muscle is reduced. These effects depend on an action on the contractile proteins, rather than on the membrane, and the mechanism is poorly understood. In humans, adrenaline and other β_2 agonists cause a marked tremor, the shakiness that accompanies fear, excitement or the excessive use of β_2 agonists (e.g. **salbutamol**) in the treatment of asthma being examples of this. It probably results from an increase in muscle spindle discharge, coupled with an effect on the contraction kinetics of the fibres, these effects combining to produce an instability in the reflex control of muscle length. β-receptor antagonists are sometimes used to control pathological tremor. The tendency to cardiac dysrhythmias associated with β_2 agonists is thought to be partly due to hypokalaemia, caused by an increase in K^+ uptake by skeletal muscle. β_2 agonists also cause long-term changes in the expression of sarcoplasmic reticulum proteins that control contraction kinetics, and thereby increase the rate and force of contraction of skeletal muscle. **Clenbuterol**, an 'anabolic' drug used illicitly by athletes to improve performance (see Ch. 58), is a β_2 agonist that acts in this way.

Histamine release by human and guinea pig lung tissue in response to anaphylactic challenge (see Ch. 17) is inhibited by catecholamines, acting on β_2 receptors.

Lymphocytes and other cells of the immune system also express adrenoceptors (mainly β adrenoceptors). Lymphocyte proliferation, lymphocyte-mediated cell killing, and production of many cytokines are inhibited by β-adrenoceptor agonists. The physiological and clinical importance of these effects has not yet been established. For a review of the effects of the sympathetic nervous system on immune function, see Elenkov et al., 2000.

Adrenoceptor agonists

- **Noradrenaline** and **adrenaline** show relatively little receptor selectivity.
- Selective α_1 agonists include **phenylephrine** and **oxymetazoline**.
- Selective α_2 agonists include **clonidine** and **α-methylnoradrenaline**. They cause a fall in blood pressure, partly by inhibition of noradrenaline release and partly by a central action. Methylnoradrenaline is formed as a false transmitter from **methyldopa**, developed as a hypotensive drug (now largely obsolete, except during pregnancy).
- Selective β_1 agonists include **dobutamine**. Increased cardiac contractility may be useful clinically, but all β_1 agonists can cause cardiac dysrhythmias.
- Selective β_2 agonists include **salbutamol**, **terbutaline** and **salmeterol**; used mainly for their bronchodilator action in asthma.
- A selective β_3 agonist, **mirabegron**, is used to treat overactive bladder; β_3 agonists promote lipolysis and have potential in the treatment of obesity.

Clinical use
The main clinical uses of adrenoceptor agonists are summarised in the clinical box (below) and Table 14.4, the

most important being the use of β-adrenoceptor agonists for the treatment of asthma (Ch. 28).

Clinical uses of adrenoceptor agonists

- Cardiovascular system:
  - cardiac arrest: **adrenaline**
  - cardiogenic shock (see Ch. 22): **dobutamine** (β_1 agonist).
- Anaphylaxis (acute hypersensitivity, see Chs 17 and 28): **adrenaline**.
- Respiratory system:
  - asthma (Ch. 28): selective β_2-receptor agonists (**salbutamol, terbutaline, salmeterol, formoterol**)
  - nasal decongestion: drops containing **xylometazoline** or **ephedrine** for short-term use.
- Miscellaneous indications:
  - **adrenaline**: with local anaesthetics to prolong their action (see Ch. 43)
  - premature labour (**salbutamol**; see Ch. 35)
  - α_2 agonists (e.g. **clonidine**): to lower blood pressure (Ch. 22) and intraocular pressure; as an adjunct during drug withdrawal in addicts (Ch. 49; Table 49.3, p. 181); to reduce menopausal flushing, especially when **oestrogen** is contraindicated as in patients with breast cancer; and to reduce frequency of migraine attacks (Ch. 15). Tourette syndrome, characterised by multiple tics and outbursts of foul language, is an unlicensed indication.
  - A β_3 agonist, **mirabegron**: to treat urgency, increased micturition frequency and incontinence (overactive bladder symptoms).

ADRENOCEPTOR ANTAGONISTS
The main drugs are listed in Table 14.2, and further information is given in Table 14.5. Most are selective for α or β receptors, and many are also subtype-selective.

α-Adrenoceptor antagonists
The main groups of α-adrenoceptor antagonists are:

- non-selective between subtypes (e.g. **phenoxybenzamine, phentolamine**)
- α_1-selective (e.g. **prazosin, doxazosin, terazosin**)
- α_2-selective (e.g. **yohimbine, idazoxan**).

In addition, *ergot derivatives* (e.g. **ergotamine, dihydroergotamine**) block α receptors as well as having many other actions, notably on 5-HT receptors. They are described in Chapter 15. Their action on α adrenoceptors is of pharmacological interest but not used therapeutically.

Non-selective α-adrenoceptor antagonists
Phenoxybenzamine is not specific for α receptors, and also antagonises the actions of acetylcholine, histamine and 5-HT. It is long lasting because it binds covalently to the receptor. **Phentolamine** is more selective, but it binds reversibly and its action is short lasting. In humans, these drugs cause a fall in arterial pressure (because of block of α-receptor-mediated vasoconstriction) and postural hypotension. The cardiac output and heart rate

Table 14.5 Adrenoceptor antagonists

Drug	Main action	Uses/function	Unwanted effects	Pharmacokinetic aspects	Notes
α-Adrenoceptor antagonists					
Phenoxybenzamine	α antagonist (non-selective, irreversible) Uptake 1 inhibitor	Phaeochromocytoma	Postural hypotension, tachycardia, nasal congestion, impotence	Absorbed orally Plasma $t_{1/2}$ ~12 h	Action outlasts presence of drug in plasma, because of covalent binding to receptor
Phentolamine	α antagonist (non-selective), vasodilator	Rarely used	As phenoxybenzamine	Usually given i.v. Metabolised by liver Plasma $t_{1/2}$ ~2 h	
Prazosin	α_1 antagonist	Hypertension	As phenoxybenzamine	Absorbed orally Metabolised by liver Plasma $t_{1/2}$ ~4 h	Doxazosin, terazosin are similar but longer acting See Ch. 22
Tamsulosin	α_{1A} antagonist ('uroselective')	Prostatic hyperplasia	Failure of ejaculation	Absorbed orally Plasma $t_{1/2}$ ~5 h	Selective for α_{1A}-adrenoceptor
Yohimbine	α_2 antagonist	Not used clinically Claimed to be aphrodisiac	Excitement, hypertension	Absorbed orally Metabolised by liver Plasma $t_{1/2}$ ~4 h	
β-Adrenoceptor antagonists					
Propranolol	β antagonist (non-selective)	Angina, hypertension, cardiac dysrhythmias, anxiety, tremor, glaucoma	Bronchoconstriction, cardiac failure, cold extremities, fatigue and depression, hypoglycaemia	Absorbed orally Extensive first-pass metabolism About 90% bound to plasma protein Plasma $t_{1/2}$ ~4 h	Timolol is similar and used mainly to treat glaucoma See Ch. 21
Alprenolol	β antagonist (non-selective) (partial agonist)	As propranolol	As propranolol	Absorbed orally Metabolised by liver Plasma $t_{1/2}$ ~4 h	Oxprenolol and pindolol are similar See Ch. 21
Metoprolol	β_1 antagonist	Angina, hypertension, dysrhythmias	As propranolol, less risk of bronchoconstriction	Absorbed orally Mainly metabolised in liver Plasma $t_{1/2}$ ~3 h	Atenolol is similar, with a longer half-life See Ch. 21
Nebivolol	β_1 antagonist Enhances nitric oxide synthesis	Hypertension	Fatigue, headache	Absorbed orally $t_{1/2}$ ~10 h	–
Butoxamine	β_2-selective antagonist Weak α agonist	No clinical uses	–	–	–
Mixed (α-/β-) antagonists					
Labetalol	α/β antagonist	Hypertension in pregnancy	Postural hypotension, brochoconstriction	Absorbed orally Conjugated in liver Plasma $t_{1/2}$ ~4 h	See Chs 21 and 22
Carvedilol	β/α_1 antagonist	Heart failure	As for other β blockers Initial exacerbation of heart failure Renal failure	Absorbed orally $t_{1/2}$ ~10 h	Additional actions may contribute to clinical benefit. See Ch. 21

are increased. This is a reflex response to the fall in arterial pressure, mediated through β receptors. The concomitant block of α₂ receptors tends to increase noradrenaline release, which has the effect of enhancing the reflex tachycardia that occurs with any blood pressure-lowering agent. Phenoxybenzamine retains a niche (but vital) use in preparing patients with *phaeochromocytoma* (Ch. 22) for surgery; its irreversible antagonism and the resultant depression in the maximum of the agonist dose–response curve (see Ch. 2, Fig. 2.4) are desirable in a situation where surgical manipulation of the tumour may release a large bolus of pressor amines into the circulation.

Labetalol and **carvedilol**[5] are mixed α₁- and β-receptor-blocking drugs, although clinically they act predominantly on β receptors. Much has been made of the fact that they combine both activities in one molecule. To a pharmacologist, accustomed to putting specificity of action high on the list of pharmacological saintly virtues, this may seem like a step backwards rather than forwards. Carvedilol is used mainly to treat hypertension and heart failure (see Chs 21 and 22); labetalol is used to treat hypertension in pregnancy.

Selective α₁ antagonists
Prazosin was the first selective α₁ antagonist. Similar drugs with longer half-lives (e.g. **doxazosin**, **terazosin**), which have the advantage of allowing once-daily dosing, are now preferred. They are highly selective for α₁ adrenoceptors and cause vasodilatation and fall in arterial pressure, but less tachycardia than occurs with non-selective α-receptor antagonists, presumably because they do not increase noradrenaline release from sympathetic nerve terminals. Postural hypotension may occur, but is less problematic than with shorter-acting prazosin.

The α₁-receptor antagonists cause relaxation of the smooth muscle of the bladder neck and prostate capsule, and inhibit hypertrophy of these tissues, and are therefore useful in treating urinary retention associated with *benign prostatic hypertrophy*. **Tamsulosin**, an α₁ₐ-receptor antagonist, shows some selectivity for the bladder, and causes less hypotension than drugs such as prazosin, which act on α₁ᵦ receptors to control vascular tone.

It is believed that α₁ₐ receptors play a part in the pathological hypertrophy not only of prostatic and vascular smooth muscle, but also in the cardiac hypertrophy that occurs in hypertension and heart failure, and the use of selective α₁ₐ-receptor antagonists to treat these chronic conditions is under investigation.

Selective α₂ antagonists
Yohimbine is a naturally occurring alkaloid; various synthetic analogues have been made, such as **idazoxan**. These drugs are used experimentally to analyse α-receptor subtypes, and yohimbine, possibly by virtue of its vasodilator effect, historically enjoyed notoriety as an aphrodisiac, but they are not used therapeutically.

Clinical uses and unwanted effects of α-adrenoceptor antagonists
The main uses of α-adrenoceptor antagonists are related to their cardiovascular actions, and are summarised in the clinical box (below). They have been tried for many

[5]Carvedilol is also a biased agonist, acting through the arrestin pathway (Ch. 3).

> ## α-Adrenoceptor antagonists
>
> - Drugs that block α₁ and α₂ adrenoceptors (e.g. **phenoxybenzamine** and **phentolamine**) were once used to produce vasodilatation in the treatment of peripheral vascular disease, but this use is now largely obsolete.
> - Selective α₁ antagonists (e.g. **prazosin**, **doxazosin**, **terazosin**) are used in treating hypertension and for benign prostatic hypertrophy. Postural hypotension, stress incontinence and impotence are unwanted effects.
> - **Tamsulosin** is α₁ₐ selective and acts mainly on the urogenital tract. It is used to treat benign prostatic hypertrophy and may cause less postural hypotension than other α₁ agonists.
> - **Yohimbine** is a selective α₂ antagonist. It is not used clinically.

purposes, but have only limited therapeutic applications. In hypertension, non-selective α-blocking drugs are unsatisfactory, because of their tendency to produce tachycardia and cardiac dysrhythmias, and gastrointestinal symptoms. Selective α₁-receptor antagonists (especially the longer-acting compounds **doxazosin** and **terazosin**) are, however, useful. They do not affect cardiac function appreciably, and postural hypotension is less troublesome than with prazosin or non-selective α-receptor antagonists. They have a place in treating severe hypertension, where they are added to treatment with first- and second-line drugs, but are not used as first-line agents (see Ch. 22). Unlike other antihypertensive drugs, they cause a modest decrease in low-density lipoprotein, and an increase in high-density lipoprotein cholesterol (see Ch. 23), although the clinical importance of these ostensibly beneficial effects is uncertain. They are also used to control urinary retention in patients with benign prostatic hypertrophy.

Phaeochromocytoma is a catecholamine-secreting tumour of chromaffin tissue, which causes severe and initially episodic hypertension. A combination of α- and β-receptor antagonists is the most effective way of controlling the blood pressure. The tumour may be surgically removable, and it is essential to block α and β receptors before surgery is begun, to avoid the effects of a sudden release of catecholamines when the tumour is disturbed. A combination of phenoxybenzamine and atenolol is effective for this purpose.

> ## Clinical uses of α-adrenoceptor antagonists
>
>
> - Severe hypertension (see Ch. 22): α₁-selective antagonists (e.g. **doxazosin**) in combination with other drugs.
> - Benign prostatic hypertrophy (e.g. **tamsulosin**, a selective α₁ₐ-receptor antagonist).
> - Phaeochromocytoma: **phenoxybenzamine** (irreversible antagonist) in preparation for surgery.

β-Adrenoceptor antagonists

The β-adrenoceptor antagonists are an important group of drugs. They were first discovered in 1958, 10 years after Ahlquist had postulated the existence of β adrenoceptors. The first compound, **dichloroisoprenaline**, had fairly low potency and was a partial agonist. Further development led to **propranolol**, which is much more potent and a pure antagonist that blocks β_1 and β_2 receptors equally. The potential clinical advantages of drugs with some partial agonist activity, and/or with selectivity for β_1 receptors, led to the development of **practolol** (selective for β_1 receptors but withdrawn because of its off-target toxicity), **oxprenolol** and **alprenolol** (non-selective with considerable partial agonist activity), and **atenolol** (β_1-selective with no agonist activity). Two newer drugs are **carvedilol** (a non-selective β-adrenoceptor antagonist with additional α_1-blocking activity) and **nebivolol** (a β_1-selective antagonist that also causes vasodilatation by inducing endothelial nitric oxide production; see Ch. 20). Both these drugs have proven more effective than conventional β-adrenoceptor antagonists in treating heart failure (see Ch. 21). The characteristics of the most important compounds are set out in Table 14.5. Most β-receptor antagonists are inactive on β_3 receptors so do not affect lipolysis.

Actions

The pharmacological actions of β-receptor antagonists can be deduced from Table 14.1. The effects produced in humans depend on the degree of sympathetic activity and are modest in subjects at rest. The most important effects are on the cardiovascular system and on bronchial smooth muscle (see Chs 21, 22 and 28).

In a healthy subject at rest, propranolol causes modest changes in heart rate, cardiac output or arterial pressure, but it markedly reduces the effect of exercise or excitement on these variables (Fig. 14.6). Drugs with partial agonist activity, such as oxprenolol, increase the heart rate at rest but reduce it during exercise. Maximum exercise tolerance is considerably reduced in normal subjects, partly because of the limitation of the cardiac response, and partly because the β-mediated vasodilatation in skeletal muscle is reduced. Coronary flow is reduced, but relatively less than the myocardial oxygen consumption, so oxygenation of the myocardium is improved, an effect of importance in the treatment of angina pectoris (see Ch. 21). In normal subjects, the reduction of the force of contraction of the heart is of no importance, but it may have important consequences for patients with heart disease (see below).

An important, and somewhat unexpected, effect of β-receptor antagonists is their antihypertensive action (see Ch. 22). Patients with hypertension (although not normotensive subjects) show a gradual fall in arterial pressure that takes several days to develop fully. The mechanism is complex and involves the following:

- reduction in cardiac output
- reduction of renin release from the juxtaglomerular cells of the kidney
- a central action, reducing sympathetic activity.

Carvedilol and nebivolol (see above) are particularly effective in lowering blood pressure, because of their additional vasodilator properties.

Blockade of the facilitatory effect of presynaptic β receptors on noradrenaline release (see Table 14.1) may also contribute to the antihypertensive effect. The antihypertensive effect of β-receptor antagonists is clinically very useful. Because reflex vasoconstriction is preserved, postural and exercise-induced hypotension are less troublesome than with many other antihypertensive drugs.

Many β-receptor antagonists have an important antidysrhythmic effect on the heart (see Ch. 21).

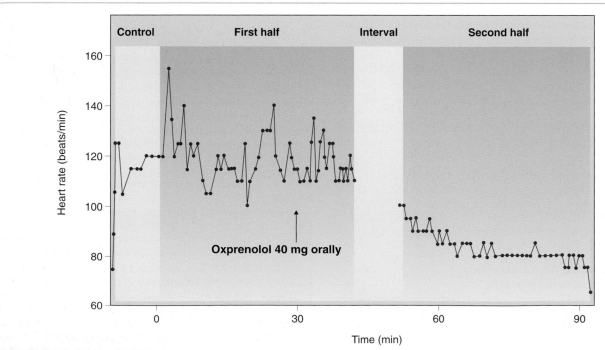

Fig. 14.6 Heart rate recorded continuously in a spectator watching a live football match, showing the effect of the β-adrenoceptor antagonist oxprenolol. *(From Taylor SH, Meeran MK 1973. In: Burley et al. (Eds) New Perspectives in Beta-Blockade. CIBA Laboratories, Horsham.)*

Airways resistance in normal subjects is only slightly increased by β-receptor antagonists, and this is of no consequence. In asthmatic subjects, however, non-selective β-receptor antagonists (such as propranolol) can cause severe bronchoconstriction, which does not, of course, respond to the usual doses of drugs such as salbutamol or adrenaline. This danger is less with β_1-selective antagonists, but none is so selective that this danger can be ignored.

Despite the involvement of β receptors in the hyperglycaemic actions of adrenaline, β-receptor antagonists cause only minor metabolic changes in normal subjects. They do not affect the onset of hypoglycaemia following an injection of insulin, but somewhat delay the recovery of blood glucose concentration. In diabetic patients, the use of β-receptor antagonists increases the likelihood of exercise-induced hypoglycaemia, because the normal adrenaline-induced release of glucose from the liver is diminished.

β-Adrenoceptor antagonists

- Non-selective between β_1 and β_2 adrenoceptors: **propranolol, alprenolol, oxprenolol**.
- β_1-selective: **atenolol, nebivolol**.
- **Alprenolol** and **oxprenolol** have partial agonist activity.
- Many clinical uses (see clinical box, below).
- Important hazards are bronchoconstriction, and bradycardia and cardiac failure (possibly less with partial agonists).
- Side effects include cold extremities, insomnia, depression, fatigue.
- Some show rapid first-pass metabolism, hence poor bioavailability.
- Some drugs (e.g. **labetalol, carvedilol**) block both α and β adrenoceptors.

Clinical use

The main uses of β-receptor antagonists are connected with their effects on the cardiovascular system, and are discussed in Chapters 21 and 22. They are as summarised in the clinical box below.

The use of β-receptor antagonists in cardiac failure deserves special mention, as clinical opinion has undergone a U-turn. Patients with heart disease may rely on a degree of sympathetic drive to the heart to maintain an adequate cardiac output, and removal of this by blocking β receptors can exacerbate cardiac failure, so using these drugs in patients with cardiac failure was considered ill-advised. In theory, drugs with partial agonist activity (e.g. oxprenolol, alprenolol) offer an advantage because they can, by their own action, maintain a degree of β_1-receptor activation, while at the same time blunting the cardiac response to increased sympathetic nerve activity or to circulating adrenaline. Clinical trials, however, have not shown a clear advantage of these drugs measurable as a reduced incidence of cardiac failure, and one such drug (**xamoterol**, since withdrawn) with particularly marked agonist activity clearly made matters worse.

Paradoxically, β-receptor antagonists are increasingly being used in low doses to treat well-compensated cardiac failure and there is strong evidence that this improves survival in carefully selected patients (Ch. 22), although at the outset there is a danger of exacerbating the problem (Bristow, 2011). **Carvedilol** is often used for this purpose. This success has led to the proposal that β-receptor antagonists might also be of value in the long-term treatment of patients with stable asthma, but this remains controversial.

Clinical uses of β-adrenoceptor antagonists

- Cardiovascular (see Chs 21 and 22):
  - angina pectoris
  - myocardial infarction, and following infarction
  - prevention of recurrent dysrhythmias (especially if triggered by sympathetic activation)
  - heart failure (in well-compensated patients)
  - hypertension (no longer first choice; Ch. 22).
- Other uses:
  - glaucoma (e.g. **timolol** eye drops)
  - thyrotoxicosis (Ch. 34), as adjunct to definitive treatment (e.g. preoperatively)
  - anxiety (Ch. 44), to control somatic symptoms (e.g. palpitations, tremor)
  - migraine prophylaxis (Ch. 15)
  - benign essential tremor (a familial disorder).

Unwanted effects

The main side effects of β-receptor antagonists result from their receptor-blocking action.

Bronchoconstriction. This is of little importance in the absence of airways disease, but in asthmatic patients the effect can be life-threatening. It is also of clinical importance in patients with other forms of obstructive lung disease (e.g. chronic bronchitis, emphysema), although the risk–benefit balance may favour cautious treatment in individual patients. As mentioned above, it has been hypothesised that β-receptor antagonists might actually be of value in treating stable asthmatic patients.

Cardiac depression. Cardiac depression can occur, leading to signs of heart failure, particularly in elderly people. Patients suffering from heart failure who are treated with β-receptor antagonists (see above) often deteriorate in the first few weeks before the beneficial effect develops.

Bradycardia. Sinus bradycardia can progress to life-threatening heart block and can occur in patients with coronary disease, particularly if they are being treated with antiarrhythmic drugs that impair cardiac conduction (see Ch. 21).

Hypoglycaemia. Glucose release in response to adrenaline is a safety device that may be important to diabetic patients and to other individuals prone to hypoglycaemic attacks. The sympathetic response to hypoglycaemia produces symptoms (especially tachycardia) that warn patients of the urgent need for carbohydrate (usually in the form of a sugary drink). β-Receptor antagonists reduce these symptoms, so incipient hypoglycaemia is more likely to go unnoticed by the patient. There is a theoretical advantage in using β_1-selective agents, because glucose release from the liver is controlled by β_2 receptors.

Fatigue. This is probably due to reduced cardiac output and reduced muscle perfusion in exercise. It is a frequent complaint of patients taking β-receptor-blocking drugs.

Cold extremities. This is common, due to a loss of β-receptor-mediated vasodilatation in cutaneous vessels. Theoretically, β_1-selective drugs are less likely to produce this effect, but it is not clear that this is so in practice.

Other adverse effects associated with β-receptor antagonists are not obviously the result of β-receptor blockade. One is the occurrence of bad dreams, which occur mainly with highly lipid-soluble drugs such as propranolol, which enter the brain easily.

▼ There are several additional factors that make β-adrenoceptor pharmacology more complicated than it appears at first sight, and may have implications for the clinical use of β-adrenoceptor antagonists:

- Several drugs that act on adrenoceptors have the characteristics of partial agonists (see Ch. 2), i.e. they block receptors and thus antagonise the actions of full agonists, but also have a weak agonist effect of their own. Some β-adrenoceptor-blocking drugs (e.g. **alprenolol**, **oxprenolol**) cause, under resting conditions, an increase in heart rate while at the same time opposing the tachycardia produced by sympathetic stimulation. This has been interpreted as a partial agonist effect, although there is evidence that mechanisms other than β-receptor activation may contribute to the tachycardia.
- The high degree of receptor specificity found for some compounds in laboratory animals is seldom found in humans.
- Though in normal hearts cardiac stimulation is mediated through β_1 receptors, in heart failure (see Ch. 21) β_2 receptors contribute significantly.
- There is evidence that β-adrenoceptor agonists and partial agonists may act not only through cAMP formation, but also through other signal transduction pathways (e.g. the mitogen-activated protein [MAP] kinase pathway; see Ch. 3), and that the relative contribution of these signals differs for different drugs. Furthermore, the pathways show different levels of constitutive activation, which is reduced by ligands that function as inverse agonists. β-Adrenoceptor antagonists in clinical use differ in respect of these properties, and drugs classified as partial agonists may actually activate one pathway while blocking another (see Baker et al., 2003).
- Genetic variants of both β_1 and β_2 receptors occur in humans, and influence the effects of agonists and antagonists (see Brodde, 2008).

DRUGS THAT AFFECT NORADRENERGIC NEURONS

Emphasis in this chapter is placed on peripheral sympathetic transmission. The same principles, however, are applicable to the central nervous system (see Ch. 37), where many of the drugs mentioned here also act. The major drugs and mechanisms are summarised in Table 14.6.

DRUGS THAT AFFECT NORADRENALINE SYNTHESIS

Only a few clinically important drugs affect noradrenaline synthesis directly. Examples are **α-methyltyrosine**, which inhibits tyrosine hydroxylase, and **carbidopa**, a hydrazine derivative of dopa, which inhibits dopa decarboxylase and is used in the treatment of parkinsonism (see Ch. 40).

Methyldopa, still used in the treatment of hypertension during pregnancy (see Ch. 22), is taken up by noradrenergic neurons, where it is converted to the false transmitter α-methylnoradrenaline. This substance is not deaminated within the neuron by MAO, so it accumulates and displaces noradrenaline from the synaptic vesicles. α-Methylnoradrenaline is released in the same way as

noradrenaline, but is less active than noradrenaline on α_1 receptors and thus is less effective in causing vasoconstriction. On the other hand, it is more active on presynaptic (α_2) receptors, so the autoinhibitory feedback mechanism operates more strongly than normal, thus reducing transmitter release below the normal levels. Both of these effects (as well as a central effect, probably caused by the same cellular mechanism) contribute to the hypotensive action. It produces side effects typical of centrally acting antiadrenergic drugs (e.g. sedation), as well as carrying a risk of immune haemolytic reactions and liver toxicity, so it is now little used, except for hypertension in late pregnancy where there is considerable experience of its use and no suggestion of harm to the unborn baby.

6-Hydroxydopamine (identical with dopamine except for an extra hydroxyl group) is a neurotoxin of the Trojan horse kind. It is taken up selectively by noradrenergic nerve terminals, where it is converted to a reactive quinone, which destroys the nerve terminal, producing a 'chemical sympathectomy'. The cell bodies survive, and eventually the sympathetic innervation recovers. The drug is useful for experimental purposes but has no clinical uses. If injected directly into the brain, it selectively destroys those nerve terminals (i.e. dopaminergic, noradrenergic and adrenergic) that take it up, but it does not reach the brain if given systemically.

MPTP (1-methyl-4-phenyl-1,2,3,5-tetrahydropyridine; see Ch. 40) is a similar selective neurotoxin acting on dopaminergic neurons.

Dihydroxyphenylserine (L-DOPS) is currently under investigation for treating hypotensive states associated with reduced noradrenaline synthesis. It penetrates the blood–brain barrier and can be regarded as a catecholamine prodrug being converted to noradrenaline directly by dopa decarboxylase, bypassing the DBH-catalysed hydroxylation step. It raises blood pressure by increasing noradrenaline release.

DRUGS THAT AFFECT NORADRENALINE STORAGE

Reserpine is an alkaloid from the shrub *Rauwolfia*, which has been used in India for centuries for the treatment of mental disorders. Reserpine, at very low concentration, blocks the transport of noradrenaline and other amines into synaptic vesicles, by blocking the vesicular monoamine transporter. Noradrenaline accumulates instead in the cytoplasm, where it is degraded by MAO. The noradrenaline content of tissues drops to a low level, and sympathetic transmission is blocked. Reserpine also causes depletion of 5-HT and dopamine from neurons in the brain, in which these amines are transmitters (see Ch. 39). Reserpine is now used only experimentally, but was at one time used as an antihypertensive drug. Its central effects, especially depression, which probably result from impairment of noradrenergic and 5-HT-mediated transmission in the brain (see Ch. 47), were a serious problem.

DRUGS THAT AFFECT NORADRENALINE RELEASE

Drugs can affect noradrenaline release in four main ways:

- by directly blocking release (noradrenergic neuron-blocking drugs)
- by evoking noradrenaline release in the absence of nerve terminal depolarisation (indirectly acting sympathomimetic drugs)

Table 14.6 Drugs that affect noradrenaline synthesis, release or uptake

Drug	Main action	Uses/function	Unwanted effects	Pharmacokinetic aspects	Notes
Drugs affecting NA synthesis					
α-Methyl-p-tyrosine	Inhibits tyrosine hydroxylase	Occasionally used in phaeochromocytoma	Hypotension, sedation	–	–
Carbidopa	Inhibits dopa decarboxylase	Used as adjunct to levodopa to prevent peripheral effects	–	Absorbed orally Does not enter brain	See Ch. 40
Methyldopa	False transmitter precursor	Hypertension in pregnancy	Hypotension, drowsiness, diarrhoea, impotence, hypersensitivity reactions	Absorbed slowly by mouth Excreted unchanged or as conjugate Plasma $t_{1/2}$ ~6 h	See Ch. 22
L-dihydroxyphenylserine (L-DOPS)	Converted to NA by dopa decarboxylase, thus increasing NA synthesis and release	Orthostatic hypotension	Not known	Absorbed orally Duration of action ~6 h	Currently in clinical trials
Drugs that release NA (indirectly acting sympathomimetic amines)					
Tyramine	NA release	No clinical uses Present in various foods	As norepinephrine	Normally destroyed by MAO in gut Does not enter brain	See Ch. 47
Amphetamine	NA release, MAO inhibitor, NET inhibitor, CNS stimulant	Used as CNS stimulant in narcolepsy, also (paradoxically) in hyperactive children Appetite suppressant Drug of abuse	Hypertension, tachycardia, insomnia Acute psychosis with overdose Dependence	Well absorbed orally Penetrates freely into brain Excreted unchanged in urine Plasma $t_{1/2}$ ~12 h, depending on urine flow and pH	See Ch. 48 Methylphenidate and atomoxetine are similar (used for CNS effects; see Ch. 49)
Ephedrine	NA release, β agonist, weak CNS stimulant action	Nasal decongestion	As amphetamine but less pronounced	Similar to amphetamine aspects	Contraindicated if MAO inhibitors are given
Drugs that inhibit NA release					
Reserpine	Depletes NA stores by inhibiting VMAT	Hypertension (obsolete)	As methyldopa Also depression, parkinsonism, gynaecomastia	Poorly absorbed orally Slowly metabolised Plasma $t_{1/2}$ ~100 h Excreted in milk	Antihypertensive effect develops slowly and persists when drug is stopped
Guanethidine	Inhibits NA release Also causes NA depletion and can damage NA neurons irreversibly	Hypertension (obsolete)	As methyldopa Hypertension on first administration	Poorly absorbed orally Mainly excreted unchanged in urine Plasma $t_{1/2}$ ~100 h	Action prevented by NET inhibitors
Drugs affecting NA uptake					
Imipramine	Blocks neuronal transporter (NET) Also has atropine-like action	Depression	Atropine-like side effects Cardiac dysrhythmias in overdose	Well absorbed orally 95% bound to plasma protein Converted to active metabolite (desmethylimipramine) Plasma $t_{1/2}$ ~4 h	Desipramine and amitriptyline are similar See Ch. 47
Cocaine	Local anaesthetic; blocks NET CNS stimulant	Rarely used local anaesthetic Major drug of abuse	Hypertension, excitement, convulsions, dependence	Well absorbed orally or intranasally	See Chs 43 and 49

COMT, catechol-O-methyltransferase; MAO, monoamine oxidase; NA, noradrenaline; VMAT, vesicular monoamine transporter.

- by acting on presynaptic receptors that indirectly inhibit or enhance depolarisation-evoked release; examples include α_2 agonists (see p. 184-187), angiotensin II, dopamine and prostaglandins
- by increasing or decreasing available stores of noradrenaline (e.g. reserpine, see p. 180; MAO inhibitors, see Ch. 47).

NORADRENERGIC NEURON-BLOCKING DRUGS

Noradrenergic neuron-blocking drugs (e.g. **guanethidine**) were first discovered in the mid-1950s when alternatives to ganglion-blocking drugs, for use in the treatment of hypertension, were being sought. The main effect of guanethidine is to inhibit the release of noradrenaline from sympathetic nerve terminals. It has little effect on the adrenal medulla, and none on nerve terminals that release transmitters other than noradrenaline. Drugs very similar to it include **bretylium**, **bethanidine** and **debrisoquin** (which is of interest mainly as a tool for studying drug metabolism; see Ch. 11).

Actions

Drugs of this class reduce or abolish the response of tissues to sympathetic nerve stimulation, but do not affect (or may potentiate) the effects of circulating noradrenaline.

The action of guanethidine on noradrenergic transmission is complex. It is selectively accumulated by noradrenergic nerve terminals, being a substrate for NET (see Table 14.6). Its initial blocking activity is due to block of impulse conduction in the nerve terminals that selectively accumulate the drug. Its action is prevented by drugs, such as *tricyclic antidepressants* (see Ch. 47), that block NET.

Guanethidine is also concentrated in synaptic vesicles by means of the vesicular transporter VMAT, possibly interfering with their ability to undergo exocytosis, and also displacing noradrenaline. In this way, it causes a gradual and long-lasting depletion of noradrenaline in sympathetic nerve endings, similar to the effect of reserpine.

Given in large doses, guanethidine causes structural damage to noradrenergic neurons, which is probably due to the fact that the terminals accumulate the drug in high concentration. It can therefore be used experimentally as a selective neurotoxin.

Guanethidine, bethanidine and debrisoquin are no longer used clinically, now that better antihypertensive drugs are available. Although extremely effective in lowering blood pressure, they produce severe side effects associated with the loss of sympathetic reflexes. The most troublesome are postural hypotension, diarrhoea, nasal congestion and failure of ejaculation.

INDIRECTLY ACTING SYMPATHOMIMETIC AMINES

Mechanism of action and structure–activity relationships

The most important drugs in the indirectly acting sympathomimetic amine category are **tyramine**, **amphetamine** and **ephedrine**, which are structurally related to noradrenaline. Drugs that act similarly and are used for their central effects (see Ch. 48) include **methylphenidate** and **atomoxetine**.

These drugs have only weak actions on adrenoceptors, but sufficiently resemble noradrenaline to be transported

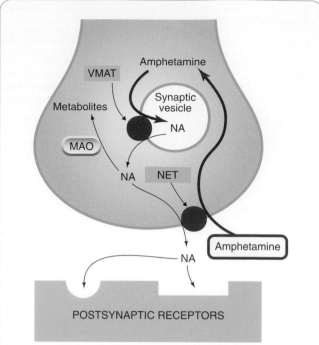

Fig. 14.7 The mode of action of amphetamine, an indirectly acting sympathomimetic amine. Amphetamine enters the nerve terminal via the noradrenaline transporter (NET) and enters synaptic vesicles via the vesicular monoamine transporter (VMAT), in exchange for NA, which accumulates in the cytosol. Some of the NA is degraded by monoamine oxidase (MAO) within the nerve terminal and some escapes, in exchange for amphetamine via the noradrenaline transporter, to act on postsynaptic receptors. Amphetamine also reduces NA reuptake via the transporter, so enhancing the action of the released NA.

into nerve terminals by NET. Once inside the nerve terminals, they are taken up into the vesicles by VMAT, in exchange for noradrenaline, which escapes into the cytosol. Some of the cytosolic noradrenaline is degraded by MAO, while the rest escapes via NET, in exchange for the foreign monoamine, to act on postsynaptic receptors (Fig. 14.7). Exocytosis is not involved in the release process, so their actions do not require the presence of Ca^{2+}. They are not completely specific in their actions, and act partly by a direct effect on adrenoceptors, partly by inhibiting NET (thereby enhancing the effect of the released noradrenaline) and partly by inhibiting MAO.

As would be expected, the effects of these drugs are strongly influenced by other drugs that modify noradrenergic transmission. Thus reserpine and 6-hydroxydopamine abolish their effects by depleting the terminals of noradrenaline. MAO inhibitors, on the other hand, strongly potentiate their effects by preventing inactivation, within the terminals, of the transmitter displaced from the vesicles. MAO inhibition particularly enhances the action of tyramine, because this substance is itself a substrate for MAO. Normally, dietary tyramine is destroyed by MAO in the gut wall and liver before reaching the systemic circulation. When MAO is inhibited this is prevented, and ingestion of tyramine-rich foods such as fermented cheese (e.g. ripe Brie) can then provoke a sudden and dangerous rise in blood pressure. Inhibitors of NET, such as **imipramine** (see Table 14.6), interfere with the effects of indirectly acting sympathomimetic amines by preventing their uptake into the nerve terminals.

These drugs, especially amphetamine, have important effects on the central nervous system (see Ch. 48) that depend on their ability to release not only noradrenaline, but also 5-HT and dopamine from nerve terminals in the brain. An important characteristic of the effects of indirectly acting sympathomimetic amines is that marked tolerance develops. Repeated doses of amphetamine or tyramine, for example, produce progressively smaller pressor responses. This is probably caused by a depletion of the releasable store of noradrenaline. A similar tolerance to the central effects also develops with repeated administration, contributing to the liability of amphetamine and related drugs to cause dependence.

Actions

The peripheral actions of the indirectly acting sympathomimetic amines include bronchodilatation, raised arterial pressure, peripheral vasoconstriction, increased heart rate and force of myocardial contraction, and inhibition of gut motility. They have important central actions, which account for their significant abuse potential and for their limited therapeutic applications (see Chs 48 and 58). Apart from ephedrine, which is still sometimes used as a nasal decongestant because it has much less central action, these drugs are no longer used for their peripheral sympathomimetic effects.

INHIBITORS OF NORADRENALINE UPTAKE

Reuptake of released noradrenaline by NET is the most important mechanism by which its action is brought to an end. Many drugs inhibit NET, and thereby enhance the effects of both sympathetic nerve activity and circulating noradrenaline. NET is not responsible for clearing circulating adrenaline, so these drugs do not affect responses to this amine.

The main class of drugs whose primary action is inhibition of NET are the *tricyclic antidepressants* (see Ch. 47), for example **imipramine**. These drugs have their major effect on the central nervous system but also cause tachycardia and cardiac dysrhythmias, reflecting their peripheral effect on sympathetic transmission. **Cocaine**, known mainly for its abuse liability (Ch. 49) and local anaesthetic activity (Ch. 43), enhances sympathetic transmission, causing tachycardia and increased arterial pressure (and with chronic use, cardiomyopathy and cardiac hypertrophy). Its central effects of euphoria and excitement (Ch. 48) are probably a manifestation of the same mechanism acting in the brain. It strongly potentiates the actions of noradrenaline in experimental animals or in isolated tissues provided the sympathetic nerve terminals are intact.

Many drugs that act mainly on other steps in sympathetic transmission also inhibit NET to some extent, presumably because the carrier molecule has structural features in common with other noradrenaline recognition sites, such as receptors and degradative enzymes.

The extraneuronal monoamine transporter EMT, which is important in clearing circulating adrenaline from the bloodstream, is not affected by most of the drugs that block NET. It is inhibited by **phenoxybenzamine**, however, and also by various *corticosteroids* (see Ch. 26). This action of corticosteroids may have some relevance to their therapeutic effect in conditions such as asthma, but is probably of minor importance.

The main sites of action of drugs that affect adrenergic transmission are summarised in Fig. 14.8.

Drugs acting on noradrenergic nerve terminals

- Drugs that inhibit noradrenaline synthesis include:
  - **α-Methyltyrosine**: blocks tyrosine hydroxylase; not used clinically
  - **carbidopa**: blocks dopa decarboxylase and is used in treatment of parkinsonism (see Ch. 40); not much effect on noradrenaline synthesis.
- **Methyldopa** gives rise to false transmitter (methylnoradrenaline), which is a potent α_2 agonist, thus causing powerful presynaptic inhibitory feedback (also central actions). Its use as an antihypertensive agent is now limited mainly to during pregnancy.
- **Reserpine** blocks noradrenaline accumulation in vesicles by VMAT, thus depleting noradrenaline stores and blocking transmission. Effective in hypertension but may cause severe depression. Clinically obsolete.
- Noradrenergic neuron-blocking drugs (e.g. **guanethidine, bethanidine**) are selectively concentrated in terminals and in vesicles (by NET and VMAT respectively), and block transmitter release, partly by local anaesthetic action. Effective in hypertension but cause severe side effects (postural hypotension, diarrhoea, nasal congestion, etc.), so now little used.
- **6-Hydroxydopamine** is selectively neurotoxic for noradrenergic neurons, because it is taken up and converted to a toxic metabolite. Used experimentally to eliminate noradrenergic neurons, not used clinically.
- Indirectly acting sympathomimetic amines (e.g. **amphetamine, ephedrine, tyramine**) are accumulated by NET and displace noradrenaline from vesicles, allowing it to escape. Effect is much enhanced by monoamine oxidase (MAO) inhibition, which can lead to severe hypertension following ingestion of tyramine-rich foods by patients treated with MAO inhibitors.
- Indirectly acting sympathomimetic agents are central nervous system stimulants. **Methylphenidate** and **atomoxetine** are used to treat attention deficit–hyperactivity disorder.
- Drugs that inhibit NET include **cocaine** and **tricyclic antidepressant** drugs. Sympathetic effects are enhanced by such drugs.

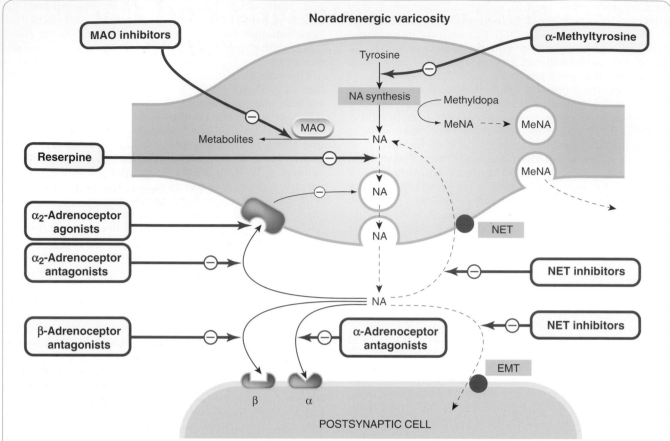

Fig. 14.8 Generalised diagram of a noradrenergic nerve terminal, showing sites of drug action. EMT, extraneuronal monoamine transporter; MAO, monoamine oxidase; MeNA, methylnoradrenaline; NA, noradrenaline; NET, neuronal noradrenaline transporter.

REFERENCES AND FURTHER READING

General

Cooper, J.R., Bloom, F.E., Roth, R.H., 2002. The Biochemical Basis of Neuropharmacology, eighth ed. Oxford University Press, New York. (*Excellent standard textbook*)

Robertson, D.W. (Ed.), 2004. Primer on the Autonomic Nervous System. Academic Press, New York. (*An excellent comprehensive textbook on all aspects, including pharmacology, of the autonomic nervous system. By no means elementary despite its title*)

Adrenoceptors

Alexander, S.P.H., et al., 2013. Concise Guide to Pharmacology. Br. J. Pharmacol. 170, 1459–1867. (*Summary articles on all major drug targets, including adrenoceptors, transporters and enzymes involved in catecholamine metabolism. A valuable reference source – not for casual reading*)

Baker, J.G., Hall, I.P., Hill, S.J., 2003. Agonist and inverse agonist actions of β-blockers at the human β₂-adrenoceptor provide evidence for agonist-directed signalling. Mol. Pharmacol. 64, 1357–1369. (*β-blockers differ in their ability to activate and block cAMP and mitogen-activated protein kinase pathways, possibly explaining why some are better than others in treating heart disease*)

Brodde, O., 2008. β₁- and β₂-Adrenoceptor polymorphisms and cardiovascular diseases. Fund. Clin. Pharmacol. 22, 107–125. (*Comprehensive review of possible genetic influences on human response to drugs acting on β-adrenoceptors*)

Elenkov, I.J., Wilder, R.L., Chrousos, G.P., et al., 2000. The sympathetic nerve – an integrative interface between two supersystems: the brain and the immune system. Pharmacol. Rev. 52, 595–638. (*Detailed catalogue of effects of catecholamines and the sympathetic nervous system on the immune system*)

Gainetdinov, R.R., Caron, M.G., 2003. Monoamine transporters: from genes to behaviour. Annu. Rev. Pharmacol. Toxicol. 43, 261–284. (*Review article focusing on the characteristics of transgenic mice lacking specific monoamine transporters*)

Gilsbach, R., Hein, L., 2012. Are the pharmacology and physiology of α₂ adrenoceptors determined by α₂-heteroreceptors and autoreceptors

respectively? Br. J. Pharmacol. 165, 90–102. (*Argues for the significance of auto- versus heteroreceptors in mediating the physiological functions of α₂-adrenoceptors and the pharmacological functions of α₂-adrenoceptor agonist drugs respectively*)

Guimaraes, S., Moura, D., 2001. Vascular adrenoceptors: an update. Pharmacol. Rev. 53, 319–356. (*Review describing the complex roles of different adrenoceptors in blood vessels*)

Kahsai, A.W., Xiao, K.H., Rajagopal, S., et al., 2011. Multiple ligand-specific conformations of the beta(2)-adrenergic receptor. Nature Chem. Biol. 7, 692–700. (*Contrary to two-state models for receptor activity, there is significant variability in receptor conformations induced by different ligands, which has significant implications for the design of new therapeutic agents*)

Philipp, M., Hein, L., 2004. Adrenergic receptor knockout mice: distinct functions of 9 receptor subtypes. Pharm. Ther. 101, 65–74.

Sacco, E., Bientinesi, R., 2012. Mirabegron: a review of recent data and its prospects in the management of overactive bladder. Ther. Adv. Urol. 4, 315–324. (*Pharmacology of a selective β₃-adrenoceptor agonist, licensed to treat symptoms of overactive bladder*)

Miscellaneous topics

Bristow, M.R., 2011. Treatment of chronic heart failure with beta-adrenergic receptor antagonists: a convergence of receptor pharmacology and clinical cardiology. Circ. Res. 109, 1176–1194. (*Argues that there is: 'ample room to improve antiadrenergic therapy, through novel approaches exploiting the nuances of receptor biology and/or intracellular signaling, as well as through pharmacogenetic targeting'*)

Eisenhofer, G., Kopin, I.J., Goldstein, D.S., 2004. Catecholamine metabolism: a contemporary view with implications for physiology and medicine. Pharmacol. Rev. 56, 331–349. (*Review that dismisses a number of fallacies concerning the routes by which catecholamines from different sources are metabolised and excreted*)

Nonogaki, K., 2000. New insights into sympathetic regulation of glucose and fat metabolism. Diabetologia 43, 533–549. (*Review of the complex adrenoceptor-mediated effects on the metabolism of liver, muscle and adipose tissue; up to date, but not a particularly easy read*)

5-Hydroxytryptamine and the pharmacology of migraine

OVERVIEW

5-Hydroxytryptamine (5-HT) is an important neuro-transmitter in the brain and periphery and also a local hormone. We describe its synthesis, storage and release and its role in the pathophysiology of three disorders (migraine, carcinoid syndrome and pulmonary hypertension). We also describe the pharmacology of the numerous drugs that act at 5-HT receptors.

5-HYDROXYTRYPTAMINE

The biologically active, low-molecular-weight, factor originally detected in extracts of gut ('enteramine') and in blood serum ('serotonin') was eventually identified chemically as *5-hydroxytryptamine*. Today, the terms '5-HT' and 'serotonin' are used interchangeably. 5-HT was subsequently found in the central nervous system (CNS) and shown to function both as a neurotransmitter and as a local hormone in the peripheral vascular system. This chapter deals with the metabolism, distribution and physiological roles of 5-HT in the periphery, and with the different types of 5-HT receptor and the drugs that act on them. Further information on the role of 5-HT in the brain, and its relationship to psychiatric disorders and the actions of psychotropic drugs, is presented in Chapters 39, 46 and 47. The use of drugs that modulate 5-HT in the gut is dealt with in Chapter 30.

DISTRIBUTION, BIOSYNTHESIS AND DEGRADATION

The highest concentrations of 5-HT occur in three organs:

- *In the wall of the intestine.* Over 90% of the total amount in the body is present in the *enterochromaffin* cells (endocrine cells with distinctive staining properties) in the gut. These cells are derived from the neural crest and resemble those of the adrenal medulla. They are found mainly in the stomach and small intestine interspersed with mucosal cells. Some 5-HT also occurs in nerve cells of the myenteric plexus, where it functions as an excitatory neurotransmitter (see Chs 12 and 30).
- *In blood.* Platelets contain high concentrations of 5-HT. They accumulate it from the plasma by an active transport system and release it from cytoplasmic granules when they aggregate (hence the high concentration of 5HT in serum from clotted blood, see Ch. 24).
- *In the CNS.* 5-HT is a transmitter in the CNS and is present in high concentrations in localised regions of the midbrain. Its functional role is discussed in Chapter 39.

Although 5-HT is present in the diet, most of this is metabolised before entering the bloodstream. Endogenous 5-HT arises from a biosynthetic pathway similar to that of noradrenaline; (see Ch. 14), except that the precursor amino acid is *tryptophan* instead of tyrosine (Fig. 15.1). Tryptophan is converted to 5-hydroxytryptophan (in chromaffin cells and neurons, but not in platelets) by the action of *tryptophan hydroxylase*, an enzyme confined to 5-HT-producing cells. The 5-hydroxytryptophan is then decarboxylated to 5-HT by a ubiquitous *amino acid decarboxylase* that also participates in the synthesis of catecholamines (Ch. 14) and histamine (Ch. 17). Platelets (and neurons) possess a high-affinity 5-HT uptake mechanism. They become loaded with 5-HT as they pass through the intestinal circulation, where the local concentration is relatively high. Because the mechanisms of synthesis, storage, release and reuptake of 5-HT are very similar to those of noradrenaline, many drugs affect both processes indiscriminately (see Ch. 14). However, *selective serotonin reuptake inhibitors* (SSRIs) have been developed and are important therapeutically as anxiolytics and antidepressants (Chs 44 and 47). 5-HT is often stored in neurons and chromaffin cells as a co-transmitter together with various peptide hormones, such as *somatostatin*, *substance P* or *vasoactive intestinal polypeptide* (Ch. 18).

Degradation of 5-HT (Fig. 15.1) occurs mainly through oxidative deamination, catalysed by *monoamine oxidase A*, followed by oxidation to *5-hydroxyindoleacetic acid* (5-HIAA), the pathway again being the same as that of noradrenaline catabolism. 5-HIAA is excreted in the urine and serves as an indicator of 5-HT production in the body. This is used, for example, in the diagnosis of carcinoid syndrome.

PHARMACOLOGICAL EFFECTS

The actions of 5-HT are numerous and complex and there is considerable species variation. This complexity reflects the profusion of 5-HT receptor subtypes. The main sites of action are as follows.

Gastrointestinal tract. Most 5-HT receptor subtypes are present in the gut with the exception of those of the 5-HT$_{5/6}$ family. Only about 10% of 5-HT in the intestine is located in neurons, where it acts as a neurotransmitter, while the remainder is located in the enterochromaffin cells, which act as sensors to transduce information about the state of the gut. 5-HT is released from enterochromaffin cells into the *lamina propria*. The responses observed are very complex and the reader is referred to Beattie & Smith (2008) for a recent comprehensive account. Broadly speaking, 5-HT receptors are present on most neuronal components of the enteric nervous system as well as smooth muscle, secretory and other cells. Their main function is to regulate peristalsis, intestinal motility, secretion and visceral sensitivity.

The importance of 5-HT in the gut is underlined by the widespread distribution of the *serotonin uptake transporter* (SERT), which rapidly and efficiently removes extracellular 5-HT, thus limiting its action. Inhibitors of

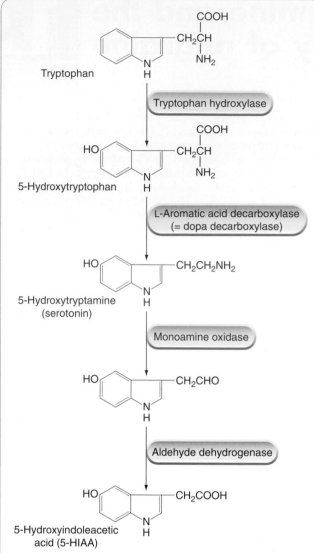

Fig. 15.1 Biosynthesis and metabolism of 5-hydroxytryptamine.

Distribution, biosynthesis and degradation of 5-hydroxytryptamine

- Tissues rich in 5-HT are:
  - gastrointestinal tract (chromaffin cells and enteric neurons)
  - platelets
  - central nervous system.
- Metabolism closely parallels that of noradrenaline.
- 5-HT is formed from dietary tryptophan, which is converted to 5-hydroxytryptophan by tryptophan hydroxylase, then to 5-HT by a non-specific decarboxylase.
- 5-HT is transported into cells by a specific serotonin uptake transporter (SERT).
- Degradation occurs mainly by monoamine oxidase, forming 5-hydroxyindoleacetic acid (5-HIAA), which is excreted in urine.

this transporter such as the SSRIs (Ch. 47) exaggerate the action of 5-HT in the gut, explaining some of the common side effects of these drugs, which include diarrhoea. Interestingly, there is evidence for genetic defects in this reuptake system in irritable bowel syndrome (Ch. 30), which might explain the rather bewildering symptoms of the disease.

Smooth muscle. In many species (although only to a minor extent in humans), smooth muscle outside of the gastrointestinal tract (e.g. uterus and bronchial tree) is also contracted by 5-HT.

Blood vessels. The effect of 5-HT on blood vessels depends on various factors, including the size of the vessel, the species and the prevailing sympathetic activity. Large vessels, both arteries and veins, are usually constricted by 5-HT, although the sensitivity varies greatly. This is the result of a direct action on vascular smooth muscle cells, mediated through $5-HT_{2A}$ receptors. Activation of $5-HT_1$ receptors causes constriction of large intracranial vessels, dilatation of which contributes to headache. 5-HT can also cause vasodilatation, partly by acting on endothelial cells to release nitric oxide (see Ch. 20) and partly by inhibiting noradrenaline release from sympathetic nerve terminals. If 5-HT is injected intravenously, the blood pressure initially rises, owing to the constriction of large vessels, and then falls, owing to arteriolar dilatation. 5-HT may play a role in the pathology of *pulmonary hypertension* (see Ch. 22).

Platelets. 5-HT causes platelet aggregation (see Ch. 24) by acting on $5-HT_{2A}$ receptors, and the platelets that collect in the vessel release further 5-HT. If the endothelium is intact, 5-HT release from adherent platelets causes vasodilatation, which helps to sustain blood flow; if it is damaged (e.g. by atherosclerosis), 5-HT causes constriction and impairs blood flow further. These effects of platelet-derived 5-HT are thought to be important in vascular disease.

Nerve endings. 5-HT stimulates nociceptive (pain-mediating) sensory nerve endings, an effect mediated mainly by $5-HT_3$ receptors. If injected into the skin, 5-HT causes pain; when given systemically, it elicits a variety of autonomic reflexes through stimulation of afferent fibres in the heart and lungs, which further complicate the cardiovascular response. Nettle stings contain 5-HT among other mediators. 5-HT also inhibits transmitter release from adrenergic neurons in the periphery.

Central nervous system. 5-HT excites some neurons and inhibits others; it may also act presynaptically to inhibit transmitter release from nerve terminals. Different receptor subtypes and different membrane mechanisms mediate these effects. The role of 5-HT in the CNS is discussed in Chapter 39.

CLASSIFICATION OF 5-HT RECEPTORS

▼ It was realised long ago that the actions of 5-HT are not all mediated by receptors of the same type, and various pharmacological classifications have come and gone. The current system is summarised in Table 15.1. This classification takes into account sequence data derived from cloning, signal transduction mechanisms and pharmacological specificity as well as the phenotypes of 5-HT receptor 'knockout' mice.

Their diversity is astonishing. Currently, there are some 14 known receptor subtypes (together with an extra gene in mouse). These are divided into seven classes ($5-HT_{1-7}$), one of which ($5-HT_3$) is a ligand-gated cation channel while the remainder are G protein-coupled receptors (GPCRs; see Ch. 3). The six GPCR families are further subdivided into some 13 receptor subtypes based on their sequence and

Table 15.1 Some significant drugs acting at the main 5-HT receptor subtypes

Receptor	Location	Main function	Signalling system	Significant drugs Agonists	Significant drugs Antagonists
5-HT$_{1A}$	CNS	Neuronal inhibition Behavioural effects: sleep, feeding, thermoregulation, anxiety	G protein (G$_i$/G$_o$) ↓ cAMP (may also modulate Ca^{2+} channels)	8-OH-DPAT, triptans, clozapine, buspirone (PA), cabergoline	Methiothepin, yohimbine, ketanserin, pizotifen, spiperone
5-HT$_{1B}$	CNS, vascular smooth muscle, many other sites	Presynaptic inhibition Behavioural effects Pulmonary vasoconstriction	G protein (G$_i$/G$_o$) ↓ cAMP (may also modulate Ca^{2+} channels)	8-OH-DPAT, triptans, clozapine, cabergoline, dihydroergotamine	Methiothepin, yohimbine, ketanserin, spiperone
5-HT$_{1D}$	CNS, blood vessels	Cerebral vasoconstriction Behavioural effects: locomotion	G protein (G$_i$/G$_o$) ↓ cAMP (may also modulate Ca^{2+} channels)	8-OH-DPAT, triptans, clozapine, cabergoline, dihydro-ergotamine/ ergotamine	Methiothepin, yohimbine, ketanserin, methysergide, spiperone
5-HT$_{1E}$	CNS	–	G protein (G$_i$/G$_o$) ↓ cAMP (may also modulate Ca^{2+} channels)	8-OH-DPAT, triptans; clozapine, dihydroergotamine	Methiothepin, yohimbine, methysergide
5-HT$_{1F}$	CNS, uterus, heart, GI tract	–	G protein (G$_i$/G$_o$) ↓ cAMP (may also modulate Ca^{2+} channels)	8-OH-DPAT, triptans; clozapine dihydro-ergotamine/ergotamine, lasmiditan	Methiothepin, yohimbine, methysergide
5-HT$_{2A}$	CNS, PNS, smooth muscle, platelets	Neuronal excitation Behavioural effects Smooth muscle contraction (gut, bronchi, etc.) Platelet aggregation Vasoconstriction/vasodilatation	G protein (G$_q$/G$_{11}$) ↑ IP$_3$, Ca^{2+}	LSD, cabergoline, methysergide (PA), 8-OH-DPAT, ergotamine (PA)	Ketanserin, clozapine, methiothepin, methysergide
5-HT$_{2B}$	Gastric fundus	Contraction	G protein (G$_q$/G$_{11}$) ↑ IP$_3$, Ca^{2+}	LSD, cabergoline, methysergide (PA), 8-OH-DPAT, ergotamine (PA)	Ketanserin, clozapine, methiothepin, yohimbine
5-HT$_{2C}$	CNS, lymphocytes	–	G protein (G$_q$/G$_{11}$) ↑ IP$_3$, Ca^{2+}	LSD, cabergoline, methysergide (PA), 8-OH-DPAT, ergotamine (PA)	Ketanserin, clozapine, methiothepin, methysergide
5-HT$_3$	PNS, CNS	Neuronal excitation (autonomic, nociceptive neurons) Emesis Behavioural effects: anxiety	Ligand-gated cation channel	2-Me-5-HT, chloromethyl biguanide	Dolesatron, granisetron, ondansetron, palonosetron, tropisetron
5-HT$_4$	PNS (GI tract), CNS	Neuronal excitation GI motility	G protein (G$_s$) ↑ cAMP	Metoclopramide, tegaserod, cisapride	Tropisetron
5-HT$_{5A}$	CNS	Modulation of exploratory behaviour (rodents)?	G protein (G$_s$) ↑ cAMP	Triptans, 8-OH-DPAT	Methiothepin, clozapine, methysergide, yohimbine, ketanserin
5-HT$_6$	CNS, leukocytes	Learning and memory?	G protein (G$_s$) ↑ cAMP	LSD, ergotamine	Methiothepin, clozapine, spiperone, methysergide, dihydro-ergotamine
5-HT$_7$	CNS, GI tract, blood vessels	Thermoregulation? Circadian rhythm?	G protein (G$_s$) ↑ cAMP	Buspirone, cisapride, 8-OH-DPAT, LSD,	Methiothepin, clozapine, methysergide, buspirone, dihydro-ergotamine, ketanserin, yohimbine

The receptor classification system is based upon the IUPHAR database at www.iuphar-db.org.
Many drugs here are not used clinically; others have been withdrawn (e.g. fenfluramine), or are not currently available in the UK (e.g. dolesatron, tropisetron), but are included as they are often referred to in the literature.
2-Me-5-HT, 2-methyl-5-hydroxytryptamine; 8-OH-DPAT, 8-hydroxy-2-(di-n-propylamino) tetraline; CNS, central nervous system; DAG, diacylglycerol; GI, gastrointestinal; IP$_3$, inositol trisphosphate; LSD, lysergic acid diethylamide; PA, partial agonist; PNS, peripheral nervous system.
The list of agonists and antagonists is not exhaustive.

Actions and functions of 5-hydroxytryptamine

- Important actions are:
  - increased gastrointestinal motility (direct excitation of smooth muscle and indirect action via enteric neurons)
  - contraction of other smooth muscle (bronchi, uterus)
  - mixture of vascular constriction (direct and via sympathetic innervation) and dilatation (endothelium dependent)
  - platelet aggregation
  - stimulation of peripheral nociceptive nerve endings
  - excitation/inhibition of central nervous system neurons.
- Postulated physiological and pathophysiological roles include:
  - in periphery: peristalsis, vomiting, platelet aggregation and haemostasis, inflammation, sensitisation of nociceptors and microvascular control
  - in CNS: many postulated functions, including control of appetite, sleep, mood, hallucinations, stereotyped behaviour, pain perception and vomiting.
- Clinical conditions associated with disturbed 5-HT include migraine, carcinoid syndrome, mood disorders and anxiety.

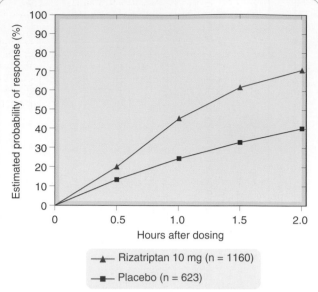

Fig. 15.2 The triptan, rizatriptan, relieves the pain associated with attacks of migraine. The graph is a Kaplan–Meir plot showing the probability of experiencing relief from the pain of the attack after treatment with placebo or with 10 mg rizatriptan. *(From Dahlof et al. 1999).*

pharmacology. Most subtypes are found in all species so far examined, but there are some exceptions (the $5\text{-}HT_{5B}$ gene is found in mouse but has not been found in humans). The sequences of $5\text{-}HT_1$ and $5\text{-}HT_2$ receptors are highly conserved among species but the $5\text{-}HT_{4\text{-}7}$ receptors are less conserved and are grouped together largely on pharmacological grounds. Most 5-HT GPCRs signal through adenylyl cyclase/cAMP, but some (the $5\text{-}HT_2$ subtype) activate phospholipase C to generate phospholipid-derived second messengers (see Ch. 3).

In addition to these main subtypes, many genetic isoforms have been found, giving rise to four or more variants of some of these receptors. The pharmacological and pathophysiological relevance of these genetic isoforms is unclear.

With the exception of $5HT_3$- selective agents, 5-HT receptor agonists and antagonists are relatively non-selective with respect to different receptor subtypes. This makes their pharmacology difficult to interpret and summarise.

Many transgenic mice lacking functional members of this receptor family have been produced (see for example Bonasera & Tecott, 2000). The functional deficits in such animals are generally quite subtle, suggesting that these receptors may serve to tune, rather than to enable, physiological responses. Table 15.1 gives an overview of the most important receptors. Some of the more significant drug targets include the following:

$5\text{-}HT_1$ receptors. Those of pharmacological significance occur mainly in the brain, the subtypes being distinguished on the basis of their regional distribution and their pharmacological specificity. They function mainly as inhibitory presynaptic receptors. The $5\text{-}HT_{1A}$ subtype is particularly important in relation to mood and behaviour (see Chs 44, 46) and $5\text{-}HT_1$ 'knockout' mice exhibit defects in sleep regulation, learning ability and other CNS functions. Receptor polymorphisms may be associated with increased susceptibility to substance abuse. The $5\text{-}HT_{1B}$ and $5\text{-}HT_{1D}$ subtypes, which are expressed in cerebral blood vessels, are believed to be important in migraine and are the target for *triptans*, such as sumatriptan an important group of drugs used to treat acute attacks (Fig. 15.2). Unfortunately, the $5\text{-}HT_{1B}$ receptor is also present in the vasculature of the heart and elsewhere,

explaining some of the unwanted effects associated with triptan therapy. The hapless '$5\text{-}HT_{1C}$' receptor – actually the first to be cloned – has been officially declared non-existent, having been ignominiously reclassified as the $5\text{-}HT_{2C}$ receptor when it was found to be linked to inositol trisphosphate production rather than adenylyl cyclase.

$5\text{-}HT_2$ receptors. These are present in the CNS but are also particularly important in the periphery. The effects of 5-HT on smooth muscle and platelets, which have been known for many years, are mediated by the $5\text{-}HT_{2A}$ receptor, as are some of the behavioural effects of agents such as **lysergic acid diethylamide** (LSD; see Table 15.1 and Ch. 48). $5\text{-}HT_2$ receptors are linked to phospholipase C and thus stimulate inositol trisphosphate formation. The $5\text{-}HT_{2A}$ subtype is functionally the most important, the others having a much more limited distribution and functional role. The role of $5\text{-}HT_2$ receptors in normal physiology is probably a minor one, but it becomes more prominent in pathological conditions such as asthma and vascular thrombosis (see Chs 28 and 24). Mice lacking $5\text{-}HT_2$ receptors exhibit defects in colonic motility ($5\text{-}HT_{2A}$), heart defects ($5\text{-}HT_{2B}$) and CNS disorders ($5\text{-}HT_{2C}$).

$5\text{-}HT_3$ receptors. $5\text{-}HT_3$ receptors are exceptional in being membrane ion channels (Ch. 3) and cause excitation directly, without involvement of any second messenger. The receptor itself consists of a pentameric assembly of distinct subunits which are designated by further subscript letters (e.g. $5\text{-}HT_{3A\text{-}E}$ in humans). $5\text{-}HT_3$ receptors occur mainly in the peripheral nervous system, particularly on nociceptive sensory neurons (see Ch. 42) and on autonomic and enteric neurons, where 5-HT exerts a strong excitatory effect. 5-HT evokes pain when injected locally; when given intravenously, it elicits a fine display of autonomic reflexes, which result from excitation of many types of vascular, pulmonary and cardiac sensory nerve fibres. $5\text{-}HT_3$ receptors also occur in the brain, particularly in the *area postrema*, a region of the medulla involved in the vomiting reflex, and selective $5\text{-}HT_3$ antagonists are used as antiemetic drugs (see Ch. 30). Polymorphisms in the subunits are associated with increased susceptibility to nausea and vomiting.

$5\text{-}HT_4$ receptors. These occur in the brain, as well as in peripheral organs such as the gastrointestinal tract, bladder and heart. Their main physiological role appears to be in the gastrointestinal tract, where they produce neuronal excitation and mediate the effect of

5-HT in stimulating peristalsis. Mice deficient in the 5-HT$_4$ receptor exhibit a complex phenotype including abnormal feeding behaviour in response to stress.

5-HT$_5$, 5-HT$_6$ and 5-HT$_7$ receptors. Little is known about these receptors. All are present in the CNS as well as other tissues. There are two genes for 5-HT$_5$ isoforms but only one codes for a functional receptor in humans although both may be functional in rodents. A recent report of selective antagonists at the 5-HT$_7$ receptor may open the way for a detailed examination of the role of this receptor in CNS pathology (Agosti, 2007).

5-Hydroxytryptamine receptors

- There are seven families (5-HT$_{1-7}$), with further subtypes of 5-HT$_1$ (A–F) and 5-HT$_2$ (A–C). Many polymorphisms and splice variants have also been observed.
- All are G protein-coupled receptors, except 5-HT$_3$, which is a ligand-gated cation channel.
  - 5-HT$_1$ receptors occur mainly in the CNS (all subtypes) and some blood vessels (5-HT$_{1B/D}$ subtypes). Some effects are mediated through inhibition of adenylyl cyclase, include neural inhibition and vasoconstriction. Specific agonists include triptans (used in migraine therapy) and **buspirone** (used in anxiety). Specific antagonists include **spiperone** and **methiothepin**.
  - 5-HT$_2$ receptors occur in the CNS and many peripheral sites (especially blood vessels, platelets, autonomic neurons). Neuronal and smooth muscle effects are excitatory and some blood vessels are dilated as a result of nitric oxide release from endothelial cells. 5-HT$_2$ receptors act through the phospholipase C/inositol trisphosphate pathway. Ligands include lysergic acid diethylamide (**LSD**; agonist in CNS, antagonist in periphery). Specific antagonists include **ketanserin**.
  - 5-HT$_3$ receptors occur in the peripheral nervous system, especially nociceptive afferent neurons and enteric neurons, and in the CNS. Effects are excitatory, mediated through direct receptor-coupled ion channels. **2-Methyl-5-HT** is a specific agonist. Specific antagonists include **ondansetron** and **tropisetron**. Antagonists are used mainly as antiemetic drugs but may also be anxiolytic.
  - 5-HT$_4$ receptors occur mainly in the enteric nervous system (also in the CNS). Effects are excitatory, through stimulation of adenylyl cyclase, causing increased gastrointestinal motility. Specific agonists include **metoclopramide** (used to stimulate gastric emptying).
  - 5-HT$_5$ receptors (one subtype in humans) are located in the CNS. Little is known about their role in humans.
  - 5-HT$_6$ receptors are located in the CNS and on leukocytes. Little is known about their role in humans.
  - 5-HT$_7$ receptors are located in the CNS and the gastrointestinal tract. Little is known about their role in humans but emerging data shows they may also be important in migraine.

DRUGS ACTING AT 5-HT RECEPTORS

Table 15.1 lists some significant agonists and antagonists at the different receptor types. Many are only partly selective. Our increasing understanding of the location and function of the different receptor subtypes has caused an upsurge of interest in developing compounds with improved receptor selectivity, and further useful new drugs are likely to appear in the near future.

Important drugs that act on 5-HT receptors in the periphery include the following:

- Although not clinically useful, selective 5-HT$_{1A}$ agonists, such as 8-hydroxy-2-(di-*n*-propylamino) tetralin (8-OH-DPAT), are potent hypotensive agents, acting through a central mechanism.
- 5-HT$_{1B/D}$ receptor agonists (e.g. the triptans) are used for treating migraine.
- 5-HT$_2$ receptor antagonists (e.g. **methysergide**, **ketanserin**) act mainly on 5-HT$_{2A}$ receptors but may also block other 5-HT receptors, as well as α adrenoceptors and histamine receptors (Ch. 26). **Dihydroergotamine** and methysergide belong to the ergot family and are used mainly for migraine prophylaxis. Other 5-HT$_2$ antagonists are used to control the symptoms of carcinoid tumours.
- 5-HT$_3$ receptor antagonists (e.g. **dolasetron**, **granisetron**, **ondansetron**, **palonosetron**, **tropisetron**) are used as antiemetic drugs (see Chs 30 and 56), particularly for controlling the severe nausea and vomiting that occurs with many forms of cancer chemotherapy.
- 5-HT$_4$ receptor agonists that stimulate coordinated peristaltic activity (known as a 'prokinetic action') could be used for treating gastrointestinal disorders (see Ch. 30). **Metoclopramide** acts in this way, as well as by blocking dopamine receptors. Similar but more selective drugs such as **cisapride** and **tegaserod** were introduced to treat irritable bowel syndrome, but were withdrawn on account of cardiovascular side effects.

5-HT is also important as a neurotransmitter in the CNS, and several important antipsychotic and antidepressant drugs act on these pathways (see Chs 39, 46 and 47). LSD is a relatively non-selective 5-HT receptor agonist or partial agonist, which acts centrally as a potent hallucinogen (see Ch. 48).

ERGOT ALKALOIDS

Ergot alkaloids have preoccupied pharmacologists for more than a century. As a group, they resist classification. Many act on 5-HT receptors, but not selectively so that their effects are complex and diverse.

▼ Ergot, an extract of the fungus *Claviceps purpurea* that infests cereal crops, contains many active substances, and it was the study of their pharmacological properties that led Dale to many important discoveries concerning acetylcholine, histamine and catecholamines. Epidemics of ergot poisoning have occurred, and still occur, when contaminated grain is used for food. The symptoms include mental disturbances and intensely painful peripheral vasoconstriction leading to gangrene. This came to be known in the Middle Ages as *St Anthony's fire*, because it was believed that it could be cured by a visit to the Shrine of St Anthony (which happened to be in an ergot-free region of France).

Ergot alkaloids are complex molecules based on lysergic acid (a naturally occurring tetracyclic compound). The important members of the group (Table 15.2) include various naturally occurring and

Table 15.2 Properties of ergot alkaloids and related compounds

Drug	Actions at receptors			Uterus	Main uses	Side effects etc.
	5-HT	α Adrenoceptor	Dopamine			
Ergotamine	Antagonist/ partial agonist (5-HT$_1$) Antagonist (other sites)	Partial agonist (blood vessels)	Inactive	Contracts ++	Migraine (largely obsolete)	Emesis, vasospasm (avoid in peripheral vascular disease and pregnancy)
Dihydroergotamine	Antagonist/ partial agonist (5-HT$_1$)	Antagonist	Inactive	Contracts +	Migraine (largely obsolete)	Less emesis than with ergotamine
Ergometrine	Weak antagonist/ partial agonist (5-HT$_1$)	Weak antagonist/ partial agonist	Weak	Contracts +++	Prevention of postpartum haemorrhage (Ch. 35)	Nausea, vomiting
Bromocriptine	Inactive	Weak antagonist	Agonist/ partial agonist	–	Parkinson's disease (Ch. 40) Endocrine disorders (Ch. 31)	Drowsiness, emesis
Methysergide	Antagonist/ partial agonist (5-HT$_2$)	–	–	–	Carcinoid syndrome Migraine (prophylaxis)	Retroperitoneal and mediastinal fibrosis Emesis

synthetic derivatives with different substituent groups arranged around a common nucleus. These compounds display diverse pharmacological actions and it is difficult to discern any clear relationship between chemical structure and pharmacological properties.

Ergot alkaloids

- These active substances are produced by a fungus that infects cereal crops and are responsible for occasional poisoning incidents. The most important compounds are:
  - **ergotamine** and **dihydroergotamine**, used in migraine prophylaxis
  - **ergometrine**, used in obstetrics to prevent postpartum haemorrhage
  - **methysergide**, used to treat carcinoid syndrome, and occasionally for migraine prophylaxis
  - **bromocriptine**, used in parkinsonism and endocrine disorders.
- Main sites of action are 5-HT receptors, dopamine receptors and adrenoceptors (mixed agonist, antagonist and partial agonist effects).
- Unwanted effects include nausea and vomiting, vasoconstriction (ergot alkaloids are contraindicated in patients with peripheral vascular disease).

Actions

Most of the effects of ergot alkaloids appear to be mediated through adrenoceptors, 5-HT or dopamine receptors, although some may be produced through other mechanisms. All alkaloids stimulate smooth muscle, some being

relatively selective for vascular smooth muscle while others act mainly on the uterus. **Ergotamine** and **dihydroergotamine** are, respectively, a partial agonist and an antagonist at α adrenoceptors. **Bromocriptine** is an agonist of dopamine receptors, particularly in the CNS (Ch. 39), and **methysergide** is an antagonist at 5-HT$_{2A}$ receptors.

The main pharmacological actions and uses of these drugs are summarised in Table 15.2. As one would expect of agents having so many actions, their physiological effects are complex and rather poorly understood. Ergotamine, dihydroergotamine and methysergide are discussed here; further information on **ergometrine** and bromocriptine is given in Chapters 33, 35 and 40.

Vascular effects. When injected into an anaesthetised animal, ergotamine activates α adrenoceptors, causing vasoconstriction and a sustained rise in blood pressure. At the same time, ergotamine reverses the pressor effect of adrenaline (epinephrine; see Ch. 14). The vasoconstrictor effect of ergotamine is responsible for the peripheral gangrene of St Anthony's fire, and probably also for some of the effects of ergot on the CNS. Methysergide and dihydroergotamine have much less vasoconstrictor effect. Methysergide is a potent 5-HT$_{2A}$ receptor antagonist, whereas ergotamine and dihydroergotamine act selectively on 5-HT$_1$ receptors. Although generally classified as antagonists, they show partial agonist activity in some tissues, and this may account for their activity when treating migraine attacks.

Clinical use. The only use of ergotamine is in the treatment of attacks of migraine unresponsive to simple analgesics (see Chs 26 and 42). Methysergide is occasionally used for migraine prophylaxis, but its main use is in treating the symptoms of carcinoid tumours. All these drugs can be used orally or by injection.

Unwanted effects. Ergotamine often causes nausea and vomiting, and it must be avoided in patients with peripheral vascular disease because of its vasoconstrictor action. Methysergide also causes nausea and vomiting, but its most serious side effect, which considerably restricts its clinical usefulness, is retroperitoneal and mediastinal fibrosis, which impairs the functioning of the gastrointestinal tract, kidneys, heart and lungs. The mechanism of this is unknown, but it is noteworthy that similar fibrotic reactions also occur in carcinoid syndrome, in which there is a high circulating level of 5-HT.

MIGRAINE AND OTHER CLINICAL CONDITIONS IN WHICH 5-HT PLAYS A ROLE

In this section, we discuss three situations where the peripheral actions of 5-HT are believed to be important, namely *migraine, carcinoid syndrome* and *pulmonary hypertension*. The use of 5-HT$_3$ antagonists for treating drug-induced emesis is discussed in Chapter 30. Modulation of 5-HT-mediated transmission in the CNS is an important mechanism of action of antidepressant and antipsychotic drugs (see Chs 39, 44 and 47).

MIGRAINE AND ANTIMIGRAINE DRUGS

Migraine[1] is a common and debilitating condition affecting 10–15% of people. Although the causes are not well understood, both genetic and environmental factors seem to be important. The frequency of attacks varies, with about three-quarters of *migraineurs* (as they are called) having more than one episode per month. Generally, the onset of attacks begins at puberty and wanes with increasing age. Women are twice as likely as men to suffer from the disorder and the attacks are often linked to the menstrual cycle or other reproductive events. It appears that rapidly falling oestrogen levels can precipitate bouts of migraine in susceptible subjects.

In the UK, some 25 million work or school days are lost each year because of the incapacitating effects of the disease, with an economic cost of more than £2 billion. The WHO has classified migraine as amongst the 20 most disabling lifetime conditions.

Migraines are differentiated from other types of headache (e.g. cluster headaches, tension headaches) based on strict diagnostic guidelines. The onset of an attack is heralded by a *premonitory phase*, with symptoms including nausea, mood changes and sensitivity to light and sound (photophobia and phonophobia). These may occur hours before the next phase, which is generally referred to as the *aura* during which phonophobia and photophobia are more common, and may be accompanied by more specific visual symptoms such as a slowly moving blind spot with associated flashing lights ('scintillating scotoma') or geometric patterns of coloured lights ('fortification spectra') or the illusion of looking through the wrong end of a telescope. The *headache* phase proper is characterised by a moderate or severe headache, starting unilaterally, but then usually spreading to both sides of the head. It may have a pulsating or throbbing quality accompanied by

nausea, vomiting and prostration. This phase may persist for hours or even days. Following resolution of the headache, is the *postdromal* phase. This may include feelings of fatigue, altered cognition or mood changes. Whilst these different phases probably represent discrete biological events, in practice they overlap and may run in parallel. A good account of these is given by Charles (2013).

PATHOPHYSIOLOGY

The causes of migraine are incompletely understood. Historically there have been three main hypotheses advanced to account for the symptoms (see Eadie, 2005).

The classic *'vascular' theory*, first proposed around 50 years ago by Wolff, implicated an initial humorally mediated intracerebral vasoconstriction as the cause of the aura, followed by an extracerebral vasodilatation causing the headache.

The *'brain' hypothesis* (see Lauritzen, 1987) linked the symptoms to the phenomenon of *cortical spreading depression*. This is a dramatic, although poorly understood, phenomenon, triggered in experimental animals by local application of K$^+$ to the cortex and also thought to occur in humans after (for example) concussion. An advancing wave of profound neural inhibition progresses slowly over the cortical surface at a rate of about 2 mm/min. In the affected area, the ionic balance is grossly disturbed, with an extremely high extracellular K$^+$ concentration, and the blood flow is reduced.

The *'inflammation' hypothesis* (see Waeber & Moskowitz, 2005) proposes that activation of trigeminal nerve terminals in the meninges and extracranial vessels is the primary event in a migraine attack. This would cause pain directly and also induce inflammatory changes through the release of neuropeptides and other inflammatory mediators from the sensory nerve terminals (neurogenic inflammation; see Chs 18 and 42). This theory is supported by experiments showing that one such peptide (*calcitonin gene-related peptide*; see Ch 18) is released into the meningeal circulation during a migraine attack and that an antagonist of this peptide, **telcagepant** – an investigational drug (discontinued because of liver toxicity) – was extremely effective in aborting attacks (Farinelli et al., 2008).

In practice, elements of all these phenomena seem to play a role in the pathogenesis of migraine. Current thinking (summarised by Charles, 2013) suggests that the symptoms associated with the premonitory phase are largely dopaminergic in origin. Antagonists of this neurotransmitter, such as **domperidone**, mitigate migraine attacks if administered in a timely fashion. Also, imaging studies have indicated changes in hypothalamic blood flow during this phase, suggesting a role in the pathogenesis of the attack as well as offering potential new targets for drug therapy. Imaging techniques have revealed widespread changes in brain perfusion during the aura phase. There may be hypoperfusion of some brain areas as well as hyperperfusion in others, suggesting that the physiological mechanisms that normally regulate the relationship between brain activity and blood flow become disengaged. Such *neurovascular uncoupling* is a feature of cortical spreading depression.

During the headache phase there are again vascular changes in (for example) the meningeal and middle cerebral arteries, but once again, these are not consistent and in any case not directly responsible for the pain and other

---

[1]The word is apparently of French origin and is probably a corruption of *hemicrania*, the Latin name for the disease.

symptoms. What does seem to be important is *central sensitisation*, which increases the migraineur's sensitivity to sound, light and other normally non-painful stimuli. This is accompanied by a release of inflammatory or nociceptive mediators such as CGRP, nitric oxide (NO) and prostaglandins. Many of the observed vascular and other changes may persist into the postdromal phase which may last for hours or days.

It is noteworthy that none of these mechanisms can explain at the biochemical level what initiates a migraine attack or define the underlying abnormality that predisposes particular individuals to suffer such attacks. In some rare types of familial migraine, inherited mutations affecting calcium channels and Na^+-K^+-ATPase have been found, suggesting that abnormal membrane function may be responsible, but in most forms of migraine there is no clear genetic cause.

Whether one inclines to the view that migraine is primarily a vascular disorder, a type of spontaneous concussion, an inflammatory disease or just a bad headache, there are two important factors that implicate 5-HT in its pathogenesis:

1. There is a sharp increase in the urinary excretion of the main 5-HT metabolite, 5-HIAA, during the attack. The blood concentration of 5-HT falls, probably because of depletion of platelet 5-HT.
2. Many of the drugs that are effective in treating migraine are 5-HT receptor agonists or antagonists. See Figure 15.3 and the clinical box below for further information.

ANTIMIGRAINE DRUGS

Drugs used for migraine

Acute attack
- Simple analgesics (e.g. **aspirin**, **paracetamol**; see Ch. 26) with or without **metoclopramide** (see Ch. 30) to hasten absorption.
- **Ergotamine** (5-HT$_{1D}$ receptor partial agonist).
- **Sumatriptan**, **zolmitriptan** (5-HT$_{1D}$ agonists).

Prophylaxis
- β-Adrenoceptor antagonists (e.g. **propranolol**, **metoprolol**; see Ch. 14).
- **Pizotifen** (5-HT$_2$ receptor antagonist).
- Other 5-HT$_2$ receptor antagonists:
  - **cyproheptadine**: also has antihistamine actions
  - **methysergide**: rarely used because of risk of retroperitoneal fibrosis.
- Tricyclic antidepressants (e.g. **amitriptyline**; see Ch. 47).
- **Clonidine**, an α$_2$ adrenoceptor agonist (see Ch. 14).
- Calcium antagonists (e.g. dihydropyridines, **verapamil**; see Ch. 21): headache is a side effect of these drugs but, paradoxically, they may reduce frequency of migraine attacks.

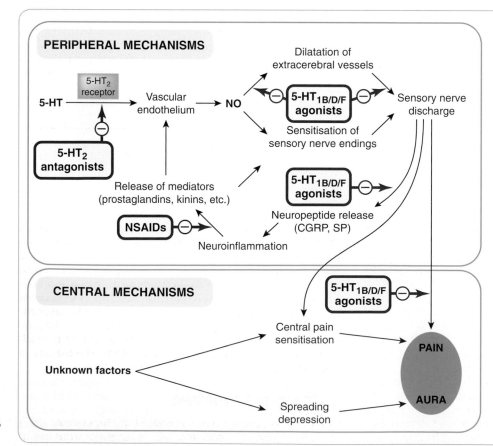

Fig. 15.3 Postulated sites of drug action in migraine. The initiating event is uncertain but may be an abnormal neuronal discharge set off by emotional or biochemical disturbances. Following the premonitory phase, this leads to localised 'spreading depression', uncoupling of neurovascular perfusion and to sensitisation of central pain pathways. Excitation (cause unknown) of nociceptive nerve terminals in the meningeal vessels, leads to the cycle of neurogenic inflammation shown in the upper part of the diagram. 5-HT, 5-hydroxytryptamine; CGRP, calcitonin gene-related peptide; NO, nitric oxide; NSAIDs, non-steroidal anti-inflammatory drugs; SP, substance P.

Table 15.3 Antimigraine drugs[a]

Use	Drug(s)	Mode of action	Side effects	Pharmacokinetic aspects	Notes
Acute	Sumatriptan	$5\text{-}HT_{1B/1D/1F}$ receptor agonist. Constricts large arteries, inhibits trigeminal nerve transmission.	Coronary vasoconstriction, dysrhythmias.	Poor oral absorption, hence delayed response. Can be given s.c. Does not cross blood–brain barrier. Plasma half-life 1.5 h.	Effective in ~70% of migraine attacks. Short duration of action is a drawback. Contraindicated in coronary disease.
Acute	Almotriptan Eletriptan Frovatriptan Naratriptan Rizatriptan Zolmitriptan	As above; additional actions on CNS.	Side effects less than with sumatriptan.	Improved bioavailability and duration of action. Able to cross blood–brain barrier.	Similar to sumatriptan; but improved pharmacokinetics and reduced cardiac side effects.
Acute	Ergotamine	$5\text{-}HT_1$ receptor partial agonist; also affects α adrenoceptors. Vasoconstrictor. Blocks trigeminal nerve transmission.	Peripheral vasoconstriction, including coronary vessels. Nausea and vomiting. Contracts uterus and may damage fetus.	Poorly absorbed. Can be given by suppository, inhalation, etc. Duration of action 12–24 h.	Effective, but use limited by side effects.
Prophylaxis	Methysergide	$5\text{-}HT_2$ receptor antagonist/partial agonist.	Nausea, vomiting, diarrhoea. Retroperitoneal or mediastinal fibrosis (rare but serious).	Used orally	Effective, but rarely used because of side effects and insidious toxicity.
Prophylaxis	Pizotifen	$5\text{-}HT_2$ receptor antagonist. Also histamine antagonist.	Weight gain, antimuscarinic side effects.	Used orally	–
Prophylaxis	Cyproheptadine	$5\text{-}HT_2$ receptor antagonist. Also blocks histamine receptors and Ca^{2+} channels.	Sedation, weight gain.	Used orally	Rarely used
Prophylaxis	Propranolol and similar drugs.	β-adrenoceptor antagonists. Mechanism of antimigraine effect not clear.	Fatigue, bronchoconstriction.	Used orally	Effective and widely used for migraine.

[a]Other drugs used for the *acute* treatment of migraine include non-steroidal anti-inflammatory drugs (NSAIDs) or opiate analgesic drugs (see Chs 42 and 47). Other drugs used for migraine *prophylaxis* include calcium channel blockers (e.g. nifedipine, see Ch. 22), antidepressants (e.g. amitriptyline; see Ch. 47), antiepileptics such as topiramate and sodium valproate (see Ch. 45) and the antihypertensive, clonidine (Ch. 14). Their efficacy is limited. Botox (botulinum toxin; type A) may be used for refractory severe cases of migraine.

The main drugs currently used to treat migraine are summarised in Table 15.3, and their postulated sites of action are shown in Figure 15.3. It is important to distinguish between drugs used *therapeutically* to treat acute attacks of migraine (appropriate when the attacks are fairly infrequent) and drugs that are used *prophylactically*. Apart from 5-HT₂ receptor antagonists, the drugs used prophylactically are a mixed bag, and their mechanisms of action are poorly understood.

The most important agents for the treatment of acute attacks are currently the triptans. These are 5-HT₁ agonists, and are usually classified as 5-HT_{1B/1D} agonists, largely because it is difficult to distinguish between actions at these two receptors. However, selective high-affinity 5-HT_{1D} subtype agonists have proved disappointing in the clinic. Sumatriptan also has high affinity for

the 5-HT_{1F} receptor (see Agosti, 2007), and **lasmiditan** an investigational non-triptan drug that is a selective 5HT_{1F} receptor agonist is highly effective in aborting migraine attacks (Tfelt-Hansen, 2012). Interestingly, this receptor subtype is scarce in the vasculature, casting doubt on the role of vascular changes in the disease. This is significant because a major drawback to triptan therapy is vasoconstriction in other peripheral vascular beds including the heart. Lasmiditan would be expected to be free of such effects; however, it commonly causes other adverse effects (e.g. dizziness and nausea) that can be severe.

CARCINOID SYNDROME

Carcinoid syndrome (see Creutzfeld & Stockmann, 1987) is a rare disorder associated with malignant tumours of enterochromaffin cells, which usually arise in the small intestine and metastasise to the liver. These tumours secrete a variety of chemical mediators: 5-HT is the most important, but neuropeptides such as substance P (Ch. 18), and other agents such as prostaglandins and bradykinin (Ch. 17), are also produced. The release of these substances into the bloodstream results in several unpleasant symptoms, including flushing, diarrhoea, bronchoconstriction and hypotension, which may cause dizziness or fainting. Fibrotic stenosis of heart valves, which can result in cardiac failure, also occurs. It is reminiscent of retroperitoneal and mediastinal fibrosis, which are adverse effects of methysergide, and appears to be related to overproduction of 5-HT.

The syndrome is readily diagnosed by measuring the urinary excretion of the main metabolite of 5-HT, 5-HIAA. This may increase by as much as 20-fold when the disease is active and is raised even when the tumour is asymptomatic. 5-HT$_2$ antagonists, such as **cyprohepta-dine**, are effective in controlling some of the symptoms of carcinoid syndrome. A complementary therapeutic approach is to use **octreotide** (a long-acting agonist at somatostatin receptors), which suppresses hormone secretion from neuroendocrine, including carcinoid, cells (see Ch. 33).

PULMONARY HYPERTENSION

Pulmonary hypertension (see also Ch. 22) is an extremely serious disease characterised by the progressive remodelling of the pulmonary vascular tree. This leads to an inexorable rise in pulmonary arterial pressure which, if untreated (and treatment is difficult), inevitably leads to right heart failure and death. The role of 5-HT in this pathology was suggested by the fact that at least one form of the condition was precipitated by the use of appetite suppressants (e.g. **dexfenfluramine** and **fenfluramine**) that were at one time widely prescribed as 'weight loss' or 'slimming' aids. These drugs apparently blocked SERT and since 5-HT promotes the growth and proliferation of pulmonary arterial smooth muscle cells and also produces a net vasoconstrictor effect in this vascular bed, the hypothesis seemed reasonable.

Though this hypothesis has undergone several important changes of emphasis, pulmonary hypertension is still considered to be a disease in which 5-HT plays an important role and which therefore may become a target for novel drug development. The interested reader is referred to MacLean & Dempsie (2010) for an accessible account of the current thinking in this area, and to Chapter 22, where this topic is also covered.

REFERENCES AND FURTHER READING

5-Hydroxytryptamine

Agosti, R.M., 2007. 5HT$_{1F}$- and 5HT$_7$-receptor agonists for the treatment of migraines. CNS Neurol. Disord. Drug Targets 6, 235–237. (*Describes research in the field of migraine treatment utilising agonists at newly cloned 5-HT receptors*)

Barnes, N.M., Sharp, T., 1999. A review of central 5-HT receptors and their function. Neuropharmacology 38, 1083–1152. (*Useful general review focusing on CNS*)

Beattie, D.T., Smith, J.A., 2008. Serotonin pharmacology in the gastrointestinal tract: a review. Naunyn Schmiedebergs Arch. Pharmacol. 377, 181–203. (*Very comprehensive review dealing with a complex topic. Easy to read*)

Bonasera, S.J., Tecott, L.H., 2000. Mouse models of serotonin receptor function: towards a genetic dissection of serotonin systems. Pharmacol. Ther. 88, 133–142. (*Review of studies on transgenic mice lacking 5-HT$_1$ or 5-HT$_2$ receptors; shows how difficult it can be to interpret such experiments*)

Branchek, T.A., Blackburn, T.P., 2000. 5-HT$_6$ receptors as emerging targets for drug discovery. Annu. Rev. Pharmacol. Toxicol. 40, 319–334. (*Emphasises future therapeutic opportunities*)

Gershon, M.D., 2004. Review article: serotonin receptors and transporters – roles in normal and abnormal gastrointestinal motility. Aliment. Pharmacol. Ther. 20 (Suppl. 7), 3–14.

Kroeze, W.K., Kristiansen, K., Roth, B.L., 2002. Molecular biology of serotonin receptors structure and function at the molecular level. Curr. Top. Med. Chem. 2, 507–528.

Spiller, R., 2008. Serotonergic agents and the irritable bowel syndrome: what goes wrong? Curr. Opin. Pharmacol. 8, 709–714. (*A very interesting account of the development – and withdrawl – of 5-HT$_{3/4}$ antagonists in irritable bowel syndrome and a discussion of the role of SERT polymorphisms in the disease. Illustrates the type of problems encountered when trying to develop useful drugs that act at 5-HT receptors*)

Migraine and other pathologies

Charles, A., 2013. The evolution of a migraine attack – a review of recent evidence. Headache 53, 413–419. (*An excellent and easily readable account of modern thinking about the causes of migraine*)

Creutzfeld, W., Stockmann, F., 1987. Carcinoids and carcinoid syndrome. Am. J. Med. 82 (Suppl. 58), 4–16.

Dahlof, C.G., Rapoport, A.M., Sheftell, F.D., Lines, C.R., 1999. Rizatriptan in the treatment of migraine. Clin. Ther. 21, 1823–1836.

Eadie, M.J., 2005. The pathogenesis of migraine – 17th to early 20th century understandings. J. Clin. Neurosci. 12, 383–388. (*Fascinating account of the historical development of theories of causes of migraine. Good if you are interested in the history of medicine!*)

Ebersberger, A., Schaible, H.-G., Averbeck, B., et al., 2001. Is there a correlation between spreading depression, neurogenic inflammation, and nociception that might cause migraine headache? Ann. Neurol. 49, 7–13. (*Their conclusion is that there is no connection – spreading depression does not produce inflammation or affect sensory neurons*)

Farinelli, I., Missori, S., Martelletti, P., 2008. Proinflammatory mediators and migraine pathogenesis: moving towards CGRP as a target for a novel therapeutic class. Expert Rev. Neurother. 8, 1347–1354.

Goadsby, P.J., 2005. Can we develop neurally acting drugs for the treatment of migraine? Nat. Rev. Drug Discov. 4, 741–750. (*Useful review of the causes and treatments of migraine*)

Lauritzen, M., 1987. Cerebral blood flow in migraine and cortical spreading depression. Acta Neurol. Scand. (Suppl. 113), 1–40. (*Review of clinical measurements of cerebral blood flow in migraine, which overturned earlier hypotheses*)

Maclean, M.R., Dempsie, Y., 2010. The serotonin hypothesis of pulmonary hypertension revisited. Adv. Exp. Med. Biol. 661, 309–322. (*An account of the evidence supporting a role for 5-HT in pulmonary hypertension by one of the leaders in this field*)

Tfelt-Hansen, P., 2012. Clinical pharmacology of current and future drugs for the acute treatment of migraine: a review and an update. Curr. Clin. Pharmacol. 7, 66–72. (*A good account of anti-migraine drugs including the latest thinking on the subject. Recommended*)

Thomsen, L.L., 1997. Investigations into the role of nitric oxide and the large intracranial arteries in migraine headache. Cephalalgia 17, 873–895. (*Revisits the old vascular theory of migraine in the light of recent advances in the nitric oxide field*)

Villalon, C.M., Centurion, D., Valdivia, L.F., et al., 2003. Migraine: pathophysiology, pharmacology, treatment and future trends. Curr. Vasc. Pharmacol. 1, 71–84.

Waeber, C., Moskowitz, M.A., 2005. Migraine as an inflammatory disorder. Neurology 64, S9–S15. (*Useful review of the 'inflammation' hypothesis of migraine*)

Books

Sjoerdsma, A.G., 2008. Starting with serotonin: how a high-rolling father of drug discovery repeatedly beat the odds. Improbable Books, Silver Spring, MD. (*Biography of an astonishing pharmacologist by his daughter. Very well reviewed*)

Purines 16

OVERVIEW

In addition to their role in the energy economy of the cell, purine nucleosides and nucleotides function as extracellular chemical mediators subserving a wide range of functions. In this chapter we describe the mechanisms responsible for their synthesis and release, the drugs that act through purinergic signalling pathways and the receptors that transduce these effects.

INTRODUCTION

Nucleosides (especially adenosine) and nucleotides (especially ADP and ATP) will already be familiar to you because of their crucial role in DNA/RNA synthesis and energy metabolism, but it may come as a surprise to learn that they also function extracellularly as signalling molecules that produce a wide range of unrelated pharmacological effects.

The finding, in 1929, that adenosine injected into anaesthetised animals caused bradycardia, hypotension, vasodilatation and inhibition of intestinal movements, foreshadowed the current interest in purines. But the true origins of the field can really be traced to the crucial observations in 1970 by Burnstock and his colleagues that provided strong evidence that ATP is a neurotransmitter (see Ch. 2). After a period during which this radical idea was treated with scepticism, it has become clear that the 'purinergic' signalling system is not only of ancient evolutionary origin but participates in many physiological control mechanisms, including the regulation of coronary blood flow and myocardial function (Chs 21 and 22), platelet aggregation and immune responses (Chs 17 and 24), as well as neurotransmission in both the central and peripheral nervous system (Chs 12 and 39).

The full complexity of purinergic control systems, and their importance in many pathophysiological mechanisms, is only now emerging, and the therapeutic relevance of the various receptor subtypes is still being unravelled. As a result there is an increasing interest in purine pharmacology and the prospect of developing 'purinergic' drugs for the treatment of pain and a variety of other disorders, particularly of thrombotic and respiratory origin. There is no doubt that such drugs will assume growing significance but, recognising that the overall picture is far from complete, we will focus our discussion in this chapter on a few prominent areas.

Figure 16.1 summarises the mechanisms by which purines are stored, released and interconverted, and the main receptor types on which they act.

PURINERGIC RECEPTORS

Purines exert their biological actions through three families of receptors. Table 16.1 lists these and summarises

what is currently known about their signalling systems, their endogenous ligands and antagonists of pharmacological interest. It should be noted, however, that the action of drugs and ligands at purinergic receptors can be confusing. In part, this is because nucleotides are rapidly degraded by ecto-enzymes and there is also evidence of interconversion by phosphate exchange. Thus ATP may produce effects at all three receptor subclasses depending upon the extent of its enzymatic conversion to ADP, AMP and adenosine.

The three main families of purine receptor are:

- Adenosine receptors (A_1, A_{2A}, A_{2B} and A_3), formerly known as P1 receptors. These are G protein-coupled receptors that act through adenylyl cyclase/cAMP, or by direct effects on Ca^{2+} and K^+ channels, as described in Ch 3.
- P2Y metabotropic receptors ($P2Y_{1-14}$), which are G protein-coupled receptors that utilise either phospholipase C activation or cAMP as their signalling system (see Ch. 3); they respond to various adenine nucleotides, generally preferring ATP over ADP or AMP. Some also recognise pyrimidines such as UTP.
- P2X ionotropic receptors ($P2X_{1-7}$) which are multimeric (in many cases heteromeric) ATP-gated cation channels.

The subtypes in each family are distinguished on the basis of their molecular structure as well as their agonist and antagonist selectivity. The P2Y group is particularly problematic: several receptors have been cloned on the basis of homology with other family members, but their ligands have yet to be identified (in other words they are 'orphan receptors'). In addition, since some members of this group also recognise pyrimidines such as UTP and UDP as well as purines, they are sometimes classed as pyrimidinoceptors. However, little is currently known about the role of pyrimidines in cell signalling.

With the exception of adenosine, **caffeine** and **theophylline**, which act at adenosine receptors, and antagonists such as **clopidogrel**, **prasugrel** and **ticagrelor,** which act at platelet $P2Y_{12}$ receptors, there are so far few therapeutic agents that act on purinergic receptors. We will therefore confine this account to some prominent and interesting aspects of purinergic pharmacology; the reading list provides further information.

ADENOSINE AS A MEDIATOR

The simplest of the purines, adenosine, is found in biological fluids throughout the body. It exists free in the cytosol of all cells and is transported in (active transport against a concentration gradient) and out mainly by a membrane transporter (of which there are several types). Little is known about the way in which this is controlled but the extracellular concentrations are usually quite low

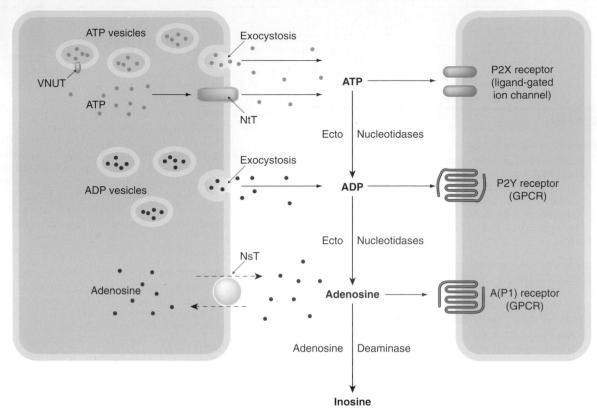

Fig. 16.1 Purines as mediators. ATP (and, in platelets, ADP) may be present in the cytosol of cells (and released following cellular damage) or concentrated into vesicles by the vesicular nucleotide transporter (VNUT). Nucleotides may be released by exocytosis or through membrane channels or transporters (NtT). Once released, ATP can be converted to ADP and to adenosine by the action of ectonucleotidases. Adenosine is present in the cytosol of all cells and is taken up and released via a specific membrane transporter(s) (NsT). Adenosine itself can be hydrolysed to inosine by the enzyme adenosine deaminase. ATP acts upon the P2X receptors (ligand-gated ion channels) and also upon P2Y receptors (GPCRs), the principal target for ADP. Adenosine itself acts on A receptors (also called P1 receptors), which are also GPCRs. Chapter 4 contains more details of exocytotic and other secretory mechanisms.

Purines as mediators

- *Adenosine* acts through A_1, A_{2A}, A_{2B} and A_3 G protein receptors, coupled to inhibition or stimulation of adenylyl cyclase. Adenosine receptors are blocked by methylxanthines such as **caffeine** and **theophylline**.
  - *Adenosine* affects many cells and tissues, including smooth muscle and nerve cells. It is not a conventional transmitter but may be important as a local hormone and 'homeostatic modulator'.
  - Important sites of action include the heart and the lung. **Adenosine** is very short-acting and is sometimes used for its antidysrhythmic effect.
  - *ADP* acts through the $P2Y_{1-14}$ 'metabotropic' G protein-receptor family. These are coupled to cAMP or $PLC\beta$.
  - Important sites of action include platelets where ADP released from granules promotes aggregation by

acting on the PY_{12} receptor. This is antagonised by the drugs **clopidogrel**, **prasugrel** and **ticagrelor**.
- *ATP* is stored in vesicles and released by exocytosis or through membrane channels. Cytoplasmic ATP may be released when cells are damaged. It also functions as an intracellular mediator, inhibiting the opening of membrane potassium channels.
  - ATP acts on P2X receptors: these are ligand-gated ion channels. It can also act on P2Y receptors.
  - **Suramin** blocks the ATP actions at most receptors.
  - Important sites of ATP action include the CNS, peripheral and central pathways and inflammatory cells.
  - ATP is rapidly converted to ADP and adenosine when released yielding products that may act on other purinergic receptors.

compared with intracellular levels. Adenosine in tissues comes partly from this intracellular source and partly from extracellular hydrolysis of released ATP or ADP (Fig. 16.1). Drugs such as **dipyridamole** block the transporter thereby indirectly increasing the concentration of extracellular adenosine. Adenosine can be inactivated by

adenosine deaminase yielding *inosine* providing yet another level of control of this biologically active molecule, and another potential drug target.

Virtually all cells express one or more adenosine receptors and so adenosine produces many pharmacological effects, both in the periphery and in the CNS. Based on its

Table 16.1 Purinergic receptors

Receptor subtype	Mechanism	Principal endogenous ligands	Notes
Adenosine (also called P1)			
A_1	G protein-coupled ($G_{i/o}$) Lowers cAMP	Adenosine (high affinity)	Caffeine, theophylline (antagonists)
A_{2A}	G protein-coupled (G_s) Raises cAMP		
A_{2B}	G protein-coupled (G_s) Raises cAMP	Adenosine (low affinity)	
A_3	G protein-coupled ($G_{i/o}$) Lowers cAMP		
P2Y 'metabotropic'[a]			
$P2Y_1$	G protein coupled (mainly $G_{q/11}$). Activates PLCβ mobilises Ca^{2+} Sometimes alters cAMP	ATP (antagonist or partial agonist) ADP (agonist)	Suramin (antagonist)
$P2Y_2$		UTP and ATP	Suramin (antagonist)
$P2Y_4$		ATP, GTP, UTP (partial agonists)	Pyrimidinoceptor
$P2Y_6$		UDP	Pyrimidinoceptor
$P2Y_{11}$		ATP > ADP	Suramin (antagonist)
$P2Y_{12}$	G protein-coupled (mainly $G_{i/o}$) Reduces cAMP	ADP>ATP	Platelet ADP receptor. Clopidigrel, prasugrel and ticagrelor (potent antagonists)
$P2Y_{13}$		ADP	Suramin, PPADS
$P2Y_{14}$		UDP-glucose	UDP
P2X 'ionotropic'			
$P2X_1$ $P2X_2$ $P2X_3$ $P2X_4$ $P2X_5$ $P2X_6$ $P2X_7$	Receptor-gated cation-selective ion channels	ATP	Suramin (antagonist)

[a]Only functional human receptors are listed. The missing numbers in the sequence indicate that these receptors have been cloned, but their ligands have not yet been identified. A further family of related receptors that binds extracellular cAMP (CAR_{1-4}) is omitted as little is known about their biology. PPADS: pyridoxalphosphate-6-azophenyl-2′,4′-disulfonic acid.

ability to minimise the metabolic requirements of cells, one of its functions may be as an 'acute' defensive agent that is released immediately when tissue integrity is threatened (e.g. by coronary or cerebral ischaemia; see Chs 21 and 40). Under less extreme conditions, variations in adenosine release may play a role in controlling blood flow and (through effects on the carotid bodies) respiration, matching them to the metabolic needs of the tissues.

ADENOSINE AND THE CARDIOVASCULAR SYSTEM

Adenosine inhibits cardiac conduction and it is likely that all four of the adenosine receptors are involved in this effect. Because of this action, adenosine is used therapeutically, being given as an intravenous bolus injection to terminate supraventricular tachycardia (Ch. 21). Because of its short duration of action (it is destroyed or taken up within a few seconds of intravenous administration) it is considered safer than alternatives such as β-adrenoceptor antagonists or **verapamil**. Longer-lasting analogues have been discovered that also show greater receptor selectivity. Adenosine uptake is blocked (and thus its action prolonged) by dipyridamole, a vasodilator and antiplatelet drug (see Ch. 24).

ADENOSINE AND ASTHMA

Adenosine receptors are found on all the cell types involved in asthma (Ch. 28) and the overall pharmacology is complex. For example, activation of the A_{2A} subtype exerts a largely protective and anti-inflammatory effect, but acting through its A_1 receptor, adenosine promotes mediator release from mast cells, and causes enhanced mucus secretion, bronchoconstriction and leukocyte activation. Methylxanthines, especially analogues of theophylline (Ch. 28), are adenosine receptor antagonists. Theophylline has been used for the treatment of asthma and part of its beneficial activity may be ascribed to its antagonism of the A_1 receptor; however, methylxanthines also increase cAMP by inhibiting phosphodiesterase, which underwrites some of their pharmacological actions independently of adenosine receptor antagonism. Certain derivatives of theophylline are claimed to show greater selectivity for adenosine receptors over phosphodiesterase.

Activation of the A_{2B} receptor also promotes mast cell mediator release, while the role of the A_3 receptor has yet to be fully elucidated. Recent thinking therefore suggests that an antagonist of the A_1 and A_{2B} receptor or an agonist of the A_{2A} receptor would represent a significant therapeutic advance (see Brown et al., 2008; Burnstock et al., 2012).

ADENOSINE IN THE CNS

Acting through A_1 and A_{2A} receptors, adenosine has an inhibitory effect on many CNS neurons, and the stimulation experienced after consumption of methylxanthines such as caffeine (see Ch. 48) occurs partly as a result of blocking this action.

ADP AS A MEDIATOR

ADP is usually stored in vesicles in cells. It exerts its direct biological effects predominantly through the P2Y family of receptors but once released it can be converted to adenosine by ectonucleotidases, of which there are several different types.

ADP AND PLATELETS

The secretory vesicles of blood platelets store both ATP and ADP in high concentrations, and release them when the platelets are activated (see Ch 24). One of the many effects of ADP is to promote platelet aggregation, so this system provides positive feedback – an important mechanism for controlling this process. The receptor involved is $P2Y_{12}$. Clopidogrel, prasugrel, and ticagrelor, are $P2Y_{12}$ antagonists and are important therapeutic agents for preventing arterial thromboembolic disorders (Ch. 24).

ATP AS A MEDIATOR

ATP exerts its action primarily through the P2X receptors. The extracellular domain of these multimeric receptors can bind three molecules of ATP. When activated, the receptor gates the cation-selective ion channels that trigger ongoing intracellular signalling. Some other actions of ATP in mammals are mediated through the P2Y receptors. **Suramin** (a drug originally developed to treat trypanasome infections) and an experimental compound *PPADS* (pyridoxalphosphate-6-azophenyl-2′,4′-disulfonic acid) antagonise ATP and have broad-spectrum inhibitory activity at most P2X receptors. Suramin may additionally antagonise P2Y receptors.

ATP is present in all cells in millimolar concentrations and is released if the cells are damaged (e.g. by ischaemia). The mechanism of release can be through exocytosis of vesicles containing ATP or through *pannexin* or *connexin* channels in the cell membrane. In addition, dying cells may release ATP, which may serve as a 'danger signal' alerting immune cells to potential tissue damage (see Ch. 6).

ATP released from cells is rapidly dephosphorylated by a range of tissue-specific nucleotidases, producing ADP and adenosine (Fig. 16.1), both of which may produce further receptor-mediated effects. The role of intracellular ATP in regulating membrane potassium channels to control vascular smooth muscle (Ch. 22) and insulin secretion (Ch. 31), is quite distinct from this transmitter function.

ATP AS A NEUROTRANSMITTER

The idea that such a workaday metabolite as ATP might be a member of the neurotransmitter elite was resisted for a long time, but is now firmly established. ATP is a transmitter in the periphery, both as a primary mediator and as a co-transmitter in noradrenergic nerve terminals. $P2X_2$, $P2X_4$ and $P2X_6$ are the predominant receptor subtypes expressed in neurons. $P2X_1$ predominates in smooth muscle.

ATP is contained in synaptic vesicles of both adrenergic and cholinergic neurons, and it accounts for many of the actions produced by stimulation of autonomic nerves that are not caused by acetylcholine or noradrenaline (see Ch. 12). These effects include the relaxation of intestinal smooth muscle evoked by sympathetic stimulation, and contraction of the bladder produced by parasympathetic nerves. Burnstock and his colleagues have shown that ATP is released on nerve stimulation in a Ca^{2+}-dependent fashion, and that exogenous ATP, in general, mimics the effects of nerve stimulation in various preparations. ATP may function as a conventional 'fast' transmitter in the CNS and in autonomic ganglia, or as an inhibitory presynaptic transmitter.

Adenosine, produced following hydrolysis of ATP, exerts presynaptic inhibitory effects on the release of excitatory transmitters in the CNS and periphery.

ATP IN NOCICEPTION

ATP causes pain when injected (for example) subdermally, as a result of activation of $P2X_2$ and/or $P2X_3$ heteromeric receptors in afferent neurons involved in the transduction of nociception (see Ch. 42). The pain can be blocked by aspirin (see Ch. 26) suggesting the involvement of prostaglandins. There is a current upsurge of interest in the potential role of purinergic receptors (mainly P2Y and P2X receptors), in various aspects of nociceptive pain transmission and in particular the development of neuropathic pain, which is difficult to treat (see Ch. 42). Interestingly, purinergic receptors are found not just on neurons, but also on glial cells, suggesting a role for these 'support' cells in modulating the chain of nociceptive transmission. It has been suggested that both types of receptors could be useful targets for analgesic and anti-migraine drugs (Tsuda et al., 2012; Magni & Ceruti, 2013).

Oddly, perhaps, the same receptors seem to be involved in taste perception on the tongue.

ATP IN INFLAMMATION

ATP is released from stimulated, damaged or dying cells and P2X receptors are widely distributed on cells of the immune system; P2Y receptors less so. Acting through these receptors, ATP can regulate neutrophil and phagocyte chemotaxis and provoke the release from macrophages and mast cells of cytokines and other mediators of the inflammatory response. Mice in which the P2X$_7$ receptor is deleted show a reduced capacity to develop chronic inflammation. Purinergic signalling also plays an important role in T-cell signalling.

Adenosine, may also exert anti-inflammatory effects and **methotrexate**, a useful anti-inflammatory drug (see Ch. 26) may owe some of its actions to the release of adenosine. A good account of the role of autocrine signalling in the immune system is given by Junger (2011).

FUTURE PROSPECTS

While there are only a few current drugs that act through purinergic receptors, the area as a whole holds promise for future therapeutic exploitation. Other disease areas not mentioned above, which seem particularly promising in this respect are gastrointestinal disorders (Burnstock, 2008; Antonioli et al., 2013) and regulation of bone remodelling (Gartland et al., 2012).

REFERENCES AND FURTHER READING

(A note of caution: the nomenclature of these receptors has changed several times and this can make for difficulties when reading some older papers. For the latest version of the nomenclature, always refer to www.guidetopharmacology.org/)

Antonioli, L., Colucci, R., Pellegrini, C., et al., 2013. The role of purinergic pathways in the pathophysiology of gut diseases: pharmacological modulation and potential therapeutic applications. Pharmacol. Ther. 139, 157–188. (*Very comprehensive survey of the distribution and function of purinergic receptors in the gut and their relevance to normal physiological function and disease*)

Brown, R.A., Spina, D., Page, C.P., 2008. Adenosine receptors and asthma. Br. J. Pharmacol. 153 (Suppl. 1), S446–S456 (*Excellent review of the pharmacology of adenosine in the lung. Very accessible*)

Brundege, J.M., Dunwiddie, T.V., 1997. Role of adenosine as a modulator of synaptic activity in the central nervous system. Adv. Pharmacol. 39, 353–391. (*Good review article*)

Burnstock, G., 2006. Purinergic P2 receptors as targets for novel analgesics. Pharmacol. Ther. 110, 433–454. (*This paper, and the reviews that follow by the same author, cover various aspects of purinergic signalling and its therapeutic application*)

Burnstock, G., 2008. Purinergic receptors as future targets for treatment of functional GI disorders. Gut 57, 1193–1194.

Burnstock, G., 2012. Purinergic signalling: Its unpopular beginning, its acceptance and its exciting future. Bioessays 34, 218–225. (*Interesting account of the entire field of purinergic signalling written by the scientist who really pioneered the field. Easy to read and informative*)

Burnstock, G., Brouns, I., Adriaensen, D., Timmermans, J.P., 2012. Purinergic signalling in the airways. Pharmacol. Rev. 64, 834–868. (*A substantial and authoritative review for those who want to delve into this area of purinergic pharmacology*)

Cunha, R.A., 2001. Adenosine as a neuromodulator and as a homeostatic regulator in the nervous system: different roles, different sources and different receptors. Neurochem. Int. 38, 107–125. (*Speculative review on the functions of adenosine in the nervous system*)

Gartland, A., Orriss, I.R., Rumney, R.M., Bond, A.P., Arnett, T., Gallagher, J.A., 2012. Purinergic signalling in osteoblasts. Front. Biosci. 17, 16–29.

Junger, W.G., 2011. Immune cell regulation by autocrine purinergic signalling. Nat. Rev. Immunol. 11, 201–212. (*An excellent, and well illustrated, overview of the role of the purinergic system in immune cells. Focuses on T cells and neutrophil autocrine signalling. Recommended reading*)

Khakh, B.S., North, R.A., 2006. P2X receptors as cell-surface ATP sensors in health and disease. Nature 442, 527–532. (*Excellent and very readable review on P2X receptors. Recommended*)

Magni, G., Ceruti, S., 2013. P2Y purinergic receptors: new targets for analgesic and antimigraine drugs. Biochem. Pharmacol. 85, 466–477. (*Very thorough review of the potential for new analgesics that act at these receptors. Useful diagrams and structural information about P2Y receptor agonists*)

Surprenant, A., North, R.A., 2009. Signalling at purinergic P2X receptors. Annu. Rev. Physiol. 71, 333–359. (*Comprehensive review of P2X receptor biology if you are interested in following up the latest cutting-edge thinking*)

Tsuda, M., Tozaki-Saitoh, H., Inoue, K., 2012. Purinergic system, microglia and neuropathic pain. Curr. Opin. Pharmacol. 12, 74–79. (*A short overview of the role of the purinergic system in microglia and the implications for the pathogenesis and treatment of neuropathic pain*)

17 Local hormones 1: histamine and the biologically active lipids

OVERVIEW

In Chapter 6 we discussed the function of cellular players in host defence and alluded to the crucial role of soluble chemical regulators of inflammation. In this chapter, and the next, we take a closer look at these substances. We begin with some small molecule mediators. While also having a physiological role, these are pressed into service by the host defence mechanism when necessary, and are therefore important targets for anti-inflammatory drug action.

INTRODUCTION

The growth of pharmacology as a discipline was attended by the discovery of many biologically active substances. Many initially attracted attention as uncharacterised smooth muscle contracting (or relaxing) 'factors', which appeared in blood or tissues during particular physiological or pathological events. Sometimes, these factors were identified comparatively quickly but others resisted analysis for many years and the development of a particular area was often tied to progress in analytical methodology. For example, 5-HT (Ch. 15) and histamine, which are quite simple compounds, were identified soon after their biological properties were described. On the other hand, structural elucidation of the more complex prostaglandins, which were first discovered in the 1930s, had to await the development of the mass spectrometer some 30 years later. Peptide and protein structures took even longer to solve. Substance P (11 amino acids) was also discovered in the 1930s, but was not characterised until 1970 when peptide sequencing techniques had been developed. By the 1980s, molecular biology had greatly enhanced our analytical proficiency. Endothelin (21 residues) for example, was discovered, fully characterised, synthesised and cloned within about a year, the complete information being published in a single paper (Yanagisawa et al., 1988).

WHAT IS A 'MEDIATOR'?

Like regular hormones, such as thyroxine (Ch. 34) or insulin (Ch. 31), a *local hormone* is simply a chemical messenger that conveys information from one cell to another.[1] Hormones such as thyroxine and insulin are released from a single endocrine gland, circulate in the blood and, in this manner, can affect other 'target' tissues. In contrast, local hormones are usually produced by local cells and operate in the immediate microenvironment. The distinction is not actually clear-cut. For example one of the 'classical' hormones, hydrocortisone, is normally released by the adrenal gland but can, it transpires, also be produced and act locally in some tissues. Conversely, some cytokines (see Ch. 18), usually described as local hormones, whilst being produced locally, can circulate in the blood and produce systemic, as well as local, effects.

When, in response to a stimulus of some kind, a local hormone produces a particular biological effect (such as contraction of smooth muscle in response to allergen challenge), it is said to be a *mediator* of this response. Traditionally, a putative mediator[2] had to satisfy certain criteria before gaining official recognition. Dale, in the 1930s, proposed a set of five rules to establish the credentials of mediators and these guidelines have been used as a point of reference ever since. Originally formulated as a test for putative neurotransmitters, these criteria cannot easily be applied to mediators of other responses and have been modified on several occasions.

Currently, the experimental criteria that establish a substance as a mediator are:

- that it is released from local cells in sufficient amounts to produce a biological action on the target cells within an appropriate time frame
- that application of an authentic sample of the mediator reproduces the original biological effect
- that interference with the synthesis, release or action (e.g. using receptor antagonists, enzyme inhibitors, 'knock-down' or 'knock out' techniques) ablates or modulates the original biological response.

HISTAMINE

In a classic study, Sir Henry Dale and his colleagues demonstrated that a local anaphylactic reaction (a type I or 'immediate hypersensitivity reaction' such as the response to egg albumin in a previously sensitised animal; see Ch. 6) was caused by antigen–antibody reactions in sensitised tissue, and found that histamine mimicked this effect both *in vitro* and *in vivo*. Later studies confirmed that histamine is present in tissues, and released (along with other mediators) during anaphylaxis.

SYNTHESIS AND STORAGE OF HISTAMINE

Histamine is a basic amine formed from histidine by histidine decarboxylase. It is found in most tissues but is present in high concentrations in tissues exposed to the

---

[1]The term 'autocrine' is sometimes used to denote a local mediator that acts on the cell from which it is released, whereas a 'paracrine' mediator acts on other neighbouring cells.

[2]To add to the lexicographical confusion that already exists over hormones and mediators, another word 'bioregulator' has recently crept into use. As this portmanteau term could cover just about any biologically active substance, it is not much use for our purposes.

outside world (lungs , skin and gastrointestinal tract). At the cellular level, it is found largely in mast cells (approximately 0.1–0.2 pmol/cell) and basophils (0.01 pmol/cell), but non-mast cell histamine occurs in 'histaminocytes' in the stomach and in histaminergic neurons in the brain (see Ch. 39). In mast cells and basophils, histamine is complexed in intracellular granules with an acidic protein and a high-molecular-weight heparin termed macroheparin.

HISTAMINE RELEASE

Histamine is released from mast cells by exocytosis during inflammatory or allergic reactions. Stimuli include complement components C3a and C5a (see Ch. 6), which interact with specific surface receptors, and the combination of antigen with cell-fixed immunoglobulin (Ig)E antibodies. In common with many secretory processes (Ch. 4), histamine release is initiated by a rise in cytosolic $[Ca^{2+}]$. Various basic drugs, such as morphine and tubocurarine, release histamine, as does **compound 48/80**, an experimental tool often used to investigate mast cell biology. Agents that increase cAMP formation (e.g. β-adrenoceptor agonists; see Ch. 14) inhibit histamine secretion. Replenishment of secreted histamine by mast cells or basophils is a slow process, which may take days or weeks, whereas turnover of histamine in the gastric histaminocyte is very rapid. Histamine is metabolised by histaminase and/or by the methylating enzyme imidazole N-methyltransferase.

HISTAMINE RECEPTORS

Four types of histamine receptor have been identified, H_{1-4}. All are G protein-coupled receptors that modulate cAMP to effect downstream signalling. Splice variants of H_3 and H_4 receptors have been reported. All four are implicated in the inflammatory response in some capacity. A good account of the role of histamine in inflammation has been given by Jutel et al. (2009).

Selective antagonists at H_1, H_2 and H_3 receptors include mepyramine, cimetidine and thioperamide, respectively. Selective agonists for H_2 and H_3 receptors are, respectively, dimaprit and (R)-methylhistamine. Histamine H_1 antagonists are the principal antihistamines used in the treatment or prevention of inflammation (notably allergic inflammation such as hay fever). Other clinical uses of subtype antagonists may be found in Chapters 28, 39 and 48. The pharmacology of H_4 receptors is less well developed.

ACTIONS

Smooth muscle effects. Histamine, acting on H_1 receptors, contracts the smooth muscle of the ileum, bronchi, bronchioles and uterus. The effect on the ileum is not as marked in humans as it is in the guinea pig (this tissue remains the *de facto* standard preparation for histamine bioassay). Histamine reduces air flow in the first phase of bronchial asthma (see Ch. 28 and Fig. 28.3).

Cardiovascular effects. Histamine dilates human blood vessels and increases permeability of postcapillary venules, by an action on H_1 receptors, the effect being partly endothelium-dependent in some vascular beds. It also increases the rate and the output of the heart by action on cardiac H_2 receptors.

Gastric secretion. Histamine stimulates the secretion of gastric acid by action on H_2 receptors. In clinical terms, this is the most important action of histamine, because it is implicated in the pathogenesis of peptic ulcer. It is considered in detail in Chapter 30.

Effects on skin. When injected intradermally, histamine causes a reddening of the skin, accompanied by a weal with a surrounding flare. This mimics the *triple response* to scratching of the skin, described by Sir Thomas Lewis over 80 years ago. The reddening reflects vasodilatation of the small arterioles and precapillary sphincters, and the weal the increased permeability of the postcapillary venules. These effects are mainly mediated through activation of H_1 receptors. The flare is an axon reflex: stimulation of sensory nerve fibres evokes antidromic impulses through neighbouring branches of the same nerve, releasing vasodilators such as calcitonin gene-related peptide (CGRP; see Chs 18 and 26). Histamine causes intense itch if injected into the skin or applied to a blister base, because it stimulates sensory nerve endings through an H_1-dependent mechanism. H_1 antagonists are used to control itch caused by allergic reactions, insect bites, etc.

Despite the fact that histamine release is manifestly capable of reproducing many of the inflammatory signs and symptoms, H_1 antagonists do not have much clinical utility in the acute inflammatory response *per se*, because other mediators are more important. Histamine is, however, important in type I hypersensitivity reactions such as allergic rhinitis and urticaria. Other significant actions of histamine in inflammation include effects on B and T cells, modulating the acquired immune response (Jutel et al., 2009).

Histamine

- Histamine is a basic amine, stored in mast cell and basophil granules, and secreted when C3a and C5a interact with specific membrane receptors or when antigen interacts with cell-fixed IgE.
- Histamine produces effects by acting on H_1, H_2, H_3 or H_4 receptors on target cells.
- The main actions in humans are:
  - stimulation of gastric secretion (H_2)
  - contraction of most smooth muscle, except blood vessels (H_1)
  - cardiac stimulation (H_2)
  - vasodilatation (H_1)
  - increased vascular permeability (H_1).
- Injected intradermally, histamine causes the 'triple response': *reddening* (local vasodilatation), *wheal* (increased permeability of postcapillary venules) and *flare* (from an 'axon' reflex in sensory nerves releasing a peptide mediator).
- The main pathophysiological roles of histamine are:
  - as a stimulant of gastric acid secretion (treated with H_2-receptor antagonists)
  - as a mediator of type I hypersensitivity reactions such as urticaria and hay fever (treated with H_1-receptor antagonists)
  - CNS functions (see Ch. 39).

The use of H_1 antagonists in these and other conditions is dealt with in Chapter 26.

EICOSANOIDS

GENERAL REMARKS

The term *eicosanoid* refers to a group of mediators that are generated from fatty acid precursors as required, and are not stored preformed in cells. They are implicated in the control of many physiological processes, are among the most important mediators and modulators of the inflammatory reaction (Figs 17.1, 17.2) and are a very significant target for drug action.

Interest in eicosanoids first arose in the 1930s after reports that semen contained a lipid substance, apparently originating from the prostate gland, which contracted uterine smooth muscle. Later, it became clear that *prostaglandin* (as the factor was named[3]) was not a single substance but a whole family of compounds that could be generated from 20-carbon unsaturated fatty acid precursors by virtually all cells.

STRUCTURE AND BIOSYNTHESIS

In mammals, the main eicosanoid precursor is arachidonic acid (5,8,11,14-eicosatetraenoic acid), a 20-carbon unsaturated fatty acid containing four unsaturated double bonds (hence the prefix *eicosa-*, referring to the 20 carbon atoms, and *tetra*-enoic, referring to the four double bonds; see Fig. 17.1). In most cell types, arachidonic acid is esterified in the phospholipid pool, and the concentration of the free acid is low.

The principal eicosanoids are prostaglandins, *thromboxanes* and *leukotrienes*, although other derivatives of arachidonate, for example the *lipoxins* and *resolvins*, are of increasing interest and importance. (The term *prostanoid* will be used here to encompass both prostaglandins and thromboxanes.)

In most instances, the initial and rate-limiting step in eicosanoid synthesis is the liberation of intracellular arachidonate, usually in a one-step process catalysed by the enzyme *phospholipase A_2* (PLA$_2$; Fig. 17.2). An alternative multi-step process involving phospholipases C or D in conjunction with diacylglycerol lipase is sometimes utilised. Several isoforms of PLA$_2$ exist, but the most important is probably the highly regulated cytosolic PLA$_2$ (cPLA$_2$). This enzyme generates not only arachidonic acid (and thus eicosanoids) but also lysoglyceryl-phosphorylcholine (lyso-PAF), the precursor of *platelet activating factor* (PAF), another inflammatory mediator (see Figs 17.1, 17.2).

Cytosolic PLA$_2$ is activated by phosphorylation and this may be triggered by many stimuli, such as thrombin action on platelets, C5a on neutrophils, bradykinin on fibroblasts and antigen–antibody reactions on mast cells. General cell damage also triggers cPLA$_2$ activation. The free arachidonic acid is metabolised separately (or sometimes jointly) by several pathways, including the following.

- *Fatty acid cyclo-oxygenase* (COX). Two main isoforms exist, COX-1 and COX-2. These are highly homologous enzymes but are regulated in different and tissue-specific ways. They enzymatically combine arachidonic (and some other unsaturated fatty acid) substrates with molecular oxygen to form unstable intermediates, which can subsequently be transformed by other enzymes to different prostanoids.
- *Lipoxygenases.* Several subtypes, which often work sequentially, synthesise leukotrienes, lipoxins or other compounds (Figs 17.1–17.3).

Chapter 26 deals in detail with the way inhibitors of these pathways (including non-steroidal anti-inflammatory drugs [NSAIDs] and glucocorticoids) produce anti-inflammatory effects.

Mediators derived from phospholipids

- The main phospholipid-derived mediators are the eicosanoids (prostanoids and leukotrienes) and platelet-activating factor (PAF).
- The eicosanoids are synthesised from arachidonic acid released directly from phospholipids by phospholipase A$_2$, or by a two-step process involving phospholipase C and diacylglycerol lipase.
- Arachidonate is metabolised by cyclo-oxygenases (COX)-1 or COX-2 to prostanoids, by 5-lipoxygenase to leukotrienes and, after further conversion, to lipoxins.
- PAF is derived from phospholipid precursors by phospholipase A$_2$, giving rise to lyso-PAF, which is then acetylated to give PAF.

PROSTANOIDS

COX-1 is present in most cells as a constitutive enzyme. It produces prostanoids that act mainly as homeostatic regulators (e.g. modulating vascular responses, regulating gastric acid secretion). COX-2 is not normally present (at least in most tissues – renal tissue is an important exception) but it is strongly induced by inflammatory stimuli and therefore believed to be more relevant as a target of anti-inflammatory drugs (see Ch. 26). Both enzymes catalyse the incorporation of two molecules of oxygen into two of the unsaturated double bonds in each arachidonate molecule, forming the highly unstable endoperoxides prostaglandin (PG)G$_2$ and PGH$_2$ (see Fig. 17.1). The suffix '2' indicates that the product contains only two double bonds. PGG$_2$ and PGH$_2$ are rapidly transformed in a tissue specific manner by endoperoxide *isomerase* or *synthase* enzymes to PGE$_2$, PGI$_2$ (prostacyclin), PGD$_2$, PGF$_{2\alpha}$ and thromboxane (TX)A$_2$, which are the principal bioactive end products of this reaction. The mix of eicosanoids thus produced varies between cell types depending on the particular endoperoxide isomerases or synthases present. In platelets, for example, TXA$_2$ predominates, whereas in vascular endothelium PGI$_2$ is the main product. Macrophages, neutrophils and mast cells synthesise a mixture of products. If eicosatrienoic acid (three double bonds) rather than arachidonic acid is the substrate, the resulting prostanoids have only a single double bond, for example PGE$_1$, while eicosapentaenoic

---

[3]The name arose through an anatomical error. In some species it is difficult to differentiate the prostaglandin-rich seminal vesicles from the prostate gland which (ironically as we now know) contains virtually none. Nevertheless the name stuck, outlasting the term *vesiglandin*, suggested later, which would have been more appropriate.

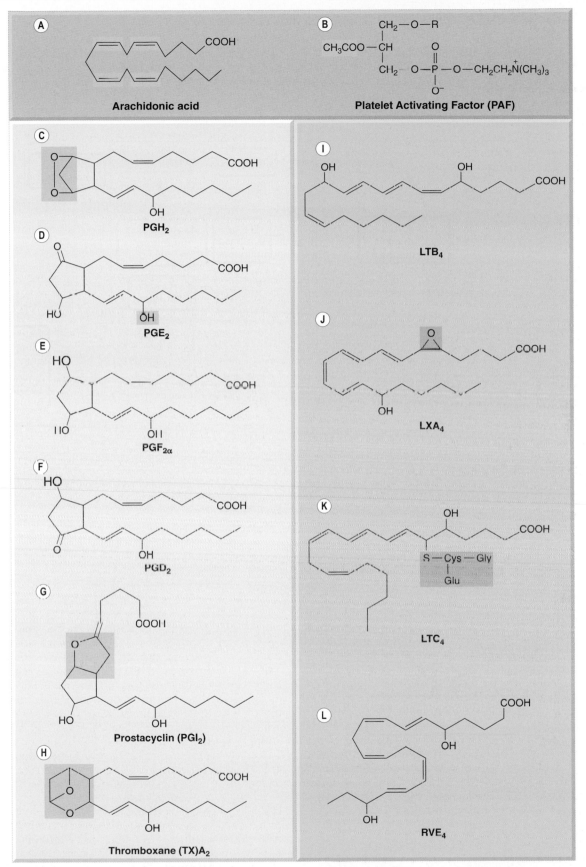

Fig. 17.1 Some key lipid mediators involved in the host defence response. [A] Arachidonic acid, an important precursor of prostanoids, leukotrienes, lipoxins and resolvins. Note the conjugated double bonds (in shaded box). [B] Platelet activating factor (PAF): the location of the acetyl group at C2 is shown in the shaded box. R is a 6- or 8-carbon saturated fatty acid attached by an ether linkage to the carbon backbone. [C] Prostaglandin (PG)H₂, one of the labile intermediates in the synthesis of prostaglandins; note unstable ring structure which can spontaneously hydrolyse in biological fluids (in shaded box). [D] PGE₂, the 15-hydroxyl group (in shaded box) is crucial for the biological activity of prostaglandins and its removal is the first step in their inactivation. [E] and [F] PGF₂α and PGD₂. [G] Prostacyclin (PGI₂); note unstable ring structure (in shaded box). [H] Thromboxane (TX)A₂; note unstable oxane structure (in shaded box). [I] Leukotriene (LT)B₄. [J] Lipoxin (LX)A₄; note unstable and highly reactive oxygen bridge structure (in shaded box). [K] Leukotriene (LT)C₄; note conjugated glutathione moiety (in shaded box). [L] Resolvin (Rv)E₄.

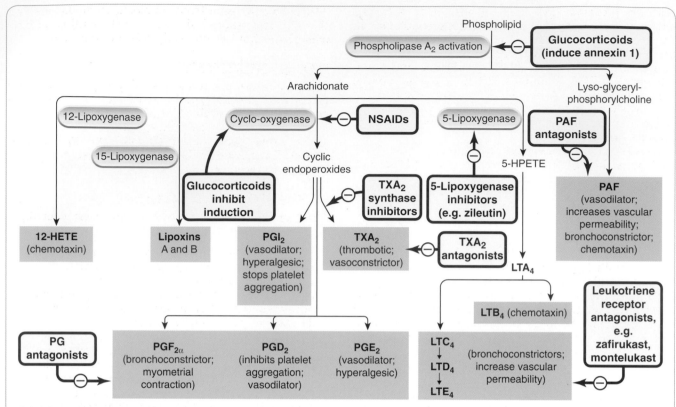

Fig. 17.2 **Summary diagram of the inflammatory mediators derived from phospholipids, with an outline of their actions and the sites of action of anti-inflammatory drugs.** The arachidonate metabolites are eicosanoids. The glucocorticoids inhibit transcription of the gene for cyclo-oxygenase-2, induced in inflammatory cells by inflammatory mediators. The effects of prostaglandin (PG)E₂ depend on which of the four receptors it activates. HETE, hydroxyeicosatetraenoic acid; HPETE, hydroperoxyeicosatetraenoic acid; LT, leukotriene; NSAID, non-steroidal anti-inflammatory drug; PAF, platelet-activating factor; PGI₂, prostacyclin; TX, thromboxane.

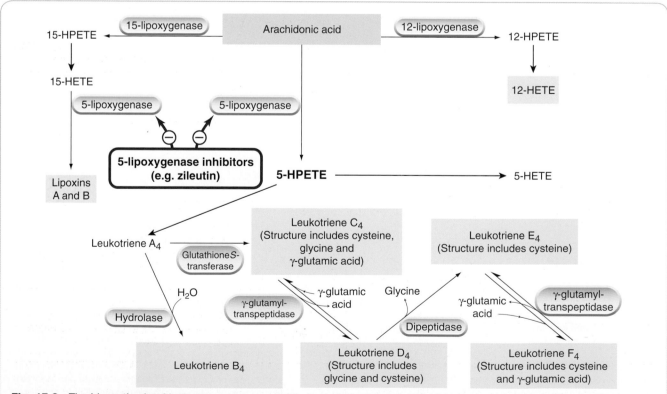

Fig. 17.3 **The biosynthesis of leukotrienes from arachidonic acid.** Compounds with biological action are shown in grey boxes. HETE, hydroxyeicosatetraenoic acid; HPETE, hydroperoxyeicosatetraenoic acid.

acid, which contains five double bonds, yields PGE_3. The latter substrate is significant because it is present in abundance in diets rich in oily fish and may, if present in sufficient amounts, represent a significant fraction of cellular fatty acids. When this occurs, the production of the pro-inflammatory PGE_2 is diminished and, more significantly, the generation of TXA_2 as well. This may partly underlie the beneficial anti-inflammatory and cardiovascular actions that are ascribed to diets rich in this type of marine product (see also Resolvins, below).

The endocannabinoid *anandamide* (see Ch. 19) is an eth-anolamine derivative of arachidonic acid and, surprisingly, it can also be oxidised by COX-2 to form a range of *prostamides*. These substances are of increasing interest. They act at prostanoid receptors but often exhibit a unique pharmacology.

CATABOLISM OF THE PROSTANOIDS

This is a multistep process. After carrier-mediated uptake, most prostaglandins are rapidly inactivated by pros-taglandin *dehydrogenase* and *reductase* enzymes. These enzymes act on the 15-hydroxyl group (see Fig. 17.1) and the 13-14 double bond, both of which are important for biological activity. The inactive products are further degraded by general fatty acid-oxidising enzymes and excreted in the urine. The dehydrogenase enzymes are present in high concentration in the lung, and 95% of infused PGE_2, PGE_1 or $PGF_{2\alpha}$ is inactivated after a single passage through the lungs, meaning that little normally reaches the arterial circulation. The half-life of most prostaglandins in the circulation is less than 1 minute.

TXA_2 and PGI_2 are slightly different. Both are inherently unstable and decay spontaneously and rapidly (within 30 s and 5 min, respectively) in biological fluids into inactive TXB_2 and 6-keto-$PGF_{1\alpha}$ respectively. Further metabolism occurs, but it is not really relevant to us here.

PROSTANOID RECEPTORS

There are five main classes of prostanoid receptor (Woodward et al., 2011), all of which are typical G protein-coupled receptors (Table 17.1). They are termed DP, FP, IP, EP and TP receptors, respectively, depending on whether their ligands are PGD, PGF, PGI, PGE or TXA species. Some have further subtypes; for example, there are four EP receptors.

ACTIONS OF THE PROSTANOIDS

The prostanoids affect most tissues and exert a bewildering variety of effects.

- PGD_2 causes vasodilatation in many vascular beds, inhibition of platelet aggregation, relaxation of gastrointestinal and uterine muscle, and modification of release of hypothalamic/pituitary hormones. It has a bronchoconstrictor effect through a secondary action on TP receptors.
- $PGF_{2\alpha}$ causes uterine contraction in humans (see Ch. 35), luteolysis in some species (e.g. cattle) and bronchoconstriction in other species (cats and dogs).
- PGI_2 causes vasodilatation, inhibition of platelet aggregation (see Ch. 24), renin release and natriuresis through effects on tubular reabsorption of Na^+.
- TXA_2 causes vasoconstriction, platelet aggregation (see Ch. 24) and bronchoconstriction (more marked in guinea pig than in humans).

Table 17.1 A simplified scheme of prostanoid receptor classification based upon their physiological effects

Receptor	Physiological ligands	Distribution	General physiological effects	Signalling system
IP	$I_2 \gg D_2$	Abundant in cardiovascular system, platelets, neurons and elsewhere	General inhibitory actions: e.g. smooth muscle relaxation, anti-inflammatory and anti-aggregatory effects	G_s ↑ cAMP
DP_1	$D_2 \gg E_2$	Low abundance; vascular smooth muscle, platelets, CNS, airways, the eye		
EP_2	$E_2 > F_{2\alpha}$	Widespread distribution		
EP_4	$E_2 > F_{2\alpha}$	Widespread distribution		
TP	$TxA_2 = H_2 > D_2$	Abundant in cardiovascular system, platelets and immune cells. Two subtypes known with opposing actions	General excitatory: e.g. smooth muscle contraction, pro-inflammatory and platelet aggregatory actions	G_q/G_{11} [PLC]* ↑ Ca^{2+}
FP	$F_{2\alpha} > D_2$	Very high expression in female reproductive organs		
EP_1	$E_2 > F_{2\alpha}$	Myometrium, intestine and lung		
EP_3	$E_2 > F_{2\alpha}$	Widespread distribution throughout body; many isoforms with different G protein coupling	General inhibitory actions: e.g. smooth muscle relaxation, anti-inflammatory and anti-aggregatory effects	G_i/G_o ↓ cAMP
DP_2	$D_2 > F_{2\alpha}$	Different structure to other prostanoid receptors. Widely distributed including immune cells		

*PLC may not be involved in EP_1 signalling.
Data derived from Woodward et al., 2011.

PGE$_2$, the predominant 'inflammatory' prostanoid has the following actions:

- on EP$_1$ receptors, it causes contraction of bronchial and gastrointestinal smooth muscle
- on EP$_2$ receptors, it causes bronchodilatation, vasodilatation, stimulation of intestinal fluid secretion and relaxation of gastrointestinal smooth muscle
- on EP$_3$ receptors, it causes contraction of intestinal smooth muscle, inhibition of gastric acid secretion (see Ch. 30), increased gastric mucus secretion, inhibition of lipolysis, inhibition of autonomic neurotransmitter release and stimulation of contraction of the pregnant human uterus (Ch. 35)
- on EP$_4$ receptors, it causes similar effects to those of EP$_2$ stimulation (these were originally thought to be a single receptor). Vascular relaxation is one consequence of receptor activation as is cervical 'ripening'. Some inhibitory effects of PGE$_2$ on leukocyte activation are probably mediated through this receptor.

A number of clinically useful drugs act at prostanoid receptors. **Misoprostil** is an EP$_2$/EP$_3$ agonist used for suppressing gastric acid secretion (see Ch. 30), **bimatoprost**,[4] **latanaprost, taluprost** and **travoprost** are FP agonists used for the treatment of glaucoma (see Ch. 13) and **iloprost** and **epoprostanol** are IP agonists used for the treatment of pulmonary hypertension (see Ch. 22).

THE ROLE OF PROSTANOIDS IN INFLAMMATION

The inflammatory response is inevitably accompanied by the release of prostanoids. PGE$_2$ predominates, although PGI$_2$ is also important. In areas of acute inflammation, PGE$_2$ and PGI$_2$ are generated by the local tissues and blood vessels, while mast cells release mainly PGD$_2$. In chronic inflammation, cells of the monocyte/macrophage series also release PGE$_2$ and TXA$_2$. Together, the prostanoids exert a sort of yin–yang effect in inflammation, stimulating some responses and decreasing others. The most striking effects are as follows.

In their own right, PGE$_2$, PGI$_2$ and PGD$_2$ are powerful vasodilators and synergise with other inflammatory vasodilators such as histamine and bradykinin. It is this combined dilator action on precapillary arterioles that contributes to the redness and increased blood flow in areas of acute inflammation. Prostanoids do not directly increase the permeability of the postcapillary venules, but potentiate the effects caused by histamine and bradykinin. Similarly, they do not themselves produce pain, but sensitise afferent C fibres (see Ch. 42) to the effects of bradykinin and other noxious stimuli. The anti-inflammatory and analgesic effects of aspirin-like drugs (NSAIDs, see Ch. 26) stem largely from their ability to block these actions.

Prostaglandins of the E series are also pyrogenic (i.e. they induce fever). High concentrations are found in cerebrospinal fluid during infection, and the increase in

temperature (attributed to cytokines) is actually finally mediated by the release of PGE$_2$. NSAIDs exert antipyretic actions (Ch. 26) by inhibiting PGE$_2$ synthesis in the hypothalamus.

However, some prostaglandins have anti-inflammatory effects which are important during the resolution phase of inflammation. For example, PGE$_2$ decreases lysosomal enzyme release and the generation of toxic oxygen metabolites from neutrophils, as well as the release of histamine from mast cells.

Prostanoids

- The term *prostanoids* encompasses the prostaglandins and the thromboxanes.
- Cyclo-oxygenases (COX) oxidise arachidonate, producing the unstable intermediates PGG$_2$ and PGH$_2$. These are enzymatically transformed to the different prostanoid species.
- There are two main COX isoforms: COX-1, a constitutive enzyme, and COX-2, which is often induced by inflammatory stimuli.
- The principal prostanoids are:
  - PGI$_2$ (prostacyclin), predominantly from vascular endothelium, acts on IP receptors, producing vasodilatation and inhibition of platelet aggregation.
  - Thromboxane (TX)A$_2$, predominantly from platelets, acts on TP receptors, causing platelet aggregation and vasoconstriction.
  - PGE$_2$ is prominent in inflammatory responses and is a mediator of fever and pain. Other effects include:
    at EP$_1$ receptors: contraction of bronchial and gastrointestinal (GI) tract smooth muscle
    at EP$_2$ receptors: relaxation of bronchial, vascular and GI tract smooth muscle
    at EP$_3$ receptors: inhibition of gastric acid secretion, increased gastric mucus secretion, contraction of pregnant uterus and of gastrointestinal smooth muscle, inhibition of lipolysis and of autonomic neurotransmitter release.
- PGF$_{2\alpha}$ acts on FP receptors, found in uterine (and other) smooth muscle, and corpus luteum, producing contraction of the uterus and luteolysis (in some species).
- PGD$_2$ is derived particularly from mast cells and acts on DP receptors, causing vasodilatation and inhibition of platelet aggregation.

LEUKOTRIENES

Leukotrienes (*leuko-* because they are made by white cells, and -*trienes* because they contain a conjugated triene system of double bonds; see Fig. 17.1) are synthesised from arachidonic acid by lipoxygenase-catalysed pathways. These soluble cytosolic enzymes are mainly found in lung, platelets, mast cells and white blood cells. The main enzyme in this group is *5-lipoxygenase*. On cell activation, this enzyme translocates to the nuclear

---

[4]Some female patients with glaucoma being treated with bimatoprost eye drops were delighted with a side effect of this drug – stimulation of eyelash growth. It wasn't long before a thriving 'off-label' market had been established for its use in beauty spas. Eventually, the FDA licensed a preparation specifically for this cosmetic indication.

Clinical uses of prostanoids

- Gynaecological and obstetric (see Ch. 35):
  - termination of pregnancy: **gemeprost** or **misoprostol** (a metabolically stable prostaglandin (PG)E analogue
  - induction of labour: **dinoprostone** or **misoprostol**
  - postpartum haemorrhage: **carboprost**.
- Gastrointestinal:
  - to prevent ulcers associated with non-steroidal anti-inflammatory drug use: **misoprostol** (see Ch. 30).
- Cardiovascular:
  - to maintain the patency of the ductus arteriosus until surgical correction of the defect in babies with certain congenital heart malformations: **alprostadil** (PGE₁)
  - to inhibit platelet aggregation (e.g. during haemodialysis): **epoprostenol** (PGI₂), especially if **heparin** is contraindicated
  - primary pulmonary hypertension: **epoprostenol** (see Ch. 22).
- Ophthalmic:
  - open-angle glaucoma: **latanoprost** eye drops.

membrane, where it associates with a crucial accessory protein, affectionately termed FLAP (**five-lipoxygenase activating protein**). The 5-lipoxygenase incorporates a hydroperoxy group at C5 in arachidonic acid to form *5-hydroperoxytetraenoic acid* (5-HPETE, Fig. 17.3), leading to the production of the unstable leukotriene (LT)A₄. This may be converted enzymatically to LTB₄ and, utilising a separate pathway involving conjugation with glutathione, to the cysteinyl-containing leukotrienes LTC₄, LTD₄, LTE₄ and LTF₄ (also referred to as the *sulfidopeptide leukotrienes*). These cysteinyl leukotrienes are produced mainly by eosinophils, mast cells, basophils and macrophages. Mixtures of these substances constitute the biological activity historically ascribed to *slow-reacting substance of anaphylaxis* (SRS-A), an elusive bronchoconstrictor factor shown many years ago to be generated in guinea-pig lung during anaphylaxis, and consequently predicted to be important in asthma.

LTB₄ is produced mainly by neutrophils. Lipoxins and other active products, some of which have anti-inflammatory properties, are also produced from arachidonate by this pathway (Figs 17.1 and 17.3).

LTB₄ is metabolised by a unique membrane-bound cytochrome P450 enzyme in neutrophils, and then further oxidised to 20-carboxy-LTB₄. LTC₄ and LTD₄ are metabolised to LTE₄, which is excreted in the urine.

LEUKOTRIENE RECEPTORS

Leukotriene receptors are termed BLT (two subtypes) if the ligand is LTB₄, and CysLT (two subtypes) for the cysteinyl leukotrienes. Their signalling mechanisms have not been completely elucidated and there may be further receptors that transduce the effects of these potent mediators.

LEUKOTRIENE ACTIONS

Cysteinyl leukotrienes have important actions on the respiratory and cardiovascular systems, and specific receptors for LTD₄ have been defined on the basis of numerous selective antagonists. The CysLT-receptor antagonists **zafirlukast** and **montelukast** are now in use in the treatment of asthma (see Ch. 28), often with a corticosteroid. Cysteinyl leukotrienes may mediate the cardiovascular changes of acute anaphylaxis. Agents that inhibit 5-lipoxygenase are therefore obvious candidates for anti-asthmatic (see Ch. 28) and anti-inflammatory agents. One such drug, **zileuton**, is available in some parts of the world but has not yet gained a definite place in therapy (see Larsson et al., 2006).

The respiratory system. Cysteinyl leukotrienes are potent spasmogens, causing dose-related contraction of human bronchiolar muscle *in vitro*. LTE₄ is less potent than LTC₄ and LTD₄, but its effect is much longer lasting. All cause an increase in mucus secretion. Given by aerosol to human volunteers, they reduce specific airway conductance and maximum expiratory flow rate, the effect being more protracted than that produced by histamine (Fig. 17.4).

The cardiovascular system. Small amounts of LTC₄ or LTD₄ given intravenously cause a rapid, short-lived fall in blood pressure, and significant constriction of small coronary resistance vessels. Given subcutaneously, they are equipotent with histamine in causing weal and flare. Given topically in the nose, LTD₄ increases nasal blood flow and increases local vascular permeability.

The role of leukotrienes in inflammation. LTB₄ is a potent chemotactic agent for neutrophils and macrophages (see Fig. 6.2). It upregulates membrane adhesion molecule expression on neutrophils, and increases the production of toxic oxygen products and the release of granule enzymes. On macrophages and lymphocytes, it stimulates proliferation and cytokine release. It is found in inflammatory exudates and tissues in many inflammatory conditions, including rheumatoid arthritis, psoriasis and ulcerative colitis.

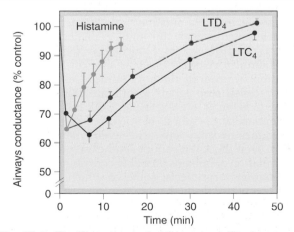

Fig. 17.4 **The time course of action on specific airways conductance of the cysteinyl leukotrienes and histamine, in six normal subjects.** Specific airways conductance was measured in a constant volume whole-body plethysmograph, and the drugs were given by inhalation. (*From Barnes et al., 1984.*)

The cysteinyl leukotrienes are present in the sputum of chronic bronchitis patients in amounts that are biologically active. On antigen challenge, they are released from samples of human asthmatic lung *in vitro*, and into nasal lavage fluid in subjects with allergic rhinitis. There is evidence that they contribute to the underlying bronchial hyper-reactivity in asthmatics, and it is thought that they are among the main mediators of both the early and late phases of asthma (see Fig. 28.2).

Leukotrienes

- 5-Lipoxygenase oxidises arachidonate to give 5-hydroperoxyeicosatetraenoic acid (5-HPETE), which is converted to leukotriene (LT)A_4. This, in turn, can be converted to either LTB_4 or to a series of glutathione adducts, the cysteinyl leukotrienes LTC_4, LTD_4 and LTE_4.
- LTB_4, acting on specific receptors, causes adherence, chemotaxis and activation of polymorphs and monocytes, and stimulates proliferation and cytokine production from macrophages and lymphocytes.
- The cysteinyl leukotrienes cause:
  - contraction of bronchial muscle
  - vasodilatation in most vessels, but coronary vasoconstriction.
- LTB_4 is an important mediator in all types of inflammation; the cysteinyl leukotrienes are of particular importance in asthma.

Di Gennaro and Haeggstrom (2012) have provided a good account of recent thinking on the role of these mediators in inflammation.

LIPOXINS AND RESOLVINS

A recently identified group of trihydroxy arachidonate metabolites termed lipoxins (Figs 17.1, 17.3) are formed by the concerted action of the 5- and the 12- or 15-lipoxygenase enzymes during inflammation. Lipoxins act on polymorphonuclear leukocytes, through a distinct G protein-coupled receptor system (which also recognises other anti-inflammatory factors such as annexin-A_1), to oppose the action of pro-inflammatory stimuli, supplying what might be called 'stop signals' to inflammation (reviewed by Ryan & Godson, 2010). Aspirin (a COX inhibitor, see Ch. 26) stimulates the synthesis of lipoxins because COX-2 can still produce hydroxy fatty acids even when inhibited by aspirin, even though it cannot synthesise prostaglandins. The formation of lipoxins probably contributes to aspirin's anti-inflammatory effects, some of which are not completely explained through inhibition of prostaglandin generation (see Gilroy & Perretti, 2005; Serhan, 2005).

Resolvins, as the name implies, are a series of compounds that fulfil a similar function, but unlike lipoxins, their precursor fatty acid is eicosapentaenoic acid. Fish oils are rich in this fatty acid and it is likely that at least some of their anti-inflammatory benefit is produced through conversion to these highly active species (see Zhang & Spite, 2012, for a recent review of this fascinating area). The leukocyte receptor for resolvins is called Chem 23. Resolvins can counteract inflammatory pain (Xu et al., 2010) and analogues are undergoing trials for the treatment of a variety of inflammatory conditions (Lee & Surh, 2012).

PLATELET-ACTIVATING FACTOR

Platelet-activating factor, also variously termed PAF-acether and AGEPC (acetyl-glyceryl-ether-phosphorylcholine), is a biologically active lipid that can produce effects at exceedingly low concentrations (less than 10_{-10} mol/l) through its G protein-coupled receptor (G_q/G_{11}; stimulates cAMP production). The name is somewhat misleading, however, because PAF has actions on a variety of different target cells, and is believed to be an important mediator in both acute and chronic allergic and inflammatory phenomena.

BIOSYNTHESIS

PAF (Fig. 17.1) is produced by platelets in response to thrombin, and by activated inflammatory cells. It is synthesised from particular phospholipids (acyl-PAF), which have an ether-linked hexadecyl or octadecyl fatty acid at C1, an unsaturated fatty acid such as arachidonic acid ester-linked at C2 and a phosphoryl choline base at C3. The action of PLA_2 on acyl-PAF produces removes the arachidonic acid from C2 leaving *lyso-PAF*, which is then acetylated by an *acetyltransferase* to yield PAF. This, in turn, can be inactivated by an *acetylhydrolase* to lyso-PAF.

ACTIONS AND ROLE IN INFLAMMATION

PAF can reproduce many of the signs and symptoms of inflammation. Injected locally, it produces vasodilatation (and thus erythema), increased vascular permeability and weal formation. Higher doses produce hyperalgesia. It is a potent chemotaxin for neutrophils and monocytes, and recruits eosinophils into the bronchial mucosa in the late phase of asthma (see Fig. 28.3). PAF contracts both bronchial and ileal smooth muscle.

PAF activates PLA_2 and stimulates arachidonate turnover in many cells. In platelets it increases TXA_2 generation, producing shape change and the release of the granule contents. This is important in haemostasis and thrombosis (see Ch. 24).

The anti-inflammatory actions of the glucocorticoids may be caused, at least in part, by inhibition of PAF synthesis (Fig. 17.2). Competitive antagonists of PAF and/or specific inhibitors of *lyso-PAF acetyltransferase* could well be useful anti-inflammatory drugs and/or antiasthmatic agents. The PAF antagonist **lexipafant** is in clinical trial in the treatment of acute pancreatitis (see Leveau et al., 2005). **Rupatidine** is a combined H_1 and PAF antagonist that is available in some parts of the world for treating allergic symptoms, but it is not clear what (if anything) its anti-PAF action adds clinically to its effect as an H_1 antagonist.

CONCLUDING REMARKS

In this chapter we have focused on histamine and lipid mediators. In some species (i.e. rodents) 5-HT (Ch. 15) has pro-inflammatory properties. Other low-molecular-weight factors also have inflammogenic actions, including some purines (Ch. 16) and nitric oxide (Ch. 20).

Platelet-activating factor (PAF)

- PAF precursors are released from activated inflammatory cells by phospholipase A_2. After acetylation, the resultant PAF is released and acts on specific receptors in target cells.
- Pharmacological actions include vasodilatation, increased vascular permeability, chemotaxis and activation of leukocytes (especially eosinophils), activation and aggregation of platelets, and smooth muscle contraction.
- PAF is implicated in bronchial hyper-responsiveness and in the delayed phase of asthma.
- A PAF antagonist, **lexipafant**, is undergoing clinical trial in pancreatitis.

REFERENCES AND FURTHER READING

Ariel, A., Serhan, C.N., 2007. Resolvins and protectins in the termination program of acute inflammation. Trends Immunol. 28, 176–183. (*Very accessible review on these unusual lipid mediators which promote inflammatory resolution and the link with fish oils*)

Barnes, N.C., Piper, P.J., Costello, J.F., 1984. Comparative effects of inhaled leukotriene C_4, leukotriene D_4, and histamine in normal human subjects. Thorax 39, 500–504.

Di Gennaro, A., Haeggstrom, J.Z., 2012. The leukotrienes: immune-modulating lipid mediators of disease. Adv. Immunol. 116, 51–92. (*Useful update on leukotriene actions in inflammation. Recommended*)

Gilroy, D.W., Perretti, M., 2005. Aspirin and steroids: new mechanistic findings and avenues for drug discovery. Curr. Opin. Pharmacol. 5, 405–411. (*A very interesting review dealing with anti-inflammatory substances that are released during the inflammatory response and that bring about resolution; it also deals with a rather odd effect of aspirin – its ability to boost the production of anti-inflammatory lipoxins. Easy to read and informative*)

Jutel, M., Akdis, M., Akdis, C.A., 2009. Histamine, histamine receptors and their role in immune pathology. Clin. Exp. Allergy 39, 1786–1800. (*Excellent review. Easy to read*)

Kim, N., Luster, A.D., 2007. Regulation of immune cells by eicosanoid receptors. ScientificWorld J. 7, 1307–1328. (*Useful overview of eicosanoids, their biology and receptor family*)

Larsson, B.M., Kumlin, M., Sundblad, B.M., et al., 2006. Effects of 5-lipoxygenase inhibitor zileuton on airway responses to inhaled swine house dust in healthy subjects. Respir. Med. 100, 226–237. (*A paper dealing with the effects of zileuton, a 5 lipoxygenase inhibitor, on the allergic response in humans; the results are not unequivocally positive, but the study is an interesting one*)

Lee, H.N., Surh, Y.J., 2012. Therapeutic potential of resolvins in the prevention and treatment of inflammatory disorders. Biochem. Pharmacol. 84, 1340–1350. (*Good review of this fast moving field. Easy to read*)

Leveau, P., Wang, X., Sun, Z., et al., 2005. Severity of pancreatitis-associated gut barrier dysfunction is reduced following treatment with the PAF inhibitor lexipafant. Biochem. Pharmacol. 69, 1325–1331. (*A paper dealing with the role of the PAF inhibitor lexipafant in pancreatitis; this is an experimental study using a rat model but provides a useful insight into the potential clinical role of such an antagonist*)

Okunishi, K., Peters-Golden, M., 2011. Leukotrienes and airway inflammation. Biochim. Biophys. Acta 1810, 1096–1102. (*Easy-to-read account of leukotrienes in airway disease and the status of drugs that interfere with their synthesis or action*)

Ryan, A., Godson, C., 2010. Lipoxins: regulators of resolution. Curr. Opin. Pharmacol. 10, 166–172.

Serhan, C.N., 2005. Lipoxins and aspirin-triggered 15 epi lipoxins are the first lipid mediators of endogenous anti-inflammation and resolution. Prostaglandins Leukot. Essent. Fatty Acids 73, 141–162. (*A paper reviewing the lipoxins – anti-inflammatory substances formed by the 5-lipoxygenase enzyme; also discusses the action of aspirin in boosting the synthesis of these compounds and the receptors on which they act. A good review that summarises a lot of work*)

Woodward, D.F., Jones, R.L., Narumiya, S., 2011. International Union of Basic and Clinical Pharmacology. LXXXIII classification of prostanoid receptors, updating 15 years of progress. Pharmacol. Rev. 63, 471–538. (*Definitive and comprehensive review by the leaders in the field*)

Xu, Z.Z., Zhang, L., Liu, T., et al., 2010. Resolvins RvE$_1$ and RvD$_1$ attenuate inflammatory pain via central and peripheral actions. Nat. Med. 16, 592–597. (*Fascinating paper reporting the ability of these anti-inflammatory lipids to reduce pain*)

Yanagisawa, M., Kurihara, H., Kimura, S., et al., 1988. A novel potent vasoconstrictor peptide produced by vascular endothelial cells. Nature 332, 411–415. (*The discovery of endothelin – a remarkable tour de force*)

Zhang, M.J., Spite, M., 2012. Resolvins: anti-inflammatory and proresolving mediators derived from omega-3 polyunsaturated fatty acids. Annu. Rev. Nutr. 32, 203–227. (*Explores the link between 'fish oils' and anti-inflammatory resolving production*)

18 Local hormones 2: peptides and proteins

OVERVIEW

Having discussed small-molecule local hormones in the previous chapter, we now turn our attention to peptides and proteins, which are orders of magnitude larger in molecular terms. This constitutes a very diverse group and, unlike others described in Chapter 17, includes compounds (e.g. cytokines) that seem to be exclusively concerned with host defence. We begin with some general introductory observations on protein and peptide synthesis and secretion. We then discuss bradykinin, neuropeptides, cytokines (interleukins, chemokines and interferons) in more detail. Finally, we conclude with a few remarks on other proteins and peptides that downregulate inflammation.

INTRODUCTION

Despite the fact that several mediators discovered early in the history of our discipline were recognised to be peptides, understanding of their pharmacology was limited until the 1970s when the techniques for purifying, sequencing and synthesising peptides and proteins were first developed. The development of high-performance liquid chromatography and solid-phase peptide synthesis, for example, have greatly accelerated the development of the area and while proteins containing 50 or more amino acids were (and are still) difficult to synthesise chemically, molecular biology techniques have provided a rapid alternative synthetic route. Indeed, the use of recombinant proteins as therapeutic agents – a development driven mainly by the emergent biotechnology industry – is rapidly gaining ground (see Ch. 59).

The use of molecular biology has helped understand peptide and protein pharmacology in many other ways as well. The availability of monoclonal antibodies for radioimmunoassay and immunocytochemistry has solved many quantitative problems. Transgenic animals with peptide or receptor genes deleted, or overexpressed, provide valuable clues about their functions, as has the use of antisense oligonucleotides and siRNA (see also Ch. 59) to silence these genes for experimental purposes. The control of precursor synthesis can be studied indirectly by measuring mRNA, for which highly sensitive and specific assays have been developed. The technique of *in situ* hybridisation enables the location and abundance of the mRNA to be mapped at microscopic resolution.

In summary, the molecular landscape has changed completely. Whereas the discovery of new 'small molecule' mediators has virtually dried up, the discovery of new protein and peptide mediators continues apace. More than 100 cytokines have been discovered since interleukin 2 (IL-2) was first characterised in 1982.

GENERAL PRINCIPLES OF PROTEIN AND PEPTIDE PHARMACOLOGY

STRUCTURE

Peptide and protein mediators generally vary from three to about 200 amino acid residues in length, the arbitrary dividing line between peptides and proteins being about 50 residues. An important difference is that proteins need to adopt a complex folded structure in order to exert their specific function, whereas short peptides are in most cases flexible. Specific residues in proteins and peptides often undergo post-translational modifications, such as *amidation, glycosylation, acetylation, carboxylation, sulfation* or *phosphorylation*. They also may contain *intramolecular* disulfide bonds, such that the molecule adopts a partially cyclic conformation, or they may comprise two or more separate chains linked by *intermolecular* disulfide bonds.

Generally speaking, larger proteins adopt restricted conformations that expose functional groups in fixed locations on their surface, which interact with multiple sites on their receptors in 'lock-and-key' mode. To envisage flexible peptides fitting into a receptor site this way is to imagine that you can unlock your front door with a length of cooked spaghetti. These features have greatly impeded the rational design of non-peptide analogues that mimic the action of proteins and peptides at their receptors (peptidomimetics). The use of random screening methods has (somewhat to the chagrin of the rationalists) nevertheless led in recent years to the discovery of many non-peptide *antagonists* – although few *agonists* – for peptide receptors.

TYPES OF PROTEIN AND PEPTIDE MEDIATOR

Protein and peptide mediators that are secreted by cells and act on surface receptors of the same or other cells can be very broadly divided into four groups:

- neurotransmitters (e.g. endogenous opioid peptides, Ch. 42) and neuroendocrine mediators (e.g. vasopressin, somatostatin, hypothalamic releasing hormones, ACTH, LH, FSH and TSH, see Chs 33–35), not discussed further in this chapter)
- hormones from non-neural sources: these comprise plasma-derived peptides, notably angiotensin (Ch. 22) and bradykinin, as well as other hormones such as insulin (Ch. 31), endothelin (Ch. 22), atrial natriuretic peptide (Ch. 21) and leptin (Ch. 32)
- growth factors: produced by many different cells and tissues that control cell growth and differentiation (especially, in adults, in the haemopoietic system; see Ch. 25)
- mediators of the immune system (cytokines, see below).

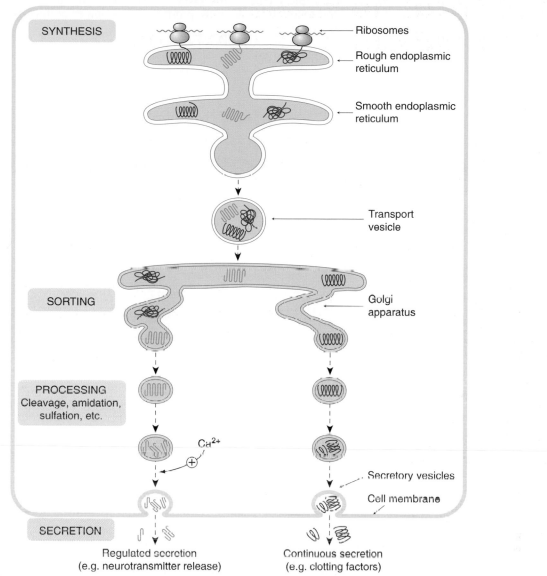

Fig. 18.1 Cellular mechanisms for peptide synthesis and release. Proteins synthesised by ribosomes are threaded through the membrane of the rough endoplasmic reticulum, from where they are conveyed in transport vesicles to the Golgi apparatus. Here, they are sorted and packaged into secretory vesicles. Processing (cleavage, glycosylation, amidation, sulfation, etc.) occurs within the transport and secretory vesicles, and the products are released from the cell by exocytosis. Constitutive secretion (e.g. of plasma proteins and clotting factors by liver cells) occurs continuously, and little material is stored in secretory vesicles. Regulated secretion (e.g. of neuropeptides or cytokines) occurs in response to increased intracellular Ca^{2+} or other intracellular signals, and material is typically stored in significant amounts in secretory vesicles awaiting release.

BIOSYNTHESIS AND REGULATION OF PEPTIDES

Peptide structure is, of course, directly coded in the genome, in a manner that the structure of (say) acetylcholine is not, so intracellular manufacture is a matter of conventional protein synthesis. This often begins with the manufacture of a precursor protein in which the desired peptide sequence is embedded. Specific proteolytic enzymes excise the active peptide, a process of sculpture rather than synthesis. The precursor protein is packaged into vesicles at the point of synthesis, and the active peptide is formed *in situ* ready for release (Fig. 18.1). Thus there is no need for specialised biosynthetic pathways, or for the uptake or recapturing

mechanisms, that are important for the synthesis and release of most non-peptide mediators (e.g. 5HT; Ch. 15).

PEPTIDE PRECURSORS

The precursor protein, or *pre-prohormone*, usually 100–250 residues in length, consists of an N-terminal *signal sequence* (peptide), followed by a variable stretch of unknown function, and a peptide-containing region that may contain several copies of active peptide fragments. Often, several different peptides are found within one precursor, but sometimes there are multiple copies of a single peptide.[1]

---

[1] In the case of the invertebrate *Aplysia*, one protein precursor contains no fewer than 28 copies of the same short peptide.

The *signal sequence*, which is strongly hydrophobic, facilitates insertion of the protein into the endoplasmic reticulum and is then cleaved off at an early stage, yielding the *prohormone*.

The active peptides are usually demarcated within the prohormone sequence by pairs of basic amino acids (Lys-Lys or Lys-Arg), which are cleavage points for the trypsin-like proteases that release the peptides. This *endoproteolytic cleavage* generally occurs in the Golgi apparatus or the secretory vesicles. The enzymes responsible are known as *prohormone convertases*. Scrutiny of the prohormone sequence often reveals likely cleavage points that demarcate previously unknown peptides. In some cases (e.g. CGRP; see below), new peptide mediators have been discovered in this way, but there are many examples where no function has yet been assigned. Whether these peptides are, like strangers at a funeral, waiting to declare their purpose or merely functionless relics, remains a mystery. There are also large stretches of the prohormone sequence of unknown function lying between the active peptide fragments.

The abundance of mRNA coding for particular pre-prohormones, which reflects the level of gene expression, is very sensitive to physiological conditions. This type of *transcriptional control* is one of the main mechanisms by which peptide expression and release are regulated over the medium to long term. Inflammation, for example, increases the expression, and hence the release, of various cytokines by immune cells (see Ch. 16). Sensory neurons respond to peripheral inflammation by increased expression of tachykinins (substance P and neurokinins A and B), which is important in the genesis of inflammatory pain (see Ch. 42).

DIVERSITY WITHIN PEPTIDE FAMILIES

Peptides commonly occur in families with similar or related sequences and actions. For example, the pro-opiomelanocortin (POMC) serves as a source of adreno-corticotrophic hormone (ACTH), melanocyte-stimulating hormones (MSH) and β-endorphin, all of which have a role in controlling the inflammatory response (as well as other processes).

GENE SPLICING AS A SOURCE OF DIVERSITY

Diversity of members of a peptide family can also arise by gene splicing or during post-translational processing of the prohormone. Genes contain coding regions (*exons*) interspersed with non-coding regions (*introns*) and when the gene is transcribed, the ensuing RNA (*heterologous nuclear RNA [hnRNA]*) is spliced to remove the introns and some of the exons, forming the final mature mRNA that is translated. Control of the splicing process allows a measure of cellular control over the peptides that are produced.

For example, the calcitonin gene codes for calcitonin itself, important in bone metabolism, Ch. 36) and also for a completely dissimilar peptide (calcitonin gene-related peptide, CGRP, involved in migraine pathogenesis, Ch. 15). Alternative splicing allows cells to produce either pro-calcitonin (expressed in thyroid cells) or pro-CGRP (expressed in many neurons) from the same gene. Substance P and neurokinin A are two closely related tachykinins belonging to the same family, and are encoded on the same gene. Alternative splicing results in the production of two precursor proteins; one of these includes both peptides, the other includes only substance P. The ratio of

the two varies widely between tissues, which correspondingly produce either one or both peptides.

POST-TRANSLATIONAL MODIFICATIONS AS A SOURCE OF PEPTIDE DIVERSITY

Many peptides, such as tachykinins and ACTH-related peptides (see Ch. 33), must undergo enzymatic amidation at the C-terminus to acquire full biological activity. Tissues may also generate peptides of varying length from the same primary sequence by the action of specific peptidases that cut the chain at different points. For example, pro-cholecystokinin (pro-CCK) contains the sequences of at least five CCK-like peptides ranging in length from 4 to 58 amino acid residues, all with the same C-terminal sequence. CCK itself (33 residues) is the main peptide produced by the intestine, whereas the brain produces mainly CCK-8. The opioid precursor prodynorphin similarly gives rise to several peptides with a common terminal sequence, the proportions of which vary in different tissues and in different neurons in the brain. In some cases (e.g. the inflammatory mediator bradykinin), peptide cleavage occurring after release generates a new active peptide (des-Arg^9-bradykinin), which acts on a different receptor, both peptides contributing differently to the inflammatory response.

PEPTIDE TRAFFICKING AND SECRETION

The basic mechanisms by which peptides are synthesised, packaged into vesicles, processed and secreted are summarised in Fig. 18.1. Two secretory pathways exist, for *constitutive* and *regulated* secretion, respectively. Constitutively secreted proteins (e.g. plasma proteins, some clotting factors) are not stored in appreciable amounts, and secretion is coupled to synthesis. Regulated secretion is, as with many hormones and transmitters, controlled by receptor-activated signals that lead to a rise in intracellular Ca^{2+} (see Ch. 4), and peptides awaiting release are stored in cytoplasmic vesicles. Specific protein–protein interactions appear to be responsible for the sorting of different proteins into different vesicles, and for choreographing their selective release. Identification of the specific 'trafficking' proteins involved in particular secretory pathways may eventually yield novel drug targets for the selective control of secretion.

Having described the general mechanisms by which peptides are synthesised, processed and released, we now describe some significant mediators that fall into this category.

BRADYKININ

Bradykinin and lysyl-bradykinin (*kallidin*) are active peptides formed by proteolytic cleavage of circulating proteins termed *kininogens* through a protease cascade pathway (see Fig. 6.1).

SOURCE AND FORMATION OF BRADYKININ

An outline of the formation of bradykinin from high-molecular-weight *kininogen* in plasma by the serine protease *kallikrein* is given in Figure 18.2. Kininogen is a plasma α-globulin that exists in both high- (M_r 110 000) and low- (M_r 70 000) molecular-weight forms. Kallikrein is derived from the inactive precursor *prekallikrein* by the

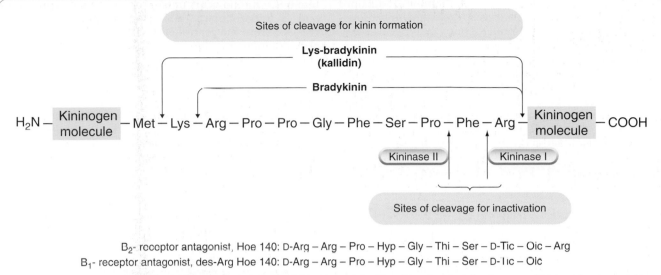

Fig. 18.2 **The structure of bradykinin and some bradykinin antagonists.** The sites of proteolytic cleavage of high-molecular-weight kininogen by kallikrein involved in the formation of bradykinin are shown in the upper half of the figure; the sites of cleavage associated with bradykinin and kallidin inactivation are shown in the lower half. The B_2-receptor antagonist icatibant (Hoe 140) has a pA_2 of 9, and the competitive B_1-receptor antagonist des-Arg Hoe 140 has a pA_2 of 8. The Hoe compounds contain unnatural amino acids: Thi, δ-Tic and Oic, which are analogues of phenylalanine and proline.

action of *Hageman factor* (factor XII; see Ch. 24 and Fig. 6.1). Hageman factor is activated by contact with negatively charged surfaces such as collagen, basement membrane, bacterial lipopolysaccharides, urate crystals and so on. Hageman factor, prekallikrein and the kininogens leak out of the vessels during inflammation because of increased vascular permeability, and exposure to negatively charged surfaces promotes the interaction of Hageman factor with prekallikrein. The activated enzyme then 'clips' bradykinin from its kininogen precursor. Kallikrein can also activate the complement system and can convert plasminogen to plasmin (see Fig. 6.1 and Ch. 24).

In addition to plasma kallikrein, there are other kinin-generating isoenzymes found in pancreas, salivary glands, colon and skin. These *tissue kallikreins* act on both high- and low-molecular-weight kininogens and generate mainly kallidin, a peptide with actions similar to those of bradykinin.

METABOLISM AND INACTIVATION OF BRADYKININ

Specific enzymes that inactivate bradykinin and related kinins are called *kininases* (Fig. 18.2). One of these, *kininase II*, is a peptidyl dipeptidase that inactivates kinins by removing the two C-terminal amino acids. This enzyme, which is bound to the luminal surface of endothelial cells, is identical to *angiotensin-converting enzyme* (ACE; see Ch. 22), which cleaves the two C-terminal residues from the inactive peptide angiotensin I, converting it to the active vasoconstrictor peptide angiotensin II. Thus kininase II inactivates a vasodilator and activates a vasoconstrictor. Potentiation of bradykinin actions by ACE inhibitors may contribute to some side effects of these drugs (e.g. cough). Kinins are also metabolised by various less specific peptidases, including a serum carboxypeptidase that removes the C-terminal arginine, generating des-Arg⁹-bradykinin, a specific agonist at one of the two main classes of bradykinin receptor.

BRADYKININ RECEPTORS

There are two bradykinin receptors, designated B_1 and B_2. Both are G protein-coupled receptors and mediate very similar effects. B_1 receptors are normally expressed at very low levels but are strongly induced in inflamed or damaged tissues by cytokines such as IL-1. B_1 receptors respond to des-Arg⁹-bradykinin but not to bradykinin itself. A number of selective peptide and non-peptide antagonists are known. It is likely that B_1 receptors play a significant role in inflammation and hyperalgesia (see Ch. 42), and antagonists could be used in cough and neurological disorders (Rodi et al., 2005).

B_2 receptors are constitutively present in many normal cells and are activated by bradykinin and kallidin, but not by des-Arg⁹-bradykinin. Peptide and non-peptide antagonists have been developed, the best known being the bradykinin analogue **icatibant**, used to treat acute attacks in patients with *hereditary angioedema* (an uncommon disorder caused by deficiency of C1-esterase inhibitor that normally restrains complement activation).

ACTIONS AND ROLE IN INFLAMMATION

Bradykinin causes vasodilatation and increased vascular permeability. Its vasodilator action is partly a result of generation of PGI_2 and release of nitric oxide (NO). It is a potent pain-producing agent at sensory neurons, and its action here is potentiated by prostaglandins (Ch. 17), which are released by bradykinin. Bradykinin also has spasmogenic actions on intestinal, uterine and bronchial smooth muscle in some species. The contraction is slow and sustained in comparison with that produced by tachykinins such as substance P (*brady-* means slow; *tachy-* means rapid).

Although bradykinin reproduces many inflammatory signs and symptoms, its role in inflammation and allergy is not clear, partly because its effects are often component parts of a complex cascade of events triggered by other mediators. However, excessive bradykinin production contributes to the diarrhoea of gastrointestinal disorders, and in allergic rhinitis it stimulates nasopharyngeal secretion. Bradykinin also contributes to the clinical picture in pancreatitis,[2] although disappointingly B_2 antagonists worsen rather than alleviate this disorder. Physiologically, the release of bradykinin by tissue kallikrein may regulate blood flow to certain exocrine glands, and influence secretions. Bradykinin also stimulates ion transport and fluid secretion by some epithelia, including intestine, airways and gall bladder.

Bradykinin

- Bradykinin (BK) is a nonapeptide 'clipped' from a plasma α-globulin, *kininogen*, by *kallikrein*.
- It is converted by *kininase I* to an octapeptide, BK_{1-8} (des-Arg^9-BK), and inactivated by the removal of an additional amino acid by *kininase II* (angiotensin-converting enzyme) in the lung.
- Pharmacological actions:
  - vasodilatation (largely dependent on endothelial cell nitric oxide and PGI_2)
  - increased vascular permeability
  - stimulation of pain nerve endings
  - stimulation of epithelial ion transport and fluid secretion in airways and gastrointestinal tract
  - contraction of intestinal and uterine smooth muscle.
- There are two main subtypes of BK receptors: B_2, which is constitutively present, and B_1, which is induced in inflammation.
- **Icatibant**, a peptide analogue of BK, is a selective competitive antagonist for B_2 receptors and is used to treat acute attacks of hereditary angioedema.

  Other, non-peptide antagonists for both B_1 and B_2 receptors are known, and may be developed for treating inflammatory disorders.

NEUROPEPTIDES

Neuropeptides constitute a large (>100) and diverse family of small to medium-sized peptides. A large number are found in the CNS, the autonomic nervous system, and peripheral sensory neurons, and they are also abundant in many peripheral tissues. They are often released as co-transmitters (Chs 38 and 39), along with non-peptide neurotransmitters.

When released from peripheral endings of nociceptive sensory neurons (see Ch. 42), neuropeptides in some species cause *neurogenic inflammation* (Maggi, 1996). The main peptides involved are *substance P, neurokinin A* and *CGRP*. Substance P and neurokinin A are small (about 1100 mw) members of the *tachykinin* family with partly homologous structures, which act on mast cells, releasing histamine and other mediators, and producing smooth muscle contraction, neural activation, mucus secretion and vasodilatation. CGRP is a member of the calcitonin

family (37 amino acids in length) shares these properties and is a particularly potent vasodilator. Tachykinins released from the central endings of nociceptive neurons also modulate transmission in the dorsal horn of the spinal cord, affecting sensitivity to pain (see Ch. 42). All these neuropeptides act on specific G protein-coupled receptors to produce their effects.

Neurogenic inflammation is implicated in the pathogenesis of several inflammatory conditions, including the delayed phase of asthma, allergic rhinitis, inflammatory bowel disease and some types of arthritis as well as migraine (Ch. 15 and Pisi et al., 2009). Antagonists at the neurokinin NK_1 receptor such as **aprepitant** and **fosaprepitant** are used to treat emesis, particularly that associated with some forms of cancer chemotherapy (see Ch. 56). Other important members of the neuropeptide family include enkephalins/endorphins (Ch. 42) and orexins (Ch. 39).

CYTOKINES

'Cytokine' is an all-purpose functional term that is applied to protein or polypeptide mediators synthesised and released by cells of the immune system during inflammation. They are crucial for the overall coordination of the inflammatory response. Cytokines act locally by autocrine or paracrine mechanisms. Unlike conventional hormones such as insulin, concentrations in blood and tissues are almost undetectable under normal circumstances, but are massively upregulated (100–1000-fold) during inflammatory episodes. All these mediators are usually active at very low (sub-nanomolar) concentrations.

On the target cell, cytokines bind to and activate specific, high-affinity receptors that, in most cases, are also upregulated during inflammation. Except for *chemokines*, which act on G protein-coupled receptors, most cytokines act on kinase-linked receptors, regulating phosphorylation cascades that affect gene expression, such as the Jak/Stat pathway (Chs 3 and 4).

In addition to their own direct actions on cells, some cytokines amplify inflammation by inducing the formation of other inflammatory mediators. Others can induce receptors for other cytokines on their target cell, or engage in synergistic or antagonistic interactions with other cytokines. Cytokines may be likened to a complex chemical signalling language, with the final response of a particular cell involved being determined by the strength and number of different messages received concurrently at the cell surface.

Various systems for classifying cytokines can be found in the literature, as can a multitude of diagrams depicting complex networks of cytokines interacting with each other and with a range of target cells. No one system of classification does justice to the complexity of cytokine biology. The terminology and nomenclature are horrendous and a comprehensive coverage of this area is beyond the scope of this book. For our purposes of this chapter, however, Table 18.1 lists some of the more significant cytokines and their biological actions. The would-be cytokine aficionado can find further classification tables in Murphy et al. (2011) and the IUPHAR/BPS Guide to Pharmacology.

More than 100 cytokines have been identified. These may be broadly categorised into four main functional groups, namely *interleukins, chemokines, interferons* and *colony-stimulating factors* (discussed separately in Ch. 25),

---

[2]A serious and painful condition in which proteolytic enzymes are released from damaged pancreatic cells, initiating cascades that release, among other things, bradykinin.

Table 18.1 Some examples of significant cytokines and their actions

Cytokine	Main cell source	Main target cell or biological effect	Comments
IL-1	Monocyte/macrophages, dendritic and other cells	Regulates cell migration to sites of infection, produces inflammation, fever and pain	Two original subtypes Il-1α and IL-1β, and IL-1ra – a receptor antagonist. Target for anti-inflammatory therapy (Ch. 26)
IL-2	T cells	Stimulates proliferation, maturation and activation of T, B and NK cells	First interleukin to be discovered
IL-4	Th2 cells	Stimulates proliferation, maturation of T and B cells and promotes IgG and E synthesis. Promotes an anti-inflammatory phenotype	A key cytokine in the regulation of the Th2 response (Ch. 26)
IL-5	Th2 cells, mast cells	Important for eosinophil activation. Stimulates proliferation, maturation of B cells and IgA synthesis	Particularly important in allergic disease
IL-6	Monocyte/macrophages and T cells	Pro-inflammatory actions including fever. Stimulation of osteoclast activity	Target for anti-inflammatory drugs (Ch. 26)
IL-8	Macrophages, endothelial cells	Neutrophil chemotaxis, phagocytosis and angiogenesis	C–X–C chemokine (CXCL8)
IL-10	Monocytes and Th2 cells	Inhibits cytokine production and downregulates inflammation	A predominately anti-inflammatory cytokine
IL-17	T cells and others	Stimulates Th17 cells, involved in allergic response and autoimmunity	Several subtypes. Target for anti-inflammatory drugs (Ch. 26)
GM–CSF	Macrophages, T cells, mast cells and others	Stimulates growth of leukocyte progenitor cells. Increases numbers of blood-borne leukocytes	Used therapeutically to stimulate myeloid cell growth (e.g. after bone marrow transplantation)
MIP-1	Macrophages/lymphocyes	Activation of neutrophils and other cells. Promotes cytokine release	C–C chemokine (CCL3). Two subtypes
TGF-β	T cells, monocytes	Induces apoptosis. Regulates cell growth	Three isoforms. Predominately anti-inflammatory action
TNF-α	Mainly macrophages but also many immune and other cells	Kills tumour cells. Stimulates macrophage cytokine expression and is a key regulator of many aspects of the immune response	A major target for anti-inflammatory drugs (Ch. 6)
TNF-β	Th1 cells	Initiates a variety of immune-stimulatory and pro-inflammatory actions in the host defence system	Now often called lymphotoxin α (LTA)
Eotaxin	Airway epithelial and other cells	Activation and chemotaxis of eosinophils. Allergic inflammation	C–C chemokine (CCL11). Three subtypes
MCP-1	Monocytes, osteoblasts/clasts, neurons and other cells	Promotes recruitment of monocytes and T cells to sites of inflammation	C–C chemokine (CC2)
RANTES	T cells	Chemotaxis of T cells. Chemotaxis and activation of other leukocytes	(CCL5)
IFN-α	Leukocytes	Activates NK cells and macrophages. Inhibits viral replication and has antitumour actions	Multiple molecular species
IFN-γ	Th1, NK cells	Stimulates Th1, and inhibits Th2, cell proliferation. Activates NK cells and macrophages	Crucial to the Th1 response (Ch. 6)

GM–CSF, granulocyte-macrophage colony-stimulating factor; IFN, interferon; Ig, immunoglobulin; IL, interleukin; MCP, monocyte chemoattractant protein; MIP, macrophage inflammatory protein; NK, natural killer (cell); RANTES, regulated on activation normal T cell expressed and secreted; TGF, transforming growth factor; Th, T-helper (cell); TNF, tumour necrosis factor.

but the demarcations are of limited use because many cytokines have multiple roles.

Using biopharmaceuticals (see Ch. 59) to interfere with cytokine action has proved to be a particularly fertile area of drug development: several successful strategies have been adopted, including direct antibody neutralisation of cytokines or the use of 'decoy' receptor proteins that remove the biologically active pool from the circulation. These are explained in detail in Chapters 26 and 59.

INTERLEUKINS AND RELATED COMPOUNDS

The name was originally coined to describe mediators that signalled between leukocytes but, like so much else in the cytokine lexicography, it has become rather redundant, not to say misleading. The primary pro-inflammatory species are *tumour necrosis factor* (TNF)-α and *interleukin 1* (IL-1). The principal members of the latter cytokine group consist of two agonists, IL-1α, IL-1β and, surprisingly, an endogenous IL-1-receptor antagonist (IL-1ra).[3] Mixtures of these are released from macrophages and many other cells during inflammation and can initiate the synthesis and release of a cascade of secondary cytokines, among which are the chemokines. TNF and IL-1 are key regulators of almost all manifestations of the inflammatory response. A long-standing debate about which of the two is really the prime mover of inflammation ended when it was found that this varies according to the disease type. In auto-*immune* disease (e.g. rheumatoid arthritis, where the adaptive immune system is activated), TNF appears to be the predominant influence and blocking its action is therapeutically effective. In auto-*inflammatory* diseases (e.g. gout, where only the innate system is involved), IL-1 seems to be the key mediator (Dinarello et al., 2012). Both TNF-α and IL-1 are important targets for anti-inflammatory biopharmaceuticals (Chs. 26 and 59).

Not all interleukins are pro-inflammatory: some, including *transforming growth factor (TGF)-β*, IL-4, IL-10 and IL-13 are potent anti-inflammatory substances. They inhibit chemokine production, and the responses driven by T-helper (Th) 1 cells, whose inappropriate activation is involved in the pathogenesis of several diseases.

CHEMOKINES

Chemokines are defined as *chemo*attractant cyto*kines* that control the migration of leukocytes, functioning as traffic coordinators during immune and inflammatory reactions. Again, the nomenclature (and the classification) is confusing, because some non-cytokine mediators also control leukocyte movement (C5a, LTB₄, fMet-Leu-Phe, etc; see Fig. 6.2) and many chemokines have more than one name. Furthermore, many chemokines have other actions, causing mast cell degranulation or promoting angiogenesis, for example.

More than 40 chemokines have been identified. They are all highly homologous peptides of 8–10 kDa, which are usually grouped according to the configuration of key cysteine residues in their polypeptide chain. Chemokines with one cysteine are known as *C chemokines*. If there are two adjacent residues they are called *C–C*

chemokines. Other members have cysteines separated by one (*C–X–C chemokines*) or three other residues (*C–XXX–C chemokines*).

The C–X–C chemokines (main example IL-8; see Fig. 6.2) act on neutrophils and are predominantly involved in acute inflammatory responses. The C–C chemokines (main examples eotaxin, MCP-1 and RANTES[4]) act on monocytes, eosinophils and other cells, and are involved predominantly in chronic inflammatory responses.

▼ Chemokines generally act through G protein-coupled receptors, and alteration or inappropriate expression of these is implicated in multiple sclerosis, cancer, rheumatoid arthritis and some cardiovascular diseases (Gerard & Rollins, 2001). Some types of virus (herpes virus, cytomegalovirus, pox virus and members of the retrovirus family) can exploit the chemokine system and subvert the host's defences (Murphy, 2001). Some produce proteins that mimic host chemokines or chemokine receptors, some act as antagonists at chemokine receptors and some masquerade as growth or angiogenic factors. The AIDS-causing HIV virus is responsible for the most audacious exploitation of the host chemokine system. This virus has a protein (gp120) in its envelope that recognises and binds T-cell receptors for CD4 and a chemokine co-receptor that allows it to penetrate the T cell (see Ch. 52).

INTERFERONS

So called because they interfere with viral replication, there are three main types of interferon, termed IFN-α, IFN-β and IFN-γ. 'IFN-α' is not a single substance but a family of approximately 20 proteins with similar activities. IFN-α and IFN-β have antiviral activity whereas IFN-α also has some antitumour action. Both are released from virus-infected cells and activate antiviral mechanisms in neighbouring cells. IFN-γ has a role in induction of Th1 responses (Fig. 6.3).

CLINICAL USE OF INTERFERONS

IFN-α is used in the treatment of chronic hepatitis B and C, and has some action against herpes zoster and in the prevention of the common cold. Antitumour action against some lymphomas and solid tumours has been reported. Dose-related side effects, including influenza-like symptoms, may occur. IFN-β is used in patients with the relapsing-remitting form of multiple sclerosis, whereas IFN-γ is used in chronic granulomatous disease, an uncommon chronic disease of childhood in which neutrophil function is impaired, in conjunction with antibacterial drugs (see clinical box below for more details).

THE 'CYTOKINE STORM'

Many cytokines release further cytokines in what is essentially a positive feedback loop. There are times when this feedback system becomes unstable, perhaps as a result of the absence of balancing anti-inflammatory factors. The result can be a massive overproduction of cytokines in response to infection or other injury. This is known as a *cytokine storm* (also called *hypercytokinemia*) and can lead to a particularly dangerous – potentially catastrophic – development called *systemic inflammatory response syndrome* (SIRS; Jaffer et al., 2010). Cytokine storms may be responsible for deaths in septic shock as well as in some pandemic diseases. A tragic case of volunteers suffering

---

[3]One might have expected evolution to generate more examples of endogenous receptor antagonists as physiological regulators, but apart from IL-1ra, they are only exploited as toxins directed against other species.

[4]MCP, monocyte chemoattractant protein; RANTES, **R**egulated on **A**ctivation **N**ormal **T** cell **E**xpressed and **S**ecreted. (Don't blame us!)

Clinical uses of interferons

- α: Chronic hepatitis B or C (ideally combined with **ribavirin**).
- Malignant disease (alone or in combination with other drugs, e.g. **cytarabine**): chronic myelogenous leukemia (CML), hairy cell leukemia, follicular lymphoma, metastatic carcinoid, multiple myeloma, malignant melanoma (as an adjunct to surgery), myelodysplastic syndrome.
- Conjugation with polyethylene glycol ('pegylation') results in preparations that are more slowly eliminated and are administered intermittently subcutaneously.
- β: Multiple sclerosis (especially the relapsing remitting form of this disease).
- γ: To reduce infection in children with chronic granulomatous disease.

Cytokines

- Cytokines are polypeptides that are rapidly induced and released during inflammation. They regulate the action of inflammatory and immune system cells.
- The cytokine superfamily includes the *interferons, interleukins, chemokines* and *colony-stimulating factors*.
- Utilising both autocrine or paracrine mechanisms, they exert complex effects on leukocytes, vascular endothelial cells, mast cells, fibroblasts, haemopoietic stem cells and osteoclasts, controlling proliferation, differentiation and/or activation.
- IL-1 and TNF-α are important primary inflammatory cytokines, inducing the formation of other cytokines.
- Chemokines, such as IL-8, are mainly involved in the regulation of cell trafficking.
- Interferons IFN-α and IFN-β have antiviral activity, and **IFN-α** is used as an adjunct in the treatment of viral infections. **IFN-γ** has significant immunoregulatory function and is used in the treatment of multiple sclerosis.

cytokine storms after receiving an experimental drug is related in Ch. 59.

PROTEINS AND PEPTIDES THAT DOWNREGULATE INFLAMMATION

Inflammation is not regulated solely by factors that cause or enhance it: it has become increasingly evident that there is another panel of mediators that function at every step to downregulate inflammation, to check its progress and limit its duration and scope. It is the dynamic balance between these two systems that regulates the onset and resolution of inflammatory episodes, and when this breaks down, may lead also to inflammatory disease or, in extreme cases, to the cytokine storm phenomenon. Some of these are peptidic in nature and we have already encountered IL-1ra, TGF-β and IL-10, which are important negative regulators of inflammation but it transpires that there are two other systems that are significant here because common anti-inflammatory drugs exploit their action.

Annexin-A1 (Anx-A1) is a 37 kDa protein produced by many cells and especially abundant in cells of the myeloid lineage. When released, it exerts potent anti-inflammatory actions, downregulating cell activation, cell transmigration and mediator release. It does this by acting through a G protein-coupled receptor called ALX/FPR2 a member of the formyl peptide receptor family: the same receptor that binds the anti-inflammatory lipoxins (see Ch. 17).

The significance of the Anx-A1 system is that it is activated by anti-inflammatory glucocorticoids (see Ch. 26), which increase Anx-A1 gene transcription and promote its release from cells. Interestingly, the anti-allergic *cromones* (cromoglicate, etc.; see Ch. 28) also promote the release of this protein from cells. Anx-A1 gene 'knockout' studies have shown that this protein is important for restraining the inflammatory response and for its timely resolution. The anti-inflammatory glucocorticoids cannot develop their full inhibitory actions without it. An account of this field is given by Perretti and D'Acquisto (2009).

The *melanocortin* system also plays an important part in regulating inflammation. There are five G protein-coupled melanocortin receptors, MC_{1-5}. Endogenous ligands for these receptors, such as *melanocyte stimulating hormone* (MSH; three types), are derived from the POMC gene, and serve a number of purposes, including regulating the development of a suntan, penile erection and the control of appetite through an action on various MC receptors.

From the point of view of host defence, the MC_3 receptor is the most important. Again, gene deletion studies have highlighted the importance of this receptor in a variety of inflammatory conditions. Interestingly, another product of the POMC gene, ACTH was formerly used as an anti-inflammatory agent but it was thought that its action was secondary to its ability to release endogenous cortisol from the adrenals (an MC_2 action, see Ch. 33). It is now known that it is a ligand at the MC_3 receptor and it is likely that it owes some of its activity to this action.

An account of the importance of this field is given by Patel et al. (2011).

CONCLUDING REMARKS

Even from the superficial sketch presented here and in Chapters 6 and 17, it must be evident that the host defence response is among the most intricate of all physiological responses. Perhaps that is not surprising, given its central importance to survival. For the same reason, it is also understandable that so many different mediators orchestrate its operation. That the activity of many of these mediators can be blocked in experimental models with little or no obvious effect on the initiation and outcome of inflammation points to redundancy amongst the many component systems and goes some way to explaining why, until the advent of highly specific antibody-based therapies for inflammatory conditions (see Chs 26 and 59), our ability to curb the worst ravages of chronic inflammatory disease was so limited.

REFERENCES AND FURTHER READING

Chung, K.F., 2005. Drugs to suppress cough. Expert. Opin. Invest. Drugs 14, 19–27. (*Useful review of cough treatments, including a section on the role of neurokinin and bradykinin receptor antagonists*)

Dinarello, C.A., Simon, A., van der Meer, J.W., 2012. Treating inflammation by blocking interleukin-1 in a broad spectrum of diseases. Nat. Rev. Drug Discov. 11, 633–652. (*An extremely comprehensive survey of the role of IL1 in disease and the therapeutic benefits that can be gained by blocking its action. Written by pioneers of the field. Good diagrams*)

Gerard, C., Rollins, B., 2001. Chemokines and disease. Nat. Immunol. 2, 108–115. (*Discusses diseases associated with inappropriate activation of the chemokine network, and discusses some therapeutic implications; describes how viruses evade the immune responses by mimicry of the chemokines or their receptors*)

Horuk, R., 2001. Chemokine receptors. Cytokine Growth Factor Rev. 12, 313–335. (*Comprehensive review focusing on chemokine receptor research; describes the molecular, physiological and biochemical properties of each chemokine receptor*)

IUPHAR/BPS. Guide to Pharmacology. www.guidetopharmacology .org/. (*Comprehensive guide to pharmacological targets and the substances that act on them*)

Jaffer, U., Wade, R.G., Gourlay, T., 2010. Cytokines in the systemic inflammatory response syndrome: a review. HSR Proc Intensive Care Cardiovasc. Anesth. 2, 161–175. (*An easy to read review dealing mainly with the role of cytokines in SIRS, but also has a good general review of cytokine biology. Some good diagrams*)

Luster, A.D., 1998. Mechanisms of disease: chemokines – chemotactic cytokines that mediate inflammation. N. Engl. J. Med. 338, 436–445. (*Excellent review; outstanding diagrams*)

Mackay, C.R., 2001. Chemokines: immunology's high impact factors. Nat. Immunol. 2, 95–101. (*Clear, elegant coverage of the role of chemokines in leukocyte–endothelial interaction, control of primary immune responses and T/B cell interaction, T cells in inflammatory diseases and viral subversion of immune responses*)

Maggi, C.A., 1996. Pharmacology of the efferent function of primary sensory neurones. In: Geppetti, P., Holzer, P. (Eds.), Neurogenic inflammation. CRC Press, London. (*Worthwhile. Covers neurogenic inflammation, the release of neuropeptides from sensory nerves and inflammatory mediators. Discusses agents that inhibit release and the pharmacological modulation of receptor-mediated release*)

Murphy, P.M., 2001. Viral exploitation and subversion of the immune system through chemokine mimicry. Nat. Immunol. 2, 116–122. (*Excellent description of viral/immune system interaction*)

Patel, H.B., Montero-Melendez, T., Greco, K.V., Perretti, M., 2011. Melanocortin receptors as novel effectors of macrophage responses in inflammation. Front. Immunol. 2, 41–46. (*Succinct and easy-to-read review of the role of melanocortins in inflammatory resolution focusing on the role of the MC_3 receptor. Useful diagrams*)

Pease, J.E., Williams, T.J., 2006. The attraction of chemokines as a target for specific anti-inflammatory therapy. Br. J. Pharmacol. 147 (Suppl. 1), S212–S221. (*Very good review of the history of chemokine research with particular emphasis on their potential role as drug targets*)

Perretti, M., D'Acquisto, F., 2009. Annexin A1 and glucocorticoids as effectors of the resolution of inflammation. Nat. Rev. Immunol. 9, 62–70. (*Explores the role of the glucocorticoid-regulated protein annexin 1 in the control of inflammatory resolution. Easy to read and good diagrams*)

Pisi, G., Olivieri, D., Chetta, A., 2009. The airway neurogenic inflammation: clinical and pharmacological implications. Inflamm. Allergy Drug Targets 8, 176–181.

Rodi, D., Couture, R., Ongali, B., et al., 2005. Targeting kinin receptors for the treatment of neurological diseases. Curr. Pharm. Des. 11, 1313–1326. (*An overview of the potential role of kinin receptor antagonists in neurological diseases, dealing particularly with those of immunological origin*)

Schulze-Topphoff, U., Prat, A., 2008. Roles of the kallikrein/kinin system in the adaptive immune system. Int. Immunopharmacol. 8, 155–160. (*Excellent overview of these mediators particularly with respect to their involvement in the adaptive response*)

Books

Murphy, K.M., Travers, P., Walport, M., 2011. Janeway's Immunobiology, eighth ed. Taylor & Francis, London. (*A classic textbook now completely updated and available as an e-book also. Excellent diagrams*)

Cannabinoids **19**

OVERVIEW

Modern pharmacological interest in cannabinoids dates from the discovery that Δ^9-tetrahydrocannabinol (THC) is the main active principle of cannabis, and took off with the discovery of specific cannabinoid receptors – termed CB receptors – and endogenous ligands (endocannabinoids), together with mechanisms for their synthesis and elimination. Drugs that act on this endocannabinoid system have considerable therapeutic potential. Here we consider plant-derived cannabinoids, cannabinoid receptors, endocannabinoids, physiological functions, pathological mechanisms, synthetic ligands and potential clinical applications. More detailed information is given by Kano et al. (2009). The pharmacology of cannabinoids in the central nervous system (CNS) is discussed in Chapters 38, 48 and 49.

PLANT-DERIVED CANNABINOIDS AND THEIR PHARMACOLOGICAL EFFECTS

Cannabis sativa, the hemp plant, has been used for its psychoactive properties for thousands of years (Ch. 48). Its medicinal use was advocated in antiquity, but serious interest resurfaced only in 1964 with the identification of Δ^9-*tetrahydrocannabinol* (THC, see Fig. 19.1) as the main psychoactive component. Cannabis extracts contain numerous related compounds, called cannabinoids, most of which are insoluble in water. The most abundant cannabinoids are THC, its precursor *cannabidiol*, and *cannabinol*, a breakdown product formed spontaneously from THC. Cannabidiol and cannabinol lack the psychoactive properties of THC, but can exhibit anticonvulsant activity and induce hepatic drug metabolism (see Ch. 9).

PHARMACOLOGICAL EFFECTS

THC acts mainly on the central nervous system (CNS), producing a mixture of psychotomimetic and depressant effects, together with various centrally mediated autonomic effects. The main subjective effects in humans consist of the following:

- Sensations of relaxation and well-being, similar to the effect of ethanol but without the accompanying recklessness and aggression. (Insensitivity to risk is an important feature of alcohol intoxication and is often a factor in road accidents. Cannabis users are less accident prone in general – although cannabis does contribute to a significant number of road deaths each year – even though their motor performance is similarly impaired.)
- Feelings of sharpened sensory awareness, with sounds and sights seeming more intense and fantastic.
- These effects are similar to, but usually less pronounced than, those produced by

psychotomimetic drugs such as lysergic acid diethylamide (LSD; see Ch. 48). Subjects report that time passes extremely slowly. The alarming sensations and paranoid delusions that often occur with LSD are seldom experienced after cannabis. However epidemiological studies support a connection between heavy cannabis use in adolescence and subsequent psychiatric disorder (Rubino et al., 2012).

Central effects that can be directly measured in human and animal studies include:

- impairment of short-term memory and simple learning tasks – subjective feelings of confidence and heightened creativity are not reflected in actual performance
- impairment of motor coordination (e.g. driving performance)
- catalepsy – the adoption of fixed unnatural postures
- hypothermia
- analgesia
- antiemetic action (see Ch. 30)
- increased appetite (see Ch. 32).

The main peripheral effects of cannabis are:

- tachycardia, which can be prevented by drugs that block sympathetic transmission
- vasodilatation, which is particularly marked in superficial blood vessels of the eye (scleral and conjunctival vessels), producing a bloodshot appearance which is characteristic of cannabis smokers
- reduction of intraocular pressure
- bronchodilatation.

PHARMACOKINETIC AND ANALYTICAL ASPECTS

The effect of cannabis, taken by smoking, takes about 1 h to develop fully and lasts for 2–3 h. A small fraction of THC is converted to 11-hydroxy-THC, which is more active than THC itself and probably contributes to the pharmacological effect of smoking cannabis, but most is converted to inactive metabolites that are subject to conjugation and enterohepatic recirculation. Being highly lipophilic, THC and its metabolites are sequestered in body fat, and detectable excretion continues for several weeks after a single dose.

ADVERSE EFFECTS

In overdose, THC is relatively safe, producing drowsiness and confusion but not life-threatening respiratory or cardiovascular depression. In this respect, it is safer than most abused substances, particularly opiates and ethanol. Even in low doses, THC and synthetic derivatives such as **nabilone** (licensed for nausea and vomiting caused by cytotoxic chemotherapy) produce euphoria and drowsiness, sometimes accompanied by sensory distortion and hallucinations. These effects, together with legal

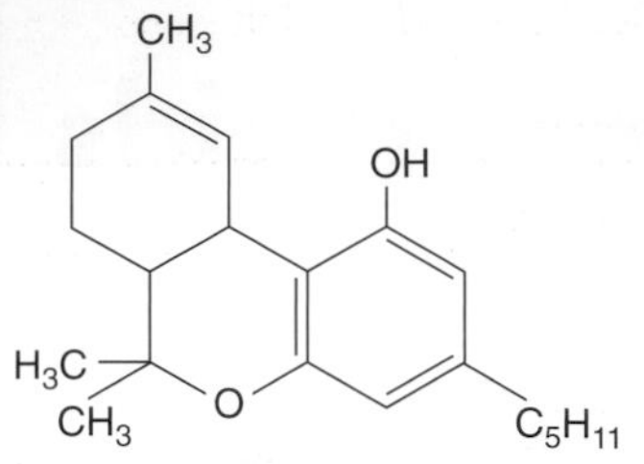

Fig. 19.1 Structures of Δ^9-tetrahydrocannabinol and two endocannabinoids.

Δ^9-Tetrahydrocannabinol (THC)

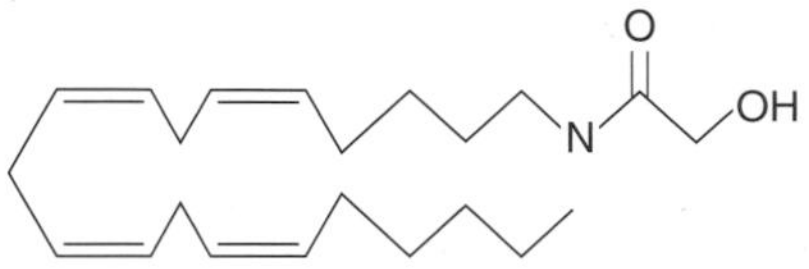

Anandamide

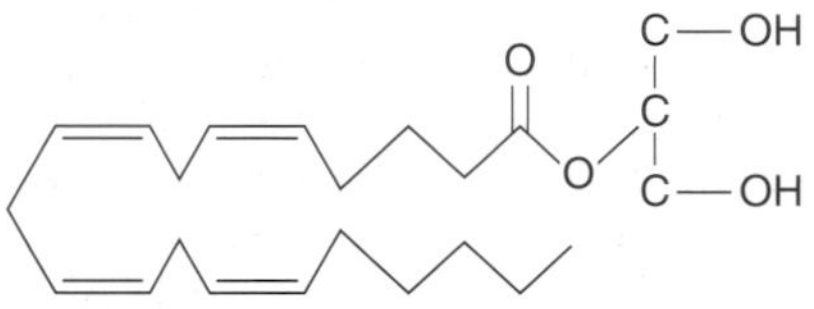

2 Arachidonoyl glycerol (2-AG)

Cannabis

- Main active constituent is Δ^9-tetrahydrocannabinol (THC) + a pharmacologically active 11-hydroxy metabolite.
- Actions on the central nervous system include both depressant and psychotomimetic effects.
- Subjective experiences include euphoria and a feeling of relaxation, with sharpened sensory awareness.
- Objective tests show impairment of learning, memory and motor performance, including impaired driving ability.
- THC also shows analgesic and antiemetic activity, as well as causing catalepsy and hypothermia in animal tests.
- Peripheral actions include vasodilatation, reduction of intraocular pressure and bronchodilatation.
- Cannabinoids are less liable than opiates, **nicotine** or **alcohol** to cause dependence but may have long-term psychological effects.

restrictions on the use of cannabis, have limited the widespread therapeutic use of cannabinoids, although recent regulatory approval in several countries for a cannabis extract as an adjunct in treating spasticitiy in multiple sclerosis may herald an expansion of potential clinical indications, several of which are being investigated.

In rodents, THC produces teratogenic and mutagenic effects, and an increased incidence of chromosome breaks in circulating white cells has been reported in humans. Such breaks are, however, by no means unique to cannabis, and epidemiological studies have not shown an increased risk of fetal malformation or cancer among cannabis users.

TOLERANCE AND DEPENDENCE

Tolerance to cannabis, and physical dependence, occur only to a minor degree and mainly in heavy users. Abstinence symptoms are similar to those of ethanol or opiate withdrawal, namely nausea, agitation, irritability, confusion, tachycardia and sweating, but are relatively mild and do not result in a compulsive urge to take the drug. Psychological dependence does occur with cannabis, but it is less compelling than with the major drugs of addiction (Ch. 49), and it has been argued whether cannabis should be classified as addictive (see Fattore et al., 2008).

CANNABINOID RECEPTORS

Cannabinoids, being highly lipid-soluble, were originally thought to act in a similar way to general anaesthetics. However, in 1988, saturable high-affinity binding of a tritiated cannabinoid was demonstrated in membranes prepared from homogenised rat brain. This led to the identification of specific cannabinoid receptors in brain. These are now termed CB_1 receptors to distinguish them from the CB_2 receptors subsequently identified in peripheral tissues. Cannabinoid receptors are typical members of the family of G protein-coupled receptors (Ch. 3). CB_1 receptors are linked via $G_{i/o}$ to inhibition of adenylyl cyclase and of voltage-operated calcium channels, and to activation of G protein-sensitive inwardly rectifying potassium (GIRK) channels, causing membrane hyperpolarisation (Fig. 19.2). These effects are similar to those mediated by opioid receptors (Ch. 42). CB_1 receptors are located in the plasma membrane of nerve endings and inhibit transmitter release from presynaptic terminals, which is caused by depolarisation and Ca^{2+} entry (Ch. 4). CB receptors also influence gene expression, both directly by activating mitogen-activated protein kinase, and indirectly by reducing the activity of protein kinase A as a result of reduced adenylyl cyclase activity (see Ch. 3).

CB_1 receptors are abundant in the brain, with similar numbers to receptors for glutamate and GABA – the main central excitatory and inhibitory neurotransmitters (Ch. 38). They are not homogeneously distributed, being concentrated in the hippocampus (relevant to effects of cannabinoids on memory), cerebellum (relevant to loss of coordination), hypothalamus (important in control of appetite and body temperature; see Ch. 32 and below), substantia nigra, mesolimbic dopamine pathways that have been implicated in psychological 'reward' (Ch. 49), and in association areas of the cerebral cortex. There is a relative paucity of CB_1 receptors in the brain stem, consistent with the lack of serious depression of respiratory or cardiovascular function by cannabinoids. At a cellular level, CB_1 receptors are mainly localised presynaptically, and inhibit transmitter release as explained in Figure 19.2. Like opioids, they can, however, increase the activity of some neuronal pathways by inhibiting inhibitory connections, including GABA-ergic interneurons in the hippocampus and amygdala.

In addition to their well-recognised location in the CNS, CB_1 receptors are also expressed in peripheral tissues, for example on endothelial cells, adipocytes and peripheral nerves. Cannabinoids promote lipogenesis

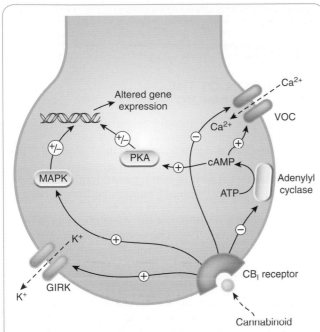

Fig. 19.2 Cellular actions of cannabinoids. CB_1 receptor activation inhibits neurotransmitter release via inhibition of Ca^{2+} entry and hyperpolarisation due to activation of potassium channels. It also alters gene expression. GIRK, G protein-sensitive inward-rectifying potassium channel; MAPK, mitogen-activated protein kinase; PKA, protein kinase A, VOC, voltage-operated calcium channel. (*Redrawn from Devane et al., 1992.*)

Table 19.1 Definite and possible endocannabinoids

Endocannabinoid	Selectivity
Definite endocannabinoids	
Anandamide	$CB_1 > CB_2$
2-Arachidonoyl glycerol	$CB_1 = CB_2$
Less well established endocannabinoid candidates	
Virodhamine	$CB_2 > CB_1$
Noladin	$CB_1 \gg CB_2$
N-Arachidonoyl dopamine	$CB_1 \gg CB_2$

through activation of CB_1 receptors, an action that could contribute to their effect on body weight (see DiPatrizio & Piomele, 2012).

The CB_2 receptor has only approximately 45% amino acid homology with CB_1 and is located mainly in lymphoid tissue (spleen, tonsils and thymus as well as circulating lymphocytes, monocytes and tissue mast cells). CB_2 receptors are also present on microglia – immune cells in the CNS which when activated contribute to chronic pain (Ch. 37). The localisation of CB_2 receptors on cells of the immune system was unexpected, but may account for inhibitory effects of cannabis on immune function. CB_2 receptors differ from CB_1 receptors in their responsiveness to cannabinoid ligands (see Table 19.1). They are linked via $G_{i/o}$ to adenylyl cyclase, GIRK channels and mitogen-activated protein kinase similarly to CB_1, but not to voltage-operated calcium channels (which are not expressed in immune cells). So far, rather little is known about their function. They are present in atherosclerotic lesions (see Ch. 22), and CB_2 agonists have antiatherosclerotic effects (Mach & Steffens, 2008).

Some endocannabinoids turned out, surprisingly,[1] to activate vanilloid receptors, ionotropic receptors that stimulate nociceptive nerve endings (see Ch. 42). Other as-yet-unidentified G protein-coupled receptors are also implicated, because cannabinoids exhibit analgesic actions and activate G proteins in the brain of CB_1 knockout mice despite the absence of CB_1 receptors.

ENDOCANNABINOIDS

The discovery of specific cannabinoid receptors led to a search for endogenous mediators. The first success was chalked up by a team that screened fractions of extracted pig brain for ability to compete with a radiolabelled cannabinoid receptor ligand (Devane et al., 1992). This led to the purification of N-*arachidonylethanolamine*, an eicosanoid mediator (see Ch. 18), the structure of which is shown in Figure 19.1. This was christened *anandamide*.[2] Anandamide not only displaced labelled cannabinoid from synaptosomal membranes in the binding assay, but also inhibited electrically evoked twitches of mouse vas deferens, a bioassay for psychotropic cannabinoids (Fig. 19.3). A few years later, a second endocannabinoid, *2-arachidonoyl glycerol* (2-AG, Fig. 19.1), was identified, and more recently three further endocannabinoid candidates with distinct CB_1/CB_2 (see Fig. 19.1) receptor selectivities have been added to the list (Table 19.1). Endocannabinoids are made 'on demand' like eicosanoids (see Ch. 18), rather than being presynthesised and stored for release when needed.

BIOSYNTHESIS OF ENDOCANNABINOIDS

Biosynthesis of anandamide and of 2-AG is summarised in Figure 19.4. A fuller account of biosynthesis and degradation is given by Di Marzo (2008).

▼ Anandamide is formed by a distinct phospholipase D (PLD) selective for N-acyl-phosphatidylethanolamine (NAPE) but with low affinity for other membrane phospholipids, and known as NAPE-PLD. NAPE-PLD is a zinc metallohydrolase that is stimulated by Ca^{2+} and also by polyamines. Selective inhibitors for NAPE-PLD are being sought. The precursors are produced by an as-yet-uncharacterised but Ca^{2+}-sensitive transacylase that transfers an acyl group from the *sn*-1 position of phospholipids to the nitrogen atom of phosphatidylethanolamine.

2-AG is also produced by hydrolysis of precursors derived from phospholipid metabolism. The key enzymes are two *sn*-1-selective diacylglycerol lipases (DAGL-α and DAGL-β), which belong to the family of serine lipases. Both these enzymes, like NAPE-PLD, are Ca^{2+} sensitive, consistent with intracellular Ca^{2+} acting as the physiological stimulus to endocannabinoid synthesis. The DAGLs are located in axons and presynaptic axon terminals during development, but postsynaptically in dendrites and cell bodies of adult neurons, consistent with a role for 2-AG in neurite growth, and with a role as a retrograde mediator (see p. 235) in adult brain.

---

[1] Surprising because capsaicin, the active principle of chilli peppers, causes intense burning pain, whereas the endocannabinoid anandamide is associated with pleasure, or even bliss … so perhaps not so surprising after all!

[2] From a Sanskrit word meaning 'bliss' + amide.

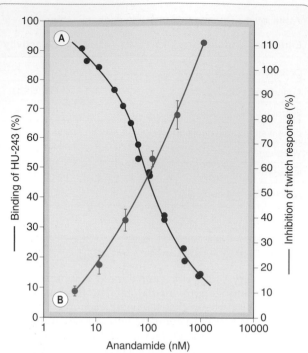

Fig. 19.3 Anandamide as an endocannabinoid.
Anandamide is an endogenous cannabinoid. **[A]** Competitive inhibition of tritiated HU-243 (a cannabinoid receptor ligand) binding to synaptosomal membranes from rat brain by natural anandamide (red circles, left hand ordinate axis). **[B]** Inhibition of vas deferens twitch response (a bioassay for cannabinoids) by natural anandamide (blue symbols, right hand ordinate). Note the similarity between the binding and bioactivity. *(Redrawn from Devane et al., 1992.)*

Little is known as yet about the biosynthesis of the more recent endocannabinoid candidates noladin, virodhamine and *N*-arachidonoyl dopamine. pH-dependent non-enzymatic interconversion of virodhamine and anandamide is one possibility, and could result in a switch between CB$_2$- and CB$_1$-mediated responses (see Table 19.1).

TERMINATION OF THE ENDOCANNABINOID SIGNAL

Endocannabinoids are rapidly taken up from the extracellular space. Being lipid-soluble, they diffuse through plasma membranes down a concentration gradient. There is also evidence for a saturable, temperature-dependent, facilitated transport mechanism for anandamide and 2-AG, dubbed the 'endocannabinoid membrane transporter', for which selective uptake inhibitors (e.g. UCM-707) have been developed. Pathways of endocannabinoid metabolism are summarised in Figure 19.4. The key enzyme for anandamide is a microsomal serine hydrolase known as fatty acid amide hydrolase (FAAH). FAAH converts anandamide to arachidonic acid plus ethanolamine and also hydrolyses 2-AG, yielding arachidonic acid and glycerol.

The phenotype of FAAH 'knockout' mice gives some clues to endocannabinoid physiology; such mice have an increased brain content of anandamide and an increased pain threshold. Selective inhibitors of FAAH have analgesic and anxiolytic properties in mice (see Ch. 44 for an explanation of how drugs are tested for anxiolytic properties in rodents). In contrast to anandamide, brain content of 2-AG is not increased in FAAH knockout animals, indicating that another route of metabolism of 2-AG is likely to be important. Other possible routes of metabolism include esterification, acylation and oxidation by cyclo-oxygenase-2 to prostaglandin ethanolamides ('prostamides'), or by 12- or 15-lipoxygenase (see Ch. 18).

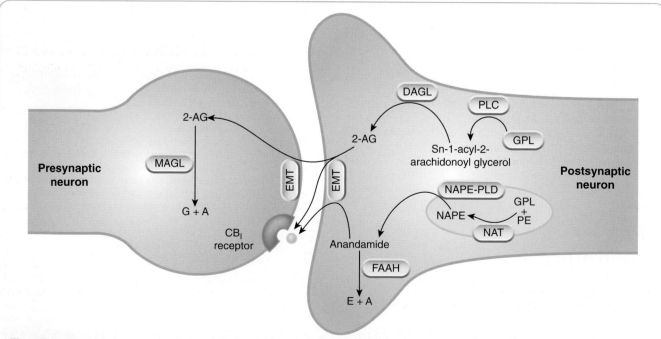

Fig. 19.4 Biosynthesis and inactivation of endocannabinoids. 2-AG, 2-arachidonoyl glycerol; A, arachidonic acid; DAGL, diacylglycerol lipase; E, ethanolamine; EMT, endocannabinoid membrane transporter; FAAH, fatty acid amide hydrolase; GPL, glycerophospholipid; MAGL, monoacyl glycerol lipase; NAPE, *N*-acyl-phosphatidylethanolamine; NAPE-PLD, *N*-acyl phosphatidylethanolamine-specific phopholipase D; NAT, *N*-acyl-transferase; PE, phosphatidylethanolamine; PLC, phospholipase C.

PHYSIOLOGICAL MECHANISMS

Stimuli that release endocannabinoids, leading to activation of CB_1 receptors and the linkage to downstream events including behavioural or psychological effects, are incompletely defined. Increased intracellular Ca^{2+} concentration is probably an important cellular trigger because, as mentioned on p. 233, Ca^{2+} activates NAPE-PLD and other enzymes involved in endocannabinoid biosynthesis.

Activation of CB receptors is implicated in a phenomenon known as *depolarisation-induced suppression of inhibition* (DSI). DSI occurs in hippocampal pyramidal cells; when these are depolarised by an excitatory input, this suppresses the GABA-mediated inhibitory input to the pyramidal cells, implying a retrograde flow of information from the depolarised pyramidal cell to inhibitory axons terminating on it. Such a reverse flow of information from post- to presynaptic cell is a feature of other instances of neuronal plasticity, such as 'wind-up' in nociceptive pathways (Fig. 42.3) and long-term potentiation in the hippocampus (Fig. 38.7). DSI is blocked by the CB_1 antagonist rimonabant. The presynaptic location of CB_1 receptors and cellular distributions of the DAGL and MAGL enzymes (Fig. 19.4) fit nicely with the idea that the endocannabinoid 2-AG could be a 'retrograde' messenger in DSI (see Fig. 39.8).

Neuromodulatory actions of endocannabinoids could influence a wide range of physiological activities, including nociception, cardiovascular, respiratory and gastrointestinal function. Interactions of endocannabinoids with hypothalamic hormones are believed to influence food intake and reproductive function. Mouse models lacking CB receptors support important and balanced roles of endocannabinoid signalling in male and female fertility and are implicated in spermatogenesis, fertilisation, preimplantation development of the early embryo, implantation and postimplantation growth of the embryo (see Battista et al., 2012). Effects of endocannabinoids on food intake are of particular interest, because of the importance of obesity (Ch. 32).

PATHOLOGICAL INVOLVEMENT

There is evidence, both from experimental animals and from human tissue, that endocannabinoid signalling is abnormal in various neurodegenerative diseases (see Ch. 40). Other diseases where abnormalities of cannabinoid signalling have been reported in human tissue as well as experimental models include hypotensive shock (both haemorrhagic and septic; see Ch. 22), advanced cirrhosis of the liver (where there is evidence that vasodilatation is mediated by endocannabinoids acting on vascular CB_1 receptors – see Bátkai et al., 2001), miscarriage (see Battista et al., 2012) and malignant disease. It seems likely that in some disorders endocannabinoid activity is a compensatory mechanism limiting the progression of disease or occurrence of symptoms, whereas in others it may be 'too much of a good thing' and actually contribute to disease progression. Consequently, there may be a place in therapeutics for drugs that potentiate or inhibit the cannabinoid system (see Di Marzo & Petrosino, 2007, for a fuller discussion).

SYNTHETIC CANNABINOIDS

Cannabinoid receptor agonists were developed in the 1970s in the hope that they would prove useful non-opioid/non-NSAID analgesics (cf. Chs 42 and 26,

> ### The endocannabinoid system
>
> - Cannabinoid receptors (CB_1, CB_2) are G protein-coupled ($G_{i/o}$).
> - Activation of CB_1 inhibits adenylyl cyclase and calcium channels, and activates potassium channels, inhibiting synaptic transmission.
> - The peripheral receptor (CB_2) is expressed mainly in cells of the immune system.
> - Selective agonists and antagonists have been developed.
> - Endogenous ligands for CB receptors are known as endocannabinoids. They are eicosanoid mediators (see Ch. 18).
> - The best-established endocannabinoids are anandamide and 2-arachidonoyl glycerol (2-AG), which have many roles, including functioning as 'retrograde' mediators passing information from postsynaptic to presynaptic neurons.
> - The main enzyme that inactivates anandamide is fatty acid amide hydrolase (FAAH).
> - A putative 'endocannabinoid membrane transporter' may transport cannabinoids from postsynaptic neurons, where they are synthesised, to the synaptic cleft, where they access CB_1 receptors, and into presynaptic terminals, where 2-AG is metabolised.
> - FAAH 'knockout' mice have an increased brain content of anandamide and an increased pain threshold; selective inhibitors of FAAH have analgesic and anxiolytic properties, implicating endocannabinoids in nociception and anxiety.

respectively, for limitations of opioids and NSAIDs), but adverse effects, particularly sedation and memory impairment, were problematic. Nevertheless, one such drug, **nabilone**, is sometimes used clinically for nausea and vomiting caused by cytotoxic chemotherapy if this is unresponsive to conventional antiemetics (Ch. 30). Furthermore synthetic cannabinoid agonists (e.g. spice) have been used as legal 'highs'. There were more than 20 of these introduced in the UK in 2012–13 in an attempt to circumvent the law on cannabis possession. The cloning of CB_2 receptors, and their absence from healthy neuronal brain cells, led to the synthesis of CB_2-selective agonists in the hope that these would lack the CNS-related adverse effects of plant cannabinoids. Several such drugs are being investigated for possible use in inflammatory and neuropathic pain.

The first selective CB_1 receptor antagonist, **rimonabant**, also has inverse agonist properties in some systems. It was licensed in Europe for treating obesity, and there were hopes that it would help promote abstinence from tobacco, but it was withdrawn because it caused psychiatric problems including depression. Synthetic inhibitors of endocannabinoid uptake and/or metabolism have shown potentially useful effects in animal models of pain, epilepsy, multiple sclerosis, Parkinson's disease, anxiety and diarrhoea.

CLINICAL APPLICATIONS

Clinical uses of drugs that act on the cannabinoid system remain controversial, but in both the UK and the USA cannabinoids have been used as antiemetics and to encourage weight gain in patients with chronic disease such as HIV-AIDS and malignancy. Cannabis extract (**sativex**) is used to treat spasticity in patients with multiple sclerosis (see Borgelt et al., 2013). Adverse events were generally mild at the doses used – see UK MS Research Group (2003). Endocannabinoids have been implicated in shock and hypotension in liver disease (Malinowska et al.,

2008), and modulation of this system is a potential therapeutic target. Other potential clinical uses are given in the clinical box below.

In addition to central CB_1 receptors, hepatocyte CB_1 receptors also implicated in obesity and in non-alcoholic fatty liver disease and research on selective peripheral antagonists continues (Klumpers et al., 2013).

Potential and actual clinical uses of cannabinoid agonists and antagonists

Cannabinoid agonists and antagonists are undergoing evaluation for a wide range of possible indications, including the following.

- Agonists:
  - glaucoma (to reduce pressure in the eye)
  - nausea/vomiting associated with cancer chemotherapy
  - cancer and AIDS (to reduce weight loss)
  - neuropathic pain
  - head injury

- Tourette's syndrome (to reduce tics – rapid involuntary movements that are a feature of this disorder)
- Parkinson's disease (to reduce involuntary movements caused as an adverse effect of **levodopa**; see Ch. 40).
- Antagonists:
  - obesity
  - tobacco dependence
  - drug addiction
  - alcoholism.

REFERENCES AND FURTHER READING

General reading

Freund, T.F., Katona, I., Piomelli, D., 2003. Role of endogenous cannabinoids in synaptic signaling. Physiol. Rev. 83, 1017–1066. (*The fine-grain anatomical distribution of the neuronal cannabinoid receptor CB_1 is described, and possible functions of endocannabinoids as retrograde synaptic signal molecules discussed in relation to synaptic plasticity and network activity patterns*)

Kano, M., Ohno-Shosaku, T., Hashimotodani, Y., et al., 2009. Endocannabinoid-mediated control of synaptic transmission. Physiol. Rev. 89, 309–380. (*Integrates current pharmacological with anatomical, electrophysiological and behavioural knowledge*)

Wilson, R.I., Nicoll, R.A., 2002. Endocannabinoid signaling in the brain. Science 296, 678–682.

Specific aspects

Battista, N., Meccariello, R., Cobellis, G., 2012. The role of endocannabinoids in gonadal function and fertility along the evolutionary axis. Mol. Cell. Endocrinol. 355, 1–14.

Bátkai, S., Járai, Z., Wagner, J.A., et al., 2001. Endocannabinoids acting at vascular CB_1 receptors mediate the vasodilated state in advanced liver cirrhosis. Nat. Med. 7, 827–832. (*Rats with cirrhosis have low blood pressure, which is elevated by a CB_1 receptor antagonist. Compared with non-cirrhotic controls, in cirrhotic human livers there was a three-fold increase in CB_1 receptors on isolated vascular endothelial cells*)

Borgelt, L.M., Franson, K.L., Nussbaum, A.M., Wang, G.S., 2013. The pharmacologic and clinical effects of medical cannabis. Pharmacotherapy 33, 195–209.

Devane, W.A., Hanu, L., Breurer, A., et al., 1992. Isolation and structure of a brain constituent that binds to the cannabinoid receptor. Science 258, 1946–1949. (*Identification of arachidonylethanolamide, extracted from pig brain, both chemically and via a bioassay, as a natural ligand for the cannabinoid receptor; the authors named it anandamide*)

Di Marzo, V., 2008. Endocannabinoids: synthesis and degradation. Rev. Physiol. Biochem. Pharmacol. 160, 1–24. (*Reviews current knowledge*)

Di Marzo, V., Petrosino, S., 2007. Endocannabinoids and the regulation of their levels in health and disease. Curr. Opin. Lipidol. 18, 129–140. (*Gastrointestinal disorders, inflammation, neurodegeneration*)

DiPatrizio, N.V., Piomele, D., 2012. The thrifty lipids: endocannabinoids and the neural control of energy conservation. Trends Neurosci. 35, 403–411. (*Endocannabinoids increase energy intake and decrease energy expenditure by controlling the activity of peripheral and central neural pathways involved in the sensing and hedonic processing of sweet and fatty foods, as well as in the storage of their energy content for future use*)

Fattore, L., Fadda, P., Spano, M.S., et al., 2008. Neurobiological mechanisms of cannabinoid addiction. Mol. Cell. Endocrinol. 286, S97–S107. (*Addiction mechanisms*)

Karst, M., Salim, K., Burstein, S., et al., 2003. Analgesic effect of the synthetic cannabinoid CT-3 on chronic neuropathic pain. A randomized controlled trial. JAMA 290, 1757–1762. (*CT-3, a potent cannabinoid, produces marked antiallodynic and analgesic effects in animals. In a preliminary randomised cross-over study in 21 patients with chronic neuropathic pain, CT-3 was effective in reducing chronic neuropathic pain compared with placebo*)

Klumpers, L.E., Fridberg, M., de Kam, M.L., et al., 2013. Peripheral selectivity of the novel cannabinoid receptor antagonist TM38837 in healthy subjects. Br. J. Clin. Pharmacol. 76, 846–857.

Mach, F., Steffens, S., 2008. The role of the endocannabinoid system in atherosclerosis. J. Neuroendocrinol. 20, 53–57. (*Review*)

Malinowska, B., Lupinski, S., Godlewski, G., et al., 2008. Role of endocannabinoids in cardiovascular shock. J. Physiol. Pharmacol. 59, 91–107.

Rubino, T., Zamberletti, E., Parolaro, D., 2012. Adolescent exposure to cannabis as a risk factor for psychiatric disorders. J. Psychopharm. 26, SI177–SI188. (*Available data support the hypothesis that heavy cannabis use in adolescence increases the risk of developing psychiatric disorders*)

Steffens, S., 2005. Low dose oral cannabinoid therapy reduces progression of atherosclerosis in mice. Nature 434, 782–786. (*Oral administration of THC (1 mg/kg per day) inhibits atherosclerosis in a mouse model by an action on CB_2 receptors. See also News and Views, p. 708 of the same issue, for comment by Roth, M.D.*)

Taber, K.H., Hurley, R.A., 2009. Endocannabinoids: stress, anxiety and fear. J. Neuropsychiat. Clin. Neurosci. 21, 108–113. (*Succinctly reviews the involvement of the endocannabinoid system in brain function, and potential therapeutic applications in treating mood/anxiety, degenerative disease and brain injury*)

UK MS Research Group, 2003. Cannabinoids for treatment of spasticity and other symptoms related to multiple sclerosis (CAMS study): multicentre randomised placebo-controlled trial. Lancet 362, 1517–1526. (*Randomised, placebo-controlled trial in 667 patients with stable multiple sclerosis and muscle spasticity. Trial duration was 15 weeks. There was no treatment effect of THC or cannabis extract on the primary outcome of spasticity assessed with a standard rating scale, but there was an improvement in patient-reported spasticity and pain, which might be clinically useful*)

Van Gaal, L.F., Rissanen, A.M., Scheen, A.J., et al.; for the RIO-Europe Study Group, 2005. Effects of the cannabinoid-1 receptor blocker rimonabant on weight reduction and cardiovascular risk factors in overweight patients: 1-year experience from the RIO-Europe study. Lancet 365, 1389–1397. (*A total of 1507 overweight patients treated with rimonabant 5 or 20 mg or with placebo daily for 1 year in addition to dietary advice: significant dose-related decrease in weight and improvement in cardiovascular risk factors in actively treated patients; adverse effects were mild*)

Nitric oxide and related mediators

20

OVERVIEW

Nitric oxide (NO) is a ubiquitous mediator with diverse functions. It is generated from L-arginine by nitric oxide synthase (NOS), an enzyme that occurs in endothelial, neuronal and inducible isoforms. In this chapter, we concentrate on general aspects of NO, especially its biosynthesis, degradation and effects. We touch on evidence that it can act as a circulating as well as a local mediator, and conclude with a brief consideration of the therapeutic potential of drugs that act on the L-arginine/NO pathway. Other gaseous mediators (carbon monoxide, hydrogen sulfide)[1] are described briefly: while they have yet to yield therapeutic drugs, their pathways are tempting drug targets.

INTRODUCTION

Nitric oxide, a free radical gas, is formed in the atmosphere during lightning storms. Less dramatically, but with far-reaching biological consequences, it is also formed in an enzyme-catalysed reaction between molecular oxygen and L-arginine. The convergence of several lines of research led to the realisation that NO is a key signalling molecule in the cardiovascular and nervous systems, and that it has a role in host defence.

A physiological function of NO emerged when biosynthesis of this gas was shown to account for the *endothelium-derived relaxing factor* described by Furchgott & Zawadzki (1980) (see Figs 20.1 and 20.2). NO is the endogenous activator of soluble guanylyl cyclase, leading to the formation of cyclic GMP (cGMP), an important 'second messenger' (Ch. 3) in many cells, including neurons, smooth muscle, monocytes and platelets. Nitrogen and oxygen are neighbours in the periodic table, and NO shares several properties with O_2, in particular a high affinity for haem and other iron–sulfur groups. This is important for activation of guanylyl cyclase, which contains a haem group, for the inactivation of NO by haemoglobin and for the regulation of diffusion of NO from endothelial cells (which express the alpha chain of haemoglobin) to vascular smooth muscle.

The role of NO in specific settings is described in other chapters: the endothelium in Chapter 22, the autonomic nervous system in Chapter 12, as a chemical transmitter and mediator of excitotoxicity in the central nervous system (CNS) in Chapters 37–39, and in the innate mediator-derived reactions of acute inflammation and the immune response in Chapter 17. Therapeutic uses of organic nitrates and of nitroprusside (NO donors) are described in Chapters 21 and 22.

BIOSYNTHESIS OF NITRIC OXIDE AND ITS CONTROL

Nitric oxide synthase (NOS) enzymes are central to the control of NO biosynthesis. There are three isoforms: an *inducible* form (iNOS or NOS2 expressed in macrophages and Kupffer cells, neutrophils, fibroblasts, vascular smooth muscle and endothelial cells in response to pathological stimuli such as invading microorganisms) and two *constitutive* forms, which are present under physiological conditions in endothelium (eNOS or NOS3)[2] and in neurons (nNOS or NOS1).[3] The constitutive enzymes generate small amounts of NO, whereas NOS2 produces much greater amounts, both because of its high activity and because of its abundance, at least in pathological states associated with cytokine release.

▼ All three NOS isoenzymes are dimers. They are structurally and functionally complex, bearing similarities to the cytochrome P450 enzymes (described in Ch. 9) that are so important in drug metabolism. Each isoform contains iron protoporphyrin IX (haem), flavin adenine dinucleotide (FAD), flavin mononucleotide (FMN) and tetrahydrobiopterin (H_4B) as bound prosthetic groups. They also bind L-arginine, reduced nicotinamide adenine dinucleotide phosphate (NADPH) and calcium–calmodulin. These prosthetic groups and ligands control the assembly of the enzyme into the active dimer. NOS3 is doubly acylated by N-myristoylation and cysteine palmitoylation; these post-translational modifications lead to its association with membranes in the Golgi apparatus and in *caveolae*, specialised cholesterol-rich microdomains in the plasma membrane derived from the Golgi apparatus. In the caveolae, NOS3 is held as an inactive complex with *caveolin*, the main membrane protein of caveolae. Dissociation from caveolin activates the enzyme.

The nitrogen atom in NO is derived from the terminal guanidino group of L-arginine. NOS enzymes combine oxygenase and reductase activities. The oxygenase domain contains haem, while the reductase domain binds calcium–calmodulin. In pathological states, the enzyme can undergo structural change leading to electron transfer between substrates, enzyme co-factors and products becoming 'uncoupled', so that electrons are transferred to molecular oxygen, leading to the synthesis of superoxide anion (O_2^-) rather than NO. This is important, as superoxide anion reacts with NO to form a toxic product (peroxynitrite anion; see p. 241).

L-Arginine, the substrate of NOS, is usually present in excess in endothelial cell cytoplasm, so the rate of production of NO is determined by the activity of the enzyme

---

[1] The pure substances (NO, CO and H_2S) are gases at room temperature and usual atmospheric pressure, and when pure NO is administered therapeutically (see p. 242 and clinical box, p. 244) it is in the form of a gas; when formed endogenously, the gases are of course dissolved in intra- and extracellular fluids.

[2] NOS3 is not restricted to endothelium. It is also present in cardiac myocytes, renal mesangial cells, osteoblasts and osteoclasts, airway epithelium and, in small amounts, platelets so the term eNOS may be somewhat misleading.
[3] It is possible that some of the NO made in healthy animals under basal conditions is derived from the action of NOS2, just as the inducible form of cyclo-oxygenase is active under basal conditions (Ch. 18) – whether this is because there is some NOS2 expressed even when there is no pathology, or because there is enough 'pathology' in healthy mammals, for example gut microflora, to induce it, is a moot point.

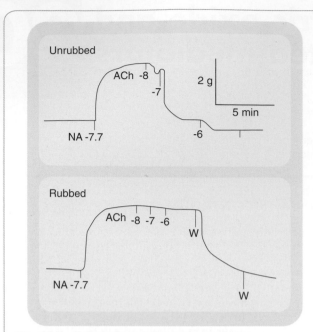

Fig. 20.1 Endothelium-derived relaxing factor.
Acetylcholine (ACh) relaxes a strip of rabbit aorta precontracted
with noradrenaline (NA) if the endothelium is intact ('unrubbed':
upper panel), but not if it has been removed by gentle rubbing
('rubbed': lower panel). The numbers are logarithms of molar
concentrations of drugs. *(From Furchgott & Zawadzki, 1980.)*

rather than by substrate availability. Nevertheless, very
high doses of L-arginine can restore endothelial NO biosynthesis in some pathological states (e.g. hypercholesterolaemia) in which endothelial function is impaired.
Possible explanations for this paradox include:

- compartmentation: i.e. existence of a distinct pool of
  substrate in a cell compartment with access to NOS,
  which can become depleted despite apparently
  plentiful total cytoplasmic arginine concentrations
- competition with endogenous inhibitors of NOS
  such as *asymmetric dimethylarginine* (ADMA; see
  p. 242 and Fig. 20.4), which is elevated in plasma
  from patients with hypercholesterolaemia
- reassembly/reactivation of enzyme in which
  transfer of electrons has become uncoupled from
  L-arginine as a result of an action of
  supraphysiological concentrations of L-arginine.

The activity of constitutive isoforms of NOS is controlled
by intracellular calcium–calmodulin (Fig. 20.3). Control is
exerted in two ways:

1. Many endothelium-dependent agonists (e.g.
   acetylcholine, bradykinin, substance P) increase the
   cytoplasmic concentration of calcium ions $[Ca^{2+}]_i$; the
   consequent increase in calcium–calmodulin activates
   NOS1 and NOS3.
2. Phosphorylation of specific residues on NOS3 controls
   its sensitivity to calcium–calmodulin; this can alter
   NO synthesis in the absence of any change in $[Ca^{2+}]_i$.

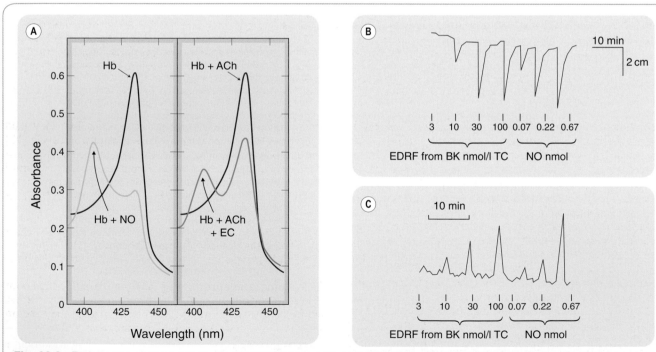

Fig. 20.2 Endothelium-derived relaxing factor (EDRF) is closely related to nitric oxide (NO). [**A**] EDRF released from aortic
endothelial cells (EC) by acetylcholine (ACh) (right panel) has the same effect on the absorption spectrum of deoxyhaemoglobin (Hb) as
does authentic NO (left panel). [**B**] EDRF is released from a column of cultured endothelial cells by bradykinin (BK 3–100 nmol) applied
through the column of cells (TC) and relaxes a de-endothelialised precontracted bioassay strip, as does authentic NO (upper trace). [**C**] A
chemical assay of NO based on chemiluminescence shows that similar concentrations of NO are present in the EDRF released from the
column of cells as in equiactive authentic NO solutions. *(From Ignarro LJ, Byrns RE, Buga GM, et al 1987 Circ Res 61, 866–879; and
Palmer RMJ, Ferrige AG, Moncada S et al 1987 Nature 327, 524–526.)*

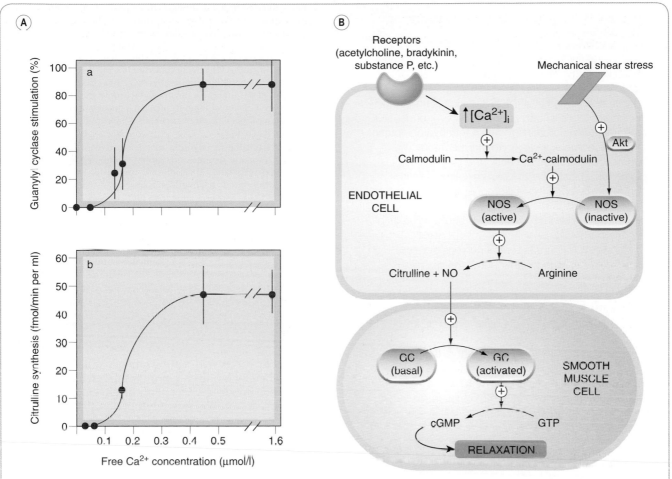

Fig. 20.3 Control of constitutive nitric oxide synthase (NOS) by calcium–calmodulin. **[A]** Dependence on Ca^{2+} of nitric oxide (NO) and citrulline synthesis from L-arginine by rat brain synaptosomal cytosol. Rates of synthesis of NO from L-arginine were determined by stimulation of guanylyl cyclase (GC) (upper panel) or by synthesis of $[^3H]$-citrulline from L-$[^3H]$-arginine (lower panel). **[B]** Regulation of GC in smooth muscle by NO formed in adjacent endothelium. Akt is a protein kinase that phosphorylates NOS, making it more sensitive to calcium–calmodulin. *(Panel [A] from Knowles RG et al. 1989 Proc Natl Acad Sci U S A 86, 5159–5162.)*

Shear stress is an important physiological stimulus to endothelial NO synthesis in resistance vessels. This is sensed by endothelial mechanoreceptors and transduced via a serine–threonine protein kinase called Akt (also known as protein kinase B). Agonists that increase cAMP in endothelial cells (e.g. β_2-adrenoceptor agonists) increase NOS3 activity, but via protein kinase A-mediated phosphorylation[4] whereas protein kinase C *reduces* NOS3 activity by phosphorylating residues in the calmodulin-binding domain, thereby reducing the binding of calmodulin. Insulin increases NOS3 activity via tyrosine kinase activation (and also increases the expression of NOS1 in diabetic mice).

In contrast to constitutive NOS isoforms, the activity of NOS2 is effectively independent of $[Ca^{2+}]_i$, being fully activated even at the low values of $[Ca^{2+}]_i$ present under resting conditions. The enzyme is induced by bacterial lipopolysaccharide and/or inflammatory cytokines, notably interferon-γ, the antiviral effect of which can be explained by this action. Tumour necrosis factor-α and

interleukin-1 do not alone induce NOS2, but they each synergise with interferon-γ in this regard (see Ch. 17). Induction of NOS2 is inhibited by glucocorticoids and by several cytokines, including transforming growth factor-β. There are important species differences in the inducibility of NOS2, which is less readily induced in human than in mouse cells.

DEGRADATION AND CARRIAGE OF NITRIC OXIDE

Nitric oxide reacts with oxygen to form N_2O_4, which combines with water to produce a mixture of nitric and nitrous acids. Nitrite ions are oxidised to nitrate by oxyhaemoglobin. These reactions are summarised as follows:

$$2NO + O_2 \rightarrow N_2O_4 \tag{20.1}$$

$$N_2O_4 + H_2O \rightarrow NO_3^- + NO_2^- + 2H^+ \tag{20.2}$$

$$NO_2^- + HbO \rightarrow NO_3^- + Hb \tag{20.3}$$

Low concentrations of NO are relatively stable in air, because the rate of reaction in (equation 20.1) depends on

---

[4]As explained in Chapter 4, β_2 agonists also act directly on smooth muscle cells, causing relaxation via cAMP.

Nitric oxide: synthesis, inactivation and carriage

- Nitric oxide (NO) is synthesised from L-arginine and molecular O_2 by nitric oxide synthase (NOS).
- NOS exists in three isoforms: inducible (NOS2), and constitutive 'endothelial' (NOS3, which is not restricted to endothelial cells) and neuronal (NOS1) forms. NOSs are dimeric flavoproteins, contain tetrahydrobiopterin and have homology with cytochrome P450. The constitutive enzymes are activated by calcium–calmodulin. Sensitivity to calcium–calmodulin is controlled by phosphorylation of specific residues on the enzymes.
- NOS2 is induced in macrophages and other cells by interferon-γ.
- NOS1 is present in the central nervous system (see Chs 37–40) and in autonomic nerves (see Ch. 12).
- NOS3 is present in platelets and other cells in addition to endothelium.
- NO diffuses to sites of action in neighbouring cells. This is regulated by the redox state of haemoglobin alpha which is present in the myoendothelial junctions that act as diffusion corridors across the internal elastic lamina (and in other cells): signalling can occur when the haem is in the Fe^{3+} state, but is stopped – like at a red traffic light – when haem is in the Fe^{2+} state.
- NO is inactivated by combination with the haem of haemoglobin or by oxidation to nitrite and nitrate, which are excreted in urine; it is also present in exhaled air, especially in patients with inflammatory lung diseases such as bronchitis.
- NO can react reversibly with cysteine residues (e.g. in globin or albumin) to form stable nitrosothiols; as a result, red cells can act as an O_2-regulated source of NO. NO released in this way escapes inactivation by haem by being exported via cysteine residues in the anion exchange protein in red cell membranes.

alpha is concentrated in these junctions and acts as a redox-sensitive stop/go signal. When the haem iron is in the oxidised Fe^{3+} state (methaemoglobin) NO can diffuse along the corridor and into the smooth muscle cell on which it acts; when the haem iron is in the Fe^{2+} state, however, NO is rapidly converted to nitrate and the diffusion pathway is effectively closed to it. Conversion of methaemoglobin to haemoglobin, preventing NO from crossing the barrier, is brought about by the enzyme cytochrome b5 reductase3 (also known as methaemoglobin reductase) – genetic or pharmacological inhibition of this enzyme increases NO bioactivity in small arteries (Straub et al., 2012).

Distinct from the inactivation reaction between NO and haem, a specific cysteine residue in globin combines reversibly with NO under physiological conditions. It is proposed that the resulting *S*-nitrosylated haemoglobin acts as a circulating oxygen-sensitive NO carrier, allowing NO to act as a circulating hormone[3]. Albumin can also be reversibly nitrosylated and could function similarly, as could the inorganic nitrite ion – indeed, foods rich in inorganic nitrate (reduced to nitrite *in vivo* by anaerobic organisms in the mouth) have potential for prevention of vascular disease; see p. 242-243. Evidence supporting the case that NO acts at a distance within the mammalian circulation is reviewed by Singel & Stamler (2005); for a sceptical view, see Schechter & Gladwyn (2003).

EFFECTS OF NITRIC OXIDE

Nitric oxide reacts with various metals, thiols and oxygen species, thereby modifying proteins, DNA and lipids. One of its most important biochemical effects (see Ch. 3) is activation of soluble guanylyl cyclase, a heterodimer present in vascular and nervous tissue as two distinct isoenzymes. Guanylyl cyclase synthesises the second messenger cGMP. NO activates the enzyme by combining with its haem group, and many physiological effects of low concentrations of NO are mediated by cGMP. These effects are prevented by inhibitors of guanylyl cyclase (e.g. 1H-[1,2,4]-oxadiazole-[4,3-α]-quinoxalin-1-one, better known as 'ODQ'), which are useful investigational tools. NO activates soluble guanylyl cyclase in intact cells (neurons and platelets) extremely rapidly, and activation is followed by desensitisation to a steady-state level. This contrasts with its effect on the isolated enzyme, which is slower but more sustained. Guanylyl cyclase contains another regulatory site, which is NO independent. This is activated by **riociguat**, recently licensed for treatment of pulmonary hypertension (see Ch. 22).

Effects of cGMP are terminated by phosphodiesterase enzymes. **Sildenafil** and **tadalafil** are inhibitors of phosphodiesterase type V that are used to treat erectile dysfunction, because they potentiate NO actions in the corpora cavernosa of the penis by this mechanism (see Ch. 35). NO also combines with haem groups in other biologically important proteins, notably cytochrome c oxidase, where it competes with oxygen, contributing to the control of cellular respiration (see Erusalimsky & Moncada, 2007). Cytotoxic and/or cytoprotective effects of higher concentrations of NO relate to its chemistry as a free radical (see Ch. 40). Some physiological and pathological effects of NO are shown in Table 20.1.

BIOCHEMICAL AND CELLULAR ASPECTS

Pharmacological effects of NO can be studied with NO gas dissolved in deoxygenated salt solution. More conveniently, but less directly, various donors of NO, such

the square of the NO concentration, so small amounts of NO produced in the lung escape degradation and can be detected in exhaled air. Exhaled NO is increased in patients with lung diseases such as bronchitis, and is used as a biomarker of airway inflammation (Ch. 28). In contrast, NO reacts very rapidly with even low concentrations of superoxide anion (O_2^-) to produce peroxynitrite anion ($ONOO^-$), which is responsible for some of its toxic effects.

▼ Haem has an affinity for NO > 10000 times greater than for oxygen. In the absence of oxygen, NO bound to haem is relatively stable, but in the presence of oxygen NO is converted to nitrate and the haem iron (Fe^{2+}) oxidised to methaemoglobin (Fe^{3+}).

Endothelium-derived NO acts locally on underlying vascular smooth muscle or on adherent monocytes or platelets. The internal elastic lamina of small arteries is a layer of elastic fibres between the endothelium and the smooth muscle, which represents a barrier to diffusion. It is penetrated by myoendothelial junctions where endothelial and smooth muscle cells kiss, forming a corridor along which NO can diffuse. Recently it has been found that haemoglobin

Table 20.1 Postulated roles of endogenous nitric oxide

System	Physiological role	Pathological role	
		Excess production	*Inadequate production or action*
Cardiovascular			
Endothelium/vascular smooth muscle	Control of blood pressure and regional blood flow	Hypotension (septic shock)	Atherogenesis, thrombosis (e.g. in hypercholesterolaemia, diabetes mellitus)
Platelets	Limitation of adhesion/aggregation	–	–
Host defence			
Macrophages, neutrophils, leukocytes	Defence against viruses, bacteria, fungi, protozoa, parasites	–	–
Nervous system			
Central	Neurotransmission, long-term potentiation, plasticity (memory, appetite, nociception)	Excitotoxicity (Ch. 39) (e.g. ischaemic stroke, Huntington's disease, AIDS dementia)	–
Peripheral	Neurotransmission (e.g. gastric emptying, penile erection)	–	Hypertrophic pyloric stenosis, erectile dysfunction

as **nitroprusside**, S-*nitrosoacetylpenicillamine* (SNAP) or S-*nitrosoglutathione* (SNOG), have been used as surrogates. This has pitfalls; for example, ascorbic acid potentiates SNAP but inhibits responses to authentic NO.[5]

Nitric oxide can activate guanylyl cyclase in the same cells that produce it, giving rise to autocrine effects, for example on the barrier function of the endothelium. NO also diffuses from its site of synthesis and activates guanylyl cyclase in neighbouring cells. The resulting increase in cGMP affects protein kinase G, cyclic nucleotide phosphodiesterases, ion channels and possibly other proteins. This inhibits the $[Ca^{2+}]_i$-induced smooth muscle contraction and platelet aggregation produced by various agonists. NO also hyperpolarises vascular smooth muscle, as a consequence of potassium-channel activation. NO inhibits monocyte adhesion and migration, adhesion and aggregation of platelets, and smooth muscle and fibroblast proliferation. These cellular effects probably underlie the antiatherosclerotic action of NO (see Ch. 23).

Large amounts of NO (released following induction of NOS or excessive stimulation of NMDA receptors in the brain) cause cytotoxic effects (either directly or via formation of peroxynitrite). These contribute to host defence, but also to the neuronal destruction that occurs when there is overstimulation of NMDA receptors by glutamate (see Chs 38 and 40). Paradoxically, NO is also cytoprotective under some circumstances (see Ch. 40).

VASCULAR EFFECTS (see also Ch. 22)

The L-arginine/NO pathway is tonically active in resistance vessels, reducing peripheral vascular resistance and hence systemic blood pressure. Mutant mice that lack the gene coding NOS3 are hypertensive, consistent with a role for NO biosynthesis in the physiological control of blood pressure. In addition, NO derived from NOS1 is implicated in the control of basal resistance vessel tone in human forearm and cardiac muscle vascular beds (Seddon et al., 2008, 2009). NO may contribute to the generalised vasodilatation that occurs during pregnancy.

NEURONAL EFFECTS (see also Ch. 12)

Nitric oxide is a non-noradrenergic non-cholinergic (NANC) neurotransmitter in many tissues (see Fig. 12.5), and is important in the upper airways, gastrointestinal tract and control of penile erection (Chs 28, 30 and 35). It is implicated in the control of neuronal development and of synaptic plasticity in the CNS (Chs 37 and 39). Mice carrying a mutation disrupting the gene coding NOS1 have grossly distended stomachs similar to those seen in human hypertrophic pyloric stenosis (a disorder characterised by pyloric hypertrophy causing gastric outflow obstruction, which occurs in approximately 1 in 150 male infants and is corrected surgically). NOS1 knockout mice resist stroke damage caused by middle cerebral artery ligation but are aggressive and oversexed (characteristics that may not be unambiguously disadvantageous, at least in the context of natural selection!).

HOST DEFENCE (see Ch. 6)

Cytotoxic and/or cytostatic effects of NO are implicated in primitive non-specific host defence mechanisms against numerous pathogens, including viruses, bacteria, fungi, protozoa and parasites, and against tumour cells. The importance of this is evidenced by the susceptibility of mice lacking NOS2 to *Leishmania major* (to which wild-type mice are highly resistant). Mechanisms whereby NO damages invading pathogens include nitrosylation of nucleic acids and combination with haem-containing enzymes, including the mitochondrial enzymes involved in cell respiration.

---

[5]Ascorbic acid releases NO from SNAP but accelerates NO degradation in solution, which could explain this divergence.

Actions of nitric oxide

- Nitric oxide (NO) acts by:
  - combining with haem in guanylyl cyclase, activating the enzyme, increasing cGMP and thereby lowering $[Ca^{2+}]_i$
  - combining with haem groups in other proteins (e.g. cytochrome c oxidase)
  - combining with superoxide anion to yield the cytotoxic peroxynitrite anion
  - nitrosation of proteins, lipids and nucleic acids.
- Effects of NO include:
  - vasodilatation, inhibition of platelet and monocyte adhesion and aggregation, inhibition of smooth muscle proliferation, protection against atheroma
  - synaptic effects in the peripheral and central nervous system
  - host defence and cytotoxic effects on pathogens
  - cytoprotection.

THERAPEUTIC ASPECTS

NITRIC OXIDE

Inhalation of high concentrations of NO (as occurred when cylinders of nitrous oxide, N_2O, for anaesthesia were accidentally contaminated) causes acute pulmonary oedema and methaemoglobinaemia, but concentrations below 50 ppm (parts per million) are not toxic. NO (5–300 ppm) inhibits bronchoconstriction (at least in guinea pigs), but the main action of low concentrations of inhaled NO in man is pulmonary vasodilatation. Inspired NO acts preferentially on ventilated alveoli, and could therefore be therapeutically useful in respiratory distress syndrome. This condition has a high mortality and is caused by diverse insults (e.g. infection). It is characterised by intrapulmonary 'shunting' (i.e. pulmonary arterial blood entering the pulmonary vein without passing through capillaries in contact with ventilated alveoli), resulting in arterial hypoxaemia, and by acute pulmonary arterial hypertension. Inhaled NO dilates blood vessels in ventilated alveoli (which are exposed to the inspired gas) and thus reduces shunting. NO is used in intensive care units to reduce pulmonary hypertension and to improve oxygen delivery in patients with respiratory distress syndrome, but it is not known whether this improves long-term survival in these severely ill patients.

NITRIC OXIDE DONORS/PRECURSORS

Nitrovasodilators have been used therapeutically for over a century. The common mode of action of these drugs is as a source of NO (Chs 21 and 22). There is interest in the potential for selectivity of nitrovasodilators; for instance, **glyceryl trinitrate** is more potent on vascular smooth muscle than on platelets, whereas SNOG (see p. 241) selectively inhibits platelet aggregation. It was shown recently that dietary nitrate (contained in beetroot juice) acutely lowers arterial blood pressure in parallel with a rise in plasma nitrite concentration and improved endothelial and platelet function. Interruption of the enterosalivary

conversion of nitrate to nitrite prevents the rise in plasma nitrite, blocks the fall in blood pressure and abolishes the inhibitory effect on platelet aggregation (see review by Lidder & Webb, 2013).

INHIBITION OF NITRIC OXIDE SYNTHESIS

▼ Drugs can inhibit NO synthesis or action by several mechanisms. Certain arginine analogues compete with arginine for NOS. Several such compounds, for example N^G-monomethyl-L-arginine (L-NMMA) and N^G-nitro-L-arginine methyl ester (L-NAME), have proved of great value as experimental tools. One such compound, ADMA, is approximately equipotent with L-NMMA. It is present in human plasma and is excreted in urine. Its plasma concentration correlates with vascular mortality in patients receiving haemodialysis for chronic renal failure, and is increased in people with hypercholesterolaemia. In addition to urinary excretion, ADMA is also eliminated by metabolism to a mixture of citrulline and methylamine by *dimethylarginine dimethylamino hydrolase* (DDAH), an enzyme that exists in two isoforms, each with a reactive cysteine residue in the active site that is subject to control by nitrosylation. Inhibition of DDAH by NO causes feedback inhibition of the L-arginine/NO pathway by allowing cytoplasmic accumulation of ADMA. Conversely, activation of DDAH could potentiate the L-arginine/NO pathway; see Figure 20.4.

Infusion of a low dose of L-NMMA into the brachial artery causes local vasoconstriction (Fig. 20.5), owing to inhibition of the basal production of NO in the infused arm, probably by inhibiting NOS1 (Seddon et al., 2008), without influencing blood pressure or causing other systemic effects, whereas intravenous L-NMMA causes vasoconstriction in renal, mesenteric, cerebral and striated muscle resistance vessels, increases blood pressure and causes reflex bradycardia.

There is therapeutic interest in selective inhibitors of different isoforms of NOS. Selective inhibitors of NOS2 versus the two constitutive forms have been described (e.g. *N*-iminoethyl-L-lysine), and have potential for the treatment of inflammatory and other conditions in which NOS2 has been implicated (e.g. asthma). 7-Nitroindazole selectively inhibits NOS1, the mechanism of selectivity being uncertain. *S*-methyl-L-thiocitrulline is a potent and

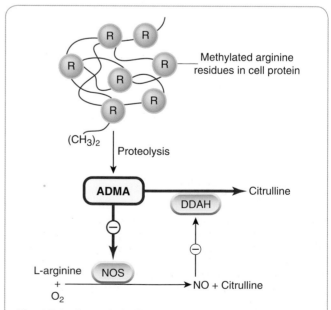

Fig. 20.4 Control of NO synthesis by asymmetric dimethylarginine (ADMA). DDAH, dimethylarginine dimethylamino hydrolase; NO, nitric oxide; NOS, nitric oxide synthase.

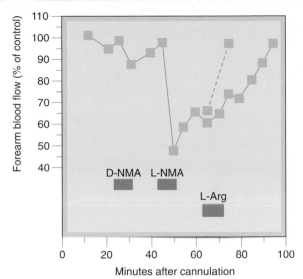

Fig. 20.5 Basal blood flow in the human forearm is influenced by nitric oxide (NO) biosynthesis. Forearm blood flow is expressed as a percentage of the flow in the non-cannulated control arm (which does not change). Brachial artery infusion of the D-isomer of the arginine analogue N^G-monomethyl-L-arginine (D-NMA) has no effect, while the L-isomer (L-NMA) causes vasoconstriction. L-Arginine (L-Arg) accelerates recovery from such vasoconstriction (dashed line). *(From Vallance P, Bhagat K, MacAllister R et al. 1989 Lancet ii, 997–1000.)*

selective inhibitor of human NOS1 (Furfine et al., 1994), and has recently provided new understanding of the importance of NOS1 in control of human resistance vessel tone *in vivo* (Seddon et al., 2008, 2009).

Inhibition of the L-arginine/nitric oxide pathway

- Glucocorticoids inhibit biosynthesis of NOS2.
- Synthetic arginine and citrulline analogues (e.g. **L-NMMA**, **L-NAME**; see text) compete with arginine and are useful experimental tools. Isoform-selective inhibitors include **S-methyl-L-thiocitrulline** (selective for NOS1).
- ADMA (asymmetric dimethylarginine) is an endogenous inhibitor of NOS.

NITRIC OXIDE REPLACEMENT OR POTENTIATION

Several means whereby the L-arginine/NO pathway could be enhanced are under investigation. Some of these rely on existing drugs of proven value in other contexts. The hope (as yet unproven) is that, by potentiating NO, they will prevent atherosclerosis or its thrombotic complications or have other beneficial effects attributed to NO. Possibilities include:

- selective NO donors as 'replacement' therapy (see clinical box, p. 244) or to protect against unwanted aspects of the action of another drug (e.g. **naproxinod**, Ch. 26)

- dietary supplementation with L-arginine or inorganic nitrate (see clinical box, p. 244)
- antioxidants (to reduce concentrations of reactive oxygen species and hence stabilise NO; Ch. 22)
- drugs that restore endothelial function in patients with metabolic risk factors for vascular disease (e.g. angiotensin-converting enzyme inhibitors, statins, insulin, oestrogens; Chs 22, 23, 31 and 35)
- β_2-adrenoceptor agonists and related drugs (e.g. **nebivolol**, a β_1-adrenoceptor antagonist that is metabolised to an active metabolite that activates the L-arginine/NO pathway)
- phosphodiesterase type V inhibitors (e.g. **sildenafil**; see clinical box, p. 244 and Ch. 35).

CLINICAL CONDITIONS IN WHICH NITRIC OXIDE MAY PLAY A PART

The wide distribution of NOS enzymes and diverse actions of NO suggest that abnormalities in the L-arginine/NO pathway could be important in disease. Either increased or reduced production could play a part, and hypotheses abound. Evidence is harder to come by but has been sought using various indirect approaches, including:

- analysing nitrate and/or cGMP in urine: these studies are bedevilled, respectively, by dietary nitrate and by membrane-bound guanylyl cyclase (which is stimulated by endogenous natriuretic peptides; see Ch. 21)
- a considerable refinement is to administer [^{15}N]-arginine and use mass spectrometry to measure the enrichment of ^{15}N over naturally abundant [^{14}N]-nitrate in urine
- measuring NO in exhaled air
- measuring effects of NOS inhibitors (e.g. L-NMMA)
- comparing responses to endothelium-dependent agonists (e.g. **acetylcholine**) and endothelium-independent agonists (e.g. **nitroprusside**)
- measuring responses to increased blood flow ('flow-mediated dilatation'), which are largely mediated by NO
- studying histochemical appearances and pharmacological responses *in vitro* of tissue obtained at operation (e.g. coronary artery surgery).

All these methods have limitations, and the dust is far from settled. Nevertheless, it seems clear that the L-arginine/NO pathway is indeed a player in the pathogenesis of several important diseases, opening the way to new therapeutic approaches. Some pathological roles of excessive or reduced NO production are summarised in Table 20.1. We touch only briefly on these clinical conditions, and would caution the reader that not all of these exciting possibilities are likely to withstand the test of time!

Sepsis can cause multiple organ failure. Whereas NO benefits host defence by killing invading organisms, excessive NO causes harmful hypotension. Disappointingly, however, L-NMMA worsened survival in one controlled clinical trial.

Chronic low-grade endotoxaemia occurs in patients with *hepatic cirrhosis*. Systemic vasodilatation is typical in such patients. Urinary excretion of cGMP is increased,

Nitric oxide in pathophysiology

- Nitric oxide (NO) is synthesised under physiological and pathological circumstances.
- Either reduced or increased NO production can contribute to disease.
- Underproduction of neuronal NO is reported in babies with hypertrophic pyloric stenosis. Endothelial NO production is reduced in patients with hypercholesterolaemia and some other risk factors for atherosclerosis, and this may contribute to atherogenesis.
- Overproduction of NO may be important in neurodegenerative diseases (see Ch. 40) and in septic shock (Ch. 22).

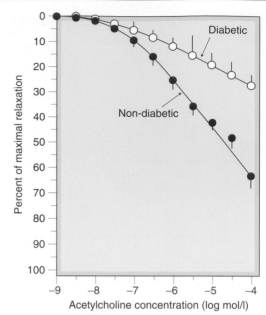

Fig. 20.6 Impaired endothelium-mediated relaxation of penile smooth muscle from diabetic men with erectile dysfunction. Mean (± SE) relaxation responses to acetylcholine in corpora cavernosa tissue (obtained at the time of performing surgical implants to treat impotence) from 16 diabetic men and 22 non-diabetic subjects. (*Data from Saenz de Tejada I, Carson MP, de las Morenas A et al. 1989 N Engl J Med 320, 1025–1030.*)

and vasodilatation may be a consequence of induction of NOS leading to increased NO synthesis.

Nitrosative stress and nitration of proteins in airway epithelium may contribute to steroid resistance in *asthma*, and the ineffectiveness of glucocorticoids in *chronic obstructive pulmonary disease* (see Ch. 28).

Nitric oxide biosynthesis is reduced in patients with *hypercholesterolaemia* and some other disorders that predispose to atheromatous vascular disease, including cigarette smoking and diabetes mellitus. In hypercholesterolaemia, evidence of blunted NO release in forearm and coronary vascular beds is supported by evidence that this can be corrected by lowering plasma cholesterol (with a statin; see Ch. 24) or by dietary supplementation with L-arginine.

Endothelial dysfunction in diabetic patients with *erectile dysfunction* occurs in tissue from the corpora cavernosum of the penis, as evidenced by blunted relaxation to acetylcholine despite preserved responses to nitroprusside (Fig. 20.6). Vasoconstrictor responses to intra-arterial L-NMMA are reduced in forearm vasculature of insulin-dependent diabetics, especially in patients with traces of albumin in their urine ('microalbuminuria': early evidence of glomerular endothelial dysfunction).

It is thought that failure to increase endogenous NO biosynthesis normally during pregnancy contributes to *eclampsia*. This is a hypertensive disorder that accounts for many maternal deaths and in which the normal vasodilatation seen in healthy pregnancy is lost.

Excessive NMDA receptor activation increases NO synthesis, which contributes to several forms of neurological damage (see Ch. 40).

NOS1 is absent in pyloric tissue from babies with idiopathic hypertrophic pyloric stenosis.

Established clinical uses of drugs that influence the L-arginine/NO system are summarised in the clinical box.

RELATED MEDIATORS

Nitric oxide (NO), promoted from pollutant to 'molecule of the year',[6] was joined, similarly implausibly, by carbon monoxide (CO) – a potentially lethal exhaust gas – and

Nitric oxide in therapeutics

- Nitric oxide (NO) donors (e.g. **nitroprusside** and organic nitrovasodilators) are well established (see Chs 21 and 22).
- Type V phosphodiesterase inhibitors (e.g. **sildenafil**, **tadalafil**) potentiate the action of NO. They are used to treat erectile dysfunction (Ch. 35).
- Other possible uses (e.g. pulmonary hypertension, gastric stasis) are being investigated.
- Inhaled NO is used in adult and neonatal respiratory distress syndrome.
- Inhibition of NO biosynthesis is being investigated in disorders where there is overproduction of NO (e.g. inflammation and neurodegenerative disease). Disappointingly, **L-NMMA** increases mortality in one such condition (sepsis).

by hydrogen sulfide (H_2S), which are also formed in mammalian tissues. There are striking similarities between these three gases, as well as some contrasts. All three are highly diffusible labile molecules that are rapidly eliminated from the body: NO as nitrite and nitrate in urine as well as NO in exhaled air (see p. 240); CO in exhaled air; H_2S as thiosulfate, sulfite and sulfate in urine (Figure 20.7) as well as in exhaled breath. All three react with haemoglobin, and all three affect cellular energetics via

[6]By the American Association for the Advancement of Science in 1992.

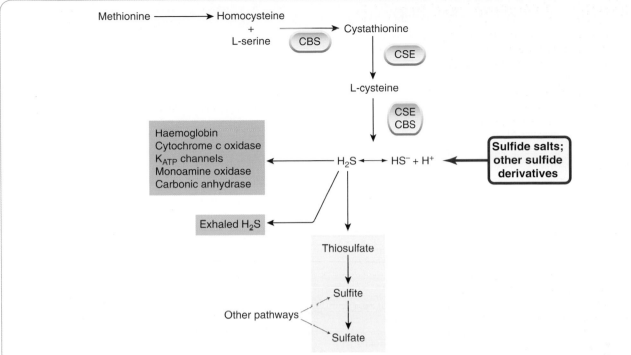

Fig. 20.7 **Synthesis, sites of action and disposition of H₂S.** Endogenous biosynthesis from sulfur-containing amino acids (methionine, cysteine) via actions of the regulated enzymes methionine cystathionine γ lyase (CSE) and cystathionine β-synthase (CBS) is shown; pharmacological H₂S donors (red-rimmed box) may be administered exogenously. Most H₂S is probably renally excreted as sulfate (yellow box). Some is eliminated in exhaled air (green box). Some molecular targets of H₂S are indicated in the blue box. (*Adapted with permission from Ritter JM 2010 Human pharmacology of hydrogen sulfide: putative gaseous mediator. Br J Clin Pharmacol 69, 573–575.*)

actions on cytochrome c oxidase. All have vasodilator effects (although chronic exposure to CO can cause vasoconstriction), and all have anti-inflammatory and cytoprotective effects at low concentrations but cause cellular injury at higher concentrations.

CARBON MONOXIDE (CO)

▼ CO is synthesised, together with biliverdin, by inducible and/or constitutive forms of haem oxygenase, and has been implicated as a signalling molecule in the cardiovascular and central nervous systems (especially olfactory pathways) and in controlling respiratory, gastrointestinal, endocrine and reproductive functions (see Wu & Wang, 2005). There is evidence that prostanoid-induced cerebral vasodilatation is mediated by CO, and that CO also interacts with NO in modulating cerebral vascular tone (Leffler et al., 2011). There are as yet no therapeutic drugs acting via this pathway, but it remains worth watching.

HYDROGEN SULFIDE (H₂S)

▼ All H₂S has been known to generations of schoolboys as the source of the odour of rotten eggs and the proposal that it too is a gaseous mediator was met with some scepticism. Its toxicology includes actions on enzymes including monoamine oxidase and carbonic anhydrase, but more recent work has demonstrated a diverse pharmacology consistent with functions as a signalling molecule under physiological conditions.

Endogenous H₂S is produced from L-cysteine by cystathionine γ-lyase (also known as cystathionase or CSE) and cystathionine β-synthase (CBS). Large amounts of CBS occur in mammalian brain (especially hippocampus and cerebellar Purkinje cells), whereas CSE activity is greatest in liver, kidney and media of blood vessels. These enzymes are under regulatory control (e.g. by lipopolysaccharide and by TNF-α) and their expression is altered in experimental diseases (including pancreatitis and diabetes mellitus). Pharmacological inhibitors of H₂S synthesis are so far only of modest potency and specificity and have been of limited use in elucidating its physiological role. Several assays of H₂S in biological fluids grossly overestimate the true concentrations. Thiosulfate excretion (Fig. 20.7) may represent a better analytical approach than plasma sulfide to estimating overall turnover of H₂S; sulfite and sulfate (to which thiosulfate is converted) are not satisfactory, as their production from other sources of sulfur swamps the contribution of H₂S.

Pharmacological effects and therapeutic potential. H₂S has potent pharmacological effects in the cardiovascular system, including vasorelaxation secondary to activation of vascular smooth muscle K_{ATP} channels (see Ch. 4), in models of inflammation and in the central nervous system. Endocrine effects include inhibition of glucose-stimulated insulin secretion; actions on K_{ATP} channels may be important here also (see Ch. 31). One of the most striking effects of H₂S is to induce a state of suspended animation, described first in nematode worms, but then also in rodents, together with hypothermia. Subsequently, a whole range of cytotoxic (high concentration) and cytoprotective (low concentration) effects of H₂S and H₂S donors have been described in a wide variety of cell types in many different tissues (reviewed by Szabo, 2007). These findings provided a rationale for studies of effects of H₂S donors in animal models of diseases as diverse as pulmonary vasoconstriction, ischaemic heart disease, pulmonary fibrosis and stroke. The results have been sufficiently encouraging to provide a rationale for studying H₂S donors in man. Several sulfide-releasing derivatives based on **diclofenac** (Ch. 26) and on **mesalazine** (Ch. 30), as well as inorganic sodium sulfide, are under investigation as potential therapeutic agents. Again, a case of 'watch this space'.

REFERENCES AND FURTHER READING

Biochemical aspects

Derbyshire, E.R., Marletta, M.A., 2012. Structure and regulation of soluble guanylate cyclase. Ann. Rev. Biochem. 81, 533–559. (*Summarises sGC structure and regulation*)

Furfine, E.S., Harmon, M.F., Paith, J.E., et al., 1994. Potent and selective inhibition of human nitric oxide synthases: selective inhibition of neuronal nitric oxide synthase by S-methyl-L-thiocitrulline and S-ethyl-L-thiocitrulline. J. Biol. Chem. 269, 26677–26683.

Hill, B.G., Dranka, B.P., Shannon, M., et al., 2010. What part of NO don't you understand? Some answers to the cardinal questions in nitric oxide biology. J. Biol. Chem. 285, 19699–19704. (*Biochemistry of NO in a biological context*)

Kim-Shapiro, D.B., Schechter, A.N., Gladwin, M.T., 2006. Unraveling the reactions of nitric oxide, nitrite, and hemoglobin in physiology and therapeutics. Arterioscler. Thromb. Vasc. Biol. 26, 697–705. (*Reviews evidence that nitrite anion may be the main intravascular NO storage molecule; cf. Singel & Stamler, 2005*)

Matsubara, M., Hayashi, N., Jing, T., Titani, K., 2003. Regulation of endothelial nitric oxide synthase by protein kinase C. J. Biochem. 133, 773–781. (*Protein kinase C inhibits NOS3 activity by altering the affinity of calmodulin for the enzyme*)

Pawloski, J.R., Hess, D.T., Stamler, J.S., 2001. Export by red cells of nitric oxide bioactivity. Nature 409, 622–626. (*Movement of NO from red blood cells via anion exchange protein AE1; see also editorial by Gross, S.S., pp. 577–578*)

Ribiero, J.M.C., Hazzard, J.M.H., Nussenzveig, R.H., et al., 1993. Reversible binding of nitric oxide by a salivary haem protein from a blood sucking insect. Science 260, 539–541. (*Action at a distance*)

Schechter, A.N., Gladwyn, M.T., 2003. Hemoglobin and the paracrine and endocrine functions of nitric oxide. N. Engl. J. Med. 348, 1483–1485. (*See also dissenting correspondence in N. Engl. J. Med. 394, 402–406*)

Shaul, P.W., 2002. Regulation of endothelial nitric oxide synthase: location, location, location. Annu. Rev. Physiol. 64, 749–774.

Singel, D.J., Stamler, J.S., 2005. Chemical physiology of blood flow regulation by red cells: the role of nitric oxide and S-nitrosohemoglobin. Annu. Rev. Physiol. 67, 99–145.

Xu, W.M., Charles, I.G., Moncada, S., 2005. Nitric oxide: orchestrating hypoxia regulation through mitochondrial respiration and the endoplasmic reticulum stress response. Cell Res. 15, 63–65.

Physiological aspects

Coggins, M.P., Bloch, K.D., 2007. Nitric oxide in the pulmonary vasculature. Arterioscler. Thromb. Vasc. Biol. 27, 1877–1885.

Diesen, D.L., Hess, D.T., Stamler, J.S., 2008. Hypoxic vasodilation by red blood cells evidence for an S-nitrosothiol-based signal. Circ. Res. 103, 545–553. (*Results suggesting that an S-nitrosothiol originating from RBCs mediates hypoxic vasodilatation by RBCs*)

Erusalimsky, J.D., Moncada, S., 2007. Nitric oxide and mitochondrial signalling from physiology to pathophysiology. Arterioscler. Thromb. Vasc. Biol. 27, 2524–2531. (*Reviews the evidence that binding of NO to cytochrome c oxidase elicits intracellular signalling events*)

Furchgott, R.F., Zawadzki, J.V., 1980. The obligatory role of endothelial cells in the relaxation of arterial smooth muscle by acetylcholine. Nature 288, 373–376. (*Classic*)

Garthwaite, J., 2008. Concepts of neural nitric oxide-mediated transmission. Eur. J. Neurosci. 27, 2783–2802. (*Diverse ways in which NO receptor activation initiates changes in neuronal excitability and synaptic strength by acting at pre- and/or postsynaptic locations*)

Nelson, R.J., Demas, G.E., Huang, P.L., et al., 1995. Behavioural abnormalities in male mice lacking neuronal nitric oxide synthase. Nature 378, 383–386. ('*A large increase in aggressive behaviour and excess, inappropriate sexual behaviour in nNOS knockout mice*')

Seddon, M.D., Chowienczyk, P.J., Brett, S.E., et al., 2008. Neuronal nitric oxide synthase regulates basal microvascular tone in humans in vivo. Circulation 117, 1991–1996. (*Paradigm shift? – very possibly; see next reference*)

Seddon, M., Melikian, N., Dworakowski, R., et al., 2009. Effects of neuronal nitric oxide synthase on human coronary artery diameter and blood flow in vivo. Circulation 119, 2656–2662. (*Local nNOS-derived NO regulates basal blood flow in the human coronary vascular bed, whereas substance P-stimulated vasodilatation is NOS3 mediated*)

Straub, A.C., Lohman, A.W., Billaud, M., et al., 2012. Endothelial cell expression of haemoglobin α regulates nitric oxide signalling. Nature 491, 473–477. (*See also accompanying editorial Gladwyn, M.T., Kim-Shapiro, D.B., 2012. Nitric oxide caught in traffic. Nature 491, 344–345*)

Toda, N., Okamura, T., 2003. The pharmacology of nitric oxide in the peripheral nervous system of blood vessels. Pharmacol. Rev. 55, 271–324.

Vallance, P., Leiper, J., 2004. Cardiovascular biology of the asymmetric dimethylarginine:dimethylarginine dimethylaminohydrolase pathway. Arterioscler. Thromb. Vasc. Biol. 24, 1023–1030.

Victor, V.M., Núñez, C., D'Ocón, P., et al., 2009. Regulation of oxygen distribution in tissues by endothelial nitric oxide. Circ. Res. 104, 1178–1183. (*Endogenously released endothelial NO inhibits cytochrome c oxidase and can modulate tissue O_2 consumption and regulates O_2 distribution to the surrounding tissues*)

Pathological aspects

Ricciardolo, F.L.M., Sterk, P.J., Gaston, B., et al., 2004. Nitric oxide in health and disease of the respiratory system. Physiol. Rev. 84, 731–765.

Clinical and therapeutic aspects

Griffiths, M.J.D., Evans, T.W., 2005. Drug therapy: inhaled nitric oxide therapy in adults. N. Engl. J. Med. 353, 2683–2695. (*Concludes that, on the available evidence, inhaled NO is not effective in patients with acute lung injury, but that it may be useful as a short-term measure in acute hypoxia ± pulmonary hypertension*)

Lidder, S., Webb, A.J., 2013. Vascular effects of dietary nitrate (as found in green leafy vegetables and beetroot) via the nitrate–nitrite–nitric oxide pathway. Br. J. Clin. Pharmacol. 75, 677–696.

Malmström, R.E., Törnberg, D.C., Settergren, G., et al., 2003. Endogenous nitric oxide release by vasoactive drugs monitored in exhaled air. Am. J. Respir. Crit. Care Med. 168, 114–120. (*In humans, acetylcholine evokes a dose-dependent increase of NO in exhaled air; NO release by vasoactive agonists can be measured online in the exhaled air of pigs and humans*)

Miller, M.R., Megson, I.L., 2007. Review – Recent developments in nitric oxide donor drugs. Br. J. Pharmacol. 151, 305–321. (*Explores some of the more promising recent advances in NO donor drug development and challenges associated with NO as a therapeutic agent*)

Pawloski, J.R., Hess, D.T., Stamler, J.S., 2005. Impaired vasodilation by red blood cells in sickle cell disease. Proc. Natl Acad. Sci. U.S.A. 102, 2531–2536. (*Sickle red cells are deficient in membrane S-nitrosothiol and impaired in their ability to mediate hypoxic vasodilation; the magnitudes of these impairments correlate with the clinical severity of disease*)

Carbon monoxide as possible mediator

Leffler, C.W., Parfenova, H., Jaggar, J.H., 2011. Carbon monoxide as an endogenous vascular modulator. Am. J. Physiol. 301, H1–H11.

Wu, L., Wang, R., 2005. Carbon monoxide: endogenous production, physiological functions and pharmacological applications. Pharmacol. Rev. 57, 585–630.

Hydrogen sulfide as possible mediator

Li, L., Moore, P.K., 2008. Putative biological roles of hydrogen sulfide in health and disease: a breath of not so fresh air? Trends Pharmacol. Sci. 29, 84–90.

Reiffenstein, R.J., Hulbert, W.C., Roth, S.H., 1992. Toxicology of hydrogen sulfide. Annu. Rev. Pharmacol. Toxicol. 32, 109–134.

Szabo, C., 2007. Hydrogen sulphide and its therapeutic potential. Nat. Rev. Drug Discov. 6, 917–935.

The heart 21

OVERVIEW

This chapter presents an overview of cardiac physiology in terms of electrophysiology, contraction, oxygen consumption and coronary blood flow, autonomic control and natriuretic peptides as a basis for understanding effects of drugs on the heart and their place in treating cardiac disease. We concentrate on drugs that act directly on the heart, namely antidysrhythmic drugs and drugs that increase the force of contraction of the heart (especially digoxin); antianginal drugs are also covered. The commonest forms of heart disease are caused by atheroma in the coronary arteries, and thrombosis on ruptured atheromatous plaques; drugs to treat and prevent these are considered in Chapters 23 and 24. Heart failure is mainly treated by drugs that work indirectly on the heart via actions on vascular smooth muscle, discussed in Chapter 22, by diuretics (Ch. 29) and β-adrenoceptor antagonists (Ch. 14).

INTRODUCTION

In this chapter we consider effects of drugs on the heart under three main headings:

1. Rate and rhythm.
2. Myocardial contraction.
3. Metabolism and blood flow.

The effects of drugs on these aspects of cardiac function are not, of course, independent of each other. For example, if a drug affects the electrical properties of the myocardial cell membrane, it is likely to influence both cardiac rhythm and myocardial contraction. Similarly, a drug that affects contraction will inevitably alter metabolism and blood flow as well. Nevertheless, from a therapeutic point of view, these three classes of effect represent distinct clinical objectives in relation to the treatment, respectively, of cardiac dysrhythmias, cardiac failure and coronary insufficiency (as occurs during angina pectoris or myocardial infarction).

PHYSIOLOGY OF CARDIAC FUNCTION

CARDIAC RATE AND RHYTHM

The chambers of the heart normally contract in a coordinated manner, pumping blood efficiently by a route determined by the valves. Coordination of contraction is achieved by a specialised conducting system. The normal *sinus rhythm* is generated by pacemaker impulses that arise in the sinoatrial (SA) node and are conducted in sequence through the atria, the atrioventricular (AV) node, bundle of His, Purkinje fibres and ventricles. Cardiac cells owe their electrical excitability to voltage-sensitive plasma membrane channels selective for various ions, including Na^+, K^+ and Ca^{2+}, the structure and function of which are described in Chapter 4. Electrophysiological features of cardiac muscle that distinguish it from other excitable tissues include:

- pacemaker activity
- absence of fast Na^+ current in SA and AV nodes, where slow inward Ca^{2+} current initiates action potentials
- long-action potential ('plateau') and refractory period
- influx of Ca^{2+} during the plateau.

Thus several of the special features of cardiac rhythm relate to Ca^{2+} currents. The heart contains *intracellular* calcium channels (i.e. ryanodine receptors and inositol trisphosphate-activated calcium channels described in Chapter 4, which are important in myocardial contraction) and voltage dependent calcium channels in the plasma membrane, which are important in controlling cardiac rate and rhythm. The main type of voltage-dependent calcium channel in adult working myocardium is the L-type channel, which is also important in vascular smooth muscle; L-type channels are important in specialised conducting regions as well as in working myocardium.

The action potential of an idealised cardiac muscle cell is shown in Figure 21.1A and is divided into five phases: 0 (fast depolarisation), 1 (partial repolarisation), 2 (plateau), 3 (repolarisation) and 4 (pacemaker).

▼ Ionic mechanisms underlying these phases can be summarised as follows.

Phase 0, rapid depolarisation, occurs when the membrane potential reaches a critical firing threshold (about −60 mV), at which the inward current of Na^+ flowing through the voltage dependent sodium channels becomes large enough to produce a regenerative ('all-or-nothing') depolarisation. This mechanism is the same as that responsible for action potential generation in neurons (see Ch. 4). Activation of sodium channels by membrane depolarisation is transient, and if the membrane remains depolarised for more than a few milliseconds, they close again (inactivation). They are therefore closed during the plateau of the action potential and remain unavailable for the initiation of another action potential until the membrane repolarises.

Phase 1, partial repolarisation, occurs as the Na^+ current is inactivated. There may also be a transient voltage-sensitive outward current.

Phase 2, the plateau, results from an inward Ca^{2+} current. Calcium channels show a pattern of voltage-sensitive activation and inactivation qualitatively similar to sodium channels, but with a much slower time course. The plateau is assisted by a special property of the cardiac muscle membrane known as *inward-going rectification*, which means that the K^+ conductance falls to a low level when the membrane is depolarised. Because of this, there is little tendency for outward K^+ current to restore the resting membrane potential during the plateau, so a relatively small inward Ca^{2+} current suffices to maintain the plateau. A persistent sodium current (I_{Nap}) also contributes to the plateau; it is a major contributor to ischaemic arrhythmias, and is a drug target (see p. 260).

Phase 3, repolarisation, occurs as the Ca^{2+} current inactivates and a delayed outwardly rectifying K^+ current (analogous to, but much slower than, the K^+ current that causes repolarisation in nerve fibres; Ch. 4) activates, causing outward K^+ current. This is augmented by

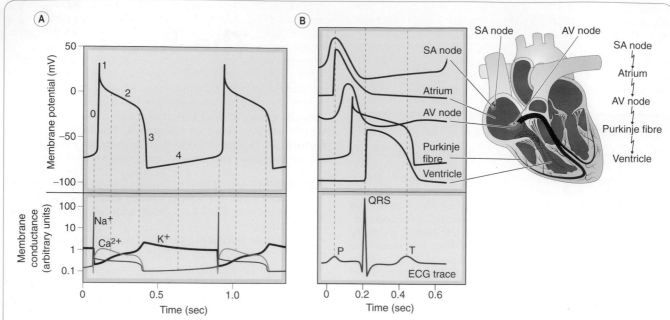

Fig. 21.1 The cardiac action potential. [A] Phases of the action potential: 0, rapid depolarisation; 1, partial repolarisation; 2, plateau; 3, repolarisation; 4, pacemaker depolarisation. The lower panel shows the accompanying changes in membrane conductance for Na⁺, K⁺ and Ca²⁺. [B] Conduction of the impulse through the heart, with the corresponding electrocardiogram (ECG) trace. Note that the longest delay occurs at the atrioventricular (AV) node, where the action potential has a characteristically slow waveform. SA, sinoatrial.

another K⁺ current, which is activated by high intracellular Ca²⁺ concentrations, [Ca²⁺]ᵢ during the plateau, and sometimes also by other K⁺ currents, including one through channels activated by acetylcholine (see p. 253) and another that is activated by arachidonic acid, which is liberated under pathological conditions such as myocardial infarction.

Phase 4, the *pacemaker potential*, is a gradual depolarisation during diastole. Pacemaker activity is normally found only in nodal and conducting tissue. The pacemaker potential is caused by a combination of increasing inward currents and declining outward currents during diastole. It is usually most rapid in cells of the SA node, which therefore acts as pacemaker for the whole heart. Cells in the SA node have a greater background conductance to Na⁺ than do atrial or ventricular myocytes, leading to a greater background inward current. In addition, inactivation of voltage-dependent calcium channels wears off during diastole, resulting in increasing inward Ca²⁺ current during late diastole. Activation of T-type calcium channels during late diastole contributes to pacemaker activity in the SA node. The negative membrane potential early in diastole activates a cation channel that is permeable to Na⁺ and K⁺, giving rise to another inward current, called I_f.[1] An inhibitor of this current, **ivabradine**, slows the heart and is used therapeutically (see below).

Several voltage- and time-dependent outward currents play a part as well: delayed rectifier K⁺ current (I_K), which is activated during the action potential, is turned off by the negative membrane potential early in diastole. Current from the electrogenic Na⁺/K⁺ pump also contributes to the outward current during the pacemaker potential.

Figure 21.1B shows the action potential configuration in different parts of the heart. Phase 0 is absent in the nodal regions, where the conduction velocity is correspondingly slow (~5 cm/s) compared with other regions such as the Purkinje fibres (conduction velocity ~200 cm/s), which propagate the action potential rapidly to the ventricles.

Regions that lack a fast inward current have a much longer refractory period than fast-conducting regions. This is because recovery of the slow inward current following its inactivation during the action potential takes a considerable time (a few hundred milliseconds), and the refractory period outlasts the action potential. With fast-conducting fibres, inactivation of the Na⁺ current recovers rapidly, and the cell becomes excitable again almost as soon as it is repolarised.

The orderly pattern of sinus rhythm can be disrupted either by heart disease or by the action of drugs or circulating hormones, and an important therapeutic use of drugs is to restore a normal cardiac rhythm where it has become disturbed. The commonest cause of cardiac dysrhythmia is ischaemic heart disease, and many deaths following myocardial infarction result from *ventricular fibrillation* rather than directly from contractile failure. Fibrillation is a state where heart chambers stop contracting in a coordinated way because the rhythm is replaced by chaotic electrical activity, causing rapid uncoordinated contractions within ventricles or atria that do not support output from the affected chambers.

DISTURBANCES OF CARDIAC RHYTHM

Clinically, dysrhythmias are classified according to:

- the site of origin of the abnormality – atrial, junctional or ventricular
- whether the rate is increased (*tachycardia*) or decreased (*bradycardia*).

They may cause palpitations (awareness of the heartbeat) or symptoms from cerebral hypoperfusion (faintness or loss of consciousness). Their diagnosis depends on the surface electrocardiogram (ECG), and details are beyond

---

[1] '*f*' for 'funny', because it is unusual for cation channels to be activated by hyperpolarisation; cardiac electrophysiologists have a peculiar sense of humour!

the scope of this book – see Opie & Gersh (2013). The commonest types of tachyarrhythmia are *atrial fibrillation*, where the heartbeat is completely irregular, and *supraventricular tachycardia* (SVT), where the heartbeat is rapid but regular. Occasional ectopic beats (ventricular as well as supraventricular) are common. Sustained ventricular tachyarrhythmias are much less common but much more serious; they include *ventricular tachycardia*, and *ventricular fibrillation* where the electrical activity in the ventricles is completely chaotic and cardiac output ceases. Bradyarrhythmias include various kinds of *heart block* (e.g. at the AV or SA node) and complete cessation of electrical activity ('asystolic arrest'). It is often unclear which of the various mechanisms discussed below are responsible. These cellular mechanisms nevertheless provide a useful starting point for understanding how antidysrhythmic drugs work. Four basic phenomena underlie disturbances of cardiac rhythm:

1. Delayed after-depolarisation.
2. Re-entry.
3. Ectopic pacemaker activity.
4. Heart block.

The main cause of delayed after-depolarisation is abnormally raised $[Ca^{2+}]_i$, which triggers inward current and hence a train of abnormal action potentials (Fig. 21.2). After-depolarisation is the result of a net inward current, known as the transient inward current. A rise in $[Ca^{2+}]_i$ activates Na^+/Ca^{2+} exchange. This transfers one Ca^{2+} ion out of the cell in exchange for entry of three Na^+ ions, resulting in a net influx of one positive charge and hence membrane depolarisation. Raised $[Ca^{2+}]_i$ also contributes to the depolarisation by opening non-selective cation channels in the plasma membrane. Consequently, hypercalcaemia (which increases the entry of Ca^{2+}) promotes after-depolarisation. Hypokalaemia also influences repolarisation, via an effect on the gating of cardiac delayed rectifier potassium channels. Many drugs, including ones whose principal effects are on other organs, delay cardiac repolarisation by binding to potassium or other cardiac channels or by influencing electrolyte concentrations (see Roden, 2004). Delayed repolarisation, evidenced by prolongation of the QT interval on the electrocardiogram, increases Ca^{2+} entry during the prolonged action potential, leading to after-depolarisation, which carries a risk of causing dangerous ventricular dysrhythmias. QT prolongation is a concern in drug development (see section on Class III drugs, p. 258, and see Ch. 57).

Normally, a cardiac action potential dies out after it has activated the ventricles because it is surrounded by refractory tissue, which it has just traversed. *Re-entry* (Fig. 21.3) describes a situation in which the impulse re-excites regions of the myocardium after the refractory period has subsided, causing continuous circulation of action potentials. It can result from anatomical anomalies or, more commonly, from myocardial damage. Re-entry underlies many types of dysrhythmia, the pattern depending on the site of the re-entrant circuit, which may be in the atria, ventricles or nodal tissue. A simple ring of tissue can give rise to a re-entrant rhythm if a transient or unidirectional conduction block is present. Normally, an impulse originating at any point in the ring will propagate in both directions and die out when the two impulses meet, but if a damaged area causes either a transient block (so that one impulse is blocked but the second can get through; Fig. 21.3) or a unidirectional block, continuous circulation of the impulse can occur. This is known as *circus movement* and was demonstrated experimentally on rings of jellyfish tissue many years ago.

Although the physiological pacemaker resides in the SA node, other cardiac tissues can take on pacemaker activity. This provides a safety mechanism in the event of failure of the SA node but can also trigger tachyarrhythmias. Ectopic pacemaker activity is encouraged by sympathetic activity and by partial depolarisation, which may occur during ischaemia. Catecholamines, acting on β_1 adrenoceptors (see p. 252), increase the rate of depolarisation during phase 4 and can cause normally quiescent parts of the heart to take on a spontaneous rhythm. Several

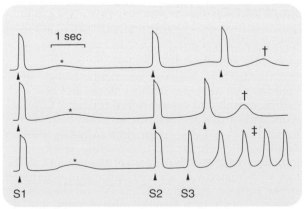

Fig. 21.2 **After-depolarisation in cardiac muscle recorded from a dog coronary sinus in the presence of noradrenaline (norepinephrine).** The first stimulus (S1) causes an action potential followed by a small after-depolarisation. As the interval S2–S3 is decreased, the after-depolarisation gets larger (†) until it triggers an indefinite train of action potentials (‡). *(Adapted from Wit AL, Cranefield PF 1977 Circ Res 41, 435.)*

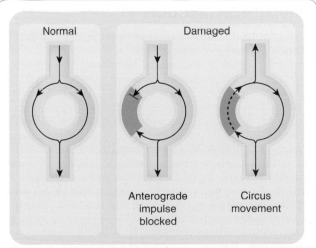

Fig. 21.3 **Generation of a re-entrant rhythm by a damaged area of myocardium.** The damaged area (brown) conducts in one direction only. This disturbs the normal pattern of conduction and permits continuous circulation of the impulse to occur.

tachyarrhythmias (e.g. paroxysmal atrial fibrillation) can be triggered by circumstances associated with increased sympathetic activity. Pain (e.g. during myocardial infarction) increases sympathetic discharge and releases adrenaline (epinephrine) from the adrenal gland. Partial depolarisation resulting from ischaemic damage also causes abnormal pacemaker activity.

Heart block results from fibrosis of, or ischaemic damage to, the conducting system (often in the AV node). In complete heart block, the atria and ventricles beat independently of one another, the ventricles beating at a slow rate determined by whatever pacemaker picks up distal to the block. Sporadic complete failure of AV conduction causes sudden periods of unconsciousness (Stokes–Adams attacks) and is treated by implanting an artificial pacemaker.

> ### Cardiac dysrhythmias
>
> - Dysrhythmias arise because of:
>   - delayed after-depolarisation, which triggers ectopic beats
>   - re-entry, resulting from partial conduction block
>   - ectopic pacemaker activity
>   - **heart block**.
> - Delayed after-depolarisation is caused by an inward current associated with abnormally raised intracellular Ca^{2+}.
> - Re-entry is facilitated when parts of the myocardium are depolarised as a result of disease.
> - Ectopic pacemaker activity is encouraged by sympathetic activity.
> - Heart block results from disease in the conducting system, especially the atrioventricular node.
> - Clinically, dysrhythmias are divided:
>   - according to their site of origin (supraventricular and ventricular)
>   - **according to whether the heart rate is increased or decreased (tachycardia or bradycardia).**

CARDIAC CONTRACTION

Cardiac output is the product of heart rate and mean left ventricular stroke volume (i.e. the volume of blood ejected from the ventricle with each heartbeat). Heart rate is controlled by the autonomic nervous system (Chs 13 and 14, and see p. 252). Stroke volume is determined by a combination of factors, including some intrinsic to the heart itself and other haemodynamic factors extrinsic to the heart. Intrinsic factors regulate myocardial contractility via $[Ca^{2+}]_i$ and ATP, and are sensitive to various drugs and pathological processes. Extrinsic circulatory factors include the elasticity and contractile state of arteries and veins, and the volume and viscosity of the blood, which together determine cardiac load (preload and afterload, see below). Drugs that influence these circulatory factors are of paramount importance in treating patients with heart failure. They are covered in Chapter 22.

MYOCARDIAL CONTRACTILITY AND VIABILITY

The contractile machinery of myocardial striated muscle is basically the same as that of voluntary striated muscle

(Ch. 4). It involves binding of Ca^{2+} to troponin C; this changes the conformation of the troponin complex, permitting cross-bridging of myosin to actin and initiating contraction. **Levosimendan** (a drug used to treat acute decompensated heart failure; Ch. 22), increases the force of contraction of the heart by binding troponin C and sensitising it to the action of Ca^{2+}.

▼ Many effects of drugs on cardiac contractility can be explained in terms of actions on $[Ca^{2+}]_i$, via effects on calcium channels in plasma membrane or sarcoplasmic reticulum, or on the Na^+/K^+ pump, which indirectly influences the Na^+/Ca^{2+} pump (see p. 259). Other factors that affect the force of contraction are the availability of oxygen and a source of metabolic energy such as free fatty acids. Myocardial *stunning* – contractile dysfunction that persists after ischaemia and reperfusion despite restoration of blood flow and absence of cardiac necrosis – is incompletely understood but can be clinically important. Its converse is known as *ischaemic preconditioning*; this refers to an improved ability to withstand ischaemia following previous ischaemic episodes. This potentially beneficial state could be clinically important. There is some evidence that it is mediated by *adenosine* (see Ch. 16), which accumulates as ATP is depleted. Exogenous adenosine affords protection similar to that caused by ischaemic preconditioning, and blockade of adenosine receptors prevents the protective effect of preconditioning (see Gross & Auchampach, 2007). There is considerable interest in developing strategies to minimise harmful effects of ischaemia while maximising preconditioning.

VENTRICULAR FUNCTION CURVES AND HEART FAILURE

The force of contraction of the heart is determined partly by its intrinsic contractility (which, as described above, depends on $[Ca^{2+}]_i$ and availability of ATP), and partly by extrinsic haemodynamic factors that affect end-diastolic volume and hence the resting length of the muscle fibres. The end-diastolic volume is determined by the end-diastolic pressure, and its effect on stroke work is expressed in the Frank–Starling law of the heart, which reflects an inherent property of the contractile system. The Frank–Starling law can be represented as a ventricular function curve (Fig. 21.4). The area enclosed by the pressure–volume curve during the cardiac cycle provides a measure of ventricular stroke work. It is approximated by the product of stroke volume and mean arterial pressure. As Starling showed, factors extrinsic to the heart affect its performance in various ways, two patterns of response to increased load being particularly important:

1. Increased cardiac filling pressure (*preload*), whether caused by increased blood volume or by venoconstriction, increases ventricular end-diastolic volume. This increases stroke volume and hence cardiac output and mean arterial pressure. Cardiac work and cardiac oxygen consumption both increase.
2. Resistance vessel vasoconstriction increases *afterload*. End-diastolic volume and hence stroke work are initially unchanged, but constant stroke work in the face of increased vascular resistance causes reduced stroke volume and hence increased end-diastolic volume. This in turn increases stroke work, until a steady state is re-established with increased end-diastolic volume and the same cardiac output as before. As with increased preload, cardiac work and cardiac oxygen consumption both increase.

Normal ventricular filling pressure is only a few centimetres of water, on the steep part of the ventricular function curve, so a large increase in stroke work can be achieved

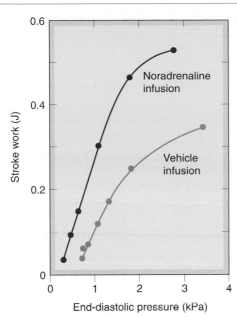

Fig. 21.4 **Ventricular function curves in the dog.** Infusion of physiological saline increases blood volume and hence end diastolic pressure. This increases stroke work ('extrinsic' control) by increasing the force of contraction of the heart. This relationship is called the Starling curve. Noradrenaline has a direct action on the heart ('intrinsic' control), increasing the slope of the Starling curve. (*Redrawn from Sarnoff SJ et al. 1960 Circ Res 8, 1108.*)

with only a small increase in filling pressure. The Starling mechanism plays little part in controlling cardiac output in healthy subjects (e.g. during exercise), because changes in contractility, mainly as a result of changes in sympathetic nervous activity, achieve the necessary regulation without any increase in ventricular filling pressure (Fig. 21.4). In contrast, the denervated heart in patients who have received a heart transplant relies on the Starling mechanism to increase cardiac output during exercise.

In heart failure, the cardiac output is insufficient to meet the needs of the body, initially only when these are increased during exercise but ultimately, as disease progresses, also at rest. It has many causes, most commonly ischaemic heart disease. In patients with heart failure (see Ch. 22), the heart may be unable to deliver as much blood as the tissues require, even when its contractility is increased by sympathetic activity. Under these conditions, the basal (i.e. at rest) ventricular function curve is greatly depressed, and there is insufficient reserve, in the sense of extra contractility that can be achieved by sympathetic activity, to enable cardiac output to be maintained during exercise without a large increase in central venous pressure (Fig. 21.4). Oedema of peripheral tissues (causing swelling of the legs) and the lungs (causing breathlessness) is an important consequence of cardiac failure. It is caused by the increased venous pressure, and retention of Na^+ (see Ch. 22).

MYOCARDIAL OXYGEN CONSUMPTION AND CORONARY BLOOD FLOW

Relative to its large metabolic needs, the heart is one of the most poorly perfused tissues in the body. Coronary flow is, under normal circumstances, closely related to

myocardial oxygen consumption, and both change over a nearly 10-fold range between conditions of rest and maximal exercise. Most drugs that influence cardiac metabolism do so indirectly by influencing coronary blood flow (although **trimetazidine**, used in some European countries, has been claimed to improve myocardial glucose utilisation through inhibition of fatty acid metabolism).

PHYSIOLOGICAL FACTORS

The main physiological factors that regulate coronary flow are:

- physical factors
- vascular control by metabolites
- neural and humoral control.

Physical factors

During systole, the pressure exerted by the myocardium on vessels that pass through it equals or exceeds the perfusion pressure, so coronary flow occurs only during diastole. Diastole is shortened more than systole during tachycardia, reducing the period available for myocardial perfusion. During diastole, the effective perfusion pressure is equal to the difference between the aortic and ventricular pressures (Fig. 21.5). If diastolic aortic pressure falls or diastolic ventricular pressure increases, perfusion pressure falls and so (unless other control mechanisms can compensate) does coronary blood flow. Stenosis of the aortic valve reduces aortic pressure but increases left ventricular pressure upstream of the narrowed valve and often causes ischaemic chest pain (angina) even in the absence of coronary artery disease.

Vascular control by metabolites/mediators

Vascular control by metabolites is the most important mechanism by which coronary flow is regulated. A reduction in arterial partial pressure of oxygen (P_{O_2}) causes marked vasodilatation of coronary vessels *in situ* but has little effect on isolated strips of coronary artery, suggesting

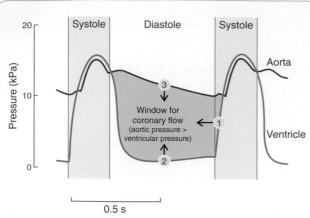

Fig. 21.5 **Mechanical factors affecting coronary blood flow.** The 'window' for coronary flow may be encroached on by: (1) shortening diastole, when heart rate increases; (2) increased ventricular end-diastolic pressure; and (3) reduced diastolic arterial pressure.

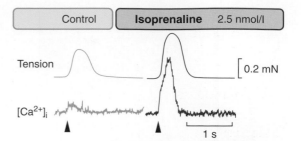

Fig. 21.6 **The calcium transient in frog cardiac muscle.** A group of cells was injected with the phosphorescent Ca^{2+} indicator aequorin, which allows $[Ca^{2+}]_i$ to be monitored optically. Isoprenaline causes a large increase in the tension and in the $[Ca^{2+}]_i$ transient caused by an electrical stimulus (▲). *(From Allen DG, Blinks JR 1978 Nature 273, 509.)*

that it is a change in the metabolites produced by the myocardial cells, rather than the change in PO_2 *per se*, that controls the state of the coronary vessels, a popular candidate for the dilator metabolite being *adenosine* (see Ch. 16).

Neural and humoral control

Coronary vessels have a dense sympathetic innervation, but sympathetic nerves (like circulating catecholamines) exert only a small direct effect on the coronary circulation. Large coronary vessels possess α adrenoceptors that mediate vasoconstriction, whereas smaller vessels have $β_2$ adrenoceptors that have a dilator effect. Coronary vessels are also innervated by purinergic, peptidergic and nitrergic nerves, and basal coronary blood flow in patients with angiographically normal coronary arteries is reduced by about one-third by selective inhibition of NOS1 (Seddon et al., 2009). Coronary vascular responses to altered mechanical and metabolic activity during exercise or pathological events overshadow neural and endocrine effects.

Coronary flow, ischaemia and infarction

- The heart has a smaller blood supply in relation to its oxygen consumption than most organs.
- Coronary flow is controlled mainly by:
  - physical factors, including transmural pressure during systole
  - **vasodilator metabolites**.
- Autonomic innervation is less important.
- Coronary ischaemia is usually the result of atherosclerosis and causes angina. Sudden ischaemia is usually caused by thrombosis and may result in cardiac infarction.
- Coronary spasm sometimes causes angina (variant angina).
- Cellular Ca^{2+} overload results from ischaemia and may be responsible for:
  - cell death
  - **dysrhythmias**.

AUTONOMIC CONTROL OF THE HEART

The sympathetic and parasympathetic systems (see Chs 12–14) each exert a tonic effect on the heart at rest and influence each of the aspects of cardiac function discussed above, namely rate and rhythm, myocardial contraction, and myocardial metabolism and blood flow.

SYMPATHETIC SYSTEM

The main effects of sympathetic activity on the heart are:

- increased force of contraction (positive *inotropic* effect; Fig. 21.6)
- increased heart rate (positive *chronotropic* effect; Fig. 21.7)
- increased *automaticity*
- repolarisation and *restoration of function* following generalised cardiac depolarisation
- reduced cardiac *efficiency* (i.e. oxygen consumption is increased more than cardiac work)
- cardiac hypertrophy (which seems to be directly mediated by stimulation of myocardial α and β adrenoceptors rather than by haemodynamic changes).

▼ These effects mainly result from activation of $β_1$ adrenoceptors. The $β_1$ effects of catecholamines on the heart, although complex, probably all occur through activation of adenylyl cyclase resulting in increased intracellular cAMP (see Ch. 3). cAMP activates protein kinase A, which phosphorylates sites on the $α_1$ subunits of calcium channels. This increases the probability that the channels will open, increasing inward Ca^{2+} current and hence force of cardiac contraction (Fig. 21.6). Activation of $β_1$ adrenoceptors also increases the Ca^{2+} sensitivity of the contractile machinery, possibly by phosphorylating troponin C; furthermore, it facilitates Ca^{2+} capture by the sarcoplasmic reticulum, thereby increasing the amount of Ca^{2+} available for release by the action potential. The net result of catecholamine action is to elevate and steepen the ventricular function curve (Fig. 21.4). The increase in heart rate results from an increased slope of the pacemaker potential (Figs 21.1 and 21.7A). Increased Ca^{2+} entry also increases automaticity because of the effect of $[Ca^{2+}]_i$ on the transient inward current, which can result in a train of action potentials following a single stimulus (see Fig. 21.2).

Activation of $β_1$ adrenoceptors repolarises damaged or hypoxic myocardium by stimulating the Na^+/K^+ pump. This can restore function if asystole has occurred following myocardial infarction, and **adrenaline** is one of the most important drugs used during cardiac arrest.

The reduction of cardiac efficiency by catecholamines is important because it means that the oxygen requirement of the myocardium increases. This limits the use of β agonists such as adrenaline and

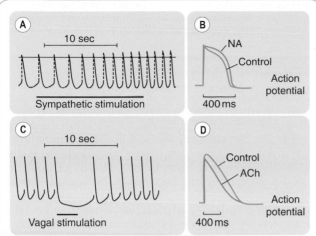

Fig. 21.7 **Autonomic regulation of the heartbeat.** [A] and [B] Effects of sympathetic stimulation and noradrenaline (NA). [C] and [D] Effects of parasympathetic stimulation and acetylcholine (ACh). Sympathetic stimulation (panel [A]) increases the slope of the pacemaker potential and increases heart rate, whereas parasympathetic stimulation (panel [C]) abolishes the pacemaker potential, hyperpolarises the membrane and temporarily stops the heart (frog sinus venosus). NA (panel [B]) prolongs the action potential, while ACh (panel [D]) shortens it (frog atrium). *(Panels [A] and [C] from Hutter OF, Trautwein W 1956 J Gen Physiol 39: 715; panel [B] from Reuter H 1974 J Physiol 242: 429; panel [D] from Giles WR, Noble SJ 1976 J Physiol 261, 103.)*

dobutamine for circulatory shock (Ch. 22). Myocardial infarction activates the sympathetic nervous system (see Fig. 21.8), which has the undesirable effect of increasing the oxygen needs of the damaged myocardium.

PARASYMPATHETIC SYSTEM

Parasympathetic activity produces effects that are, in general, opposite to those of sympathetic activation. However, in contrast to sympathetic activity, the parasympathetic nervous system has little effect on contractility, its main effects being on rate and rhythm, namely:

- cardiac slowing and reduced automaticity
- inhibition of AV conduction.

▼ These effects result from activation of muscarinic (M$_2$) acetylcholine receptors, which are abundant in nodal and atrial tissue but sparse in the ventricles. These receptors are negatively coupled to adenylyl cyclase and thus reduce cAMP formation, acting to inhibit the opening of L-type Ca^{2+} channels and reduce the slow Ca^{2+} current, in opposition to β$_1$ adrenoceptors. M$_2$ receptors also open a type of K$^+$ channel known as GIRK (G protein-activated inward rectifying K$^+$ channel). The resulting increase in K$^+$ permeability produces a hyperpolarising current that opposes the inward pacemaker current, slowing the heart and reducing automaticity (see Fig. 21.7C). Vagal activity is often increased during myocardial infarction, both in association with vagal afferent stimulation and as a side effect of opioids used to control the pain, and parasympathetic effects are important in predisposing to acute dysrhythmias.

Vagal stimulation decreases the force of contraction of the atria associated with marked shortening of the action potential (Fig. 21.7D). Increased K$^+$ permeability and reduced Ca^{2+} current both contribute to conduction block at the AV node, where propagation

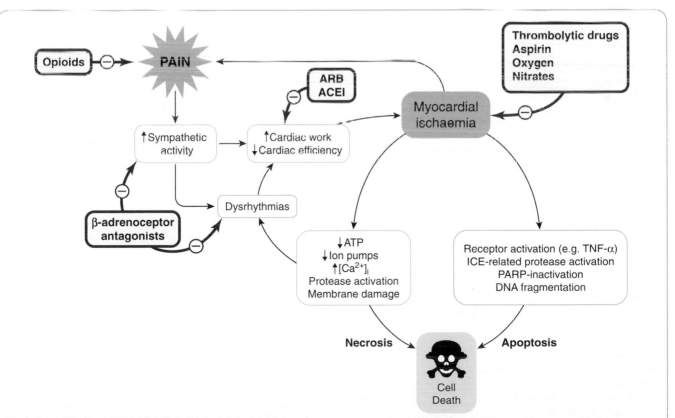

Fig. 21.8 **Effects of myocardial ischaemia.** This leads to cell death by one of two pathways: necrosis or apoptosis. ACEI, angiotensin-converting enzyme inhibitor; ARB, angiotensin AT$_1$ receptor antagonist; ICE, interleukin-1-converting enzyme; PARP, poly-[ADP-ribose]-polymerase; TNF-α, tumour necrosis factor-α.

depends on the Ca^{2+} current. Shortening the atrial action potential reduces the refractory period, which can lead to re-entrant arrhythmias. Coronary vessels lack cholinergic innervation; consequently, the parasympathetic nervous system has little effect on coronary artery tone (see Ch. 13).

Autonomic control of the heart

- Sympathetic activity, acting through β_1 adrenoceptors, increases heart rate, contractility and automaticity, but reduces cardiac efficiency (in relation to oxygen consumption).
- The β_1 adrenoceptors act by increasing cAMP formation, which increases Ca^{2+} currents.
- Parasympathetic activity, acting through muscarinic M_2 receptors, causes cardiac slowing, decreased force of contraction (atria only) and inhibition of atrioventricular conduction.
- M_2 receptors inhibit cAMP formation and also open potassium channels, causing hyperpolarisation.

CARDIAC NATRIURETIC PEPTIDES

Cardiac natriuretic peptides are an important family of mediators (see Potter et al., 2009, for a review). Atrial cells contain secretory granules, and store and release *atrial natriuretic peptide* (ANP). This has powerful effects on the kidney and vascular system. Release of ANP occurs during volume overload in response to stretching of the atria, and intravenous saline infusion is sufficient to stimulate its release. B-natriuretic peptide (BNP) is released from ventricular muscle and opposes ventricular fibrosis; its plasma concentration is increased in patients with heart failure and is used as an aid to diagnosis. C-natriuretic peptide (CNP) is stored in endothelium and in addition to vascular actions influences development of long bones.

The main effects of natriuretic peptides are to increase Na^+ and water excretion by the kidney; relax vascular smooth muscle (except efferent arterioles of renal glomeruli; see below); increase vascular permeability; and inhibit the release and/or actions of several vasoconstrictor or salt-retaining hormones and mediators, including aldosterone, angiotensin II, endothelin and antidiuretic hormone. They exert their effects by combining with membrane receptors (natriuretic peptide receptors, NPRs, which exist in at least two subtypes, designated A and B).[2]

▼ Both NPR-A and NPR-B incorporate a catalytic guanylyl cyclase moiety (see Ch. 3), and, when activated, increase intracellular cGMP. Organic nitrates (discussed later) and endogenous nitric oxide (Ch. 20) also increase cGMP, though they interact with soluble rather than membrane-bound guanylyl cyclase. Renal glomerular afferent arterioles are dilated by ANP but efferent arterioles are constricted, so filtration pressure is increased, leading to increased glomerular filtration and enhanced Na^+ excretion. Elsewhere in the vasculature,

natriuretic peptides cause vasorelaxation and reduce blood pressure. Their therapeutic potential, which remains controversial (see Richards, 2009), is considered in Chapter 22.

ISCHAEMIC HEART DISEASE

Atheromatous deposits are ubiquitous in the coronary arteries of adults living in developed countries. They are asymptomatic for most of the natural history of the disease (see Ch. 23), but can progress insidiously, culminating in acute myocardial infarction and its complications, including dysrhythmia and heart failure. Details of ischaemic heart disease are beyond the scope of this book, and excellent accounts (e.g. Mann et al., 2014) are available for those seeking pathological and clinical information. Here, we merely set the scene for understanding the place of drugs that affect cardiac function in treating this most common form of heart disease.

Important consequences of coronary atherosclerosis include:

- angina (chest pain caused by cardiac ischaemia)
- myocardial infarction.

ANGINA

Angina occurs when the oxygen supply to the myocardium is insufficient for its needs. The pain has a characteristic distribution in the chest, arm and neck, and is brought on by exertion, cold or excitement. A similar type of pain occurs in skeletal muscle when it is made to contract while its blood supply is interrupted, and Lewis showed many years ago that chemical factors released by ischaemic muscle are responsible. Possible candidates include K^+, H^+ and adenosine (Ch. 16), all of which sensitise or stimulate nociceptors (see Ch. 42). It is possible that the same mediator that causes coronary vasodilatation is responsible, at higher concentration, for initiating pain.

Three kinds of angina are recognised clinically: stable, unstable and variant.

Stable angina. This is predictable chest pain on exertion. It is produced by an increased demand on the heart and is usually caused by a fixed narrowing of the coronary vessels by atheroma, although as explained above narrowing of the aortic valve ('aortic stenosis') can cause angina by reducing coronary blood flow even in the absence of coronary artery narrowing. Symptomatic therapy is directed at reducing cardiac work with organic nitrates, β-adrenoceptor antagonists and/or calcium antagonists, together with treatment of the underlying atheromatous disease, usually including a statin (Ch. 23), and prophylaxis against thrombosis with an antiplatelet drug, usually **aspirin** (Ch. 24).

Unstable angina. This is characterised by pain that occurs with less and less exertion, culminating in pain at rest. The pathology is similar to that involved in myocardial infarction, namely platelet–fibrin thrombus associated with a ruptured atheromatous plaque, but without complete occlusion of the vessel. Treatment is as for myocardial infarction. Antiplatelet drugs (aspirin and/or an ADP antagonist such as **clopidogrel** or **prasugrel**) reduce the risk of myocardial infarction in this setting, and antithrombotic drugs add to this benefit (Ch. 24) at the cost of increased risk of haemorrhage, and organic nitrates relieve ischaemic pain.

---

[2]The nomenclature of natriuretic peptides and their receptors is peculiarly obtuse. The peptides are named 'A' for arterial, 'B' for brain – despite being present mainly in cardiac ventricle – and 'C' for A, B, C …; NPRs are named NPR-A, which preferentially binds ANP; NPR-B, which binds C natriuretic peptide preferentially; and NPR-C for 'clearance' receptor, because until recently clearance via cellular uptake and degradation by lysosomal enzymes was the only definite known function of this binding site.

Variant angina. This is relatively uncommon. It occurs at rest and is caused by coronary artery spasm, often in association with atheromatous disease. Therapy is with coronary artery vasodilators (e.g. organic nitrates, calcium antagonists).

MYOCARDIAL INFARCTION

Myocardial infarction occurs when a coronary artery has been blocked by thrombus. This may be fatal and is a common cause of death, usually as a result of mechanical failure of the ventricle or from dysrhythmia. Cardiac myocytes rely on aerobic metabolism. If the supply of oxygen remains below a critical value, a sequence of events leading to cell death ensues, detected clinically by an elevation of circulating *troponin* (the gold-standard biochemical marker of myocardial injury). The sequences leading from vascular occlusion to cell death via necrosis or apoptosis (see Ch. 5) are illustrated in Figure 21.8. The relative importance of these two pathways in causing myocardial cell death is unknown, but apoptosis may be an adaptive process in hypoperfused regions, sacrificing some jeopardised myocytes but thereby avoiding the disturbance of membrane function and risk of dysrhythmia inherent in necrosis. Consequently, it is currently unknown if pharmacological approaches to promote or inhibit this pathway could be clinically beneficial.

Prevention of irreversible ischaemic damage following an episode of coronary thrombosis is an important therapeutic aim. Opening the occluded artery is key, and it is important that this is achieved promptly, irrespective of the means by which it is done. If logistically possible, *angioplasty* (performed using a catheter with an inflatable balloon near its tip, with a glycoprotein IIb/IIIa antagonist – see Chapter 24 – to prevent reocclusion) is somewhat more effective than thrombolytic drugs. The main therapeutic drugs (see Fig. 21.8) include drugs to improve cardiac function by maintaining oxygenation and reducing cardiac work as well as treating pain and preventing further thrombosis. They are used in combination, and include:

- combinations of thrombolytic, antiplatelet (aspirin and clopidogrel) and antithrombotic (a heparin preparation) drugs to open the blocked artery and prevent reocclusion (see Ch. 24)
- oxygen if there is arterial hypoxia
- opioids (given with an antiemetic) to prevent pain and reduce excessive sympathetic activity
- organic nitrate
- β-adrenoceptor antagonists
- angiotensin-converting enzyme inhibitors (ACEIs) or angiotensin AT_1 receptor antagonists (ARBs; see Ch. 22).

β-Adrenoceptor antagonists reduce cardiac work and thereby the metabolic needs of the heart, and are used as soon as the patient is stable. ACEIs and ARBs also reduce cardiac work and improve survival as does opening the coronary artery (with angioplasty or thrombolytic drug) and antiplatelet treatment.

DRUGS THAT AFFECT CARDIAC FUNCTION

Drugs that have a major action on the heart can be divided into three groups.

1. *Drugs that affect myocardial cells directly.* These include:
   a. autonomic neurotransmitters and related drugs
   b. antidysrhythmic drugs
   c. cardiac glycosides and other inotropic drugs
   d. miscellaneous drugs and hormones; these are dealt with elsewhere (e.g. **doxorubicin**, Ch. 56; thyroxine, Ch. 34; glucagon, Ch. 31).
2. *Drugs that affect cardiac function indirectly.* These have actions elsewhere in the vascular system. Some antianginal drugs (e.g. nitrates) fall into this category, as do many drugs that are used to treat heart failure (e.g. diuretics and ACEIs).
3. *Calcium antagonists.* These affect cardiac function by a direct action on myocardial cells and also indirectly by relaxing vascular smooth muscle.

ANTIDYSRHYTHMIC DRUGS

A classification of antidysrhythmic drugs based on their electrophysiological effects was proposed by Vaughan Williams in 1970. It provides a good starting point for discussing mechanisms, although many useful drugs do not fit neatly into this classification (Table 21.1). Furthermore, emergency treatment of serious dysrhythmias is usually by physical means (e.g. pacing or electrical cardioversion by applying a direct current shock to the chest or via an implanted device) rather than drugs.

There are four classes (see Table 21.2).

- Class I: drugs that block voltage-sensitive sodium channels. They are subdivided: Ia, Ib and Ic.
- Class II: β-adrenoceptor antagonists.
- Class III: drugs that substantially prolong the cardiac action potential.
- Class IV: calcium antagonists.

The phase of the action potential on which each of these classes of drug have their main effect is shown in Figure 21.9.

MECHANISMS OF ACTION

Class I drugs

Class I drugs block sodium channels, just as local anaesthetics do, by binding to sites on the α subunit (see Chs 4 and 43). Because this inhibits action potential propagation in many excitable cells, it has been referred to as

Table 21.1 Antidysrhythmic drugs unclassified in the Vaughan Williams system

Drug	Use
Atropine	Sinus bradycardia
Adrenaline (epinephrine)	Cardiac arrest
Isoprenaline	Heart block
Digoxin	Rapid atrial fibrillation
Adenosine	Supraventricular tachycardia
Calcium chloride	Ventricular tachycardia due to hyperkalaemia
Magnesium chloride	Ventricular fibrillation, digoxin toxicity

Table 21.2 Summary of antidysrhythmic drugs (Vaughan Williams classification)

Class	Example(s)	Mechanism
Ia	Disopyramide	Sodium-channel block (intermediate dissociation)
Ib	Lidocaine	Sodium-channel block (fast dissociation)
Ic	Flecainide	Sodium-channel block (slow dissociation)
II	Propranolol	β-Adrenoceptor antagonism
III	Amiodarone, sotalol	Potassium-channel block
IV	Verapamil	Calcium-channel block

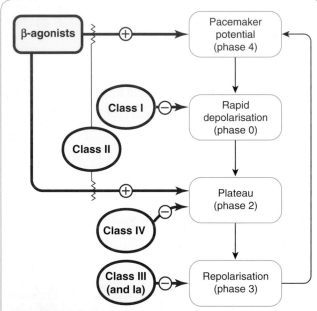

Fig. 21.9 Effects of antidysrhythmic drugs on the different phases (as defined in **Fig. 21.1**) of the cardiac action potential.

'membrane-stabilising' activity, a phrase best avoided now that the ionic mechanism is understood. The characteristic effect on the action potential is to reduce the maximum rate of depolarisation during phase 0.

▼ The reason for further subdivision of these drugs into classes Ia, Ib and Ic is that the earliest examples, **quinidine** and **procainamide** (class Ia), have different effects from many of the more recently developed drugs, even though all share the same basic mechanism of action. A partial explanation for these functional differences comes from electrophysiological studies of the characteristics of the sodium-channel block produced by different class I drugs.

The central concept is of *use-dependent channel block*. It is this characteristic that enables all class I drugs to block the high-frequency excitation of the myocardium that occurs in tachyarrhythmias, without preventing the heart from beating at normal frequencies. Sodium channels exist in three distinct functional states: resting, open and inactivated (see Ch. 4). Channels switch rapidly from resting to open in response to depolarisation; this is known as

activation. Maintained depolarisation, as in ischaemic muscle, causes channels to change more slowly from open to inactivated, and the membrane, which is then refractory, must then be repolarised for a time to restore the channel to the resting state before it can be activated again. Class I drugs bind to channels most strongly when they are in either the open or the inactivated state, less strongly to channels in the resting state. Their action therefore shows the property of 'use dependence' (i.e. the more frequently the channels are activated, the greater the degree of block produced).

Class Ib drugs, for example **lidocaine**, associate and dissociate rapidly within the timeframe of the normal heartbeat. The drug binds to open channels during phase 0 of the action potential (affecting the rate of rise very little, but leaving many of the channels blocked by the time the action potential reaches its peak). Dissociation occurs in time for the next action potential, provided the cardiac rhythm is normal. A premature beat, however, will be aborted because the channels are still blocked. Furthermore, class Ib drugs bind selectively to inactivated channels and thus block preferentially when the cells are depolarised, for example in ischaemia.

Class Ic drugs, such as **flecainide** and **encainide**, associate and dissociate much more slowly, thus reaching a steady-state level of block that does not vary appreciably during the cardiac cycle. They markedly inhibit conduction through the His–Purkinje system.

Class Ia, the oldest group (e.g. **quinidine**, **procainamide**, **disopyramide**), lies midway in its properties between Ib and Ic but, in addition, prolongs repolarisation, albeit less markedly than class III drugs (see below).

Class II drugs

Class II drugs comprise the β-adrenoceptor antagonists (e.g. **metoprolol**).

Adrenaline can cause dysrhythmias by its effects on the pacemaker potential and on the slow inward Ca^{2+} current (see p. 252-253). Ventricular dysrhythmias following myocardial infarction are partly the result of increased sympathetic activity (see Fig. 21.8), providing a rationale for using β-adrenoceptor antagonists in this setting. AV conduction depends critically on sympathetic activity; β-adrenoceptor antagonists increase the refractory period of the AV node and can therefore prevent recurrent attacks of supraventricular tachycardia (SVT). The β-adrenoceptor antagonists are also used to prevent paroxysmal attacks of atrial fibrillation when these occur in the setting of sympathetic activation.

Class III drugs

The class III category was originally based on the unusual behaviour of a single drug, **amiodarone** (see p. 258), although others with similar properties (e.g. **sotalol**) have since been described. Both amiodarone and sotalol have more than one mechanism of antidysrhythmic action. The special feature that defines them as class III drugs is that they substantially prolong the cardiac action potential. The mechanism of this effect is not fully understood, but it involves blocking some of the potassium channels involved in cardiac repolarisation, including the outward (delayed) rectifier. Action potential prolongation increases the refractory period, accounting for powerful and varied antidysrhythmic activity, for example by interrupting re-entrant tachycardias and suppressing ectopic activity. However, drugs that prolong the cardiac action potential (detected clinically as prolonged QT interval on the ECG; see above) can paradoxically also have *proarrhythmic* effects, notably a polymorphic form of ventricular tachycardia called (somewhat whimsically) *torsade de pointes* (because the appearance of the ECG trace is said to be reminiscent of this ballet sequence). This occurs particularly in patients taking other drugs that can prolong QT, including several antipsychotic drugs; those with disturbances of electrolytes involved in repolarisation (e.g. hypokalaemia, hypercalcaemia); or individuals with hereditary prolonged QT (Ward–Romano syndrome).[3] The mechanism of the dysrhythmia is not fully understood; possibilities include increased dispersion of repolarisation (i.e. lack of spatial homogeneity) and increased Ca^{2+} entry during the prolonged action potential, leading to increased after-depolarisation.

Class IV drugs

Class IV agents act by blocking voltage-sensitive calcium channels. Class IV drugs in therapeutic use as antidysrhythmic drugs (e.g. **verapamil**) act on L-type channels. Class IV drugs slow conduction in the SA and AV nodes where action potential propagation depends on slow inward Ca^{2+} current, slowing the heart and terminating SVT by causing partial AV block. They shorten the plateau of the action potential and reduce the force of contraction. Decreased Ca^{2+} entry reduces after-depolarisation and thus suppresses premature ectopic beats. Functionally distinct classes of L-type voltage-gated calcium channels are expressed in heart and vascular smooth muscle, and L-type calcium-channel blockers that act mainly on vascular smooth muscle (e.g. **nifedipine**) indirectly increase sympathetic tone via their hypotensive effect, causing reflex tachycardia.

DETAILS OF INDIVIDUAL DRUGS

Quinidine, procainamide and disopyramide (class Ia)

Quinidine and **procainamide,** now mainly of historical interest, are pharmacologically similar. **Disopyramide** resembles quinidine, possessing an atropine-like effect, distinct from its class Ia action, which can cause blurred vision, dry mouth, constipation and urinary retention. It has more negative inotropic action than quinidine but is less likely to cause hypersensitivity reactions.

Lidocaine (class Ib)

Lidocaine, also well known as a local anaesthetic (see Ch. 43), is given by intravenous infusion, to treat and prevent ventricular dysrhythmias in the immediate aftermath of myocardial infarction. It is almost completely extracted from the portal circulation by hepatic first-pass metabolism (Ch. 9), and so cannot usefully be swallowed (although if administered into the mouth to produce local anaesthesia it can be absorbed directly into the systemic circulation and cause systemic effects). Its plasma half-life is normally about 2 h, but its elimination is slowed if hepatic blood flow is reduced, for example by reduced cardiac output following myocardial infarction or by drugs that reduce cardiac output (e.g. β-adrenoceptor antagonists). Dosage must be reduced accordingly to

prevent accumulation and toxicity. Indeed, its clearance has been used to estimate hepatic blood flow, analogous to the use of *para*-aminohippurate clearance to measure renal blood flow.

The adverse effects of lidocaine are mainly due to its actions on the central nervous system and include drowsiness, disorientation and convulsions. Because of its relatively short half-life, the plasma concentration can be adjusted fairly rapidly by varying the infusion rate.

Flecainide and encainide (class Ic)

Flecainide and **encainide** suppress ventricular ectopic beats. They are long-acting and reduce the frequency of ventricular ectopic beats when administered orally. However, in clinical trials, they unexpectedly increased the incidence of sudden death associated with ventricular fibrillation after myocardial infarction, so they are no longer used in this setting. This counterintuitive result had a profound impact on the way clinicians and drug regulators view the use of seemingly reasonable intermediate end points (in this case, reduction of frequency of ventricular ectopic beats) as evidence of efficacy in clinical trials. Currently, the main use of flecainide is in prophylaxis against paroxysmal atrial fibrillation.

> **Clinical uses of class I antidysrhythmic drugs**
>
> - **Class Ia** (e.g. **disopyramide**)
>   - ventricular dysrhythmias
>   - prevention of recurrent paroxysmal atrial fibrillation triggered by vagal overactivity.
> - **Class Ib** (e.g. intravenous **lidocaine**)
>   - treatment and prevention of ventricular tachycardia and fibrillation during and immediately after myocardial infarction.
> - **Class Ic**
>   - to prevent paroxysmal atrial fibrillation (**flecainide**)
>   - recurrent tachyarrhythmias associated with abnormal conducting pathways (e.g. Wolff–Parkinson–White syndrome).

β-Adrenoceptor antagonists (class II)

β-Adrenoceptor antagonists are described in Chapter 14. Their clinical use for rhythm disorders is shown in the clinical box. **Propranolol**, like several other drugs of this type, has some class I action in addition to blocking β adrenoceptors. This may contribute to its antidysrhythmic effects, although probably not very much, because an isomer with little β-antagonist activity has little antidysrhythmic activity, despite similar activity as a class I agent.

Adverse effects include worsening bronchospasm in patients with asthma, a negative inotropic effect, bradycardia and fatigue. It was hoped that the use of $β_1$-selective drugs (e.g. **metoprolol, atenolol**) would reduce the risk of bronchospasm, but their selectivity is insufficient to achieve this goal in clinical practice, although the once-a-day convenience of several such drugs has led to their widespread use in patients without lung disease.

---

[3]A 3-year-old girl began to have blackouts, which decreased in frequency with age. Her ECG showed a prolonged QT interval. When 18 years of age, she lost consciousness running for a bus. When she was 19, she became quite emotional as a participant in a live television audience and died suddenly. The molecular basis of this rare inherited disorder is now known. It is caused by a mutation in either the gene coding for a particular potassium channel – called *HERG* – or another gene, *SCN5A*, which codes for the sodium channel and disruption of which results in a loss of inactivation of the Na^+ current (see Welsh & Hoshi, 1995, for a commentary).

> ### Clinical uses of class II antidysrhythmic drugs (e.g. propranolol, timolol)
>
> - To reduce mortality following myocardial infarction.
> - To prevent recurrence of tachyarrhythmias (e.g. paroxysmal atrial fibrillation) provoked by increased sympathetic activity.

Class III

Amiodarone is highly effective at suppressing dysrhythmias (see the clinical box below). Like other drugs that interfere with cardiac repolarisation, it is important to monitor plasma electrolyte concentrations (especially of K^+). Unfortunately, several peculiarities complicate its use. It is extensively bound in tissues, has a long elimination half-life (10–100 days) and accumulates in the body during repeated dosing. For this reason, a loading dose is used, and for life-threatening dysrhythmias this is given intravenously via a central vein (it causes phlebitis if given into a peripheral vessel). Adverse effects are numerous and important; they include photosensitive skin rashes and a slate-grey/bluish discoloration of the skin; thyroid abnormalities (hypo- and hyper-, connected with its iodine content); pulmonary fibrosis, which is late in onset but may be irreversible; corneal deposits; and neurological and gastrointestinal disturbances, including hepatitis. Surprisingly (since it delays repolarisation and prolongs the QT interval) reports of torsades de pointes and ventricular tachycardia are very unusual. **Dronedarone** is a related benzofuran with somewhat different effects on individual ion channels. It lacks iodine and was designed to be less lipophilic than amiodarone in hopes of reducing thyroid and pulmonary toxicities. Its elimination $t_{1/2}$ is shorter than that of amiodarone and while it increased mortality in patients with severe heart failure (Køber et al., 2008), it improved survival in high-risk patients with atrial fibrillation (Hohnloser et al., 2009) and is approved for this indication.

Sotalol is a non-selective β-adrenoceptor antagonist, this activity residing in the L isomer. Unlike other β antagonists, it prolongs the cardiac action potential and the QT interval by delaying the slow outward K^+ current. This class III activity is present in both L and D isomers. Racemic sotalol (the form prescribed) appears to be somewhat less effective than amiodarone in preventing chronic

> ### Clinical uses of class III antidysrhythmic drugs
>
> - **Amiodarone**: tachycardia associated with the Wolff–Parkinson–White syndrome. It is also effective in many other supraventricular and ventricular tachyarrhythmias but has serious adverse effects.
> - (Racemic) **sotalol** combines class III with class II actions. It is used in paroxysmal supraventricular dysrhythmias and suppresses ventricular ectopic beats and short runs of ventricular tachycardia.

life-threatening ventricular tachyarrhythmias. It can cause torsades de pointes; it is valuable in patients in whom β-adrenoceptor antagonists are not contraindicated. Close monitoring of plasma K^+ is important.

Verapamil and diltiazem (class IV)

Verapamil is given by mouth. (Intravenous preparations are available but are dangerous and almost never needed.) It has a plasma half-life of 6–8 h and is subject to quite extensive first-pass metabolism, which is more marked for the isomer that is responsible for its cardiac effects. A slow-release preparation is available for once-daily use, but it is less effective when used for prevention of dysrhythmia than the regular preparation because the bioavailability of the cardioactive isomer is reduced through the presentation of a steady low concentration to the drug-metabolising enzymes in the liver. If verapamil is added to **digoxin** in patients with poorly controlled atrial fibrillation, the dose of digoxin should be reduced and plasma digoxin concentration checked after a few days, because verapamil both displaces digoxin from tissue-binding sites and reduces its renal elimination, hence predisposing to digoxin accumulation and toxicity.

▼ Verapamil is contraindicated in patients with Wolff–Parkinson–White syndrome (a pre-excitation syndrome caused by a rapidly conducting pathway between atria and ventricles, anatomically distinct from the physiological conducting pathway, that predisposes to re-entrant tachycardia), and is ineffective and dangerous in ventricular dysrhythmias. Adverse effects of verapamil and diltiazem are described below in the section on calcium channel antagonists.

Diltiazem is similar to verapamil but has relatively more effect on smooth muscle while producing less bradycardia (said to be 'rate neutral').

Adenosine (unclassified in the Vaughan Williams classification)

Adenosine is produced endogenously and is an important chemical mediator (Ch. 16) with effects on breathing, cardiac and smooth muscle, vagal afferent nerves and on platelets, in addition to the effects on cardiac conducting tissue that underlie its therapeutic use. The A_1 receptor is responsible for its effect on the AV node. These receptors are linked to the same cardiac potassium channel that is activated by acetylcholine, and adenosine hyperpolarises cardiac conducting tissue and slows the rate of rise of the pacemaker potential accordingly. It is administered intravenously to terminate SVT if this rhythm persists despite manoeuvres such as carotid artery massage to increase vagal tone. It has largely replaced verapamil for this purpose, because it is safer owing to its effect being short-lived. This is a consequence of its pharmacokinetics: it is taken up via a specific nucleoside transporter by red blood cells and is metabolised by enzymes on the lumenal surface of vascular endothelium. Consequently, the effects of a bolus dose of adenosine last only 20–30 s. Once SVT has terminated, the patient usually remains in sinus rhythm, even though adenosine is no longer present in plasma. Its short-lived unwanted effects include chest pain, shortness of breath, dizziness and nausea. **Theophylline** and other xanthines (Chs 28 and 48) block adenosine receptors and inhibit the actions of intravenous adenosine, whereas **dipyridamole** (a vasodilator and antiplatelet drug; see p. 261 and Ch. 24) blocks the nucleoside uptake mechanism, potentiating adenosine and prolonging its adverse effects. Both these interactions are clinically important.

DRUGS THAT INCREASE MYOCARDIAL CONTRACTION

CARDIAC GLYCOSIDES

Cardiac glycosides come from foxgloves (*Digitalis* spp.) and related plants. Withering wrote on the use of the foxglove in 1775: 'it has a power over the motion of the heart to a degree yet unobserved in any other medicine …' Foxgloves contain several cardiac glycosides with similar actions. Their basic chemical structure consists of three components: a sugar moiety, a steroid and a lactone ring. The lactone is essential for activity, the other parts of the molecule mainly determining potency and pharmacokinetic properties. Therapeutically the most important cardiac glycoside is **digoxin**.

Endogenous cardiotonic steroids (CTSs), also called digitalis-like factors, have been mooted for nearly half a century. There is evidence in mammals of an endogenous digitalis-like factor closely similar to **ouabain**, a short-acting cardiac glycoside (see Schoner & Scheiner-Bobis, 2007). CTSs were first considered important in the regulation of renal sodium transport and arterial pressure, but they have now been implicated in the regulation of cell growth, differentiation, apoptosis, fibrosis, the modulation of immunity and of carbohydrate metabolism, and the control of various central nervous functions (Bagrov et al., 2009).

Actions and adverse effects

The main actions of glycosides are on the heart, but some of their adverse effects are extracardiac, including nausea, vomiting, diarrhoea and confusion. The cardiac effects are:

- cardiac slowing and reduced rate of conduction through the AV node, due to increased vagal activity
- increased force of contraction
- disturbances of rhythm, especially:
  - block of AV conduction
  - increased ectopic pacemaker activity.

Adverse effects are common and can be severe. One of the main drawbacks of glycosides in clinical use is the narrow margin between effectiveness and toxicity.

Mechanism

The mechanism whereby cardiac glycosides increase the force of cardiac contraction (positive inotropic effect) is inhibition of the Na^+/K^+ pump in the cardiac myocytes. Cardiac glycosides bind to a site on the extracellular aspect of the α subunit of the Na^+-K^+-ATPase, and are useful experimental tools for studying this important transport system. The molecular mechanism underlying increased

vagal tone (negative chronotropic effect) is unknown, but could also be due to inhibition of the Na^+/K^+ pump.

Rate and rhythm

Cardiac glycosides slow AV conduction by increasing vagal outflow. Their beneficial effect in established rapid atrial fibrillation results partly from this. If ventricular rate is excessively rapid, the time available for diastolic filling is inadequate, so slowing heart rate increases stroke volume and cardiac efficiency even if atrial fibrillation persists. Digoxin can terminate paroxysmal atrial tachycardia by its effect on AV conduction, although adenosine (see p. 258) is usually preferred for this indication.

Toxic concentrations of glycosides disturb sinus rhythm. This can occur at plasma concentrations of digoxin within, or only slightly above, the therapeutic range. Slowing of AV conduction can progress to AV block. Glycosides can also cause ectopic beats. Because Na^+/K^+ exchange is electrogenic, inhibition of the pump by glycosides causes depolarisation, predisposing to disturbances of cardiac rhythm. Furthermore, the increased $[Ca^{2+}]_i$ causes increased after-depolarisation, leading first to coupled beats (bigeminy), in which a normal ventricular beat is followed by an ectopic beat; ventricular tachycardia and eventually ventricular fibrillation may ensue.

Force of contraction

Glycosides cause a large increase in twitch tension in isolated preparations of cardiac muscle. Unlike catecholamines, they do not accelerate relaxation (compare Fig. 21.6 with Fig. 21.10). Increased tension is caused by an increased $[Ca^{2+}]_i$ transient (Fig. 21.10). The action potential is only slightly affected and the slow inward current little changed, so the increased $[Ca^{2+}]_i$ transient probably reflects a greater release of Ca^{2+} from intracellular stores. The most likely mechanism is as follows (see also Ch. 4):

1. Glycosides inhibit the Na^+/K^+ pump.
2. Increased $[Na^+]_i$ slows extrusion of Ca^{2+} via the Na^+/Ca^{2+} exchange transporter. Increasing $[Na^+]_i$ reduces the inwardly directed gradient for Na^+; the smaller this gradient, the slower is extrusion of Ca^{2+} by Na^+/Ca^{2+} exchange.
3. Increased $[Ca^{2+}]_i$ is stored in the sarcoplasmic reticulum, and thus increases the amount of Ca^{2+} released by each action potential.

The effect of extracellular potassium

Effects of cardiac glycosides are increased if plasma $[K^+]$ decreases, because of reduced competition at the K^+-

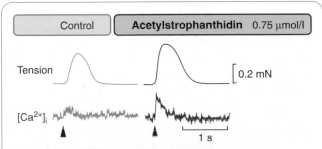

Fig. 21.10 **Effect of a cardiac glycoside (acetylstrophanthidin) on the Ca^{2+} transient and tension produced by frog cardiac muscle.** The effect was recorded as in Figure 21.6. (From Allen DG, Blinks JR 1978 Nature 273, 509.)

binding site on the Na⁺-K⁺-ATPase. This is clinically important, because many diuretics, which are often used to treat heart failure (Ch. 29), decrease plasma [K^+] thereby increasing the risk of glycoside-induced dysrhythmia.

Pharmacokinetic aspects

Digoxin is administered by mouth or, in urgent situations, intravenously. It is a polar molecule; elimination is mainly by renal excretion and involves P-glycoprotein (Ch. 8), leading to clinically significant interactions with other drugs used to treat heart failure, such as **spironolactone**, and with antidysrhythmic drugs such as **verapamil** and **amiodarone**. Elimination half-time is approximately 36 h in patients with normal renal function, but considerably longer in elderly patients and those with overt renal failure, for whom the dose must be reduced. A loading dose is used in urgent situations. The therapeutic range of plasma concentrations, below which digoxin is unlikely to be effective and above which the risk of toxicity increases substantially, is rather narrow (1–2.6 nmol/l). Determination of plasma digoxin concentration is useful when lack of efficacy or toxicity is suspected.

Clinical uses of cardiac glycosides (e.g. digoxin)

- To slow ventricular rate in rapid persistent atrial fibrillation.
- Treatment of heart failure in patients who remain symptomatic despite optimal use of diuretics and angiotensin-converting enzyme inhibitors (Ch. 22).

OTHER DRUGS THAT INCREASE MYOCARDIAL CONTRACTION

Certain β_1-adrenoceptor agonists, for example **dobutamine**, are used to treat acute but potentially reversible heart failure (e.g. following cardiac surgery or in some cases of cardiogenic or septic shock) on the basis of their positive inotropic action. Dobutamine, for reasons that are not well understood, produces less tachycardia than other β_1 agonists. It is administered intravenously. **Glucagon** also increases myocardial contractility by increasing synthesis of cAMP, and has been used in patients with acute cardiac dysfunction caused by overdosage of β-adrenoceptor antagonists.

Inhibitors of the heart-specific subtype (type III) of phosphodiesterase, the enzyme responsible for the intracellular degradation of cAMP, increase myocardial contractility. Consequently, like β-adrenoceptor agonists, they increase intracellular cAMP but cause dysrhythmias for the same reason. Compounds in this group include **amrinone** and **milrinone**. They improve haemodynamic indices in patients with heart failure but paradoxically worsen survival, presumably because of dysrhythmias. As with the encainide/flecainide example (see p. 257) this disparity has had a sobering effect on clinicians and drug regulatory authorities.

ANTIANGINAL DRUGS

The mechanism of anginal pain is discussed above. Angina is managed by using drugs that improve perfusion of the myocardium or reduce its metabolic demand, or both.

Two of the main groups of drugs, organic nitrates and calcium antagonists, are vasodilators and produce both these effects. The third group, β-adrenoceptor antagonists, slow the heart and hence reduce metabolic demand. Organic nitrates and calcium antagonists are described below. The β-adrenoceptor antagonists are covered in Chapter 14, and their antidysrhythmic actions are described above. **Ivabradine** slows the heart by inhibiting the sinus node I_f current (see p. 248), and is an alternative to β-adrenoceptor antagonists in patients in whom these are not tolerated or are contraindicated. **Ranolazine** was recently introduced as an adjunct to other anti-anginal drugs: it inhibits late sodium current and hence indirectly reduces intracellular calcium and force of contraction, without affecting heart rate; more potent and selective inhibitors of the persistent sodium current are in development. Newer anti-anginal drugs are described by Jones et al. (2013).

ORGANIC NITRATES

The ability of organic nitrates (see also Chs 20 and 22) to relieve angina was discovered by Lauder Brunton, a distinguished British physician, in 1867. He had found that angina could be partly relieved by bleeding, and also knew that **amyl nitrite**, which had been synthesised 10 years earlier, caused flushing and tachycardia, with a fall in blood pressure, when its vapour was inhaled. He thought that the effect of bleeding resulted from hypotension, and found that amyl nitrite inhalation worked much better. Amyl nitrite has now been replaced by **glyceryl trinitrate** (GTN).[4] Several related organic nitrates, of which the most important is **isosorbide mononitrate**, have a prolonged action. **Nicorandil**, a potassium channel activator with additional nitrovasodilator activity, is sometimes combined with other antianginal treatment in resistant cases.

Actions

Organic nitrates relax smooth muscle (especially vascular smooth muscle, but also other types including oesophageal and biliary smooth muscle). They relax veins, with a consequent reduction in central venous pressure (reduced preload). In healthy subjects, this reduces stroke volume; venous pooling occurs on standing and can cause postural hypotension and dizziness. Therapeutic doses have less effect on small resistance arteries than on veins, but there is a marked effect on larger muscular arteries. This reduces pulse wave reflection from arterial branches (as appreciated in the 19th century by Murrell but neglected for many years thereafter), and consequently reduces central (aortic) pressure and cardiac afterload (see Ch. 22 for the role of these factors in determining cardiac work). The direct dilator effect on coronary arteries opposes coronary artery spasm in variant angina. With larger doses, resistance arteries and arterioles dilate, and arterial pressure falls. Nevertheless, coronary flow is increased as a result of coronary vasodilatation. Myocardial oxygen consumption is reduced because of the reductions in both cardiac preload and afterload. This, together with the increased coronary blood flow, causes a large increase in the oxygen content of coronary sinus blood. Studies in experimental animals have shown that glyceryl trinitrate diverts blood

---

[4]Nobel discovered how to stabilise GTN with kieselguhr, enabling him to exploit its explosive properties in dynamite, the manufacture of which earned him the fortune with which he endowed the eponymous prizes.

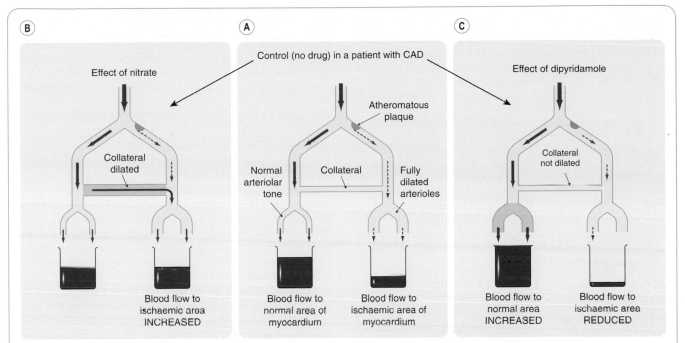

Fig. 21.11 Comparison of the effects of organic nitrates and an arteriolar vasodilator (dipyridamole) on the coronary circulation. **[A]** Control. **[B]** Nitrates dilate the collateral vessel, thus allowing more blood through to the underperfused region (mostly by diversion from the adequately perfused area). **[C]** Dipyridamole dilates arterioles, increasing flow through the normal area at the expense of the ischaemic area (in which the arterioles are anyway fully dilated). CAD, coronary artery disease.

from normal to ischaemic areas of myocardium. The mechanism involves dilatation of collateral vessels that bypass narrowed coronary artery segments (Fig. 21.11).

▼ It is interesting to compare this effect with that of other vasodilators, notably **dipyridamole**, which dilate arterioles but not collaterals. Dipyridamole is at least as effective as nitrates in increasing coronary flow in normal subjects but actually *worsens* angina. This is probably because arterioles in an ischaemic region are fully dilated by the ischaemia, and drug-induced dilatation of the arterioles in normal areas has the effect of diverting blood away from the ischaemic areas (Fig. 21.11), producing what is termed a vascular steal. This effect is exploited in a pharmacological 'stress test' for coronary arterial disease, in which dipyridamole is administered intravenously to patients in whom this diagnosis is suspected but who cannot exercise, while monitoring myocardial perfusion and the ECG.

In summary, the antianginal action of nitrates involves:

- reduced cardiac work, because of reduced cardiac preload (venodilatation) and afterload (reduced arterial wave reflection), leading to reduced myocardial oxygen requirement
- redistribution of coronary flow towards ischaemic areas via collaterals
- relief of coronary spasm.

▼ In addition to its effects on smooth muscle, nitric oxide (NO) increases the rate of relaxation of cardiac muscle (dubbed a '*lusiotropic*' action). It is probable that organic nitrates mimic this action, which could be important in patients with impaired diastolic function, a common accompaniment of hypertension and of heart failure.

Mechanism of action

Organic nitrates are metabolised with release of NO. At concentrations achieved during therapeutic use, this involves an enzymic step and possibly a reaction with tissue sulfhydryl (–SH) groups. Nitric oxide activates soluble guanylyl cyclase (see Ch. 20), increasing formation

of cGMP, which activates protein kinase G (Ch. 4) and leads to a cascade of effects in smooth muscle culminating in dephosphorylation of myosin light chains, sequestration of intracellular Ca^{2+} and consequent relaxation.

Tolerance and unwanted effects

Repeated administration of nitrates to smooth muscle preparations *in vitro* results in diminished relaxation, possibly partly because of depletion of free –SH groups, although attempts to prevent tolerance by agents that restore tissue –SH groups have not been clinically useful. Tolerance to the antianginal effect of nitrates does not occur to a clinically important extent with ordinary formulations of short-acting drugs (e.g. glyceryl trinitrate), but does occur with longer-acting drugs (e.g. isosorbide mononitrate) or when glyceryl trinitrate is administered by prolonged intravenous infusion or by frequent application of slow-release transdermal patches (see below).

The main adverse effects of nitrates are a direct consequence of their main pharmacological actions, and include postural hypotension and headache. This was the cause of 'Monday morning sickness' among workers in explosives factories. Tolerance to these effects develops quite quickly but wears off after a brief nitrate-free interval (which is why the symptoms appeared on Mondays and not later in the week). Formation of *methaemoglobin*, an oxidation product of haemoglobin that is ineffective as an oxygen carrier, seldom occurs when nitrates are used clinically but is induced deliberately with **amyl nitrite** in the treatment of *cyanide poisoning*, because methaemoglobin binds and inactivates cyanide ions.

Pharmacokinetic and pharmaceutical aspects

Glyceryl trinitrate is rapidly inactivated by hepatic metabolism. It is well absorbed from the mouth and is taken as a tablet under the tongue or as a sublingual spray, producing its effects within a few minutes. If swallowed, it is ineffective because of first-pass metabolism. Given sublingually, the trinitrate is converted to di- and mononitrates. Its effective duration of action is approximately 30 min. It is appreciably absorbed through the skin, and a more sustained effect can be achieved by applying it as a transdermal patch. Once a bottle of the tablets has been opened, its shelf-life is quite short because the volatile active substance evaporates; spray preparations avoid this problem.

Isosorbide mononitrate is longer acting than glyceryl trinitrate because it is absorbed and metabolised more slowly but has similar pharmacological actions. It is swallowed rather than taken sublingually, and is taken twice a day for prophylaxis (usually in the morning and at lunch, to allow a nitrate-free period during the night, when patients are not exerting themselves, to avoid tolerance). It is also available in slow-release form for once-daily use in the morning.

Organic nitrates

- Important compounds include **glyceryl trinitrate** and longer-acting **isosorbide mononitrate**.
- These drugs are powerful vasodilators, acting on veins to reduce cardiac preload and reducing arterial wave reflection to reduce afterload.
- Act via nitric oxide, to which they are metabolised. Nitric oxide stimulates formation of cGMP and hence activates protein kinase G, affecting both contractile proteins (myosin light chains) and Ca^{2+} regulation.
- Tolerance occurs experimentally and is important clinically with frequent use of long-acting drugs or sustained-release preparations.
- Effectiveness in angina results partly from reduced cardiac load and partly from dilatation of collateral coronary vessels, causing more effective distribution of coronary flow. Dilatation of constricted coronary vessels is particularly beneficial in variant angina.
- Serious unwanted effects are uncommon; headache and postural hypotension may occur initially. Overdose can, rarely, cause methaemoglobinaemia.

Clinical uses of organic nitrates

- Stable angina:
  - prevention (e.g. daily **isosorbide mononitrate**, or **glyceryl trinitrate** sublingually immediately before exertion)
  - treatment (sublingual **glyceryl trinitrate**).
- Unstable angina: intravenous **glyceryl trinitrate**.
- Acute heart failure: intravenous **glyceryl trinitrate**.
- Chronic heart failure: **isosorbide mononitrate**, with **hydralazine** in patients of African origin (Ch. 22).
- Uses related to relaxation of other smooth muscles (e.g. uterine, biliary) are being investigated.

POTASSIUM CHANNEL ACTIVATORS

Nicorandil combines activation of the potassium K_{ATP} channel (see Ch. 4) with nitrovasodilator (nitric oxide donor) actions. It is both an arterial and a venous dilator, and causes the expected unwanted effects of headache, flushing and dizziness. It is used for patients who remain symptomatic despite optimal management with other drugs, often while they await surgery or angioplasty.

β-ADRENOCEPTOR ANTAGONISTS

β-Adrenoceptor antagonists (see Ch. 14) are important in prophylaxis of stable angina, and in treating patients with unstable angina. They work for these indications by reducing cardiac oxygen consumption. In addition, they reduce the risk of death following myocardial infarction, probably via their antidysrhythmic action. Any effects on coronary vessel diameter are of minor importance, although these drugs are avoided in variant angina because of the theoretical risk that they will increase coronary spasm. Their astonishingly diverse clinical uses are summarised in the clinical boxes above (p. 258) and in Chapter 14.

CALCIUM ANTAGONISTS

The term 'calcium antagonist' is used for drugs that block cellular entry of Ca^{2+} through calcium channels rather than its intracellular actions (Ch. 4). Some authors use the term 'Ca^{2+} entry blockers' to make this distinction clearer. Therapeutically important calcium antagonists act on L-type channels. L-type calcium antagonists comprise three chemically distinct classes: *phenylalkylamines* (e.g. verapamil), *dihydropyridines* (e.g. **nifedipine**, **amlodipine**) and *benzothiazepines* (e.g. **diltiazem**).

Mechanism of action: types of calcium channel

The properties of voltage-gated calcium channels have been studied by voltage clamp and patch clamp techniques (see Ch. 3). Drugs of each of the three chemical classes mentioned above all bind the α_1 subunit of the L-type calcium channel but at distinct sites. These interact allosterically with each other and with the gating machinery of the channel to prevent its opening (see below and Fig. 21.12), thus reducing Ca^{2+} entry. Many calcium antagonists show properties of use dependence (i.e. they block more effectively in cells in which the calcium channels are most active; see the discussion of class I antidysrhythmic drugs above). For the same reason, they also show voltage-dependent blocking actions, blocking more strongly when the membrane is depolarised, causing calcium channel opening and inactivation.

▼ Dihydropyridines affect calcium channel function in a complex way, not simply by physical plugging of the pore. This became clear when some dihydropyridines, exemplified by BAY K 8644, were found to bind to the same site but to do the opposite; that is, to promote the opening of voltage-gated calcium channels. Thus BAY K 8644 *increases* the force of cardiac contraction, and *constricts* blood vessels; it is competitively antagonised by nifedipine. Calcium channels can exist in one of three distinct states, termed 'modes' (Fig. 21.12). When a channel is in mode 0, it does not open in response to depolarisation; in mode 1, depolarisation produces a low opening probability, and each opening is brief. In mode 2, depolarisation produces a very high opening probability, and single openings are prolonged. Under normal conditions, about 70% of the channels at any one moment exist in mode 1, with only 1% or less in mode 0; each channel switches randomly and quite slowly between the three modes. Dihydropyridine antagonists bind selectively to channels in

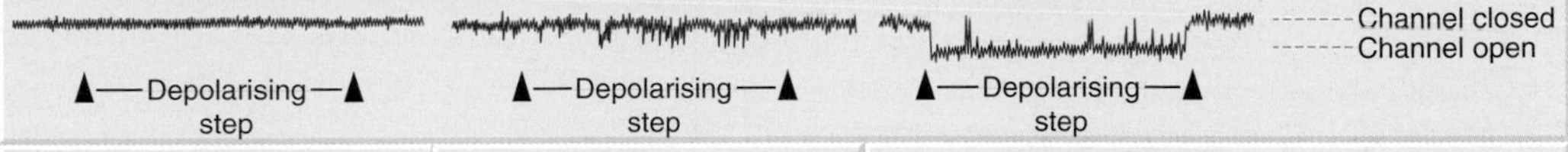

Mode	**Mode 0**	**Mode 1**	**Mode 2**	
	▲—Depolarising—▲ step	▲—Depolarising—▲ step	▲—Depolarising—▲ step	- - - - Channel closed - - - - Channel open
Opening probability	Zero	Low	High	
Favoured by	DHP antagonists		DHP agonists	
% of time normally spent in this mode	<1%	~70%	~30%	

Fig. 21.12 Mode behaviour of calcium channels. The traces are patch clamp recordings (see Ch. 3) of the opening of single calcium channels (downward deflections) in a patch of membrane from a cardiac muscle cell. A depolarising step is imposed close to the start of each trace, causing an increase in the opening probability of the channel. When the channel is in mode 1 (centre), this causes a few brief openings to occur; in mode 2 (right), the channel stays open for most of the time during the depolarising step; in mode 0 (left), it fails to open at all. Under normal conditions, in the absence of drug, the channel spends most of its time in modes 1 and 2, and only rarely enters mode 0. DHP, dihydropyridine. *(Redrawn from Hess et al. 1984 Nature 311, 538–544.)*

mode 0, thus favouring this non-opening state, whereas agonists bind selectively to channels in mode 2 (Fig. 21.12). This type of two-directional modulation resembles the phenomenon seen with the GABA/benzodiazepine interaction (Ch. 44), and invites speculation about possible endogenous dihydropyridine-like mediator(s) with a regulatory effect on Ca^{2+} entry.

Mibefradil blocks T- as well as L type channels at therapeutic concentrations, but was withdrawn from therapeutic use because it caused adverse drug interactions by interfering with drug metabolism. **Ethosuximide** (a carbonic anhydrase inhibitor used to treat absence seizures, Ch. 45) also blocks T channels in thalamic and reticular neurones.

Pharmacological effects

The main effects of calcium antagonists, as used therapeutically, are on cardiac and smooth muscle. Verapamil preferentially affects the heart, whereas most of the dihydropyridines (e.g. nifedipine) exert a greater effect on smooth muscle than on the heart. Diltiazem is intermediate in its actions.

Cardiac actions

The antidysrhythmic effects of verapamil and diltiazem have been discussed above. Calcium antagonists can cause AV block and cardiac slowing by their actions on conducting tissues, but this is offset by a reflex increase in sympathetic activity secondary to their vasodilator action. For example, nifedipine typically causes reflex tachycardia; diltiazem causes little or no change in heart rate and verapamil slows the heart rate. Calcium antagonists also have a negative inotropic effect, from their inhibition of Ca^{2+} entry during the action potential plateau. Verapamil has the most marked negative inotropic action, and is contraindicated in heart failure, whereas amlodipine does not worsen cardiovascular mortality in patients with severe but stable chronic heart failure.

Vascular smooth muscle

Calcium antagonists cause generalised arterial/arteriolar dilatation, thereby reducing blood pressure, but do not much affect the veins. They affect all vascular beds, although regional effects vary considerably between different drugs. They cause coronary vasodilatation and are used in patients with coronary artery spasm (variant angina). Other types of smooth muscle (e.g. biliary tract, urinary tract and uterus) are also relaxed by calcium antagonists, but these effects are less important therapeutically than their actions on vascular smooth muscle.

Protection of ischaemic tissues

There are theoretical reasons (see Fig. 21.8) why calcium antagonists might exert a cytoprotective effect in ischaemic tissues (see Ch. 40) and thus be of use in treating heart attack and stroke. However, randomised clinical trials have been disappointing, with little or no evidence of beneficial (or harmful) effects of calcium antagonists on cardiovascular morbidity or mortality in patient groups other than patients with hypertension, in whom calcium antagonists have beneficial effects comparable with those of other drugs that lower blood pressure to similar extents (see Ch. 22). **Nimodipine** is partly selective for cerebral vasculature and there is some evidence that it reduces cerebral vasospasm following subarachnoid haemorrhage.

Pharmacokinetics

Calcium antagonists in clinical use are well absorbed from the gastrointestinal tract, and are given by mouth except for some special indications, such as following subarachnoid haemorrhage, for which intravenous preparations are available. They are extensively metabolised. Pharmacokinetic differences between different drugs and different pharmaceutical preparations are clinically important, because they determine the dose interval and also the intensity of some of the unwanted effects, such as headache and flushing. Amlodipine has a long elimination half-life and is given once daily, whereas nifedipine, diltiazem and verapamil have shorter elimination half-lives and are either given more frequently or are formulated in various slow-release preparations to permit once-daily dosing.

Unwanted effects

Most of the unwanted effects of calcium antagonists are extensions of their main pharmacological actions. Short-acting dihydropyridines cause flushing and headache because of their vasodilator action, and in chronic use, dihydropyridines often cause ankle swelling related to arteriolar dilatation and increased permeability of postcapillary venules. Verapamil can cause constipation, probably because of effects on calcium channels in gastrointestinal nerves or smooth muscle. Effects on cardiac rhythm (e.g. heart block) and force of contraction (e.g. worsening heart failure) are discussed above.

Apart from these predictable effects, calcium-channel antagonists, as a class, have few idiosyncratic adverse effects.

Calcium antagonists

- Block Ca^{2+} entry by preventing opening of voltage-gated L-type calcium channels.
- There are three main L-type antagonists, typified by **verapamil**, **diltiazem** and dihydropyridines (e.g. **nifedipine**).
- Mainly affect heart and smooth muscle, inhibiting the Ca^{2+} entry caused by depolarisation in these tissues.
- Selectivity between heart and smooth muscle varies: **verapamil** is relatively cardioselective, **nifedipine** is relatively smooth muscle selective, and diltiazem is intermediate.
- Vasodilator effect (mainly dihydropyridines) is mainly on resistance vessels, reducing afterload. Calcium antagonists dilate coronary vessels, which is important in variant angina.

- Effects on heart (**verapamil**, **diltiazem**): antidysrhythmic action (mainly atrial tachycardias), because of impaired atrioventricular conduction; reduced contractility.
- Clinical uses:
  - antidysrhythmic (mainly **verapamil**)
  - angina (e.g. **diltiazem**)
  - **hypertension (mainly dihydropyridines).**
- Unwanted effects include headache, constipation (**verapamil**) and ankle oedema (dihydropyridines). There is a risk of causing cardiac failure or heart block, especially with **verapamil**.

Clinical uses of calcium antagonists

- Dysrhythmias (**verapamil**):
  - to slow ventricular rate in rapid atrial fibrillation
  - to prevent recurrence of supraventricular tachycardia (SVT) (intravenous administration of **verapamil** to terminate SVT attacks has been replaced by use of **adenosine**).

- Hypertension: usually a dihydropyridine drug (e.g. **amlodipine** or slow-release **nifedipine**; Ch. 22).
- To prevent angina (e.g. **dihydropyridine** or **diltiazem**).

REFERENCES AND FURTHER READING

Further reading

Fink, M., Noble, D., 2010. Pharmacodynamic effects in the cardiovascular system: the modeller's view. Basic Clin. Pharmacol. Toxicol. 106, 243–249.

Jones, D.A., Timmis, A., Wragg, A., 2013. Novel drugs for treating angina. BMJ 347, 34–37. (*Useful summary of drugs currently available, including recent introductions*)

Mann, D.L., Zipes, D.P., Libby, P., Bonow, R.O., 2014. Braunwald's Heart Disease: A Textbook of Cardiovascular Medicine, tenth ed. Saunders/Elsevier, Philadelphia.

Opie, L.H., Gersh, B.J., 2013. Drugs for the Heart, eighth ed. Saunders/ Elsevier, Philadelphia.

Specific aspects
Physiological and pathophysiological aspects

Bagrov, A.Y., Shapiro, J.I., Fedorova, O.V., 2009. Endogenous cardiotonic steroids: physiology, pharmacology, and novel therapeutic targets. Pharmacol. Rev. 61, 9–38. (*Reviews physiological interactions between CTS and other regulatory systems that may be important in the pathophysiology of essential hypertension, pre-eclampsia, end-stage renal disease, congestive heart failure and diabetes*)

Gross, G.J., Auchampach, J.A., 2007. Reperfusion injury: does it exist? J. Mol. Cell. Cardiol. 42, 12–18. (*Mounting evidence supports the concept of reperfusion injury, based on work conducted with adenosine and opioid receptor ligands, and the discovery of 'postconditioning' [POC] and of the reperfusion injury salvage kinase [RISK] signalling pathway*)

Noble, D., 2008. Computational models of the heart and their use in assessing the actions of drugs. J. Pharmacol. Sci. 107, 107–117. (*Models of cardiac cells are sufficiently well developed to answer questions concerning the actions of drugs such as ranolazine, a recently introduced blocker of persistent sodium current, on repolarisation and the initiation of arrhythmias*)

Potter, L.R., Yoder, A.R., Flora, D.R., et al., 2009. Natriuretic peptides: their structures, receptors, physiologic functions and therapeutic applications. Handb. Exp. Pharmacol. 191, 341–366. (*Reviews the history, structure, function and clinical applications of natriuretic peptides and their receptors*)

Richards, A.M., 2009. Therapeutic potential of infused cardiac natriuretic peptides in myocardial infarction. Heart 95, 1299–1300. (*Editorial on this controversial issue*)

Rockman, H.A., Koch, W.J., Lefkowitz, R.J., 2002. Seven-transmembrane-spanning receptors and heart function. Nature 415, 206–212.

Schoner, W., Scheiner-Bobis, G., 2007. Endogenous and exogenous cardiac glycosides: their roles in hypertension, salt metabolism, and cell growth. Am. J. Physiol. Cell Physiol. 293, C509–C536. (*Review: touches on anticancer potential also*)

Seddon, M., Melikian, N., Dworakowski, R., et al., 2009. Effects of neuronal nitric oxide synthase on human coronary artery diameter and blood flow in vivo. Circulation 119, 2656–2662. (*Local nNOS-derived NO regulates basal blood flow in the human coronary vascular bed, whereas substance P-stimulated vasodilatation is eNOS mediated*)

Welsh, M.J., Hoshi, T., 1995. Molecular cardiology — ion channels lose the rhythm. Nature 376, 640–641. (*Commentary on Ward–Romano syndrome*)

Therapeutic aspects

COMMIT Collaborative Group, 2005. Early intravenous then oral metoprolol in 45852 patients with acute myocardial infarction: randomised placebo-controlled trial. Lancet 366, 1622–1632. (*Early β blockade reduced ventricular fibrillation and reinfarction, benefits that were offset by increased cardiogenic shock in patients with signs of heart failure; see accompanying comment by Sabatine, M.S., pp. 1587–1589 in the same issue*)

Fox, K., Ford, I., Steg, P.G., et al., 2008. Ivabradine for patients with stable coronary artery disease and left-ventricular systolic dysfunction (BEAUTIFUL): a randomised, double-blind, placebo-controlled trial. Lancet 372, 807–816. (*Ivabradine does not improve cardiac outcomes in all patients with stable coronary artery disease and left-ventricular systolic dysfunction, but improved outcome in patients with heart rates >70 bpm. See also adjacent paper: Fox, K., et al., 2008. Heart rate as a prognostic risk factor in patients with coronary artery disease and left-ventricular systolic dysfunction (BEAUTIFUL): a subgroup analysis of a randomised controlled trial. Lancet 372, 817–821*)

Hohnloser, S.H., Crijns, H.J., van Eickels, M., et al., 2009. Effect of dronedarone on cardiovascular events in atrial fibrillation. N. Engl. J. Med. 360, 668–678. (*4628 patients with atrial fibrillation who had additional risk factors for death; those randomised to dronedarone had fewer hospitalisations due to cardiovascular events and longer survival*)

ISIS-4 Collaborative Group, 1995. ISIS-4: a randomised factorial trial assessing early oral captopril, oral mononitrate, and intravenous magnesium sulphate in 58050 patients with suspected acute myocardial infarction. Lancet 345, 669–685. (*Impressive trial: disappointing results! Magnesium was ineffective; oral nitrate did not reduce 1-month mortality*)

Køber, L., Torp-Pedersen, C., McMurray, J.J.V., et al., 2008. Increased mortality after dronedarone therapy for severe heart failure. N. Engl. J. Med. 358, 2678–2687.

Rahimtoola, S.H., 2004. Digitalis therapy for patients in clinical heart failure. Circulation 109, 2942–2946. (*Review*)

Roden, D.M., 2004. Drug therapy: drug-induced prolongation of the QT interval. N. Engl. J. Med. 350, 1013–1022. (*Adverse effect of great concern in drug development*)

Ruskin, J.N., 1989. The cardiac arrhythmia suppression trial (CAST). N. Engl. J. Med. 321, 386–388. (*Enormously influential trial showing increased mortality with active treatment despite suppression of dysrhythmia*)

The vascular system

22

OVERVIEW

This chapter is concerned with the pharmacology of blood vessels. The walls of arteries, arterioles, venules and veins contain smooth muscle whose contractile state is controlled by circulating hormones and by mediators released locally from sympathetic nerve terminals (Ch. 13) and endothelial cells. These work mainly by regulating Ca^{2+} in vascular smooth muscle cells, as described in Chapter 4. In the present chapter, we first consider the control of vascular smooth muscle by the endothelium and by the renin–angiotensin system, followed by the actions of vasoconstrictor and vasodilator drugs. Finally, we briefly consider clinical uses of vasoactive drugs in some important diseases, namely hypertension (pulmonary as well as systemic), heart failure, shock, peripheral vascular disease and Raynaud's disease. The use of vasoactive drugs to treat angina is covered in Chapter 21.

INTRODUCTION

Actions of drugs on the vascular system can be broken down into effects on:

- total systemic ('peripheral') vascular resistance, one of the main determinants of arterial blood pressure
- the resistance of individual vascular beds, which determines the local distribution of blood flow to and within different organs; such effects are relevant to the drug treatment of angina (Ch. 21), Raynaud's phenomenon, pulmonary hypertension and circulatory shock
- aortic compliance and pulse wave reflection, which are relevant to the treatment of hypertension, cardiac failure and angina
- venous tone and blood volume (the 'fullness' of the circulation), which together determine the central venous pressure and are relevant to the treatment of cardiac failure and angina; diuretics (which reduce blood volume) are discussed in Chapter 29
- atheroma (Ch. 23) and thrombosis (Ch. 24)
- new vessel formation (angiogenesis) – important, for example, in diabetic retinopathy (Ch. 31) and in treating malignant disease (Ch. 56).

Drug effects considered in this chapter are caused by actions on vascular smooth muscle cells. Like other muscles, vascular smooth muscle contracts when cytoplasmic Ca^{2+} ($[Ca^{2+}]_i$) rises, but the coupling between $[Ca^{2+}]_i$ and contraction is less tight than in striated or cardiac muscle (Ch. 4). Vasoconstrictors and vasodilators act by increasing or reducing $[Ca^{2+}]_i$, and/or by altering the sensitivity of the contractile machinery to $[Ca^{2+}]_i$.

Figure 4.10 (see Ch. 4) summarises cellular mechanisms that are involved in the control of smooth muscle contraction and relaxation. The control of vascular smooth muscle tone by various mediators is described in other chapters (noradrenaline in Ch. 14, 5-HT in Ch. 15, prostanoids in Ch. 17, nitric oxide (NO) in Ch. 20, cardiac natriuretic peptides in Ch. 21, antidiuretic hormone in Ch. 33). Here we focus on endothelium-derived mediators and on the renin–angiotensin–aldosterone system, before describing the actions of vasoactive drugs and their uses in some important clinical disorders (hypertension, heart failure, shock, peripheral vascular disease and Raynaud's disease).

VASCULAR STRUCTURE AND FUNCTION

Blood is ejected with each heartbeat from the left ventricle into the aorta, whence it flows rapidly to the organs via large conduit arteries. Successive branching leads via muscular arteries to arterioles (endothelium surrounded by a layer of smooth muscle only one cell thick) and capillaries (naked tubes of endothelium), where gas and nutrient exchanges occur. Capillaries coalesce to form postcapillary venules, venules and progressively larger veins leading, via the vena cava, to the right heart. Deoxygenated blood ejected from the right ventricle travels through the pulmonary artery, pulmonary capillaries and pulmonary veins back to the left atrium.[1] Small muscular arteries and arterioles are the main resistance vessels, while veins are capacity vessels that contain a large fraction of the total blood volume. In terms of cardiac function, therefore, arteries and arterioles regulate the *afterload*, while veins and pulmonary vessels regulate the *preload* of the ventricles (see Ch. 21).

Viscoelastic properties of large arteries determine arterial compliance (i.e. the degree to which the volume of the arterial system increases as the pressure increases). This is an important factor in a circulatory system that is driven by an intermittent pump such as the heart. Blood ejected from the left ventricle is accommodated by distension of the aorta, which absorbs the pulsations and delivers a relatively steady flow to the tissues. The greater the compliance of the aorta, the more effectively are fluctuations damped out,[2] and the smaller the oscillations of arterial pressure with each heartbeat (i.e. the difference

---

[1] William Harvey (physician to King Charles I) inferred the circulation of the blood on the basis of superbly elegant quantitative experiments long before the invention of the microscope enabled visual confirmation of the tiny vessels he had predicted. This intellectual triumph did his medical standing no good at all, and Aubrey wrote that 'he fell mightily in his practice, and was regarded by the vulgar as crack-brained'. *Plus ça change …*
[2] This cushioning action is called the 'windkessel' effect. The same principle was used to deliver a steady rather than intermittent flow from old-fashioned fire pumps.

265

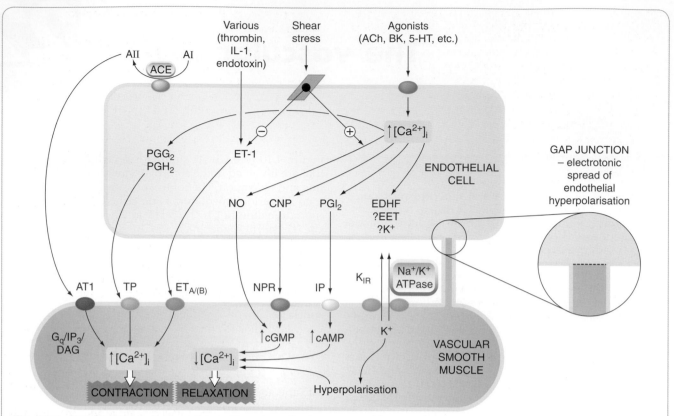

Fig. 22.1 Endothelium-derived mediators. The schematic shows some of the more important endothelium-derived contracting and relaxing mediators; many (if not all) of the vasoconstrictors also cause smooth muscle mitogenesis, while vasodilators commonly inhibit mitogenesis. 5-HT, 5-hydroxytryptamine; A, angiotensin; ACE, angiotensin-converting enzyme; ACh, acetylcholine; AT_1, angiotensin AT_1 receptor; BK, bradykinin; CNP, C-natriuretic peptide; DAG, diacylglycerol; EDHF, endothelium-derived hyperpolarising factor; EET, epoxyeicosatetraenoic acid; ET-1, endothelin-1; $ET_{A/(B)}$, endothelin A (and B) receptors; G_q, G protein; IL-1, interleukin-1; IP, I prostanoid receptor; IP_3, inosinol 1,4,5-trisphosphate; K_{IR}, inward rectifying potassium channel; Na^+/K^+ ATPase, electrogenic pump; NPR, natriuretic peptide receptor; PG, prostaglandin; TP, T prostanoid receptor.

between the systolic and diastolic pressure, known as the 'pulse pressure'). Reflection[3] of the pressure wave from branch points in the vascular tree also sustains arterial pressure during diastole. In young people this helps to preserve a steady perfusion of vital organs, such as the kidney, during diastole.

However, excessive reflection can pathologically augment aortic systolic pressure, because the less compliant the aorta the greater the pulse wave velocity. Consequently returning (reflected) pressure waves collide with the forward-going pulse wave from the next heart beat earlier in the cardiac cycle. This results from stiffening of the aorta due to loss of elastin during ageing, especially in people with hypertension. Elastin is replaced by inelastic collagen. Cardiac work (see Ch. 21) can be reduced by increasing arterial compliance or by reducing arterial wave reflection (both of which decease the pulse pressure), even if the cardiac output and mean arterial pressure are unchanged. Over the age of around 55 years, pulse pressure and aortic stiffness are important risk factors for cardiac disease.

CONTROL OF VASCULAR SMOOTH MUSCLE TONE

Two important physiological systems that regulate vascular tone, namely the vascular endothelium and the renin–angiotensin system, deserve special attention.

THE VASCULAR ENDOTHELIUM

A new chapter in our understanding of vascular control opened with the discovery that vascular endothelium acts not only as a passive barrier between plasma and extracellular fluid, but also as a source of numerous potent mediators. These actively control the underlying smooth muscle as well as influencing platelet and mononuclear cell function: the roles of the endothelium in haemostasis and thrombosis are discussed in Chapter 24. Several distinct classes of mediator are involved (Fig. 22.1).

- *Prostanoids* (see Ch. 17). The discovery by Bunting, Gryglewski, Moncada and Vane (1976) of prostaglandin PGI_2 (prostacyclin) ushered in this era. This mediator, acting on IP receptors (Ch. 17), relaxes smooth muscle and inhibits platelet aggregation by activating adenylyl cyclase. Endothelial cells from microvessels also synthesise

---

[3]Think of the waves in your bath as you sit up: down the tub, a splash down the overflow but most comes back as reflections from the foot end under the taps and interacts with the forward waves.

Vascular smooth muscle

- Vascular smooth muscle is controlled by mediators secreted by sympathetic nerves (Chs 21 and 14) and vascular endothelium, and by circulating hormones.
- Smooth muscle cell contraction is initiated by a rise in $[Ca^{2+}]_i$, which activates myosin light-chain kinase, causing phosphorylation of myosin, or by sensitisation of the myofilaments to Ca^{2+} by inhibition of myosin phosphatase (see Ch. 4).
- Agents cause contraction via one or more mechanism:
  - release of intracellular Ca^{2+} via inositol trisphosphate
  - depolarising the membrane, opening voltage-gated calcium channels and causing Ca^{2+} entry
  - increasing sensitivity to Ca^{2+} via actions on myosin light-chain kinase and/or myosin phosphatase (Ch. 4, Fig. 4.9).
- Agents cause relaxation by:
  - inhibiting Ca^{2+} entry through voltage-gated calcium channels either directly (e.g. **nifedipine**) or indirectly by hyperpolarising the membrane (e.g. potassium channel activators such as the active metabolite of **minoxidil**)
  - increasing intracellular cAMP or cGMP; cAMP inactivates myosin light-chain kinase and facilitates Ca^{2+} efflux, cGMP opposes agonist-induced increases in $[Ca^{2+}]_i$.

PGE$_2$, which is a direct vasodilator and inhibits noradrenaline release from sympathetic nerve terminals, while lacking the effect of PGI$_2$ on platelets. Prostaglandin endoperoxide intermediates (PGG$_2$, PGH$_2$) are endothelium-derived contracting factors acting via thromboxane (TX) TP receptors.

- *Nitric oxide (NO)* (see Ch. 20). *Endothelium-derived relaxing factor* (EDRF) was described by Furchgott and Zawadzki in 1980, and identified as NO by the groups of Moncada and of Ignarro (see Fig. 20.2). These discoveries enormously expanded our understanding of the role of the endothelium. NO activates guanylyl cyclase. It is released continuously in resistance vessels, giving rise to vasodilator tone and contributing to the physiological control of blood pressure. As well as causing vascular relaxation, it inhibits vascular smooth muscle cell proliferation, inhibits platelet adhesion and aggregation, and inhibits monocyte adhesion and migration; consequently, it may protect blood vessels from atherosclerosis and thrombosis (see Chs 23 and 24).
- *Peptides.* The endothelium secretes several vasoactive peptides (see Ch. 18 for general mechanisms of peptide secretion). *C-natriuretic peptide* (Ch. 21) and *adrenomedulin* (a vasodilator peptide originally discovered in an adrenal tumour – phaeochromocytoma – but expressed in many tissues, including vascular endothelium) are vasodilators working, respectively, through cGMP and cAMP. *Angiotensin II*, formed by angiotensin-converting enzyme (ACE) on the surface of endothelial cells (see p. 270), and *endothelin* are

potent endothelium-derived vasoconstrictor peptides.

- *Endothelium-derived hyperpolarisation factors (EDHFs).* PGI$_2$ and NO each hyperpolarise vascular smooth muscle, and this can contribute to their relaxant effects. Endothelium-dependent dilatation and hyperpolarisation in response to several mediators (including acetylcholine and bradykinin) persists in some vessels in the absence of prostaglandin and NO synthesis. Several endothelium-derived mediators have been implicated, including *epoxyeicosatrienoic acids* (EETs – derived from endothelial cytochrome P450 enzymes), various lipoxygenase (LOX) products, *hydrogen peroxide* (H_2O_2), *carbon monoxide* (CO), *hydrogen sulphide* (H_2S), and *C-natriuretic peptide* (CNP) – see Félétou & Vanhoutte (2009). These authors define an additional 'endothelium-derived hyperpolarising factor' (EDHF) distinct from these mediators, and dependent on calcium-activated potassium (K_{Ca}) channels in endothelial cells. As the name implies, these channels are activated by an increase in endothelial cell $[Ca^{2+}]_i$.

In addition to secreting vasoactive mediators, endothelial cells express several enzymes and transport mechanisms that act on circulating hormones and are important targets of drug action. Angiotensin-converting enzyme (ACE) is a particularly important example (see p. 270, including Figs 22.4 and 22.5).

Many endothelium-derived mediators are mutually antagonistic, conjuring an image of opposing rugby football players swaying back and forth in a scrum; in moments of exasperation, one sometimes wonders whether all this makes sense or whether the designer simply could not make up their mind! An important distinction is made between mechanisms that are tonically active in resistance vessels under basal conditions, as is the case with the noradrenergic nervous system (Ch. 14), NO (Ch. 20) and endothelin (see p. 268-269), and those that operate mainly in response to injury, inflammation, etc., as with PGI$_2$. Some of the latter group may be functionally redundant, perhaps representing vestiges of mechanisms that were important to our evolutionary forebears, or they may simply be taking a breather on the touchline and are ready to rejoin the fray if called on by the occurrence of some vascular insult. Evidence for such a 'back-up' role comes, for example, from mice that lack the IP receptor for PGI$_2$, and that have a normal blood pressure and do not develop spontaneous thrombosis, but are more susceptible to vasoconstrictor and thrombotic stimuli than their wild-type litter mates (Murata et al., 1997).

THE ENDOTHELIUM IN ANGIOGENESIS

As touched on in Chapter 8, the barrier function of vascular endothelium differs markedly in different organs, and its development during angiogenesis is controlled by several growth factors, including *vascular endothelial growth factor (VEGF)* and various tissue-specific factors such as endocrine gland VEGF. These are involved in repair processes and in pathogenesis (e.g. tumour growth and in neovascularisation in the eye – an important cause of blindness in patients with diabetes mellitus). These factors and their receptors are potentially fruitful targets for drug development and new therapies (including gene therapies; Ch. 59).

Table 22.1   Distribution of endothelins and endothelin receptors in various tissues[a]

	Endothelin			Endothelin receptor	
Tissues	*1*	*2*	*3*	*ET_A*	*ET_B*
Vascular tissue Endothelium	++++				+
Smooth muscle	+			++	
Brain	+++		+	+	+++
Kidney	++	++	+	+	++
Intestines	+	+	+++	+	+++
Adrenal gland	+		+++	+	++

[a]Levels of expression of endothelins or the receptor mRNA and/or immunoreactive endothelins: ++++, highest; +++, high; ++, moderate; +, low.
Adapted from Masaki T 1993 Endocr Rev 14, 256–268.

ENDOTHELIN

Discovery, biosynthesis and secretion

Hickey et al. described a vasoconstrictor factor produced by cultured endothelial cells in 1985. This was identified as *endothelin*, a 21-residue peptide, by Yanagisawa et al. (1988), who achieved the isolation, analysis and cloning of the gene for this peptide, which at that time was the most potent vasoconstrictor known,[4] in an impressively short space of time.

▼ Three genes encode different sequences (ET-1, ET-2 and ET-3), each with a distinctive 'shepherd's crook' structure produced by two internal disulfide bonds. These isoforms are differently expressed in organs such as brain and adrenal glands (Table 22.1), suggesting that endothelins have functions beyond the cardiovascular system and this is supported by observations of mice in which the gene coding for ET-1 is disrupted (see below). ET-1 is the only endothelin present in endothelial cells, and is also expressed in many other tissues. Its synthesis and actions are summarised schematically in Figure 22.2. ET-2 is much less widely distributed: it is present in kidney and intestine. ET-3 is present in brain, lung, intestine and adrenal gland. ET-1 is synthesised from a 212-residue precursor molecule (prepro-ET), which is processed to 'big ET-1' and finally cleaved by an endothelin-converting enzyme to yield ET-1. Cleavage occurs not at the usual Lys–Arg or Arg–Arg position (see Ch. 18), but at a Trp–Val pair, implying a very atypical endopeptidase. The converting enzyme is a metalloprotease and is inhibited by **phosphoramidon** (a pharmacological tool but not used therapeutically). Big ET-1 is converted to ET-1 intracellularly and also on the surface of endothelial and smooth muscle cells.

Stimuli of endothelin synthesis include many vasoconstrictor mediators released by trauma or inflammation, including activated platelets, endotoxin, thrombin, various cytokines and growth factors, angiotensin II, antidiuretic hormone (ADH), adrenaline, insulin, hypoxia and low shear stress. Inhibitors of ET synthesis include NO, natriuretic peptides, PGE_2, PGI_2, heparin and high shear stress.

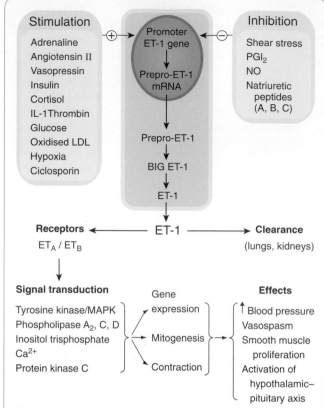

Fig. 22.2   Endothelin-1 (ET-1) synthesis and actions. The schematic shows some of the more important actions only. IL-1, interleukin-1; LDL, low-density lipoprotein; MAPK, mitogen-activated protein kinase; NO, nitric oxide; PGI_2, prostaglandin I_2.

Release of ET-1 is poorly understood. Preformed ET-1 can be stored in endothelial cells, although probably not in granules. ET-1 concentration in plasma is too low (<5 pmol/l) to activate endothelin receptors, but concentrations in the extracellular space between endothelium and vascular smooth muscle are presumably much higher, since endothelin receptor antagonists (see below) cause vasodilatation when infused directly into the brachial artery, implying tonic ET-1-mediated vasoconstrictor activity in resistance vasculature. ET-1 has a plasma half-life of less than 5 min, despite a much longer duration of action, and clearance occurs mainly in the lung and kidneys.

Endothelin receptors and responses

There are two types of endothelin receptor, designated ET_A and ET_B (Table 22.2), both of which are G protein-coupled (Ch. 3). The predominant overall response is vasoconstriction.

▼ Endothelin-1 preferentially activates ET_A receptors. Messenger RNA for the ET_A receptor is expressed in many human tissues, including vascular smooth muscle, heart, lung and kidney. It is not expressed in endothelium. ET_A-mediated responses include vasoconstriction, bronchoconstriction and aldosterone secretion. ET_A receptors are coupled to phospholipase C, which stimulates Na^+/H^+ exchange, protein kinase C and mitogenesis, as well as causing vasoconstriction through inositol trisphosphate-mediated Ca^{2+} release (Ch. 3). There are several partially selective ET_A-receptor antagonists, including BQ-123 (a cyclic pentapeptide) and several

---

[4]Subsequently an 11-amino acid peptide (*urotensin*) was isolated from the brains of bony fish and found to be 50–100 times more potent than endothelin in some blood vessels. It and its receptor are expressed in human tissue but its function, if any, in man remains enigmatic.

Table 22.2 Endothelin receptors

Receptor	Affinity	Pharmacological response
ET$_A$	ET-1 = ET-2 > ET-3	Vasoconstriction, bronchoconstriction, stimulation of aldosterone secretion
ET$_B$	ET-1 = ET-2 = ET-3	Vasodilatation, inhibition of *ex vivo* platelet aggregation

From Masaki T 1993 Endocr Rev 14, 256–268.

orally active non-peptide drugs (e.g. **bosentan**, a mixed ET$_A$/ET$_B$ antagonist used in treating pulmonary arterial hypertension – see p. 282-283). ET$_B$ receptors are activated to a similar extent by each of the three endothelin isoforms, but *sarafotoxin S6c* (a 21-residue peptide that shares the shepherd's crook structure of the endothelins and was isolated from the venom of the burrowing asp) is a selective agonist and has proved useful as a pharmacological tool for studying the ET$_B$ receptor. Messenger RNA for the ET$_B$ receptor is mainly expressed in brain (especially cerebral cortex and cerebellum), with moderate expression in aorta, heart, lung, kidney and adrenals. In contrast to the ET$_A$ receptor, it is highly expressed in endothelium, where it may initiate *vasodilatation* by stimulating NO and PGI$_2$ production, but it is also present in vascular smooth muscle, where it initiates vasoconstriction like the ET$_A$ receptor. ET$_B$ receptors play a part in clearing ET-1 from the circulation, and ET antagonists with appreciable affinity for ET$_B$ receptors consequently increase plasma concentrations of ET-1, complicating interpretation of experiments with these drugs.

Functions of endothelin

Endothelin-1 is a local mediator rather than a circulating hormone, although it stimulates secretion of several hormones (see Table 22.1). Administration of an ET$_A$-receptor antagonist or of phosphoramidon into the brachial artery increases forearm blood flow, and ET$_A$ receptor antagonists lower arterial blood pressure, suggesting that ET-1 contributes to vasoconstrictor tone and the control of peripheral vascular resistance in man. Endothelins have several other possible functions, including roles in:

- release of various hormones, including atrial natriuretic peptide, aldosterone, adrenaline, and hypothalamic and pituitary hormones
- natriuresis and diuresis via actions of collecting duct-derived ET-1 on ET$_B$ receptors on tubular epithelial cells
- thyroglobulin synthesis (the concentration of ET-1 in thyroid follicles is extremely high)
- control of uteroplacental blood flow (ET-1 is present in very high concentrations in amniotic fluid)
- renal and cerebral vasospasm (Fig. 22.3)
- development of the cardiorespiratory systems (if the ET-1 gene is disrupted in mice, pharyngeal arch tissues develop abnormally and homozygotes die of respiratory failure at birth), and ET receptor antagonists are teratogenic, causing cardiorespiratory developmental disorders.

THE RENIN–ANGIOTENSIN SYSTEM

The renin–angiotensin system synergises with the sympathetic nervous system, for example by increasing the release of noradrenaline from sympathetic nerve

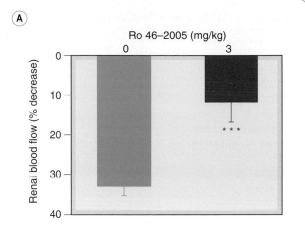

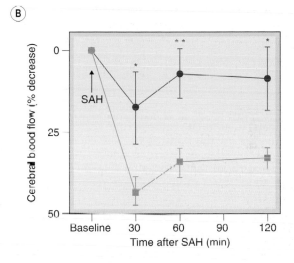

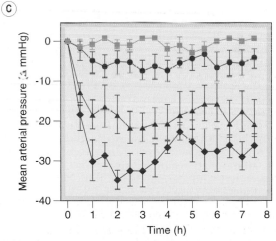

Fig. 22.3 *In vivo* effects of a potent non-peptide endothelin-1 ET$_A$- and ET$_B$-receptor antagonist, Ro 46-2005, in three animal models. [**A**] Prevention by Ro 46-2005 of post-ischaemic renal vasoconstriction in rats. [**B**] Prevention by Ro 46-2005 of the decrease in cerebral blood flow after subarachnoid haemorrhage (SAH) in rats treated with placebo (blue) or with Ro 46-2005 (red). [**C**] Effect of orally administered Ro 46-2005 on mean arterial pressure in sodium-depleted squirrel monkeys treated with placebo (blue) or increasing doses of antagonist (red: ♦ < ▲ < ⬇). (From Clozel M et al. 1993 Nature 365, 759–761.)

The role of the endothelium in controlling vascular smooth muscle

- Endothelial cells release vasoactive mediators including prostacyclin (PGI_2), nitric oxide (NO) and distinct but incompletely characterised hyperpolarising factor(s) 'EDHF' (vasodilators), and endothelin and endoperoxide thromboxane receptor agonists (vasoconstrictors).
- Many vasodilators (e.g. acetylcholine and bradykinin) act via endothelial NO production. The NO derives from arginine and is produced when $[Ca^{2+}]_i$ increases in the endothelial cell, or the sensitivity of endothelial NO synthase to Ca^{2+} is increased (see Fig. 20.3).
- NO relaxes smooth muscle by increasing cGMP formation.
- Endothelin is a potent and long-acting vasoconstrictor peptide released from endothelial cells by many chemical and physical factors. It is not confined to blood vessels, and it has several functional roles.

terminals. It stimulates aldosterone secretion and plays a central role in the control of Na⁺ excretion and fluid volume, as well as of vascular tone.

The control of renin secretion (Fig. 22.4) is only partly understood. It is a proteolytic enzyme that is secreted by the *juxtaglomerular apparatus* (see Ch. 29, Fig. 29.2) in response to various physiological stimuli including reduced renal perfusion pressure, or reduced Na⁺ concentration in distal tubular fluid which is sensed by the *macula densa* (a specialised part of the distal tubule apposed to the juxtaglomerular apparatus). Renal sympathetic nerve activity, β-adrenoceptor agonists and PGI_2 all stimulate renin secretion directly, whereas angiotensin II causes feedback inhibition. Atrial natriuretic peptide (Ch. 21) also inhibits renin secretion. Renin is cleared rapidly from plasma. It acts on *angiotensinogen* (a plasma globulin made in the liver), splitting off a decapeptide, *angiotensin I*.

Angiotensin I is inactive, but is converted by *angiotensin-converting enzyme* (ACE) to an octapeptide, *angiotensin II*, which is a potent vasoconstrictor. Angiotensin II is a substrate for enzymes (aminopeptidase A and N) that remove single amino acid residues, giving rise, respectively, to angiotensin III and angiotensin IV (Fig. 22.5). Angiotensin III stimulates aldosterone secretion and is involved in thirst. Angiotensin IV also has distinct actions, probably via its own receptor, including release of *plasminogen activator inhibitor-1* from the endothelium (Ch. 24). Receptors for angiotensin IV have a distinctive distribution, including the hypothalamus.

Angiotensin-converting enzyme is a membrane-bound enzyme on the surface of endothelial cells, and is particularly abundant in the lung, which has a vast surface area of vascular endothelium.[5] The common isoform of ACE is also present in other vascular tissues, including heart, brain, striated muscle and kidney, and is not restricted to endothelial cells.[6] Consequently, local formation of

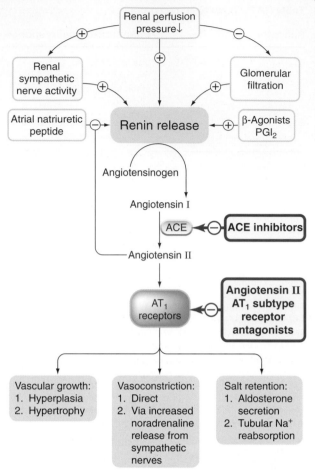

Fig. 22.4 **Control of renin release and formation, and action of angiotensin II.** Sites of action of drugs that inhibit the cascade are shown. ACE, angiotensin-converting enzyme; AT_1, angiotensin II receptor subtype 1.

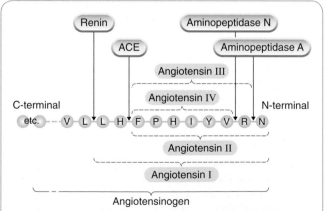

Fig. 22.5 **Formation of angiotensins I–IV from the N-terminal of the precursor protein angiotensinogen.**

angiotensin II can occur in different vascular beds, and it provides local control independent of blood-borne angiotensin II. ACE inactivates bradykinin (see Ch. 18) and

[5]Approximately that of a football field.

[6]A different isoform of ACE is also present in testis, and male mice lacking this ACE have markedly reduced fertility.

Table 22.3 Classification of vasoactive drugs that act indirectly

Site	Mechanism	Examples	See chapter
Vasoconstrictors			
Sympathetic nerves	Noradrenaline (norepinephrine) release	Tyramine	14
	Blocks noradrenaline reuptake	Cocaine	14
Endothelium	Endothelin release	Angiotensin II (in part)	This chapter
Vasodilators			
Sympathetic nerves	Inhibits noradrenaline release	Prostaglandin E_2, guanethidine	12, 14
Endothelium	Nitric oxide release	Acetylcholine, substance P	20
Central nervous system	Vasomotor inhibition	Anaesthetics	40
Enzymes	Angiotensin-converting enzyme inhibition	Captopril	This chapter

several other peptides. This may contribute to the pharmacological actions of ACE inhibitors, as discussed below. The main actions of angiotensin II are mediated via AT_1 and/or AT_2 receptors, which belong to the family of G protein-coupled receptors. Effects mediated by AT_1 receptors include:

- generalised vasoconstriction, especially marked in efferent arterioles of the renal glomeruli
- increased noradrenaline release, reinforcing sympathetic effects
- proximal tubular reabsorption of Na^+
- secretion of aldosterone from the adrenal cortex (see Ch. 33)
- growth of cardiac and vascular cells.[7]

AT_2 receptors are expressed during fetal life and in distinct brain regions in adults. They may be involved in growth, development and exploratory behaviour. Cardiovascular effects of AT_2 receptors (inhibition of cell growth and lowering of blood pressure) are relatively subtle and oppose those of AT_1 receptors.

The renin–angiotensin–aldosterone pathway contributes to the pathogenesis of heart failure, and several leading classes of therapeutic drug act on it at different points (see Fig. 22.4).

VASOACTIVE DRUGS

Drugs can affect vascular smooth muscle by acting either directly on smooth muscle cells, or indirectly, for example on endothelial cells, on sympathetic nerve terminals or on the central nervous system (CNS) (Table 22.3). Mechanisms of directly acting vasoconstrictors and vasodilators are summarised in Figure 4.10 (Ch. 4). Many indirectly acting drugs are discussed in other chapters (see Table 22.3). We concentrate here on agents that are not covered elsewhere.

VASOCONSTRICTOR DRUGS

The α_1-adrenoceptor agonists and drugs that release noradrenaline from sympathetic nerve terminals or inhibit its reuptake (sympathomimetic amines) are discussed in Chapter 14. Some eicosanoids (e.g. *thromboxane A₂*; see Chs 17 and 24) and several peptides, notably *endothelin*, *angiotensin* and *ADH*, are also predominantly vasoconstrictor. **Sumatriptan** and ergot alkaloids acting on certain 5-hydroxytryptamine receptors ($5-HT_2$ and $5-HT_{1D}$) also cause vasoconstriction (Ch. 15).

ANGIOTENSIN II

The physiological role of the renin–angiotensin system is described above. Angiotensin II is roughly 40 times as potent as noradrenaline in raising blood pressure. Like α_1-adrenoceptor agonists, it constricts mainly cutaneous, splanchnic and renal vasculature, with less effect on blood flow to brain and skeletal muscle. It has no routine clinical uses, its therapeutic importance lying in the fact that other drugs (e.g. **captopril** and **losartan**, see p. 274–276) affect the cardiovascular system by reducing its production or action.

ANTIDIURETIC HORMONE

Antidiuretic hormone (ADH, also known as vasopressin) is a posterior pituitary peptide hormone (Ch. 33). It is important for its antidiuretic action on the kidney (Ch. 29) but is also a powerful vasoconstrictor in skin and some other vascular beds. Its effects are initiated by two distinct receptors (V_1 and V_2). Water retention is mediated through V_2 receptors, occurs at low plasma concentrations of ADH and involves activation of adenylyl cyclase in renal collecting ducts. Vasoconstriction is mediated through V_1 receptors (two subtypes, see Ch. 33), requires higher concentrations of ADH and involves activation of phospholipase C (see Ch. 3). ADH causes generalised vasoconstriction, including the coeliac, mesenteric and coronary vessels. It also affects other (e.g. gastrointestinal and uterine) smooth muscle and causes abdominal cramps for this reason. It is sometimes used to treat patients with bleeding oesophageal varices and portal hypertension before more definitive treatment, although many

[7]These effects are initiated by the G protein-coupled AT_1 receptor acting via the same intracellular tyrosine phosphorylation pathways as are used by cytokines, for example the Jak/Stat pathway (Ch. 3).

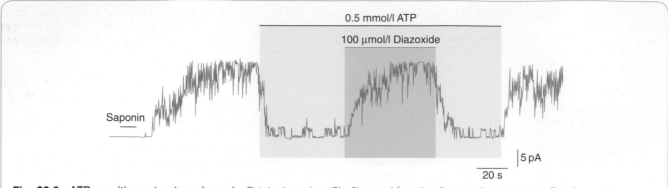

Fig. 22.6 **ATP-sensitive potassium channels.** Patch clamp (see Ch. 3) record from insulin-secreting pancreatic B cell: saponin permeabilised the cell, with loss of intracellular ATP, causing the channels to open (upward deflection) until they were inhibited by ATP. Addition of diazoxide, a vasodilator drug (which also inhibits insulin secretion; see text) reopens the channels. In smooth muscle, this causes hyperpolarisation and relaxation. *(Redrawn from Dunne et al. 1990 Br J Pharmacol 99, 169.)*

gastroenterologists prefer to use **octreotide** (unlicensed indication; see Ch. 33) for this. It may also have a place in treating hypotensive shock (see p. 281).

ENDOTHELIN

Endothelins are discussed above in the context of their physiological roles; as explained above, they have vasodilator and vasoconstrictor actions, but vasoconstriction predominates. Intravenous administration causes transient vasodilatation followed by profound and long-lived vasoconstriction. The endothelins are even more potent vasoconstrictors than angiotensin II. As yet, they have no clinical uses, and ET antagonists are licensed only for the rare disease primary pulmonary hypertension (see p. 282).

Vasoconstrictor substances

- The main groups are sympathomimetic amines (direct and indirect; Ch. 14), certain eicosanoids (especially thromboxane A$_2$; Ch. 17), peptides (angiotensin II, antidiuretic hormone [ADH] and endothelin; Ch. 19) and a group of miscellaneous drugs (e.g. ergot alkaloids; Ch. 15).
- Clinical uses include local applications (e.g. nasal decongestion, co-administration with local anaesthetics). Sympathomimetic amines and **ADH** are used in circulatory shock. **Adrenaline** is life-saving in anaphylactic shock and in cardiac arrest. **ADH** or **terlipressin** (an analogue) has been infused intravenously to stop bleeding from oesophageal varices prior to surgery in patients with portal hypertension caused by liver disease.

VASODILATOR DRUGS

Vasodilator drugs play a major role in the treatment of common conditions, including hypertension, cardiac failure and angina pectoris, as well as several less common but severe diseases, including pulmonary hypertension and Raynaud's disease.

DIRECT ACTING VASODILATORS

Targets on which drugs act to relax vascular smooth muscle include plasma membrane voltage-dependent calcium channels, sarcoplasmic reticulum channels (Ca^{2+} release or reuptake) and enzymes that determine Ca^{2+} sensitivity of the contractile proteins (see Fig. 4.10).[8]

Calcium antagonists

L-type calcium antagonists are discussed in Chapter 21. As well as their actions on the heart they cause generalised arterial vasodilatation, although individual agents exhibit distinct patterns of regional potency. Dihydropyridines (e.g. **nifedipine**) act preferentially on vascular smooth muscle, whereas **verapamil** acts directly on the heart (negative chronotropic and inotropic effects) in addition to causing vasodilatation; **diltiazem** is intermediate in specificity. Consequently, rapid-acting dihydropyridines usually produce reflex tachycardia, whereas verapamil and diltiazem do not.

Drugs that activate potassium channels

Some drugs (e.g. **minoxidil**, **diazoxide**) relax smooth muscle by opening K$_{ATP}$ channels (see Fig. 22.6). This hyperpolarises the cells and switches off voltage-dependent calcium channels. Potassium channel activators work by antagonising the action of intracellular ATP on these channels.

Minoxidil (acting through an active sulphate metabolite) is an especially potent and long-acting vasodilator, used as a drug of last resort in treating severe hypertension unresponsive to other drugs. It causes hirsutism (the active metabolite is actually used as a rub-on cream to treat baldness, see Ch. 27). It causes marked salt and water retention, so is usually prescribed with a loop diuretic. It causes reflex tachycardia, and a β-adrenoceptor antagonist is used to prevent this. **Nicorandil** (Ch. 21) combines K$_{ATP}$ channel activation with NO donor activity, and is used in refractory angina. **Levosimendan** combines K$_{ATP}$ channel activation with sensitisation of the cardiac contractile mechanism to Ca^{2+} by binding troponin C (Ch. 21), and is used in decompensated heart failure (see p. 281).

---

[8]A pyridine drug, Y27632, causes vasorelaxation by inhibiting a Rho-associated protein kinase, thereby selectively inhibiting smooth muscle contraction by inhibiting Ca^{2+} sensitisation.

Drugs that act via cyclic nucleotides

Cyclase activation

Many drugs relax vascular smooth muscle by increasing the cellular concentration of either cGMP or cAMP. For example, NO, nitrates and the natriuretic peptides act through cGMP (see Chs 20 and 21); BAY41-2272, a pyrazolopyridine, activates soluble guanylyl cyclase via an NO-independent site (see Ch. 20). The β_2 agonists, adenosine and PGI_2 increase cytoplasmic cAMP (see Ch. 14). Dopamine has mixed vasodilator and vasoconstrictor actions. It selectively dilates renal vessels, where it increases cAMP by activating adenylyl cyclase. Dopamine, when administered as an intravenous infusion, produces a mixture of cardiovascular effects resulting from agonist actions on α and β adrenoceptors, as well as on dopamine receptors. Blood pressure increases slightly, but the main effects are vasodilatation in the renal circulation and increased cardiac output. Dopamine was widely used in intensive care units in patients in whom renal failure associated with decreased renal perfusion appeared imminent; despite its beneficial effect on renal haemodynamics, clinical trials have shown that it does not improve survival in these circumstances and this use is obsolete.. **Nesiritide**, a recombinant form of human B-type natriuretic peptide (BNP) (see Ch. 21), was widely used in the USA for the treatment of acutely decompensated heart failure, but efficacy data have not been impressive (O'Connor et al., 2011).

Nitroprusside (nitroferricyanide) is a powerful vasodilator with little effect outside the vascular system, which acts by releasing NO (Ch 20). Unlike the organic nitrates, which preferentially dilate capacitance vessels and muscular arteries, it acts equally on arterial and venous smooth muscle. Its clinical usefulness is limited because it must be given intravenously. In solution, particularly when exposed to light, nitroprusside hydrolyses with formation of cyanide. The intravenous solution must therefore be made up freshly from dry powder and protected from light. Nitroprusside is rapidly converted to thiocyanate in the body, its plasma half-life being only a few minutes, so it must be given as a continuous infusion with careful monitoring to avoid hypotension. Prolonged use causes thiocyanate accumulation and toxicity (weakness, nausea and inhibition of thyroid function); consequently, nitroprusside is useful only for short-term treatment (usually up to 72 h maximum). It is used in intensive care units for hypertensive emergencies, to produce controlled hypotension during surgery, and to reduce cardiac work during the reversible cardiac dysfunction that occurs after cardiopulmonary bypass surgery.

Phosphodiesterase inhibition

Phosphodiesterases (PDEs; see Ch. 3) include at least 14 distinct isoenzymes. Methylxanthines (e.g. **theophylline**) and **papaverine** are non-selective PDE inhibitors (and have additional actions). Methylxanthines exert their main effects on bronchial smooth muscle and on the CNS, and are discussed in Chapters 28 and 48. In addition to inhibiting PDE, some methylxanthines are also purine receptor antagonists (Ch. 16). Papaverine is produced by opium poppies (see Ch. 42) and is chemically related to **morphine**. However, pharmacologically it is quite unlike morphine, its main action being to relax smooth muscle. Its mechanism is poorly understood but seems to involve a combination of PDE inhibition and block of calcium channels. Selective PDE type III inhibitors (e.g. **milrinone**)

increase cAMP in cardiac muscle. They have a positive inotropic effect but, despite short-term haemodynamic improvement, increase mortality in patients with heart failure, possibly by causing dysrhythmias. **Dipyridamole**, as well as enhancing the actions of adenosine (see Ch. 16), also causes vasodilatation by inhibiting phosphodiesterase. It is used to prevent stroke, but can provoke angina. Selective *PDE type V* inhibitors (e.g. **sildenafil**) inhibit the breakdown of cGMP. Penile erection is caused by nitrergic nerves in the pelvis. These release NO (Ch. 20), which activates guanylyl cyclase in smooth muscle in the corpora cavernosa. Taken by mouth about an hour before sexual stimulation, sildenafil increases penile erection by potentiating this pathway. It has revolutionised treatment of erectile dysfunction (see Ch. 35) and has therapeutic potential in other situations, including pulmonary hypertension (see clinical box, p. 282) by potentiating NO.

> ### Vasodilator drugs
>
> - Vasodilators act:
>   - to increase local tissue blood flow
>   - to reduce arterial pressure
>   - to reduce central venous pressure.
> - Net effect is to reduce cardiac preload (reduced filling pressure) and afterload (reduced vascular resistance), hence reduction of cardiac work.
> - Main uses are:
>   - antihypertensive therapy (e.g. AT_1 antagonists, calcium antagonists and α_1-adrenoceptor antagonists)
>   - treatment/prophylaxis of angina (e.g. calcium antagonists, nitrates)
>   - treatment of cardiac failure (e.g. angiotensin-converting enzyme inhibitors, AT_1 antagonists)
>   - treatment of erectile dysfunction.

VASODILATORS WITH UNKNOWN MECHANISM OF ACTION

Hydralazine

Hydralazine acts mainly on arteries and arterioles, causing a fall in blood pressure accompanied by reflex tachycardia and increased cardiac output. It interferes with the action of inositol trisphosphate on Ca^{2+} release from the sarcoplasmic reticulum. Its original clinical use was in hypertension, and is still used for short-term treatment of severe hypertension in pregnancy but it can cause an immune disorder resembling systemic lupus erythematosus,[9] so alternative agents are now usually preferred for long-term treatment of hypertension. It has a place in treating heart failure in patients of African origin in combination with a long-acting organic nitrate (see clinical box, p. 281).

Ethanol

Ethanol (see Ch. 49) dilates cutaneous vessels, causing the familiar drunkard's flush. Several general anaesthetics (e.g. **propofol**) cause vasodilatation as an unwanted effect (Ch. 41).

---

[9]An autoimmune disease affecting one or more tissues, including joints, blood platelets, skin and pleural membranes. It is characterised by auto-antibodies including antibodies directed against DNA.

INDIRECTLY ACTING VASODILATOR DRUGS

The two main groups of indirectly acting vasodilator drugs are inhibitors of the main vasoconstrictor systems, namely the sympathetic nervous system (see Ch. 14 for a discussion of drugs that interfere with sympathetic neurotransmission) and the renin–angiotensin–aldosterone system.

The central control of sympathetically mediated vasoconstriction is believed to involve α_2 adrenoceptors and also another class of receptor, termed the *imidazoline I_1 receptor*, present in the brain stem in the rostral ventrolateral medulla. **Clonidine** (an α_2-adrenoceptor agonist, now largely obsolete as an antihypertensive drug) and **moxonodine**, an I_1-receptor agonist, lower blood pressure by reducing sympathetic activity centrally. In addition, many vasodilators (e.g. acetylcholine, bradykinin, substance P) exert some or all of their effects by stimulating biosynthesis of vasodilator prostaglandins or of NO (or of both) by vascular endothelium (see above and Ch. 20),

thereby causing functional antagonism of the constrictor tone caused by sympathetic nerves and angiotensin II.

Many useful drugs act by blocking the renin–angiotensin–aldosterone system (RAAS; see Table 22.4 for a summary of selective antagonists), which can be inhibited at several points:

- renin release: β-adrenoceptor antagonists inhibit renin release (although their other actions can result in a small increase in peripheral vascular resistance)
- renin activity: renin inhibitors inhibit conversion of angiotensinogen to angiotensin I
- ACE: ACE inhibitors (ACEIs, see below) block conversion of angiotensin I to angiotensin II
- angiotensin II receptors: AT_1-receptor antagonists (ARBs, see below)
- aldosterone receptors: aldosterone-receptor antagonists (see below).

Table 22.4 Summary of drugs that inhibit the renin–angiotensin–aldosterone system

Class	Drug[a]	Pharmacokinetics	Adverse effects[b]	Uses	Notes
ACE inhibitors	Captopril	Short acting $t_{1/2}$ ~2 h Dose 2–3 times daily	Cough Hypotension Proteinuria Taste disturbance	Hypertension Heart failure After MI	ACEIs are cleared mainly by renal excretion
	Enalapril	Pro-drug – active metabolite enalaprilat $t_{1/2}$ ~11 h Dose 1–2 times daily	Cough Hypotension Reversible renal impairment (in patients with renal artery stenosis)	As captopril	Lisinopril, perindopril, ramipril, trandalopril are similar Some are licensed for distinct uses (e.g. stroke, left ventricular hypertrophy)
Angiotensin receptor blockers (ARBs)	Valsartan	$t_{1/2}$ ~6 h	Hypotension Reversible renal impairment (in patients with renal artery stenosis)	Hypertension Heart failure	ARBs are cleared by hepatic metabolism
	Losartan	Long-acting metabolite $t_{1/2}$ ~8 h	As valsartan	As valsartan Diabetic nephropathy	Irbesartan is similar, with $t_{1/2}$ ~10–15 h
	Candesartan	$t_{1/2}$ 5–10 h Long acting because receptor complex is stable	As valsartan	As valsartan	Given as prodrug ester (candesartan cilexetil)
Renin inhibitor	Aliskiren	Low oral bioavailability $t_{1/2}$ 24 h	As valsartan, also diarrhoea	Essential hypertension	Contraindicated in patients with renal disease, diabetes
Aldosterone antagonists	Eplerenone	$t_{1/2}$ 3–5 h	As valsartan, especially hyperkalemia Nausea, diarrhoea	Heart failure after MI	
	Spironolactone	Prodrug converted to canrenone, which has $t_{1/2}$ ~24 h	As eplerenone Also oestrogenic effects (gynaecomastia, menstrual irregularity, erectile dysfunction)	Primary hyperaldosteronism Heart failure Oedema and ascites (e.g. in hepatic cirrhosis)	

[a]All drugs listed are orally active.
[b]Adverse effects common to all drugs listed include hyperkalemia (especially in patients with impaired renal function) and teratogenesis.
ACEI, angiotensin-converting enzyme inhibitor; MI, myocardial infarction.

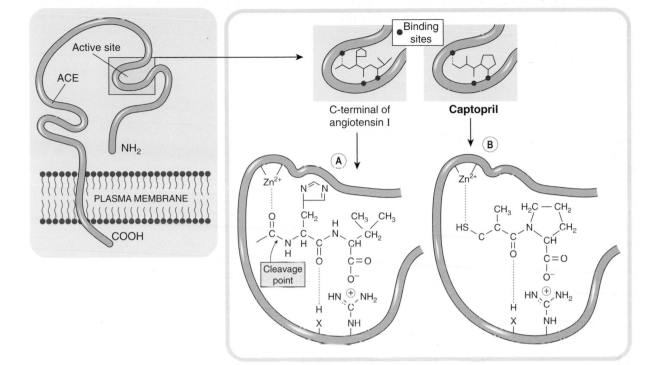

Fig. 22.7 The active site of angiotensin-converting enzyme. [**A**] Binding of angiotensin I. [**B**] Binding of the inhibitor captopril, which is an analogue of the terminal dipeptide of angiotensin I.

Renin inhibitors

Aliskiren, an orally active non-peptide renin inhibitor, was developed and registered as an antihypertensive drug. It is a triumph of drug design and lowers blood pressure, but has been clinically somewhat unsuccessful with adverse effects that include diarrhoea (common), acute renal failure and, rarely, angioedema and severe allergic reactions.

Angiotensin-converting enzyme inhibitors

The first ACEI to be marketed was **captopril** (Fig. 22.7), an early example of successful drug design based on a chemical knowledge of the target molecule. Various small peptides had been found to be weak inhibitors of the enzyme.[10] Captopril was designed to combine the steric properties of such peptide antagonists in a non-peptide molecule that was active when given by mouth. Captopril has a short plasma half-life (about 2 h) and must be given 2 or 3 times daily. Many of the ACE inhibitors developed subsequently (Table 22.4), which are widely used in the clinic, have a longer duration of action and are administered once daily.

Pharmacological effects

ACE inhibitors cause only a small fall in arterial pressure in healthy human subjects who are consuming the amount of salt contained in a usual Western diet, but a much larger fall in hypertensive patients, particularly those in whom renin secretion is enhanced (e.g. in patients receiving diuretics). ACEIs affect capacitance and resistance vessels, and reduce cardiac load as well as arterial pressure. They act preferentially on angiotensin-sensitive vascular beds, which include those of the kidney, heart and brain. This selectivity may be important in sustaining adequate perfusion of these vital organs in the face of reduced perfusion pressure. Critical renal artery stenosis[11] represents an exception to this, where ACE inhibition results in a fall in glomerular filtration rate (see below).

Clinical uses of ACE inhibitors are summarised in the clinical box.

> ### Clinical uses of angiotensin-converting enzyme inhibitors
>
>
> - Hypertension.
> - Cardiac failure.
> - Following myocardial infarction (especially when there is ventricular dysfunction).
> - In people at high risk of ischaemic heart disease.
> - Diabetic nephropathy.
> - Chronic renal insufficiency to prevent progression.

Unwanted effects

Adverse effects (Table 22.4) directly related to ACE inhibition are common to all drugs of this class. These include

---

[10]The lead compound was a nonapeptide derived from the venom of *Bothrops jacaraca* – a South American snake. It was originally characterised as a bradykinin-potentiating peptide (ACE inactivates bradykinin, Ch. 17).

[11]Severe narrowing of the renal artery caused, for example, by atheroma (Ch. 23).

hypotension, especially after the first dose and especially in patients with heart failure who have been treated with loop diuretics, in whom the renin–angiotensin system is highly activated. A dry cough, possibly the result of accumulation of bradykinin (Ch. 17), is the commonest persistent adverse effect. Kinin accumulation may also underlie *angioedema* (painful swelling in tissues which can be life-threatening if it involves the airway). Patients with severe bilateral renal artery stenosis predictably develop renal failure if treated with ACEIs, because glomerular filtration is normally maintained, in the face of low afferent arteriolar pressure, by angiotensin II, which selectively constricts *efferent* arterioles; hyperkalaemia may be severe owing to reduced aldosterone secretion. Such renal failure is reversible provided that it is recognised promptly and treatment with ACEI discontinued.

Angiotensin II receptor antagonists

Losartan, candesartan, valsartan and **irbesartan** (sartans) are non-peptide, orally active AT_1 receptor antagonists (ARBs). ARBs differ pharmacologically from ACEIs (Fig. 22.8) but appear to behave superficially similarly to ACEIs apart from not causing cough – consistent with the 'bradykinin accumulation' explanation of this side effect, mentioned above; however, ACE inhibitors have a more robust evidence base than ARBs, reducing cardiovascular morbidity and mortality (including stroke) compared with placebo in hypertension. For ethical and historical reasons placebo-controlled outcome data are not available for ARBs, which were introduced after incontrovertible evidence was available for the efficacy of other drug classes. The situation has been further clouded by evidence of fabricated clinical trial data in several studies of valsartan, and the jury is still out.

ACE is not the only enzyme capable of forming angiotensin II, *chymase* (which is not inhibited by ACE inhibitors) providing one alternative route. It is not known if alternative pathways of angiotensin II formation are important *in vivo*, but if so, then ARBs could be more effective than ACE inhibitors in such situations. It is not known whether any of the beneficial effects of ACE inhibitors are bradykinin/NO mediated, so it is unwise to assume that ARBs will necessarily share all the therapeutic properties of ACE inhibitors, although there is considerable overlap in the clinical indications for ARBs and ACEIs (Table 22.4).

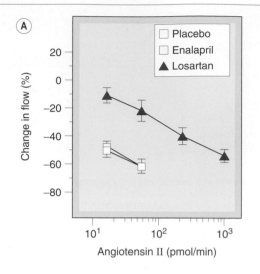

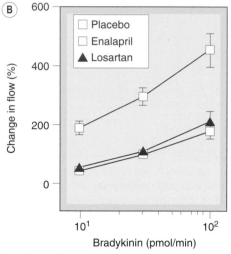

Fig. 22.8 Comparison of effects of angiotensin-converting enzyme inhibition and angiotensin receptor blockade in the human forearm vasculature. [**A**] Effect of brachial artery infusion of angiotensin II on forearm blood flow after oral administration of placebo, enalapril (10 mg) or losartan (100 mg). [**B**] Effect of brachial artery infusion of bradykinin, as in [**A**]. *(From Cockcroft JR et al. 1993 J Cardiovasc Pharmacol 22, 579–584.)*

CLINICAL USES OF VASOACTIVE DRUGS

It is beyond the scope of this book to provide a detailed account of the clinical uses of vasoactive drugs, but it is nonetheless useful to consider briefly the treatment of certain important disorders, namely:

- systemic hypertension
- heart failure
- shock
- peripheral vascular disease
- Raynaud's disease
- pulmonary hypertension.

SYSTEMIC HYPERTENSION

Systemic hypertension is a common disorder that, if not effectively treated, increases the risk of coronary thrombosis, strokes and renal failure. Until about 1950, there was no effective treatment, and the development of antihypertensive drugs has been a major therapeutic success story. Systemic blood pressure is an excellent 'surrogate marker' for increased cardiovascular risk in that there is good evidence from randomised controlled trials that common antihypertensive drugs (diuretics, ACEIs, calcium antagonists) combined with lifestyle changes not only lower blood pressure but also prolong life and reduce the extra risks of heart attacks and strokes associated with high blood pressure.

Correctable causes of hypertension include phaeochromocytoma,[12] steroid-secreting tumours of the adrenal cortex and narrowing (coarctation) of the aorta, but most cases involve no obvious cause and are grouped as

---

[12]Catecholamine-secreting tumours of chromaffin tissue, usually the adrenal medulla (Ch. 13).

Types of vasodilator drug

Directly acting vasodilators

- Calcium antagonists (e.g. **nifedipine**, **diltiazem**, **verapamil**): block Ca^{2+} entry in response to depolarisation. Common adverse effects include ankle swelling and (especially with verapamil) constipation.
- K_{ATP} channel activators (e.g. **minoxidil**): open membrane potassium channels, causing hyperpolarisation. Ankle swelling and increased hair growth are common.
- Drugs that increase cytoplasmic cyclic nucleotide concentrations by:
  - increasing adenylyl cyclase activity, for example prostacyclin (**epoprostenol**), β_2-adrenoceptor agonists, **adenosine**
  - increasing guanylyl cyclase activity: nitrates (e.g. **glyceryl trinitrate**, **nitroprusside**)
  - inhibiting phosphodiesterase activity (e.g. **sildenafil**).

Indirectly acting vasodilators

- Drugs that interfere with the sympathetic nervous system (e.g. α_1-adrenoceptor antagonists). Postural hypotension is a common adverse effect.
- Drugs that block the renin–angiotensin system:
  - renin inhibitors (e.g. **aliskiren**)
  - angiotensin-converting enzyme inhibitors (e.g. **ramipril**); dry cough may be troublesome
  - AT_1 receptor antagonists (e.g. **losartan**).
- Drugs or mediators that stimulate endothelial NO release (e.g. acetylcholine, bradykinin).
- Drugs that block the endothelin system:
  - endothelin synthesis (e.g. **phosphoramidon**)
  - endothelin receptor antagonists (e.g. **bosentan**).

Vasodilators whose mechanism is uncertain

- Miscellaneous drugs including alcohol, **propofol** (Ch. 41) and **hydralazine**.

Clinical uses of angiotensin II subtype 1 receptor antagonists (sartans)

The AT_1 antagonists are extremely well tolerated but are teratogenic. Their uses include the following:
- Hypertension, especially in:
  - young patients (who have higher renin than older ones)
  - diabetic patients
  - hypertension complicated by left ventricular hypertrophy.
- Heart failure.
- Diabetic nephropathy.

essential hypertension (so-called because it was originally, albeit incorrectly, thought that the raised blood pressure was 'essential' to maintain adequate tissue perfusion). Increased cardiac output may be an early feature, but by the time essential hypertension is established (commonly in middle life) there is usually increased peripheral resistance and the cardiac output is normal. Blood pressure control is intimately related to the kidneys, as demonstrated in humans requiring renal transplantation: hypertension 'goes with' the kidney from a hypertensive donor, and donating a kidney from a normotensive to a hypertensive corrects hypertension in the recipient (see also Ch. 29). Persistently raised arterial pressure leads to hypertrophy of the left ventricle and remodelling of resistance arteries, with narrowing of the lumen, and predisposes to atherosclerosis in larger conduit arteries.

Figure 22.9 summarises physiological mechanisms that control arterial blood pressure and shows sites at which antihypertensive drugs act, notably the sympathetic nervous system, the renin–angiotensin–aldosterone system and endothelium-derived mediators. Remodelling of resistance arteries in response to raised pressure reduces the ratio of lumen diameter to wall thickness and increases the peripheral vascular resistance. The role of cellular growth factors (including angiotensin II) and inhibitors of growth (e.g. NO) in the evolution of these structural changes is of great interest to vascular biologists, and is potentially important for ACEIs and ARBs.

Reducing arterial blood pressure greatly improves the prognosis of patients with hypertension. Controlling hypertension (which is asymptomatic) without producing unacceptable side effects is therefore an important clinical need, which is, in general, well catered for by modern drugs. Treatment involves non-pharmacological measures (e.g. increased exercise, reduced dietary salt and saturated fat with increased fruit and fibre, and weight and alcohol reduction) followed by the staged introduction of drugs, starting with those of proven benefit and least likely to produce side effects. Some of the drugs that were used to lower blood pressure in the early days of antihypertensive therapy, including *ganglion blockers, adrenergic neuron blockers* and **reserpine** (see Ch. 14), produced a fearsome array of adverse effects and are now obsolete. The preferred regimens have changed progressively as better-tolerated drugs have become available. The strategy recommended in the British Hypertension Society guidelines, is to start treatment with either an ACEI or an ARB in patients who are likely to have normal or raised plasma renin (i.e. younger white people), and with either a thiazide diuretic or a calcium antagonist in older people and people of African origin (who are more likely to have low plasma renin). If the target blood pressure is not achieved but the drug is well tolerated, then a drug of the other group is added. It is best not to increase the dose of any one drug excessively, as this often causes adverse effects and engages homeostatic control mechanisms (e.g. renin release by a diuretic) that limit efficacy.

β-Adrenoceptor antagonists are less well tolerated than ACEIs or ARBs, and the evidence supporting their routine use is less strong than for other classes of antihypertensive drugs. They are useful for hypertensive patients with some additional indication for β blockade, such as angina or heart failure.

Addition of a third or fourth drug (e.g. to ARB/diuretic or ARB/calcium antagonist combination) is often needed, and a long-acting α_1-adrenoceptor antagonist (Ch. 14) such as **doxazosin** is one option in this setting. The α_1 antagonists additionally improve symptoms of prostatic hyperplasia (also known as benign prostatic hypertrophy)

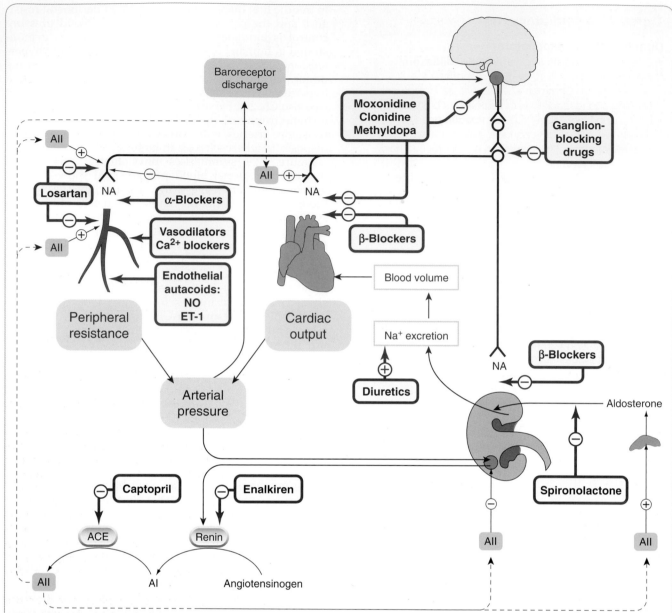

Fig. 22.9 Main mechanisms involved in arterial blood pressure regulation (black lines), and the sites of action of antihypertensive drugs (hatched boxes + orange lines). ACE, angiotensin-converting enzyme; AI, angiotensin I; AII, angiotensin II; ET-1, endothelin-1; NA, noradrenaline; NO, nitric oxide.

(Chs 14 and 29), which is common in older men, albeit at the expense of some postural hypotension, which is the main unwanted effect of these agents. Doxazosin is used once daily and has a mild but theoretically desirable effect on plasma lipids (reducing the ratio of low- to high-density lipoproteins; see Ch. 23). **Spironolactone** (a competitive antagonist of aldosterone; Ch. 32) has staged something of a comeback in treating severe hypertension. Careful monitoring of plasma K$^+$ concentration is required, because spironolactone inhibits urinary K$^+$ excretion as well as causing oestrogen-related adverse effects, but it is usually well tolerated in low doses. **Methyldopa** is now used mainly for hypertension during pregnancy because of the lack of documented adverse effects on the baby (in contrast to ACEIs, ARBs and standard β-adrenoceptor antagonists, which are contraindicated

during pregnancy). **Clonidine** (a centrally acting α$_2$ agonist) is now seldom used. **Moxonidine**, a centrally acting agonist at imidazoline I$_1$ receptors that causes less drowsiness than α$_2$ agonists, is licensed for mild or moderate hypertension, but there is little evidence from clinical end-point trials to support its use. **Minoxidil**, combined with a diuretic and β-adrenoceptor antagonist, is sometimes effective where other drugs have failed in severe hypertension resistant to other drugs. **Fenoldopam**, a selective dopamine D$_1$ receptor agonist, is approved in the USA for the short-term management in hospital of severe hypertension. Its effect is similar in magnitude to that of intravenous nitroprusside, but it lacks thiocyanate-associated toxicity and is slower in onset and offset.

Commonly used antihypertensive drugs and their main adverse effects are summarised in Table 22.5.

Table 22.5 Common antihypertensive drugs and their adverse effects

Drug	Adverse effects[a]		
	Postural hypotension	*Impotence*	*Other*
Thiazide (e.g. bendroflumethiazide) and related (e.g. chlortalidone) diuretics	±	++	Urinary frequency, gout, glucose intolerance, hypokalemia, hyponatremia
ACE inhibitors (e.g. enalapril)	±	−	Cough, first-dose hypotension, teratogenicity, reversible renal dysfunction (in presence of renal artery stenosis)
AT_1 antagonists (e.g. losartan)	−	−	Teratogenicity, reversible renal dysfunction (in presence of renal artery stenosis)
Ca^{2+} antagonists (e.g. nifedipine)	−	±	Ankle oedema
β-adrenoceptor antagonists (e.g. metoprolol)	−	+	Bronchospasm, fatigue, cold hands and feet, bradycardia
$α_1$-adrenoceptor antagonists (e.g. doxazosin)	++	−	First-dose hypotension

[a]± indicates that the adverse effect occurs in special circumstances only (e.g. postural hypotension occurs with a thiazide diuretic only if the patient is dehydrated for some other reason, is taking some additional drug or suffers from some additional disorder).

HEART FAILURE

Heart failure is a clinical syndrome characterised by symptoms of breathlessness and/or fatigue, usually with signs of fluid overload (oedema, crackles heard when listening to the chest). The underlying physiological abnormality (see also Ch. 21) is a cardiac output that is inadequate to meet the metabolic demands of the body, initially during exercise but, as the syndrome progresses, also at rest. It may be caused by disease of the myocardium itself (most commonly secondary to coronary artery disease but also other pathologies including cardiotoxic drugs such as **doxorubicin** – Ch. 56 – or **trastuzumab** – Ch. 59), or by circulatory factors such as volume overload (e.g. leaky valves, or arteriovenous shunts caused by congenital defects) or pressure overload (e.g. stenosed – i.e. narrowed – valves, arterial or pulmonary hypertension). Some of these underlying causes are surgically correctable, and in some either the underlying disease (e.g. hyperthyroidism; Ch. 34), or an aggravating factor such as anaemia (Ch. 25) or atrial fibrillation (Ch. 21), is treatable with drugs. Here, we focus on drugs used to treat heart failure *per se*, irrespective of the underlying cause.

When cardiac output is insufficient to meet metabolic demand, an increase in fluid volume occurs, partly because increased venous pressure causes increased formation of tissue fluid, and partly because reduced renal blood flow activates the renin–angiotensin–aldosterone system, causing Na^+ and water retention. Irrespective of the cause, the outlook for adults with cardiac failure is grim: 50% of those with the most severe grade are dead in 6 months, and of those with 'mild/moderate' disease, 50% are dead in 5 years. Non-drug measures, including dietary salt restriction and exercise training in mildly affected patients,[13] are important, but drugs are needed to improve symptoms of oedema, fatigue and breathlessness, and to improve prognosis.

A simplified diagram of the sequence of events is shown in Figure 22.10. A common theme is that several of the feedbacks that are activated are 'counter-regulatory' – i.e. they make the situation worse not better. This occurs because the body fails to distinguish the haemodynamic state of heart failure from haemorrhage, in which release of vasoconstrictors such as angiotensin II and ADH would be appropriate.[14] ACEIs and ARBs, β-adrenoceptor and aldosterone antagonists interrupt these counter-regulatory neurohormonal mechanisms and have each been shown to prolong life in heart failure, although prognosis remains poor despite optimal management.

Drugs used to treat heart failure act in various complementary ways to do the following.

Increase natriuresis. Diuretics, especially loop diuretics (Ch. 29), are important in increasing salt and water excretion, especially if there is pulmonary oedema. In chronic heart failure, drugs that have been shown to improve survival were all studied in patients treated with diuretics.

Inhibit the renin–angiotensin–aldosterone system. The renin–angiotensin–aldosterone system is inappropriately activated in patients with cardiac failure, especially when they are treated with diuretics. The β-adrenoceptor antagonists inhibit renin secretion and are used in clinically stable patients with chronic heart failure (see clinical box, p. 281). ACEIs and ARBs block the formation of angiotensin II and inhibit its action, respectively, thereby reducing vascular resistance, improving tissue perfusion and reducing cardiac afterload. They also cause natriuresis by inhibiting secretion of aldosterone and by reducing the direct stimulatory effect of angiotensin II on reabsorption of Na^+ and HCO_3^- in the early part of the proximal convoluted tubule. Most important of all, they prolong life.

[13]Bed rest used to be recommended but results in deconditioning, and regular exercise has been shown to be beneficial in patients who can tolerate it.

[14]Natural selection presumably favoured mechanisms that would benefit young hunter–gatherers at risk of haemorrhage; middle-aged or elderly people at high risk of heart failure are past their reproductive prime.

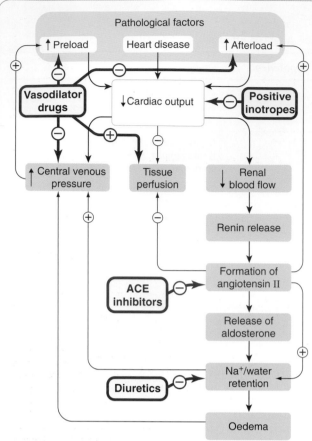

Fig. 22.10 Simplified scheme showing the pathogenesis of heart failure, and the sites of action of some of the drugs used to treat it. The symptoms of heart failure are produced by reduced tissue perfusion, oedema and increased central venous pressure. ACE, angiotensin-converting enzyme.

▼ Differences in the pharmacology of ACE inhibitors and ARBs led to the hypothesis that co-administration of these drugs ('dual block-ade') could confer additional benefit over increasing the dose of either given as a single agent. However, two large randomised con-trolled trials comparing monotherapy with ACEI or ARB with com-bined therapy both showed that the combined treatment produced more symptoms attributable to hypotension, and no survival benefit compared with monotherapy in patients with acute myocardial inf-arction (Pfeffer et al., 2003).

Angiotensin II is not the only stimulus to aldosterone secretion, and during chronic treatment with ACEIs, cir-culating aldosterone concentrations return towards pre-treatment values (a phenomenon known as 'aldosterone escape'). This provides a rationale for combining **spironol-actone** (an aldosterone antagonist; see Ch. 33) with ACEI treatment, which further reduces mortality. **Eplerenone** is an aldosterone antagonist with less oestrogen-like adverse effects than sprironolactone; it too has been shown to improve survival in patients with heart failure when added to conventional therapy. Patients with impaired renal function were excluded from these trials, and careful monitoring of plasma K^+ concentration is important when they are treated with an ACEI or an ARB in combination with an aldosterone antagonist.

Block β adrenoceptors. Heart failure is accompanied by potentially harmful activation of the sympathetic nervous system as well as of the renin–angiotensin system, provid-ing a rationale for using β-adrenoceptor antagonists. Most

clinicians were very wary of this approach because of the negative inotropic action of these drugs, but when started in low doses that are increased slowly, **metoprolol**, **carvedilol** and **bisoprolol** each improve survival when added to optimal treatment in clinically stable patients with chronic heart failure.

Antagonise ADH. ADH (see above and Ch. 33) is released in heart failure and may contribute to undesira-ble vasoconstriction (via V_{1A} receptors) and hyponatrae-mia (via V_2 receptors).[15] Two non-peptide vasopressin receptor antagonists ('vaptans') are available and more are in development (Finley et al., 2008). **Conivaptan** is a non-selective V_{1A}/V_2 antagonist licensed for treatment of the syndrome of inappropriate ADH secretion (SIADH) and intravenously for short-term treatment of hypervol-aemic (or euvolaemic) heart failure. **Tolvaptan** is a selec-tive V_2 receptor antagonist approved for oral treatment of clinically significant hypervolaemic (or euvolaemic) hyponatraemia. Neither has been shown to improve long-term survival in heart failure, and their possible place in therapy is currently the subject of intense investigation (Jessup et al., 2009).

Relax vascular smooth muscle. Glyceryl trinitrate (Ch. 21) is infused intravenously to treat acute cardiac failure. Its venodilator effect reduces venous pressure, and its effects on arterial compliance and wave reflection reduce cardiac work. The combination of **hydralazine** (to reduce afterload) with a long-acting organic nitrate (to reduce preload) in patients with chronic heart failure improved survival in a North American randomised con-trolled trial, but the results suggested that the benefit was restricted to patients of African origin. This ethnic group is genetically very heterogeneous, and it is unknown what other groups will benefit from such treatment.

Increase the force of cardiac contraction. Cardiac gly-cosides (Ch. 21) are used either in patients with heart failure who also have chronic rapid atrial fibrillation (in whom it improves cardiac function by slowing ventricular rate and hence ventricular filling in addition to any benefit from its positive inotropic action), or in patients who remain symptomatic despite treatment with a diuretic and ACEI. **Digoxin** does not reduce mortality in heart failure patients in sinus rhythm who are otherwise opti-mally treated, but does improve symptoms and reduce the need for hospital admission. In contrast, PDE inhibi-tors (see Ch. 21) increase cardiac output, but increase mortality in heart failure, probably through cardiac dys-rhythmias. **Dobutamine** (a $β_1$-selective adrenoceptor agonist; see Ch. 21) is used intravenously when a rapid response is needed in the short term, for example follow-ing heart surgery.

SHOCK AND HYPOTENSIVE STATES

Shock is a medical emergency characterised by inadequate perfusion of vital organs, usually because of a very low arterial blood pressure. This leads to anaerobic metabolism and hence to increased lactate production. Mortality is very high, even with optimal treatment in an intensive care unit. Shock can be caused by various insults, including haemor-rhage, burns, bacterial infections, anaphylaxis (Ch. 17) and

---

[15]Inappropriate secretion of ADH causes hyponatraemia because the kidney retains water while continuing to excrete sodium ions, whereas drinking, which is largely determined by habit in addition to thirst, continues. This leads to reduction of the plasma sodium concentration as a result of dilution.

Drugs used in chronic heart failure

- Loop diuretics, for example **furosemide** (Ch. 29).
- Angiotensin-converting enzyme inhibitors (e.g. **ramipril**).
- Angiotensin II subtype 1 receptor antagonists (e.g. **valsartan**, **candesartan**).
- β-adrenoceptor antagonists (e.g. **metoprolol**, **bisoprolol**, **carvedilol**), introduced in low dose in stable patients.
- Aldosterone receptor antagonists (e.g. **spironolactone**, Ch. 29; and **eplerenone**).
- **Digoxin** (see Ch. 21), especially for heart failure associated with established rapid atrial fibrillation. It is also indicated in patients who remain symptomatic despite optimal treatment.
- Organic nitrates (e.g. **isosorbide mononitrate**) reduce preload, and **hydralazine** reduces afterload. Used in combination, these prolong life in African-Americans.

myocardial infarction (Fig. 22.11). The common factor is reduced effective circulating blood volume (hypovolae-mia) caused either directly by bleeding or by movement of fluid from the plasma to the gut lumen or extracellular fluid. The physiological (homeostatic) response to this is complex: vasodilatation in a vital organ (e.g. brain, heart or kidney) favours perfusion of that organ, but at the expense of a further reduction in blood pressure, which leads to reduced perfusion of other organs. Survival depends on a balance between vasoconstriction in non-essential vascular beds and vasodilatation in vital ones. The dividing line between the normal physiological response to blood loss and clinical shock is that in shock tissue hypoxia produces secondary effects that magnify rather than correct the primary disturbance. Therefore patients with established shock have profound and inappropriate vasodilatation in non-essential organs, and this is difficult to correct with vasoconstrictor drugs. The release of mediators (e.g. hista-mine, 5-hydroxytryptamine, bradykinin, prostaglandins, cytokines including interleukins and tumour necrosis factor, NO and undoubtedly many more as-yet-unidenti-fied substances) that cause capillary dilatation and leaki-ness is the opposite of what is required to improve function in this setting. Mediators promoting vasodilatation in shock converge on two main mechanisms:

1. Activation of ATP-sensitive potassium channels in vascular smooth muscle by reduced cytoplasmic ATP and increased lactate and protons.
2. Increased synthesis of NO, which activates myosin light-chain phosphatase and activates K_{Ca} channels.

A third important mechanism seems to be a relative *defi-ciency* of ADH, which is secreted acutely in response to haemorrhage but subsequently declines, probably because of depletion from the neurohypophysis (see Ch. 33) – contrast this with the situation in *chronic* heart failure discussed above where *excess* (rather than deficient) ADH may contribute to problems.

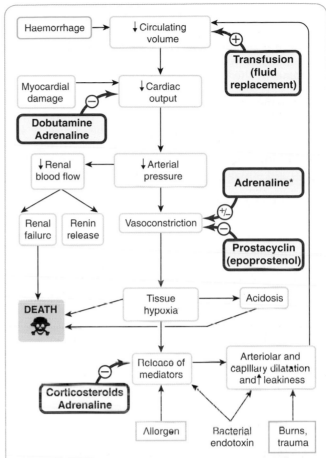

Fig. 22.11 Simplified scheme showing the pathogenesis of hypovolaemic shock. *Adrenaline causes vasodilatation in some vascular beds, vasoconstriction in others.

Patients with shock are not a homogeneous popula-tion, making it hard to perform valid clinical trials, and in contrast to hypertension and heart failure there is very little evidence to support treatment strategies based on hard clinical end points (such as improved survival). *Volume replacement* is of benefit if there is hypovolaemia; *antibiotics* are essential if there is persistent bacterial infection; **adrenaline** can be life-saving in anaphylactic shock and is also used by intensivists in managing circu-latory shock of other aetiologies. Hypoperfusion leads to multiple organ failure (including renal failure), and intensive therapy specialists spend much effort support-ing the circulations of such patients with cocktails of vasoactive drugs in attempts to optimise flow to vital organs. Trials of antagonists designed to block or neutral-ise endotoxin, interleukins, tumour necrosis factor and the inducible form of NO synthase, and of recombinant human protein C (**drotecogin**, Ch. 24) have shown them to be ineffective or actually harmful. **Vasopressin** may be effective in increasing blood pressure even when there is resistance to adrenaline; *corticosteroids* suppress the for-mation of NO and of prostaglandins but are not of proven benefit once shock is established; **epoprostenol** (PGI₂) may be useful in patients with inappropriate platelet activation (e.g. *meningococcal sepsis*); positive inotropic agents, including adrenaline and **dobutamine**, may help in individual patients, as may **levosimendan** (Mebazaa et al., 2007).

PERIPHERAL VASCULAR DISEASE

When atheroma involves peripheral arteries, the first symptom is usually pain in the calves on walking (claudication), followed by pain at rest, and in severe cases gangrene of the feet or legs. Other vascular beds (e.g. coronary, cerebral and renal) are often also affected by atheromatous disease in patients with peripheral vascular disease. Treatment is mainly surgical, combined with drugs that reduce the risk of ischaemic heart disease and strokes. Drug treatment includes antiplatelet drugs (e.g. **aspirin**, **clopidogrel**; see Ch. 24), a statin (e.g. **simvastatin**; see Ch. 23) and an ACEI (e.g. **ramipril**; see p. 274-275).

RAYNAUD'S DISEASE

Inappropriate vasoconstriction of small arteries and arterioles gives rise to Raynaud's phenomenon (blanching of the fingers during vasoconstriction, followed by blueness owing to deoxygenation of the static blood and redness from reactive hyperaemia following return of blood flow). This can be mild, but if severe causes ulceration and gangrene of the fingers. It can occur in isolation (Raynaud's disease) or in association with a number of other diseases, including several so-called connective tissue diseases (e.g. systemic sclerosis, systemic lupus erythematosus). Treatment of Raynaud's phenomenon hinges on stopping smoking (crucially) and on avoiding the cold; β-adrenoceptor antagonists are contraindicated. Vasodilators (e.g. **nifedipine**; see Ch. 21) are of some benefit in severe cases, and evidence from several small studies suggests that other vasodilators (e.g. PGI_2, CGRP) can have surprisingly prolonged effects, but are difficult to administer.

PULMONARY HYPERTENSION

After birth, pulmonary vascular resistance is much lower than systemic vascular resistance, and systolic pulmonary artery pressure in adults is normally approximately 20 mmHg.[16]

---

[16]In fetal life, pulmonary vascular resistance is high; failure to adapt appropriately at birth is associated with prematurity, lack of pulmonary surfactant and hypoxaemia. The resulting pulmonary hypertension is treated by paediatric intensive care specialists with measures including replacement of surfactant and ventilatory support, sometimes including inhaled NO – see Chapter 20.

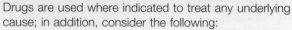

Drugs used in pulmonary hypertension

Drugs are used where indicated to treat any underlying cause; in addition, consider the following:
- Oral anticoagulants (Ch. 24).
- Diuretics (Ch. 29).
- **Oxygen**.
- **Digoxin** (Ch. 21).
- Calcium-channel blockers.
- Endothelin receptor antagonists (e.g. **bosentan**, **ambrisentan**, **sitaxentan**) by mouth for less severe stages of disease.

- Prostanoid analogues (**iloprost**, **treprostinil**, **beraprost**) by parenteral routes of administration, e.g. subcutaneous or inhaled, for more severe stages of disease.
- **Epoprostenol** (Ch. 17). This is given as a long-term intravenous infusion, and improves survival (Fig. 22.12).
- Inhaled **NO** is administered in intensive care, for example for pulmonary hypertensive crises in newborn babies.
- Phosphodiesterase V inhibitor: **sildenafil** is licensed for this indication.

Clinical disorders for which vasoactive drugs are important

- Systemic hypertension:
  – secondary to underlying disease (e.g. renal or endocrine)
  – primary 'essential' hypertension, an important risk factor for atheromatous disease (Ch. 23). Treatment reduces the excess risk of stroke or myocardial infarction, the main classes of drugs being (a) angiotensin-converting enzyme (ACE) inhibitors or AT_1 receptor antagonists; (b) β-adrenoceptor antagonists; (c) calcium antagonists; and (d) diuretics.
- Cardiac failure. Several diseases (most commonly ischaemic heart disease) impair the ability of the heart to deliver an output adequate to meet metabolic needs. Symptoms of oedema can be improved with diuretics. Life expectancy is reduced but can be improved by treatment of haemodynamically stable patients with:
  – ACE inhibitors and/or AT_1 receptor antagonists
  – β-adrenoceptor antagonists (e.g. **carvedilol**, **bisoprolol**)
  – aldosterone antagonists (e.g. **spironolactone**).

- Shock. Several diseases (e.g. overwhelming bacterial infections, Ch. 51; anaphylactic reactions, Ch. 28) lead to inappropriate vasodilatation, hypotension and reduced tissue perfusion with raised circulating concentrations of lactic acid. Pressors (e.g. **adrenaline**) are used.
- Peripheral vascular disease. Atheromatous plaques in the arteries of the legs are often associated with atheroma in other vascular territories. Statins (Ch. 23) and antiplatelet drugs (Ch. 24) are important.
- Raynaud's disease. Inappropriate vasoconstriction in small arteries in the hands causes blanching of the fingers followed by blueness and pain. **Nifedipine** or other vasodilators are used.
- Pulmonary hypertension, which can be:
  – idiopathic (a rare disorder): **epoprostenol**, **iloprost**, **bosentan** and **sildenafil** are of benefit in selected patients
  – associated with hypoxic lung disease.

Pulmonary artery pressure is much less easy to measure than is systemic pressure, often requiring cardiac catheterisation, so only severe and symptomatic pulmonary hypertension usually gets diagnosed. Pulmonary hypertension usually causes some regurgitation of blood from the right ventricle to the right atrium. This tricuspid regurgitation can be used to estimate the pulmonary artery pressure indirectly by ultrasonography. Pulmonary hypertension may be *idiopathic* (i.e. of unknown cause, analogous to essential hypertension in the systemic circulation), or associated with some other disease. Increased pulmonary pressure can result from an increased cardiac output (such as occurs, for example, in patients with hepatic cirrhosis – where vasodilatation may accompany intermittent subclinical exposure to bacterial endotoxin – or in patients with congenital connections between the systemic and pulmonary circulations). Vasoconstriction and/or structural narrowing of the pulmonary resistance arteries increase pulmonary arterial pressure, even if cardiac output is normal. In some situations, both increased cardiac output and increased pulmonary vascular resistance are present.

In contrast to systemic hypertension, pulmonary hypertension associated with other diseases is much more common than idiopathic pulmonary hypertension, which is a rare, severe and progressive disease. Endothelial dysfunction (see p. 266–268, and also Chs 23 and 24) is implicated in its aetiology. Drugs (e.g. anorexic drugs including **dexfenfluramine**, now withdrawn) and toxins (e.g. *monocrotaline*) can cause pulmonary hypertension. Occlusion of the pulmonary arteries, for example with *recurrent pulmonary emboli* (Ch. 24), is a further cause, and *anticoagulation* (see Ch. 24) is an important part of treatment. Aggregates of deformed red cells in patients with *sickle cell anaemia* (Ch. 25) can also occlude small pulmonary arteries.

Increased pulmonary vascular resistance may, alternatively, result from vasoconstriction and/or structural changes in the walls of pulmonary resistance arteries.

Many of the diseases (e.g. systemic sclerosis) associated with Raynaud's phenomenon mentioned in the section above are also associated with pulmonary hypertension. Vasoconstriction may precede cellular proliferation and medial hypertrophy which causes wall thickening in the pulmonary vasculature. Treatment with vasodilators (e.g. nifedipine) is used. Vasodilators with an antiproliferative action (e.g. epoprostenol, see Fig. 22.12), drugs that potentiate NO such as **riociguat**, an allosteric activator of soluble guanylyl cyclase (see Ch. 20), recently approved for this indication in Europe and the USA, or antagonise endothelin – for example bosentan and **ambrisentan** – are more promising.

Drugs used in treating pulmonary arterial hypertension and clinical disorders for which vasoactive drugs are important are shown in the clinical boxes.

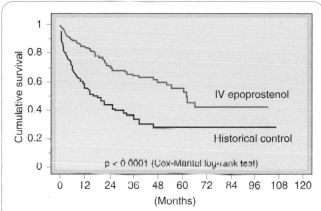

Fig. 22.12 Survival in primary pulmonary hypertension. Survival in 178 patients treated with intravenous epoprostenol versus a historical control group of 135 patients matched for disease severity. (*Adapted from Sitbon O et al. 2002 Prog Cardiovasc Dis 45, 115.*)

REFERENCES AND FURTHER READING

Vascular endothelium (see Ch. 20 for further reading on nitric oxide)
Prostacyclin
Bunting, S., Gryglewski, R., Moncada, S., Vane, J.R., 1976. Arterial walls generate from prostaglandin endoperoxides a substance (*prostaglandin X*) which relaxes strips of mesenteric and celiac arteries and inhibits platelet aggregation. Prostaglandins 12, 897–913. (*Classic*)
Murata, T., Ushikubi, F., Matsuoka, T., et al., 1997. Altered pain perception and inflammatory response in mice lacking prostacyclin receptor. Nature 388, 678–682. (*I prostanoid receptor-deficient mice are viable, reproductive and normotensive; however, their susceptibility to thrombosis is increased … the results establish that prostacyclin is an endogenous antithrombotic agent*)

Endothelium-derived hyperpolarising factor
Félétou, M., Vanhoutte, P.M., 2009. EDHF: an update. Clin. Sci. 117, 139–155. (*Reviews briefly the many endothelial mediators that can cause hyperpolarisation and vascular muscle relaxation*)

Angiogenesis
Carmeliet, P., Jain, R.K., 2000. Angiogenesis in cancer and other diseases. Nature 407, 249–257. (*New approaches to treatment of cancer and other diseases, via a growing number of pro- and antiangiogenic molecules; see also (in same issue) Yancopoulos, G.D., et al., 2000. Vascular specific growth factors and blood vessel formation, pp. 242–248*)

Endothelin
Hickey, K.A., Rubanyi, G., Paul, R.J., Highsmith, R.F., 1985. Characterization of a coronary vasoconstrictor produced by cultured endothelial cells. Am. J. Physiol. 248 (Pt 1), C550–C556. (*Key discovery*)
Kirchengast, M., Luz, M., 2005. Endothelin receptor antagonists – clinical realities and future directions. J. Cardiovasc Pharmacol. 5, 182–191. (*Critically reviews clinical data on endothelin receptor antagonism in cardiovascular indications against the background of preclinical research*)
Yanagisawa, M., Kurihara, H., Kimura, S., et al., 1988. A novel potent vasoconstrictor peptide produced by vascular endothelial cells. Nature 332, 411–415. (*Tour de force*)

Renin–angiotensin system
Heart Outcomes Prevention Evaluation Study Investigators, 2000. Effects of an angiotensin-converting enzyme inhibitor, ramipril, on cardiovascular events in high-risk patients. N. Engl. J. Med. 342, 145–153. (*Ramipril significantly lowers rates of death, myocardial infarction and stroke in a wide range of high-risk patients*)
Lang, C.C., Struthers, A.D., 2013. Targeting the renin-angiotensin-aldosterone system in heart failure. Nat. Rev. Cardiol. 10, 125–134.
ONTARGET Investigators, 2008. Telmisartan, ramipril or both in patients at high risk for vascular events. N. Engl. J. Med. 358, 1547–1559.
Pfeffer, M.A., McMurray, J.J.V., Velasquez, E.J., et al., 2003. The Valsartan in Acute Myocardial Infarction Trial I. Valsartan, captopril or both in myocardial infarction complicated by heart failure, left ventricular dysfunction, or both. N. Engl. J. Med. 349, 1839–1906.

Antidiuretic hormone

Holmes, C.L., Russell, J.A., 2004. Vasopressin. Semin. Respir. Crit. Care Med. 25, 705–711. ('*A deficiency of vasopressin exists in some shock states and replacement of physiological levels of vasopressin can restore vascular tone. Vasopressin is therefore emerging as a rational therapy for vasodilatory shock.' Reviews rationale, evidence and uncertainties for using vasopressin in shock*)

Vasodilator drugs (see Ch. 21 for further reading on calcium antagonists)

Chan, C.K.S., Burke, S.L., Zhu, H., et al., 2005. Imidazoline receptors associated with noradrenergic terminals in the rostral ventrolateral medulla mediate the hypotensive responses of moxonidine but not clonidine. Neuroscience 132, 991–1007. (*The hypotensive and bradycardic actions of moxonidine but not clonidine are mediated through imidazoline receptors and depend on noradrenergic CNS pathways; noradrenergic innervation may be associated with imidazoline receptor protein*)

Heart failure

Finley, J.J., Konstam, M.A., Udelson, J.E., 2008. Arginine vasopressin antagonists for the treatment of heart failure and hyponatraemia. Circulation 118, 410–421.

Gheorghiade, M., Pang, P.S., 2009. Acute heart failure syndromes. JACC. 53, 557–573.

Jessup, M., Abraham, W.T., Casey, D.E., et al., 2009. 2009 Focused Update: ACCF/AHA Guidelines for the diagnosis and management of heart failure in adults: a report of the American College of Cardiology Foundation/American Heart Association Task Force on Practice Guidelines: developed in collaboration with the International Society for Heart and Lung Transplantation. Circulation 119, 1977–2016.

Taylor, A.L., Ziesche, S., Yancy, C., et al., 2004. Combination of isosorbide dinitrate and hydralazine in blacks with heart failure. N. Engl. J. Med. 351, 2049–2057. (*Addition of a fixed dose of isosorbide dinitrate plus hydralazine to standard therapy for heart failure including neurohormonal blockers increased survival among black patients with advanced heart failure*)

Shock

Landry, D.W., Oliver, J.A., 2001. Mechanisms of disease: the pathogenesis of vasodilatory shock. N. Engl. J. Med. 345, 588–595. (*Reviews mechanisms promoting inappropriate vasodilation in shock, including activation of ATP-sensitive potassium channels, increased synthesis of NO and depletion of ADH*)

Other references

Mebazaa, A., Nieminen, M.S., Packer, M., et al., for the SURVIVE investigators, 2007. Levosimendan vs dobutamine for patients with acute decompensated heart failure. JAMA 297, 1883–1891. (*Randomised, double-blind trial comparing the efficacy and safety of intravenous levosimendan versus dobutamine in 1327 patients hospitalised with acute decompensated heart failure. Addition of levosimendam did not improve survival of patients treated with dobutamine*)

O'Connor, C.M., Starling, R.C., Hernandez, A.F., et al., 2011. Effect of nesiritide in patients with acute decompensated heart failure. N. Engl. J. Med. 365, 32–43. (*see also Topol, E.T., 2011. The lost decade of nesiritide. N. Engl. J. Med. 365, 81–82*)

Further reading

Badesch, D.B., Abman, S.H., Ahearn, G.S., et al., 2004. Medical therapy for pulmonary arterial hypertension – ACCP evidence-based clinical practice guidelines. Chest 126 (Suppl.), 35S–62S. (*Evidence-based treatment recommendations for physicians involved in the care of these complex patients*)

Beppu, H., Ichinose, F., Kawai, N., et al., 2004. BMPR-II heterozygous mice have mild pulmonary hypertension and an impaired pulmonary vascular remodeling response to prolonged hypoxia. Am. J. Physiol. Lung Cell. Mol. Physiol. 287, L1241–L1247. ('*Heterozygous mutations of the bone morphogenetic protein type II receptor, BMPR-II, gene have been identified in patients with primary pulmonary hypertension … in mice, mutation of one copy of the BMPR-II gene causes pulmonary hypertension but impairs the ability of the pulmonary vasculature to remodel in response to prolonged hypoxic breathing*')

Higenbottam, T., Laude, L., Emery, C., Essener, M., 2004. Pulmonary hypertension as a result of drug therapy. Clin. Chest Med. 25, 123–131. (*Reviews anorectic drug-induced pulmonary arterial hypertension and considers mechanisms*)

Humbert, M., Sitbon, O., Simonneau, G., 2004. Drug therapy: treatment of pulmonary arterial hypertension. N. Engl. J. Med. 351, 1425–1436.

Lee, A.J., Chiao, T.B., Tsang, M.P., 2005. Sildenafil for pulmonary hypertension. Ann. Pharmacother. 39, 869–884. (*Sildenafil is a promising and well-tolerated treatment for pulmonary hypertension; well-designed trials are needed*)

Liang, K.V., Williams, A.W., Greene, E.L., Redfield, M.M., 2008. Acute decompensated heart failure and the cardiorenal syndrome. Crit. Care Med. 36 (Suppl. 1), S75–S88. (*Review from Mayo Clinic*)

McLaughlin, V.V., Sitbon, O., Badesch, D.B., et al., 2005. Survival with first-line bosentan in patients with primary pulmonary hypertension. Eur. Respir. J. 25, 244–249. (*Bosentan improved survival in patients with advanced primary pulmonary hypertension*)

Napoli, C., Loscalzo, J., 2004. Nitric oxide and other novel therapies for pulmonary hypertension. J. Cardiovasc. Pharmacol. Ther. 9, 1–8. (*Focus on endothelial NO, NO replacement and related therapies*)

Rich, S., McLaughlin, V.V., 2005. Chapter 67. In: Zipes, D.P., Libby, P., Bonow, R.O., Braunwald, E. (Eds.), Braunwald's Heart Disease, seventh ed. Elsevier, Philadelphia, pp. 1807–1842.

Ritter, J.M., 2011. Angiotensin converting enzyme inhibitors and angiotensin receptor blockers in hypertension. Br. Med. J. 342, 868–873. (*Compares the clinical use of these classes of agents*)

Task-force on Diagnosis and Treatment of Pulmonary Arterial Hypertension of the European Society of Cardiology, 2004. Guidelines on diagnosis and treatment of pulmonary arterial hypertension. Eur. Heart J. 25, 2243–2278.

Atherosclerosis and lipoprotein metabolism

23

OVERVIEW

Atheromatous disease is ubiquitous and underlies the commonest causes of death (myocardial infarction caused by thrombosis – Ch. 24 – on ruptured atheromatous plaque in a coronary artery) and disability (stroke, heart failure) in industrial societies. Hypertension is one of the most important risk factors for atheroma, and is discussed in Chapter 22. Here, we consider other risk factors, especially dyslipidaemia,[1] which, like hypertension, is amenable to drug therapy. We describe briefly the processes of atherogenesis and of lipid transport as a basis for understanding the actions of lipid-lowering drugs. Important agents (statins, fibrates, cholesterol absorption inhibitors, nicotinic acid derivatives, fish oil derivatives) are described, with emphasis on the statins, which reduce the incidence of arterial disease and prolong life.

INTRODUCTION

In this chapter we summarise the pathological process of atherogenesis and approaches to the prevention of atherosclerotic disease. Lipoprotein transport forms the basis for understanding drugs used to treat dyslipidaemia. We emphasise the **statins**, which have been a major success story, not only lowering plasma cholesterol but also reducing cardiovascular events by approximately 25–50% and prolonging life. However, some patients cannot tolerate them, and others fail to respond. Evidence that other drugs that influence dyslipidaemia improve clinical outcomes is less secure than for the statins, and two recent setbacks described below call into question the reliability of changes in circulating lipid concentrations in response to drugs as surrogates predicting clinical improvement. In the absence of hard evidence of clinical improvement, other classes of lipid-lowering drugs remain second line to statins, so there is rather a lot of 'small print' in this section.

ATHEROGENESIS

Atheroma is a focal disease of the intima of large and medium-sized arteries. Lesions evolve over decades, during most of which time they are clinically silent, the occurrence of symptoms signalling advanced disease. Presymptomatic lesions are often difficult to detect non-invasively, although ultrasound is useful in accessible arteries (e.g. the carotids), and associated changes such as reduced aortic compliance and arterial calcification can be detected by measuring, respectively, aortic pulse wave velocity and coronary artery calcification. There were no good animal models until transgenic mice (see Ch. 7) deficient in apolipoproteins or receptors that play key roles in lipoprotein metabolism transformed the scene. Nevertheless, most of our current understanding of atherogenesis comes from human epidemiology and pathology, and from clinical investigations.

Epidemiological studies have identified numerous risk factors for atheromatous disease. Some of these cannot be altered (e.g. a family history of ischaemic heart disease), but others are modifiable (see Table 23.1) and are potential targets for therapeutic drugs. Clinical trials have shown that improving risk factors can reduce the consequences of atheromatous disease. Many risk factors (e.g. type 2 diabetes, dyslipidaemia, cigarette smoking) cause endothelial dysfunction (see Ch. 22), evidenced by reduced vasodilator responses to acetylcholine or to increased blood flow (so-called 'flow-mediated dilatation', responses that are inhibited by drugs that block nitric oxide [NO] synthesis; Ch. 20). Healthy endothelium produces NO and other mediators that protect against atheroma, so it is likely that metabolic cardiovascular risk factors act by causing endothelial dysfunction.

Atherogenesis involves:

1. *Endothelial dysfunction*, with altered NO (Ch. 20) biosynthesis, predisposes to atherosclerosis.
2. *Injury* of dysfunctional endothelium, which leads to expression of adhesion molecules. This encourages monocyte attachment and migration of monocytes from the lumen into the intima. Lesions have a predilection for regions of disturbed flow such as the origins of aortic branches.
3. *Low-density lipoprotein (LDL) cholesterol* transport into the vessel wall. Endothelial cells and monocytes/macrophages generate free radicals that oxidise LDL (oxLDL), resulting in lipid peroxidation.
4. *oxLDL* uptake by macrophages via 'scavenger' receptors. Such macrophages are called *foam cells* because of their 'foamy' histological appearance, resulting from accumulation of cytoplasmic lipid, and are characteristic of atheroma. Uptake of oxLDL activates macrophages and releases proinflammatory cytokines.
5. Subendothelial accumulation of foam cells and T lymphocytes to form *fatty streaks*.
6. Protective mechanisms, for example cholesterol *mobilisation from the artery wall* and transport in plasma as high-density lipoprotein (HDL) cholesterol, termed 'reverse cholesterol transport'.
7. Cytokine and growth factor release by activated platelets, macrophages and endothelial cells, causing proliferation of smooth muscle and deposition of connective tissue components. This *inflammatory fibroproliferative response* leads to a dense fibrous cap overlying a lipid-rich core, the whole structure comprising the atheromatous plaque.

---

[1]The term dyslipidaemia is preferred to hyperlipidaemia because a low plasma concentration of high-density lipoprotein cholesterol is believed to be harmful and is a potential therapeutic target.

Table 23.1 Modifiable risk factors for atheromatous disease

Raised low-density lipoprotein cholesterol
Reduced high-density lipoprotein cholesterol
Hypertension (Ch. 22)
Diabetes mellitus (Ch. 31)
Cigarette smoking (Ch. 49)
Obesity (Ch. 32)
Physical inactivity
Raised C-reactive protein[a]
Raised coagulation factors (e.g. factor VII, fibrinogen)
Raised homocysteine
Raised lipoprotein(a)[b]

[a]Strongly associated with atheromatous disease but unknown if this is causal.
[b]Potentially modifiable but strongly genetically determined: nicotinic acid does lower lipoprotein(a).

8. Plaque *rupture*, which provides a substrate for *thrombosis* (see Ch. 24, Figs 24.1 and 24.10). The presence of large numbers of macrophages predisposes to plaque rupture, whereas vascular smooth muscle and matrix proteins stabilise the plaque.

To understand how drugs prevent atheromatous disease, it is necessary briefly to review lipoprotein transport.

LIPOPROTEIN TRANSPORT

Lipids and cholesterol are transported in the bloodstream as complexes of lipid and protein known as *lipoproteins*. These consist of a central core of hydrophobic lipid (including triglycerides and cholesteryl esters) encased in a hydrophilic coat of polar phospholipid, free cholesterol and *apoprotein*. There are four main classes of lipoprotein, differing in the relative proportion of the core lipids and in the type of apoprotein (various kinds of apoA and apoB). Apoproteins bind to specific receptors that mediate uptake of lipoprotein particles into liver, blood or other tissues. Lipoproteins differ in size and density, and this latter property, measured originally by ultracentrifugation but now commonly estimated by simpler methods, is the basis for their classification into:

- HDL particles (contain apoA1 and apoA2), diameter 7–20 nm
- LDL particles (contain apoB-100), diameter 20–30 nm
- very-low-density lipoprotein (VLDL) particles (contain apoB-100), diameter 30–80 nm
- chylomicrons (contain apoB-48), diameter 100–1000 nm.

Each class of lipoprotein has a specific role in lipid transport, and there are different pathways for exogenous and endogenous lipids, as well as a pathway for reverse cholesterol transport (Fig. 23.1). In the *exogenous pathway*, cholesterol and triglycerides absorbed from the ileum are

transported as chylomicrons in lymph and then blood, to capillaries in muscle and adipose tissue. Here, triglycerides are hydrolysed by lipoprotein lipase, and the tissues take up the resulting free fatty acids and glycerol. The chylomicron remnants, still containing their full complement of cholesteryl esters, pass to the liver, bind to receptors on hepatocytes and undergo endocytosis. Cholesterol liberated in hepatocytes is stored, oxidised to bile acids, secreted unaltered in bile, or can enter the endogenous pathway.

In the *endogenous pathway*, cholesterol and newly synthesised triglycerides are transported from the liver as VLDL to muscle and adipose tissue, where triglyceride is hydrolysed to fatty acids and glycerol; these enter the tissues as described above. During this process, the lipoprotein particles become smaller but retain a full complement of cholesteryl esters and become LDL particles. LDL provides the source of cholesterol for incorporation into cell membranes and for synthesis of steroids (see Chs 33 and 35) but is also key in atherogenesis. Cells take up LDL by endocytosis via *LDL receptors* that recognise apoB-100. Cholesterol can return to plasma from the tissues in HDL particles (reverse cholesterol transport). Cholesterol is esterified with long-chain fatty acids in HDL particles, and the resulting cholesteryl esters are transferred to VLDL or LDL particles by a transfer protein present in the plasma and known as *cholesteryl ester transfer protein* (CETP). Lipoprotein(a), or Lp(a), is a species of LDL that is associated with atherosclerosis and is localised in atherosclerotic lesions. Lp(a) contains a unique apoprotein, apo(a), with structural similarities to plasminogen (Ch. 24). Lp(a) competes with plasminogen for its receptor on endothelial cells. Plasminogen is the substrate for plasminogen activator, which is secreted by, and bound to endothelial cells, generating the fibrinolytic enzyme *plasmin* (see Fig. 24.10). The effect of the binding of Lp(a) is that less plasmin is generated, fibrinolysis is inhibited and thrombosis promoted.

▼ There is current interest in lipid transfer proteins that have been implicated in atherogenesis (Stein & Stein, 2005). *ACAT* (acyl coenzyme A: cholesterol acyltransferase), which is expressed in two forms, catalyses the intracellular synthesis of cholesteryl ester in macrophages, adrenal cortex, gut and liver. **Tamoxifen**, used in the treatment and prevention of breast cancer (Chs 35 and 56), is a potent ACAT inhibitor (de Medina et al., 2004). *CETP* is involved in transfer of cholesterol between different classes of lipoprotein particle in plasma. Microsomal triglyceride transport protein (MTP) is a lipid-transfer protein present in the lumen of the endoplasmic reticulum responsible for binding and transfer of lipids between membranes. Inhibition of MTP interferes with apoB secretion and LDL assembly.

DYSLIPIDAEMIA

Dyslipidaemia may be primary or secondary. The *primary* forms are due to a combination of diet and genetics (often but not always polygenic). They are classified into six phenotypes (the Frederickson classification; Table 23.2). An especially great risk of ischaemic heart disease occurs in a subset of primary type IIa hyperlipoproteinaemia caused by single-gene defects of LDL receptors; this is known as *familial hypercholesterolaemia* (FH), and the plasma cholesterol concentration in affected adults is typically >8 mmol/l in heterozygotes and 12–25 mmol/l in homozygotes. Study of FH enabled Brown & Goldstein (1986) to define the LDL receptor pathway of cholesterol homeostasis (for which they shared a Nobel Prize). Drugs used to treat primary dyslipidaemia are described below.

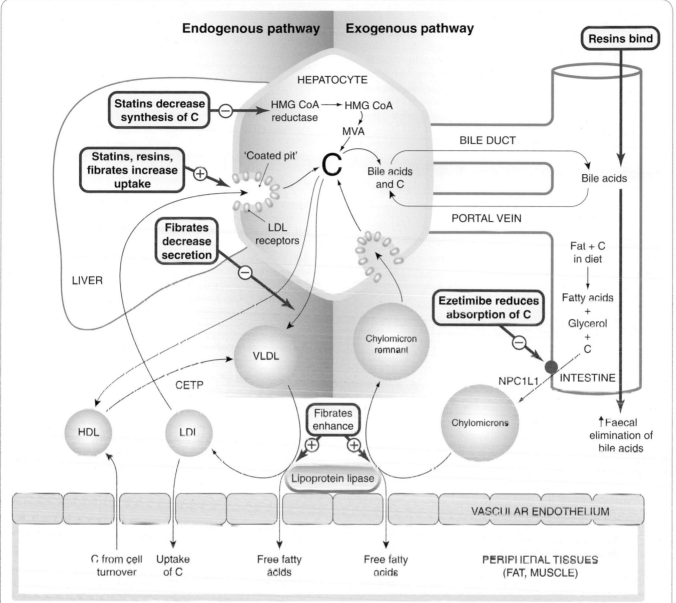

Fig. 23.1 Schematic diagram of cholesterol transport in the tissues, with sites of action of the main drugs affecting lipoprotein metabolism. C, cholesterol; CETP, cholesteryl ester transport protein; HDL, high-density lipoprotein; HMG-CoA reductase, 3-hydroxy-3 methylglutaryl-coenzyme A reductase; LDL, low-density lipoprotein; MVA, mevalonate; NPC1L1, a cholesterol transporter in the brush border of enterocytes; VLDL, very-low-density lipoprotein.

Table 23.2 Frederickson/World Health Organization classification of hyperlipoproteinaemia

Type	Lipoprotein elevated	Cholesterol	Triglycerides	Atherosclerosis risk	Drug treatment
I	Chylomicrons	+	+++	NE	None
IIa	LDL	++	NE	High	Statin ± ezetimibe
IIb	LDL + VLDL	++	++	High	Fibrates, statin, nicotinic acid
III	βVLDL	++	++	Moderate	Fibrates
IV	VLDL	+	++	Moderate	Fibrates
V	Chylomicrons + VLDL	I	++	NE	Fibrate, niacin, fish oil and statin combinations

+, increased concentration; LDL, low-density lipoprotein; NE, not elevated; VLDL, very-low-density lipoprotein; βVLDL, a qualitatively abnormal form of VLDL identified by its pattern on electrophoresis.

Secondary forms of dyslipidaemia are a consequence of other conditions, such as diabetes mellitus, alcoholism, nephrotic syndrome, chronic renal failure, hypothyroidism, liver disease and administration of drugs, for example **isotretinoin** (an isomer of vitamin A given by mouth as well as topically in the treatment of severe acne, see Ch. 27), **tamoxifen, ciclosporine** (Ch. 26) and *protease inhibitors* used to treat infection with human immunodeficiency virus (Ch. 52). Secondary forms are treated where possible by correcting the underlying cause.

Lipoprotein metabolism and dyslipidaemia

Lipids, including cholesterol and triglycerides, are transported in the plasma as lipoproteins, of which there are four classes:

- Chylomicrons transport triglycerides and cholesterol from the gastrointestinal tract to the tissues, where triglyceride is split by lipoprotein lipase, releasing free fatty acids and glycerol. These are taken up in muscle and adipose tissue. Chylomicron remnants are taken up in the liver, where cholesterol is stored, secreted in bile, oxidised to bile acids or converted into:
  – very-low-density lipoproteins (VLDLs), which transport cholesterol and newly synthesised triglycerides to the tissues, where triglycerides are removed as before, leaving:
  – intermediate-density and low-density lipoprotein (LDL) particles with a large component of cholesterol; some LDL cholesterol is taken up by the tissues and some by the liver, by endocytosis via specific LDL receptors.
- High-density lipoprotein (HDL) particles adsorb cholesterol derived from cell breakdown in tissues (including arteries) and transfer it to VLDL and LDL particles via cholesterol ester transport protein (CETP).
- Dyslipidaemias can be primary, or secondary to a disease (e.g. hypothyroidism). They are classified according to which lipoprotein particle is abnormal into six phenotypes (the Frederickson classification). The higher the LDL cholesterol and the lower the HDL cholesterol, the higher the risk of ischaemic heart disease.

PREVENTION OF ATHEROMATOUS DISEASE

Drug treatment is often justified, to supplement healthy habits. Treatment of hypertension (Ch. 22) and, to a lesser extent, diabetes mellitus (Ch. 31) reduces the incidence of symptomatic atheromatous disease, and antithrombotic drugs (Ch. 24) reduce arterial thrombosis. Reducing LDL is also effective and is the main subject of this present chapter, but several other steps in atherogenesis are also potential targets for pharmacological attack.

▼ *Angiotensin-converting enzyme inhibitors* (Ch. 22) improve endothelial function and prolong life in patients with atheromatous disease. Other drugs that also increase NO biosynthesis or availability are under investigation.

Measures to increase HDL: moderate alcohol consumption increases HDL, and epidemiological evidence favours moderate alcohol consumption in older people.[2] Regular exercise also increases circulating HDL; drug treatment to increase HDL is of uncertain benefit. Fibrates and nicotinic acid derivatives – see below – modestly increase HDL, and reduce LDL and triglycerides. In subjects with low HDL, inhibition of cholesteryl ester transfer protein (CETP) with **torcetrapib** markedly increased HDL, but also increased blood pressure and was associated with a 60% *increase* in all-cause mortality (leading to abrupt discontinuation of its development). It is unclear if this is a class effect, but **anacetrapib** markedly increases HDL without increasing blood pressure; whether it reduces mortality should be answered when one large trial completes in 2017. *ApoA-I Milano* is a variant of apolipoprotein A-I identified in individuals in rural Italy with very low levels of HDL but almost no cardiovascular disease. Infusion of recombinant ApoA-I Milano–phospholipid complexes causes rapid regression of atherosclerosis in animal models, and administered intravenously caused regression of atherosclerosis in patients with acute coronary syndrome. It is expensive to produce and must be administered intravenously, but the strategy continues to be a focus of intense interest (see review by Duffy & Rader, 2009).

Antioxidants (e.g. vitamin C and vitamin E) are of interest, both because of evidence that they improve endothelial function in patients with increased oxidant stress, and because of epidemiological evidence that a diet rich in antioxidants is associated with reduced risk of coronary artery disease. Results from clinical trials have been negative, however, and several antioxidants reduce HDL. **Oestrogen**, used to prevent symptoms of the menopause (Ch. 35) and to prevent postmenopausal osteoporosis, has antioxidant properties and exerts other vascular effects that could be beneficial. Epidemiological evidence suggested that women who use such hormone replacement might be at reduced risk of atheromatous disease, but controlled trials showed significant *adverse* effects on cardiovascular mortality (Ch. 35).

Anti-inflammatory approaches: drug treatment to lower *C-reactive protein* has been mooted, but it is possible that elevated C-reactive

Atheromatous disease

- Atheroma is a focal disease of large and medium-sized arteries. Atheromatous plaques occur in most people, progress insidiously over many decades, and underlie the commonest causes of death (myocardial infarction) and disability (e.g. stroke) in industrialised countries.
- Fatty streaks are the earliest structurally apparent lesion and progress to fibrous and/or fatty plaques. Symptoms occur only when blood flow through the vessel is reduced below that needed to meet the metabolic demands of tissues downstream from the obstruction.
- Important modifiable risk factors include hypertension (Ch. 22), dyslipidaemia (this chapter) and smoking (Ch. 49).
- The pathophysiology is of chronic inflammation in response to injury. Endothelial dysfunction leads to loss of protective mechanisms, monocyte/macrophage and T-cell migration, uptake of low-density lipoprotein (LDL) cholesterol and its oxidation, uptake of oxidised LDL by macrophages, smooth muscle cell migration and proliferation, and deposition of collagen.
- Plaque rupture leads to platelet activation and thrombosis (Ch. 24).

---

[2]'Sinful, ginful, rum-soaked men, survive for three score years and ten' – or longer, we rather hope …

protein is a marker of vascular inflammation rather than playing an active part in disease progression. Other anti-inflammatory measures are being investigated; for example, *acyl coenzyme A, cholesterol acyltransferase (ACAT) inhibitors*.

LIPID-LOWERING DRUGS

Several drugs decrease plasma LDL. Drug therapy is used in addition to dietary measures and correction of other modifiable cardiovascular risk factors.

The main agents used clinically are:

- statins: 3-hydroxy-3-methylglutaryl-coenzyme A (HMG-CoA) reductase inhibitors
- fibrates
- inhibitors of cholesterol absorption
- nicotinic acid or its derivatives
- fish oil derivatives.

STATINS: HMG-COA REDUCTASE INHIBITORS

The rate-limiting enzyme in cholesterol synthesis is HMG-CoA reductase, which catalyses the conversion of HMG-CoA to mevalonic acid (see Fig. 23.1). **Simvastatin, lovastatin** and **pravastatin** are specific, reversible, competitive HMG-CoA reductase inhibitors with K_i values of approximately 1 nmol/l. **Atorvastatin** and **rosuvastatin** are long-lasting inhibitors. Decreased hepatic cholesterol synthesis upregulates LDL receptor synthesis, increasing LDL clearance from plasma into liver cells. The main biochemical effect of statins is therefore to reduce plasma LDL. There is also some reduction in plasma triglyceride and increase in HDL. Several large randomised placebo controlled trials of the effects of HMG-CoA reductase inhibitors on morbidity and mortality have been positive.

▼ The Scandinavian Simvastatin Survival Study (4S) recruited patients with ischaemic heart disease and plasma cholesterol of 5.5–8.0 mmol/l; simvastatin lowered serum LDL by 35% and death by 30% (Fig. 23.2). There was a 42% reduction in death from coronary disease. Other large trials have confirmed reduced mortality

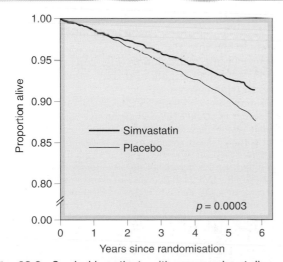

Fig. 23.2 **Survival in patients with coronary heart disease and serum cholesterol 5.5–8.0 mmol/l treated either with placebo or with simvastatin.** The relative risk of death in the simvastatin group was 0.70 (95% confidence intervals 0.58–0.85). *(Based on 4S Study 1994 Lancet 344, 1383–1389.)*

both in patients with established ischaemic heart disease and in healthy people at risk of coronary disease, with a wide range of plasma cholesterol values and other risk factors, and treated with different statins. Intensive lowering of LDL with atorvastatin 80 mg had a greater effect on event rate than did a 10 mg dose, but with a greater incidence of abnormally raised plasma transaminase activity (evidence of liver damage). In secondary prevention trials of statins, cardiovascular event rate has been approximately linearly related to the achieved plasma LDL over a concentration range from approximately 1.8–4.9 mmol/l, and the event rate falls on the same line in placebo- and statin-treated patients, suggesting that plasma LDL is a valid surrogate marker of cardiovascular risk in this context.

Other actions of statins

Products of the mevalonate pathway react with protein ('lipidation', which is the addition to a protein of hydrophobic groups such as prenyl or farnesyl moieties). Several important membrane-bound enzymes (e.g. endothelial NO synthase; see Ch. 20) are modified in this way. The fatty groups serve as anchors, localising the enzyme in organelles such as caveoli and Golgi apparatus. Consequently, there is currently great interest in actions of statins that are unrelated, or indirectly related, to their effect on plasma LDL (sometimes referred to as *pleiotropic* effects). Some of these actions are undesirable (e.g. HMG-CoA reductase guides migrating primordial germ cells, and statin use is contraindicated during pregnancy), but some offer therapeutic promise, for example in Alzheimer's disease, where a role for statins is controversial, and prevention of prostate cancer. Such potentially beneficial actions include:

- improved endothelial function
- reduced vascular inflammation
- reduced platelet aggregability
- increased neovascularisation of ischaemic tissue
- increased circulating endothelial progenitor cells
- stabilisation of atherosclerotic plaque
- antithrombotic actions
- enhanced fibrinolysis
- inhibition of germ cell migration during development
- immune suppression
- protection against sepsis.

The extent to which these effects contribute to the anti-atheromatous actions of statins is unknown.

Pharmacokinetics

Short-acting statins are given by mouth at night to reduce peak cholesterol synthesis in the early morning. They are well absorbed and extracted by the liver, their site of action, and are subject to extensive presystemic metabolism via cytochrome P450 and glucuronidation pathways. Simvastatin is an inactive lactone prodrug; it is metabolised in the liver to its active form, the corresponding β-hydroxy fatty acid.

Adverse effects

Statins are well tolerated; mild unwanted effects include muscle pain (myalgia), gastrointestinal disturbance, raised concentrations of liver enzymes in plasma, insomnia and rash. More serious adverse effects are rare but include skeletal muscle damage (myositis, which when severe is described as rhabdomyolysis) and angio-oedema. Myositis is a class effect of statins, occurs also with other lipid-lowering drugs (especially fibrates) and is dose-related.[3] It is more common in patients with low lean body mass or uncorrected hypothyroidism.

Clinical uses of HMG-CoA reductase inhibitors (statins, e.g. simvastatin, atorvastatin)

- Secondary prevention of myocardial infarction and stroke in patients who have symptomatic atherosclerotic disease (e.g. angina, transient ischaemic attacks, or following myocardial infarction or stroke).
- Primary prevention of arterial disease in patients who are at high risk because of elevated serum cholesterol concentration, especially if there are other risk factors for atherosclerosis such as diabetes (Ch. 31) or renal failure (Ch. 29). Tables (available for example in the British National Formulary) are used to target treatment to those at greatest risk.
- **Atorvastatin** lowers serum cholesterol in patients with homozygous familial hypercholesterolaemia.
- In severe drug-resistant dyslipidaemia (e.g. heterozygous familial hypercholesterolaemia), **ezetimibe** is combined with statin treatment.
- Contraindicated in pregnancy.

FIBRATES

Several fibric acid derivatives (fibrates) are available, including **bezafibrate**, **ciprofibrate**, **gemfibrozil**, **fenofibrate** and **clofibrate**. These markedly reduce circulating VLDL, and hence triglyceride, with a modest (approximately 10%) reduction in LDL and an approximately 10% increase in HDL. Their mechanism of action is complex (see Fig. 23.1). They are agonists at PPARα nuclear receptors[4] (Ch. 3); in humans, the main effects are to increase transcription of the genes for lipoprotein lipase, apoA1 and apoA5. They increase hepatic LDL uptake. In addition to effects on lipoproteins, fibrates reduce plasma C-reactive protein and fibrinogen, improve glucose tolerance and inhibit vascular smooth muscle inflammation by inhibiting the expression of the transcription factor nuclear factor κB (see Ch. 3). As with the pleiotropic effects of statins (see p. 289), there is great interest in these actions, although again it is unknown if they are clinically important.

▼ In one study, gemfibrozil reduced coronary heart disease by approximately one-third compared with placebo in middle-aged men with primary hyperlipoproteinaemia, but fibrates have not been shown to improve survival. A trial in some 2500 men with coronary heart disease and low HDL together with low LDL showed that gemfibrozil increased HDL and reduced coronary disease and stroke. Event rates were linked to changes in HDL but not to triglycerides or to LDL, suggesting that increasing HDL with a fibrate reduces vascular risk.

---

[3]**Cerivastatin**, a potent statin introduced at relatively high dose, was withdrawn because of rhabdomyolysis occurring particularly in patients treated with gemfibrozil – discussed later in the chapter.
[4]Standing for peroxisome proliferator-activated receptors – don't ask! (Peroxisomes are organelles that are not present in human cells, so something of a misnomer!) Thiazolidinedione drugs used in treating diabetes act on related PPARγ receptors; see Ch. 31.

Adverse effects

Rhabdomyolysis is unusual but can be severe, giving rise to acute renal failure associated with excretion of muscle proteins, especially myoglobin, by the kidney. It occurs particularly in patients with renal impairment, because of reduced protein binding and impaired drug elimination. Fibrates should be avoided in such patients and also in alcoholics, who are predisposed to hypertriglyceridaemia but are at risk of severe muscle inflammation and injury.[5] Rhabdomyolysis can also be caused (rarely) by statins (see p. 289), and the combined use of fibrates with this class of drugs is therefore generally inadvisable (although it is sometimes undertaken by specialists). Gastrointestinal symptoms, pruritus and rash are more common than with statins. Clofibrate predisposes to gallstones, and its use is therefore limited to patients who have had a cholecystectomy (i.e. removal of the gall bladder).

Clinical uses of fibrates (e.g. gemfibrozil, fenofibrate)

- Mixed dyslipidaemia (i.e. raised serum triglyceride as well as cholesterol), provided this is not caused by excessive alcohol consumption. **Fenofibrate** is uricosuric, which may be useful where hyperuricaemia coexists with mixed dyslipidaemia.
- In patients with low high-density lipoprotein and high risk of atheromatous disease (often type 2 diabetic patients; see Ch. 31).
- Combined with other lipid-lowering drugs in patients with severe treatment-resistant dyslipidaemia. This may, however, increase the risk of rhabdomyolysis.

DRUGS THAT INHIBIT CHOLESTEROL ABSORPTION

Historically, bile acid-binding resins (e.g. **colestyramine**, **colestipol**) were the only agents available to reduce cholesterol absorption and were among the few means to lower plasma cholesterol. Taken by mouth, they sequester bile acids in the intestine and prevent their reabsorption and enterohepatic recirculation (Fig. 23.1). The concentration of HDL is unchanged, and they cause an unwanted increase in triglycerides.

▼ The American Lipid Research Clinics' trial of middle-aged men with primary hypercholesterolaemia showed that addition of a resin to dietary treatment caused a fall in plasma cholesterol and a 20–25% fall in coronary heart disease over 7 years, but no studies have shown improved survival. Decreased absorption of exogenous cholesterol and increased metabolism of endogenous cholesterol into bile acids in the liver lead to increased expression of LDL receptors on hepatocytes, and hence to increased clearance of LDL from the blood and a reduced concentration of LDL in plasma. Resins are bulky, unpalatable and often cause diarrhoea. They interfere with the absorption of fat-soluble vitamins, and of *thiazide diuretics* (Chs 22, 29 and 58), digoxin (Ch. 21) and warfarin (Ch. 24), which should therefore be taken at least 1 h before or 4–6 h after the resin. With the introduction of statins, their use in treating dyslipidaemia was

---

[5]For several reasons, including a tendency to lie immobile for prolonged periods followed by generalised convulsions – 'rum fits' – and delirium tremens.

relegated largely to additional treatment in patients with severe disease (e.g. FH) and (a separate use) treating bile salt-associated symptoms of pruritus (itch) and diarrhoea – see clinical box below. **Colesevelam** (introduced recently) is less bulky (daily dose up to 4 g compared with a dose up to 36 g for colestyramine) but more expensive. Subsequently, plant sterols and stanols have been marketed; these are isolated from wood pulp and used to make margarines or yoghurts. They reduce plasma cholesterol to a small extent and are tastier than resins.[6] Phytosterol and phytostanol esters interfere with the micellar presentation of sterols to the enterocyte surface, reducing cholesterol absorption and hence the exogenous pathway.

EZETIMIBE

Ezetimibe is one of a group of azetidinone cholesterol absorption inhibitors, and is used as an adjunct to diet and statins in hypercholesterolaemia. It inhibits absorption of cholesterol (and of plant stanols) from the duodenum by blocking a transport protein (NPC1L1) in the brush border of enterocytes, without affecting the absorption of fat-soluble vitamins, triglycerides or bile acids. Because of its high potency compared with resins (a daily dose of 10 mg), it should represent a useful advance as a substitute for resins as supplementary treatment to statins in patients with severe dyslipidaemia. The results of a trial evaluating its effect on cardiovascular outcome is ongoing and long-awaited.

Ezetimibe is administered by mouth and is absorbed into intestinal epithelial cells, where it localises to the brush border, which is its presumed site of action. It is also extensively (>80%) metabolised to an active metabolite. Enterohepatic recycling results in slow elimination. The terminal half-life is approximately 22 h. It enters milk (at least in animal studies) and is contraindicated for women who are breastfeeding. It is generally well tolerated but can cause diarrhoea, abdominal pain or headache; rash and angio-oedema have been reported.

> **Clinical use of drugs that reduce cholesterol absorption: Ezetimibe or bile acid-binding resins (e.g. colestyramine)**
>
> - As an addition to a statin when response has been inadequate (**ezetimibe**).
> - For hypercholesterolaemia when a statin is contraindicated.
> - Uses unrelated to atherosclerosis, including:
>   - pruritus in patients with partial biliary obstruction (bile acid-binding resin)
>   - bile acid diarrhoea, for example caused by diabetic neuropathy (bile acid-binding resin).

NICOTINIC ACID

▼ Nicotinic acid is a vitamin, and as such is essential for many important metabolic processes. Quite separately from this, it has been used in gram quantities as a lipid-lowering agent. It is converted to nicotinamide, which inhibits hepatic VLDL secretion (see

Fig. 23.1), with consequent reductions in circulating triglyceride and LDL including Lp(a), and an increase in HDL. The mechanism is poorly understood but is believed to be initiated by an effect on lipolysis via a G protein-coupled orphan receptor called HM74A and present in adipocyte membranes. Adverse effects include flushing, palpitations and gastrointestinal disturbance. Disappointingly, addition of nicotinic acid to a statin does not improve cardiovascular outcome, but does increase serious adverse effects (HSP2-THRIVE trial).

FISH OIL DERIVATIVES

▼ Omega-3 marine triglycerides reduce plasma triglyceride concentrations but increase cholesterol. Plasma triglyceride concentrations are less strongly associated with coronary artery disease than is cholesterol, but there is epidemiological evidence that eating fish regularly does reduce ischaemic heart disease, and dietary supplementation with ω-3 polyunsaturated fatty acids (PUFAs) improves survival in patients who have recently had a myocardial infarction (GISSI-Prevenzione Investigators, 1999). The mechanism may be the potent antiarrhythmic effects of PUFA. The mechanism of action of fish oil on plasma triglyceride concentrations is unknown. Fish oil is rich in PUFA, including eicosapentaenoic and docosahexaenoic acid and it has other potentially important effects including inhibition of platelet function, prolongation of bleeding time, anti-inflammatory effects and reduction of plasma fibrinogen. Eicosapentaenoic acid substitutes for arachidonic acid in cell membranes and gives rise to 3-series prostaglandins, thromboxanes and 5-series leukotrienes (Ch. 17). This probably accounts for their effects on haemostasis, because thromboxane A_3 is much less active as a platelet-aggregating agent than is thromboxane A_2, whereas PGI_3 is similar in potency to PGI_2 as an inhibitor of platelet function. The alteration in leukotriene biosynthesis probably partly underlies the anti-inflammatory effects of fish oil; the production of resolvins from eicosa-pentaenoic acid (Ch. 17) is also important. Fish oil is contraindicated in patients with type IIa hyperlipoproteinaemia because of the increase in LDL that it causes. A preparation of omega 3-acid ethyl esters is licensed in the UK for prevention of recurrent events after myocardial infarction in addition to treatment of hypertriglyceridaemia; it causes less increase in LDL and fewer problems with fishy odour, weight gain and dyspepsia than the older fish oil preparations.

Other novel therapies in development include drugs that inhibit squalene synthesis, microsomal transport protein (MTP) inhibitors and drugs that alter apoB. Among drugs that alter apoB, **mipomersen**, approved in the USA but not in Europe for the 'orphan' indication of homozygous familial hypercholesterolaemia (FH), is an antisense oligonucleotide complementary to the coding region for apoB-100 of mRNA, which thereby inhibits synthesis of apoB-100 and LDL. Chemical modifications (see Ch. 59) make mipomersen resistant to degradation by nucleases, allowing it to be administered once weekly, as an adjunct to other treatment for homozygous FH. It accumulates in the liver, which is the site of its intended action but also of toxicity – hepatotoxicty being one ongoing concern of the regulators.

Lomitapide has also recently been approved as an adjunct to other treatment for homozygous FH. It is a small molecule inhibitor of microsomal triglyceride transfer protein (MTP). MTP plays a key role in the assembly and release of apoB-containing lipoproteins into the circulation and inhibition of this protein significantly lowers plasma lipid levels. This action contrasts with other lipid lowering drugs, which mainly work by increasing LDL uptake rather than by reducing hepatic lipoprotein secretion. Lomitapide is administered orally once a day and the dose individualised according to how it is tolerated.

---

[6]This is not, however, saying much.

Drugs in dyslipidaemia

The main drugs used in patients with dyslipidaemias are:
- HMG-CoA reductase inhibitors (statins, e.g. **simvastatin**): inhibit synthesis of cholesterol, increasing expression of low-density lipoprotein (LDL) receptors on hepatocytes and hence increasing hepatic LDL cholesterol (LDL-C) uptake. They reduce cardiovascular events and prolong life in people at risk, and clinically are the most important class of drugs used in dyslipidaemias. Adverse effects include myalgias (rarely, severe muscle damage) and raised liver enzymes.
- Fibrates (e.g. **gemfibrozil**): activate PPARα receptors, increase activity of lipoprotein lipase, decrease hepatic very-low-density lipoprotein production and enhance clearance of LDL by the liver. They markedly lower serum triglycerides, and modestly increase high-density lipoprotein cholesterol. Adverse effects include muscle damage.
- Agents that interfere with cholesterol absorption, usually as an adjunct to diet plus statin:
  - **ezetimibe**
  - stanol-enriched foods
  - bile acid-binding resins (e.g. **colestyramine**, **colesevelam**).
- Fish oil derivatives – omega-3-acid ethyl esters.
- **Mipomerson** and **lomitopide** were recently introduced as adjuncts in treating patients with the rare homozygous form of familial hypercholesterolaemia.

REFERENCES AND FURTHER READING

Atherosclerosis and dyslipidaemia

Brown, M.S., Goldstein, J.L., 1986. A receptor-mediated pathway for cholesterol homeostasis. Science 232, 34–47. (*Classic from these Nobel Prize winners; see also Goldstein, J.L., Brown, M.S., 1990. Regulation of the mevalonate pathway. Nature 343, 425–430*)

Durrington, P.N., 2005. Hyperlipidaemia: Diagnosis and Management, third ed. Hodder Arnold, London. (*Extremely readable, authoritative book*)

Ross, R., 1999. Atherosclerosis – an inflammatory disease. N. Engl. J. Med. 340, 115–126.

Stein, O., Stein, Y., 2005. Lipid transfer proteins (LTP) and atherosclerosis. Atherosclerosis 178, 217–230. (*Lipid transfer proteins – ACAT, CETP, LCAT and PLTP – and the therapeutic potential of modulating them*)

Statins

Hague, W., Emberson, J., Ridker, P.M., 2001. For the Air Force/Texas Coronary Atherosclerosis Prevention Study Investigators. Measurement of C-reactive protein for the targeting of statin therapy in the primary prevention of acute events. N. Engl. J. Med. 344, 1959–1965. (*Statins may be effective in preventing coronary events in people with unremarkable serum lipid concentrations but with elevated C-reactive protein, a marker of inflammation and risk factor for coronary disease*)

Liao, J.K., Laufs, U., 2005. Pleiotropic effects of statins. Annu. Rev. Pharmacol. Toxicol. 45, 89–118. ('*Many pleiotropic effects are mediated by inhibition of isoprenoids, which serve as lipid attachments for intracellular signalling molecules. In particular, inhibition of small GTP-binding proteins, Rho, Ras, and Rac, whose proper membrane localisation and function are dependent on isoprenylation, may play an important role in mediating the pleiotropic effects of statins*')

Merx, M.W., Liehn, E.A., Graf, J., et al., 2005. Statin treatment after onset of sepsis in a murine model improves survival. Circulation 112, 117–124. (*Statins offer the potential of effective sepsis treatment*)

Van Doren, M., Broihier, H.T., Moore, L.A., et al., 1998. HMG-CoA reductase guides migrating primordial germ cells. Nature 396, 466–469. (*Regulated expression of HMG-CoA reductase provides spatial guide to migrating primordial germ cells*)

Vasa, M., Fichtlscherer, S., Adler, K., et al., 2001. Increase in circulating endothelial progenitor cells by statin therapy in patients with stable coronary artery disease. Circulation 103, 2885–2890. (*May participate in repair after ischaemic injury*)

Other therapies
Nicotinic acid

Canner, P.L., Furberg, C.D., Terrin, M.L., et al., 2005. Benefits of niacin by glycemic status in patients with healed myocardial infarction (from the Coronary Drug Project). Am. J. Cardiol. 95, 254–257. (*The Coronary Drug Project, conducted during 1966 to 1974, was a randomised, double-blind, placebo-controlled trial in 8341 men with previous myocardial infarction; nicotinic acid significantly reduced total mortality during 6.2 years' treatment plus an additional 9 years of post-trial follow-up*)

HPS2-THRIVE Collaborative Group, 2013. HPS2-THRIVE randomized placebo-controlled trial in 25 673 high-risk patients of ER niacin/laropiprant: trial design, pre-specified muscle and liver outcomes, and reasons for stopping study treatment. Eur. Heart J. 34, 1279–1291.

Fibrates

Bloomfield Rubins, H., Davenport, J., Babikian, V., et al., 2001. Reduction in stroke with gemfibrozil in men with coronary heart disease and low HDL cholesterol. The Veterans Affairs HDL Intervention Trial (VA-HIT). Circulation 103, 2828–2833. (*Evidence that increasing HDL reduces stroke*)

Gervois, P., Torra, I.P., Fruchart, J.C., et al., 2000. Regulation of lipid and lipoprotein metabolism by PPAR activators. Clin. Chem. Lab. Med. 38, 3–11. (*Review*)

Fish oil

GISSI-Prevenzione Investigators (Gruppo Italiano per lo Studio della Sopravvivenza nell'Infarto Miocardico), 1999. Dietary supplementation with n-3 polyunsaturated fatty acids and vitamin E after myocardial infarction: results of the GISSI-Prevenzione trial. Lancet 354, 447–455. (*11 324 patients surviving myocardial infarction were randomly assigned supplements of n-3 PUFA, 1 g daily, vitamin E, both or neither for 3.5 years. The primary end point was death, non-fatal myocardial infarction and stroke combined. Dietary supplementation with n-3 PUFA led to a clinically important and statistically significant benefit. Vitamin E had no benefit*)

Ezetimibe

Kosoglou, T., Statkevich, P., Johnson-Levonas, A.O., et al., 2005. Ezetimibe – a review of its metabolism, pharmacokinetics and drug interactions. Clin. Pharmacokinetics 44, 467–494.

Lomitapide

Cuchel, M., Meagher, E.A., du Toit Theron, H., et al., 2013. Efficacy and safety of a microsomal triglyceride transfer protein inhibitor in patients with homozygous familial hypercholesterolaemia: a single-arm, open-label, phase 3 study. Lancet 381, 40–46. (*See also accompanying editorial: Raal, F.J., pp. 7–8*)

Mipomersen

Merki, E., Graham, M.J., Mullick, A.E., 2008. Antisense oligonucleotide directed to human apolipoprotein B-100 reduces lipoprotein(a) levels and oxidized phospholipids on human apolipoprotein B-100 particles in lipoprotein(a) transgenic mice. Circulation 118, 743–753.

Potential therapies

Duffy, D., Rader, D.J., 2009. Update on strategies to increase HDL quantity and function. Nature. Rev. Cardiol. 6, 455–463.

de Medina, P., Payrá, B.L., Bernad, J., et al., 2004. Tamoxifen is a potent inhibitor of cholesterol esterification and prevents the formation of foam cells. J. Pharmacol. Exp. Ther. 308, 1542–1548. (*Molecular modelling revealed similarity between tamoxifen and ACAT inhibitor*)

Wierzbicki, A.S., 2004. Lipid lowering therapies in development. Expert Opin. Invest. Drugs 13, 1405–1408.

Haemostasis and thrombosis

OVERVIEW

This chapter summarises the main features of blood coagulation, platelet function and fibrinolysis. These processes underlie haemostasis and thrombosis, and provide a basis for understanding haemor-rhagic disorders (e.g. haemophilia) and thrombotic diseases both of arteries (e.g. thrombotic stroke, myocardial infarction) and of veins (e.g. deep vein thrombosis, pulmonary embolism). Anticoagulants, antiplatelet drugs and fibrinolytic drugs are espe-cially important because of the prevalence of throm-botic disease.

INTRODUCTION

Haemostasis is the arrest of blood loss from damaged blood vessels and is essential to life. A wound causes vasoconstriction, accompanied by:

- adhesion and activation of platelets
- formation of fibrin.

Platelet activation leads to the formation of a haemostatic plug, which stops the bleeding and is subsequently rein-forced by fibrin. The relative importance of each process depends on the type of vessel (arterial, venous or capil-lary) that has been injured.

Thrombosis is the pathological formation of a 'haemo-static' plug within the vasculature in the absence of bleed-ing ('haemostasis in the wrong place'). Over a century ago, Rudolph Virchow defined three predisposing factors – 'Virchow's triad': *injury to the vessel wall* – for example, when an atheromatous plaque ruptures or becomes eroded; *altered blood flow* – for example, in the left atrial appendage of the heart during atrial fibrillation, or in the veins of the legs while sitting awkwardly on a long journey; and *abnormal coagulability* of the blood – as occurs, for example, in the later stages of pregnancy or during treatment with certain oral contraceptives (see Ch. 35). Increased coagulability of the blood can be inherited and is referred to as *thrombophilia*. A *thrombus*, which forms *in vivo*, should be distinguished from a *clot*, which forms in blood *in vitro* (for example in a glass tube). Clots are amor-phous, consisting of a diffuse fibrin meshwork in which red and white blood cells are trapped indiscriminately. By contrast, arterial and venous thrombi each have a distinct structure.

An *arterial thrombus* (see Fig. 24.1) is composed of so-called white thrombus consisting mainly of platelets in a fibrin mesh. It is usually associated with atherosclerosis and can interrupt blood flow, causing ischaemia or death (infarction) of tissue downstream. Venous thrombus is composed of 'red thrombus' and consists of a small white head and a large jelly-like red tail, similar in composition to a blood clot, which streams away in the flow. Thrombus

can break away from its attachment and float through the circulation, forming an embolus; venous emboli usually lodge in a pulmonary artery ('pulmonary embolism'), while thrombus that embolises from the left heart or a carotid artery usually lodges in an artery in the brain or other organs, causing death, stroke or other disaster.

Drug therapy to promote haemostasis (e.g. antifibrino-lytic and haemostatic drugs; see p. 307) is indicated when this essential process is defective (e.g. coagulation factors in haemophilia or following excessive anticoagulant therapy), or when it proves difficult to staunch haemor-rhage following surgery or for menorrhagia. Drug therapy to treat or prevent thrombosis or thromboembolism is extensively used because such diseases are common as well as serious. Drugs affect haemostasis and thrombosis in three distinct ways, by influencing:

- blood coagulation (fibrin formation)
- platelet function
- fibrin removal (fibrinolysis).

BLOOD COAGULATION

COAGULATION CASCADE

Blood coagulation means the conversion of liquid blood to a clot. The main event is the conversion by thrombin of soluble *fibrinogen* to insoluble strands of *fibrin*, the last step in a complex enzyme cascade. The components (called factors) are present in blood as inactive precursors (zymogens) of proteolytic enzymes and co-factors. They are activated by proteolysis, the active forms being desig-nated by the suffix 'a'. Factors XIIa, XIa, Xa, IXa and thrombin (IIa) are all serine proteases. Activation of a small amount of one factor catalyses the formation of larger amounts of the next factor, which catalyses the formation of still larger amounts of the next, and so on; consequently, the cascade provides a mechanism of amplification.[1] As might be expected, this accelerating enzyme cascade has to be controlled by inhibitors, because otherwise all the blood in the body would solidify within minutes of the initiation of haemostasis. One of the most important inhibitors is *antithrombin III*, which neutralises all the serine proteases in the cascade. Vascular endothelium also actively limits thrombus extension (see p. 295-296).

Two pathways of fibrin formation were described tra-ditionally (termed 'intrinsic' – because all the components are present in the blood – and 'extrinsic' – because some components come from outside the blood). The intrinsic or 'contact' pathway is activated when shed blood comes into contact with an artificial surface such as glass, but physiologically the system functions as a single *in vivo*

---

[1]Coagulation of 100 ml of blood requires 0.2 mg of factor VIII, 2 mg of factor X, 15 mg of prothrombin and 250 mg of fibrinogen.

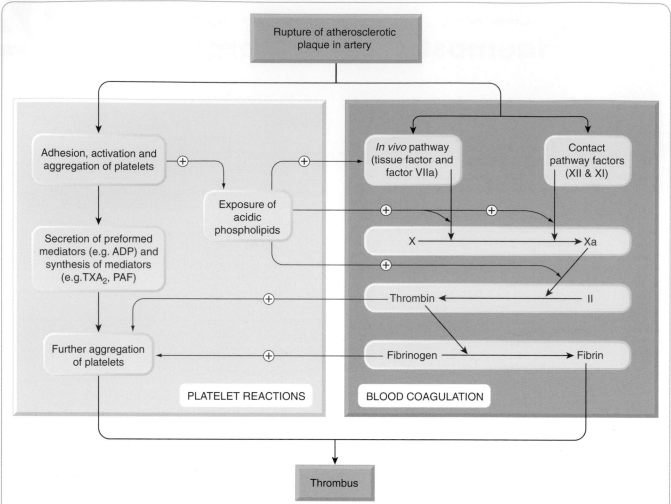

Fig. 24.1   The main events in the formation of an arterial thrombus. Exposure of acidic phospholipids during platelet activation provides a surface on which factors IXa and VIIa interact with factor X; factor Xa then interacts with factor II, as illustrated in more detail in Figure 24.4. Activation of factor XII also initiates the fibrinolytic pathway, which is shown in Figure 24.10. (A similar series of events occurs when there is vascular damage, leading to haemostasis.) PAF, platelet-activating factor; TXA$_2$, thromboxane A$_2$.

pathway (Fig. 24.2). Tissue damage exposes blood to *tissue factor*, initiating the process and leading to production of a small amount of thrombin. This acts through several positive feedbacks (on Va, VIIIa and on platelets) that amplify and propagate the process with production of more thrombin.

▼ 'Tissue factor' is the cellular receptor for factor VII, which, in the presence of Ca^{2+}, undergoes an active site transition. This results in rapid autocatalytic activation of factor VII to VIIa. The tissue factor–VIIa complex activates factors IX and X. Acidic phospholipids function as *surface catalysts*. They are provided during platelet activation, which exposes acidic phospholipids (especially phosphatidylserine), and these activate various clotting factors, closely juxtaposing them in functional complexes. Platelets also contribute by secreting coagulation factors, including factor Va and fibrinogen. Coagulation is sustained by further generation of factor Xa by IXa–VIIIa–Ca^{2+}–phospholipid complex. This is needed because the tissue factor–VIIa complex is rapidly inactivated in plasma by tissue factor pathway inhibitor and by antithrombin III. Factor Xa, in the presence of Ca^{2+}, phospholipid and factor Va, activates prothrombin to thrombin, the main enzyme of the cascade. The *contact* (intrinsic) pathway commences when factor XII (Hageman factor) adheres to a negatively charged surface and converges with the *in vivo* pathway at the stage of factor X activation (see Fig. 24.2). The proximal part of this

pathway is not crucial for blood coagulation *in vivo*.[2] The two pathways are not entirely separate even before they converge, and various positive feedbacks promote coagulation.

THE ROLE OF THROMBIN

Thrombin (factor IIa) cleaves fibrinogen, producing fragments that polymerise to form fibrin. It also activates factor XIII, a *fibrinoligase*, which strengthens fibrin-to-fibrin links, thereby stabilising the coagulum. In addition to coagulation, thrombin also causes platelet aggregation, stimulates cell proliferation and modulates smooth muscle contraction. Paradoxically, it can inhibit as well as promote coagulation (see p. 295-296). Effects of thrombin on platelets and smooth muscle are initiated by interaction with specific protease-activated receptors (PARs; see Ch. 3), which belong to the superfamily of G protein-coupled receptors. PARs initiate cellular responses that contribute not only to haemostasis and thrombosis, but also to inflammation

---

[2]Mr Hageman (the patient deficient in factor XII after whom it was named) died not from excessive bleeding but from a pulmonary embolism: factor XII deficiency does not give rise to a bleeding disorder.

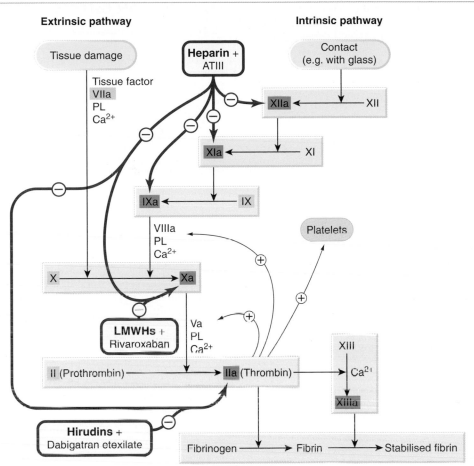

Fig. 24.2 **The coagulation cascade: sites of action of anticoagulant drugs.** Oral anticoagulants interfere with post-translational γ-carboxylation of factors II, VII, IX and X (shown in blue boxes); see Figure 24.4. Heparins activate antithrombin III. ATIII, antithrombin III; LMWHs, low-molecular-weight heparins; PL, negatively charged phospholipid supplied by activated platelets.

Haemostasis and thrombosis

- Haemostasis is the arrest of blood loss from damaged vessels and is essential to survival. The main phenomena are:
  - platelet adhesion and activation
  - blood coagulation (fibrin formation).
- Thrombosis is a pathological condition resulting from inappropriate activation of haemostatic mechanisms:
  - venous thrombosis is usually associated with stasis of blood; a venous thrombus has a small platelet component and a large component of fibrin
  - arterial thrombosis is usually associated with atherosclerosis, and the thrombus has a large platelet component.
- A portion of a thrombus may break away, travel as an embolus and lodge downstream, causing ischaemia and/or infarction.

VASCULAR ENDOTHELIUM IN HAEMOSTASIS AND THROMBOSIS

Vascular endothelium, the container of the circulating blood, can change focally from a non-thrombogenic to a thrombogenic structure in response to different demands. Normally, it provides a non-thrombogenic surface by virtue of membrane *heparan sulfate*, a glycosaminoglycan related to heparin, which is, like heparin, a co-factor for antithrombin III. Endothelium thus plays an essential role in preventing intravascular platelet activation and coagulation. However, it also plays an active part in haemostasis, synthesising and storing several key haemostatic components; von Willebrand factor,[3] tissue factor and plasminogen activator inhibitor (PAI)-1 are particularly important. PAI-1 is secreted in response to *angiotensin IV*, receptors for which are present on endothelial cells, providing a link between the renin–angiotensin system (see Ch. 22) and thrombosis. These prothrombotic factors are involved, respectively, in platelet adhesion and in coagulation and clot stabilisation. However, the endothelium is

and perhaps angiogenesis. The signal transduction mechanism is unusual: receptor activation requires proteolysis by thrombin of the extracellular N-terminal domain of the receptor, revealing a new N-terminal sequence that acts as a 'tethered agonist' (see Fig. 3.7).

[3]von Willebrand factor is a glycoprotein that is missing in a hereditary haemorrhagic disorder called von Willebrand's disease, which is the least uncommon of the inherited bleeding disorders. It is synthesised by vascular endothelial cells (the presence of immunoreactive von Willebrand factor is an identifying feature of these cells in culture) and is also present in platelets.

also implicated in thrombus limitation. Thus it generates prostaglandin (PG) I$_2$ (prostacyclin; Ch. 17) and nitric oxide (NO; Ch. 20); converts ADP, which causes platelet aggregation, to adenosine, which inhibits it (Ch. 16); synthesises *tissue plasminogen activator* (tPA; see p. 304-306); and expresses *thrombomodulin*, a receptor for thrombin. After combination with thrombomodulin, thrombin activates an anticoagulant, *protein C*. Activated protein C, helped by its co-factor protein S, inactivates factors Va and VIIa. This is known to be physiologically important, because a naturally occurring mutation of the gene coding for factor V (factor V Leiden), which confers resistance to activated protein C, results in the commonest recognised form of inherited thrombophilia.

Endotoxin and some cytokines, including tumour necrosis factor, tilt the balance of prothrombotic and antithrombotic endothelial functions towards thrombosis by causing loss of heparan (see above) and increased expression of tissue factor, and impair endothelial NO function. If other mechanisms limiting coagulation are also faulty or become exhausted, *disseminated intravascular coagulation* can result. This is a serious complication of sepsis and of certain malignancies, and the main treatment is to correct the underlying disease.

Blood coagulation (fibrin formation)

The clotting system consists of a cascade of proteolytic enzymes and co-factors.

- Inactive precursors are activated sequentially, each giving rise to more of the next.
- The last enzyme, thrombin, derived from prothrombin (II), converts soluble fibrinogen (I) to an insoluble meshwork of fibrin in which blood cells are trapped, forming the clot.
- There are two limbs in the cascade:
  - the *in vivo* (extrinsic) pathway
  - the contact (intrinsic) pathway.
- Both pathways result in activation of factor X to Xa, which converts prothrombin to thrombin.
- Calcium ions and a negatively charged phospholipid (PL) are essential for three steps, namely the actions of:
  - factor IXa on X
  - factor VIIa on X
  - factor Xa on II.
- PL is provided by activated platelets adhering to the damaged vessel.
- Some factors promote coagulation by binding to PL and a serine protease factor; for example, factor Va in the activation of II by Xa, or VIIIa in the activation of X by IXa.
- Blood coagulation is controlled by:
  - enzyme inhibitors (e.g. antithrombin III)
  - fibrinolysis.

DRUGS THAT ACT ON THE COAGULATION CASCADE

Drugs are used to modify the cascade either when there is a defect in coagulation or when there is unwanted coagulation.

COAGULATION DEFECTS

Genetically determined deficiencies of clotting factors are not common. Examples are classic haemophilia, caused by lack of factor VIII, and an even rarer form of haemophilia (haemophilia B or Christmas disease) caused by lack of factor IX (also called Christmas factor). Intravenous factor replacement is given by specialists to prevent or to limit bleeding in such patients. Some patients develop factor inhibitors, and their management is particularly demanding (for example by induction of immune tolerance, see Ch. 6). Plasma-derived concentrates are giving way to pure recombinant proteins (for example of factors VIII and IX; recombinant factor II is in development) – this is a rapidly evolving field. A human recombinant form of factor VIIa is also available for bleeding in patients with severe bleeding disorders but can cause intravascular coagulation.

Acquired clotting defects are more common than hereditary ones. The causes include liver disease, vitamin K deficiency (universal in neonates) and excessive oral anticoagulant therapy, each of which may require treatment with vitamin K.

VITAMIN K

Vitamin K (for *Koagulation* in German) is a fat-soluble vitamin (Fig. 24.3) occurring naturally in plants (vitamin K$_1$) and as a series of bacterial menaquinones (vitamin K$_2$) formed in the gut (see Shearer & Newman, 2008, for a review). It is essential for the formation of clotting factors II, VII, IX and X, which are glycoproteins with γ-carboxyglutamic acid (Gla) residues. The interaction of factors Xa and prothrombin (factor II) with Ca^{2+} and phospholipid is shown in Figure 24.4. γ-Carboxylation occurs after the synthesis of the amino acid chain, and the carboxylase enzyme requires reduced vitamin K as a co-factor (Fig. 24.5). Binding does not occur in the absence of γ-carboxylation. Similar considerations apply to the proteolytic activation of factor X by IXa and by VIIa (see Fig. 24.2).

There are several other vitamin K-dependent Gla proteins, including proteins C and S and osteocalcin in bone.

Administration and pharmacokinetic aspects

Natural vitamin K$_1$ (**phytomenadione**) may be given orally or by injection. If given by mouth, it requires bile salts for absorption, and this occurs by a saturable energy-requiring process in the proximal small intestine. A

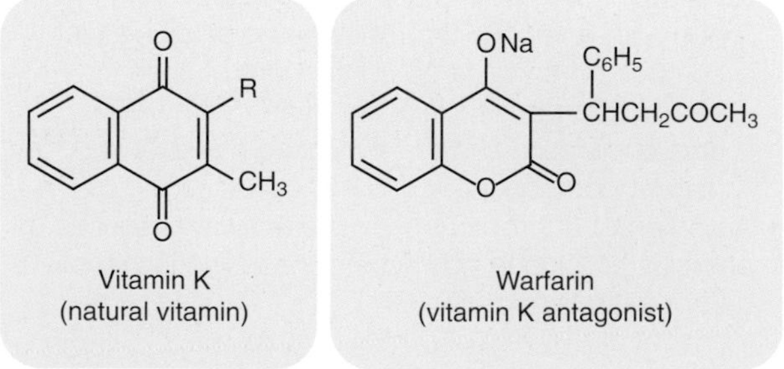

Vitamin K (natural vitamin)	Warfarin (vitamin K antagonist)

Fig. 24.3 Vitamin K and warfarin. Warfarin, a vitamin K antagonist, is an oral anticoagulant. It competes with vitamin K (note the similarity in their structures) for the reductase enzyme (VKORC1) that activates vitamin K and is the site of its action (see Fig. 24.5).

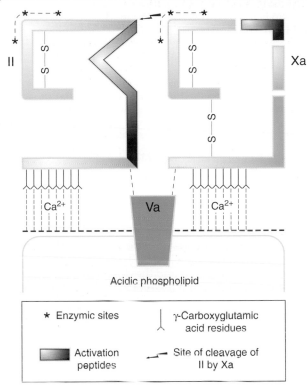

Fig. 24.4 Activation of prothrombin (factor II) by factor Xa. The complex of factor Va with a negatively charged phospholipid surface (supplied by aggregating platelets) forms a binding site for factor Xa and prothrombin (II), which have peptide chains (shown schematically) that are similar to one another. Platelets thus serve as a localising focus. Calcium ions are essential for binding. Xa activates prothrombin, liberating thrombin (shown in grey). *(Modified from Jackson CM 1978 Br J Haematol 39, 1.)*

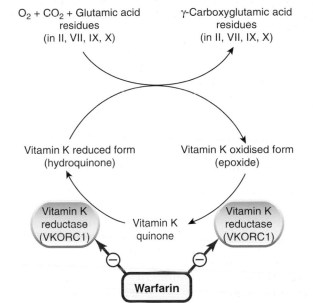

Fig. 24.5 Mechanism of vitamin K and of warfarin. After the peptide chains in clotting factors II, VII, IX and X have been synthesised, reduced vitamin K (the hydroquinone) acts as a co-factor in the conversion of glutamic acid to γ carboxyglutamic acid. During this reaction, the reduced form of vitamin K is converted to the epoxide, which in turn is reduced to the quinone and then the hydroquinone by vitamin K epoxide reductase component 1 (VKORC1), the site of action of warfarin.

synthetic preparation, **menadiol sodium phosphate**, is also available. It is water-soluble and does not require bile salts for its absorption. This synthetic compound takes longer to act than phytomenadione. There is very little storage of vitamin K in the body. It is metabolised to more polar substances that are excreted in the urine and the bile.

Clinical uses of vitamin K are summarised in the clinical box.

> ### Clinical uses of vitamin K
>
> - Treatment and/or prevention of bleeding:
>   - from excessive oral anticoagulation (e.g. by **warfarin**)
>   - in babies: to prevent *haemorrhagic disease of the newborn*.
> - For vitamin K deficiencies in adults:
>   - *sprue, coeliac disease, steatorrhoea*
>   - lack of bile (e.g. with *obstructive jaundice*).

THROMBOSIS

Thrombotic and thromboembolic disease is common and has severe consequences, including myocardial infarction,

stroke, deep vein thrombosis and pulmonary embolus. The main drugs used for platelet-rich 'white' arterial thrombi are the antiplatelet drugs and fibrinolytic drugs, which are considered below. The main drugs used to prevent or treat 'red' venous thrombi are:

- injectable anticoagulants (**heparin** and newer thrombin inhibitors)
- oral anticoagulants (**warfarin** and related compounds; orally active thrombin inhibitors).

Heparins and thrombin inhibitors act immediately, whereas warfarin and other vitamin K antagonists take several days to exert their effect. Consequently, if warfarin is used to treat patients with venous thrombosis, an agent that acts immediately is also administered until the effect of warfarin has become established.

HEPARIN (INCLUDING LOW-MOLECULAR-WEIGHT HEPARINS)

Heparin was discovered in 1916 by a second-year medical student at Johns Hopkins Hospital. He was attempting to extract thromboplastic (i.e. coagulant) substances from various tissues during a vacation project, but found instead a powerful anticoagulant activity.[4] This was named heparin, because it was first extracted from liver.

---

[4]This kind of good fortune also favoured Vane and his colleagues in their discovery of PGI$_2$ (Ch. 17), where they were looking for one kind of biological activity and found another. More specific chemical assays (Ch. 7), for all their strengths, cannot throw up this kind of unexpected discovery.

Heparin is not a single substance but a family of sulfated glycosaminoglycans (mucopolysaccharides). It is present together with histamine in the granules of mast cells. Commercial preparations are extracted from beef lung or hog intestine and, because preparations differ in potency, assayed biologically against an agreed international standard: doses are specified in units of activity rather than of mass.

Heparin fragments (e.g. **enoxaparin, dalteparin**) or a synthetic pentasaccharide (**fondaparinux**), referred to as low-molecular-weight heparins (LMWHs), are longer acting than unfractionated heparin and are usually preferred, the unfractionated product being reserved for special situations such as patients with renal failure in whom LMWHs are contraindicated.

Mechanism of action

Heparin inhibits coagulation, both *in vivo* and *in vitro*, by activating antithrombin III. Antithrombin III inhibits thrombin and other serine proteases by binding to the active site. Heparin modifies this interaction by binding, via a unique pentasaccharide sequence, to antithrombin III, changing its conformation and increasing its affinity for serine proteases.

To inhibit thrombin, it is necessary for heparin to bind to the enzyme as well as to antithrombin III; to inhibit factor Xa, it is necessary only for heparin to bind to antithrombin III (Fig. 24.6). Antithrombin III deficiency is very rare but can cause thrombophilia and resistance to heparin therapy.

The LMWHs increase the action of antithrombin III on factor Xa but not its action on thrombin, because the molecules are too small to bind to both enzyme and inhibitor, essential for inhibition of thrombin but not for that of factor Xa (Fig. 24.6).

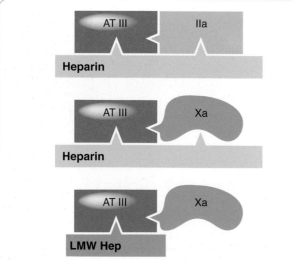

Fig. 24.6 Action of heparins. The schematic shows interactions of heparins, antithrombin III (AT III) and clotting factors. To increase the inactivation of thrombin (IIa) by AT III, heparin needs to interact with both substances (top), but to speed up its effect on factor Xa it need only interact with AT III (middle). Low-molecular-weight heparins (LMW Hep) increase the action of AT III on factor Xa (bottom), but cannot increase the action of AT III on thrombin because they cannot bind both simultaneously.

Administration and pharmacokinetic aspects

Heparin is not absorbed from the gut because of its charge and high molecular weight, and it is therefore given intravenously or subcutaneously (intramuscular injections would cause haematomas).

▼ After intravenous injection of a bolus dose, there is a phase of rapid elimination followed by a more gradual disappearance owing both to saturable processes (involving binding to sites on endothelial cells and macrophages) and to slower non-saturable processes including renal excretion. As a result, once the dose exceeds the saturating concentration, a greater proportion is dealt with by these slower processes, and the apparent half-life increases with increasing dose (saturation kinetics; see Ch. 10).

Heparin acts immediately following intravenous administration, but the onset is delayed by up to 60 min when it is given subcutaneously. The elimination half-life is approximately 40–90 min. In urgent situations, it is therefore usual to start treatment with a bolus intravenous dose, followed by a constant-rate infusion. The *activated partial thromboplastin time* (APTT), or some other *in vitro* clotting test, is measured and the dose of heparin adjusted to achieve a value within a target range (e.g. 1.5–2.5 times control).

Low-molecular-weight heparins are given subcutaneously. They have a longer elimination half-life than unfractionated heparin, and this is independent of dose (first-order kinetics), so the effects are more predictable and dosing less frequent (once or twice a day). LMWHs do not prolong the APTT. Unlike unfractionated heparin, the effect of a standard dose is sufficiently predictable that monitoring is not required routinely. LMWHs are eliminated mainly by renal excretion, and unfractionated heparin is preferred in renal failure, but with this exception LMWHs are at least as safe and effective as unfractionated heparin and are more convenient to use, because patients can be taught to inject themselves at home and there is generally no need for blood tests and dose adjustment.

Unwanted effects

Haemorrhage. The main hazard is haemorrhage, which is treated by stopping therapy and, if necessary, giving **protamine sulfate**. This heparin antagonist is a strongly basic protein that forms an inactive complex with heparin; it is given intravenously. The dose is estimated from the dose of heparin that has been administered recently, and it is important not to give too much, as this can itself cause bleeding. If necessary, an *in vitro* neutralisation test is performed on a sample of blood from the patient to provide a more precise indication of the required dose.

Thrombosis. This is an uncommon but serious adverse effect of heparin and, as with warfarin necrosis, may be misattributed to the natural history of the disease for which heparin is being administered.

▼ Paradoxically, it is associated with *heparin-induced thrombocytopenia* (HIT). A transitory early decrease in platelet numbers is not uncommon after initiating heparin treatment, and is not clinically important. More serious thrombocytopenia occurring 2–14 days after the start of therapy is uncommon and is referred to as type II HIT. This is caused by IgM or IgG antibodies against complexes of heparin and a platelet-derived chemokine, platelet factor 4. Circulating immune complexes bind to circulating platelets, and cause thrombocytopenia. Antibody also binds to platelet factor 4 attached to the surface of endothelial cells, leading to immune injury of the vessel wall, thrombosis and disseminated intravascular coagulation. LMWHs are less likely than unfractionated heparin to cause thrombocytopenia and thrombosis by this mechanism. HIT is usually treated by substituting **danaparoid** or a direct thrombin inhibitor such as **lepirudin** instead of the heparin preparation that caused the problem. Danaparoid is a low-molecular-weight heparinoid consisting of a mixture of heparan, dermatan and chondroitin sulfates, with well-established antithrombotic activity.

Osteoporosis with spontaneous fractures has been reported with long-term (6 months or more) treatment with heparin (usually during pregnancy, when warfarin is contraindicated or problematic). Its explanation is unknown.

Hypoaldosteronism (with consequent hyperkalaemia) is uncommon, but increases with prolonged treatment. It is recommended to check plasma K^+ concentration if treatment is to be continued for >7 days.

Hypersensitivity reactions are rare with heparin but more common with protamine. (Protamine sensitivity also occurs in patients treated with protamine zinc insulin; Ch. 31. Protamine is extracted from fish roe, and sensitivity to protamine occurs in some people with fish allergy.)

DIRECT THROMBIN INHIBITORS AND RELATED DRUGS

Hirudins are polypeptides that act as direct thrombin inhibitors. They are derived from the anticoagulant present in saliva from the medicinal leech. Unlike the heparins, they do not depend on activation of antithrombin. **Lepirudin** is a recombinant hirudin that binds irreversibly to both the fibrin-binding and catalytic sites on thrombin and is used for thromboembolic disease in patients with type II HIT. It is administered intravenously, the dose being adjusted depending on the APTT, and can cause bleeding or hypersensitivity reactions (rash or fever). **Bivalirudin**, another hirudin analogue, is used in combination with **aspirin** and **clopidogrel** (see p. 302-303) in patients undergoing percutaneous coronary artery surgery. Treatment is initiated with an intravenous bolus followed by an infusion during and up to 4 h after the procedure. It can cause bleeding and hypersensitivity reactions.

Orally active direct inhibitors. This field had more than one false dawn, but rapid progress has been made recently, and indications for such drugs have expanded considerably. In time orally active direct inhibitors could come to replace warfarin, a venerable but troublesome drug that is a common cause of serious adverse effects. **Dabigatran** is a synthetic serine protease inhibitor; **dabigatran etexilate**, a prodrug with a hydrophobic tail, is orally active and is licensed for prevention of venous thromboembolism following hip or knee replacement and for the prevention of stroke and systemic embolism in atrial fibrillation (Ch. 20). It works rapidly and is administered 1–4 hours after surgery and then once daily for up to a month (depending on the type of surgery), or twice daily indefinitely for the prevention of stroke. The dose is reduced in patients aged over 75 or receiving concomitant verapamil or amiodarone. **Rivaroxaban**, an orally active direct inhibitor of factor Xa rather than of thrombin, but similar to dabigatran in other respects, is licensed for the same indications and in addition for the treatment (as well as prophylaxis) of deep vein thrombosis. **Apixiban** is similar. These drugs are administered in standard doses without laboratory monitoring of their anticoagulant effects. Their commonest adverse effects are predictable (bleeding, anaemia); rivaroxaban also commonly causes nausea. Other indications are being investigated, and if they prove safe and effective for a range of indications, this could transform the clinical management of the large group of patients currently maintained on warfarin (see the clinical box on the clinical use of anticoagulants, p. 301).

▼ Various other approaches are being explored. These include several naturally occurring anticoagulants (tissue factor pathway inhibitor, thrombomodulin and protein C) synthesised by recombinant technology. A particularly ingenious approach is the development of thrombin agonists that are selective for the anticoagulant properties of thrombin. One such modified thrombin, differing by a single amino acid substitution, has substrate specificity for protein C. It produces anticoagulation in monkeys without prolonging bleeding times, suggesting that it may be less likely than standard anticoagulants to cause bleeding (Bah et al., 2009).

WARFARIN

▼ Oral anticoagulants were discovered as an indirect result of a change in agricultural policy in North America in the 1920s. Sweet clover was substituted for corn in cattle feed, and an epidemic of deaths of cattle from haemorrhage ensued. This turned out to be caused by bishydroxycoumarin in spoiled sweet clover, and it led to the discovery of warfarin (named for the Wisconsin Alumni Research Foundation). One of the first uses to which this was put was as a rat poison, but for more than 50 years it was the standard anticoagulant for the treatment and prevention of thromboembolic disease.

Warfarin (Fig. 24.3) is the most important oral anticoagulant; alternatives with a similar mechanism of action, for example **phenindione**, are now used only in rare patients who experience idiosyncratic adverse reactions to warfarin. Warfarin and other vitamin K antagonists require frequent blood tests to individualise dose, and are consequently inconvenient as well as having a low margin of safety.

Mechanism of action

Vitamin K antagonists act only *in vivo* and have no effect on clotting if added to blood *in vitro*. They interfere with the post-translational γ-carboxylation of glutamic acid residues in clotting factors II, VII, IX and X. They do this by inhibiting *vitamin K epoxide reductase component 1* (VKORC1), thus inhibiting the reduction of vitamin K epoxide to its active hydroquinone form (Fig. 24.5). Inhibition is competitive (reflecting the structural similarity between warfarin and vitamin K; Fig. 24.3). The *VKORC1* gene is polymorphic (see Ch. 11), and different haplotypes have different affinities for warfarin. Genotyping to determine the haplotype, combined with genotyping *CYP2C9* (see below), while not yet routine, can reduce the variability in response to warfarin by around one-third. The effect of warfarin takes several days to develop because of the time taken for degradation of preformed carboxylated clotting factors. Onset of action thus depends on the elimination half-lives of the relevant factors. Factor VII, with a half-life of 6 h, is affected first, then IX, X and II, with half-lives of 24, 40 and 60 h, respectively.

Administration and pharmacokinetic aspects

Warfarin is absorbed rapidly and completely from the gut after oral administration. It has a small distribution volume, being strongly bound to plasma albumin (see Ch. 8). The peak concentration in the blood occurs within an hour of ingestion, but because of the mechanism of action this does not coincide with the peak pharmacological effect, which occurs about 48 h later. The effect on prothrombin time (PT, see below) of a single dose starts after approximately 12–16 h and lasts 4–5 days. Warfarin is metabolised by CYP2C9, which is polymorphic (see

Ch. 11). Partly in consequence of this, its half-life is very variable, being of the order of 40 h in many individuals.

Warfarin crosses the placenta and is not given in the first months of pregnancy because it is teratogenic (see Table 57.2, Ch. 57), nor in the later stages because it can cause intracranial haemorrhage in the baby during delivery. It appears in milk during lactation. This could theoretically be important because newborn infants are naturally deficient in vitamin K. However, infants are routinely prescribed vitamin K to prevent haemorrhagic disease, so warfarin treatment of the mother does not generally pose a risk to the breastfed infant.

The therapeutic use of warfarin requires a careful balance between giving too little, leaving unwanted coagulation unchecked, and giving too much, thereby causing haemorrhage. Therapy is complicated not only because the effect of each dose is maximal some 2 days after its administration, but also because numerous medical and environmental conditions modify sensitivity to warfarin, including interactions with other drugs (see Ch. 9). The effect of warfarin is monitored by measuring prothrombin time (PT), which is expressed as an *international normalised ratio* (INR).

▼ The PT is the time taken for clotting of citrated plasma after the addition of Ca^{2+} and standardised reference thromboplastin; it is expressed as the ratio (PT ratio) of the PT of the patient to the PT of a pool of plasma from healthy subjects on no medication. Because of the variability of thromboplastins, different results are obtained in different laboratories. To standardise PT measurements internationally, each thromboplastin is assigned an international sensitivity index (ISI), and the patient's PT is expressed as an INR, where INR = (PT ratio)^{ISI}. This kind of inter-laboratory normalisation procedure shocks purists but provides similar results when a patient moves from, say, Birmingham to Baltimore. Pragmatic haematologists argue that the proof of the pudding is in the eating!

The dose of warfarin is usually adjusted to give an INR of 2–4, the precise target depending on the clinical situation. The duration of treatment also varies, but for several indications (e.g. to prevent thromboembolism in chronic atrial fibrillation), treatment is long term, with the logistical challenge of providing a worldwide network of anticoagulant clinics and demands on the patient in terms of repeat visits and blood tests.

FACTORS THAT POTENTIATE WARFARIN

Various diseases and drugs potentiate warfarin, increasing the risk of haemorrhage.

Disease

Liver disease interferes with the synthesis of clotting factors; conditions in which there is a high metabolic rate, such as fever and thyrotoxicosis, increase the effect of anticoagulants by increasing degradation of clotting factors.

Drugs (see also Ch. 9)

Many drugs potentiate warfarin.

Agents that inhibit hepatic drug metabolism. Examples include **co-trimoxazole, ciprofloxacin, metronidazole, amiodarone** and many antifungal azoles. Stereoselective effects (warfarin is a racemate, and its isomers are metabolised differently from one another) are described in Chapter 9.

Drugs that inhibit platelet function. Aspirin increases the risk of bleeding if given during warfarin therapy, although this combination can be used safely with careful

monitoring. Other non-steroidal anti-inflammatory drugs (NSAIDs) also increase the risk of bleeding, partly by their effect on platelet thromboxane synthesis (Ch. 26) and, in the case of some NSAIDs, also by inhibiting warfarin metabolism as above. Some antibiotics, including **moxalactam** and **carbenicillin**, inhibit platelet function.

Drugs that displace warfarin from binding sites on plasma albumin. Some of the NSAIDs and **chloral hydrate** cause a transient increase in the concentration of free warfarin in plasma by competing with it for binding to plasma albumin. This mechanism seldom causes clinically important effects, unless accompanied by inhibition of warfarin metabolism, as with **phenylbutazone** (Ch. 9).

Drugs that inhibit reduction of vitamin K. Such drugs include the *cephalosporins*.

Drugs that decrease the availability of vitamin K. Broad-spectrum antibiotics and some *sulfonamides* (see Ch. 50) depress the intestinal flora that normally synthesise vitamin K_2; this has little effect unless there is concurrent dietary deficiency.

FACTORS THAT LESSEN THE EFFECT OF WARFARIN

Physiological state/disease

There is a decreased response to warfarin in conditions (e.g. pregnancy) where there is increased coagulation factor synthesis. Similarly, the effect of oral anticoagulants is lessened in hypothyroidism, which is associated with reduced degradation of coagulation factors.

Drugs (see also Ch. 9)

Several drugs reduce the effectiveness of warfarin; this leads to increased doses being used to achieve the target INR. Furthermore, the dose of warfarin must be reduced when the interacting drug is discontinued, to avoid haemorrhage.

Vitamin K. This vitamin is a component of some parenteral feeds and vitamin preparations.

Drugs that induce hepatic P450 enzymes. Enzyme induction (e.g. by **rifampicin, carbamazepine**) increases the rate of degradation of warfarin. Induction may wane only slowly after the inducing drug is discontinued, making it difficult to adjust the warfarin dose appropriately.

Drugs that reduce absorption. Drugs that bind warfarin in the gut, for example **colestyramine**, reduce its absorption.

UNWANTED EFFECTS OF WARFARIN

Haemorrhage (especially into the bowel or the brain) is the main hazard. Depending on the urgency of the situation, treatment may consist of withholding warfarin (for minor problems), administration of vitamin K, or fresh plasma or coagulation factor concentrates (for life-threatening bleeding).

Oral anticoagulants are *teratogenic*, causing disordered bone development which is believed to be related to binding to the vitamin K-dependent protein osteocalcin.

Hepatotoxicity occurs but is uncommon.

Necrosis of soft tissues (e.g. breast or buttock) owing to thrombosis in venules is a rare but serious effect that occurs shortly after starting treatment and is attributed to inhibition of biosynthesis of protein C, which has a shorter elimination half-life than do the vitamin K-dependent coagulation factors; this results in a procoagulant state

Drugs affecting blood coagulation

Procoagulant drugs: vitamin K

- Reduced vitamin K is a co-factor in the post-translational γ-carboxylation of glutamic acid (Glu) residues in factors II, VII, IX and X. The γ-carboxylated glutamic acid (Gla) residues are essential for the interaction of these factors with Ca²⁺ and negatively charged phospholipid.

Injectable anticoagulants (e.g. heparin, low-molecular-weight heparins)

- Potentiate antithrombin III, a natural inhibitor that inactivates Xa and thrombin.
- Act both *in vivo* and *in vitro*.
- Anticoagulant activity results from a unique pentasaccharide sequence with high affinity for antithrombin III.
- **Heparin** therapy is monitored via activated partial thromboplastin time (APTT), and dose individualised. Unfractionated heparin (UFH) is used for patients with impaired renal function.
- **Low-molecular-weight heparins** (LMWHs) have the same effect on factor X as heparin but less effect on thrombin; therapeutic efficacy is similar to **heparin** but monitoring and dose individualisation are not needed. Patients can administer them subcutaneously at home. They are preferred over UFH except for patients with impaired renal function.

Oral anticoagulants (e.g. warfarin, direct thrombin and Xa inhibitors)

- **Warfarin** is the main vitamin K antagonist.
- Vitamin K antagonists act on vitamin K epoxide reductase component 1 (VKORC1) to inhibit the reduction of vitamin K epoxide, thus inhibiting the γ-carboxylation of Glu in II, VII, IX and X.
- Vitamin K antagonists act only *in vivo*, and their effect is delayed until preformed clotting factors are depleted.
- Many factors modify the action of vitamin K antagonists; genetic factors (polymorphisms of CYP2C6 and VKORC1) and drug interactions are especially important.
- There is wide variation in response to vitamin K antagonists; their effect is monitored by measuring the international normalised ratio (INR) and the dose individualised accordingly.
- Orally active direct thrombin inhibitors (e.g. **dabigatran etexilate**) or factor Xa inhibitors (e.g. **rivaroxaban, apixiban**) are used increasingly and do not require laboratory monitoring/dose titration. They are licensed for preventing stroke in patients with atrial fibrillation and for preventing deep vein thrombosis after orthopaedic surgery.

Clinical uses of anticoagulants

Heparin (often as **low-molecular-weight heparin**) is used acutely. **Warfarin** or a direct thrombin or Xa inhibitor is used for more prolonged therapy. Anticoagulants are used to prevent:
- deep vein thrombosis (e.g. perioperatively)
- extension of established deep vein thrombosis
- pulmonary embolism
- thrombosis and embolisation in patients with atrial fibrillation (Ch. 21)
- thrombosis on prosthetic heart valves
- clotting in extracorporeal circulations (e.g. during haemodialysis)
- progression of myocardial damage in patients with unstable angina and during treatment of ST-elevation myocardial infarction.

PLATELET ADHESION AND ACTIVATION

Platelets maintain the integrity of the circulation: a low platelet count results in *thrombocytopenic purpura*.[5]

When platelets are activated, they undergo a sequence of reactions that are essential for haemostasis, important for the healing of damaged blood vessels, and play a part in inflammation (see Ch. 17). These reactions, several of which are redundant (in the sense that if one pathway of activation is blocked another is available) and several autocatalytic, include:

- *adhesion* following vascular damage (via von Willebrand factor bridging between subendothelial macromolecules and glycoprotein [GP] Ib receptors on the platelet surface)[6]
- *shape change* (from smooth discs to spiny spheres with protruding pseudopodia)
- *secretion* of the granule contents (including platelet agonists, such as ADP and 5-hydroxytryptamine, and coagulation factors and growth factors, such as platelet-derived growth factor)
- *biosynthesis of labile mediators* such as platelet-activating factor and thromboxane (TX)A₂ (see Ch. 17 and Fig. 24.7)
- *aggregation*, which is promoted by various agonists, including collagen, thrombin, ADP, 5-hydroxytryptamine and TXA₂, acting on specific receptors on the platelet surface; activation by agonists leads to expression of GPIIb/IIIa receptors that bind fibrinogen, which links adjacent platelets to form aggregates
- *exposure of acidic phospholipid* on the platelet surface, promoting thrombin formation (and hence further platelet activation via thrombin receptors and fibrin formation via cleavage of fibrinogen; see above).

soon after starting treatment. Treatment with a heparin is usually started at the same time as warfarin, avoiding this problem except in individuals experiencing HIT as an adverse effect of heparin (see p. 298).

The clinical use of anticoagulants is summarised in the box.

[5]Purpura means a purple rash caused by multiple spontaneous bleeding points in the skin. When this is caused by reduced circulating platelets, bleeding can occur into other organs, including the gut and brain.
[6]Various platelet membrane glycoproteins act as receptors or binding sites for adhesive proteins such as von Willebrand factor or fibrinogen.

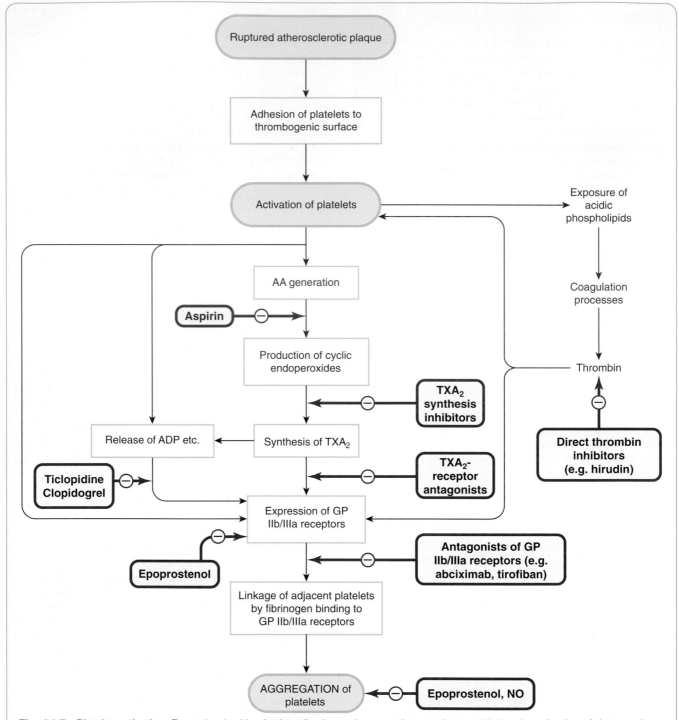

Fig. 24.7   Platelet activation. Events involved in platelet adhesion and aggregation are shown, with the sites of action of drugs and endogenous mediators. AA, arachidonic acid; ADP, adenosine bisphosphate; GP, glycoprotein; NO, nitric oxide; TXA$_2$, thromboxane A$_2$.

These processes are essential for haemostasis but may be inappropriately triggered if the artery wall is diseased, most commonly with atherosclerosis, resulting in thrombosis (Fig. 24.7).

ANTIPLATELET DRUGS

Platelets play such a critical role in thromboembolic disease that it is no surprise that antiplatelet drugs are of great therapeutic value. Clinical trials of aspirin radically

altered clinical practice, and more recently drugs that block ADP receptors and GPIIb/IIIa have also been found to be therapeutically useful. Sites of action of antiplatelet drugs are shown in Figure 24.7.

ASPIRIN

Low-dose aspirin (see Ch. 26) in chronic use profoundly (>95%) inhibits platelet TXA$_2$ synthesis, by irreversible acetylation of a serine residue in the active site of

Platelet function

- Healthy vascular endothelium prevents platelet adhesion.
- Platelets adhere to diseased or damaged areas and become activated, changing shape and exposing negatively charged phospholipids and glycoprotein (GP) IIb/IIIa receptors, and synthesise and/or release various mediators, for example thromboxane A_2 and ADP, which activate other platelets, causing aggregation.
- Aggregation entails fibrinogen binding to and bridging between GPIIb/IIIa receptors on adjacent platelets.
- Activated platelets constitute a focus for fibrin formation.
- Chemotactic factors and growth factors necessary for repair, but also implicated in atherogenesis, are released during platelet activation.

cyclo-oxygenase I (COX-I). Oral administration is relatively selective for platelets because of presystemic drug elimination (Ch. 9). Unlike nucleated cells, platelets cannot synthesise proteins, so after administration of aspirin, TXA_2 synthesis does not recover fully until the affected cohort of platelets is replaced in 7–10 days. Clinical trials have demonstrated the efficacy of aspirin in several clinical settings (e.g. Fig. 24.8). For acute indications

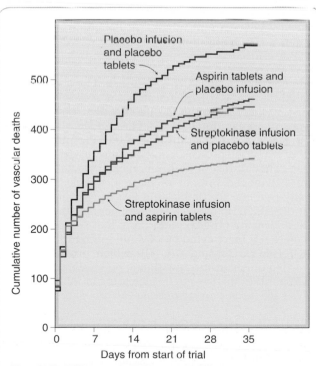

Fig. 24.8 Efficacy of aspirin and streptokinase for myocardial infarction. The curves show cumulative vascular mortality in patients treated with placebo, aspirin alone, streptokinase alone or a combined aspirin–streptokinase regimen. (ISIS-2 Trial 1988 Lancet ii, 350–360.)

(thrombotic stroke in evolution, acute myocardial infarction) treatment is started with a single dose of approximately 300 mg in order to achieve rapid substantial (>95%) inhibition of platelet thromboxane synthesis, followed by regular daily doses of 75 mg. Adverse effects of aspirin, mainly on the gastrointestinal tract, are, however, clearly dose-related, so a low dose (often 75 mg once daily) is usually recommended for thromboprophylaxis. Thromboprophylaxis is reserved for people at high cardiovascular risk (e.g. survivors of myocardial infarction), in whom the cardiovascular benefit of aspirin usually outweighs the risk of gastrointestinal bleeding.

▼ Treatment failure can occur despite taking aspirin, and there is current interest in the possibility that some patients exhibit a syndrome of 'aspirin resistance', although the mechanism and possible importance of this remains controversial (see Goodman et al., 2008). Other non-steroidal drugs that inhibit platelet TXA_2 synthesis > 95% (e.g. **sulfinpyrazone**, for which there is also supportive clinical trial evidence, and **naproxen** – see Ch. 26) may have antithrombotic effects, but where inhibition of platelet TXA_2 synthesis does not reach this threshold there is evidence that such drugs are *proaggregatory*, related to inhibition of COX-2, possibly due to inhibition of antiaggregatory PGI_2 in blood vessels.

DIPYRIDAMOLE

Dipyridamole inhibits platelet aggregation by several mechanisms, including inhibition of phosphodiesterase, block of adenosine uptake into red cells (see Ch. 16) and inhibition of TXA_2 synthesis (see Ch. 26). Clinical effectiveness has been uncertain, but one study showed that a modified-release form of dipyridamole reduced the risk of stroke and death in patients with transient ischaemic attacks by around 15% – similar to aspirin (25 mg twice daily).[7] The beneficial effects of aspirin and dipyridamole were additive. The main side effects of dipyridamole are dizziness, headache and gastrointestinal disturbances; unlike aspirin, it does not increase the risk of bleeding.

ADENOSINE (P2Y$_{12}$) RECEPTOR ANTAGONISTS

Ticlopidine was the first to be introduced, but causes neutropenia and thrombocytopenia. The main agents are currently **clopidogrel, prasugrel** and **ticagrelor** each of which is combined with low-dose aspirin in patients with unstable coronary artery disease, usually for up to 1 year.

Clopidogrel and prasugrel inhibit ADP induced platelet aggregation by irreversible inhibition of $P2Y_{12}$ receptors (Ch. 16) to which they link via a disulfide bond, whereas ticagrelor is a reversible but non-competitive inhibitor of the $P2Y_{12}$ receptor.

Pharmacokinetics and unwanted effects

Clopidogrel is well absorbed when administered by mouth, and in urgent situations is given orally as a loading dose of 300 mg followed by maintenance dosing of 75 mg once daily. It is a prodrug and is converted into its active sulfhydryl metabolite by CYP enzymes in the liver including CYP2C19. Patients with variant alleles of *CYP2C19* (poor metabolisers) are at increased risk of therapeutic failure. There is a potential for interaction with other drugs, such as **omeprazole** (Ch. 30), that are metabolised by CYP2C19 and current labelling recommends against use with proton pump inhibitors for this reason. Prasugrel

---

[7]This dose regimen of aspirin is unconventional, being somewhat lower than the 75 mg once daily commonly used in thromboprophylaxis.

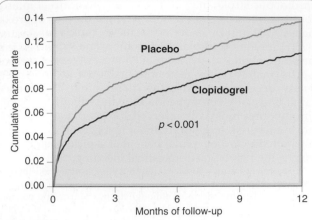

Fig. 24.9 **Effect of adding clopidogrel to aspirin.** The curves show cumulative hazard rates for major vascular events in patients with acute coronary syndromes treated either with placebo + aspirin or clopidogrel + aspirin. *(Modified from CURE Investigators 2001 N Engl J Med 345, 494–502.)*

is given as a loading dose followed by maintenance once daily dosing with dose adjustment in older and underweight patients. Ticagrelor is given as a loading dose followed by twice daily maintenance.

These drugs predictably increase the risk of haemorrhage. Clopidogrel can cause dyspepsia, rash or diarrhoea. The serious blood dyscrasias caused by ticlopidine are very rare with clopidogrel. Prasugrel can cause rash or, rarely hypersensitivity reactions and angioedema. Ticagrelor can cause dyspnea (perhaps related to the role of adenosine signalling in the carotid bodies, Ch. 28) or, less commonly, gastrointestinal symptoms.

Clinical use

Clopidogrel was slightly more effective than aspirin as a single agent in reducing a composite outcome of ischaemic stroke, myocardial infarction or vascular death in one large trial; it can be used instead of aspirin in patients with symptomatic atheromatous disease, but is usually reserved for patients who are intolerant of aspirin. Clinical trials of adding clopidogrel to aspirin in patients with acute coronary syndromes (see Fig. 24.9) and (in a megatrial of over 45 000 patients) in patients with acute myocardial infarction (COMMIT Collaborative Group, 2005) demonstrated that combined treatment reduces mortality. Treatment with clopidogrel for this indication is given for 4 weeks. Prasugrel is more effective than clopidogrel in acute coronary syndromes, but more often causes serious bleeding. Pretreatment with clopidogrel and aspirin followed by longer-term therapy is also effective in patients with ischaemic heart disease undergoing percutaneous coronary interventions. Treatment of acute coronary syndrome with ticagrelor as compared with clopidogrel significantly reduces the rate of death for unknown reasons.

GLYCOPROTEIN IIB/IIIA RECEPTOR ANTAGONISTS

Antagonists of the GPIIb/IIIa receptor have the theoretical attraction that they inhibit all pathways of platelet activation (because these all converge on activation of GPIIb/IIIa receptors). A hybrid murine–human monoclonal antibody Fab fragment directed against the GPIIb/

IIIa receptor, which rejoices in the catchy little name of **abciximab**,[8] is licensed for use in high-risk patients undergoing coronary angioplasty, as an adjunct to heparin and aspirin. It reduces the risk of restenosis at the expense of an increased risk of bleeding. Immunogenicity limits its use to a single administration.

Tirofiban is a synthetic non-peptide and **eptifibatide** is a cyclic peptide based on the Arg–Gly–Asp ('RGD') sequence that is common to ligands for GPIIb/IIIa receptors. Neither is absorbed if administered by mouth. Given intravenously as an adjunct to aspirin and a heparin preparation, they reduce early events in acute coronary syndrome, but long-term oral therapy with GPIIb/IIIa receptor antagonists is not effective and may be harmful. Unsurprisingly, they increase the risk of bleeding.

OTHER ANTIPLATELET DRUGS

Epoprostenol (PGI₂), an agonist at prostanoid IP receptors (see Ch. 17), causes vasodilatation as well as inhibiting platelet aggregation. It is added to blood entering the dialysis circuit in order to prevent thrombosis during haemodialysis, especially in patients in whom heparin is contraindicated. It is also used in severe pulmonary hypertension (Ch. 22) and circulatory shock associated with meningococcal septicaemia. It is unstable under physiological conditions and has a half-life of around 3 min, so it is administered as an intravenous infusion. Adverse effects related to its vasodilator action include flushing, headache and hypotension.

The clinical use of antiplatelet drugs is summarised in the clinical box (p. 306).

FIBRINOLYSIS (THROMBOLYSIS)

When the coagulation system is activated, the fibrinolytic system is also set in motion via several endogenous *plasminogen activators*, including tissue plasminogen activator (tPA), urokinase-type plasminogen activator, kallikrein and neutrophil elastase. tPA is inhibited by a structurally related lipoprotein, *lipoprotein(a)*, increased concentrations of which constitute an independent risk factor for myocardial infarction (Ch. 23). Plasminogen is deposited on the fibrin strands within a thrombus. Plasminogen activators are serine proteases and are unstable in circulating blood. They diffuse into thrombus and cleave plasminogen, a zymogen present in plasma, to release plasmin locally (see Fig. 24.10). Plasmin is a trypsin-like protease that digests fibrin as well as fibrinogen, factors II, V and VIII, and many other proteins; any that escapes into the circulation is inactivated by plasmin inhibitors, including PAI-1 (see p. 295 and Ch. 22), which protect us from digesting ourselves from within.

Drugs affect this system by increasing or inhibiting fibrinolysis (*fibrinolytic* and *antifibrinolytic* drugs, respectively).

FIBRINOLYTIC DRUGS

Figure 24.10 summarises the interaction of the fibrinolytic system with the coagulation cascade and platelet activation, and the action of drugs that modify this. Several

---

[8]The convention for naming monoclonals is: momab = -**mo**use **mo**noclonal **a**nti**b**ody; -umab = human; -zumab = humanised; -ximab = chimeric – a kind of medieval mouse–man nightmare.

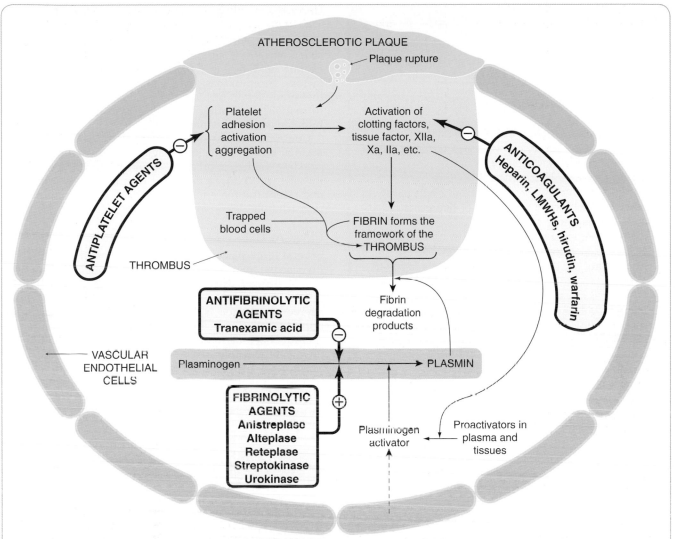

Fig. 24.10 Fibrinolytic system. The schematic shows interactions with coagulation and platelet pathways and sites of action of drugs that modify these systems. LMWHs, low-molecular-weight heparins. For more details of platelet activation and the coagulation cascade, refer to Figures 24.1, 24.2 and 24.7.

Antiplatelet drugs

- **Aspirin** inhibits cyclo-oxygenase irreversibly. In chronic use low doses very effectively (>95%) inhibit platelet thromboxane (TX)A$_2$ synthesis and reduce the risk of thrombosis. Treatment is started with a larger dose (300 mg) in acute settings in order to achieve rapid inhibition of platelet thromboxane synthesis.
- ADP antagonists are combined with low dose aspirin in treating patients with ustable coronary artery disease. **Clopidogrel** is a prodrug. Given by mouth, it irreversibly inhibits P2Y$_{12}$ receptors and thereby inhibits platelet responses to ADP. Its clinical effect is additive with **aspirin**. **Prasugrel** has as similar mechanism. **Ticagrelor** is reversible but non-competitive. **Prasugrel** and **ticagrelor** are more effective than licensed doses of **clopidogrel**.

- Antagonists of GPIIb/IIIa receptors include a monoclonal antibody (**abciximab**) and several synthetic molecules (e.g. **tirofiban**). They inhibit diverse agonists, for example ADP and TXA$_2$, because different pathways of activation converge on GPIIb/IIIa receptors. They are administered intravenously for short-term treatment.
- **Dipyridamole** inhibits phosphodiesterase and adenosine uptake. It is used in addition to aspirin in some patients with stroke or transient ischaemic attack.
- **Epoprostenol** (synthetic PGI$_2$) is chemically unstable. Given as an intravenous infusion, it acts on I prostanoid (IP) receptors on vascular smooth muscle and platelets (Ch. 17), stimulating adenylyl cyclase and thereby causing vasodilatation and inhibiting aggregation caused by any pathway (e.g. ADP or TXA$_2$).

Clinical uses of antiplatelet drugs

The main drug is **aspirin**. Other drugs with distinct actions (e.g. **dipyridamole**, **clopidogrel**, **ticagrelor**) can have additive effects, or be used in patients who are intolerant of **aspirin**. Uses of antiplatelet drugs relate mainly to arterial thrombosis and include:

- *acute myocardial infarction*
- prevention of myocardial infarction in patients at high risk, including a history of *myocardial infarction, angina or intermittent claudication* (see Ch. 22)
- following *coronary artery bypass grafting*
- *unstable coronary syndromes* (a P2Y12 antagonist such as **clopidogrel, prasugrel** or **ticagrelor** is added to **aspirin**)
- following coronary artery *angioplasty* and/or *stenting* (intravenous glycoprotein IIb/IIIa antagonists, e.g. **abciximab**, are used in some patients in addition to **aspirin**)
- *transient cerebral ischaemic attack* ('ministrokes') or *thrombotic stroke*, to prevent recurrence (**dipyridamole** can be added to **aspirin**)
- *atrial fibrillation*, if oral anticoagulation is contraindicated; or, by specialists, in high-risk situations in combination with anticoagulant.

    Other antiplatelet drugs such as **epoprostenol** (PGI$_2$; see Ch. 17) have specialised clinical applications (e.g. in *haemodialysis* or *haemofiltration*, Ch. 29, or in *pulmonary hypertension*, Ch. 22).

---

fibrinolytic (thrombolytic) drugs are used clinically, principally to reopen the occluded arteries in patients with acute myocardial infarction[9] or stroke, less commonly in patients with life-threatening venous thrombosis or pulmonary embolism.

Streptokinase is a plasminiogen activating protein extracted from cultures of streptococci. Infused intravenously, it reduces mortality in acute myocardial infarction, and this beneficial effect is additive with aspirin (Fig. 24.8). Its action is blocked by antibodies, which appear 4 days or more after the initial dose: its use should not be repeated after this time has elapsed.

Alteplase and **duteplase** are, respectively, single- and double-chain recombinant tPA. They are more active on fibrin-bound plasminogen than on plasma plasminogen, and are therefore said to be 'clot selective'. Recombinant tPA is not antigenic, and can be used in patients likely to have antibodies to streptokinase. Because of their short half-lives, they must be given as intravenous infusions. **Reteplase** is similar but has a longer elimination half-life, allowing for bolus administration and making for simplicity of administration. It is available for clinical use in myocardial infarction.

---

[9]Fibrinolytic drugs are now less widely used in acute myocardial infarction since many units throughout the world provide an emergency angioplasty service (the blocked artery is identified angiographically, opened with a balloon catheter and, if necessary, kept open by means of a stent, Ch. 21). The important thing is to open up the thrombosed artery as swiftly as possible. If facilities are available to do this mechanically, this is at least as good as using a lytic drug.

UNWANTED EFFECTS AND CONTRAINDICATIONS

The main hazard of all fibrinolytic agents is bleeding, including gastrointestinal haemorrhage and haemorrhagic stroke. If serious, this can be treated with **tranexamic acid** (see p. 307), fresh plasma or coagulation factors. Streptokinase can cause allergic reactions and low-grade fever. Streptokinase causes a burst of plasmin formation, generating kinins (see Ch. 17), and can cause hypotension by this mechanism.

Contraindications to the use of these agents are active internal bleeding, haemorrhagic cerebrovascular disease, bleeding diatheses, pregnancy, uncontrolled hypertension, invasive procedures in which haemostasis is important, and recent trauma – including vigorous cardiopulmonary resuscitation.

CLINICAL USE

Several large placebo-controlled studies in patients with myocardial infarction have shown convincingly that fibrinolytic drugs reduce mortality if given within 12 h of the onset of symptoms, and that the sooner they are administered the better is the result. Similar considerations apply to their use in thrombotic stroke. Scanning to exclude haemorrhagic stroke is advisable, though not always practicable in an emergency situation. Available fibrinolytic drugs, used in combination with aspirin, provide similar levels of benefit, generally less than that obtained by mechanical (mainly angioplasty) unblocking procedures. Other uses of fibrinolytic agents are listed in the clinical box.

Fibrinolysis and drugs modifying fibrinolysis

- A fibrinolytic cascade is initiated concomitantly with the coagulation cascade, resulting in the formation within the coagulum of plasmin, which digests fibrin.
- Various agents promote the formation of plasmin from its precursor plasminogen, for example **streptokinase**, and tissue plasminogen activators (tPAs) such as **alteplase, duteplase** and **reteplase**. Most are infused; reteplase can be given as a bolus injection.
- Some drugs (e.g. **tranexamic acid**) inhibit fibrinolysis.

Clinical uses of fibrinolytic drugs

The main drugs are **streptokinase** and tissue plasminogen activators (tPAs), for example **alteplase**.

- The main use is in acute myocardial infarction, within 12 h of onset (the earlier the better!).
- Other uses include:
  - *acute thrombotic stroke* within 3 h of onset (tPA), in selected patients
  - clearing *thrombosed shunts* and *cannulae*
  - *acute arterial thromboembolism*
  - life-threatening *deep vein thrombosis* and *pulmonary embolism* (streptokinase, given promptly).

ANTIFIBRINOLYTIC AND HAEMOSTATIC DRUGS

Tranexamic acid inhibits plasminogen activation and thus prevents fibrinolysis. It can be given orally or by intravenous injection. It is used to treat various conditions in which there is bleeding or risk of bleeding, such as haemorrhage following prostatectomy or dental extraction, in menorrhagia (excessive menstrual blood loss) and for life-threatening bleeding following thrombolytic drug administration. It is also used in patients with the rare disorder of hereditary angio-oedema.

REFERENCES AND FURTHER READING

Blood coagulation and anticoagulants

Bah, A., Carrell, C.J., Chen, Z.W., et al., 2009. Stabilization of the E* form turns thrombin into an anticoagulant. J. Biol. Chem. 284, 20034–20040. (*The anticoagulant profile caused by a mutation of the thrombin gene is due to stabilisation of the inactive E* form of thrombin that is selectively shifted to the active E form upon thrombomodulin and protein C binding*)

Hirsh, J., O'Donnell, M., Weitz, J.I., 2005. New anticoagulants. Blood 105, 453–463. (*Review article on limitations of existing anticoagulants, vitamin K antagonist and heparins that have led to the development of newer anticoagulant therapies*)

Shearer, M.J., Newman, P., 2008. Metabolism and cell biology of vitamin K. Thromb. Haemost. 100, 530–547. (*Review*)

Endothelium, platelets and antiplatelet agents

Chew, D.P., Bhatt, D., Sapp, S., et al., 2001. Increased mortality with oral platelet glycoprotein IIb/IIIa antagonists: a meta-analysis of phase III multicenter trials. Circulation 103, 201–206.

COMMIT Collaborative Group, 2005. Addition of clopidogrel to aspirin in 45852 patients with acute myocardial infarction: randomised placebo-controlled trial. Lancet 366, 1607–1621. (*Clopidogrel reduced the risk of death, myocardial infarction or stroke combined, and of mortality alone; see accompanying comment by Sabatine, M.S., pp. 1587–1589 in the same issue*)

Goodman, T., Ferro, A., Sharma, P., 2008. Pharmacogenetics of aspirin resistance: a comprehensive systematic review. Br. J. Clin. Pharmacol. 66, 222–232. (*Supports a genetic association between the PlA1/A2 molecular variant and aspirin resistance in healthy subjects, with the effect diminishing in the presence of cardiovascular disease*)

Patrono, C., Coller, B., FitzGerald, G.A., et al., 2004. Platelet-active drugs: the relationships among dose, effectiveness, and side effects. Chest 126, 234S–264S.

Wallentin, L., Becker, R.C., Budaj, A., et al., 2009. Ticagrelor versus clopidogrel in patients with acute coronary syndromes. N. Engl. J. Med. 361, 1045–1057.

Wiviott, S.D., Braunwald, E., McCabe, C.H., et al., 2007. For the TRITON-TIMI 38 Investigators. Prasugrel versus clopidogrel in patients with acute coronary syndromes. N. Engl. J. Med. 357, 2001–2015. (*Prasugrel reduced ischaemic events, including stent thrombosis, but with an increased risk of major bleeding, including fatal bleeding. Overall mortality did not differ significantly between treatment groups*)

Clinical and general aspects

Aster, R.H., 1995. Heparin-induced thrombocytopenia and thrombosis. N. Engl. J. Med. 332, 1374–1376. (*Succinct and lucid editorial; see also accompanying paper, pp. 1330–1335*)

Diener, H., Cunha, L., Forbes, C., et al., 1996. European Stroke Prevention Study 2. Dipyridamole and acetylsalicylic acid in the secondary prevention of stroke. J. Neurol. Sci. 143, 1–14 (*Slow-release dipyridamole 200 mg twice daily was as effective as aspirin 25 mg twice daily, and the effects of aspirin and dipyridamole were additive*)

Goldhaber, S.Z., 2004. Pulmonary embolism. Lancet 363, 1295–1305.

Kyrle, P.A., Eichinger, S., 2005. Deep vein thrombosis. Lancet 365, 1163–1174.

Levine, M., 1995. A comparison of low-molecular-weight heparin administered primarily at home with unfractionated heparin administered in the hospital for proximal deep vein thrombosis. N. Engl. J. Med. 334, 677–681. (*Concludes that LMWH can be used safely and effectively at home; this has potentially very important implications for patient care*)

Markus, H.S., 2005. Current treatments in neurology: stroke. J. Neurol. 252, 260–267.

25 Haemopoietic system and treatment of anaemia

OVERVIEW

This chapter summarises the different kinds of anaemia, caused by nutrient deficiencies, bone marrow depression or increased red cell destruction, and covers the main haematinic agents used to treat them. We describe haemopoietic growth factors for red and white blood cells, and conclude by mentioning two drugs (hydroxycarbamide and eculizumab) used in treating, respectively, sickle cell anaemia and paroxysmal nocturnal haemoglobinuria.

INTRODUCTION

In this chapter we briefly review the haemopoietic system and different types of anaemia due to blood loss, deficiency of nutrients, depression of the bone marrow or increased destruction of red cells (haemolytic anaemias). Nutritional deficiencies of *iron, vitamin B₁₂ or folic acid* are common and important and most of the chapter is devoted to these haematinic agents (i.e. nutrients needed for healthy haemopoiesis and related drugs). Treatment of many forms of bone marrow depression is mainly supportive, but *haemopoietic growth factors* (especially *epoietins* – preparations of the natural hormone erythropoietin) have a place, especially in patients with chronic renal failure, and are covered briefly, as are other haemopoietic factors, known as *colony-stimulating factors* (CSFs), which are used to increase numbers of circulating white blood cells. Treatment of haemolytic anaemias is again mainly supportive, but we mention two drugs (**hydroxycarbamide** and **eculizumab**) that provide mechanistic insights as well as clinical benefit in two specific haemolytic disorders.

THE HAEMOPOIETIC SYSTEM

The main components of the haemopoietic system are the blood, bone marrow, lymph nodes and thymus, with the spleen, liver and kidneys as important accessory organs. Blood consists of formed elements (red and white blood cells and platelets) and plasma. This chapter deals mainly with red cells, which have the principal function of carrying oxygen. Their oxygen-carrying power depends on their haemoglobin content. The most important site of formation of red blood cells in adults is the bone marrow, whereas the spleen acts as their slaughterhouse. Red cell loss in healthy adults is precisely balanced by production of new cells. The liver stores vitamin B₁₂ and is involved in the process of breakdown of the haemoglobin liberated when red blood cells are destroyed. The kidney manufactures *erythropoietin*, a hormone that stimulates red cell

production and is used in the anaemia of chronic kidney disease (Ch. 29) as well as (notoriously) in competitive cycling (Ch. 58). CSFs regulate the production of leukocytes and are also used therapeutically (e.g. in the supportive management of patients with haematological malignancies undergoing chemotherapy, Ch. 56). *Thrombopoietin* stimulates platelet formation; attempts to develop it for therapeutic use are a cautionary tale, which is mentioned briefly below. Drugs used to treat leukaemias are described in Chapter 56.

TYPES OF ANAEMIA

Anaemia is characterised by a reduced haemoglobin content in the blood. It may cause fatigue but, especially if it is chronic, is often surprisingly asymptomatic. The commonest cause is blood loss resulting from menstruation, drug treatment (e.g. with **aspirin** or other nonsteroidal anti-inflammatory drugs; Ch. 26) or pathological processes such as colonic carcinoma or (especially in developing countries) parasitic infestation (Ch. 55). Pregnancy and child-bearing are other important physiological drains on iron reserves. There are several different types of anaemia based on indices of red cell size and haemoglobin content and microscopical examination of a stained blood smear:

- *hypochromic, microcytic anaemia* (small red cells with low haemoglobin; caused by chronic blood loss giving rise to iron deficiency)
- *macrocytic anaemia* (large red cells, few in number)
- *normochromic normocytic anaemia* (fewer normal-sized red cells, each with a normal haemoglobin content)
- mixed pictures.

Further evaluation may include determination of concentrations of ferritin, iron, vitamin B₁₂ and folic acid in serum, and microscopic examination of smears of bone marrow. This leads to more precise diagnostic groupings of anaemias into:

- Deficiency of nutrients necessary for haemopoiesis, most importantly:
  - iron
  - folic acid and vitamin B₁₂
  - pyridoxine and vitamin C.
- Depression of the bone marrow, commonly caused by:
  - drug toxicity (e.g. anticancer drugs, **clozapine**)
  - exposure to radiation, including radiotherapy
  - diseases of the bone marrow (e.g. idiopathic aplastic anaemia, leukaemias)
  - reduced production of, or responsiveness to, erythropoietin (e.g. chronic renal failure, rheumatoid arthritis, AIDS).

- Excessive destruction of red blood cells (i.e. haemolytic anaemia); this has many causes, including *haemoglobinopathies* (such as sickle cell anaemia), adverse reactions to drugs and inappropriate immune reactions.

HAEMATINIC AGENTS

It is important to note that the use of haematinic agents is often only an adjunct to treatment of the underlying cause of the anaemia – for example, surgery for colon cancer (a common cause of iron deficiency) or antihelminthic drugs for patients with hookworm (a frequent cause of anaemia in parts of Africa and Asia; Ch. 55). Sometimes treatment consists of stopping an offending drug, for example a non-steroidal anti-inflammatory drug that is causing blood loss from the gastrointestinal tract (Ch. 26).

IRON

Iron is a transition metal with two important properties relevant to its biological role, namely its ability to exist in several oxidation states, and to form stable coordination complexes.

The body of a 70 kg man contains about 4 g of iron, 65% of which circulates in the blood as haemoglobin. About one-half of the remainder is stored in the liver, spleen and bone marrow, chiefly as *ferritin* and *haemosiderin*. The iron in these molecules is available for haemoglobin synthesis. The rest, which is not available for haemoglobin synthesis, is present in myoglobin, cytochromes and various enzymes.

The distribution and turnover of iron in an average adult man are shown in Table 25.1 and Figure 25.1. The corresponding values in a woman are approximately 45% less. Because most of the iron in the body is either part of – or destined to be part of – haemoglobin, the most obvious clinical result of iron deficiency is anaemia, and the only indication for therapy with iron is for treatment or prophylaxis of iron deficiency anaemia.

Table 25.1 The distribution of iron in the body of a healthy 70 kg man

Protein	Tissue	Iron content (mg)
Haemoglobin	Erythrocytes	2600
Myoglobin	Muscle	400
Enzymes (cytochromes, catalase, guanylyl cyclase, etc.)	Liver and other tissues	25
Transferrin	Plasma and extracellular fluid	8
Ferritin and haemosiderin	Liver Spleen Bone marrow	410 48 300

Data from Jacobs A, Worwood M 1982 Chapter 5. In: Hardisty RM, Weatherall DJ (Eds) Blood and Its Disorders. Blackwell Scientific, Oxford

Haemoglobin is made up of four protein chain subunits (globins), each of which contains one haem moiety. Haem consists of a tetrapyrrole porphyrin ring containing ferrous (Fe^{2+}) iron. Each haem group can carry one oxygen molecule, which is bound reversibly to Fe^{2+} and to a histidine residue in the globin chain. This reversible binding is the basis of oxygen transport.

IRON TURNOVER AND BALANCE

The normal daily requirement for iron is approximately 5 mg for men, and 15 mg for growing children and for menstruating women. A pregnant woman needs between 2 and 10 times this amount because of the demands of the fetus and increased requirements of the mother.[1] The average diet in Western Europe provides 15–20 mg of iron daily, mostly in meat. Iron in meat is generally present as haem, and about 20–40% of haem iron is available for absorption.

▼ Humans are adapted to absorb haem iron. It is thought that one reason why modern humans have problems in maintaining iron balance (there are an estimated 500 million people with iron deficiency in the world) is that the change from hunting to grain cultivation 10 000 years ago led to cereals, which contain little utilisable iron, replacing meat in the diet. Non-haem iron in food is mainly in the ferric state, and this needs to be converted to ferrous iron for absorption. Iron salts have low solubility at the neutral pH of the small intestine; however, in the stomach iron dissolves and binds to a mucoprotein carrier. In the presence of ascorbic acid, fructose and various amino acids, iron is detached from the carrier, forming soluble low-molecular weight complexes that enable it to remain in soluble form in the intestine. Ascorbic acid stimulates iron absorption partly by forming soluble iron–ascorbate chelates and partly by reducing ferric

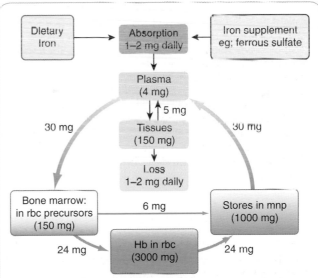

Fig. 25.1 Distribution and turnover of iron in the body. The quantities by the arrows indicate the usual amounts transferred each day. The transfer of 6 mg from red cell precursors to phagocytes represents aborted cells that fail to develop into functional red blood cells. Hb, haemoglobin; mnp, mononuclear phagocytes (mainly in liver, spleen and bone marrow); rbc, red blood cells.

[1] Each pregnancy 'costs' the mother 680 mg of iron, equivalent to 1300 ml of blood, owing to the demands of the fetus, plus requirements of the expanded blood volume and blood loss at delivery.

iron to the more soluble ferrous form. **Tetracycline** forms an insoluble iron chelate, impairing absorption of both substances.

The amount of iron in the diet and the various factors affecting its availability are thus important determinants in absorption, but the regulation of iron absorption is a function of the intestinal mucosa, influenced by the body's iron stores. Because there is no mechanism whereby iron excretion is regulated, the absorptive mechanism has a central role in iron balance as it is the sole mechanism by which body iron is controlled.

Iron absorption takes place in the duodenum and upper jejunum, and is a two-stage process involving uptake across the brush border into the mucosal cells, followed by transfer into the plasma.. The second stage, which is rate-limiting, is energy-dependent. Haem iron in the diet is absorbed as intact haem, and the iron is released in the mucosal cell by the action of haem oxidase. Non-haem iron is absorbed in the ferrous state. Within the cell, ferrous iron is oxidised to ferric iron, which is bound to an intracellular carrier, a transferrin-like protein; the iron is then either held in storage in the mucosal cell as *ferritin* (if body stores of iron are high) or passed on to the plasma (if iron stores are low).

▼ Iron is carried in the plasma bound to *transferrin*, a β-globulin with two binding sites for ferric iron. The binding sites are normally only approximately 30% saturated. Plasma contains 4 mg of iron at any one time, but the daily turnover is about 30 mg (Fig. 25.1). Most of the iron that enters the plasma is derived from mononuclear phagocytes, following the degradation of time-expired erythrocytes. Intestinal absorption and mobilisation of iron from storage depots contribute only small amounts. Most of the iron that leaves the plasma each day is used for haemoglobin synthesis by red cell precursors (erythroblasts). These have receptors that bind transferrin, releasing it again when its cargo of iron has been captured.

Iron is stored in two forms: soluble ferritin and insoluble *haemosiderin*. Ferritin is present in all cells, the mononuclear phagocytes of liver, spleen and bone marrow containing especially high concentrations. It is also present in plasma. The precursor of ferritin, *apoferritin*, is a protein of molecular weight 450 000, composed of 24 identical polypeptide subunits that enclose a cavity in which up to 4500 iron atoms can be stored. Apoferritin takes up ferrous iron, oxidises it and deposits the ferric iron in its core. In this form, it constitutes ferritin, the primary storage form of iron, from which the iron is most readily available. The lifespan of this iron-laden protein is only a few days. Haemosiderin is a degraded form of ferritin in which the iron cores of several ferritin molecules have aggregated, following partial disintegration of the outer protein shells.

Ferritin in plasma contains very little iron. It is, however, in equilibrium with the storage ferritin in cells, and its concentration in plasma (normal range 40–100 ng/ml) provides a clinically useful indicator of total body iron stores since values below 40 ng/ml signal mild iron deficiency despite normal haemoglobin, red cell morphology, serum iron concentration and transferrin saturation, with values below 20 and 10 ng/ml signalling moderate and severe anaemia respectively.

The body has no means of actively excreting iron. Small amounts leave the body through shedding of mucosal cells containing ferritin, and even smaller amounts leave in the bile, sweat and urine. A total of about 1 mg is lost daily. Iron balance is therefore critically dependent on the active absorption mechanism in the intestinal mucosa. This absorption is influenced by the iron stores in the body, but the precise mechanism of this control is uncertain. Iron balance is summarised in Figure 25.1. Since red cells contain approximately 0.6 mg iron per ml of blood, loss of only a few millilitres of blood per day substantially increases dietary iron requirement.

ADMINISTRATION OF IRON

Iron is usually given orally, e.g. as **ferrous sulfate**. Other salts for oral administration are **ferrous succinate, gluconate** or **fumarate**.

Parenteral iron (e.g. **iron-dextran, iron-sucrose**) may be necessary in individuals who are not able to absorb oral iron because of malabsorption syndromes, or as a result of surgical procedures or inflammatory conditions involving the gastrointestinal tract. It is also used for patients who do not tolerate oral preparations, and patients with chronic renal failure or with chemotherapy-induced anaemia who are receiving treatment with erythropoietin (see p. 313-315). Iron-dextran can be given by deep intramuscular injection or slow intravenous infusion; iron-sucrose is given by slow intravenous infusion. A small initial dose is given because of the risk of anaphylactoid reaction.

Unwanted effects

The unwanted effects of oral iron administration are dose-related and include nausea, abdominal cramps and diarrhoea. Parenteral iron can cause anaphylactoid reactions (Ch. 57). Iron is an important nutrient for several pathogens and there is concern that excessive iron could worsen the clinical course of infection. Iron treatment is usually avoided during infection for this reason.

Acute iron toxicity, usually seen in young children who have swallowed attractively coloured iron tablets in mistake for sweets, can result in severe necrotising gastritis with vomiting, haemorrhage and diarrhoea, followed by circulatory collapse.

> ## Clinical uses of iron salts
>
> To treat iron deficiency anaemia, which can be caused by:
>
> - *chronic blood loss* (e.g. with menorrhagia, hookworm, colon cancer)
> - *increased demand* (e.g. in pregnancy and early infancy)
> - *inadequate dietary intake* (uncommon in developed countries)
> - *inadequate absorption* (e.g. following gastrectomy, or in diseases such as coeliac disease, where the intestinal mucosa is damaged by an immunologically based intolerance to the wheat protein gluten).

Iron overload

Chronic iron toxicity or iron overload occurs in chronic haemolytic anaemias requiring frequent blood transfusions, such as the *thalassaemias* (a large group of genetic disorders of globin chain synthesis) and *haemochromatosis* (a genetic iron storage disease with increased iron absorption, resulting in damage to liver, islets of Langerhans, joints and skin).[2]

The treatment of acute and chronic iron toxicity involves the use of iron chelators such as **desferrioxamine**. These drugs form a complex with ferric iron which, unlike unbound iron, is excreted in the urine. Desferrioxamine is not absorbed from the gut. For treating chronic iron overload (e.g. in thalassaemia), it must be given by slow

---

[2]'Bronze diabetes' – where chronic iron overload is treated by repeated bleeding, one of the few modern uses of this once near-universal 'remedy'; polycythaemia vera (caused by mutations in erythroid progenitors that increase their proliferation) is another.

subcutaneous infusion several times a week. For acute iron overdose, it is given intramusculalrly or intravenously (as well as intragastrically to sequester unabsorbed iron. **Deferiprone** is an orally absorbed iron chelator, used as an alternative treatment for iron overload in patients with thalassaemia major who are unable to take desferrioxamine. Agranulocytosis and other blood dyscrasias are serious potential adverse effects. **Deferasirox** is similar, but can cause gastrointestinal bleeding.

Iron

- Iron is important for the synthesis of haemoglobin, myoglobin, cytochromes and other enzymes.
- Ferric iron (Fe^{3+}) must be converted to ferrous iron (Fe^{2+}) for absorption in the gastrointestinal tract.
- Absorption involves active transport into mucosal cells in the duodenum and jejunum (the upper ileum), from where it can be transported into the plasma and/or stored intracellularly as ferritin.
- Total body iron is controlled exclusively by absorption; in iron deficiency, more is transported into plasma than is stored as ferritin in jejunal mucosa.
- Iron loss occurs mainly by sloughing of ferritin-containing mucosal cells.
- Iron in plasma is bound to transferrin, and most is used for erythropoiesis. Some is stored as ferritin in other tissues. Iron from time-expired erythrocytes enters the plasma for reuse.
- The main therapeutic preparation is **ferrous sulfate**; **iron-sucrose** can be given as an intravenous infusion.
- Unwanted effects include gastrointestinal disturbances. Severe toxic effects occur if large doses are ingested; such acute poisoning can be treated with **desferrioxamine**, an iron chelator as can chronic iron overload in diseases such as thalassaemia.

FOLIC ACID AND VITAMIN B$_{12}$

Vitamin B_{12} and folic acid are essential constituents of the human diet, being necessary for DNA synthesis and consequently for cell proliferation. Their biochemical actions are interdependent (see key point box, p. 301), and treatment with folic acid corrects some, but not all, of the features of vitamin B_{12} deficiency. Deficiency of either vitamin B_{12} or folic acid affects tissues with a rapid cell turnover, particularly bone marrow, but vitamin B_{12} deficiency also causes important neuronal disorders, which are not corrected (or may even be made worse) by treatment with folic acid. Deficiency of either vitamin causes *megaloblastic haemopoiesis*, in which there is disordered erythroblast differentiation and defective erythropoiesis in the bone marrow. Large abnormal erythrocyte precursors appear in the marrow, each with a high RNA:DNA ratio as a result of decreased DNA synthesis. The circulating abnormal erythrocytes ('macrocytes' – i.e. large red blood cells) are large fragile cells, often distorted in shape.

Mild leukopenia and thrombocytopenia (i.e. low white blood cell and platelet counts) usually accompany the anaemia, and the nuclei of polymorphonuclear (PMN) leukocytes are structurally abnormal (hypersegmented – as young PMNs mature, their nuclei acquire 'lobes' in the form of discrete bulges, leading to hypersegmentation in post-mature cells. The nuclei of megaloblasts – the precursors of macrocytic red cells in patients with B_{12} or folate deficiency – are old before their time, compared with the cells' low haemoglobin content). Neurological disorders caused by deficiency of vitamin B_{12} include peripheral neuropathy and dementia, as well as *subacute combined degeneration*[3] of the spinal cord. Folic acid deficiency is caused by dietary deficiency, especially during increased demand (e.g. during pregnancy – particularly important because of the link between folate deficiency and neural tube defects in the baby [see Ch. 57] or because of chronic haemolysis in patients with haemoglobinopathies such as *sickle cell anaemia* – see p. 315). Vitamin B_{12} deficiency, however, is usually due to decreased absorption (see p. 312).

FOLIC ACID

Some aspects of folate structure and metabolism are dealt with in Chapters 50 and 56, because several important antibacterial and anticancer drugs are antimetabolites that interfere with folate synthesis in microorganisms or tumour cells. Liver and green vegetables are rich sources of folate. In healthy non-pregnant adults, the daily requirement is about 0.2 mg daily, but this is increased during pregnancy.

Mechanism of action

Reduction of folic acid, catalysed by *dihydrofolate reductase* in two stages yields *dihydrofolate* (FH$_2$) and *tetrahydrofolate* (FH$_4$), co-factors which transfer methyl groups (1-carbon transfers) in several important metabolic pathways. FH$_4$ is essential for DNA synthesis because of its role as co-factor in the synthesis of purines and pyrimidines. It is also necessary for reactions involved in amino acid metabolism.

FH$_4$ is important for the conversion of deoxyuridylate monophosphate (DUMP) to deoxythymidylate monophosphate (DTMP). This reaction is rate-limiting in mammalian DNA synthesis and is catalysed by thymidylate synthetase, with FH$_4$ acting as methyl donor.

Pharmacokinetic aspects

Therapeutically, folic acid is given orally and is absorbed in the ileum. Methyl-FH$_4$ is the form in which folate is usually carried in blood and which enters cells. It is functionally inactive until it is demethylated in a vitamin B_{12}-dependent reaction (see p. 312). Folate is taken up into hepatocytes and bone marrow cells by active transport. Within the cells, folic acid is reduced and formylated before being converted to the active polyglutamate form. **Folinic acid**, a synthetic FH$_4$, is converted much more rapidly to the polyglutamate form.

Unwanted effects

Unwanted effects do not occur even with large doses of folic acid – except possibly in the presence of vitamin B_{12}

---

[3]'Combined' because the lateral as well as the dorsal columns are involved, giving rise to motor as well as sensory symptoms.

deficiency, when it is possible that administration of folic acid may improve the anaemia while exacerbating the neurological lesion. It is therefore important to determine whether a megaloblastic anaemia is caused by folate or vitamin B_{12} deficiency and treat accordingly.

Clinical uses of folic acid and vitamin B_{12} (hydroxocobalamin)

Folic acid

- Treatment of megaloblastic anaemia resulting from folate deficiency, which can be caused by:
  - *poor diet* (common in alcoholic individuals)
  - *malabsorption syndromes*
  - drugs (e.g. **phenytoin**).
- Treatment or prevention of toxicity from **methotrexate**, a folate antagonist (see Chs 26 and 56).
- Prophylactically in individuals at hazard from developing folate deficiency, for example:
  - *pregnant women* and *before conception* (especially if there is a risk of birth defects)
  - *premature infants*
  - patients with *severe chronic haemolytic anaemias*, including haemoglobinopathies (e.g. sickle cell anaemia).

Vitamin B_{12} (hydroxocobalamin)

- Treatment of *pernicious anaemia* and other causes of vitamin B_{12} deficiency.
- Prophylactically after surgical operations that remove the site of production of intrinsic factor (the stomach) or of vitamin B_{12} absorption (the terminal ileum).

VITAMIN B_{12}

Vitamin B_{12}, also called cobalamin, corrects pernicious anaemia. The vitamin B_{12} preparation used therapeutically is **hydroxocobalamin**. The principal dietary sources are meat (particularly liver, where it is stored), eggs and dairy products. For activity, cobalamins must be converted to *methylcobalamin* (methyl-B_{12}) or *5′-deoxyadenosyl-cobalamin* (ado-B_{12}). The average European diet contains 5–25 μg of vitamin B_{12} per day, and the daily requirement is 2–3 μg. Absorption requires *intrinsic factor* (a glycoprotein secreted by gastric parietal cells). Vitamin B_{12}, complexed with intrinsic factor, is absorbed by active transport in the terminal ileum. Healthy stomach secretes a large excess of intrinsic factor, but in patients with pernicious anaemia (an autoimmune disorder where the lining of the stomach atrophies), or following total gastrectomy, the supply of intrinsic factor is inadequate to maintain vitamin B_{12} absorption in the long term. Surgical removal of the terminal ileum, for example to treat Crohn's disease (see Ch. 30), can also impair B_{12} absorption.

Vitamin B_{12} is carried in the plasma by binding proteins called *transcobalamins*. It is stored in the liver, the total amount in the body being about 4 mg. This store is so large compared with the daily requirement, that if vitamin B_{12} absorption stops suddenly – as after a total gastrectomy – it takes 2–4 years for evidence of deficiency to become manifest.

Mechanism of action

▼ Vitamin B_{12} is required for two main biochemical reactions in humans.

The conversion of methyl-FH_4 to FH_4. The metabolic activities of vitamin B_{12} and folic acid are linked in the synthesis of DNA. It is also through this pathway that folate/vitamin B_{12} treatment can lower plasma homocysteine concentration. Because increased homocysteine concentrations may have undesirable vascular effects (Ch. 23, Table 23.1), this has potential therapeutic and public health implications. The reaction involves conversion of both methyl-FH_4 to FH_4 and homocysteine to methionine. The enzyme that accomplishes this (*homocysteine–methionine methyltransferase*) requires vitamin B_{12} as co-factor and methyl-FH_4 as methyl donor. The methyl group from methyl-FH_4 is transferred first to B_{12}, and then to homocysteine to form methionine. Vitamin B_{12} deficiency thus traps folate in the inactive methyl-FH_4 form, thereby depleting the folate polyglutamate coenzymes needed for DNA synthesis. Vitamin B_{12}-dependent methionine synthesis also affects the synthesis of folate polyglutamate coenzymes by an additional mechanism. The preferred substrate for polyglutamate synthesis is formyl-FH_4, and the conversion of FH_4 to formyl-FH_4 requires a formate donor such as methionine.

Isomerisation of methylmalonyl-CoA to succinyl-CoA. This isomerisation reaction is part of a route by which propionate is converted to succinate. Through this pathway, cholesterol, odd-chain fatty acids, some amino acids and thymine can be used for gluconeogenesis or for energy production via the tricarboxylic acid cycle. Coenzyme B_{12} (ado-B_{12}) is an essential co-factor, so methylmalonyl-CoA accumulates in vitamin B_{12} deficiency. This distorts the pattern of fatty acid synthesis in neural tissue and may be the basis of neuropathy in vitamin B_{12} deficiency.

Administration of vitamin B_{12}

When vitamin B_{12} is used therapeutically (as **hydroxocobalamin**), it is usually given by injection[4] because, as explained above, vitamin B_{12} deficiency commonly results from malabsorption. Patients with pernicious anaemia require life-long therapy, with maintenance injections every 3 months following a loading dose. Hydroxocobalamin does not cause unwanted effects.

HAEMOPOIETIC GROWTH FACTORS

Every 60 seconds, a human being must generate about 120 million granulocytes and 150 million erythrocytes, as well as numerous mononuclear cells and platelets. The cells responsible for this remarkable productivity are derived from a relatively small number of self-renewing, pluripotent stem cells laid down during embryogenesis. Maintenance of haemopoiesis necessitates a balance between self-renewal of the stem cells on the one hand, and differentiation into the various types of blood cell on the other. The factors involved in controlling this balance are the *haemopoietic growth factors*, which direct the division and maturation of the progeny of these cells down eight

---

[4]At least in Anglo-Saxon countries; in France, very large doses of vitamin B_{12} are given by mouth to achieve sufficient absorption for therapeutic efficacy despite the absence of intrinsic factor. Either method is a great improvement on eating the prodigious quantities of raw liver required by Minot and Murphy's 'liver diet' of 1925!

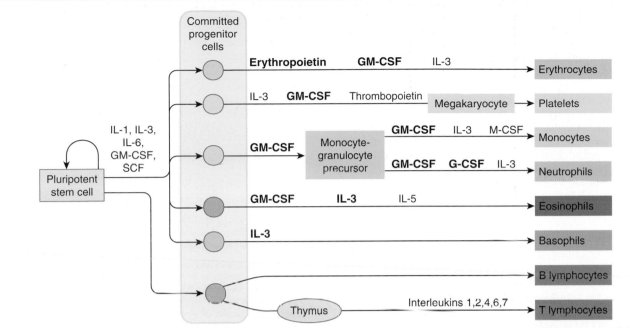

Fig. 25.2 Haemopoietic growth factors in blood cell differentiation. Various preparations of the factors shown in bold are in clinical use (see text). Most T cells generated in the thymus die by apoptosis; those that emerge are either CD4 or CD8 T cells. The colours used for the mature blood cells reflect how they appear in common staining preparations (and after which some are named). CSF, colony-stimulating factor; G-CSF, granulocyte CSF; GM-CSF, granulocyte–macrophage CSF; IL-1, interleukin-1; IL-3, interleukin-3 or multi-CSF; M-CSF, macrophage CSF; SCF, stem cell factor. (See also Ch. 6.)

Vitamin B₁₂ and folic acid

Both vitamin B_{12} and folic acid are needed for DNA synthesis. Deficiencies particularly affect erythropoiesis, causing macrocytic megaloblastic anaemia.

Folic acid

- There is active uptake of folic acid into cells and reduction to tetrahydrofolate (FH_4) by dihydrofolate reductase; extra glutamates are then added.
- Folate polyglutamate is a co-factor (a carrier of 1 carbon units) in the synthesis of purines and pyrimidines (especially thymidylate).

Vitamin B₁₂ (hydroxocobalamin)

- Vitamin B_{12} needs intrinsic factor (a glycoprotein) secreted by gastric parietal cells for absorption in the terminal ileum.
- It is stored in the liver.
- It is required for:
  - conversion of methyl-FH_4 (inactive form of FH_4) to active formyl-FH_4, which, after polyglutamation, is a co-factor in the synthesis of purines and pyrimidines
  - isomerisation of methylmalonyl-CoA to succinyl-CoA.
- Deficiency occurs most often in pernicious anaemia, which results from malabsorption caused by lack of intrinsic factor from the stomach. It causes neurological disease as well as anaemia.
- Vitamin B_{12} is given by injection to treat pernicious anaemia.

possible lines of development (Fig. 25.2). These cytokine growth factors are highly potent glycoproteins, acting at concentrations of 10^{-12} to 10^{-10} mol/l. They are present in plasma at very low concentrations under basal conditions, but on stimulation their concentrations can increase within hours by 1000-fold or more. *Erythropoietin* regulates the red cell line, and the signal for its production is blood loss and/or low tissue oxygen tension. *Colony-stimulating factors* (CSFs) regulate the myeloid divisions of the white cell line, and the main stimulus for their production is infection (see also Ch. 6).

Recombinant erythropoietin (**epoietin**),[5] and recombinant granulocyte CSF (**filgrastim, lenograstim, pegfilgrastim**) are used clinically (see below); *thrombopoietin* has been manufactured in recombinant form but there are concerns about effects on tumour progression (it activates a cell surface protein that is an oncogene product) and it has been associated with severe immunologically mediated adverse effects. Some of the other haemopoietic growth factors (e.g. interleukin-3, interleukin-5 and various other cytokines) are covered in Chapter 6.

ERYTHROPOIETIN

Erythropoietin is a glycoprotein produced in juxtatubular cells in the kidney and also in macrophages; it stimulates committed erythroid progenitor cells to proliferate

---

[5]The first therapeutic agent to be produced by recombinant technology, by Amgen in 1989 – a huge commercial success, heralding the emergence of the biotechnology industry – albeit with some anxious moments (see Fig. 25.3).

and generate erythrocytes (Fig. 25.2). Recombinant human erythropoietins are made in cultured mammalian cells (because their pharmacokinetic properties depend critically on the degree of glycosylation, a post-translational modification that occurs in mammalian but not so predictably in bacterial cells) and used to treat anaemia caused by erythropoietin deficiency, for example in patients with chronic kidney disease, AIDS or cancer. Epoietin (recombinant human erythropoietin) exists in several forms (alpha, beta, theta and zeta). **Darbepoetin**, a hyperglycosylated form, has a longer half-life and can be administered less frequently; **methoxy polyethylene glycol-epoetin beta** is another preparation with long half-life. Epoietin and darbopoietin are given intravenously or subcutaneously, the response being greater after subcutaneous injection and faster after intravenous injection.

Epoietins are reaching the end of patent protection and the first 'biosimilar' products have been licensed. Unlike the situation for small-molecule chemical entities where criteria for bioequivalence are relatively uncontroversial – Chapter 8 – biologically produced macromolecules may vary markedly with seemingly minor changes in manufacture, and have many opportunities to form immunologically distinct products during cell culture.

Unwanted effects

Transient influenza-like symptoms are common. Hypertension is also common and can cause encephalopathy with headache, disorientation and sometimes convulsions. Iron deficiency can be induced because more iron is required for the enhanced erythropoiesis. Blood viscosity increases as the haematocrit (i.e. the fraction of the blood that is occupied by red blood cells) rises, increasing the risk of thrombosis, especially during dialysis. There have been reports of a devastating chronic condition known as pure red cell aplasia (PRCA), connected with development of neutralising antibodies directed against erythropoietin which inactivate the endogenous hormone as well as the recombinant product (Berns, 2013). This has been a huge concern with indirect implications for quality control between batches of biological products and, indirectly, for the licensing of biosimilar products.

▼ Before 1998, only three cases of PRCA in association with epoietin treatment had been published. In that year, in response to concerns about transmitting bovine spongiform encephalopathy ('mad cow disease'), the formulation of the leading brand was changed, human serum albumin (used to stabilise the product) being replaced by polysorbate 80 and glycine. The incidence of PRCA increased abruptly, with approximately 250 documented cases by 2002, many of whom died or became completely dependent on blood transfusions. A large proportion had been treated with the new formulation. The mechanism whereby the manufacturing change led to the change in immunogenicity remains a matter of debate (Locatelli et al., 2007), but the packaging and storage were changed in 2003, since when the incidence of PRCA has declined (Fig. 25.3). The moral is that immunogenicity is unpredictable and can be caused by seemingly minor changes in manufacture or storage (Kuhlmann & Marre, 2010).

Clinical use

Iron or folate deficiency must be corrected before starting treatment. Parenteral iron preparations are often needed (see p. 310). Haemoglobin must be monitored and maintained within the range 10–12 g/dl to avoid the unwanted

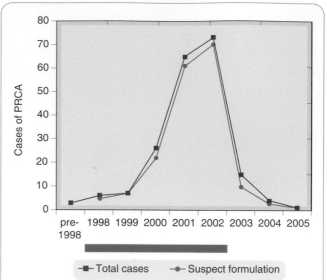

Fig. 25.3 **Incidence of pure red cell aplasia (PRCA) in relation to introduction in 1998 of a changed formulation of the leading brand of epoietin.** The incidence increased markedly and the suspect formulation (blue) accounted for almost all of the cases that were positive for anti-erythropoietin antibody (red); the formulation and instructions for its administration and storage were changed again in 2003 with an abrupt subsequent decline in PRCA. The period when the suspect formulation was in use is indicated by the blue rectangle. *(Redrawn from Kuhlmann & Marre 2010.)*

effects described above. The clinical use of epoietin is given in the box below.

COLONY-STIMULATING FACTORS (CSFs)

CSFs are cytokines that stimulate the formation of maturing colonies of leukocytes, observable in tissue culture. They not only stimulate particular committed progenitor cells to proliferate (Fig. 25.2) but also cause irreversible differentiation. The responding precursor cells have membrane receptors for specific CSFs and may express receptors for more than one factor, thus permitting collaborative interactions between factors.

Granulocyte CSF is produced mainly by monocytes, fibroblasts and endothelial cells, and controls primarily the development of neutrophils, increasing their proliferation and maturation, stimulating their release from bone marrow storage pools and enhancing their function. Recombinant forms (filgrastim, which is not glycosylated, and glycosylated lenograstim) are used therapeutically. Pegfilgrastim is a derivative of filgrastim conjugated with polyethylene glycol ('pegylated'), which has the effect of increasing its duration of action.

Thrombopoietin, made in liver and kidney, stimulates proliferation and maturation of megakaryocytes to form platelets. Recombinant thrombopoietin has been a tempting but horribly deceptive therapeutic target. Thrombocytopenia is a predictable and limiting toxicity of many chemotherapeutic regimens in oncology (Ch. 56), and a means to mitigate this would be a valuable prize. Recombinant thrombopoietin, seemingly the logical answer to this need, was manufactured and increased platelet counts in healthy volunteers and patients with mild chemotherapy-induced thrombocytopenia. But in early trials on healthy subjects, repeated dosing of a pegylated product caused the appearance of neutralising antibodies and consequently prolonged thrombocytopenia (Li et al., 2001), driving home the message from experience with erythropoietin (see Fig. 25.3) that subtle differences between biological products and natural mediators can lead to very serious immunologically mediated adverse effects. **Eltrombopag** (oral) and **romiplostim** (injectable) are recently approved thrombopoietin agonists.

Administration and unwanted effects

Filgrastim and lenograstim are given either subcutaneously or by intravenous infusion. Pegfilgrastim is administered subcutaneously. Gastrointestinal effects, fever, bone pain, myalgia and rash are recognised adverse effects; less common effects include pulmonary infiltrates and enlargement of liver or spleen.

HAEMOLYTIC ANAEMIA

Anaemia associated with increased red cell destruction can arise from genetic causes (e.g. sickle cell disease, thalassaemia, paroxysmal nocturnal haemoglobinuria) or a variety of non-genetic causes such as autoimmunity, infections and adverse drug reactions.

▼ *Sickle cell anaemia* is caused by a mutation in the gene that codes the β-globin chain of haemoglobin, resulting in a single amino acid substitution. The abnormal haemoglobin (haemoglobin S) can polymerise when deoxygenated, changing the physical properties of the red cells (which deform to a sickle shape, hence the name) and damaging cell membranes. This can block the microcirculation, causing painful crises, and haemolysis can reduce the availability of nitric oxide (Ch. 20). Polymerisation, and the severity of the disease, are markedly reduced when other forms of haemoglobin (A and F) are present.

Paroxysmal nocturnal haemoglobinuria (PNH) is a rare and previously untreatable form of haemolytic anaemia caused by clonal expansion of haemopoietic stem cells with somatic mutations that prevent formation of glycophosphatidylinositol (GPI), which anchors many proteins to the cell surface, rendering the cell susceptible to complement-mediated haemolysis. In addition to anaemia, patients with PNH suffer from other features, including thrombosis, attacks of abdominal pain and pulmonary hypertension (Ch. 22).

DRUGS USED TO TREAT HAEMOLYTIC ANAEMIAS

Hydroxycarbamide (also known as **hydroxyurea**) is a cytotoxic drug that has been used for decades to lower the red cell and platelet counts in patients with *polycythaemia rubra vera* (a myeloproliferative disorder affecting especially the red cell lineage) or to treat chronic myeloid leukaemia. It is additionally used to treat sickle cell disease.

Mechanism of action

Hydroxycarbamide inhibits DNA synthesis by inhibiting *ribonucleotide reductase* and is S-phase specific (Ch. 5). Consequently, it is relatively selective for the rapidly dividing population of red cell precursors that produce haemoglobin F, while reducing those producing haemoglobin S. Hydroxycarbamide metabolism gives rise to nitric oxide, which may contribute to its beneficial effect in sickle cell disease. Some of its beneficial effect in reducing painful crises could relate to anti-inflammatory effects secondary to its cytotoxic action.

Administration and unwanted effects

Hydroxycarbamide is administered by mouth once daily in rather lower starting dose than is used for treating malignant disease; reduced doses are used in patients

Haemopoietic growth factors

Erythropoietin

- Regulates red cell production.
- Is given intravenously, subcutaneously, intraperitoneally.
- Can cause transient flu-like symptoms, hypertension, iron deficiency and increased blood viscosity.
- Is available, as epoietin, to treat patients with anaemia caused by chronic renal failure.

Granulocyte colony-stimulating factor

- Stimulates neutrophil progenitors.
- Is available as **filgrastim**, **pegfilgrastim** or **lenograstim**; it is given parenterally.

Clinical uses of epoietin

- Anaemia of chronic *renal failure*.
- Anaemia during *chemotherapy* for cancer.
- Prevention of the anaemia that occurs in *premature infants* (unpreserved formulations are used because benzyl alcohol, used as a preservative, has been associated with a fatal toxic syndrome in neonates).
- To increase the yield of autologous blood before *blood donation*.
- Anaemia of *AIDS* (exacerbated by **zidovudine**).
- Anaemia of *chronic inflammatory conditions* such as rheumatoid arthritis (investigational).

Clinical uses of the colony-stimulating factors

Colony-stimulating factors are used in specialist centres:

- To reduce the severity/duration of neutropenia induced by cytotoxic drugs during:
  - intensive *chemotherapy* necessitating autologous *bone marrow rescue*
  - following *bone marrow transplant*.
- To harvest *progenitor cells*.
- To expand the number of harvested progenitor cells *ex vivo* before reinfusing them.
- For persistent neutropenia in *advanced HIV infection*.
- In *aplastic anaemia*.

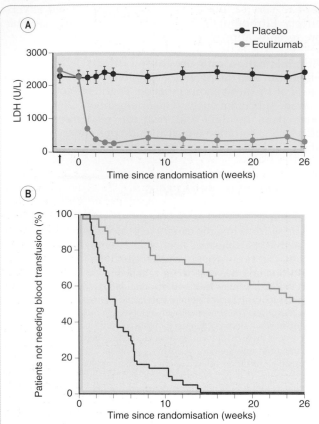

Fig. 25.4 Effect of eculizumab in patients with paroxysmal nocturnal haemoglobinuria (PNH). [**A**] Effect on plasma lactate dehydrogenase (LDH) activity, a measure of haemolyisis. The horizontal dotted line shows the upper limit of normal. The arrow shows the baseline level at screening (n = 44 in placebo group, n = 43 in eculizumab group, *P* <0.001). [**B**] Kaplan–Meier curves for the time to first transfusion during treatment in the same patients shown in [**A**] (*P* <0.001). (*Redrawn from Hillmen et al. 2006.*)

with impaired renal function. The blood count and haemoglobin F are monitored and the dose adjusted accordingly. Once stabilised, treatment may be continued indefinitely.

Myelosuppression, nausea and rashes are the commonest adverse effects. Animal studies demonstrated teratogenicity, and potential adverse effects on spermatogenesis.

Eculizumab, now licensed for the treatment of PNH, is a humanised monoclonal antibody which blocks the terminal complement protein C5 (Ch. 17). In a double-blind, randomised, controlled trial in 87 patients, treatment with eculizumab dramatically reduced haemolysis and transfusion requirement during 6 months of treatment (Fig. 25.4). Patients must be inoculated against meningococcal infection before treatment. It is administered by intravenous infusion weekly for 4 weeks and then approximately every 2 weeks. Serious adverse effects include infection, notably meningococcal infection, but are uncommon. The commonest adverse effects are headache and back pain.

In most forms of haemolytic anaemia, treatment is symptomatic (e.g. analgesia for painful crises in patients with sickle cell disease) and supportive (e.g. attention to fluid balance, oxygen therapy, blood transfusion when essential, treatment of iron overload, provision of adequate folate to support increased red cell turnover and, in some cases, antibiotics and immunisation). Acute haemolytic anaemia associated with autoantibodies may respond to treatment with glucocorticoids (Ch. 33).

REFERENCES AND FURTHER READING

General

Fishbane, S., 2009. Erythropoiesis-stimulating agent treatment with full anemia correction: a new perspective. Kidney Int. 75, 358–365.

Fishman, S.M., Christian, P., West, K.P., 2000. The role of vitamins in the prevention and control of anaemia. Public Health Nutr. 3, 125–150.

Kurzrock, R., 2005. Thrombopoietic factors in chronic bone marrow failure states: the platelet problem revisited. Clin. Cancer Res. 11, 1361–1367. (*Slow progress, see Li et al. below*)

Iron and iron deficiency

Andrews, N.C., 1999. Disorders of iron metabolism. N. Engl. J. Med. 341, 1986–1995.

Provan, D., Weatherall, D., 2000. Red cells, II: acquired anaemias and polycythaemia. Lancet 355, 1260–1268.

Toh, B.-H., van Driel, I.R., Gleeson, P.A., 1997. Pernicious anaemia. N. Engl. J. Med. 337, 1441–1448. (*Immunopathogenesis of pernicious anaemia; excellent figures*)

EPO and pure red cell aplasia

Berns, J.S., 2013. <http://www.uptodate.com/contents/ pure-red-cell-aplasia-due-to-anti-erythropoietin-antibodies>.

Kuhlmann, M., Marre, M., 2010. Lessons learned from biosimilar epoitins and insulins. Br. J. Diab. Vasc. Dis. 10, 90–97.

Locatelli, F., Del Vecchio, L., Pozzoni, P., 2007. Pure red-cell aplasia "epidemic" – mystery completely revealed? Perit. Dial. Int. 27 (Suppl. 2), S303–S307.

Colony-stimulating factors

Lieschke, G.J., Burges, A.W., 1992. Granulocyte colony-stimulating factor and granulocyte–macrophage colony-stimulating factor. N. Engl. J. Med. 327, 1–35, 99–106. (*Worthwhile, comprehensive reviews*)

Mohle, R., Kanz, L., 2007. Hematopoietic growth factors for hematopoietic stem cell mobilization and expansion. Semin. Hematol. 44, 193–202.

Haemolytic anaemias

Charache, S., Terrin, M.L., Moore, R.D., et al., 1995. Effect of hydroxyurea on the frequency of painful crises in sickle-cell-anemia. N. Engl. J. Med. 332, 1317–1322. (*Important randomised, controlled trial evidence of efficacy and safety over mean follow-up of 21 months*)

Hillmen, P., Young, N.S., Schubert, J., et al., 2006. The complement inhibitor eculizumab in paroxysmal nocturnal hemoglobinuria. N. Engl. J. Med. 355, 1233–1243. (*Eculizumab is an effective therapy for PNH*)

Platt, O.S., 2008. Hydroxyurea for the treatment of sickle cell anaemia. N. Engl. J. Med. 358, 1362–1369. (*Clinical vignette and discussion of this form of treatment*)

Thrombopoietin and prolonged thrombocytopenia

Li, J., Yang, C., Xia, Y., et al., 2001. Thrombocytopenia caused by the development of antibodies to thrombopoietin. Blood 98, 3241–3248.

Anti-inflammatory and immunosuppressant drugs

OVERVIEW

This chapter deals with drugs used to treat inflammatory and immune disorders. While generally associated with conditions such as rheumatoid arthritis, inflammation forms a significant component of many, if not most, of the diseases encountered in the clinic; consequently anti-inflammatory drugs are extensively employed in virtually all branches of medicine.

The chief drugs used to treat inflammation may be divided into five major groups:

- Drugs that inhibit the cyclo-oxygenase (COX) enzyme – the non-steroidal anti-inflammatory drugs (NSAIDs) and the coxibs.
- Antirheumatoid drugs – the disease-modifying antirheumatic drugs (DMARDs), including some immunosuppressants.
- The glucocorticoids.
- Anticytokines and other biological agents.
- Other drugs that do not fit into these groups, including antihistamines and drugs used to control gout.

We first describe the therapeutic effects, mechanism of action and unwanted effects common to all NSAIDs, and then deal in a little more detail with aspirin, paracetamol and drugs that are selective for COX-2. The antirheumatoid drugs comprise a rather heterogeneous group and include immunosuppressant drugs that are also used to treat other autoimmune diseases, and prevent rejection of organ transplants. The glucocorticoids are covered in Chapter 33, but are briefly discussed in this chapter. We then consider the biopharmaceutical 'revolution' which has changed the therapeutic landscape of severe disease. Finally, we consider drugs that do not fit easily into these categories: those used to treat gout and the histamine H_1 receptor antagonists used to treat acute allergic conditions.

CYCLO-OXYGENASE INHIBITORS

This group includes the 'traditional' (in the historical sense) NSAIDs[1] as well as the coxibs, which are more selective for COX-2. NSAIDs, sometimes called the aspirin-like drugs or antipyretic analgesics, are among the most widely used of all agents. There are now more than 50 different examples on the global market; common examples are listed in Table 26.1 and some NSAID structures depicted in Figure 26.1.

These drugs provide symptomatic relief from fever, pain and swelling in chronic joint disease such as occurs in osteo- and rheumatoid arthritis, as well as in more acute inflammatory conditions such as fractures, sprains, sports and other soft tissue injuries. They are also useful in the treatment of postoperative, dental and menstrual pain, as well as headaches and migraine. Several NSAIDs are available over the counter and they are widely used to treat minor aches and pains and other ailments. There are also many different NSAID formulations available, including tablets, injections and gels. Virtually all these drugs, particularly the 'traditional' NSAIDs, can have significant unwanted effects, especially in the elderly. Newer agents provoke fewer adverse actions.

While there are differences between individual NSAIDs, their primary pharmacology is related to their shared ability to inhibit the fatty acid COX enzyme, thereby inhibiting the production of prostaglandins and thromboxane. As explained in Chapter 17, there are two common isoforms of this enzyme, COX-1 and COX-2, but there may be other isoforms as yet uncharacterised. While COX-1 and COX-2 are closely related (>60% sequence identity) and catalyse the same reaction, there are important differences between the expression and role of these two isoforms. COX-1 is a constitutive enzyme expressed in most tissues, including blood platelets. It has a 'housekeeping' role in the body, being involved principally in tissue homeostasis. It is, for example, responsible for the production of prostaglandins involved in gastric cytoprotection (see Ch. 30), platelet aggregation (Ch 24), renal blood flow autoregulation (Ch. 29) and the initiation of parturition (Ch. 35).

In contrast, COX-2 is induced mainly in inflammatory cells when they are activated by, for example, the inflammatory cytokines – interleukin (IL)-1 and tumour necrosis factor (TNF)-α (see Ch. 18). Thus the COX-2 isoform is considered to be mainly responsible for the production of prostanoid mediators of inflammation (Vane & Botting, 2001). There are, however, some significant exceptions. COX-2 is constitutively expressed in the kidney, generating prostacyclin, which plays a part in renal homeostasis (see Ch 29), and in the central nervous system (CNS), where its function is not clear.

Most 'traditional' NSAIDs inhibit both COX-1 and COX-2, although their relative potency against the two isoforms differs. It is believed that the anti-inflammatory action (and probably most analgesic and antipyretic actions) of the NSAIDs are related to inhibition of COX-2, while their unwanted effects – particularly those affecting the gastrointestinal tract – are largely a result of their inhibition of COX-1. Compounds with a selective inhibitory action on COX-2 are now in clinical use, but while these drugs show fewer gastrointestinal side effects, they are by no means as well tolerated as was once hoped. This is partly because many patients have already been exposed to less selective drugs and have already suffered some

---

[1] Here, we use the term NSAID to include the coxibs but this is not a convention always followed in the literature.

Table 26.1 Comparison of some common anti-inflammatory cyclo-oxygenase inhibitors

Drug	Type	Indication	COX selectivity	Comments
Aceclofenac	Phenylacetate	RA, OA, AS	–	–
Acemetacin	Indole ester	RD, OA, MS, PO	–	Ester of indometacin
Aspirin	Salicylate	Mainly CV usage	Weakly COX-1 selective	Component of many OTC preparations
Celecoxib	Coxib	RA, OA, AS	Moderately COX-2 selective	Fewer gastrointestinal effects
Dexibruprofen	Propionate	OA, MS, D, H&M	–	Active enantiomer of ibuprofen
Dexketoprofen	Propionate	PO, D, H&M	–	Isomer of ketoprofen
Diclofenac	Phenylacetate	RA, OA, G, MS, PO, H&M	Weakly COX-2 selective	Moderate potency. Various salts
Etodolac	Pyranocarboxylate	RA, OA	Moderately COX-2 selective	Possibly fewer gastrointestinal effects
Etoricoxib	Coxib	RA, OA, G, AS	Very COX-2 selective	–
Fenoprofen	Propionate	RA, OA, MS, PO	Non-selective	Pro-drug; activated in liver
Flurbiprofen	Propionate	RA, OA, MS, PO, D, H&M	Very COX-1 selective	–
Ibuprofen	Propionate	RA, OA, MS, PO, D, H&M	Weakly COX-1 selective	Suitable for children
Indometacin	Indole	RA, OA, G, MS, PO, D	Weakly COX-1 selective	Suitable for moderate to severe disease
Ketoprofen	Propionate	RA, OA, G, MS, PO, D	Weakly COX-1 selective	Suitable for mild disease
Ketorolac	Pyrrolizine	PO	Highly COX-1 selective	–
Mefenamic acid	Fenamate	RA, OA, PO, D	–	Moderate activity
Meloxicam	Oxicam	RA, OA, AS	Moderately COX-2 selective	Possibly fewer gastrointestinal effects
Nabumetone	Naphthylalkenone	RA, OA	–	Prodrug activated in liver
Naproxen	Propionate	RA, OA, G, MS, PO, D	Weakly COX-1 selective	Possibly CV safe?
Parecoxib	Coxib	PO	–	Prodrug activated in liver
Piroxicam	Oxicam	RA, OA, AS	Weakly COX-2 selective	–
Sulindac	Indene	RA, OA, G, MS	Weakly COX-2 selective	Prodrug
Tenoxicam	Oxicam	RA, OA, MS	–	–
Tiaprofenic acid	Propionate	RA, OA, MS	–	–
Tolfenamic acid	Fenamate	H&M	–	–

AS, ankylosing spondylitis; CV, cardiovascular; D, dysmenorrhoea; G, acute gout; H&M, headache and migraine; MS, musculoskeletal injuries and pain; OA, osteoarthritis; OTC, over-the-counter; PO, postoperative pain; RA, rheumatoid arthritis. (Data from British National Formulary 2013 and COX selectivity data, where tested, from Warner & Mitchell, 2004 and 2008.)

gastrointestinal damage. As COX-2 also seems to be important in healing and resolution, one can see how problems might still occur. There is also a concern about the cardiovascular effects of all NSAIDs when these are taken chronically. Some notes on the relative selectivity of some NSAIDs and coxibs are given in Table 26.1.

▼ Though NSAIDs differ in toxicity and degree of patient acceptability and tolerance, their pharmacological actions are broadly similar, with certain important exceptions. **Aspirin** has other qualitatively different pharmacological actions (see below), and **paracetamol** is an interesting exception to the general NSAID 'stereotype'.

While it is an excellent analgesic (see Ch. 42) and antipyretic, its anti-inflammatory activity is slight and seems to be restricted to a few special cases (e.g. inflammation following dental extraction; see Skjelbred et al., 1984). Paracetamol has been shown to inhibit prostaglandin biosynthesis in some experimental settings (e.g. in the CNS during fever) but not in others (see also Ch. 42).

MECHANISM OF ACTION

In 1971 Vane and his colleagues demonstrated that the NSAIDs inhibit prostaglandin biosynthesis by a direct

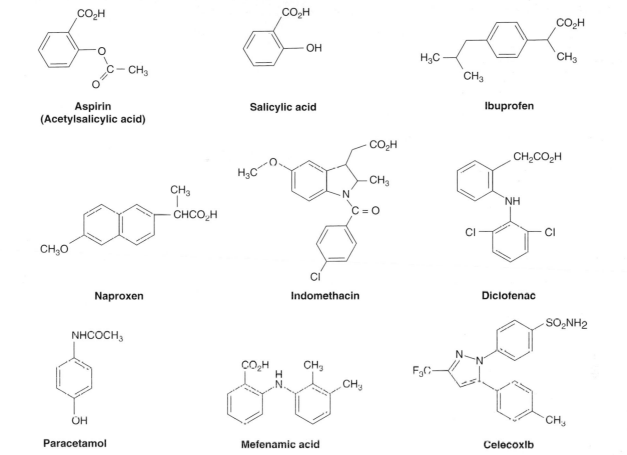

Fig. 26.1 **Significant structural features of some non-steroidal anti-inflammatory drugs (NSAIDs) and coxibs.** Aspirin contains an acetyl group that is responsible for the inactivation of the COX enzyme. Salicylic acid is the end product when aspirin is de-acetylated. Oddly it has anti-inflammatory activity in its own right. Paracetamol is a commonly used analgesic agent also of simple structure. Most 'classic' NSAIDs are carboxylic acids. Coxibs (celecoxib shown here as an example), however, often contain sulfonamide or sulfone groups. These are thought to be important in determining the selectivity of the molecule as they impede access to the hydrophobic channel in the COX-1 enzyme (see Fig. 26.2).

Cyclo-oxygenase inhibitors

These drugs have three major therapeutic actions, stemming from the suppression of prostanoid synthesis in inflammatory cells mainly through inhibition of the COX-2 isoform. They are as follows:

- *An anti-inflammatory action*: the decrease in prostaglandin E_2 and prostacyclin reduces vasodilatation and, indirectly, oedema. Accumulation of inflammatory cells is not directly reduced.
- *An analgesic effect*: decreased prostaglandin generation means less sensitisation of nociceptive nerve endings to inflammatory mediators such as bradykinin and 5-hydroxytryptamine. Relief of headache is probably a result of decreased prostaglandin-mediated vasodilatation.
- *An antipyretic effect*: interleukin-1 releases prostaglandins in the central nervous system, where they elevate the hypothalamic set point for temperature control, thus causing fever. NSAIDs prevent this.

Some important NSAIDs are **aspirin**, **ibuprofen**, **naproxen**, **indometacin**, **piroxicam** and **paracetamol**. Newer agents with more selective inhibition of COX-2 (and thus fewer adverse effects on the gastrointestinal tract) include **celecoxib** and **etoricoxib**.

action on the COX enzyme and established the hypothesis that this single action explained their therapeutic actions and most side effects (see Fig. 26.2). This has since been confirmed by numerous studies.

▼ COX enzymes are bifunctional, having two distinct catalytic activities. The first, dioxygenase step incorporates two molecules of oxygen into the arachidonic (or other fatty acid substrate) chain at C11 and C15, giving rise to the highly unstable *endoperoxide interme- diate* PGG_2 with a hydroperoxy group at C15. A second, peroxidase function of the enzyme converts this to PGH_2 with a hydroxy group at C15 (see Ch. 17), which can then be transformed in a cell-specific manner by separate *isomerase*, *reductase* or *synthase* enzymes into other prostanoids. Both COX-1 and COX-2 are haem-containing

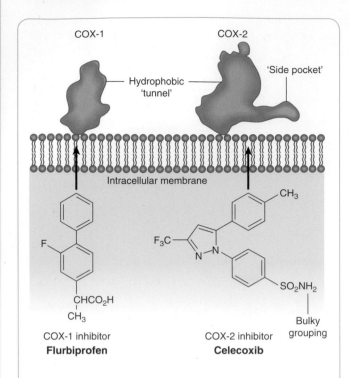

Fig. 26.2 Schematic diagram comparing the binding sites of cyclo-oxygenase (COX)-1 and COX-2. The illustration shows the differences in NSAID binding sites in the two isoforms. Note that the COX-2 binding site is characterised by a 'side pocket' that can accommodate the realtively 'bulky' groups, such as the sulfonamide moiety of celecoxib, which would impede its access to the COX-1 site. Other NSAIDs, such as flurbiprofen (shown here), can enter the active site of either enzyme. (*After Luong et al. 1996.*)

enzymes that exist as homodimers attached to intracellular membranes. Interestingly, only one monomer is catalytically active at one time. Structurally, COX-1 and COX-2 are similar; both contain a hydrophobic channel into which the arachidonic or other substrate fatty acids dock so that the oxygenation reaction can proceed.

Most NSAIDs inhibit only the initial dioxygenation reaction. They are generally rapid 'competitive reversible' inhibitors of COX-1, but there are differences in their kinetics. Inhibition of COX-2 is more time-dependent and the inhibition is often irreversible. To block the enzymes, NSAIDs enter the hydrophobic channel, forming hydrogen bonds with an arginine residue at position 120, thus preventing substrate fatty acids from entering into the catalytic domain. However, a single amino acid change (isoleucine to valine at position 523) in the structure of the entrance of this channel in COX-2 results in a 'bulge' in the channel that is not found in COX-1. This is important in understanding why some drugs, especially those with large sulfur-containing side groups, are more selective for the COX-2 isoform (Fig. 26.2). Aspirin is, however, an anomaly. It enters the active site and acetylates a serine at position 530, irreversibly inactivating COX. This is the basis for aspirin's long-lasting effects on platelets. Interestingly, aspirin-inactivated COX can still generate some hydroxyacids, but cannot produce PGG_2. Binding of NSAIDs to one COX monomer can inhibit the catalytic activity of the entire dimeric complex.

Other actions besides inhibition of COX may contribute to the anti-inflammatory effects of some NSAIDs. Reactive oxygen radicals produced by neutrophils and macrophages are implicated in tissue damage in some conditions, and some NSAIDs (e.g. **sulindac**) have oxygen radical-scavenging effects as well as COX inhibitory activity, so

may decrease tissue damage. Aspirin also inhibits expression of the transcription factor NFκB (see Ch. 3), which has a key role in the transcription of the genes for inflammatory mediators.

PHARMACOLOGICAL ACTIONS

All the NSAIDs have actions very similar to those of aspirin, the archetypal NSAID which was introduced into clinical medicine in the 1890s. Their pharmacological profile is listed in the box.

THERAPEUTIC ACTIONS

ANTI-INFLAMMATORY EFFECTS

As described in Chapters 17 and 18, many mediators coordinate inflammatory and allergic reactions. The NSAIDs reduce those components in which prostaglandins, mainly derived from COX-2, play a significant part. These include the vasodilatation (by reducing the synthesis of vasodilator prostaglandins) and the oedema of inflammation because vasodilatation facilitates and potentiates the action of mediators that increase the permeability of postcapillary venules, such as histamine; Ch. 17).

▼ While NSAIDs suppress the signs and symptoms of inflammation, they have little or no action on underlying chronic disease itself. As a class, they are generally without direct effect on other aspects of inflammation, such as cytokine/chemokine release, leukocyte migration, lysosomal enzyme release and toxic oxygen radical production, which contribute to tissue damage in chronic inflammatory conditions such as rheumatoid arthritis, vasculitis and nephritis.

ANTIPYRETIC EFFECTS

A centre in the hypothalamus controls the balance between heat production and heat loss thereby regulating normal body temperature. Fever occurs when there is a disturbance of this hypothalamic 'thermostat', which raises body temperature. NSAIDs 'reset' this thermostat. Once there has been a return to the normal 'set point', the temperature-regulating mechanisms (dilatation of superficial blood vessels, sweating, etc.) then operate to reduce temperature. Normal body temperature in healthy humans is not affected by NSAIDs.[2]

▼ The NSAIDs exert their antipyretic action largely through inhibition of prostaglandin production in the hypothalamus. During infection, bacterial endotoxins cause the release from macrophages of IL-1 (Ch. 17). In the hypothalamus this cytokine stimulates the generation of E-type prostaglandins that elevate the temperature set point. COX-2 may have a role here, because IL-1 induces this enzyme in the hypothalamic vascular endothelium. There is some evidence that prostaglandins are not the only mediators of fever, hence NSAIDs may have an additional antipyretic effect by mechanisms as yet unknown.

ANALGESIC EFFECTS

The NSAIDs are effective against mild or moderate pain, especially that arising from inflammation or tissue damage. Two sites of action have been identified.

Peripherally, NSAIDs decrease production of prostaglandins that sensitise nociceptors to inflammatory mediators such as bradykinin (see Chs 18 and 42) and they are therefore effective in arthritis, bursitis, pain of muscular

---

[2]With possible exception of paracetamol, which has been used clinically to lower body temperature during surgery.

and vascular origin, toothache, dysmenorrhoea, the pain of postpartum states and the pain of cancer metastases in bone. All conditions are associated with increased local prostaglandin synthesis probably as a result of COX-2 induction. Alone, or in combination with opioids, they decrease postoperative pain and in some cases can reduce the requirement for opioids by as much as one-third. Their ability to relieve headache may be related to the reduction in vasodilator prostaglandins acting on the cerebral vasculature.

In addition to these peripheral effects, there is a second, less well characterised central action, possibly in the spinal cord. Peripheral inflammatory lesions increase COX-2 expression and prostaglandin release within the cord, facilitating transmission from afferent pain fibres to relay neurons in the dorsal horn (see Ch. 42).

UNWANTED EFFECTS

Overall, the burden of unwanted side effects amongst NSAIDs is high, probably reflecting the fact that they are used extensively in the more vulnerable elderly population, and often for extended periods of time. When used for joint diseases (which usually necessitates fairly large doses and sustained treatment), there is a high incidence of side effects – particularly in the gastrointestinal tract but also in the liver, kidney, spleen, blood and bone marrow.

Because prostaglandins are involved in gastric cytoprotection, platelet aggregation, renal vascular autoregulation and induction of labour, all NSAIDs share a broadly similar profile of unwanted mechanism-dependent side effects on these processes, although there may be other additional unwanted effects peculiar to individual members of the group. COX-2-selective drugs have less, but not negligible, gastrointestinal toxicity.

Gastrointestinal disturbances

Adverse gastrointestinal (GI) events are the commonest unwanted effects of the NSAIDs. They are believed to result mainly from inhibition of gastric COX-1, which synthesises prostaglandins that normally inhibit acid secretion and protect the mucosa (see Ch. 30, Fig. 30.2).

Symptoms typically include gastric discomfort ('dyspepsia'), constipation, nausea and vomiting, and in some cases gastric bleeding and ulceration. It has been estimated that 34–46% of users of NSAIDs will sustain some gastrointestinal damage which, while it may be asymptomatic, can carry a risk of serious haemorrhage and/or perforation. These severe GI effects are said to result in the hospitalisation of over 100 000 people per year in the USA, some 15% of whom die from this iatrogenic disease (Fries, 1998). Damage is seen whether the drugs are given orally or systemically. However, in some cases (aspirin being a good example), local damage to the gastric mucosa caused directly by the drug itself may compound the damage. Oral administration of 'replacement' prostaglandin analogues such as **misoprostol** (see Ch. 30) diminishes the gastric damage produced by these agents and is often co-prescribed or combined in a single pill.

Based on extensive experimental evidence, it had been predicted that COX-2-selective agents would provide good anti-inflammatory and analgesic actions with less gastric damage. Indeed, some older drugs that were better tolerated in the clinic (e.g. **meloxicam**) turned out to have some COX-2 selectivity. Two large prospective studies compared the gastrointestinal side effects of two highly

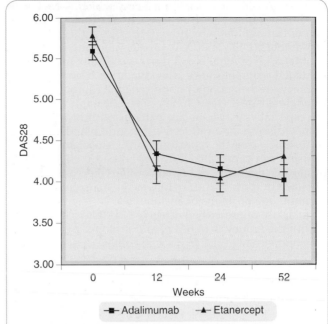

Fig. 26.3 **The effect of anticytokine biologics on rheumatoid arthritis.** In this figure, adalimumab (a humanised monoclonal antibody that neutralises TNF) and etanercept (a fusion protein decoy receptor that binds to TNF) were used to treat patients with active rheumatoid arthritis. The Y-axis measures a composite disease activity scores obtained from clinical assessment of 28 joints (DAS28: the lower the score, the less swollen and painful the joints). *(From Johanputra et al. 2012.)*

selective COX-2 inhibitors, **celecoxib** and **rofecoxib,** with those of standard comparator NSAIDs in patients with arthritis. The coxibs showed some benefit, although the results were not as clear-cut as had been hoped. The actual situation following therapy is complex because the degree to which the two COX isoforms are inhibited depends not only upon the intrinsic activity of the drug but also the inhibitory kinetics and the pharmacokinetics. Warner and Mitchell (2008) have suggested that the degree to which NSAIDs inhibit COX-1 when they inhibit COX-2 by 80% is the best measure of 'selectivity'.

Damage to the small intestine may also occur following NSAID treatment. It is not clear if a COX-dependent mechanism is involved.

Skin reactions

Rashes are common idiosyncratic unwanted effects of NSAIDs, particularly with **mefenamic acid** (10–15% frequency) and **sulindac** (5–10% frequency). They vary from mild erythematous, urticarial and photosensitivity reactions to more serious and potentially fatal diseases including *Stevens–Johnson syndrome* (a blistering rash that extends into the gut, see Ch. 57), and *toxic epidermal necrolysis*[3] (fortunately very rare). The mechanism is unclear.

Adverse renal effects

Therapeutic doses of NSAIDs in healthy individuals pose little threat to kidney function, but in susceptible patients

---

[3] A horrible condition where skin peels away in sheets as if scalded.

they cause acute renal insufficiency, which is reversible on discontinuing the drug (see Ch. 57, Table 57.1). This occurs through the inhibition of the biosynthesis of those prostanoids (PGE_2 and PGI_2; prostacyclin) involved in the maintenance of renal blood flow, specifically in the PGE_2-mediated compensatory vasodilatation that occurs in response to the action of noradrenaline (norepinephrine) or angiotensin II (see Ch. 29). Neonates and the elderly are especially at risk, as are patients with heart, liver or kidney disease, or a reduced circulating blood volume.

Chronic NSAID consumption, especially NSAID 'abuse',[4] can cause analgesic nephropathy characterised by chronic nephritis and renal papillary necrosis (Ch. 29). **Phenacetin** (now withdrawn) was the main culprit; paracetamol, one of its major metabolites, is much less toxic. Regular use of prescribed doses of NSAIDs is less hazardous for the kidney than heavy and prolonged use of over-the-counter analgesics in a social context.

Cardiovascular side effects

Though aspirin is widely for its beneficial antiplatelet action (see below) other NSAIDs generally lack this action, and produce various adverse cardiovascular side effects. As well as opposing the effects of some antihypertensive drugs, NSAIDs also raise blood pressure in patients not taking antihypertensive drugs, and therefore predispose to adverse cardiovascular events such as stroke and myocardial infarction.

▼ This was first recognised during trials of the COX-2 inhibitor rofecoxib. Uncertainty about the cardiovascular risk posed by this drug during clinical trials led to the addition of a 'warning label' in 2002, but the results from a later long-term trial designed to assess the anticancer activity of rofecoxib showed that the risk of cardiovascular events increased significantly after 18 months of drug treatment. As a result of this, the drug was withdrawn by its manufacturer in 2004.

With the exception of low-dose aspirin, adverse cardiovascular effects may be common to all NSAIDs, especially following prolonged (months–years) use or in patients with pre-existing cardiovascular risk. Some drugs (e.g. **naproxen**) appear to be better tolerated in this respect than others (see Ray et al., 2009).

The reasons for the adverse cardiovascular effects are unclear and controversial. Since prostaglandins are important in the control of renal function, including the regulation by cells of the *macula densa* region, of renin release and hence blood pressure, inhibition of COX-2 at this site may be the culprit. The hypertensive effect is dose- and time-dependent and rarely occurs with short-term (i.e. days) administration.

Other unwanted effects

Approximately 5% of patients exposed to NSAIDs may experience aspirin-sensitive asthma. The exact mechanism is unknown, but inhibition of COX is implicated (see Ch. 28) and the presence of a sensitising, pre-existing viral infection may be the culprit. Aspirin is the worst offender, but there is cross-reaction with other NSAIDs, except possibly COX-2 inhibitors (see Ch. 28). Other, much less common, unwanted effects of NSAIDs include CNS effects, bone marrow disturbances and liver disorders, the last being more likely if there is already renal

---

General unwanted effects of cyclo-oxygenase inhibitors

Unwanted effects, many stemming from inhibition of the constitutive housekeeping enzyme COX-1 isoform, are common, particularly in the elderly, and include the following:

- *Dyspepsia, nausea, vomiting* and *other gastrointestinal effects*. Gastric and intestinal damage may occur in chronic users, with risk of haemorrhage, ulceration and perforation which can be life-threatening. The cause is suppression of gastroprotective prostaglandins in the gastric mucosa.
- *Skin reactions*. Mechanism unknown.
- *Reversible renal insufficiency*. Seen mainly in individuals with compromised renal function when the compensatory prostaglandin I_2/E_2-mediated vasodilatation is inhibited.
- *Adverse cardiovascular effects*. These can occur with many NSAIDs and coxibs and may be related to inhibition of COX-2 in the *macula densa* or elsewhere leading to hypertension.
- *'Analgesic-associated nephropathy'*. This can occur following long-term high-dose regimes of NSAIDs and is often irreversible.
- *Liver disorders, bone marrow depression*. Relatively uncommon.
- *Bronchospasm*. Seen in 'aspirin-sensitive' asthmatics. Does not occur with coxibs.

---

impairment.[5] Paracetamol overdose causes liver failure. All NSAIDs (except COX-2 inhibitors) prevent platelet aggregation and therefore may prolong bleeding. Again, aspirin is the main problem in this regard.

SOME IMPORTANT NSAIDS AND COXIBS

Table 26.1 lists commonly used NSAIDs and the clinical uses of the NSAIDs are summarised in the clinical box. We now look at some of the more significant drugs in a little more detail.

ASPIRIN

Aspirin (acetylsalicylic acid) was among the earliest drugs synthesised, and is still one of the most commonly consumed drugs worldwide.[6] It is also a common ingredient in many over-the-counter proprietary medicines. The drug itself is relatively insoluble, but its sodium and calcium salts dissolve readily in aqueous solutions.

While aspirin was originally an old anti-inflammatory workhorse, it is seldom used for this purpose now, having been supplanted by other, better tolerated NSAIDs.

---

[4]So called because the availability of NSAIDs (often in combination with other substances, such as caffeine) in over-the-counter proprietary medicines, has tempted some people to consume them in prodigious quantities, for every conceivable malady. Swiss workers manufacturing watches used to share analgesics in the same way as sweets or cigarettes!

[5]An odd side effect of the NSAID diclofenac came to light when a team of scientists investigated the curious decline in the vulture population of the Indian subcontinent. Dead cattle form an important part of the diet of these birds, and some animals had been treated with diclofenac for veterinary reasons. Apparently, residual amounts of the drug in the carcasses proved uniquely toxic to this species.
[6]Indeed, many people do not seem to regard it as a 'drug' at all. Many studies of platelet aggregation have been ruined by the failure of volunteers to declare their consumption of aspirin.

Clinical uses of NSAIDs

NSAIDs are widely used but cause serious adverse effects (especially gastrointestinal, renal, pulmonary and cardiovascular effects related to their main pharmacological actions, as well as idiosyncratic effects). Elderly patients and those with pre-existing disorders are at particular risk. The main uses are:

- *Antithrombotic*: e.g. **aspirin** (Ch. 24) for patients at high risk of arterial thrombosis (e.g. following myocardial infarction). (Other NSAIDs that cause less profound inhibition of platelet thromboxane synthesis than does **aspirin**, *increase* the risk of thrombosis and should be avoided in high-risk individuals if possible.)
- *Analgesia* (e.g. for headache, dysmenorrhoea, backache, bony metastases, postoperative pain):
  - short-term use: e.g. **aspirin**, **paracetamol**, **ibuprofen**
  - chronic pain: more potent, longer-lasting drugs (e.g. **naproxen**, **piroxicam**) often combined with a low-potency opioid (e.g. **codeine**, Ch. 42)
  - to reduce the requirement for narcotic analgesics (the NSAID **ketorolac** is sometimes given postoperatively for this purpose).
- *Anti-inflammatory*: e.g. **ibuprofen**, **naproxen** for symptomatic relief in rheumatoid arthritis, gout, soft tissue disorders.
- *Antipyretic*: **paracetamol**.

Today, in addition to its widespread use as an over-the-counter remedy, it is used clinically mainly as a cardiovascular drug because of its ability to provide a prolonged inhibition of platelet COX-1 and hence reduce aggregation (see Ch. 24).

▼ While inhibition of platelet function is a feature of most NSAIDs, the effect of aspirin is longer lasting. This is because it irreversibly acetylates COX enzymes, and while these proteins can be replaced in most cells, platelets, lacking a nucleus, are not able to accomplish *de novo* protein synthesis, and remain inactivated for their lifetime (approximately 10 days). Since a proportion of platelets is replaced each day from the bone marrow, this inhibition gradually abates but a small daily dose of aspirin (e.g. 75 mg/day) is all that is required to suppress platelet function to levels which benefit patients at risk for myocardial infarction and other cardiovascular problems (Ch. 24). The view that even patients not at risk would benefit from taking the drug prophylactically (primary prevention) was challenged in a meta-analysis (Baigent et al., 2009) suggesting that in the normal population, the risk from gastrointestinal bleeding just outweighs the protective action. In cases where there is a previous history of cardiovascular episodes the case for prophylactic aspirin (secondary prevention) seems unassailable.

The use of aspirin has also been canvassed for other conditions. These include:

- colonic and rectal cancer: aspirin (and some COX-2 inhibitors) may reduce some types of colorectal and other cancers although one always has to be aware of the GI risk (Schror, 2011)
- Alzheimer's disease (Ch. 40): epidemiological evidence suggested aspirin might be beneficial but so far, clinical trial results have been disappointing (see Heneka et al., 2011)
- radiation-induced diarrhoea.

Pharmacokinetic aspects

Aspirin, being a weak acid, is protonated in the acid environment of the stomach, thus facilitating its passage across the mucosa. Most absorption, however, occurs in the ileum, because of the extensive surface area of the microvilli.

▼ Aspirin is rapidly (within 30 min) hydrolysed by esterases in plasma and tissues, particularly the liver, yielding *salicylate*. This compound itself has anti-inflammatory actions (indeed, it was the original anti-inflammatory from which aspirin was derived); the mechanism is not clearly understood, although it may depend upon inhibition of the NFκB system (Ch. 3) and only secondarily on COX inhibition. Oral salicylate is no longer used for treating inflammation, although it is a component of some topical preparations. Approximately 25% of the salicylate is oxidised; some is conjugated to give the glucuronide or sulfate before excretion, and about 25% is excreted unchanged, the rate of excretion being higher in alkaline urine (see Ch. 8).

The plasma half-life of aspirin will depend on the dose, but the duration of action is not directly related to the plasma half-life because of the irreversible nature of the action of the acetylation reaction by which it inhibits COX activity.

Aspirin

Aspirin (acetylsalicylic acid) is the oldest non-steroidal anti-inflammatory drug. It acts by irreversibly inactivating COX-1 and COX-2.

- In addition to its anti-inflammatory actions, **aspirin** inhibits platelet aggregation, and its main clinical use now is in the therapy of cardiovascular disease.
- It is given orally and is rapidly absorbed; 75% is metabolised in the liver.
- Elimination of its metabolite salicylate follows first-order kinetics with low doses (half-life 4 h), and saturation kinetics with high doses (half-life over 15 h).
- Unwanted effects:
  - with therapeutic doses: some gastric bleeding (usually slight and asymptomatic) is common
  - with larger doses: dizziness, deafness and tinnitus ('salicylism'); compensated respiratory alkalosis may occur
  - with toxic doses (e.g. from self-poisoning): uncompensated metabolic acidosis may occur, particularly in children
  - aspirin has been linked with a rare but serious postviral encephalitis (Reye's syndrome) in children
  - If given concomitantly with warfarin, aspirin can cause a potentially hazardous increase in the risk of bleeding.

Unwanted effects

Salicylates (e.g. aspirin, **diflunisal** and **sulfasalazine**) may produce both local and systemic toxic effects. Aspirin shares many of the general unwanted effects of NSAIDs outlined above. In addition, there are certain specific unwanted effects that occur with aspirin and other salicylates. Reye's syndrome, a rare disorder of children that is characterised by hepatic encephalopathy following an acute viral illness, carries a 20–40% mortality. Since the withdrawal of aspirin for paediatric use, the incidence of Reye's syndrome has fallen dramatically. *Salicylism*, characterised by tinnitus, vertigo, decreased hearing and sometimes also nausea and vomiting, occurs with overdosage of any salicylate.

▼ Acute salicylate poisoning (a medical emergency that occurs mainly in children and attempted suicides) causes major disturbance of acid–base and electrolyte balance. Salicylates uncouple oxidative phosphorylation (mainly in skeletal muscle), leading to increased oxygen consumption and thus increased production of carbon dioxide. This stimulates respiration, which is also stimulated by a direct action of the drugs on the respiratory centre. The resulting hyperventilation causes a respiratory alkalosis that is normally compensated by renal mechanisms involving increased bicarbonate excretion. Larger doses actually cause a depression of the respiratory centre, less CO_2 is exhaled and therefore increases in the blood. Because this is superimposed on a reduction in plasma bicarbonate, an uncompensated respiratory acidosis will occur. This may be complicated by a metabolic acidosis, which results from the accumulation of metabolites of pyruvic, lactic and acetoacetic acids (an indirect consequence of uncoupled oxidative phosphorylation). Hyperthermia secondary to the increased metabolic rate is also likely to be present, and dehydration may follow repeated vomiting. In the CNS, initial stimulation with excitement is followed eventually by coma and respiratory depression. Bleeding can also occur, mainly as a result of depressed platelet aggregation.

Drug interactions

Aspirin may cause a potentially hazardous increase in the effect of warfarin, partly by displacing it from plasma protein binding sites (Ch. 56) thereby increasing its effective concentration and partly because its effect on platelets further interferes with haemostasis (see Ch. 24). Aspirin also antagonises the effect of some antihypertensive and uricosuric agents such as probenecid and sulfinpyrazone. Because low doses of aspirin may, on their own, reduce urate excretion (Ch. 29), it should not be used in gout.

PARACETAMOL

Paracetamol (called acetaminophen in the USA) is one of the most commonly used non-narcotic analgesic–antipyretic agents and is a component of many over-the-counter proprietary preparations. In some ways, the drug constitutes an anomaly: while it has excellent analgesic and antipyretic activity, which can be traced to inhibition of prostaglandin synthesis in the CNS, it has very weak anti-inflammatory activity and does not share the gastric or platelet side effects of the other NSAIDs. For this reason, paracetamol is sometimes not classified as an NSAID at all.

▼ One potential solution to this puzzle was suggested by the discovery of a further COX isoform, COX-3 (an alternate splice product of COX-1) in the CNS of some species. Paracetamol, as well as some other drugs with similar properties (e.g. **antipyrine** and **dipyrone**), were selective inhibitors of this enzyme (Chandrasekharan et al., 2002). However, alternative explanations have also been proposed based upon consideration of the local redox environment in the CNS or the effect of paracetamol metabolites on Trp channels (see reading list and Ch. 42).

Pharmacokinetic aspects

Paracetamol is well absorbed when given orally, with peak plasma concentrations reached in 30–60 min. The plasma half-life of therapeutic doses is 2–4 h, but with toxic doses it may be extended to 4–8 h. Paracetamol is inactivated in the liver, being conjugated to give the glucuronide or sulfate.

Unwanted effects

With therapeutic doses, side effects are few and uncommon, although allergic skin reactions sometimes occur. It is possible that regular intake of large doses over a long period may cause kidney damage.

> ## Paracetamol
>
> **Paracetamol** is a commonly used drug that is available over the counter. It has potent analgesic and antipyretic actions but rather weaker anti-inflammatory effects than other NSAIDs. Its COX inhibitory action seems to be specific to the CNS enzyme.
>
> - It is given orally and metabolised in the liver (half-life 2–4 h).
> - Toxic doses cause nausea and vomiting, then, after 24–48 h, potentially fatal liver damage by saturating normal conjugating enzymes, causing the drug to be converted by mixed function oxidases to N-acetyl-p-benzoquinone imine. If not inactivated by conjugation with glutathione, this compound reacts with cell proteins and kills the cell.
> - Agents that increase glutathione (intravenous **acetylcysteine** or oral **methionine**) can prevent liver damage if given early.

Toxic doses (10–15 g) cause potentially fatal hepatotoxicity. This occurs when normal conjugation reactions are saturated, and the drug is metabolised instead by mixed function oxidases. The resulting toxic metabolite, N-acetyl-p-benzoquinone imine, is normally inactivated by conjugation with glutathione, but when this is depleted the toxic intermediate accumulates in the liver and the kidney tubules and causes necrosis.

▼ The initial symptoms of acute paracetamol poisoning are nausea and vomiting, the hepatotoxicity being a delayed manifestation that occurs 24–48 h later. Further details of the toxic effects are given in Chapter 57. If the patient is seen sufficiently soon after ingestion, the liver damage can be prevented by administering agents that increase glutathione formation in the liver (**acetylcysteine** intravenously, or **methionine** orally). If more than 12 h have passed since the ingestion of a large dose, the antidotes, which themselves can cause adverse effects (nausea, allergic reactions), are less likely to be useful. Regrettably, ingestion of large amounts of paracetamol is a common method of suicide.

COXIBS

Three coxibs are currently available for clinical use in the UK; others may be available elsewhere. Several have been withdrawn following claims of cardiovascular and other toxicity. Coxibs are generally offered to patients for whom treatment with conventional NSAIDs would pose a high probability of serious gastrointestinal side effects. However, gastrointestinal disturbances may still occur with coxibs, perhaps because COX-2 has been implicated in the healing of pre-existing ulcers, so inhibition could delay recovery from earlier lesions. As is the case with all NSAID treatment, cardiovascular risk should be assessed prior to long-term treatment.

Celecoxib and etoricoxib

Celecoxib and **etoricoxib** are licensed in the UK for symptomatic relief in the treatment of osteoarthritis and rheumatoid arthritis and some other conditions.

▼ Both are administered orally and have similar pharmacokinetic profiles, being well absorbed with peak plasma concentrations being achieved within 1–3 h. They are extensively (>99%) metabolised in the liver, and plasma protein binding is high (>90%).

Common unwanted effects may include headache, dizziness, skin rashes and peripheral oedema caused by fluid retention. Because of the potential role of COX-2 in the healing of ulcers, patients with pre-existing disease should avoid the drugs, if possible.

Parecoxib

Parecoxib is a prodrug of **valdecoxib**. The latter drug has now been withdrawn, but parecoxib is licensed for the short-term treatment of postoperative pain. It is given by intravenous or intramuscular injection, and is rapidly and virtually completely (>95%) converted into the active valdecoxib by enzymatic hydrolysis in the liver.

▼ Maximum blood levels are achieved within approximately 30–60 min, depending on the route of administration. Plasma protein binding is high. The active metabolite, valdecoxib, is converted in the liver to various inactive metabolites, and has a plasma half-life of about 8 h. Skin reactions, some of them serious, have been reported with valdecoxib, and patients should be monitored carefully. The drug should also be given with caution to patients with impaired renal function, and renal failure has been reported in connection with this drug. Postoperative anaemia may also occur.

ANTIRHEUMATOID DRUGS

Rheumatoid arthritis is one of the commonest chronic inflammatory conditions in developed countries, and a common cause of disability. Affected joints become swollen, painful, deformed and immobile. One in three patients with rheumatoid arthritis is likely to become severely disabled. The disease also has cardiovascular and other systemic manifestations and carries an increased risk of mortality. The degenerative joint changes, which are driven by an autoimmune reaction, are characterised by inflammation, proliferation of the synovium and erosion of cartilage and bone. The primary inflammatory cytokines, IL-1 and TNF-α, have a major role in the disease (Ch. 17). A simplified scheme showing the development of rheumatoid arthritis and the sites of action of therapeutic drugs, is given in Figure 26.4.

The drugs most frequently used in initial therapy are the 'disease-modifying antirheumatic drugs' (DMARDs

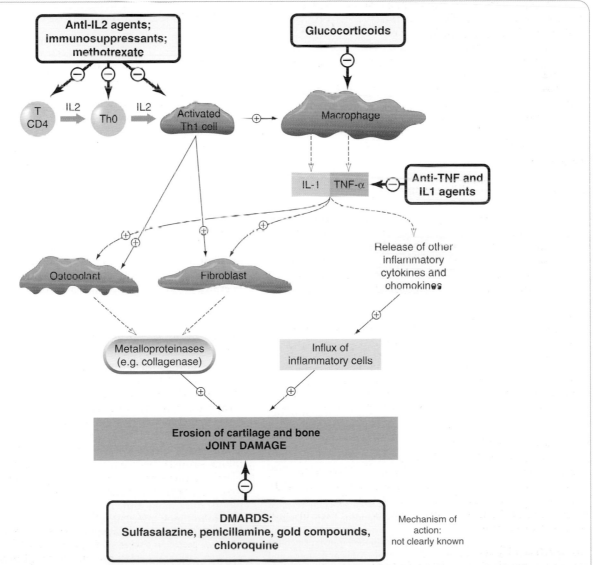

Fig. 26.4 A schematic diagram of the cells and mediators involved in the pathogenesis of rheumatoid joint damage, indicating the sites of action of antirheumatoid drugs. DMARD, disease-modifying antirheumatic drug. For details of the anti-TNF, IL-1 and IL-2 receptor agents, see Chapter 6 and Table 26.3.

Table 26.2 Comparison of some common 'disease-modifying' and immunosuppressive drugs used in the treatment of the arthritides

Type	Drug	Indication	Severity	Comments
Gold complexes	Sodium aurothiomalate	RA	–	Many side effects. Long latency of action
Antimalarials	Chloroquine	RA, SLE	Moderate	Used when other therapies fail
	Hydroxy-chloroquine sulfate	RA, SLE	Moderate	Also useful for some skin disorders
Immunomodulators	Methotrexate	RA, PS, JRA	Moderate to severe	A 'first-choice' drug. Also used in Crohn's disease and cancer treatment. Often used in combination with other drugs
	Azathioprine	RA, IBS	–	Used when other therapies fail. Also used in transplant rejection, IBS and eczema
	Ciclosporin	RA, AD, PA	Severe	Used when other therapies fail, in some skin diseases and transplant rejection
	Cyclophosphamide	RA	Severe	Used when other therapies fail
	Leflunomide	RA, PA	Moderate to severe	Also used in psoriatic arthritis
NSAID	Sulfasalazine	RA, PA, JRA	–	A 'first-choice' drug. Also used in ulcerative colitis
Penicillin metabolite	Penicillamine	RA	Severe	Many side effects. Long latency of action

AD, atopic dermatitis; IBS, inflammatory bowel disease; JRA, juvenile rheumatoid arthritis; NSAID, non-steroidal anti-inflammatory drug; PA, psoriatic arthritis; PS, psoriasis; RA, rheumatoid arthritis; SLE, systemic lupus erythematosus.
Data from various sources, including the British National Formulary, 2013.

– especially **methotrexate**) and the NSAIDs. Unlike the NSAIDs, which only reduce the symptoms, DMARDs may halt or reverse the underlying disease itself. Although such claims are often over-optimistic, these drugs are nevertheless useful in the treatment of discrete groups of patients, and Rau (2005) has argued for their continuing use despite the availability of the newer anticytokine agents (see below). Some immunosuppressants (e.g. **azathioprine**, **ciclosporin**) are also used, as are the glucocorticoids (covered in Chs 3 and 33).

Davis and Matteson (2012) have reviewed the question of how to classify and treat this miserable and disabling disease.

DISEASE-MODIFYING ANTIRHEUMATIC DRUGS

The term 'DMARD' is a latex concept that can be stretched to cover a heterologous group of agents with unrelated chemical structures and different mechanisms of action. Included in this category are methotrexate, **sulfasalazine**, **gold compounds**, **penicillamine**, **chloroquine** and other anti-malarials (see Table 26.2) and various immunosuppressant drugs.

▼ The antirheumatoid action of most of these agents was discovered through a mixture of serendipity and clinical intuition. When they were introduced, nothing was known about their mechanism of action and decades of *in vitro* experiments have generally resulted in further bewilderment rather than understanding. DMARDs generally improve symptoms and can reduce disease activity in rheumatoid arthritis, as measured by reduction in the number of swollen and tender joints, pain score, disability score, X-ray appearance and serum concentration of acute-phase proteins and of *rheumatoid factor* (an immunoglobulin IgM antibody against host IgG).

The DMARDs are often referred to as *second-line drugs*, with the implication that they are only resorted to when

other therapies (e.g. NSAIDs) failed, but DMARD therapy may be initiated as soon as a definite diagnosis has been reached. Their clinical effects are usually slow (months) in onset, and it is usual to provide NSAID 'cover' during this induction phase. If therapy is successful (and the success rate is variable), concomitant NSAID (or glucocorticoid) therapy can be reduced. Some DMARDs (e.g. methotrexate) have a place in the treatment of other chronic inflammatory diseases, whereas others (e.g. penicillamine) are not thought to have a general anti-inflammatory action. Putative mechanisms of action of DMARDs have been reviewed by Bondeson (1997) and Cutolo (2002).

METHOTREXATE

Methotrexate is a folic acid antagonist with cytotoxic and immunosuppressant activity (Ch. 56). It has a useful and reliable antirheumatoid action and is a common first-choice drug. It has a more rapid onset of action than other DMARDs, but treatment must be closely monitored because of potential blood dyscrasias (some fatal) and liver cirrhosis. It is, however, superior to most other DMARDs in terms of efficacy and patient tolerance, and is often given in conjunction with the anticytokine drugs.

Its mechanism of action is unrelated to its effect on folic acid (which is routinely co-administered to prevent blood dyscrasia) but may well be connected with its ability to block adenosine uptake (see Ch. 16 and Chan & Cronstein, 2010).

SULFASALAZINE

Sulfasalazine, another common first-choice DMARD in the UK, produces remission in active rheumatoid arthritis and is also used for chronic inflammatory bowel disease (see Ch. 30). It may act by scavenging the toxic oxygen metabolites produced by neutrophils. The drug is a complex of a sulfonamide (sulfapyridine) and salicylate. It is split into its component parts by bacteria in the colon, the 5-aminosalicylic acid being the putative radical scavenger. It is poorly absorbed after oral administration.

▼ The drug is generally well tolerated but common side effects include gastrointestinal disturbances, malaise and headache. Skin reactions and leukopenia can occur but are reversible on stopping the drug. The absorption of folic acid is sometimes impaired; this can be countered by giving folic acid supplements. A reversible decrease in sperm count has also been reported. As with other sulfonamides, bone marrow depression and anaphylactic-type reactions may occur in a few patients. Haematological monitoring may be necessary.

PENICILLAMINE

Penicillamine is *dimethylcysteine*; it is produced by hydrolysis of penicillin and appears in the urine after treatment with that drug. The D-isomer is used in the therapy of rheumatoid disease. About 75% of patients with rheumatoid arthritis respond to penicillamine. Therapeutic effects are seen within weeks but do not reach a plateau for several months. Penicillamine is thought to modify rheumatoid disease partly by decreasing the immune response and IL-1 generation, and/or partly by preventing the maturation of newly synthesised collagen. However, the precise mechanism of action is still a matter of conjecture. The drug has a highly reactive thiol group and also has metal-chelating properties, which are put to good use in the treatment of *Wilson's disease* (pathological copper deposition causing neurodegeneration and liver disease) and heavy metal poisoning.

▼ Penicillamine is given orally, but only half the dose is absorbed. It reaches peak plasma concentrations in 1–2 h and is excreted in the urine. Dosage is started low and increased only gradually to minimise the unwanted effects, which occur in about 40% of patients and may necessitate cessation of therapy. Rashes and stomatitis are the most common unwanted effects but may resolve if the dosage is lowered. Anorexia, fever, nausea and vomiting, and disturbances of taste (the last related to the chelation of zinc) are seen, but often disappear with continued treatment. Proteinuria occurs in 20% of patients and should be monitored. Haematological monitoring is also required when treatment is initiated. Thrombocytopenia may require lowering the dose. Leukopenia or aplastic anaemia are absolute contraindications, as are autoimmune conditions (e.g. thyroiditis, myasthenia gravis). Because penicillamine is a metal chelator, it should not be given with gold compounds.

GOLD COMPOUNDS

Gold is administered as an organic complex, **sodium aurothiomalate**. The anti-inflammatory effect develops slowly over 3–4 months. Pain and joint swelling subside, and the progression of bone and joint damage diminishes. The mechanism of action is not clear. Sodium aurothiomalate is given by deep intramuscular injection. Gold complexes gradually accumulate in synovial cells in joints as well as other tissues, such as liver cells, kidney tubules, the adrenal cortex and macrophages, and remain for some time after treatment is stopped. Excretion is mostly renal, but some is eliminated in the gastrointestinal tract. The half-life is 7 days initially but increases with treatment, so the drug is usually given first at weekly, then at monthly intervals.

▼ Unwanted effects with aurothiomalate are seen in about one-third of patients treated, and serious toxic effects in about 1 patient in 10. Important unwanted effects include skin rashes (which can be severe), mouth ulcers, non-specific flu-like symptoms, proteinuria, thrombocytopenia and blood dyscrasias. Anaphylactic reactions can occur. If therapy is stopped when the early symptoms appear, the incidence of serious toxic effects is relatively low.

ANTIMALARIAL DRUGS

Hydroxychloroquine and chloroquine are 4-aminoquinoline drugs used mainly in the prevention and treatment of malaria (Ch. 54), but they are also used as DMARDs. Chloroquine is usually reserved for cases where other treatments have failed. They are also used to treat another autoimmune disease, lupus erythematosus, but are contraindicated in patients with psoriatic arthropathy because they exacerbate the skin lesions. The related antimalarial, **mepacrine**, is also sometimes used for discoid lupus. The antirheumatic effects do not appear until a month or more after the drug is started, and only about half the patients treated respond. The administration, pharmacokinetic aspects and unwanted effects of chloroquine are dealt with in Ch. 54; screening for ocular toxicity is particularly important.

IMMUNOSUPPRESSANT DRUGS

▼ Immunosuppressants are used in the therapy of autoimmune disease and also to prevent and/or treat transplant rejection. Because they impair the immune response, they carry the hazard of a decreased response to infections and may facilitate the emergence of malignant cell lines. However, the relationship between these adverse effects and potency in preventing graft rejection varies with different drugs. The clinical use of immunosuppressants is summarised in the clinical box.

Most of these drugs act during the induction phase of the immunological response, reducing lymphocyte proliferation (see Ch. 6), although others also inhibit aspects of the effector phase. There are three main groups:

- drugs that inhibit IL-2 production or action (e.g. ciclosporin, **tacrolimus**)
- drugs that inhibit cytokine gene expression (e.g. corticosteroids)
- drugs that inhibit purine or pyrimidine synthesis (e.g. azathioprine, **mycophenolate mofetil**).

CICLOSPORIN

Ciclosporin is a naturally occurring compound first identified in a fungus. It is a cyclic peptide of 11 amino acid residues (including some not found in animals) with potent immunosuppressive activity but no effect on the acute inflammatory reaction *per se*. Its unusual activity, which (unlike most earlier immunosuppressants) does not involve cytotoxicity, was discovered in 1972 and was crucial for the development of transplant surgery (for a detailed review, see Borel et al., 1996). The drug has numerous actions but those of relevance to immunosuppression are:

- decreased clonal proliferation of T cells, primarily by inhibiting IL-2 synthesis and possibly also by decreasing expression of IL-2 receptors
- reduced induction and clonal proliferation of cytotoxic T cells from CD8+ precursor T cells
- reduced function of the effector T cells responsible for cell-mediated responses (e.g. decreased delayed-type hypersensitivity)
- some reduction of T cell-dependent B cell responses.

Clinical uses of immunosuppressant drugs

Immunosuppressant drugs are used by specialists, often in combination with glucorticoid and/or cytotoxic drugs:

- To slow the progress of rheumatoid and other arthritic diseases including psoriatic arthritis, ankylosis spondylitis, juvenile arthritis: *disease-modifying antirheumatic drugs* (DMARDs), e.g. **methotrexate, leflunomide, ciclosporin**; *cytokine modulators* (e.g. **adalimumab, etanercept, infliximab**) are used when the response to methotrexate or other DMARDs has been inadequate.
- To suppress rejection of transplanted organs, e.g. **ciclosporin, tacrolimus, sirolimus**.
- To suppress graft-versus-host disease following bone marrow transplantation, e.g. **ciclosporin**.
- In autoimmune disorders including idiopathic thrombocytopenic purpura, some forms of haemolytic anaemias and of glomerulonephritis and myasthenia gravis.
- In severe inflammatory bowel disease (e.g. **ciclosporin** in ulcerative colitis, **infliximab** in Crohn's disease).
- In severe skin disease (e.g. **pimecrolimus**, **tacrolimus** for atopic eczema uncontrolled by maximal topical glucocorticoids; **etanercept**, **infliximab** for very severe plaque psoriasis which has failed to respond to **methotrexate** or **ciclosporin**).

Immunosuppressants

- Clonal proliferation of T-helper cells can be decreased through inhibition of transcription of interleukin (IL)-2: **ciclosporin, tacrolimus, sirolimus** and **pimecrolimus** and glucocorticoids act in this way.
- **Ciclosporin** and **tacrolimus** bind to cytosolic proteins (immunophilins) and produce their effects on gene transcription by inhibiting calcineurin or activating protein kinases.
- **Ciclosporin** and **tacrolimus** are given orally or intravenously; a common adverse effect is nephrotoxicity.
- For glucocorticoids, see separate box.
- DNA synthesis is inhibited by:
  - **azathioprine**, through its active metabolite mercaptopurine
  - **mycophenolate mofetil**, through inhibition of *de novo* purine synthesis.
  T cell signal transduction events are blocked by **basiliximab** and **daclizumab**, which are monoclonal antibodies against the α chain of the IL-2 receptor.

The main action is a relatively selective inhibitory effect on IL-2 gene transcription, although a similar effect on interferon (IFN)-γ and IL-3 has also been reported. Normally, interaction of antigen with a T-helper (Th) cell receptor results in increased intracellular Ca^{2+} (Chs 2 and

6), which in turn stimulates a phosphatase, calcineurin. This activates various transcription factors that initiate IL-2 expression. Ciclosporin binds to cyclophilin, a cytosolic protein member of the immunophilin family (a group of proteins that act as intracellular receptors for such drugs). The drug–immunophilin complex binds to, and inhibits, calcineurin which acts in opposition to the many protein kinases involved in signal transduction (see Ch. 3), thereby preventing activation of Th cells and production of IL-2 (Ch. 6).

Ciclosporin itself is poorly absorbed by mouth but can be given orally in a more readily absorbed formulation, or by intravenous infusion. After oral administration, peak plasma concentrations are usually attained in about 3–4 h. The plasma half-life is approximately 24 h. Metabolism occurs in the liver, and most of the metabolites are excreted in the bile. Ciclosporin accumulates in most tissues at concentrations three to four times that seen in the plasma. Some of the drug remains in lymphomyeloid tissue and remains in fat depots for some time after administration has stopped.

The commonest and most serious unwanted effect of ciclosporin is nephrotoxicity, which is thought to be unconnected with calcineurin inhibition. It may be a limiting factor in the use of the drug in some patients (see also Ch. 57). Hepatotoxicity and hypertension can also occur. Less important unwanted effects include anorexia, lethargy, hirsutism, tremor, paraesthesia (tingling sensation), gum hypertrophy (especially when co-prescribed with calcium antagonists for hypertension; Ch. 22) and gastrointestinal disturbances. Ciclosporin has no depressant effects on the bone marrow.

TACROLIMUS

Tacrolimus is a macrolide antibiotic of fungal origin with a very similar mechanism of action to ciclosporin, but higher potency. The main difference is that the internal receptor for this drug is not cyclophilin but a different immunophilin termed FKBP (FK-binding protein, so-called because tacrolimus was initially termed FK506). The tacrolimus–FKBP complex inhibits calcineurin with the effects described above. It is not used for arthritis but mainly in organ transplantation and severe atopic eczema. **Pimecrolimus** (used to treat atopic eczema) acts in a similar way. **Sirolimus** (used to prevent organ rejection after transplantation, and also in coating on cardiac stents to prevent restenosis; Ch. 22) also combines with an immunophilin, but activates a protein kinase to produce its immunosuppressant effect.

▼ Tacrolimus can be given orally, by intravenous injection or as an ointment for topical use in inflammatory disease of the skin. It is 99% metabolised by the liver and has a half-life of approximately 7 h. The unwanted effects of tacrolimus are similar to those of ciclosporin but are more severe. The incidence of nephrotoxicity and neurotoxicity is higher, but that of hirsutism is lower. Gastrointestinal disturbances and metabolic disturbances (hyperglycaemia) can occur. Thrombocytopenia and hyperlipidaemia have been reported but decrease when the dosage is reduced.

AZATHIOPRINE

Azathioprine interferes with purine synthesis and is cytotoxic. It is widely used for immunosuppression, particularly for control of autoimmune diseases such as rheumatoid arthritis and to prevent tissue rejection in transplant surgery. This drug is metabolised to mercaptopurine, an analogue that inhibits DNA synthesis (see Ch. 56). Because it inhibits clonal proliferation during the induction phase of the immune response (see Ch. 6) through a cytotoxic action on dividing cells, both cell-mediated and antibody-mediated immune reactions are depressed by this drug. As is the case with mercaptopurine itself, the main unwanted effect is depression of the bone marrow. Other toxic effects are nausea and vomiting, skin eruptions and a mild hepatotoxicity.

CYCLOPHOSPHAMIDE

Cyclophosphamide is a potent immunosuppressant that is mainly used to treat cancer. Its mechanism of action is explained in Chapter 56. It has substantial toxicity and is therefore generally reserved for serious cases of rheumatoid arthritis in which all other therapies have failed.

MYCOPHENOLATE MOFETIL

Mycophenolate mofetil is a semisynthetic derivative of a fungal antibiotic, and is used for preventing organ rejection. In the body, it is converted to mycophenolic acid, which restrains proliferation of both T and B lymphocytes and reduces the production of cytotoxic T cells by inhibiting inosine monophosphate dehydrogenase. This enzyme is crucial for *de novo* purine biosynthesis in both T and B cells (other cells can generate purines through another pathway), so the drug has a fairly selective action.

▼ Mycophenolate mofetil is given orally and is well absorbed. Magnesium and aluminium hydroxides impair absorption, and colestyramine reduces plasma concentrations. The metabolite mycophenolic acid undergoes enterohepatic cycling and is eliminated by the kidney as the inactive glucuronide. Unwanted gastrointestinal effects are common.

LEFLUNOMIDE

Leflunomide, used mainly to treat rheumatoid arthritis and occasionally to prevent transplant rejection, has a relatively specific inhibitory effect on activated T cells. It is transformed to a metabolite that inhibits *de novo* synthesis of pyrimidines by inhibiting dihydro-orotate dehydrogenase. It is orally active and well absorbed from the gastrointestinal tract. It has a long plasma half-life, and the active metabolite undergoes enterohepatic circulation. Unwanted effects include diarrhoea, alopecia, raised liver enzymes and indeed, a risk of hepatic failure. The long half-life increases the risk of cumulative toxicity.

GLUCOCORTICOIDS

The therapeutic action of the glucocorticoids involves both their inhibitory effects on the immune response and their anti-inflammatory actions. These are described in Chapter 33, and their sites of action on cell-mediated immune reactions are indicated in Figure 26.4. Glucocorticoids are immunosuppressant chiefly because, like ciclosporin, they restrain the clonal proliferation of Th cells, through decreasing transcription of the gene for IL-2. However, they also decrease the transcription of many other cytokine genes (including those for TNF-α, IFN-γ, IL-1 and many other interleukins) in both the induction and effector phases of the immune response. The synthesis and release of anti-inflammatory proteins (e.g. annexin 1, protease inhibitors) is also increased. These effects are mediated through inhibition of the action of transcription factors, such as activator protein-1 and NFκB (Ch. 3).

ANTICYTOKINE DRUGS AND OTHER BIOPHARMACEUTICALS

The drugs in this section probably represent the greatest technological and conceptual breakthrough in the treatment of severe chronic inflammation for decades (see Maini, 2005). By their use, treatment can, for the first time, be targeted at specific aspects of the disease processes. These drugs are biopharmaceuticals, that is to say, they are engineered recombinant antibodies and other proteins (see Ch. 59). As such, they are difficult and expensive to produce, and this limits their use. In the UK (in the National Health Service), they are generally restricted to patients who do not respond adequately to other DMARD therapy and they are usually administered under specialist supervision only. Some of these drugs are administered in combination with methotrexate, which apparently provides a synergistic anti-inflammatory action.

The characteristics and indications of some current biopharmaceuticals are shown in Table 26.3. The effect of two of these agents on rheumatoid arthritis is shown in Figure 26.3 (see p. 321). Many neutralise soluble cytokines. **Adalimumab, certolizumab pegol, golimumab, etanercept** and **infliximab** target TNF-α; anakinra targets IL-1 and **tocilizumab**, IL-6. **Abatacept** and **natalizumab** target T cells, either disrupting activation, proliferation or emigration. **Rituximab** and **belimumab** target B cells. While they are not used for treating arthritis, **basiliximab**, **belatacept** and **daclizumab** are included in the table as they act to prevent the rejection of transplanted organs in a similar way – by suppressing T cell proliferation.

There is debate over the precise nature of the target of the anti-TNF agents. Some target both soluble and membrane-bound forms of TNF whereas others are more selective. Antibodies that target membrane-bound TNF (e.g. infliximab and adalimumab) may kill the host cell by complement-induced lysis. This produces a different quality of effect than simple immunoneutralisation of the soluble mediator (by, for example, etanercept). This fact is probably the reason why some of these drugs exhibit a slightly different pharmacological profile despite apparently acting through the same mechanism (see Arora et al., 2009, for further details).

▼ As proteins, none of these drugs can be given orally. Administration is usually by subcutaneous injection or intravenous infusion and their pharmacokinetic profiles vary enormously. Dosing regimes differ but anakinra is usually given daily, efalizumab and etanercept once or twice per week, adalimumab, certolizumab pegol, infliximab and rituximab every 2 weeks, and abatacept, belimumab, golimumab, natalizumab and tocilizumab every month. Sometimes a loading dose of these drugs is given as a preliminary to regular administration.

A proportion of patients (about 30%) do not respond to many of these anticytokine drugs for reasons that are not entirely clear and therapy is generally discontinued if no therapeutic benefit is evident within 2–4 weeks.

Cytokines are crucial to the regulation of host defence systems (see Ch. 18), and leukocytes are key players in their functioning and execution. One might predict, therefore, that anticytokine or antileukocyte therapy – like any treatment that interferes with immune function – may precipitate latent disease (e.g. tuberculosis and hepatitis

Table 26.3 Biologics used in the treatment of inflammatory disease

Target	Drug	Type	Mode of action	Indication
Soluble TNF	Adalimumab	Humanised monoclonal ab	Imuno-neutralisation	RA (moderate–severe), PA, AS, PP, CD
	Certolizumab pegol	Pegylated ab fragment		RA[a] (moderate–severe)
	Golimumab	Humanised monoclonal ab		RA (moderate–severe), PA, PS
	Infliximab	Chimeric neutralising ab		RA[a] (moderate–severe), PA, AS, PP
	Etanercept	Fusion protein decoy receptor	Neutralisation	RA[a] (moderate–severe), PA, AS, PP
Soluble IL-1	Anakinra	Recombinant version of IL-1 ra	Neutralisation	RA[a] (moderate–severe)
Soluble IL-6	Tocilizumab	Humanised monoclonal ab	Neutralisation	RA[a] (moderate–severe)
T cells	Abatacept	Fusion protein	Prevents co-stimulation of T cells	RA[a] (moderate–severe)
	Basiliximab	Chimeric monoclonal ab	IL-2 receptor antagonist	Immunosuppression for transplantation surgery
	Belatacept	Fusion protein	Prevents activation of T cells	
	Daclizumab	Humanised monoclonal ab	IL-2 receptor antagonist	
	Natalizumab	Humanised monoclonal ab	VLA-4 on lymphocytes (neutralises)	Severe multiple sclerosis
B cells	Belimumab	Humanised monoclonal ab	Immuno-neutralises B-cell-activating factor	SLE
	Rituximab	Chimeric monoclonal ab	Causes B cells lysis	RA[a] (moderate–severe), some malignancies

[a]Used in conjunction with methotrexate. ab, antibody; AS, ankylosing spondylitis; CD, Crohn's disease; PA, psoriatic arthritis; PP, plaque psoriasis (e.g. skin); RA, rheumatoid arthritis; SLE, systemic lupus erythematosus.

B) or encourage opportunistic infections. Reports suggest that this may be a problem with adalimumab, etanercept, infliximab, natalizumab and rituximab. The area has been reviewed by Bongartz et al. (2006). Another unexpected, but fortunately rare, effect seen with these drugs is the onset of psoriasis-like syndrome (Fiorino et al., 2009). Hypersensitivity, injection site reactions or mild gastrointestinal symptoms may be seen with any of these drugs.

DRUGS USED IN GOUT

Gout is a metabolic disease in which urate crystals are deposited in tissues, usually because plasma urate concentration is raised. Sometimes this is linked to overindulgence in alcoholic beverages, especially beer, or purine-rich foods such as offal (urate is a product of purine metabolism). Increased cell turnover in haematological malignancies, particularly after treatment with cytotoxic drugs (see Ch. 56), or impaired excretion of uric acid are other causes. It is characterised by extremely painful intermittent attacks of acute arthritis produced by the deposition of the crystals in the synovial tissue of distal joints, such as the big toe, and elsewhere, such as the external ear – the common theme is that these are cool, favouring crystal deposition. An inflammatory response is evoked, involving activation of the kinin, complement and plasmin systems (see Ch. 18 and Ch. 6, Fig. 6.1), generation of prostaglandins, lipoxygenase products such as leukotriene B4 (Ch. 17, Fig. 17.1), and local accumulation of neutrophil granulocytes. These engulf the crystals by phagocytosis, releasing tissue-damaging toxic oxygen metabolites and subsequently causing lysis of the cells with release of proteolytic enzymes. Urate crystals also induce the production of IL-1 and possibly other cytokines.

Drugs used to treat gout act in the following ways:

- by decreasing uric acid synthesis (**allopurinol**, the main prophylactic drug)
- by increasing uric acid excretion (*uricosuric agents*: **probenecid**, **sulfinpyrazone**; see Ch 29)
- by inhibiting leukocyte migration into the joint (**colchicine**)
- by a general anti-inflammatory and analgesic effect (NSAIDs and occasionally glucocorticoids).

Their clinical uses are summarised in the clinical box (see below).

ALLOPURINOL

Allopurinol is an analogue of hypoxanthine that reduces the synthesis of uric acid by competitive inhibition of xanthine oxidase (Fig. 26.5). The drug is first converted by xanthine oxidase to alloxanthine, which persists in the tissue for a considerable time, and is an effective non-competitive inhibitor of the enzyme. Some inhibition of *de novo* purine synthesis also occurs.

Allopurinol reduces the concentration of the relatively insoluble urates and uric acid in tissues, plasma and urine,

Drugs used in gout and hyperuricaemia

- To treat acute gout:
  - an NSAID, e.g. **ibuprofen**, **naproxen**
  - **colchicine** is useful if NSAIDs are contraindicated
  - a glucocorticoid, e.g. **hydrocortisone** (oral, intramuscular or intra-articular) is another alternative to an NSAID.
- For prophylaxis (must not generally be started until the patient is asymptomatic):
  - **allopurinol**
  - a uricosuric drug (e.g. **probenecid**, **sulfinpyrazone**), for patients allergic to **allopurinol**
  - **rasburicase** by intravenous infusion for prevention and treatment of acute hyperuricaemia in patients with haematological malignancy at risk of rapid lysis.

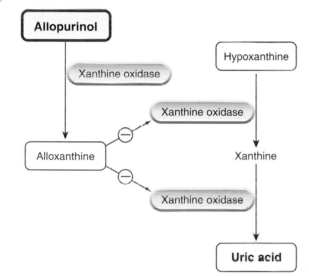

Fig. 26.5 Inhibition of uric acid synthesis by allopurinol. See text for details.

while increasing the concentration of their more soluble precursors, the xanthines and hypoxanthines. The deposition of urate crystals in tissues (tophi) is reversed, and the formation of renal stones is inhibited. Allopurinol is the drug of choice in the long-term treatment of gout, but it actually exacerbates inflammation and pain in an acute attack (see below). **Febuxostat** has a similar pharmacology.

Allopurinol is given orally and is well absorbed. Its half-life is 2–3 h: its active metabolite alloxanthine (Fig. 26.5) has a half-life of 18–30 h. Renal excretion is a balance between glomerular filtration and probenecid-sensitive tubular reabsorption.

Unwanted effects are otherwise few. Gastrointestinal disturbances, allergic reactions (mainly rashes) and some blood problems can occur but usually disappear if the drug is stopped. Potentially fatal skin diseases such as toxic epidermal necrolysis and Stevens–Johnson syndrome

are rare – but devastating. Re-challenge under these circumstances is never justified. Acute attacks of gout occur commonly during the early stages of therapy (possibly as a result of physicochemical changes in the surfaces of urate crystals as these start to re-dissolve), so treatment with allopurinol is never initiated during an acute attack and is usually combined with an NSAID initially.

▼ Allopurinol increases the effect of mercaptopurine, an antimetabolite used in cancer chemotherapy (Ch. 56), and also that of azathioprine (Table 26.2), which is metabolised to mercaptopurine. Allopurinol also enhances the effect of another anticancer drug, cyclophosphamide (Ch. 56). The effect of **warfarin** is increased because its metabolism is inhibited.

URICOSURIC AGENTS

Uricosuric drugs increase uric acid excretion by a direct action on the renal tubule (see Ch. 29). They remain useful as prophylaxis for patients with severe recurrent gout who have severe adverse reactions to allopurinol. Common drugs include probenecid and sulfinpyrazone (which also has NSAID activity). **Benzbromarone** is also available on a named patient basis for treatment of patients with renal impairment. Treatment with uricosuric drugs is initiated together with an NSAID, as in the case of allopurinol. Aspirin and salicylates antagonise the action of uricosuric drugs and should not be used concurrently.

Although not strictly speaking in this group, **rasburicase**, a preparation containing the enzyme uric acid oxidase, is sometimes used for aggressive treatment of gout. It oxidises uric acid in the blood to allantoin, which is more soluble and thus more readily excreted.

COLCHICINE

Colchicine is an alkaloid extracted from the autumn crocus. It has a beneficial effect in gouty arthritis and can be used both to prevent and to relieve acute attacks. It prevents migration of neutrophils into the joint apparently by binding to tubulin, resulting in the depolymerisation of the microtubules and reduced cell motility. Colchicine-treated neutrophils develop a 'drunken walk'. Colchicine may also prevent the production, by neutrophils that have phagocytosed urate crystals, of a putative inflammatory glycoprotein. Other mechanisms may also be important in bringing about its effects. At higher doses than are used to treat gout, colchicine inhibits mitosis, carrying a risk of serious bone marrow depression.

Colchicine is given orally, and is excreted partly in the gastrointestinal tract and partly in the urine.

The acute unwanted effects of colchicine during therapy are largely gastrointestinal and include nausea, vomiting and abdominal pain. Severe diarrhoea[7] may be a problem and with large doses, or prolonged treatment, its antimitotic action may cause serious side effects, including gastrointestinal haemorrhage, kidney damage, bone marrow depression and peripheral neuropathy.

ANTAGONISTS OF HISTAMINE

Antihistamines were introduced by Bovet and his colleagues in the 1930s, before the discovery of the four

---

[7]Because the therapeutic margin is so small, it used to be said by rheumatologists that 'patients must run before they can walk'.

histamine receptor subtypes described in Ch. 17. The generic term 'antihistamine' conventionally refers only to the H$_1$-receptor antagonists that are used for treating various inflammatory and allergic conditions, and it is these drugs that are discussed in this section

Details of some typical systemic H$_1$-receptor antagonists are shown in Table 26.4. In addition to these, there are several others that are primarily used topically (e.g. in nasal sprays or eye drops) in the treatment of hay fever and other allergic symptoms. These include **antazoline**, **azelastine**, **epinastine**, **olapatadine** and **emadastine**. In addition to their H$_1$ antagonist activities, some antihistamines (e.g. **ketotifen**) may also have 'mast cell stabilising' and other anti-inflammatory properties unrelated to histamine antagonism (see Assanasen & Naclerio, 2002).

PHARMACOLOGICAL ACTIONS

Conventionally, the antihistamines are divided into 'first-generation' drugs, which cross the blood–brain barrier and often have sedating actions, and 'second-generation' drugs, which do not. Some of the original second-generation agents (e.g. **terfenadine**) exhibited some cardiac toxicity (torsade de pointes, see Ch. 21). While the risk was extremely low, it was increased when the drug was taken with grapefruit juice or with agents that inhibit cytochrome P450 in the liver (see Chs 9 and 57). These drugs were therefore withdrawn and replaced by 'third-generation' 'cardio-safe' drugs (often active metabolites of the original drugs, e.g. **fexofenadine**).

▼ Pharmacologically, many of the actions of the H$_1$-receptor antagonists follow from the actions of histamine outlined in Chapter 17. *In vitro*, for example, they decrease histamine-mediated contraction of the smooth muscle of the bronchi, the intestine and the uterus. They inhibit histamine-induced increases in vascular permeability and bronchospasm in the guinea pig *in vivo*, but are unfortunately of little value in allergic bronchospasm in humans. The clinical uses of H$_1$-receptor antagonists are summarised in the clinical box.

The CNS 'side effects' of some older H$_1$-receptor antagonists are sometimes more clinically useful than the peripheral H$_1$-antagonist effects. Some are fairly strong sedatives and may be used for this action (e.g. **chlorphenamine**; see Table 26.4). Several are antiemetic and are used to prevent motion sickness (e.g. **promethazine**; see Ch. 30).

Several H$_1$-receptor antagonists show weak blockade of α_1 adrenoceptors (e.g. promethazine). Cyproheptadine is a 5-HT antagonist as well as an H$_1$-receptor antagonist and **rupatadine** is also a PAF antagonist.

Table 26.4 Comparison of some commonly used systemic H$_1$ antagonists

Drug	Common use	Comments
Sedating		
Alimemazine	U	Strong sedative action. Used for anaesthetic premedication
Chlorphenamine	AE, H, U	–
Cinnarizine	–	Used to treat nausea, vomiting, motion sickness
Clemastine	H, U	–
Cyclizine	–	Used to treat nausea, vomiting, motion sickness
Cyproheptadine	H, U	Also used for migraine
Hydroxyzine	U	May cause QT interval prolongation
Ketotifen	H	–
Promethazine	H, U, AE	Strong sedative action. Also used to control nausea and vomiting
Non-sedating		
Acrivastine	H, U	–
Bilastine	H, U	–
Cetirizine	H, U	–
Desloratidine	H, U	Metabolite of loratadine. Long-lasting action
Fexofenadine	H, U	'Cardio-safe' metabolite of terfenidine
Levocetirizine	H, U	Isomer of cetirizine
Loratidine	H, U	–
Mizolastine	H, U	May cause QT interval prolongation
Rupatidine	H, U	Also antagonises PAF (see Ch. 17)

AE, allergic emergency (e.g. anaphylactic shock); H, hay fever; S, sedation; U, urticaria and/or pruritus.

> **Clinical uses of histamine H$_1$-receptor antagonists**
>
> - Allergic reactions (see Ch. 16):
>   - non-sedating drugs (e.g. **fexofenadine**, **cetirizine**) are used for allergic rhinitis (hay fever) and urticaria
>   - topical preparations may be used for insect bites
>   - injectable formulations are useful as an adjunct to **adrenaline** (**epinephrine**) for severe drug hypersensitivity reactions and emergency treatment of anaphylaxis.
> - As antiemetics (see Ch. 30):
>   - prevention of motion sickness (e.g. **cyclizine**, **cinnarizine**)
>   - other causes of nausea, especially labyrinthine disorders.
> - For sedation (see Ch. 44, e.g. **promethazine**).

PHARMACOKINETIC ASPECTS

Most orally active H$_1$-receptor antagonists are well absorbed and remain effective for 3–6 h, although there are some prominent exceptions (e.g. **loratidine**, which is converted to a long-acting metabolite). Most appear to be widely distributed throughout the body, but some do not penetrate the blood–brain barrier, for example the non-sedating drugs mentioned above (see Table 26.4). They are mainly metabolised in the liver and excreted in the urine.

When antihistamines are used to treat allergies, the sedative CNS effects are generally unwanted, but there are other occasions (e.g. in small children approaching bedtime) when such effects are more desirable. Even under these circumstances, other CNS effects, such as dizziness and fatigue, are unwelcome.

Many antihistamines have peripheral anti-muscarinic side effects. The commonest of these is dryness of the mouth, but blurred vision, constipation and retention of urine can also occur. Unwanted effects that are not mechanism-based are also seen; gastrointestinal disturbances are fairly common, while allergic dermatitis can follow topical application.

POSSIBLE FUTURE DEVELOPMENTS

Undoubtedly the most exciting area of current development is in 'biologicals' (see Ch. 59). The success of the anti-TNF agents has been very gratifying and the skilful use of recombinant and protein engineering to produce antibodies that neutralise inflammogens or block key leukocyte receptors or adhesion molecules is likely to continue. The main problem with this sector is not so much the efficacy of the drugs (although a proportion of patients, mysteriously, fail to respond) but rather their cost and lack of oral availability. This places a severe strain on budgets and prevents them from being used as a first-line therapy. Hopefully, ways will be found to reduce the cost of production and development in this important technology.

Clearly a low-cost alternative to a neutralising anti-TNF antibody would be a welcome development. *TNF converting enzyme* (TACE; at least two forms) cleaves membrane-bound TNF thus releasing the soluble active form, and so might be an attractive target. A number of putative small-molecule inhibitors of this enzyme are effective in animal models but have not transferred well to the clinic (see Moss et al., 2008 and Sharma et al., 2013 for a review).

The emerging evidence that all NSAIDs (and coxibs) may have cardiovascular side effects has raised further questions about our existing therapeutic arsenal.[8] One of the few real innovations in the beleaguered NSAID area has been the design and synthesis of nitric oxide (NO)-NSAIDs – conventional NSAIDs that have NO-donating groups attached. The ability of these drugs to release NO following hydrolysis in plasma and tissue fluid is aimed at reducing the risk of ulcerogenic events and increasing the anti-inflammatory activity, presumably due to the beneficial effects of low concentrations of NO (see Ch. 20). Some of these drugs (e.g. naproxcinod, a derivative of naproxen) have been tested in man but have not yet received regulatory approval. Yedgar et al. (2007) discuss some alternative approaches to manipulating the production or action of eicosanoid mediators of inflammation.

---

[8]This does not, of course, apply to low-dose aspirin.

REFERENCES AND FURTHER READING

NSAIDs and coxibs

Baigent, C.L., Blackwell, L., Collins, R., et al., 2009. Aspirin in the primary and secondary prevention of vascular disease: collaborative meta-analysis of individual participant data from randomised trials. Lancet 373, 1849–1860. (*An important study of the use of aspirin in the prevention of cardiovascular disease*)

Boutaud, O., Aronoff, D.M., Richardson, J.H., et al., 2002. Determinants of the cellular specificity of acetaminophen as an inhibitor of prostaglandin H_2 synthases. Proc. Natl Acad. Sci. U.S.A. 99, 7130–7135. (*Proposes a solution to the paracetamol mystery: read together with Ouellet et al., 2001, below*)

Chandrasekharan, N.V., Dai, H., Roos, K.L., et al., 2002. COX-3, a cyclooxygenase-1 variant inhibited by acetaminophen and other analgesic/antipyretic drugs: cloning, structure, and expression. Proc. Natl Acad. Sci. U.S.A. 99, 13926–13931. (*A new COX isozyme is described: COX-3. In humans, the COX-3 mRNA is expressed most abundantly in cerebral cortex and heart. It is selectively inhibited by analgesic/antipyretic drugs such as paracetamol and is inhibited by some other NSAIDs*)

Conaghan, P.G., 2012. A turbulent decade for NSAIDs: update on current concepts of classification, epidemiology, comparative efficacy, and toxicity. Rheumatol. Int. 32, 1491–1502. (*Excellent update on NSAIDs, coxibs and associated toxicity*)

FitzGerald, G.A., Patrono, C., 2001. The coxibs, selective inhibitors of cyclooxygenase-2. N. Engl. J. Med. 345, 433–442. (*Excellent coverage of the selective COX-2 inhibitors*)

Flower, R.J., 2003. The development of COX-2 inhibitors. Nat. Rev. Drug Discov. 2, 179–191. (*Reviews the work that led up to the development of the COX-2 inhibitors; several useful diagrams*)

Fries, J.F., 1998. Quality-of-life considerations with respect to arthritis and nonsteroidal anti-inflammatory drugs. Am. J. Med. 104, 14S–20S, discussion 21S–22S.

Heneka, M.T., Kummer, M.P., Weggen, S., et al., 2011. Molecular mechanisms and therapeutic application of NSAIDs and derived compounds in Alzheimer's disease. Curr. Alzheimer Res. 8, 115–131.

Henry, D., Lim, L.L., Garcia Rodriguez, L.A., et al., 1996. Variability in risk of gastrointestinal complications with individual non-steroidal anti-inflammatory drugs: results of a collaborative meta-analysis BMJ 312, 1563–1566. (*Substantial analysis of the gastrointestinal effects of non-selective NSAIDs*)

Luong, C., Miller, A., Barnett, J., et al., 1996. Flexibility of the NSAID binding site in the structure of human cyclooxygenase-2. Nat. Struct. Biol. 3, 927–933. (*An important research paper detailing the crystal structure of COX-2 and the relevance of this to NSAID and coxib action. Essential reading if you are seriously interested in this topic*)

Ouellet, M., Percival, M.D., 2001. Mechanism of acetaminophen inhibition of cyclooxygenase isoforms. Arch. Biochem. Biophys. 387, 273–280. (*Proposes a solution to the paracetamol mystery: read together with Boutaud et al., 2002, above*)

Ray, W.A., Varas-Lorenzo, C., Chung, C.P., et al., 2009. Cardiovascular risks of non-steroidal anti-inflammatory drugs in patients after hospitalization for serious coronary heart disease. Circ. Cardiovasc. Qual. Outcomes 2, 155–163. (*This paper, together with an editorial on pages 146–147 of the same issue, present and comment on the findings from observational studies on the cardiovascular risk of a range of coxibs and NSAIDs*)

Schror, K., 2011. Pharmacology and cellular/molecular mechanisms of action of aspirin and non-aspirin NSAIDs in colorectal cancer. Best Pract. Res. Clin. Gastroenterol. 25, 473–484.

Skjelbred, P., Løkken, P., Skoglund, L.A., 1984. Post-operative administration of acetaminophen to reduce swelling and other inflammatory events. Curr. Ther. Res. 35, 377–385. (*A study showing that paracetamol can have anti-inflammatory properties under some circumstances*)

Vane, J.R., 1971. Inhibition of prostaglandin synthesis as a mechanism of action for aspirin-like drugs. Nat. New Biol. 231, 232–239. (*The definitive, seminal article that proposed cyclo-oxygenase inhibition as a mechanism of action for the aspirin-like drugs*)

Vane, J.R., Botting, R.M. (Eds.), 2001. Therapeutic roles of selective COX-2 inhibitors. William Harvey Press, London, p. 584. (*Outstanding multi-author book covering all aspects of the mechanisms of action, actions, adverse effects and clinical role of COX-2 inhibitors in a range of tissues; excellent coverage though a bit dated now)*

Wallace, J.L., 2000. How do NSAIDs cause ulcer disease? Baillière's Best Pract. Res. Clin. Gastroenterol. 14, 147–159. (*Proposes an interesting idea concerning the role of the two COX isoforms in gastric homeostasis*)

Warner, T.D., Mitchell, J.A., 2004. Cyclooxygenases: new forms, new inhibitors, and lessons from the clinic. FASEB J. 18, 790–804. (*Excellent review of COX-1/-2 inhibitors and the relative merits of coxibs and the physiological role of COX-2*)

Warner, T.D., Mitchell, J.A., 2008. COX-2 selectivity alone does not define the cardiovascular risks associated with non-steroidal anti-inflammatory drugs. Lancet 371, 270–273. (*Thoughtful article about cardiovascular risk of NSAIDs*)

Yedgar, S., Krimsky, M., Cohen, Y., Flower, R.J., 2007. Treatment of inflammatory diseases by selective eicosanoid inhibition: a double-edged sword? Trends Pharmacol. Sci. 28, 459–464. (*A very accessible article that deals with the drawbacks of current NSAID therapy and reviews some potential solutions to the problems*)

Antirheumatoid drugs

Alldred, A., Emery, P., 2001. Leflunomide: a novel DMARD for the treatment of rheumatoid arthritis. Expert Opin. Pharmacother. 2, 125–137. (*Useful review and update of this DMARD*)

Bondeson, J., 1997. The mechanisms of action of disease-modifying antirheumatic drugs: a review with emphasis on macrophage signal transduction and the induction of proinflammatory cytokines. Gen. Pharmacol. 29, 127–150. (*Detailed review examining possible modes of action of these drugs*)

Borel, J.F., Baumann, G., Chapman, I., et al., 1996. *In vivo* pharmacological effects of ciclosporin and some analogues. Adv. Pharmacol. 35, 115–246. (*Borel was instrumental in the development of ciclosporin*)

Chan, E.S., Cronstein, B.N., 2010. Methotrexate – how does it really work? Nat. Rev. Rheumatol. 6, 175–178. (*An in-depth investigation of the actions of what is probably the most widely employed DMARD. Good diagrams*)

Cutolo, M., 2002. Effects of DMARDs on IL-1Ra levels in rheumatoid arthritis: is there any evidence? Clin. Exp. Rheumatol. 20 (5 Suppl. 27), S26–S31. (*Reviews the actions of DMARDs on the generation and release of the endogenous IL-1 antagonist. An interesting slant on the mechanism of action of these drugs*)

Rau, R., 2005. Have traditional DMARDs had their day? Effectiveness of parenteral gold compared to biologic agents. Clin. Rheumatol. 24, 189–202. (*Argues for a continuing place of DMARDs in the clinic despite the introduction of the new biologicals*)

Smolen, J.S., Kalden, J.R., Scott, D.L., et al., 1999. Efficacy and safety of leflunomide compared with placebo and sulphasalazine in active rheumatoid arthritis: a double-blind, randomised, multicentre trial. Lancet 353, 259–260. (*Gives details of the results of a clinical trial showing the efficacy of leflunomide*)

Snyder, S.H., Sabatini, D.M., 1995. Immunophilins and the nervous system. Nat. Med. 1, 32–37. (*Good coverage of mechanism of action of ciclosporin and related drugs*)

Anticytokine drugs and other biologicals

Arora, T., Padaki, R., Liu, L., et al., 2009. Differences in binding and effector functions between classes of TNF antagonists. Cytokine 45, 124–131. (*A research paper detailing the significance of the membrane-bound versus soluble TNF neutralising actions of the drugs*)

Bongartz, T., Sutton, A.J., Sweeting, M.J., et al., 2006. Anti-TNF antibody therapy in rheumatoid arthritis and the risk of serious infections and malignancies: systematic review and meta-analysis of rare harmful effects in randomized controlled trials. JAMA 295, 2275–2285. (*The title is self-explanatory*)

Breedeveld, F.C., 2000. Therapeutic monoclonal antibodies. Lancet 355, 735–740. (*Good review on the clinical potential of monoclonal antibodies*)

Carterton, N.L., 2000. Cytokines in rheumatoid arthritis: trials and tribulations. Mol. Med. Today 6, 315–323. (*Good review of agents modulating the action of TNF-α and IL-1; simple, clear diagram of cellular action of these cytokines, and summaries of the clinical trials of the agents in tabular form*)

Choy, E.H.S., Panayi, G.S., 2001. Cytokine pathways and joint inflammation in rheumatoid arthritis. N. Engl. J. Med. 344, 907–916. (*Clear description of the pathogenesis of rheumatoid arthritis, emphasising the cells and mediators involved in joint damage; excellent diagrams of the interaction of inflammatory cells and of the mechanism of action of anticytokine agents*)

Feldmann, M., 2002. Development of anti-TNF therapy for rheumatoid arthritis. Nat. Rev. Immunol. 2, 364–371. (*Excellent review covering the role of cytokines in rheumatoid arthritis and the effects of anti-TNF therapy*)

Fiorino, G., Allez, M., Malesci, A., Danese, E., 2009. Review article: anti TNF-alpha induced psoriasis in patients with inflammatory bowel disease. Aliment. Pharmacol. Ther. 29, 921–927. (*Deals with this rare and unexpected side effect of anti-TNF therapy*)

Jobanputra, P., Maggs, F., Deeming, A., et al., 2012. A randomised efficacy and discontinuation study of etanercept versus adalimumab (RED SEA) for rheumatoid arthritis: a pragmatic, unblinded, non-inferiority study of first TNF inhibitor use: outcomes over 2 years. BMJ Open 2, 1–9.

Maini, R.N., 2005. The 2005 International Symposium on Advances in Targeted Therapies: what have we learned in the 2000s and where are we going? Ann. Rheum. Dis. 64 (Suppl. 4), 106–108. (*An updated review dealing with the role of cytokines in the pathogenesis of rheumatoid arthritis and the results of clinical trials with anti-TNF and anti-IL-1 therapy*)

O'Dell, J.R., 1999. Anticytokine therapy – a new era in the treatment of rheumatoid arthritis. N. Engl. J. Med. 340, 310–312. (*Editorial with excellent coverage of the role of TNF-α in rheumatoid arthritis; summarises the differences between infliximab and etanercept*)

Antihistamines

Assanasen, P., Naclerio, R.M., 2002. Antiallergic anti-inflammatory effects of H₁-antihistamines in humans. Clin. Allergy Immunol. 17, 101–139. (*An interesting paper that reviews several alternative mechanisms whereby antihistamines may regulate inflammation*)

Leurs, R., Blandina, P., Tedford, C., Timmerm, N.H., 1998. Therapeutic potential of histamine H₃ receptor agonists and antagonists. Trends Pharmacol. Sci. 19, 177–183. (*Describes the available H₃ receptor agonists and antagonists, and their effects in a variety of pharmacological models, with discussion of possible therapeutic applications*)

Simons, F.E.R., Simons, K.J., 1994. Drug therapy: the pharmacology and use of H₁-receptor-antagonist drugs. N. Engl. J. Med. 23, 1663–1670. (*A bit dated now but contains effective coverage of the topic from the clinical viewpoint*)

New directions

Davis, J.M. 3rd, Matteson, E.L., 2012. My treatment approach to rheumatoid arthritis. Mayo Clin. Proc. 87, 659–673. (*Written from the viewpoint of a practical clinician, this review explains the latest guidance on classifying pathotypes of rheumatoid arthritis and adjusting the many different types of treatment to suit the patient*)

Moss, M.L., Sklair-Tavron, L., Nudelman, R., 2008. Drug insight: tumor necrosis factor-converting enzyme as a pharmaceutical target for rheumatoid arthritis. Nat. Clin. Pract. Rheumatol. 4, 300–309. (*Accessible review dealing with this potentially important new concept. Some good diagrams*)

Sharma, M., Mohapatra, J., Acharya, A., Deshpande, S.S., Chatterjee, A., Jain, M.R., 2013. Blockade of tumor necrosis factor-alpha converting enzyme (TACE) enhances IL-1-beta and IFN-gamma via caspase-1 activation: a probable cause for loss of efficacy of TACE inhibitors in humans? Eur. J. Pharmacol. 701, 106–113. (*A discussion of the prospects and pitfalls of low molecular weight TNF inhibitors*)

Skin 27

OVERVIEW

With a surface area of about 1.6–1.8 m² and a weight of about 4.5 kg in the average adult, skin qualifies as the largest and heaviest organ in the body. It is also an important target for drug therapy as well as cosmetic and other agents. Here, we look at the structure of human skin and briefly review some common skin disorders. We then discuss some of the many types of drugs that act upon, or through, this organ.

INTRODUCTION

Skin is a complex organ with many roles.[1] Firstly, it acts as a barrier. Being impermeable to water it prevents the loss of moisture from the body as well as the ingress of water and many other substances into the body. It also cushions the underlying tissue against thermal and mechanical damage and shields it from ultraviolet radiation and infection. Even if they can thrive in the slightly acidic environment of the skin's surface, microorganisms cannot easily cross the outer barrier of the skin, but should they do so, skin is well endowed with specialised immunological surveillance systems comprising *Langerhans cells*, a type of dendritic cell, as well as mast cells and other immunocompetent cell types.

A second function is thermoregulation. Approximately 10% of the total blood volume is contained within the dense capillary networks of the skin. Skin arterioles, controlled by the sympathetic nervous system, regulate blood flow and heat loss from the skin. Sweat glands (*eccrine glands*) in the skin secrete an aqueous fluid under cholinergic control which, upon evaporation, increases heat loss.

In the presence of sunlight, vitamin D₃ (cholecalciferol) is synthesised in the *stratum basale* and *stratum spinosum* of skin. Absence of this vitamin through lack of exposure to the ultraviolet (UV B) component of sunlight can lead to deficiency symptoms (see Ch. 36). Melanin, produced by melanocytes in the basal dermal layer, gives skin its characteristic colour. The production of melanin granules is stimulated by sunlight.

Skin is also a profoundly sensory organ. It is densely innervated with sensory neurons, including specific sensory nerve endings that signal itch (a sensation unique to skin with an interesting pharmacology), pain, heat and cold as well as specialised receptors that detect touch (*Meissner's corpuscles*) and pressure (*Pacinian corpuscles*). The cell bodies of cutaneous nerves reside in the dorsal root ganglia.

Being highly visible, skin and its specialised appendages such as hair and nails play an important part in social and sexual signalling. As such it is an important target for cosmetic preparations, suntan lotions, anti-ageing compounds and more. Because unsightly skin can cause problems of social adjustment or even frank psychiatric illness, the distinction between a therapeutic agent and a cosmetic preparation can become blurred. In fact the market for 'cosmeceuticals' as they are called is huge: in 2012, over $8 billion was spent on these compounds (many of which have no proof of efficacy) in the USA alone (Nolan et al., 2012).

Here we look briefly at some common conditions affecting the skin and at some of the drugs used to treat them (see Table 27.1). In most cases, these drugs also have other uses and their mechanisms of action are described elsewhere in the book so the appropriate cross-references are given in the table. Inflammation is a common feature of skin diseases, and anti-inflammatory drugs, discussed in detail in Chapter 26, are often used. In some other instances, the drugs themselves, or their particular utility, are almost unique to skin pharmacology so they will be explained in a little more detail. Drugs used to treat skin infections and cancers are discussed in Chapters 51 and 56.

Topical application of drugs onto the skin can be used as a route for systemic administration (see Ch. 8), and is also used to treat the underlying tissues. For example, NSAIDs applied topically can reduce the inflammation of underlying joints and connective tissue with less unwanted effects than those seen after systemic administration (Klinge & Sawyer, 2013). However, we will not deal in depth with this topic here.

STRUCTURE OF SKIN

Skin comprises three main layers: the outermost layer, the *epidermis*, a middle layer, the *dermis*, and the innermost layer, the *subdermis*, sometimes called the *hypodermis* or *subcutis* (see Fig. 27.1).

The epidermis consists largely of keratinocytes. There are four layers of cells. The *stratum basale* is the innermost layer and lies adjacent to the *dermoepidermal junction*. It comprises mainly dividing keratinocytes interspersed with melanocytes. The latter cells produce granules of melanin in *melanosomes*, which are transferred to the dividing keratinocytes. As the keratinocytes divide and mature they progress towards the skin surface. In the next layer, they form the *stratum spinosum* ('spiny' layer), so called because *desmosomes* (intercellular protein links) begin to appear on the cells. Gradually, these cells begin to flatten adopting a *squamous* (scaly) morphology. They lose their nuclei and the cytoplasm acquires a granular appearance. Lying immediately above this is a thin translucent layer of tissue called the *stratum lucidum*. The

---

[1]As the American humourist and songwriter Alan Sherman so succinctly put it, 'Skin's the thing that if you've got it outside/It keeps your insides in'.

Table 27.1 Drug treatment of some common skin disorders

Disease	Class	Examples	Comments	Chapter
Acne	Antibacterials	Erythromycin, clindamycin	For mild-moderate acne. Sometimes systemic treatment is also used	50, 51
	Retinoids	Retinoin, isoretinoin, adapalene	For more severe disease. Sometimes systemic treatment is also used	–
Alopecia	Androgen antagonists	Finasteride, minoxidil	Generally in men only	35
Hirsutism	Hormone antagonists	Eflornithine, co-cypyrindiol	Usually in women only	35
Infections	Antibacterials	Mupirocin, neomycin sulfate, polymixins, retapamulin, sulfadiazine, fusidic acid, metronidazole	Usually given topically but some drugs may be given orally	50, 51
	Antivirals	Aciclovir, peniciclovir		52
	Antifungal	Amorolfine, clotrimazole, econazole, griseofulvin, ketconazole,miconazole, nystatin, terbinafine, tioconazole	–	53
	Antiparasite	Topical insecticides (e.g. permethrin).	–	54
Pruritus	Antihistamines, topical anaesthetics and related drugs	Crotamiton, diphenhydramine, doxepin	Antihistamines may be given topically or orally. Sometimes a 'sedating' antihistamine is useful	26, 33
Eczema	Glucocorticoids	Mild-potent (i.e. hydrocortisone, betamethasone esters)	May be combined with antibacterial or antifungal agent if infection is present	26, 33
	Retinoids	Alitretinoin	Given orally. Only used if glucocorticoid therapy has failed	–
Psoriasis	Vitamin D analogues	Calcipotriol, calcitriol, tacalcitol	DMARDS and anticytokine drugs used for severe cases	26, 36
	Retinoids	Tazarotene, acitretin	Oral retinoids sometimes used	–
	Glucocorticoids	Moderate–potent (i.e. hydrocortisone butyrate, clobestasol proprinate)	May be combined with antibacterial or antifungal agent if infection is present	26, 33
Rosacea	Antibacterials	Tetracycline, erythromycin, doxycycline, metronidazole	Glucocorticoids are contraindicated	50, 51
Urticaria	Antihistamines	Diphenhydramine, doxepin	Usually given orally. Sometimes a 'sedating' antihistamine is useful	26
Warts	Keratolytic agents and others	Salicylic acid, podophyllotoxin, imiquimod	–	–

DMARDs, disease-modifying antirheumatic drugs.

outermost layer of skin is the *stratum corneum*. By now, the keratinocytes are no longer viable. They have become fused together (cornified) and most tissues have 10–30 layers of these hardened sheets of tissue. The *corneocytes*, as they are now called, are surrounded with a hydrated proteinaceous envelope. Lipid bilayers occupy the extracellular space providing a hydrophilic waterproof layer. The water and lipid content of skin is critical to its function. If the moisture content of the hydrated layer falls, the skin loses its supple properties and cracks. The keratinocytes are normally replenished about every 45 days (Bergstresser & Taylor, 1977). Because of this, healthy skin constantly sheds the outer layer of cornified cells. If this does not occur, patches of dry skin begin to appear.

Below the epidermis lies the dermis. This layer varies in thickness. In some tissues it is very thick (e.g. the palms and the soles of the feet) and in others, very thin (e.g. the

eyelids). Histologically, the dermis comprises a *papillary layer* and a deeper *reticular layer*. The main cell types are fibroblasts. These produce and secrete important structural elements of the skin such as glycoproteins, which contribute to the hydration of the tissue, and collagen and elastin that provide strength and elasticity. Other types of cells associated with the immune system are also present (see Ch. 6). The dermis is richly endowed with blood vessels and lymphatics and densely innervated.

Hair follicles, *sebaceous glands* and *sweat glands* are embedded in the dermis. Hair follicles are lined with specialised cells that produce keratin and associated melanocytes that produce pigment for the growing hair shaft. Associated with each hair follicle is an *erector pili* muscle that causes the hair shaft to become erect. Cold, fear and other strong emotional stimuli trigger this response giving the sensation of 'goose bumps'. Sebaceous glands associated with hair follicles coat the hair with waxy substance. The

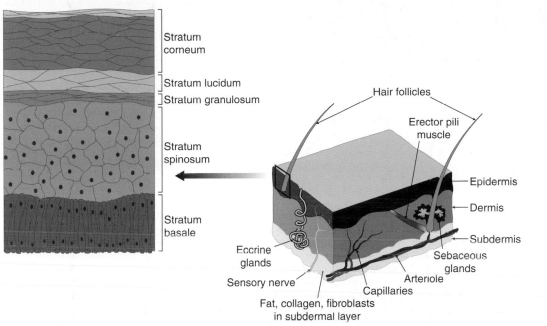

Fig. 27.1 A simplified diagram showing the structure of the skin. The skin comprises three main layers coloured differently in the right-hand drawing: epidermis (dark red/brown); dermis (pink), and subdermis (yellow). On the left is an enlarged diagram of the complex outer, epidermal, layer. Not shown are the apocrine glands within the hair follicles.

Skin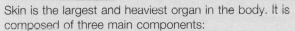

Skin is the largest and heaviest organ in the body. It is composed of three main components:

- *The epidermis.* This is the outermost layer and is comprised of four layers of keratinocytes with interspersed melanocytes. Keratinocytes divide in the basal layer and migrate upwards to the skin surface where they form cornified layers. Lipids in the extracellular spaces confer water-repellent properties.
- *The dermis.* The middle layer is of variable thickness. It consists of fibroblasts that produce structural components such as collagen and elastin as well as immunocompetent cells. Hair follicles and sweat glands are also embedded in this layer and it is densely innervated with nerves, blood vessels and lymphatics.
- *The subdermis* (*hypodermis* or *hypocutis*). This comprises connective tissue and varying amounts of adipose tissue.

Skin has four main functions:

- *A barrier.* Skin prevents the egress or ingress of water, other chemicals and microorganisms. It also acts as a mechanical and thermal barrier and a shock absorber.
- *Thermoregulation.* Vasodilatation of the rich capillary network of the skin, in combination with sweating, increases the loss of heat whilst vasoconstriction has the reverse effect.
- *Vitamin D synthesis.* In the presence of sunlight, vitamin D_3 is synthesised by cells in the epidermal layer.
- *A sensory organ.* Skin contains abundant sensory receptors for touch, heat, cold, pain and itch. Information arising from these dermal receptors is one of the chief ways in which we interact with the outside world.

growth of hair and the activity of these glands is controlled by androgens.

There are two types of sweat glands: *apocrine* glands are associated with hair, especially in the armpits and perineum. They empty their proteinaceous secretion into the hair follicle. *Eccrine* glands, on the other hand, are distributed over much of the skin surface.

The innermost layer of skin is the hypodermis or cutis. This comprises connective tissue and also adipose tissue, which may be particularly thick at some anatomical locations (e.g. the abdomen).

COMMON DISEASES OF THE SKIN

▼ Here we briefly review some common skin disorders, focusing on those for which specific drug treatment is available.

ACNE

▼ The most common form of the disease occurs during puberty, and mainly in boys. Changes in circulating androgens stimulate the sebaceous glands associated with hair follicles, which become enlarged and blocked with sebum and debris. The confined material

337

may become infected, causing an inflammatory reaction that compounds the problem. Normally acne disappears after puberty but some forms may persist or manifest in later life and require long-term treatment. If severe, acne can cause irreversible scarring and considerable psychological misery.

ROSACEA

▼ The diagnostic feature of rosacea is the presence of a chronic hyperaemia of the facial skin. There is often a characteristic pattern with the erythema spreading across the nose, the cheeks and forehead. The erythema is caused by vasodilatation and dilated blood vessels close to the surface of the skin are usually visible. The affected skin may become dry and flaky; there may be a stinging or burning sensation, and a tendency to flush in response to various stimuli, including exertion, emotional stress, heat, sunlight and spicy foods.

There is a genetic basis for the disorder. It is more prevalent in women than men and may be exacerbated during the menopause. The disease cannot be cured and the symptoms can be very long lasting and difficult to control, with both drug and other therapies playing a role. There is a debate about the cause of rosacea. However, a hypothesis that is gaining ground is that rosacea is a disorder of the innate immune system and that antimicrobial peptides in the skin are indirectly responsible for the symptoms (see Antal et al., 2011; Yamasaki & Gallo, 2011). Antibiotic treatment is usually the first choice where clinical management demands drugs.

BALDNESS AND HIRSUTISM

▼ There are two main types of baldness, *male pattern baldness (androgenic alopecia)* and *alopecia areata*. Androgenic alopecia is caused by rising androgen levels and so particularly affects men after puberty; it starts with bi-temporal recession and progresses. Androgens inhibit the growth of hair on the scalp but stimulate it elsewhere (e.g. the face, chest, back etc.). Alopecia areata is a condition where hair falls out in patches that come and go. Eventually, these patches may coalesce, leading to total baldness. The disease seems to be of autoimmune origin.

Hirsutism is common in men (who seldom complain) but less socially acceptable in women. Once again, rising androgen levels are the cause, stimulating the growth of hair on areas of the body where it does not normally occur in women (e.g. the face); this is commoner in some ethnic groups and seldom pathological but can be a symptom of androgenising endocrine tumours (such as *Sertoli–Leydig cell tumours*, which are rare functioning ovarian tumours).

ECZEMA

▼ This is a generic term and refers to a common (approximately 5–20% of children) condition where the skin becomes dry, itchy, flaky and inflamed. The distribution is distinctive, namely on flexor surfaces (e.g. wrists, elbows and behind the knees, in contrast to psoriasis). There are several potential causes. *Atopic eczema* is often seen in patients who also suffer from asthma or seasonal rhinitis (hay fever), although the long-held notion that eczema is primarily an immunological disorder has rather little to support it. It tends to run in families, indicating a genetic susceptibility. *Contact dermatitis* arises when the skin becomes 'sensitised' to a particular antigen. Nickel sensitivity is a classic example: contact with the metal either provokes the production of antibodies or modifies structural elements of the epidermis so that autoantibodies are produced. This is more often seen in women because it is a common component of (less-expensive) jewellery.[2] The pathophysiology is now believed to stem from disordered barrier function leading to epidermal water loss, and a vicious cycle of itching and scratching with release of inflammatory mediators. Penetration of allergens and interaction with IgE-bearing Langerhans cells can add a Th2-mediated immunological component. *Xerotic eczema* refers to eczema that is produced when the skin dries out. This is more common in the winter months, especially amongst older people.

PRURITUS

▼ Itch is a common symptom of skin diseases, but can also occur with systemic disorders, such as jaundice, or neurological disorders such as shingles (herpes zoster). Some drugs (e.g. opioids) also can cause itching. There is a complex relationship between the neural systems that detect and transduce pain and itch (see Greaves & Khalifa, 2004; Ikoma et al., 2006) and there may be a dedicated population of nociceptors that function as 'itch transducers'.

Skin diseases commonly causing itch include eczema, urticaria and psoriasis. These are largely caused by the release of inflammatory mediators in the skin from mast cells (e.g. histamine, leukotrienes, proteases and cytokines).

URTICARIA

▼ This term refers to a range of inflammatory changes in the skin characterised by the presence of raised wheals or bumps. They are normally surrounded by a red margin and are intensely itchy. There are many known causes, including exposure to the sun (*solar urticaria*[3]), heat or cold, insect bites or stings, foodstuffs or infection as well as some drugs. Many cases are allergic in nature while others have no known cause. A bizarre manifestation of urticaria seen in some people is *dermographia* – literally 'writing on the skin'. This is an exaggerated form of the 'triple response' caused by injecting histamine into the skin (see Ch. 17) and may be provoked by scratching or in some cases simply rubbing or stroking the skin.

Urticaria is associated with inflammatory changes in the dermis including mast cell degranulation and the accompanying release of mediators. It may co-exist with a related condition, *angioedema*, which primarily affects the blood vessels of the subdermal layer. Urticaria can resolve relatively rapidly or can persist for weeks (*chronic urticaria*). The disorder can be difficult to manage and glucocorticoids, which suppress most inflammatory responses, are usually ineffective.

PSORIASIS

▼ Psoriasis is an autoimmune condition affecting about 2–3% of Europeans. There is a genetic component and several susceptibility loci have been identified, most of which are connected with the operation of the immune system. Cytokines such as TNF, IL-17 and IL-23 are involved in the inflammatory mechanism and anticytokine biologics can be used to treat severe manifestations of the disease (see Ch. 6). Histologically, it manifests as inflammation accompanied by hyper-proliferation of keratinocytes. This leads to an accumulation of scaly dead skin at the sites of the disease. The most common form is *plaque psoriasis*. This presents as areas of scaly silvery-white skin surrounded by red margins. The distribution is usually quite characteristic, with plaques first appearing on the knees and elbows. The lesions are sometimes itchy (in fact the word psoriasis originates from Greek and literally means 'itchy skin', though in contrast to eczema, itch is by no means a predominant symptom) and may be painful.

Psoriasis can also affect the fingernails, giving a 'pitted' appearance, and/or the joints (typically but not exclusively the distal interphalangeal joints) or other connective tissue (*psoriatic arthritis*).

Psoriasis is generally a life-long condition but one that can appear and disappear for no apparent reason. Stress is said to be a precipitating factor as is dry skin. Several drugs (e.g. β-adrenoceptor antagonists, non-steroidal anti-inflammatory drugs [NSAIDs] and lithium) are purported precipitants (Basavaraj et al., 2010).

---

[2]However, the number of men suffering from the condition is rising because of the popularity of body piercing. If body art is your thing, insist on high-quality nickel-free jewellery.

[3]Not to be confused with miliaria (prickly heat), which is caused by blocked sweat glands.

WARTS

▼ Warts are caused by infection with one of the many types of human papilloma virus (HPV). They are characterised by small raised lesions with an irregular shape. As infection of the epidermis by the virus causes *hyperkeratinisation*, they also have a 'rough' feel. The many varieties of HPV are usually specific for particular tissues, so different strains give rise to different types of warts at diverse anatomical locations. The most common type is usually found on hands and feet (e.g. as *verrucas*). Other types of HPV specifically infect the anogenital region, giving *anogenital warts*.

Most warts are benign in nature and disappear spontaneously after a period of time (usually weeks–months). However, some types of HPV are linked to cancers such as cervical cancer. It is hoped that, in time, immunisation against HPV will reduce the incidence of this disease.

OTHER INFECTIONS

▼ In addition to acne and rosacea, there are a number of other important bacterial skin infections that can be treated with appropriate antibiotics, either topical or systemic. These include superficial skin infections such as *erysipelas* and *impetigo*, and *cellulitis*, which is a more deep-seated infection mainly involving the dermis and subdermis.

Fungal infections of the skin are a common problem. *Tinea*, *candida* and other infections (see Ch. 53) affect skin at several sites (e.g. *tinea pedis* – 'athlete's foot'). These infections are easy to catch and can be difficult to eradicate completely.

The most common viral infections affecting the skin are *herpes simplex* (cold sores) and *herpes zoster* (shingles), which are treated with antiviral drugs (see Ch. 52). The most common parasite infections of the skin are head lice (*Pediculus humanis capitus*) crab lice (*Pthirus pubis*) and scabies (*Sarcoptes scabiei*).

DRUGS ACTING ON SKIN

FORMULATION

Targeting drugs to the skin is both easy and difficult. Unlike most therapeutic settings, drugs can be applied directly to the diseased tissue. There is a caveat, however: since skin is a highly effective barrier, it can prevent the entry of many medicinal agents and this can pose a problem. To reach its site of action (often the lower layer of the epidermis or the dermis) the drug has to pass through the epidermal layer with its highly enriched lipid and aqueous environment. The transdermal delivery of drugs is therefore a highly specialised topic (see Ch. 8). Generally speaking, absorption may be facilitated if the molecule is more hydrophobic in nature: thus, for example, glucocorticoids are often derivatised with fatty acid esters to render them more easily absorbed. The use of a waterproof *occlusion dressing* to cover the skin after applying the drug improves absorption by keeping the epidermis fully hydrated.

The vehicle in which the drug is dissolved is also important. Creams and ointments – essentially stable oil/water emulsions – can be tailored to individual drugs. For example a water-in-oil emulsion is preferable for a hydrophobic drug such as **ciclosporin** whilst an oil-in-water is better for a water-soluble drug such as an NSAID. The appearance and odour of the formulated drug are also important. Most patients would rather take a tablet than apply skin creams that may be greasy, smelly or unsightly (see Tan et al., 2012).

The actual physical condition of the skin is important in maintaining its barrier function and various agents can be used to protect the skin and promote repair. These include *emollients*, which re-hydrate the skin and *barrier creams* that help to prevent damage from irritants. Use of such agents is often indicated alongside treatment with drugs.

Many new ideas for formulating drugs for passage across the skin are under investigation, including the use of 'nanocarriers' and other sophisticated chemical measures (see Schroeter et al., 2010).

Drugs and the skin

Formulation. Because the skin comprises a unique combination of hydrophobic/hydrophilic structures, many drugs are not absorbed and special formulations may be necessary to promote penetration.

Many drugs used for skin conditions are also used to treat disorders in other organs. The main groups are:

- *Glucocorticoids.* Widely used to treat psoriasis, eczema and pruritus because of their anti-inflammatory properties. They are usually specially formulated to enhance topical penetration.
- *Antimicrobial agents.* Used topically or systemically to treat skin infections (e.g. acne, impetigo, cellulitis and rosacea).
- *Hormone antagonists.* Androgen antagonists are used topically or systemically to treat male pattern baldness or hirsutism in women.

Some drugs are used almost exclusively for skin disorders. These include:

- *Retinoids.* These are derivatives of vitamin A and include **tretinoin**, **isotretinoin**, **alitretinoin**, **tazarotene** and **adapalene**. They are used to treat acne, eczema and psoriasis. They are usually given topically, but can be given systemically.
- *Vitamin D derivatives.* Drugs such as **calcitriol**, **calcipotriol** and **tacalcitol** are used to treat psoriasis.

PRINCIPAL DRUGS USED IN SKIN DISORDERS

Many drugs in the dermatological arsenal are also used to treat other diseases and their mechanism of action is the same. The use of agents described below to treat specific skin disorders is shown in Table 27.1. We refer the reader to other chapters in the book where information about these agents may be found (see Table 27.1). Other drugs, such as analogues of vitamins A and D, are rather specific to skin pharmacology.

ANTIMICROBIAL AGENTS

Chapters 50–55 deal in depth with the mechanism of action of this group of drugs. Antibiotics can be applied topically in diseases such as impetigo and acne, or given systemically in the case of cellulitis or rosacea. Fungal infections of the skin are generally treated with topical fungicidal drugs but oral preparations of **ketoconazole** may be used under some circumstances. Herpes simplex infections may be treated with topical or systemic **acyclovir** or **penciclovir** (see Ch. 52).

GLUCOCORTICOIDS AND OTHER ANTI-INFLAMMATORY AGENTS

As one might predict, antihistamines are useful when controlling mild pruritus at least in some circumstances, e.g. eczema, insect bites and mild inflammation. Another topical drug which is useful in treating pruritus is **crotamiton**. This acts rapidly and has long lasting antipruritic effects. The mechanism of action is not known.

The main agents for treating inflammation of the skin are the glucocorticoids. These drugs are widely used to treat psoriasis, eczema and pruritus. Their general mechanism of action is described in Chapters 3 and 33. Preparations used in dermatological practice are often formulated as fatty acid esters of the active drugs. This promotes their absorption through the highly hydrophobic layers of the skin and also alters their efficacy: for example, the potency of **hydrocortisone** on the skin is greatly enhanced by formulating it as a butyrate ester.

▼ Whilst schemes around the world vary, the convention is to classify these drugs by potency. For example:

- *Mild*: e.g. hydrocortisone
- *Moderate*: e.g. **alclomethasone diproprionate, clobetasone butyrate, fludroxycortide** and **fluocortolone**
- *Potent*: e.g. **beclomethasone diproprionate, betamethasone** (various esters) **fluoccinolone acetonide, flucocinonide, fluticasone proprionate, mometasone fuorate** and **triamcinolone acetonide**
- *Very potent*: e.g. **clobetasol proprionate** and **diflucortolone valerate**.

The choice of glucocorticoid depends upon the severity of the disease and, because the thickness of skin varies from one location to the other, its anatomical site. They are sometimes used in combination with antibacterial or fungicidal drugs if they are to be used at the site of an infection.

The action of glucocorticoids on the skin is similar in mechanism to their effect elsewhere in the body. They are potent inhibitors of the release of inflammatory mediators from mast cells, of neutrophil activation and emigration, and immune cell activation (see Chs 26, 33). Their topical application produces vasoconstriction in the skin causing a characteristic 'blanching' reaction.[4] The mechanism is unknown.

Unwanted effects. Generally speaking, short-term treatment with low potency steroid preparations are safe; hydrocortisone formulations are available from pharmacies without prescription.

There are potentially serious side effects associated with prolonged usage or the more potent members of the class, however. These include:

- *Steroid 'rebound'.* If topical steroid therapy is suddenly discontinued, the underlying disease often returns in a more aggressive form. The biological basis of this is probably that the gluococorticoid receptor is downregulated during topical treatment and can no longer respond to normal circulating glucocorticoids. Gradually tapering the drug can avoid this problem.
- *Skin atrophy.* Catabolic effects of glucocorticoids (Ch. 33) can lead to atrophy of the skin that is only partially reversible upon stopping treatment.

- *Systemic effects.* Systemic absorption can cause depression of the hypothalamic–pituitary–adrenal axis, as described in Ch. 33. This is avoidable provided that the drug regime is well managed (Castela et al., 2012).
- *Spread of infection.* Because glucocorticoids suppress the immune system, there is a danger that they may encourage or reactivate infection. For this reason they are contraindicated in acne, where there is a co-existent infection.
- *'Steroid rosacea' (skin reddening and pimples)* is a recognised problem when treating facial skin with glucocorticoids.
- *Production of stretch marks (striae atrophica)* and *telangiectasia* (small superficial dilated blood vessels).

For more serious cases of eczema or psoriasis or where glucocorticoids are ineffective, topical or systemic application of immunosuppressants such as **ciclosporin, pimecrolimus** or **tacrolimus** may be used (Ch. 26). Biopharmaceuticals such as **adalimumab** and **infliximab** are also used in severe cases and the use of these 'cytokine modulators' in these diseases is set to increase (see Pastore et al., 2008; Williams, 2012).

DRUGS USED TO CONTROL HAIR GROWTH

Hair growth in both sexes is driven by androgens as is male-pattern baldness. Because of this, androgen antagonists, or compounds that modulate androgen metabolism, can be used to treat both hirsutism in women and androgenic alopecia in men.

Co-cyprindol is mixture of an antiandrogen **cyproterone acetate** and a female sex hormone **ethinylestrodiol**. Antagonising androgenic actions reduces sebum production by sebaceous glands and also hair growth (which is androgen-dependent) so it can be used for treating acne as well as hirsutism in women. Unwanted effects include venous thromboembolism and it is contraindicated in women with a family history of cardiovascular disease.

Finasteride inhibits the enzyme (5α-reductase) that converts testosterone to the more potent androgen, dihydrotestosterone (see Ch. 35). It is used for the treatment of androgenic alopecia as well as prostatic hypertrophy. It is applied topically but the treatment takes months to produce real changes. Unwanted effects resulting from its action on androgen metabolism include a reduction in libido, possibly impotence and tenderness of the breasts.

Eflornithine was originally developed as an antiprotozoal drug (see Ch. 54). It can be used topically to treat hirsutism because it irreversibly inhibits *ornithine decarboxylase* in hair follicles. This interrupts cell replication and the growth of new hair follicles. Unwanted effects include skin reactions and acne.

Minoxidil is a vasodilator drug that was originally developed for treating hypertension (see Ch. 22). Applied topically, it is converted in hair follicles to a more potent metabolite, minoxidil sulfate (some preparations contain this salt). Perhaps because of its ability to increase blood supply to hair follicles, it stimulates growth of new hair and the progression of the new follicle through successive phases of the cell cycle (Ch. 9). Existing follicles, usually stalled in their resting (telogen) phase, must first be 'shed' to make way for new, rapidly growing follicles, so there is initial hair loss – an unwelcome and slightly alarming

---

[4]This observation was used by Cornell and Stoughton in 1985 as the basis for the first quantitative assay of glucocorticoid potency in man.

action of the drug. Other unwanted effects are few but some local irritation may occur.

RETINOIDS

Disturbances in vitamin A metabolism are known to result in skin pathology. The vitamin is normally acquired in ester form from dietary sources. It is converted to *retinol* in the gut and this seems to be a storage form of the vitamin.

Vitamin A has many biological roles. As *retinal* it is an essential component of rhodopsin and hence crucial for normal vision. However, it can also undergo an irreversible oxidation to *retinoic acid*, which lacks any effects on the visual system, but has potent effects on skin homeostasis.

The retinoid drugs are derivatives of retinoic acid (see Fig. 27.2). The principal examples are **tretinoin, isotretinoin, alitretinoin, tazarotene** and **adapalene**. They are widely used for the treatment of acne, eczema and psoriasis. Topical application is the usual route of administration but oral therapy is sometimes used for severe cases.

Most workers believe that retinoids act by binding to RXR and RAR nuclear receptors (see Ch. 3 and Fig. 27.2) in their target cells, which include keratinocytes and the cells of sebaceous glands, although some have questioned this mechanism (Arechalde & Saurat, 2000). The main dermatological actions of retinoids include modulation of epidermal cell growth and reduction in sebaceous gland activity and sebum production. They also have pleiotropic actions on the adaptive and innate immune system that produce a net anti-inflammatory effect (Fisher & Voorhees, 1996; Orfanos et al., 1997).

Unwanted effects. Retinoids may cause dry or flaky skin, stinging or burning sensations and also joint pains (after oral administration). Most are teratogenic and can be used in women only in the presence of suitable contraception.

VITAMIN D ANALOGUES

Vitamin D is actually a mixture of several related substances. Although classed as a 'vitamin' and therefore by implication an essential dietary factor, vitamin D$_3$ (cholecalciferol) is synthesised by the skin in the presence of sufficient sunlight (in fact, *phototherapy* is an important therapeutic modality in some skin disorders for this and other reasons). Other forms of the vitamin (e.g. D$_2$) can be obtained from the diet. The vitamin plays a crucial role in calcium and phosphate metabolism and bone formation (see Ch. 36). It also has complex regulatory actions on the immune system, reducing the activity of the adaptive system but increasing the activity of the innate immune system.

The biologically active metabolite calcitriol (see Ch. 36) is synthesised in the body by a multi-step process that requires transformations in the liver and kidney. At the molecular level, vitamin D and its analogues act though the VDR group of nuclear receptors in keratinocytes, fibroblasts, Langerhans cells and sebaceous gland cells to modulate gene transcription. Amongst the effects seen after treatment, are antiproliferative and pro-differentiation actions on keratinocytes, increased apoptosis of plaque keratinocytes (Tiberio et al., 2009) and the inhibition of T cell activation (Tremezaygues & Reichrath, 2011).

The main analogues used are **calcitriol** itself, **calcipotriol**, and **tacalcitol**. Their principal clinical use is treating

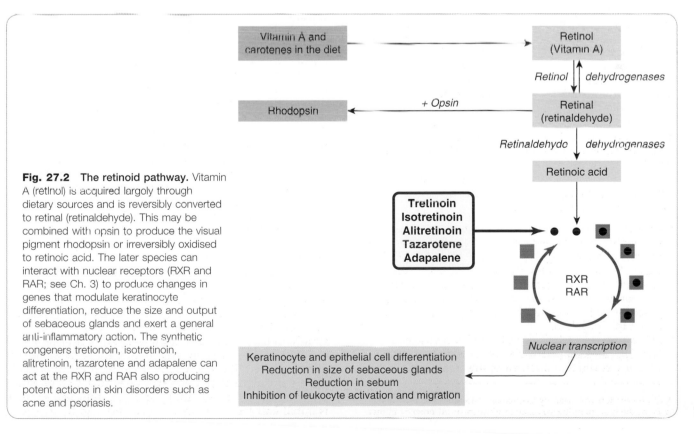

Fig. 27.2 The retinoid pathway. Vitamin A (retinol) is acquired largely through dietary sources and is reversibly converted to retinal (retinaldehyde). This may be combined with opsin to produce the visual pigment rhodopsin or irreversibly oxidised to retinoic acid. The later species can interact with nuclear receptors (RXR and RAR; see Ch. 3) to produce changes in genes that modulate keratinocyte differentiation, reduce the size and output of sebaceous glands and exert a general anti-inflammatory action. The synthetic congeners tretionoin, isotretinoin, alitretinoin, tazarotene and adapalene can act at the RXR and RAR also producing potent actions in skin disorders such as acne and psoriasis.

psoriasis. Oral administration is possible but they are generally administered topically, sometimes in combination with a glucocorticoid.

Unwanted effects. There is always a concern about the possible effects of the drugs on bone and they should be avoided in patients who have problems related to calcium or bone metabolism. Topical application can lead to skin irritation.

AGENTS ACTING BY OTHER MECHANISMS

Many ancillary agents are used in dermatology, including topical antiseptics, emollients, soothing lotions and other substances. Amongst this group are '**coal tars**', which are poorly defined mixtures containing thousands of aromatic hydrocarbons generated during the conversion of coal to coke or gas. They have been used in dermatological practice for decades. Though their mechanism of action is unknown, they can bring about a useful therapeutic benefit in eczema, psoriasis and some other skin conditions, and are often the first agents to be tried. Given their origin, one might expect coal tars to be carcinogenic, although in fact this does not appear to be the case (Roelofzen et al., 2010). Preparations containing coal tars are applied topically.

Amongst other drugs unique to skin pharmacology are **salicylic acid** and **podophyllotoxin**. Topical salicylic acid has a *keratolytic* effect in situations when excess skin is being produced (e.g. warts), causing epidermal layers to be shed. It is a common ingredient of numerous proprietary wart removers. Podophyllotoxin is a toxin extracted from plants of the podophyllum family. It is usually reserved for treating anogenital warts. It is applied topically and prevents the excess growth of skin probably because it inhibits tubulin polymerisation and hence arrests the normal cell cycle.

Another agent used for anogenital warts is **imiquimod**. This drug is an immune modifier and is also used for the topical treatment some types of skin cancer (e.g. basal cell carcinoma). Its mechanism of action is not known but it may increase immune surveillance mechanisms. Unwanted effects include local skin reactions.

CONCLUDING REMARKS

Despite the plethora of preparations available to treat skin disorders, there is clearly still an unfilled therapeutic need in several areas (e.g. rosacea) and, as always, reducing the unwanted effects of existing drugs (e.g. the glucocorticoids) is a further worthwhile objective that would greatly enhance their clinical utility.

It is perhaps surprising that 'itch' is still such a problem. Various new drug targets (e.g. NK_1-receptor antagonists, see Ch. 18) have been identified for treating the chronic disease (reviewed in Benecke et al., 2013).

The search for new drugs to treat psoriasis has largely focused upon the actions of biopharmaceuticals (see Gniadecki & Calverley, 2002; Pastore et al., 2008) with relatively little attention given to new small-molecule drugs.

In terms of improving the side effects of existing drugs some of the most interesting ideas arise from reconsidering the design of the glucocorticoids, vitamin D analogues and especially the retinoids. All these drugs act predominantly through nuclear receptors and recent thinking suggests that differentiating the mechanisms of transrepression and transactivation of genes by these drugs may be an achievable goal. Clearly, the prospect of separating the calcaemic from the anti-inflammatory effects of vitamin D analogues is very attractive (Tremezaygues & Reichrath, 2011). Likewise an improvement of the selectivity of retinoids would also be very welcome (Orfanos et al., 1997). Progress towards separating the therapeutic from the unwanted effects of the glucocorticoids is already apparently yielding fruit (see Ch. 28 for a discussion of this).

REFERENCES AND FURTHER READING

Antal, A.S., Dombrowski, Y., Koglin, S., Ruzicka, T., Schauber, J., 2011. Impact of vitamin D3 on cutaneous immunity and antimicrobial peptide expression. Dermatoendocrinol. 3, 18–22. (*This paper explores the idea that, in addition to their protective role, antimicrobial peptides (cathelicidins) in the skin may actually cause some skin diseases such as rosacea. The paper also suggests that the inhibitory action of vitamin D analogues on cathelicidin production is a potential mechanism of action of these drugs*)

Arechalde, A., Saurat, J.H., 2000. Management of psoriasis: the position of retinoid drugs. Biodrugs 13, 327–333. (*Discusses the therapeutic action of retinoids, especially tazarotene, and concludes that the mechanism of action is not exclusively through binding to RXR and RAR receptors*)

Basavaraj, K.H., Ashok, N.M., Rashmi, R., Praveen, T.K., 2010. The role of drugs in the induction and/or exacerbation of psoriasis. Int. J. Dermatol. 49, 1351–1361. (*The title here is self-explanatory. Also explores the mechanisms by which drugs provoke the disease*)

Benecke, H., Lotts, T., Stander, S., 2013. Investigational drugs for pruritus. Expert. Opin. Investig. Drugs 22, 1167–1179. (*Could be read in conjunction with the paper by Ikoma et al. – below*)

Bergstresser, P.R., Taylor, J.R., 1977. Epidermal 'turnover time' – a new examination. Br. J. Dermatol. 96, 503–509.

Castela, E., Archier, E., Devaux, S., et al., 2012. Topical corticosteroids in plaque psoriasis: a systematic review of risk of adrenal axis suppression and skin atrophy. J. Eur. Acad. Dermatol. Venereol. 26 (Suppl. 3), 47–51. (*This is a systemic literature review of the area and an analysis of data from many studies*)

Dunn, L.K., Gaar, L.R., Yentzer, B.A., O'Neill, J.L., Feldman, S.R., 2011. Acitretin in dermatology: a review. J. Drugs Dermatol. 10, 772–782.

Fisher, G.J., Voorhees, J.J., 1996. Molecular mechanisms of retinoid actions in skin. FASEB J. 10, 1002–1013. (*Easy-to-read review of retinoid action in the skin and a discussion of in vitro and in vivo models of retinoid action*)

Garnock-Jones, K.P., Perry, C.M., 2009. Alitretinoin: in severe chronic hand eczema. Drugs 69, 1625–1634.

Gniadecki, R., Calverley, M.J., 2002. Emerging drugs in psoriasis. Expert Opin. Emerg. Drugs 7, 69–90. (*Deals mainly with biological and anticytokine drugs as potential new therapies*)

Greaves, M.W., Khalifa, N., 2004. Itch: more than skin deep. Int. Arch. Allergy Immunol. 135, 166–172.

Ikoma, A., Steinhoff, M., Stander, S., Yosipovitch, G., Schmelz, M., 2006. The neurobiology of itch. Nat. Rev. Neurosci. 7, 535–547. (*A comprehensive review of the neural pathways and local mediators of pruritus and itch. Excellent diagrams. Highly recommended*)

James, K.A., Burkhart, C.N., Morrell, D.S., 2009. Emerging drugs for acne. Expert Opin. Emerg. Drugs 14, 649–659.

Klinge, S.A., Sawyer, G.A., 2013. Effectiveness and safety of topical versus oral nonsteroidal anti-inflammatory drugs: a comprehensive review. Phys. Sportsmed. 41, 64–74.

Naldi, L., Raho, G., 2009. Emerging drugs for psoriasis. Expert Opin. Emerg. Drugs 14, 145–163.

Nolan, K.A., Marmur, E.S., 2012. Over-the-counter topical skincare products: a review of the literature. J. Drugs Dermatol. 11, 220–224.

Orfanos, C.E., Zouboulis, C.C., Almond-Roesler, B., Geilen, C.C., 1997. Current use and future potential role of retinoids in dermatology. Drugs 53, 358–388.

Pastore, S., Gubinelli, E., Leoni, L., Raskovic, D., Korkina, L., 2008. Biological drugs targeting the immune response in the therapy of psoriasis. Biologics 2, 687–697.

Raut, A.S., Prabhu, R.H., Patravale, V.B., 2013. Psoriasis clinical implications and treatment: a review. Crit. Rev. Ther. Drug Carrier Syst. 30, 183–216.

Ritter, J.M., 2012. Drugs and the skin: psoriasis. Br. J. Clin. Pharmacol. 74, 393–395. (*Succinct and easily readable introduction to the treatment of psoriasis focusing on the role of cytokines in the disease mechanism and the utility of new biologicals. Good diagram. Highly recommended*)

Roelofzen, J.H., Aben, K.K., Oldenhof, U.T., et al., 2010. No increased risk of cancer after coal tar treatment in patients with psoriasis or eczema. J. Invest. Dermatol. 130, 953–961.

Ryan, C., Abramson, A., Patel, M., Menter, A., 2012. Current investigational drugs in psoriasis. Expert Opin. Investig. Drugs 21, 473–487.

Schoepe, S., Schacke, H., May, E., Asadullah, K., 2006. Glucocorticoid therapy-induced skin atrophy. Exp. Dermatol. 15, 406–420. (*Good review of one of what is one of the main adverse effects of glucocorticoid therapy for skin disorders, together with a discussion of how this can be minimised*)

Schroeter, A., Engelbrecht, T., Neubert, R.H., Goebel, A.S., 2010. New nanosized technologies for dermal and transdermal drug delivery. A review. J. Biomed. Nanotechnol. 6, 511–528.

Tan, X., Feldman, S.R., Chang, J., Balkrishnan, R., 2012. Topical drug delivery systems in dermatology: a review of patient adherence issues. Expert Opin. Drug Deliv. 9, 1263–1271.

Tiberio, R., Bozzo, C., Pertusi, G., et al., 2009. Calcipotriol induces apoptosis in psoriatic keratinocytes. Clin. Exp. Dermatol. 34, 972–974.

Tremezaygues, L., Reichrath, J., 2011. Vitamin D analogs in the treatment of psoriasis: Where are we standing and where will we be going? Dermatoendocrinol. 3, 180–186. (*A very useful account of the biosynthesis and role of vitamin D and the action of its analogues in the regulation of skin inflammation. Recommended*)

Williams, S.C., 2012. New biologic drugs get under the skin of psoriasis. Nat. Med. 18, 638. (*One-pager. Short account of the latest candidate biologicals used in the treatment of psoriasis*)

Yamasaki, K., Gallo, R.L., 2011. Rosacea as a disease of cathelicidins and skin innate immunity. J. Investig. Dermatol. Symp. Proc. 15, 12–15. (*Could be read in conjunction with the paper by Antal et al. – above*)

28 Respiratory system

OVERVIEW

Basic aspects of respiratory physiology (regulation of airway smooth muscle, pulmonary vasculature and glands) are considered as a basis for a discussion of pulmonary disease and its treatment. We devote most of the chapter to asthma, dealing first with pathogenesis and then the main drugs used in its treatment and prevention – inhaled bronchodilators and anti-inflammatory agents. We also discuss chronic obstructive pulmonary disease (COPD). There are short sections on allergic emergencies, surfactants and the treatment of cough. Other important pulmonary diseases, such as bacterial infections (e.g. tuberculosis and acute pneumonias) and malignancies, are addressed in Chapters 51 and 56, respectively, or are not yet amenable to drug treatment (e.g. occupational and interstitial lung diseases). Antihistamines, important in treatment of hay fever, are covered in Chapter 26. Pulmonary hypertension is covered in Chapter 22.

THE PHYSIOLOGY OF RESPIRATION

CONTROL OF BREATHING

Respiration is controlled by spontaneous rhythmic discharges from the respiratory centre in the medulla, modulated by input from pontine and higher central nervous system (CNS) centres and vagal afferents from the lungs. Various chemical factors affect the respiratory centre, including the partial pressure of carbon dioxide in arterial blood ($P_A CO_2$) by an action on medullary chemoreceptors, and of oxygen ($P_A O_2$) by an action on the chemoreceptors in the carotid bodies.

Some voluntary control can be superimposed on the automatic regulation of breathing, implying connections between the cortex and the motor neurons innervating the muscles of respiration. Bulbar poliomyelitis and certain lesions in the brain stem result in loss of the automatic regulation of respiration without loss of voluntary regulation.[1]

REGULATION OF MUSCULATURE, BLOOD VESSELS AND GLANDS OF THE AIRWAYS

Irritant receptors and non-myelinated afferent nerve fibres respond to chemical irritants and cold air, and also to inflammatory mediators. Efferent pathways controlling

the airways include cholinergic parasympathetic nerves and non-noradrenergic non-cholinergic (NANC) inhibitory nerves (see Ch. 12). Inflammatory mediators (see Ch. 17) and other bronchoconstrictor mediators also have a role in diseased airways.

The tone of bronchial muscle influences airway resistance, which is also affected by the state of the mucosa and activity of the submucosal mucus-secreting glands in patients with asthma and bronchitis. Airway resistance can be measured indirectly by instruments that record the volume or flow of forced expiration. FEV_1 is the forced expiratory volume in 1 second. The peak expiratory flow rate (PEFR) is the maximal flow (expressed as l/min) after a full inhalation; this is simpler to measure at the bedside than FEV_1, which it follows closely.

EFFERENT PATHWAYS

Autonomic innervation

The autonomic innervation of human airways is reviewed by van der Velden & Hulsmann (1999).

Parasympathetic innervation. Parasympathetic innervation of bronchial smooth muscle predominates. Parasympathetic ganglia are embedded in the walls of the bronchi and bronchioles, and the postganglionic fibres innervate airway smooth muscle, vascular smooth muscle and glands. Three types of muscarinic (M) receptors are present (see Ch. 13, Table 13.2). M_3 receptors are pharmacologically the most important. They are found on bronchial smooth muscle and glands, and mediate bronchoconstriction and mucus secretion. M_1 receptors are localised in ganglia and on postsynaptic cells, and facilitate nicotinic neurotransmission, whereas M_2 receptors are inhibitory autoreceptors mediating negative feedback on acetylcholine release by postganglionic cholinergic nerves. Stimulation of the vagus causes bronchoconstriction – mainly in the larger airways. The possible clinical relevance of the heterogeneity of muscarinic receptors in the airways is discussed below.

A distinct population of NANC nerves (see Ch. 12) also regulates the airways. Bronchodilators released by these nerves include *vasoactive intestinal polypeptide* (Table 12.2) and *nitric oxide* (NO; Ch. 20).

Sympathetic innervation. Sympathetic nerves innervate tracheobronchial blood vessels and glands, but not human airway smooth muscle. However, β adrenoceptors are abundantly expressed on human airway smooth muscle (as well as mast cells, epithelium, glands and alveoli) and β agonists relax bronchial smooth muscle, inhibit mediator release from mast cells and increase mucociliary clearance. In humans, β adrenoceptors in the airways are of the $β_2$ variety.

In addition to the autonomic innervation, non-myelinated sensory fibres linked to irritant receptors in the lungs release tachykinins such as *substance P,*

---

[1]Referred to as Ondine's curse. Ondine was a water nymph who fell in love with a mortal. When he was unfaithful to her, the king of the water nymphs put a curse on him – that he must stay awake in order to breathe. When exhaustion finally supervened and he fell asleep, he died.

neurokinin A and *neurokinin B* (see Chs 19 and 42), producing *neurogenic inflammation.*

SENSORY RECEPTORS AND AFFERENT PATHWAYS

Slowly adapting *stretch receptors* control respiration via the respiratory centre. Unmyelinated sensory *C fibres* and rapidly adapting *irritant receptors* associated with myelinated vagal fibres are also important.

Physical or chemical stimuli, acting on irritant receptors on myelinated fibres in the upper airways and/or C-fibre receptors in the lower airways, cause coughing, bronchoconstriction and mucus secretion. Such stimuli include cold air and irritants such as ammonia, sulfur dioxide, cigarette smoke and the experimental tool *capsaicin* (Ch. 42), as well as endogenous inflammatory mediators.

Regulation of airway muscle, blood vessels and glands

Afferent pathways

- Irritant receptors and C fibres respond to exogenous chemicals, inflammatory mediators and physical stimuli (e.g. cold air).

Efferent pathways

- Parasympathetic nerves cause bronchoconstriction and mucus secretion through M_3 receptors.
- Sympathetic nerves innervate blood vessels and glands, but not airway smooth muscle.
- β_2-Adrenoceptor agonists relax airway smooth muscle. This is pharmacologically important.
- Inhibitory non-noradrenergic non-cholinergic (NANC) nerves relax airway smooth muscle by releasing nitric oxide and vasoactive intestinal peptide.
- Excitation of sensory nerves causes neuroinflammation by releasing tachykinins: substance P and neurokinin A.

PULMONARY DISEASE AND ITS TREATMENT

Common symptoms of pulmonary disease include shortness of breath, wheeze, chest pain and cough with or without sputum production or haemoptysis (blood in the sputum). Ideally, treatment is of the underlying disease, but sometimes symptomatic treatment, for example of cough, is all that is possible. The lung is an important target organ of many diseases addressed elsewhere in this book, including infections (Chs 51–55), malignancy (Ch. 56) and occupational and rheumatological diseases; drugs (e.g. **amiodarone**, **methotrexate**) can damage lung tissue and cause pulmonary fibrosis. Heart failure leads to pulmonary oedema (Ch. 22). Thromboembolic disease (Ch. 24) and pulmonary hypertension (Ch. 22) affect the pulmonary circulation. In this present chapter, we concentrate on two important diseases of the airways: asthma and chronic obstructive pulmonary disease (COPD).

BRONCHIAL ASTHMA

Asthma is the commonest chronic disease in children in economically developed countries, and is also common in adults. It is increasing in prevalence and severity.[2] It is an inflammatory condition in which there is recurrent reversible airways obstruction in response to irritant stimuli that are too weak to affect non-asthmatic subjects. The obstruction usually causes wheeze and merits drug treatment, although the natural history of asthma includes spontaneous remissions. Reversibility of airways obstruction in asthma contrasts with COPD, where the obstruction is either not reversible or at best incompletely reversible by bronchodilators.

CHARACTERISTICS OF ASTHMA

Asthmatic patients experience intermittent attacks of wheezing, shortness of breath – with difficulty especially in breathing out – and sometimes cough. As explained above, acute attacks are reversible, but the underlying pathological disorder can progress in older patients to a chronic state superficially resembling COPD.

Acute severe asthma (also known as *status asthmaticus*) is not easily reversed and causes hypoxaemia. Hospitalisation is necessary, as the condition, which can be fatal, requires prompt and energetic treatment.

Asthma is characterised by:

- inflammation of the airways
- bronchial hyper-reactivity
- reversible airways obstruction.

Bronchial hyper-reactivity (or hyper-responsiveness) is abnormal sensitivity to a wide range of stimuli, such as irritant chemicals, cold air and stimulant drugs, all of which can result in bronchoconstriction. In allergic asthma, these features may be initiated by sensitisation to allergen(s), but, once established, asthma attacks can be triggered by various stimuli such as viral infection, exercise (in which the stimulus may be cold air and/or drying of the airways) and atmospheric pollutants such as sulfur dioxide. Immunological desensitisation to allergens such as pollen or dust mites is popular in some countries but is not superior to conventional inhaled drug treatment.

PATHOGENESIS OF ASTHMA

The pathogenesis of asthma involves both genetic and environmental factors, and the asthmatic attack itself consists, in many subjects, of two main phases: an immediate and a late (or delayed) phase (see Fig. 28.1).

Numerous cells and mediators play a part, and the full details of the complex events involved are still a matter of debate (Walter & Holtzman, 2005). The following simplified account is intended to provide a basis for understanding the rational use of drugs in the treatment of asthma.

Asthmatics have activated T cells, with a T-helper (Th)2 profile of cytokine production (see Ch. 18 and Table 6.2) in their bronchial mucosa. How these cells are activated is not fully understood, but allergens (Fig. 28.2) are one mechanism. The Th2 cytokines that are released do the following:

---

[2]William Osler, 19th-century doyen of American and British clinicians, wrote that 'the asthmatic pants into old age' – this at a time when the most effective drug that he could offer was to smoke stramonium cigarettes, a herbal remedy the antimuscarinic effects of which were offset by direct irritation from the smoke. Its use persisted in English private schools into the 1950s, as one author can attest – much to the envy of his fellows!

- Attract other inflammatory granulocytes, especially eosinophils, to the mucosal surface. Interleukin (IL)-5 and granulocyte–macrophage colony-stimulating factor prime eosinophils to produce cysteinyl leukotrienes (see Ch. 17), and to release granule proteins that damage the epithelium. This damage is one cause of bronchial hyper-responsiveness.
- Promote immunoglobulin (Ig)E synthesis and responsiveness in some asthmatics (IL-4 and IL-13 'switch' B cells to IgE synthesis and cause expression of IgE receptors on mast cells and eosinophils; they also enhance adhesion of eosinophils to endothelium).

Some asthmatics, in addition to these mechanisms, are also *atopic* – i.e. they make allergen-specific IgE that binds

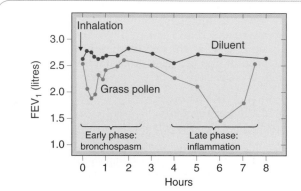

Fig. 28.1   Two phases of asthma demonstrated by the changes in forced expiratory volume in 1 second (FEV$_1$) after inhalation of grass pollen in an allergic subject. *(From Cockcroft DW 1983 Lancet ii, 253.)*

to mast cells in the airways. Inhaled allergen cross-links IgE molecules on mast cells, triggering degranulation with release of histamine and leukotriene B$_4$, both of which are powerful bronchoconstrictors to which asthmatics are especially sensitive because of their airway hyper-responsiveness. This provides a mechanism for acute exacerbation of asthma in atopic individuals exposed to allergen. The effectiveness of **omalizumab** (an anti-IgE antibody; see p. 351) serves to emphasise the importance of IgE in the pathogenesis of asthma as well as in other allergic diseases. Noxious gases (e.g. sulfur dioxide, ozone) and airway dehydration can also cause mast cell degranulation.

Clinicians often refer to atopic or 'extrinsic' asthma and non-atopic or 'intrinsic' asthma; we prefer the terms allergic and non-allergic.

The immediate phase of an asthma attack

In allergic asthma the immediate phase (i.e. the initial response to allergen provocation) occurs abruptly and is mainly caused by spasm of the bronchial smooth muscle. Allergen interaction with mast cell-fixed IgE causes release of histamine, leukotriene B$_4$ and prostaglandin (PG)D$_2$ (Ch. 17).

Other mediators released include IL-4, IL-5, IL-13, macrophage inflammatory protein-1α and tumour necrosis factor (TNF)-α.

Various chemotaxins and chemokines (see Ch. 18) attract leukocytes – particularly eosinophils and mononuclear cells – setting the stage for the late phase (Fig. 28.3).

The late phase

The late phase or delayed response (see Figs 28.1 and 28.3) may be nocturnal. It is, in essence, a progressing inflammatory reaction, initiation of which occurred during the first phase, the influx of Th2 lymphocytes

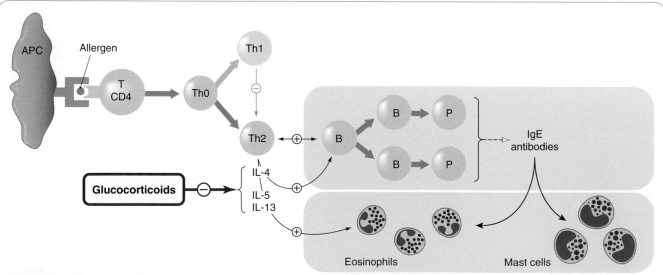

Fig. 28.2   The part played by T lymphocytes in allergic asthma. In genetically susceptible individuals, allergen (green circle) interacts with dendritic cells and CD4⁺ T cells, leading to the development of Th0 lymphocytes, which give rise to a clone of Th2 lymphocytes. These then (1) generate a cytokine environment that switches B cells/plasma cells to the production and release of immunoglobulin (Ig)E; (2) generate cytokines, such as interleukin (IL)-5, which promote differentiation and activation of eosinophils; and (3) generate cytokines (e.g. IL-4 and IL-13) that induce expression of IgE receptors. Glucocorticoids inhibit the action of the cytokines specified. APC, antigen-presenting dendritic cell; B, B cell; P, plasma cell; Th, T-helper cell.

Asthma

- Asthma is defined as recurrent reversible airway obstruction, with attacks of wheeze, shortness of breath and often nocturnal cough. Severe attacks cause hypoxaemia and are life-threatening.
- Essential features include:
  - airways inflammation, which causes
  - bronchial hyper-responsiveness, which in turn results in
  - recurrent reversible airway obstruction.
- Pathogenesis involves exposure of genetically disposed individuals to allergens; activation of Th2 lymphocytes and cytokine generation promote:
  - differentiation and activation of eosinophils

- IgE production and release
- expression of IgE receptors on mast cells and eosinophils
- Important mediators include leukotriene B_4 and cysteinyl leukotrienes (C_4 and D_4); interleukins IL-4, IL-5, IL-13; and tissue-damaging eosinophil proteins.
- Antiasthmatic drugs include:
  - bronchodilators
  - anti-inflammatory agents.
- Treatment is monitored by measuring forced expiratory volume in 1 second (FEV_1) or peak expiratory flow rate and, in acute severe disease, oxygen saturation and arterial blood gases.

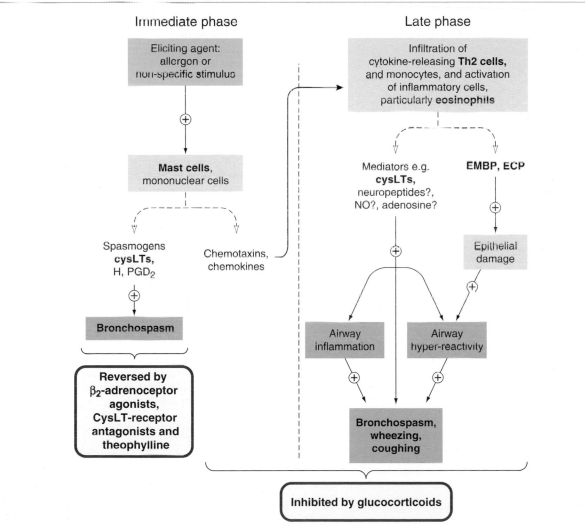

Fig. 28.3 Immediate and late phases of asthma, with the actions of the main drugs. CysLTs, cysteinyl leukotrienes (leukotrienes C_4 and D_4); ECP, eosinophil cationic protein; EMBP, eosinophil major basic protein; H, histamine; iNO, induced nitric oxide. (For more detail of the Th2-derived cytokines and chemokines, see Ch. 17 and Ch. 6, Fig. 6.4.)

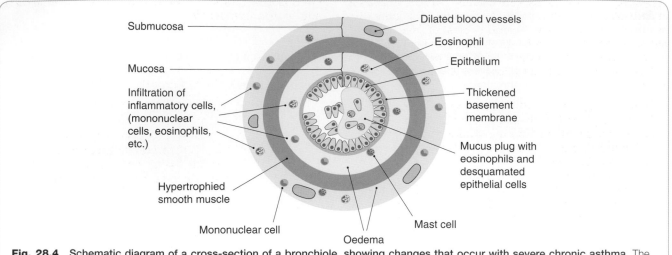

Fig. 28.4 Schematic diagram of a cross-section of a bronchiole, showing changes that occur with severe chronic asthma. The individual elements depicted are not, of course, drawn to scale.

being of particular importance. The inflammatory cells include activated eosinophils. These release cysteinyl leukotrienes, interleukins IL-3, IL-5 and IL-8, and the toxic proteins *eosinophil cationic protein, major basic protein* and *eosinophil-derived neurotoxin*. These play an important part in the events of the late phase, the toxic proteins causing damage and loss of epithelium. Other putative mediators of the inflammatory process in the delayed phase are adenosine (acting on the A_1 receptor; see Ch. 16), induced NO (see Ch. 20) and neuropeptides (see Ch. 18).

Growth factors released from inflammatory cells act on smooth muscle cells, causing hypertrophy and hyperplasia, and the smooth muscle can itself release proinflammatory mediators and growth factors (Chs 5 and 18). Figure 28.4 shows schematically the changes that take place in the bronchioles. Epithelial cell loss means that irritant receptors and C fibres are more accessible to irritant stimuli – an important mechanism of bronchial hyper-reactivity.

'Aspirin-sensitive' asthma

▼ Non-steroidal anti-inflammatory drugs (NSAIDs), especially **aspirin**, can precipitate asthma in sensitive individuals. Such aspirin-sensitive asthma (Ch. 26) is relatively uncommon (<10% of asthmatic subjects), and is often associated with nasal polyps. Individuals sensitive to one NSAID are usually also sensitive to other chemically unrelated cyclo-oxygenase (COX) inhibitors, including sometimes **paracetamol** (Ch. 26). Abnormal leukotriene production and sensitivity are implicated. Patients with aspirin-sensitive asthma produce more cysteinyl leukotriene and have greater airway hyper-responsiveness to inhaled cysteinyl leukotrienes than aspirin-tolerant asthmatics. Such airway hyper-responsiveness reflects elevated expression of cysteinyl leukotriene receptors on inflammatory cells, and this is downregulated by aspirin desensitisation. In addition, aspirin and similar drugs directly activate eosinophils and mast cells in these patients through IgE-independent mechanisms.

DRUGS USED TO TREAT AND PREVENT ASTHMA

There are two categories of antiasthma drugs: *bronchodilators* and *anti-inflammatory agents*. Bronchodilators reverse

the bronchospasm of the immediate phase; anti-inflammatory agents inhibit or prevent the inflammatory components of both phases (Fig. 28.3). These two categories are not mutually exclusive: some drugs classified as bronchodilators also have some anti-inflammatory effect.

How best to use these drugs to treat asthma is complex. A guideline on the management of asthma (BTS/SIGN, 2012) specifies five therapeutic steps for adults and children with chronic asthma. Very mild disease may be controlled with short-acting bronchodilator (**salbutamol** or **terbutaline**) alone (step 1), but if patients need this more than once a day, a regular inhaled corticosteroid should be added (step 2). If the asthma remains uncontrolled, step 3 is to add a long-acting bronchodilator (**salmeterol** or **formoterol**); this minimises the need for increased doses of inhaled corticosteroid. **Theophylline** and leukotriene antagonists, such as **montelukast**, also exert a corticosteroid-sparing effect, but this is less reliable. One or other is added (step 4) for patients who remain symptomatic and/or the dose of inhaled corticosteroid increased to the maximum recommended. Step 5 is addition of a regular oral corticosteroid (e.g. **prednisolone**). Corticosteroids are the mainstay of therapy because they are the only asthma drugs that potently inhibit T-cell activation, and thus the inflammatory response, in the asthmatic airways. **Cromoglicate** (see p. 351) has only a weak effect and is now seldom used.

BRONCHODILATORS

The main drugs used as bronchodilators are β_2-adrenoceptor agonists; others include **theophylline**, cysteinyl leukotriene receptor antagonists and muscarinic receptor antagonists.

β-Adrenoceptor agonists

The β_2-adrenoceptor agonists are dealt with in Chapter 14. Their primary effect in asthma is to dilate the bronchi by a direct action on the β_2 adrenoceptors of smooth muscle. Being physiological antagonists of bronchoconstrictors (see Ch. 2), they relax bronchial muscle whatever spasmogen is involved. They also inhibit mediator release from mast cells and TNF-α release from monocytes, and increase mucus clearance by an action on cilia.

β₂-adrenoceptor agonists are usually given by inhalation of aerosol, powder or nebulised solution (i.e. solution that has been converted into a cloud or mist of fine droplets), but some products may be given orally or by injection. A metered-dose inhaler is used for aerosol preparations.

Two categories of β₂-adrenoceptor agonists are used in asthma.

- Short-acting agents: **salbutamol** and **terbutaline**. These are given by inhalation; the maximum effect occurs within 30 min and the duration of action is 3–5 h; they are usually used on an 'as needed' basis to control symptoms.
- Longer-acting agents: e.g. **salmeterol** and **formoterol**. These are given by inhalation, and the duration of action is 8–12 h. They are not used 'as needed' but are given regularly, twice daily, as adjunctive therapy in patients whose asthma is inadequately controlled by glucocorticoids.

Antiasthma drugs: bronchodilators

- β₂-Adrenoceptor agonists (e.g. **salbutamol**) are first-line drugs (for details, see Ch. 14):
  they act as physiological antagonists of the spasmogenic mediators but have little or no effect on the bronchial hyper-reactivity
  - salbutamol is given by inhalation; its effects start immediately and last 3–5 h, and it can also be given by intravenous infusion in status asthmaticus
  - **salmeterol** or **formoterol** are given regularly by inhalation; their duration of action is 8–12 h.
- Theophylline (often formulated as **aminophylline**):
  - is a methylxanthine
  - inhibits phosphodiesterase and blocks adenosine receptors
  - has a narrow therapeutic window: unwanted effects include cardiac dysrhythmia, seizures and gastrointestinal disturbances
  - is given intravenously (by slow infusion) for status asthmaticus, or orally (as a sustained-release preparation) as add-on therapy to inhaled corticosteroids and long-acting β₂ agonists (step 4)
  - is metabolised in the liver by P450; liver dysfunction and viral infections increase its plasma concentration and half-life (normally approximately 12 h)
  - interacts importantly with other drugs; some (e.g. some antibiotics) increase the half-life of **theophylline**, others (e.g. anticonvulsants) decrease it.
- Cysteinyl leukotriene receptor antagonists (e.g. **montelukast**) are third-line drugs for asthma. They:
  - compete with cysteinyl leukotrienes at CysLT₁ receptors
  - are used mainly as add-on therapy to inhaled corticosteroids and long-acting β₂ agonists (step 4).

Unwanted effects
The unwanted effects of β₂-adrenoceptor agonists result from systemic absorption and are given in Chapter 14. In the context of their use in asthma, the commonest adverse effect is *tremor*; other unwanted effects include *tachycardia* and *cardiac dysrhythmia*.

Clinical use of β₂-adrenoceptor agonists as bronchodilators

- Short-acting drugs (**salbutamol** or **terbutaline**, usually by inhalation) to prevent or treat wheeze in patients with reversible obstructive airways disease.
- Long-acting drugs (**salmeterol, formoterol**) to prevent bronchospasm (e.g. at night or with exercise) in patients requiring long-term bronchodilator therapy.

Methylxanthines (see Chs 16 and 48)
Theophylline (1,3-dimethylxanthine), which is also used as theophylline ethylenediamine (known as **aminophylline**), is the main therapeutic drug of this class, and has long been used as a bronchodilator.[3] Here we consider it in the context of respiratory disease, its only current therapeutic use.

Mechanism of action
The mechanism of theophylline is still unclear. The relaxant effect on smooth muscle has been attributed to inhibition of phosphodiesterase (PDE) isoenzymes, with resultant increase in cAMP and/or cGMP (see Ch. 4, Fig. 4.10). However, the concentrations necessary to inhibit the isolated enzymes exceed the therapeutic range of plasma concentrations.

Competitive antagonism of adenosine at adenosine A_1 and A_2 receptors (Ch. 16) may contribute, but the PDE inhibitor **enprofylline**, which is a potent bronchodilator, is not an adenosine antagonist.

Type IV PDE is implicated in inflammatory cells, and methylxanthines may have some anti-inflammatory effect. (**Roflumilast**, a type IV PDE inhibitor, is mentioned below in the context of COPD.)

Theophylline activates *histone deacetylase* (HDAC) and may thereby reverse resistance to the anti-inflammatory effects of corticosteroids (Barnes, 2006).

Methylxanthines stimulate the CNS (Ch. 48) and respiratory stimulation may be beneficial in patients with COPD and reduced respiration causing retention of CO_2. **Caffeine** has a special niche in treating hypoventilation of prematurity (see Ch. 48).

Unwanted effects
When theophylline is used in asthma, its other actions (CNS, cardiovascular, gastrointestinal and diuretic) result in unwanted side effects (e.g. insomnia, nervousness). The therapeutic plasma concentration range is 30–100 μmol/l, and adverse effects are common with concentrations greater than 110 μmol/l; thus there is a relatively narrow therapeutic window. Serious cardiovascular and CNS effects can occur when the plasma concentration exceeds 200 μmol/l. The most serious cardiovascular effect is *dysrhythmia* (especially during intravenous administration of aminophylline), which can be fatal. *Seizures* can occur

---

[3]Over 200 years ago, William Withering recommended 'coffee made very strong' as a remedy for asthma. Coffee contains caffeine, a related methylxanthine.

with theophylline concentrations at or slightly above the upper limit of the therapeutic range, and can be fatal in patients with impaired respiration due to severe asthma. Monitoring the concentration of theophylline in plasma is useful for optimising the dose.

Clinical use of theophylline

- In addition to steroids, in patients whose asthma does not respond adequately to β₂-adrenoceptor agonists.
- In addition to steroids in COPD.
- Intravenously (as **aminophylline**, a combination of **theophylline** with **ethylenediamine** to increase its solubility in water) in acute severe asthma.

Pharmacokinetic aspects

Theophylline is given orally as a sustained-release preparation. Aminophylline can be given by slow intravenous injection of a loading dose followed by intravenous infusion.

Theophylline is well absorbed from the gastrointestinal tract. It is metabolised by P450 enzymes in the liver; the mean elimination half-life is approximately 8 h in adults but there is wide inter-individual variation. The half-life is increased in liver disease, cardiac failure and viral infections, and is decreased in heavy cigarette smokers (as a result of enzyme induction). Unwanted drug interactions are clinically important: its plasma concentration is decreased by drugs that induce P450 enzymes (including **rifampicin**, **phenytoin** and **carbamazepine**). The concentration is increased by drugs that inhibit P450 enzymes, such as **erythromycin**, **clarithromycin**, **ciprofloxacin**, **diltiazem** and **fluconazole**. This is important in view of the narrow therapeutic window; antibiotics such as clarithromycin are often started when asthmatics are hospitalised because of a severe attack precipitated by a chest infection, and if the dose of theophylline is unaltered, severe toxicity can result.

Muscarinic receptor antagonists

Muscarinic receptor antagonists are dealt with in Chapter 13. The main compound used as a bronchodilator is **ipratropium**. It is seldom used on a regular basis in asthma but can be useful for cough caused by irritant stimuli in such patients.

Ipratropium is a quaternary derivative of atropine. It does not discriminate between muscarinic receptor subtypes (see Ch. 13), and it is possible that its blockade of M₂ autoreceptors on the cholinergic nerves increases acetylcholine release and reduces the effectiveness of its antagonism at the M₃ receptors on smooth muscle. It is not particularly effective against allergen challenge, but it inhibits the augmentation of mucus secretion that occurs in asthma and may increase the mucociliary clearance of bronchial secretions. It has no effect on the late inflammatory phase of asthma.

Ipratropium is given by aerosol inhalation. As a quaternary nitrogen compound, it is highly polar and is not well absorbed into the circulation (Ch. 8), limiting systemic effects. The maximum effect occurs approximately 30 min after inhalation and persists for 3–5 h. It has few unwanted

effects and is, in general, safe and well tolerated. It can be used with β₂-adrenoceptor agonists. See the clinical box, below, for clinical uses. **Tiotropium** is similar; it is a longer-acting drug used in maintenance treatment of COPD (see below).

Clinical use of inhaled muscarinic receptor antagonists (e.g. ipratropium)

- For asthma, as an adjunct to β₂-adrenoceptor agonists and steroids.
- For some patients with COPD, especially long-acting drugs (e.g. **tiotropium**).
- For bronchospasm precipitated by β₂-adrenoceptor antagonists.

Cysteinyl leukotriene receptor antagonists

Cysteinyl leukotrienes (LTC₄, LTD₄ and LTE₄) act on *CysLT₁* and *CysLT₂* receptors (see Ch. 17), both of which are expressed in respiratory mucosa and infiltrating inflammatory cells, but the functional significance of each is unclear. The 'lukast' drugs (**montelukast** and **zafirlukast**) antagonise only CysLT₁.

Lukasts reduce acute reactions to aspirin in sensitive patients, but have not been shown to be particularly effective for aspirin-sensitive asthma (see p. 348) in the clinic. They inhibit exercise-induced asthma and decrease both early and late responses to inhaled allergen. They relax the airways in mild asthma but are less effective than salbutamol, with which their action is additive. They reduce sputum eosinophilia, but there is no clear evidence that they modify the underlying inflammatory process in chronic asthma.

The lukasts are taken by mouth, in combination with an inhaled corticosteroid. They are generally well tolerated, adverse effects consisting mainly of headache and gastrointestinal disturbances.

Histamine H₁-receptor antagonists

Although mast cell mediators play a part in the immediate phase of allergic asthma (Fig. 28.3) and in some types of exercise-induced asthma, histamine H₁-receptor antagonists have no routine place in therapy, although they may be modestly effective in mild atopic asthma, especially when this is precipitated by acute histamine release in patients with concomitant allergy such as severe hay fever.

ANTI-INFLAMMATORY AGENTS
Glucocorticoids

Glucocorticoids (see Ch. 33) are the main drugs used for their anti-inflammatory action in asthma. They are not bronchodilators, but prevent the progression of chronic asthma and are effective in acute severe asthma (see clinical box, p. 351).[4]

---

[4]In 1900, Solis-Cohen reported that dried bovine adrenals had antiasthma activity. He noted that the extract did not serve acutely 'to cut short the paroxysm' but was 'useful in averting recurrence of paroxysms'. Mistaken for the first report on the effect of adrenaline, his astute observation was probably the first on the efficacy of steroids in asthma.

Actions and mechanism

The basis of the anti-inflammatory action of glucocorticoids is discussed in Chapter 33. An important action, of relevance for asthma, is that they restrain clonal proliferation of Th cells by reducing the transcription of the gene for IL-2 and decrease formation of cytokines, in particular the Th2 cytokines that recruit and activate eosinophils and are responsible for promoting the production of IgE and the expression of IgE receptors. Glucocorticoids also inhibit the generation of the vasodilators PGE_2 and PGI_2, by inhibiting induction of COX-2 (Ch. 17, Fig. 17.1). By inducing *annexin-1*,[5] they could inhibit production of leukotrienes and platelet-activating factor, although there is currently no direct evidence that annexin-1 is involved in the therapeutic action of glucocorticoids in human asthma.

Corticosteroids inhibit the allergen-induced influx of eosinophils into the lung. Glucocorticoids upregulate β_2 adrenoceptors, decrease microvascular permeability and indirectly reduce mediator release from eosinophils by inhibiting the production of cytokines (e.g. IL-5 and granulocyte–macrophage colony stimulating factor) that activate eosinophils. Reduced synthesis of IL-3 (the cytokine that regulates mast cell production) may explain why long-term steroid treatment eventually reduces the number of mast cells in the respiratory mucosa, and hence suppresses the early-phase response to allergens and exercise.

Glucocorticoids are sometimes ineffective, even in high doses, for reasons that are incompletely understood. Many individual mechanisms could contribute to glucocorticoid resistance. The phenomenon has been linked to the number of glucocorticoid receptors, but in some situations other mechanisms are clearly in play – for example, reduced activity of *histone deacetylase* (HDAC) may be important in cigarette smokers.

The main compounds used are beclometasone, **budesonide, fluticasone, mometasone** and **ciclesonide**. These are given by inhalation with a metered-dose or dry powder inhaler, the full effect on bronchial hyper-responsiveness being attained only after weeks or months of therapy. Oral glucocorticoids (Ch. 33) are reserved for patients with the severest disease.

Unwanted effects

Serious unwanted effects are uncommon with inhaled steroids. Oropharyngeal candidiasis (thrush; Ch. 53) can occur (T lymphocytes are important in protection against fungal infection), as can sore throat and croaky voice, but use of 'spacing' devices, which decrease oropharyngeal deposition of the drug and increase airway deposition, reduces these problems. Regular high doses of inhaled glucocorticoids can produce some adrenal suppression, particularly in children, and necessitate carrying a 'steroid card' (Ch. 33). This is less likely with fluticasone, mometasone and ciclesonide, as these drugs are poorly absorbed from the gastrointestinal tract and undergo almost complete presystemic metabolism. The unwanted effects of oral glucocorticoids are given in Chapter 33 and Figure 33.7.

Cromoglicate and nedocromil

These two drugs, of similar chemical structure and properties, are now hardly used for the treatment of asthma.

Clinical use of glucocorticoids in asthma

- Patients who require regular bronchodilators should be considered for glucocorticoid treatment (e.g. with inhaled **beclometasone**).
- More severely affected patients are treated with high-potency inhaled drugs (e.g. **budesonide**).
- Patients with acute exacerbations of asthma may require intravenous **hydrocortisone** and oral **prednisolone**.
- A 'rescue course' of oral prednisolone may be needed at any stage of severity if the clinical condition is deteriorating rapidly.
- Prolonged treatment with oral prednisolone, in addition to inhaled bronchodilators and steroids, is needed by a few severely asthmatic patients.

Although very safe, they have only weak anti-inflammatory effects and short duration of action. They are given by inhalation as aerosols or dry powders, and can also be used topically for allergic conjunctivitis or rhinitis. They are not bronchodilators, having no direct effects on smooth muscle, nor do they inhibit the actions of any of the known smooth muscle stimulants. Given prophylactically, they reduce both the immediate- and late-phase asthmatic responses and reduce bronchial hyper-reactivity.

Their mechanism of action is not fully understood. Cromoglicate is a 'mast cell stabiliser', preventing histamine release from mast cells. However, this is not the basis of its action in asthma, because compounds that are more potent than cromoglicate at inhibiting mast cell histamine release are ineffective against asthma.

Cromoglicate depresses the exaggerated neuronal reflexes that are triggered by stimulation of the 'irritant receptors'; it suppresses the response of sensory C fibres to capsaicin and may inhibit the release of T-cell cytokines. Various other effects, of uncertain importance, on the inflammatory cells and mediators involved in asthma have been described.

Anti-IgE treatment

Omalizumab is a humanised monoclonal anti-IgE antibody. It is effective in patients with allergic asthma as well as in allergic rhinitis. It is of considerable theoretical interest (see review by Holgate et al., 2005), but it is expensive and its place in therapeutics is unclear.

SEVERE ACUTE ASTHMA (STATUS ASTHMATICUS)

Severe acute asthma is a medical emergency requiring hospitalisation. Treatment includes oxygen (in high concentration, usually $\geq 60\%$), inhalation of nebulised salbutamol, and intravenous hydrocortisone followed by a course of oral prednisolone. Additional measures occasionally used include nebulised ipratropium, intravenous salbutamol or aminophylline, and antibiotics (if bacterial infection is present). Monitoring is by PEFR or FEV_1, and by measurement of arterial blood gases and oxygen saturation.

---

[5]Previously known as lipocortin-1 – the nomenclature was changed in order to comply with the latest genomics data, which indicate there are approximately 30 members of this family!

**Antiasthma drugs:
anti-inflammatory agents**

Glucocorticoids (for details, see Ch. 32)

- These reduce the inflammatory component in chronic asthma and are life-saving in status asthmaticus (acute severe asthma).
- They do not prevent the immediate response to allergen or other challenges.
- The mechanism of action involves decreased formation of cytokines, particularly those generated by Th2 lymphocytes, decreased activation of eosinophils and other inflammatory cells.
- They are given by inhalation (e.g. **beclometasone**); systemic unwanted effects are uncommon at moderate doses, but oral thrush and voice problems can occur. Systemic effects can occur with high doses but are less likely with **mometasone** because of its presystemic metabolism. In deteriorating asthma, an oral glucocorticoid (e.g. **prednisolone**) or intravenous **hydrocortisone** is also given.

ALLERGIC EMERGENCIES

Anaphylaxis (Ch. 6) and *angio-oedema* are emergencies involving acute airways obstruction; **adrenaline** (epinephrine) is potentially life-saving. It is administered intramuscularly (or occasionally intravenously, as in anaphylaxis occurring in association with general anaesthesia). Patients at risk of acute anaphylaxis, for example from food or insect sting allergy, may self-administer intramuscular adrenaline using a spring-loaded syringe. Oxygen, an antihistamine such as **chlorphenamine** and hydrocortisone are also indicated.

Angio-oedema is the intermittent occurrence of focal swelling of the skin or intra-abdominal organs caused by plasma leakage from capillaries. Most often, it is mild and 'idiopathic', but it can occur as part of acute allergic reactions, when it is generally accompanied by urticaria – 'hives' – caused by histamine release from mast cells. If the larynx is involved, it is life-threatening; swelling in the peritoneal cavity can be very painful and mimic a surgical emergency. It can be caused by drugs, especially *angiotensin-converting enzyme inhibitors* – perhaps because they block the inactivation of peptides such as bradykinin (Ch. 18) – and by aspirin and related drugs in patients who are aspirin sensitive (see Ch. 26). The hereditary form is associated with lack of C1 esterase inhibitor – C1 esterase is an enzyme that degrades the complement component C1 (see Ch. 6). **Tranexamic acid** (Ch. 24) or **danazol** (Ch. 35) may be used to prevent attacks in patients with hereditary angioneurotic oedema, and administration of partially purified C1 esterase inhibitor or fresh plasma, with antihistamines and glucocorticoids, can terminate acute attacks. **Icatibant**, a peptide bradykinin B_2 receptor antagonist (Ch. 18), is effective for acute attacks of hereditary angio-oedema. It is administered subcutaneously and can cause nausea, abdominal pain and nasal stuffiness.

CHRONIC OBSTRUCTIVE PULMONARY DISEASE

Chronic obstructive pulmonary disease (COPD) is a major global health problem – current projections suggest that it will be the third commonest cause of death by 2012. Cigarette smoking is the main cause, and is increasing in the developing world. Air pollution, also aetiologically important, is also increasing, and there is a huge unmet need for effective drugs. Despite this, COPD has received much less attention than asthma. A resurgence of interest in new therapeutic approaches (see Barnes, 2008) has yet to bear fruit but there are a number of promising avenues.

Clinical features. The clinical picture starts with attacks of morning cough during the winter, and progresses to chronic cough with intermittent exacerbations, often initiated by an upper respiratory infection, when the sputum becomes purulent. There is progressive breathlessness. Some patients have a reversible component of airflow obstruction identifiable by an improved FEV_1 following a dose of bronchodilator. Pulmonary hypertension (Ch. 22) is a late complication, causing symptoms of heart failure (*cor pulmonale*). Exacerbations may be complicated by respiratory failure (i.e. reduced $P_{A}O_2$) requiring hospitalisation and intensive care. Tracheostomy and artificial ventilation, while prolonging survival, may serve only to return the patient to a miserable life.

Pathogenesis. There is fibrosis of small airways, resulting in obstruction, and/or destruction of alveoli and of elastin fibres in the lung parenchyma. The latter features are hallmarks of emphysema,[6] thought to be caused by proteases, including elastase, released during the inflammatory response. It is emphysema that causes respiratory failure, because it destroys the alveoli, impairing gas transfer. There is chronic inflammation (bronchitis), predominantly in small airways and lung parenchyma, characterised by increased numbers of macrophages, neutrophils and T lymphocytes. The inflammatory mediators have not been as clearly defined as in asthma. Lipid mediators, inflammatory peptides, reactive oxygen and nitrogen species, chemokines, cytokines and growth factors are all implicated (Barnes, 2004).

Principles of treatment. Stopping smoking (Ch. 46) slows the progress of COPD. Patients should be immunised against influenza and *Pneumococcus*, because superimposed infections with these organisms are potentially lethal. Glucocorticoids are generally ineffective, in contrast to asthma, but a trial of glucocorticoid treatment is worthwhile because asthma may coexist with COPD and have been overlooked. This contrast with asthma is puzzling, because in both diseases multiple inflammatory genes are activated, which might be expected to be turned off by glucocorticoids. Inflammatory gene activation results from acetylation of nuclear histones around which DNA is wound. Acetylation opens up the chromatin structure, allowing gene transcription and synthesis of inflammatory proteins to proceed. HDAC de-acetylates histones, and suppresses production of proinflammatory cytokines. Corticosteroids recruit HDAC to activated genes, switching off inflammatory gene transcription

---

[6]Emphysema is a pathological condition sometimes associated with COPD, in which lung parenchyma is destroyed and replaced by air spaces that coalesce to form bullae – blister-like air-filled spaces in the lung tissue.

(Barnes et al., 2004). There is a link between the severity of COPD (but not of asthma) and reduced HDAC activity in lung tissue (Ito et al., 2005); furthermore, HDAC activity is inhibited by smoking-related oxidative stress, which may explain the lack of effectiveness of glucocorticoids in COPD.

Long-acting bronchodilators give modest benefit, but do not deal with the underlying inflammation. No currently licensed treatments reduce the progression of COPD or suppress the inflammation in small airways and lung parenchyma. Several new treatments that target the inflammatory process are in clinical development (Barnes, 2013). Some, such as chemokine antagonists, are directed against the influx of inflammatory cells into the airways and lung parenchyma, whereas others target inflammatory cytokines such as TNF-α. PDE IV inhibitors show promise and **roflumilast** is licensed as an adjunct to bronchodilators for patients with severe COPD and frequent exacerbations. Other drugs that inhibit cell signalling (see Chs 3 and 5) include inhibitors of p38 mitogen-activated protein kinase, nuclear factor κB and phosphoinositide-3 kinase-γ. More specific approaches include antioxidants, inhibitors of inducible NO synthase and leukotriene B$_4$ antagonists. Other treatments have the potential to combat mucus hypersecretion, and there is a search for serine protease and matrix metallo-protease inhibitors to prevent lung destruction and the development of emphysema.

Specific aspects of treatment. Short- and long-acting inhaled bronchodilators can provide useful palliation in patients with a reversible component. The main short-acting drugs are ipratropium and salbutamol; long-acting drugs include **tiotropium** and **salmeterol** or **formoterol** (Chs 13 and 14). Theophylline (Ch. 16) can be given by mouth but is of uncertain benefit. Its respiratory stimulant effect may be useful for patients who tend to retain CO$_2$. Other respiratory stimulants (e.g. doxapram) are sometimes used briefly in acute respiratory failure (e.g. postoperatively) but have largely been replaced by mechanical ventilatory support (intermittent positive-pressure ventilation).

Long-term oxygen therapy administered at home prolongs life in patients with severe disease and hypoxaemia (at least if they refrain from smoking – an oxygen fire is not a pleasant way to go).

Acute exacerbations. Acute exacerbations of COPD are treated with inhaled O$_2$ in a concentration (initially, at least) of only 24% O$_2$, i.e. only just above atmospheric O$_2$ concentration (approximately 20%). The need for caution is because of the risk of precipitating CO$_2$ retention as a consequence of terminating the hypoxic drive to respiration. Blood gases and tissue oxygen saturation are monitored, and inspired O$_2$ subsequently adjusted accordingly. Broad-spectrum antibiotics with activity against *Haemophilus influenzae* (e.g. cefuroxime; Ch. 51), are used if there is evidence of infection. Inhaled bronchodilators may provide some symptomatic improvement.

A systemically active glucocorticoid (intravenous hydrocortisone or oral prednisolone) is also administered routinely, although efficacy is modest. Inhaled steroids do not influence the progressive decline in lung function in patients with COPD, but do improve the quality of life, probably as a result of a modest reduction in hospital admissions.

SURFACTANTS

Pulmonary surfactants act, not by binding to specific targets, but by lowering the surface tension of fluid lining the alveoli, allowing air to enter. They are effective in the prophylaxis and management of *respiratory distress syndrome* in newborn babies, especially premature babies in whom endogenous surfactant production is deficient. Examples include **beractant** and **poractant alpha**, which are derivatives of the physiological pulmonary surfactant protein. They are administered directly into the tracheobronchial tree via an endotracheal tube. (The mothers of premature infants are sometimes treated with glucocorticoids before birth in an attempt to accelerate maturation of the fetal lung and minimise incidence of this disorder.)

COUGH

Cough is a protective reflex that removes foreign material and secretions from the bronchi and bronchioles. It is a very common adverse effect of angiotensin-converting enzyme inhibitors, in which case the treatment is usually to substitute an alternative drug, often an angiotensin receptor antagonist, less likely to cause this adverse effect (Ch. 22). It can be triggered by inflammation in the respiratory tract, for example by undiagnosed asthma or chronic reflux with aspiration, or by neoplasia. In these cases, cough suppressant (antitussive) drugs are sometimes useful, for example for the dry painful cough associated with bronchial carcinoma, but are to be avoided in cases of chronic pulmonary infection, as they can cause undesirable thickening and retention of sputum, and in asthma because of the risk of respiratory depression.

DRUGS USED FOR COUGH

Opioid analgesics are the most effective antitussive drugs in clinical use (Ch. 42). They act by an ill defined effect in the brain stem, depressing an even more poorly defined 'cough centre' and suppress cough in doses below those required for pain relief. Those used as cough suppressants have minimal analgesic actions and addictive properties. New opioid analogues that suppress cough by inhibiting release of excitatory neuropeptides through an action on μ receptors (see Table 42.2) on sensory nerves in the bronchi are being assessed.

Codeine (methylmorphine) is a weak opioid (see Ch. 42) with considerably less addiction liability than a strong opioid, and is a mild cough suppressant. It decreases secretions in the bronchioles, which thickens sputum, and inhibits ciliary activity. Constipation is common. **Dextromethorphan** (a non-selective serotonin-uptake inhibitor and sigma-1-receptor agonist) and **pholcodine** have less adverse effects than codeine. Respiratory depression is a risk with all centrally acting cough suppressants. **Morphine** is used for palliative care in cases of lung cancer associated with distressing cough.

REFERENCES AND FURTHER READING

General

Barnes, P.J., 2011. Pathophysiology of allergic inflammation. Immunol. Rev. 242, SI31–SI50.

Bezemer, G.F.G., Sagar, S., van Bergenhenegouwen, J., et al., 2012. Dual role of toll-like receptors in asthma and chronic obstructive pulmonary disease. Pharmacol. Rev. 64, 337–358. (*Update on the role of TLRs in asthma and in COPD which discusses targeting these for airway diseases. TLR agonist, adjuvant and antagonist therapies could all be argued to be effective. Because of a possible dual role of TLRs in airway diseases with shared symptoms and risk factors but different immunological mechanisms, caution should be taken while designing pulmonary TLR-based therapies*)

Korkmaz, B., Horwitz, M.S., Jenne, D.E., Gauthier, F., 2010. Neutrophil elastase, proteinase 3, and cathepsin G as therapeutic targets in human diseases. Pharmacol. Rev. 62, 726–759. (*Describes the functions of these proteases, their role in human diseases and discusses identifying new therapeutics; also describes how non-human primate experimental models could assist*)

Melo, R.C.N., Liu, L., Xenakis, J.J., 2013. Eosinophil-derived cytokines in health and disease: unraveling novel mechanisms of selective secretion. Allergy 68, 274–284.

van der Velden, V.H.J., Hulsmann, A.R., 1999. Autonomic innervation of human airways: structure, function, and pathophysiology in asthma. Neuroimmunomodulation 6, 145–159. (*Review*)

Velasquez, R., Teran, L.M., 2011. Chemokines and their receptors in the allergic airway inflammatory process. Clin. Rev. Allerg. Immunol. 41, 76–88.

Asthma

Berry, M., Hargadon, B., Morgan, A., et al., 2005. Alveolar nitric oxide in adults with asthma: evidence of distal lung inflammation in refractory asthma. Eur. Respir. J. 25, 986–991. (*Alveolar NO as a measure of distal airway inflammation*)

BTS/SIGN (British Thoracic Society/Scottish Intercollegiate Guideline Network), 2012. British Guideline on Management of Asthma. <www.brit-thoracic.org.uk> (accessed April 2013).

Pelaia, G., Cuda, G., Vatrella, A., et al., 2005. Mitogen-activated protein kinases and asthma. J. Cell. Physiol. 202, 642–653. (*Reviews involvement of mitogen-activated protein kinases in asthma pathogenesis, and discusses their possible role as molecular targets for antiasthma drugs*)

Wadsworth, S.J., Sandford, A.J., 2013. Personalised medicine and asthma diagnostics/management. Curr. Allergy Asthma Rep. 13, 118–129.

Walter, M.J., Holtzman, M.J., 2005. A centennial history of research on asthma pathogenesis. Am. J. Respir. Cell Mol. Biol. 32, 483–489.

Chronic obstructive pulmonary disease

Barnes, P.J., 2004. Mediators of chronic obstructive pulmonary disease. Pharmacol. Rev. 56, 515–548. (*'The identification of inflammatory mediators and understanding their interactions is important for the development of anti-inflammatory treatments for this important disease'*)

Barnes, P.J., 2008. Frontrunners in novel pharmacotherapy of COPD. Curr. Opin. Pharmacol. 8, 300–307. (*Discusses candidates that may inhibit inflammation and reduce progression of COPD; most promising are theophylline-like drugs(!), new anti-oxidants and non-antibiotic macrolides*)

Barnes, P.J., 2013. New anti-inflammatory targets for chronic obstructive pulmonary disease. Nat. Rev. Drug Discov. 12, 543–559.

Barnes, P.J., Ito, K., Adcock, I.M., 2004. Corticosteroid resistance in chronic obstructive pulmonary disease: inactivation of histone deacetylase. Lancet 363, 731–733. (*Hypothesis that in patients with COPD, HDAC is impaired by cigarette smoking and oxidative stress, leading to reduced responsiveness to corticosteroids; see also Ito et al., 2005, below*)

Ito, K., Ito, M., Elliott, W.M., et al., 2005. Decreased histone deacetylase activity in chronic obstructive pulmonary disease. N. Engl. J. Med. 352, 1967–1976. (*There is a link between the severity of COPD and the reduction in HDAC activity in the peripheral lung tissue; HDAC is a key molecule in the repression of production of proinflammatory cytokines in alveolar macrophages*)

Cough

Morice, A.H., Kastelik, J.A., Thompson, R., 2001. Cough challenge in the assessment of cough reflex. Br. J. Clin. Pharmacol. 52, 365–375.

Reynolds, S.M., Mackenzie, A.J., Spina, D., Page, C.P., 2004. The pharmacology of cough. Trends Pharmacol. Sci. 25, 569–576. (*Discusses the pathophysiological mechanisms of cough and implications for developing new antitussive drugs*)

Drugs and therapeutic aspects

Barnes, P.J., 2006. How corticosteroids control inflammation. Br. J. Pharmacol. 148, 245–254.

Ben-Noun, L., 2000. Drug-induced respiratory disorders: incidence, prevention and management. Drug Safety 23, 143–164. (*Diverse pulmonary adverse drug effects*)

Cazzola, M., Page, C.P., Calzetta, L., Matera, M.G., 2012. Pharmacology and therapeutics of bronchodilators. Pharmacol. Rev. 64, 450–504.

Conti, M., Beavo, J., 2007. Biochemistry and physiology of cyclic nucleotide phosphodiesterases: essential components in cyclic nucleotide signaling. Ann. Rev. Biochem. 76, 481–511.

Giri, S.N., 2003. Novel pharmacological approaches to manage interstitial lung fibrosis in the twenty first century. Annu. Rev. Pharmacol. Toxicol. 43, 73–95. (*Reviews approaches including maintaining intracellular nicotinamide adenine dinucleotide [NAD+] and ATP, blocking transforming growth factor-β and integrins, platelet-activating factor receptor antagonists and NO synthase inhibitors*)

Holgate, S.T., Djukanovic, R., Casale, T., Bousquet, J., 2005. Anti-immunoglobulin E treatment with omalizumab in allergic diseases: an update on anti-inflammatory activity and clinical efficacy. Clin. Exp. Allergy 35, 408–416. (*Reviews mechanism and clinical studies*)

Lewis, J.F., Veldhuizen, R., 2003. The role of exogenous surfactant in the treatment of acute lung injury. Annu. Rev. Physiol. 65, 613–642.

29

The kidney and urinary system

OVERVIEW

We set the scene with a brief outline of renal physiology based on the functional unit of the kidney – the nephron – before describing drugs that affect renal function. Emphasis is on diuretics – drugs that increase the excretion of Na$^+$ ions and water, and reduce arterial blood pressure. We also consider briefly other drugs used to treat patients with renal failure and urinary tract disorders.

INTRODUCTION

The main drugs that work by altering renal function – the diuretics – are crucial for the management of cardiovascular disease (Chs 21 and 22) as well as patients with renal disease. The kidneys are the main organ by which drugs and their metabolites are eliminated from the body (Ch. 9), and so the dosing regimens of many drugs must be adapted in patients with impaired renal function. Furthermore, the kidneys are a target for various kinds of drug toxicity (Ch. 57), due in part to the very high concentrations of drugs and drug metabolites in some renal tissues. Antihypertensive drugs (commonly indicated in kidney disease) are covered in Chapter 22, immunosuppressant drugs (effective in several of the diseases that can cause renal failure, and crucial following renal transplantation) in Chapter 26 and antibacterial drugs (used to treat renal and urinary tract infections) in Chapter 51. Drugs, as well as surgical procedures, are also used to treat lower urinary tract disorders which commonly cause urinary retention or incontinence. Patients with anaemia due to chronic renal failure benefit from **epoietin** (Ch. 25).

OUTLINE OF RENAL FUNCTION

The main function of the kidney is to maintain the constancy of the 'interior environment' by eliminating waste products and by regulating the volume, electrolyte content and pH of the extracellular fluid in the face of varying dietary intake and other environmental (e.g. climatic) demands.

The kidneys receive about a quarter of the cardiac output. From the several hundred litres of plasma that flow through them each day, they filter (in a 70 kg human) approximately 120 litres per day, 11 times the total extracellular fluid volume. This filtrate is similar in composition to plasma, apart from the absence of protein. As it passes through the renal tubule, about 99% of the filtered water, and much of the filtered Na$^+$, is reabsorbed, and some substances are secreted into it from the blood. Eventually, approximately 1.5 litres is voided as urine per 24 h under usual conditions (Table 29.1).

Each kidney consists of an outer cortex, an inner medulla and a hollow pelvis, which empties into the ureter. The functional unit is the nephron, of which there are approximately 1.4×10^6 in each kidney (approximately half this number in people with hypertension), with considerable variation between individuals and an age-related decline.

THE STRUCTURE AND FUNCTION OF THE NEPHRON

Each nephron consists of a *glomerulus*, *proximal tubule*, *loop of Henle*, *distal convoluted tubule* and *collecting duct* (Fig. 29.1). The glomerulus comprises a tuft of capillaries projecting into a dilated end of the renal tubule. Most nephrons lie largely or entirely in the cortex. The remaining 12%, called the *juxtamedullary nephrons*, have their glomeruli and convoluted tubules next to the junction of the medulla and cortex, and their loops of Henle pass deep into the medulla.

THE BLOOD SUPPLY TO THE NEPHRON

Nephrons possess the special characteristic of having two capillary beds in series with each other (see Fig. 29.1). The afferent arteriole of each cortical nephron branches to form the glomerulus; glomerular capillaries coalesce into the efferent arteriole which, in turn, branches to form a second capillary network in the cortex, around the convoluted tubules and loops of Henle, before converging on venules and thence on renal veins. By contrast, efferent arterioles of juxtamedullary nephrons lead to vessel loops (*vasa recta*) that pass deep into the medulla with the thin loops of Henle, and play a key role in counter-current exchange (see below).

THE JUXTAGLOMERULAR APPARATUS

A conjunction of afferent arteriole, efferent arteriole and distal convoluted tubule near the glomerulus forms the juxtaglomerular apparatus (Fig. 29.2). At this site, there are specialised cells in both the afferent arteriole and in the tubule. The latter, termed *macula densa* cells, respond to changes in the rate of flow and the composition of tubule fluid, and they control *renin* release from specialised granular renin-containing cells in the afferent arteriole (Ch. 22). Various chemical mediators also influence renin secretion, including β_2 agonists, vasodilator prostaglandins and feedback inhibition from angiotensin II acting on AT_1 receptors (see Fig. 22.4). The role of the juxtaglomerular apparatus in the control of Na$^+$ balance is dealt with below.

GLOMERULAR FILTRATION

Fluid is driven from the capillaries into the tubular capsule (Bowman's capsule) by hydrodynamic force opposed by

355

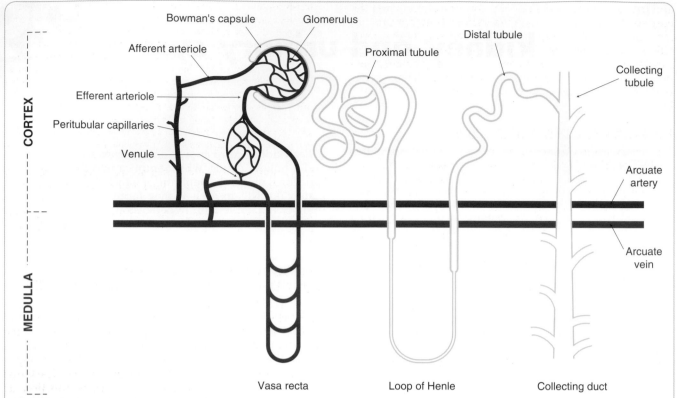

Fig. 29.1 **Simplified diagram of a juxtamedullary nephron and its blood supply.** The tubules and the blood vessels are shown separately for clarity. In the kidney, the peritubular capillary network surrounds the convoluted tubules, and the distal convoluted tubule passes close to the glomerulus, between the afferent and efferent arterioles. (This last is shown in more detail in Fig. 29.2.)

Table 29.1 **Reabsorption of fluid and solute in the kidney[a]**

	Filtered/day	Excreted/day[b]	Percentage reabsorbed
Na⁺ (mmol)	25 000	150	99+
K⁺ (mmol)	600	90	93+
Cl⁻ (mmol)	18 000	150	99+
HCO₃⁻ (mmol)	4900	0	100
Total solute (mosmol)	54 000	700	87
H₂O (litres)	180	~1.5	99+

[a]Typical values for a healthy young adult: renal blood flow, 1200 ml/min (20–25% of cardiac output); renal plasma flow, 660 ml/min; glomerular filtration rate, 125 ml/min.

[b]These are typical figures for an individual eating a Western diet. The kidney excretes more or less of each of these substances to maintain the constancy of the internal milieu, so on a low-sodium diet (for instance in the Yanomami Indians of the upper Amazon basin), NaCl excretion may be reduced to below 10 mmol/day! At the other extreme, individuals living in some fishing communities in Japan eat (and therefore excrete) several hundred mmol/day.

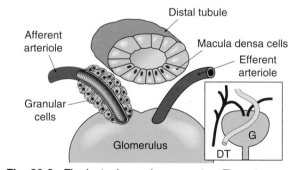

Fig. 29.2 **The juxtaglomerular apparatus.** The cutaway sections show the granular renin-containing cells round the afferent arteriole, and the macula densa cells in the distal convoluted tubule. The inset shows the general relationships between the structures. DT, distal tubule; G, glomerulus.

TUBULAR FUNCTION

The apex (lumenal surface) of each tubular cell is surrounded by a tight junction, as in all epithelia. This is a specialised region of membrane that separates the intercellular space from the lumen. The movement of ions and water across the epithelium can occur *through* cells (the transcellular pathway) and *between* cells through the tight junctions (the paracellular pathway). A common theme is that energy is expended to pump Na⁺ out of the cell by Na⁺-K⁺-ATPase situated in the basolateral cell membrane

the oncotic pressure of the plasma proteins, to which the glomerular capillaries are impermeable. All the low-molecular-weight constituents of plasma appear in the filtrate, while albumin and larger proteins are retained in the blood.

and the resulting gradient of Na⁺ concentration drives the entry of Na⁺ from the lumen via various transporters that facilitate Na⁺ entry coupled with movement of other ions, either in the same direction as Na⁺ in which case they are called *symporters* or *co-transporters* or in the opposite direction in which case they are called *antiporters*. These transporters vary in different parts of the nephron, as described below.

THE PROXIMAL CONVOLUTED TUBULE

The epithelium of the proximal convoluted tubule is 'leaky', i.e. the tight junctions in the proximal tubule are not so 'tight' after all, being permeable to ions and water, and permitting passive flow in either direction. This prevents the build-up of large concentration gradients; thus, although approximately 60–70% of Na⁺ reabsorption occurs in the proximal tubule, this transfer is accompanied by passive absorption of water so that fluid leaving the proximal tubule remains approximately isotonic to the glomerular filtrate.

Some of the transport processes in the proximal tubule are shown in Figures 29.3–29.5. The most important mechanism for Na⁺ entry into proximal tubular cells from the filtrate occurs by Na⁺/H⁺ exchange (Fig. 29.5). Intracellular carbonic anhydrase is essential for production of H⁺ for secretion into the lumen. Na⁺ is reabsorbed from tubular fluid into the cytoplasm of proximal tubular cells in exchange for cytoplasmic H⁺. It is then transported out of the cells into the interstitium by a Na⁺-K⁺-ATPase (sodium pump) in the basolateral membrane. This is the main active transport mechanism of the nephron in terms of energy consumption. Reabsorbed Na⁺ then diffuses into blood vessels.

▼ Bicarbonate is normally completely reabsorbed in the proximal tubule. This is achieved by combination with protons, yielding carbonic acid, which dissociates to form carbon dioxide and water – a reaction catalysed by carbonic anhydrase present in the lumenal brush border of the proximal tubule cells (Fig. 29.5A) – followed by passive reabsorption of the dissolved carbon dioxide.[1] The selective removal of sodium bicarbonate, with accompanying water, in the early proximal tubule causes a secondary rise in the concentration of chloride ions. Diffusion of chloride down its concentration gradient via the paracellular shunt leads, in turn, to a lumen-positive potential difference that favours reabsorption of sodium. The other mechanism involved in movement via the paracellular route is that sodium ions are secreted by Na⁺-K⁺-ATPase into the lateral intercellular space, slightly raising its osmolality because of the 3 Na⁺:2 K⁺ stoichiometry of the transporter. This leads to osmotic movement of water across the tight junction, in turn causing sodium reabsorption by convection (so-called solvent drag).

Many organic acids and bases are actively secreted into the tubule from the blood by specific transporters (see below, Fig. 29.3 and Ch. 9).

After passage through the proximal tubule, tubular fluid (now 30–40% of the original volume of the filtrate) passes on to the loop of Henle.

THE LOOP OF HENLE, MEDULLARY COUNTER-CURRENT MULTIPLIER AND EXCHANGER

The loop of Henle consists of a descending and an ascending portion (Figs 29.1 and 29.4), the ascending portion having both thick and thin segments. This part of the nephron enables the kidney to excrete urine that is either more or less concentrated than plasma, and hence to regulate the osmotic balance of the body as a whole. The loops of Henle of the juxtamedullary nephrons function as counter-current multipliers, and the vasa recta as counter-current exchangers. NaCl is actively reabsorbed in the thick ascending limb, causing hypertonicity of the interstitium. In the descending limb, water moves out and the tubular fluid becomes progressively more concentrated as it approaches the bend.

▼ The *descending limb* is permeable to water, which exits passively because the interstitial fluid of the medulla is kept hypertonic by the counter-current concentrating system. In juxtamedullary nephrons with long loops, there is extensive movement of water out of the tubule so that the fluid eventually reaching the tip of the loop has a high osmolality – normally approximately 1200 mosmol/kg, but up to 1500 mosmol/kg under conditions of dehydration – compared with plasma and extracellular fluid, which is approximately 300 mosmol/kg.[2] The hypertonic milieu of medulla, through which the collecting ducts of all nephrons pass on the way to the renal pelvis, is important in providing a mechanism by which the osmolarity of the urine is controlled.

The *ascending limb* has very low permeability to water, i.e. the tight junctions really are 'tight', enabling the build-up of a substantial concentration gradient across the wall of the tubule. It is here, in the thick ascending limb of the loop of Henle, that 20–30% of filtered Na⁺ is reabsorbed. There is active reabsorption of NaCl, unaccompanied by water, reducing the osmolarity of the tubular fluid and making the interstitial fluid of the medulla hypertonic. The osmotic gradient in the medullary interstitium is the key consequence of the counter-current multiplier system, the main principle being that small horizontal osmotic gradients 'stack up' to produce a large vertical gradient. Urea contributes to the gradient because it is more slowly reabsorbed than water and may be added to fluid in the

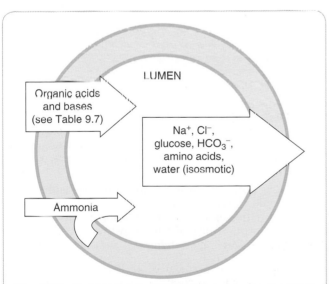

Fig. 29.3 Transport processes in the proximal convoluted tubule. The main driving force for the absorption of solutes and water from the lumen is the Na⁺-K⁺-ATPase in the basolateral membrane of the tubule cells. Many drugs are secreted into the proximal tubule (see Ch. 9). *(Redrawn from Burg 1985, pp 145-175 in The Kidney, third ed., Brenner BM, Rector FC (eds), WB Saunders, Philadelphia.)*

LUMEN

Organic acids and bases (see Table 9.7)

Na⁺, Cl⁻, glucose, HCO₃⁻, amino acids, water (isosmotic)

Ammonia

---

[1] The reaction is reversible, and the enzyme (as any catalyst) does not alter the equilibrium, just speeds up the rate with which it is attained. The concentrations inside the cell are such that carbon dioxide combines with water to produce carbonic acid: the same enzyme (carbonic anhydrase) catalyses this as well (Fig. 29.5A).

[2] These figures are for humans; some other species, notably the desert rat, can do much better, with urine osmolalities up to 5000 mosmol/kg.

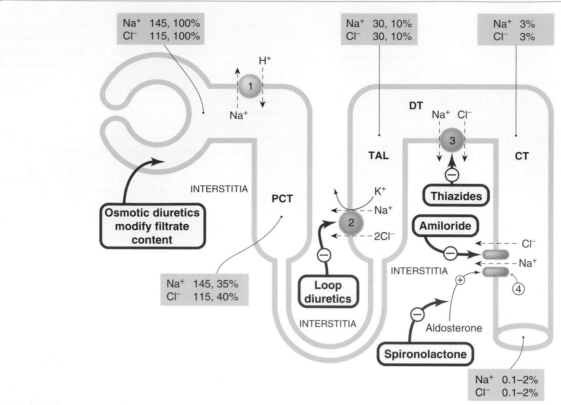

Fig. 29.4 **Schematic showing the absorption of sodium and chloride in the nephron and the main sites of action of drugs.** Cells are depicted as a pink border round the yellow tubular lumen. Mechanisms of ion absorption at the apical margin of the tubule cell: (1) Na^+/H^+ exchange; (2) $Na^+/K^+/2Cl^-$ co-transport; (3) Na^+/Cl^- co-transport; (4) Na^+ entry through sodium channels. Sodium is pumped out of the cells into the interstitium by the Na^+-K^+-ATPase in the basolateral margin of the tubular cells (not shown). The numbers in the boxes give the concentration of ions as millimoles per litre of filtrate, and the percentage of filtered ions still remaining in the tubular fluid at the sites specified. CT, collecting tubule; DT, distal tubule; PCT, proximal convoluted tubule; TAL, thick ascending loop. *(Data from Greger 2000.)*

descending limb, so its concentration rises along the nephron until it reaches the collecting tubules, where it diffuses out into the interstitium. It is thus 'trapped' in the inner medulla.

Ions move into cells of the thick ascending limb of the loop of Henle across the apical membrane by a $Na^+/K^+/2Cl^-$ co-transporter, driven by the Na^+ gradient produced by Na^+-K^+-ATPase in the basolateral membrane (Fig. 29.5B). Most of the K^+ taken into the cell by the $Na^+/K^+/2Cl^-$ co-transporter returns to the lumen through apical potassium channels, but some K^+ is reabsorbed, along with Mg^{2+} and Ca^{2+}.

Reabsorption of salt from the thick ascending limb is not balanced by reabsorption of water, so tubular fluid is hypotonic with respect to plasma as it enters the distal convoluted tubule (Fig. 29.4). The thick ascending limb is therefore sometimes referred to as the 'diluting segment'.

THE DISTAL TUBULE

In the early distal tubule, NaCl reabsorption, coupled with impermeability of the *zonula occludens* to water, further dilutes the tubular fluid. Transport is driven by Na^+-K^+-ATPase in the basolateral membrane. This lowers cytoplasmic Na^+ concentration, and consequently Na^+ enters the cell from the lumen down its concentration gradient, accompanied by Cl^-, by means of a Na^+/Cl^- co-transporter (Fig. 29.5C).

The excretion of Ca^{2+} is regulated in this part of the nephron, *parathormone* and *calcitriol* both increasing Ca^{2+} reabsorption (see Ch. 36).

THE COLLECTING TUBULE AND COLLECTING DUCT

Distal convoluted tubules empty into collecting tubules, which coalesce to form collecting ducts (Fig. 29.1). Collecting tubules include principal cells, which reabsorb Na^+ and secrete K^+ (Fig. 29.5D), and two populations of intercalated cells, α and β, which secrete acid and base, respectively.

The tight junctions in this portion of the nephron are impermeable to water and ions. The movement of ions and water in this segment is under independent hormonal control: absorption of NaCl by *aldosterone* (Ch. 22), and absorption of water by *antidiuretic hormone* (ADH), also termed *vasopressin* (Ch. 33).

Aldosterone enhances Na^+ reabsorption and promotes K^+ excretion. It promotes Na^+ reabsorption by:

- a rapid effect, stimulating Na^+/H^+ exchange by an action on membrane aldosterone receptors[3]

---

[3]A mechanism distinct from regulation of gene transcription, which is the normal transduction mechanism for steroid hormones (Ch. 3).

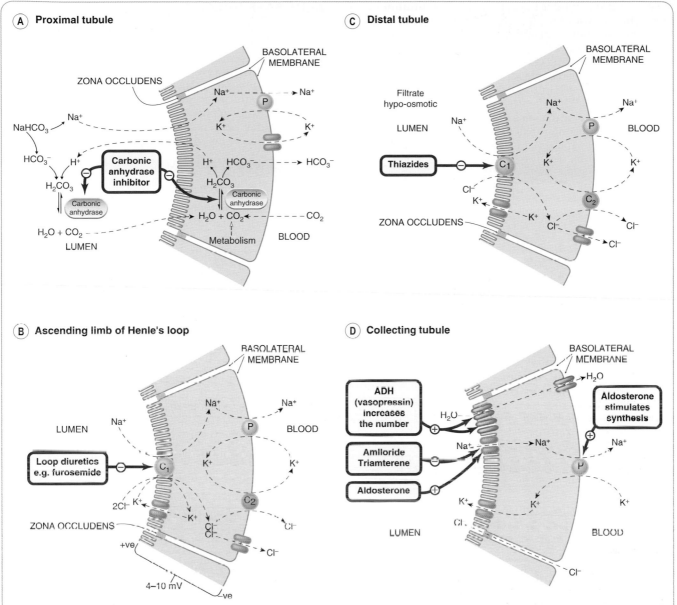

Fig. 29.5 **Drug effects on renal tubular ion transport.** **[A]** Bicarbonate ion reabsorption in the proximal convoluted tubule, showing the action of carbonic anhydrase inhibitors. **[B]** Ion transport in the thick ascending limb of Henle's loop, showing the site of action of loop diuretics. **[C]** Salt transport in the distal convoluted tubule, showing the site of action of thiazide diuretics. **[D]** Actions of hormones and drugs on the collecting tubule. The cells are impermeable to water in the absence of antidiuretic hormone (ADH), and to Na$^+$ in the absence of aldosterone. Aldosterone acts on a nuclear receptor within the tubule cell and on membrane receptors. *(Adapted from Greger 2000.)*

- a delayed effect, via nuclear receptors (see Ch. 3), directing the synthesis of a specific protein mediator that activates sodium channels in the apical membrane (Fig. 29.5D).

ADH and nephrogenic diabetes insipidus. ADH is secreted by the posterior pituitary (Ch. 33) and acts on V$_2$ receptors in the basolateral membranes of cells in the collecting tubules and ducts, increasing expression of *aquaporin* (water channels; see Ch. 8) in the apical membranes (Fig. 29.5D). This renders this part of the nephron permeable to water, allowing passive reabsorption of water as the collecting duct traverses the hyperosmotic region of the

medulla, and hence the excretion of concentrated urine. Conversely, in the absence of ADH, collecting duct epithelium is impermeable to water, so hypotonic fluid that leaves the distal tubule remains hypotonic as it passes down the collecting ducts, leading to the excretion of dilute urine. Defective ADH secretion (Ch. 33) or action on the kidney results in *diabetes insipidus*, an uncommon disorder in which patients excrete large volumes of dilute urine.

Ethanol (Ch. 49) inhibits the secretion of ADH, causing a water diuresis (possibly familiar to some of our readers) as a kind of transient diabetes insipidus. **Nicotine** enhances ADH secretion (perhaps contributing to the appeal of an after-dinner cigar?).

Several drugs inhibit the action of ADH: **lithium** (used in psychiatric disorders; see Ch. 46), **demeclocycline** (a tetracycline used not as an antibiotic, but rather to treat inappropriate secretion of ADH from tumours or in other conditions), **colchicine** (Ch. 26) and *vinca alkaloids* (Ch. 56). Recently, more specific antagonists of ADH (e.g. **conivaptan**, **tolvaptan**) have been introduced for treatment of hyponatraemia (see Ch. 22). All these drugs can cause acquired forms of *nephrogenic* diabetes insipidus, caused by a failure of the renal collecting ducts to respond to ADH. Nephrogenic diabetes insipidus can also be caused by two genetic disorders affecting the V_2 receptor or aquaporin.

Renal tubular function

- Protein-free glomerular filtrate enters via Bowman's capsule.
- Na^+-K^+-ATPase in the basolateral membrane is the main active transporter. It provides the Na^+-gradients (low cytoplamic Na^+ concentrations) for passive transporters in the apical membranes which facilitate Na^+ entry (reabsorption) from the tubular fluid down a concentration gradient.
- 60–70% of the filtered Na^+ and >90% of HCO_3^- is absorbed in the proximal tubule.
- Carbonic anhydrase is key for $NaHCO_3$ reabsorption in the proximal tubule and also for distal tubular urine acidification.
- The thick ascending limb of Henle's loop is impermeable to water; 20–30% of the filtered $NaCl$ is actively reabsorbed in this segment.
- Ions are reabsorbed from tubular fluid by a $Na^+/K^+/2Cl^-$ co-transporter in the apical membranes of the thick ascending limb.
- $Na^+/K^+/2Cl^-$ co-transport is inhibited by loop diuretics.
- Filtrate is diluted as it traverses the thick ascending limb as ions are reabsorbed, so that it is hypotonic when it leaves.
- The tubular counter-current multiplier actively generates a concentration gradient – small horizontal differences in solute concentration between tubular fluid and interstitium are multiplied vertically. The deeper in the medulla, the more concentrated is the interstitial fluid.
- Medullary hypertonicity is preserved passively by counter-current exchange in the vasa recta.
- Na^+/Cl^- co-transport (inhibited by thiazide diuretics) reabsorbs 5–10% of filtered Na^+ in the distal tubule.
- K^+ is secreted into tubular fluid in the distal tubule and the collecting tubules and collecting ducts.
- In the absence of antidiuretic hormone (ADH), the collecting tubule and collecting duct have low permeability to salt and water. ADH increases water permeability.
- Na^+ is reabsorbed from the collecting duct through epithelial sodium channels.
- These epithelial Na^+ channels are activated by aldosterone and inhibited by **amiloride** and by **trimterene**. K^+ or H^+ is secreted into the tubule in exchange for Na^+ in this distal region.

ACID–BASE BALANCE

The kidneys (together with the lungs; Ch. 28) regulate the H^+ concentration of body fluids. Acid or alkaline urine can be excreted according to need, the usual requirement being to form acid urine to eliminate phosphoric and sulfuric acids generated during the metabolism of nucleic acid and of sulfur-containing amino acids consumed in the diet. Consequently, metabolic acidosis is a common accompaniment of renal failure. Altering urine pH to alter drug excretion is mentioned below.

POTASSIUM BALANCE

Extracellular K^+ concentration – critically important for excitable tissue function (see Ch. 4) – is tightly controlled through regulation of K^+ excretion by the kidney. Urinary K^+ excretion matches dietary intake, usually approximately 50–100 mmol in 24 h in Western countries. Most diuretics cause K^+ loss (see below). This can cause problems if they are co-administered with cardiac glycosides or class III antidysrhythmic drugs whose toxicity is increased by low plasma K^+ (Ch. 21) – clinically important drug interactions.

Potassium ions are transported into collecting duct and collecting tubule cells from interstitial fluid by Na^+-K^+-ATPase in the basolateral membrane, and leak into the lumen through a K^+-selective ion channel. Na^+ passes from tubular fluid through sodium channels in the apical membrane down the electrochemical gradient created by the Na^+-K^+-ATPase; a lumen-negative potential difference across the cell results, increasing the driving force for K^+ secretion into the lumen. Thus K^+ secretion is coupled to Na^+ reabsorption.

Consequently, K^+ is lost when:

- more Na^+ reaches the collecting duct, as occurs with any diuretic acting proximal to the collecting duct
- Na^+ reabsorption in the collecting duct is increased directly (e.g. in hyperaldosteronism).

Conversely, K^+ is retained when:

- Na^+ reabsorption in the collecting duct is decreased, for example by **amiloride** or **triamterene**, which block the sodium channel in this part of the nephron, or **spironolactone** or **eplerenone**, which antagonise aldosterone (see below).

EXCRETION OF ORGANIC MOLECULES

There are distinct mechanisms (see Ch. 9, Table 9.7) for secreting organic anions and cations into the proximal tubular lumen. Secreted anions include several important drugs, for example *thiazides*, **furosemide**, **salicylate** (Ch. 26), and most *penicillins* and *cephalosporins* (Ch. 51). Similarly, several secreted organic cations are important drugs, for example **triamterene**, **amiloride**, **atropine** (Ch. 13), **morphine** (Ch. 42) and **quinine** (Ch. 54). Both anion and cation transport mechanisms are, like other renal ion transport processes, indirectly powered by active transport of Na^+ and K^+, the energy being derived from Na^+-K^+-ATPase in the basolateral membrane.

Organic anions in the interstitial fluid are exchanged with cytoplasmic α-ketoglutarate by an antiport (i.e. an exchanger that couples uptake and release of α-ketoglutarate with, in the opposite direction, uptake and release of a different organic anion) in the basolateral membrane, and diffuse passively into the tubular lumen (Fig. 29.3).

Organic cations diffuse into the cell from the interstitium and are then actively transported into the tubular lumen in exchange for H^+.

NATRIURETIC PEPTIDES

Endogenous A, B and C natriuretic peptides (ANP, BNP and CNP; see Chs 21 and 22) are involved in the regulation of Na^+ excretion. They are released from the heart in response to stretch (A and B), from endothelium (C) and from brain (B). They activate guanylyl cyclase (Ch. 3), and cause natriuresis both by renal haemodynamic effects (increasing glomerular capillary pressure by dilating afferent and constricting efferent arterioles) and by direct tubular actions. The tubular actions include the inhibition of angiotensin II-stimulated Na^+ and water reabsorption in the proximal convoluted tubule, and of the action of ADH in promoting water reabsorption in the collecting tubule.

Within the kidney, the post-translational processing of ANP prohormone differs from that in other tissues, resulting in an additional four amino acids being added to the amino terminus of ANP to yield a related peptide, *urodilutin*, that promotes Na^+ excretion by acting on receptors on the lumenal side of the collecting duct cells.

PROSTAGLANDINS AND RENAL FUNCTION

Prostaglandins (PGs; see Ch. 17) generated in the kidney influence its haemodynamic and excretory functions. The main renal prostaglandins in humans are vasodilator and natriuretic, namely PGE_2 in the medulla and PGI_2 (prostacyclin) in glomeruli. Factors that stimulate their synthesis include ischaemia, angiotensin II, ADH and bradykinin.

Prostaglandin biosynthesis is low under basal conditions. However, when vasoconstrictors (e.g. angiotensin II, noradrenaline) are released, local release of PGE_2 and PGI_2 compensates, preserving renal blood flow by their vasodilator action.

The influence of renal prostaglandins on salt balance and haemodynamics can be inferred from the effects of non-steroidal anti-inflammatory drugs (NSAIDs, which inhibit prostaglandin production by inhibiting cyclo-oxygenase; see Ch. 26). NSAIDs have little or no effect on renal function in healthy people, but predictably cause acute renal failure in clinical conditions in which renal blood flow depends on vasodilator prostaglandin biosynthesis. These include cirrhosis of the liver, heart failure, nephrotic syndrome, glomerulonephritis and extracellular volume contraction (see Ch. 57, Table 57.1). NSAIDs increase blood pressure in patients treated for hypertension by impairing PG-mediated vasodilatation and salt excretion. They exacerbate salt and water retention in patients with heart failure (see Ch. 22), partly by this same direct mechanism.[4]

---

[4]Additionally, NSAIDs make many of the diuretics used to treat heart failure less effective by competing with them for the organic anion transport (OAT) mechanism mentioned above; loop diuretics and thiazides act from within the lumen by inhibiting exchange mechanisms – see later in this chapter – so blocking their secretion into the lumen reduces their effectiveness by reducing their concentrations at their sites of action.

DRUGS ACTING ON THE KIDNEY

DIURETICS

Diuretics increase the excretion of Na^+ and water. They decrease the reabsorption of Na^+ and an accompanying anion (usually Cl^-) from the filtrate, increased water loss being secondary to the increased excretion of NaCl (natriuresis). This can be achieved:

- by a direct action on the cells of the nephron
- indirectly, by modifying the content of the filtrate.

Because a very large proportion of salt (NaCl) and water that passes into the tubule via the glomerulus is reabsorbed (Table 29.1), even a small decrease in reabsorption can cause a marked increase in Na^+ excretion. A summary diagram of the mechanisms and sites of action of various diuretics is given in Figure 29.4 and more detailed information on different classes of drugs in Figure 29.5.

Most diuretics with a direct action on the nephron act from within the tubular lumen and reach their sites of action by being secreted into the proximal tubule (**spironolactone** is an exception).

DIURETICS ACTING DIRECTLY ON CELLS OF THE NEPHRON

The main therapeutically useful diuretics act on the:

- thick ascending loop of Henle
- early distal tubule
- collecting tubules and ducts.

For a more detailed review of the actions and clinical uses of the diuretics, see Greger et al. (2005).

Loop diuretics

Loop diuretics (Fig. 29.5B) are the most powerful diuretics (see Fig. 29.6 for a comparison with thiazides), capable of causing the excretion of 15–25% of filtered Na^+. Their action is often described – in a phrase that conjures up a rather uncomfortable picture – as causing 'torrential urine flow'. The main example is **furosemide**; **bumetanide** is an alternative agent. These drugs act on the thick ascending limb, inhibiting the $Na^+/K^+/2Cl^-$ carrier in the lumenal membrane by combining with its Cl^- binding site.

Loop diuretics also have incompletely understood vascular actions. Intravenous administration of furosemide to patients with pulmonary oedema caused by acute heart failure (see Ch. 22) causes a therapeutically useful vasodilator effect independent of the onset of diuresis. Possible mechanisms that have been invoked include decreased vascular responsiveness to vasoconstrictors such as angiotensin II and noradrenaline; increased formation of vasodilating prostaglandins (see above); decreased production of the endogenous ouabain-like natriuretic hormone (Na^+-K^+-ATPase inhibitor; see Ch. 21), which has vasoconstrictor properties; and potassium-channel opening effects in resistance arteries (see Greger et al., 2005).

Loop diuretics increase the delivery of Na^+ to the distal nephron, causing loss of H^+ and K^+. Because Cl^- but not HCO_3^- is lost in the urine, the plasma concentration of HCO_3^- increases as plasma volume is reduced – a form of metabolic alkalosis therefore referred to as 'contraction alkalosis'.

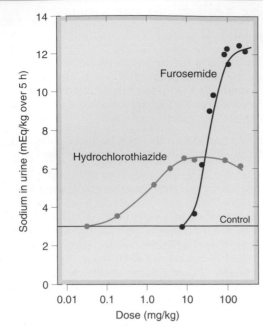

Fig. 29.6 Dose–response curves for furosemide and hydrochlorothiazide, showing differences in potency and maximum effect 'ceiling'. Note that these doses are not used clinically. (*Adapted from Timmerman RJ et al 1964 Curr Ther Res 6, 88.*)

Loop diuretics increase excretion of Ca^{2+} and Mg^{2+} and decrease excretion of uric acid.

Pharmacokinetic aspects

Loop diuretics are absorbed from the gastrointestinal tract, and are usually given by mouth. They may also be given intravenously in urgent situations (e.g. acute pulmonary oedema) or when intestinal absorption is impaired, for example as a result of reduced intestinal perfusion in patients with severe chronic congestive heart failure, who can become resistant to the action of orally administered diuretics. Given orally, they act within 1 h; given intravenously, they produce a peak effect within 30 min. Loop diuretics are strongly bound to plasma protein, and so do not pass directly into the glomerular filtrate. They reach their site of action – the lumenal membrane of the cells of the thick ascending limb – by being secreted in the proximal convoluted tubule by the organic acid transport mechanism; the fraction thus secreted is excreted in the urine.

In nephrotic syndrome,[5] loop diuretics become bound to albumin in the tubular fluid, and consequently are not available to act on the $Na^+/K^+/2Cl^-$ carrier – another cause of diuretic resistance. Molecular variation in the $Na^+/K^+/2Cl^-$ carrier may also be important in some cases of diuretic resistance (Shankar & Brater, 2003).

The fraction of the diuretic not excreted in the urine is metabolised, mainly in liver – **bumetanide** by cytochrome P450 pathways and **furosemide** being glucuronidated. The

plasma half-life of both these drugs is approximately 90 min (longer in renal failure), and the duration of action 3–6 h. The clinical use of loop diuretics is given in the box.

> **Clinical uses of loop diuretics (e.g. furosemide)**
>
> - Loop diuretics are used (cautiously!), in conjunction with dietary salt restriction and often with other classes of diuretic, in the treatment of salt and water overload associated with:
>   - *acute pulmonary oedema*
>   - *chronic heart failure*
>   - *cirrhosis* of the liver complicated by ascites
>   - *nephrotic syndrome*
>   - *renal failure*.
> - Treatment of *hypertension* complicated by renal impairment (thiazides are preferred if renal function is preserved).
> - Treatment of *hypercalcaemia* after replacement of plasma volume with intravenous NaCl solution.

Unwanted effects

Unwanted effects directly related to the renal action of loop diuretics are common.[6] Excessive Na^+ and water loss are common, especially in elderly patients, and can cause hypovolaemia and hypotension. Potassium loss, resulting in low plasma K^+ (hypokalaemia), and metabolic alkalosis are common. Hypokalaemia increases the effects and toxicity of several drugs (e.g. **digoxin** and type III antidysrhythmic drugs, Ch. 21), so this is potentially a clinically important source of drug interaction. If necessary, hypokalaemia can be averted or treated by concomitant use of K^+-sparing diuretics (see below), sometimes with supplementary potassium replacement. Hypomagnesaemia is less often recognised but can also be clinically important. Hyperuricaemia is common and can precipitate acute gout (see Ch. 26). Excessive diuresis leads to reduced renal perfusion and pre-renal renal impairment (an early warning of this is a rise in serum urea concentration).

Unwanted effects *unrelated to the renal actions* of the drugs are infrequent. Dose-related hearing loss (compounded by concomitant use of other ototoxic drugs such as aminoglycoside antibiotics) can result from impaired ion transport by the basolateral membrane of the stria vascularis in the inner ear. It occurs only at much higher doses than usually needed to produce diuresis. Adverse reactions unrelated to the main pharmacological effect (e.g. rashes, bone marrow depression) can occur.

Diuretics acting on the distal tubule

Diuretics acting on the distal tubule include thiazides (e.g. **bendroflumethiazide**, **hydrochlorothiazide**) and related drugs (e.g. **chlortalidone**, **indapamide** and **metolazone**; see Fig. 29.5C).

---

[5]Several diseases that damage renal glomeruli impair their ability to retain plasma albumin, causing massive loss of albumin in the urine and a reduced concentration of albumin in the plasma, which can in turn cause peripheral oedema. This is referred to as nephrotic syndrome.

[6]Such unwanted effects are re-enacted in extreme form in Bartter syndrome type 1, a rare autosomal recessive single gene disorder of the $Na^+/K^+/2Cl^-$ transporter, whose features include polyhydramnios – caused by fetal polyuria – and, postnatally, renal salt loss, low blood pressure, hypokalaemic metabolic alkalosis and hypercalciuria.

Thiazides are less powerful than loop diuretics, at least in terms of peak increase in rate of urine formation, and are preferred in treating uncomplicated hypertension (Ch. 22). They are better tolerated than loop diuretics, and in clinical trials have been shown to reduce risks of stroke and heart attack associated with hypertension. In the largest trial (ALLHAT, 2002), chlortalidone performed as well as newer antihypertensive drugs (an angiotensin-converting enzyme [ACE] inhibitor and a calcium antagonist). Thiazides bind the Cl^- site of the distal tubular Na^+/Cl^- co-transport system, inhibiting its action and causing natriuresis with loss of sodium and chloride ions in the urine. The resulting contraction in blood volume stimulates renin secretion, leading to angiotensin formation and aldosterone secretion (Ch. 22, see Figs 22.4 and 22.9). This homeostatic mechanism limits the effect of the diuretic on the blood pressure, resulting in an *in vivo* dose–hypotensive response relationship with only a gentle gradient during chronic dosing.

Effects of thiazides on Na^+, K^+, H^+ and Mg^{2+} balance are qualitatively similar to those of loop diuretics, but smaller in magnitude. In contrast to loop diuretics, however, thiazides reduce Ca^{2+} excretion, which may be advantageous in older patients at risk of osteoporosis. This could favour thiazides over loop diuretics in terms of bone metabolism (Aung & Htay 2011)

Although thiazides are milder than loop diuretics when used alone, co-administration with loop diuretics has a synergistic effect, because the loop diuretic delivers a greater fraction of the filtered load of Na^+ to the site of action of the thiazide in the distal tubule.

Thiazide diuretics have a vasodilator action (see Chs 4 and 22). When used in the treatment of hypertension (Ch. 22), the initial fall in blood pressure results from the decreased blood volume caused by diuresis, but vasodilatation contributes to the later phase.

Thiazide diuretics have a paradoxical effect in diabetes insipidus, where they *reduce* the volume of urine by interfering with the production of hypotonic fluid in the distal tubule, and hence reduce the ability of the kidney to excrete hypotonic urine (i.e. they reduce free water clearance).

Pharmacokinetic aspects

Thiazides and thiazide-related drugs are effective orally. All are excreted in the urine, mainly by tubular secretion, and they compete with uric acid for the organic anion transporter (OAT; see Ch. 9). Bendroflumethiazide has its maximum effect at about 4–6 h and duration is 8–12 h. Chlortalidone has a longer duration of action.

The clinical use of thiazide diuretics is given in the clinical box.

Clinical uses of thiazide diuretics (e.g. bendroflumethiazide)

- *Hypertension*.
- Mild *heart failure* (loop diuretics are usually preferred).
- Severe resistant *oedema* (**metolazone**, especially, is used, together with loop diuretics).
- To prevent recurrent stone formation in *idiopathic hypercalciuria*.
- *Nephrogenic diabetes insipidus*.

Unwanted effects

Apart from an increase in *urinary frequency*, the commonest unwanted effect of thiazides not obviously related to their main renal action is *erectile dysfunction*. This emerged in an analysis of reasons given by patients for withdrawing from blinded treatment in the Medical Research Council mild hypertension trial, where (to the surprise of the investigators) erectile dysfunction was substantially more common than in men allocated to a β-adrenoceptor antagonist or to placebo. Thiazide-associated erectile dysfunction is reversible; it is less common with the low doses used in current practice but remains a problem. *Potassium loss* can be important, as can loss of Mg^{2+}. Excretion of uric acid is decreased, and hypochloraemic alkalosis can occur.

Impaired glucose tolerance (see Ch. 31), due to inhibition of insulin secretion, is thought to result from activation of K_{ATP} channels in pancreatic islet cells.[7] **Diazoxide**, a non-diuretic thiazide, also activates K_{ATP} channels, causing vasodilatation and impaired insulin secretion. **Indapamide** is said to lower blood pressure with less metabolic disturbance than related drugs, possibly because it is marketed at a lower equivalent dose.

Hyponatraemia is potentially serious, especially in the elderly. Hypokalaemia can be a cause of adverse drug interaction (see above under Loop diuretics) and can precipitate encephalopathy in patients with severe liver disease.

Adverse reactions unrelated to the main pharmacology (e.g. rashes, blood dyscrasias) are not common but can be serious.

Aldosterone antagonists

Spironolactone and **eplerenone** (Weinberger, 2004) have very limited diuretic action when used singly, because distal Na^+/K^+ exchange – the site on which they act (Fig. 29.5D) – accounts for reabsorption of only 2% of filtered Na^+. They do, however, have marked antihypertensive effects (Ch. 22), prolong survival in selected patients with heart failure (Ch. 22) and can prevent hypokalaemia when combined with loop diuretics or with thiazides. They compete with aldosterone for its intracellular receptor (see Ch. 33), thereby inhibiting distal Na^+ retention and K^+ secretion (see Fig. 29.5D).

Pharmacokinetic aspects

Spironolactone is well absorbed from the gut. Its plasma half-life is only 10 min, but its active metabolite, **canrenone**, has a plasma half-life of 16 h. The action of spironolactone is largely attributable to canrenone. Consistent with this, its onset of action is slow, taking several days to develop. Eplerenone has a shorter elimination half-life than canrenone and has no active metabolites. It is administered by mouth once daily.

Unwanted effects

Aldosterone antagonists predispose to hyperkalaemia, which is potentially fatal. Potassium supplements should not be co-prescribed other than in exceptional circumstances and then with close monitoring, and close

---

[7]The chemically related sulfonylurea group of drugs used to treat diabetes mellitus (Ch. 31) act in the opposite way, by closing K_{ATP} channels and enhancing insulin secretion.

monitoring of plasma creatinine and electrolytes is also needed if these drugs are used for patients with impaired renal function, especially if other drugs that can increase plasma potassium, such as *ACE inhibitors, angiotensin receptor antagonists* (sartans) (Ch. 22) or *β-adrenoceptor antagonists* (Ch. 14) are also prescribed – as they often are for patients with heart failure. Gastrointestinal upset is quite common. Actions of spironolactone/ canrenone on progesterone and androgen receptors in tissues other than the kidney can result in gynaecomastia, menstrual disorders and testicular atrophy. Eplerenone has lower affinity for these receptors, and such oestrogen-like side effects are less common with licensed doses of this drug.

The clinical use of potassium-sparing diuretics is given in the clinical box.

Clinical uses of potassium-sparing diuretics (e.g. amiloride, spironolactone)

- With K⁺-losing (i.e. loop or thiazide) diuretics to prevent K⁺ loss, where hypokalaemia is especially hazardous (e.g. patients requiring **digoxin** or **amiodarone**; see Ch. 21).
- **Spironolactone** or **eplerenone** is used in:
  - *heart failure*, to improve survival (see Ch. 21)
  - *primary hyperaldosteronism* (Conn's syndrome)
  - *resistant essential hypertension* (especially low-renin hypertension)
  - *secondary hyperaldosteronism* caused by hepatic cirrhosis complicated by ascites.

Triamterene and amiloride

Like aldosterone antagonists, **triamterene** and **amiloride** have only limited diuretic efficacy, because they also act in the distal nephron, where only a small fraction of Na⁺ reabsorption occurs. They act on the collecting tubules and collecting ducts, inhibiting Na⁺ reabsorption by blocking lumenal sodium channels (see Ch. 4) and decreasing K⁺ excretion (see Fig. 29.5D).

They can be given with loop diuretics or thiazides in order to maintain potassium balance.

Pharmacokinetic aspects
Triamterene is well absorbed in the gastrointestinal tract. Its onset of action is within 2 h, and its duration of action 12–16 h. It is partly metabolised in the liver and partly excreted unchanged in the urine. Amiloride is less well absorbed and has a slower onset, with a peak action at 6 h and duration of about 24 h. Most of the drug is excreted unchanged in the urine.

Unwanted effects
The main unwanted effect, hyperkalaemia, is related to the pharmacological action of these drugs and can be dangerous, especially in patients with renal impairment or receiving other drugs that can increase plasma K⁺ (see above). Gastrointestinal disturbances have been reported but are infrequent. Triamterene has been identified in

kidney stones, but its aetiological role is uncertain. Idiosyncratic reactions, for example rashes, are uncommon.

Carbonic anhydrase inhibitors
Carbonic anhydrase inhibitors (Fig. 29.5A) – for example **acetazolamide** – increase excretion of bicarbonate with accompanying Na⁺, K⁺ and water, resulting in an increased flow of an alkaline urine and metabolic acidosis. These agents, although not now used as diuretics, are still used in the treatment of glaucoma to reduce the formation of aqueous humour (Ch. 13), in some types of infantile epilepsy (Ch. 45), and to accelerate acclimatisation to high altitude.

Urinary loss of bicarbonate depletes extracellular bicarbonate, and the diuretic effect of carbonic anhydrase inhibitors is consequently self-limiting. Acetazolamide is a sulfonamide and unwanted effects as occur with other sulfonamides such as rashes, blood dyscrasias and interstitial nephritis can occur.

DIURETICS THAT ACT INDIRECTLY BY MODIFYING THE CONTENT OF THE FILTRATE
Osmotic diuretics
Osmotic diuretics are pharmacologically inert substances (e.g. **mannitol**) that are filtered in the glomerulus but not reabsorbed by the nephron (see Fig. 29.4).[8] To cause a diuresis, they must constitute an appreciable fraction of the osmolarity of tubular fluid. Within the nephron, their main effect is exerted on those parts of the nephron that are freely permeable to water: the proximal tubule, descending limb of the loop and (in the presence of ADH; see above) the collecting tubules. Passive water reabsorption is reduced by the presence of non-reabsorbable solute within the tubule; consequently a larger volume of fluid remains within the proximal tubule. This has the secondary effect of reducing Na⁺ reabsorption.

Therefore the main effect of osmotic diuretics is to increase the amount of water excreted, with a smaller increase in Na⁺ excretion. They are sometimes used in acute renal failure, which can occur as a result of haemorrhage, injury or systemic infections. In acute renal failure, glomerular filtration rate is reduced, and absorption of NaCl and water in the proximal tubule becomes almost complete, so that more distal parts of the nephron virtually 'dry up', and urine flow ceases. Protein is deposited in the tubules and may impede the flow of fluid. Osmotic diuretics (e.g. **mannitol** given intravenously in a dose of 12–15 g) can limit these effects, at least if given in the earliest stages, albeit while increasing intravascular volume and risking left ventricular failure.

They are also used for the emergency treatment of acutely raised intracranial or intraocular pressure. Such treatment has nothing to do with the kidney, but relies on the increase in plasma osmolarity by solutes that do not enter the brain or eye, which results in efflux of water from these compartments.

Unwanted effects include transient expansion of the extracellular fluid volume (with a risk of precipitating left ventricular failure) and hyponatraemia. Headache, nausea and vomiting can occur.

---

[8] In hyperglycaemia, glucose acts as an osmotic diuretic once plasma glucose exceeds the renal reabsorptive capacity (usually approximately 12 mmol/l), accounting for the cardinal symptom of polyuria in diabetes mellitus; see Chapter 31.

Diuretics

- Normally <1% of filtered Na^+ is excreted.
- Diuretics increase the excretion of salt (NaCl or $NaHCO_3$) and water.
- Loop diuretics, thiazides and K^+-sparing diuretics are the main therapeutic drugs.
- Loop diuretics (e.g. **furosemide**) cause copious urine production. They inhibit the $Na^+/K^+/2Cl^-$ co-transporter in the thick ascending loop of Henle. They are used to treat heart failure and other diseases complicated by salt and water retention. Hypovolaemia and hypokalaemia are important unwanted effects.
- Thiazides (e.g. **bendroflumethiazide**) are less potent than loop diuretics. They inhibit the Na^+/Cl^- co-transporter in the distal convoluted tubule. They are used to treat hypertension. Erectile dysfunction is an important adverse effect. Hypokalaemia and other metabolic effects can occur.
- Potassium-sparing diuretics:
  - act in the distal nephron and collecting tubules; they are very weak diuretics but effective in some forms of hypertension and heart failure, and they can prevent hypokalaemia caused by loop diuretics or thiazides
  - **spironolactone** and **eplerenone** compete with aldosterone for its receptor
  - **amiloride** and **triamterene** act by blocking the sodium channels controlled by aldosterone's protein mediator.

DRUGS THAT ALTER THE pH OF THE URINE

It is possible, by the use of pharmacological agents, to produce urinary pH values ranging from approximately 5 to 8.5.

Carbonic anhydrase inhibitors increase urinary pH by blocking bicarbonate reabsorption (see above). **Citrate** (given by mouth as a mixture of sodium and potassium salts) is metabolised via the Krebs cycle with generation of bicarbonate, which is excreted, alkalinising the urine. This may have some antibacterial effects, as well as improving dysuria (a common symptom of bladder infection, consisting of a burning sensation while passing urine). Additionally, some citrate is excreted in the urine as such and inhibits urinary stone formation. Alkalinisation is important in preventing certain weak acid drugs with limited aqueous solubility, such as *sulfonamides* (see Ch. 51), from crystallising in the urine; it also decreases the formation of uric acid and cystine stones by favouring the charged anionic form that is more water-soluble (Ch. 8).

Alkalinising the urine increases the excretion of drugs that are weak acids (e.g. salicylates and some barbiturates). Sodium bicarbonate is sometimes used to treat salicylate overdose (Ch. 9).

Urinary pH can be decreased with **ammonium chloride**, but this is now rarely, if ever, used clinically except in a specialised test to discriminate between different kinds of renal tubular acidosis.

DRUGS THAT ALTER THE EXCRETION OF ORGANIC MOLECULES

Uric acid metabolism and excretion are relevant in the treatment and prevention of gout (Ch. 26), and a few points about its excretion are made here.

Uric acid is derived from the catabolism of purines, and is present in plasma mainly as ionised urate. In humans, it passes freely into the glomerular filtrate, and most is then reabsorbed in the proximal tubule while a small amount is secreted into the tubule by the anion-secreting mechanism. The net result is excretion of approximately 8–12% of filtered urate. The secretory mechanism is generally inhibited by low doses of drugs that affect uric acid transport (see below), whereas higher doses are needed to block reabsorption. Such drugs therefore tend to cause retention of uric acid at low doses, while promoting its excretion at higher doses. Normal plasma urate concentration is approximately 0.24 mmol/l. In some individuals, the plasma concentration is high, predisposing to gout (see Ch. 26). Drugs that increase the elimination of urate (*uricosuric agents*, e.g. **probenecid** and **sulfinpyrazone**) may be useful in such patients, although these have largely been supplanted by **allopurinol**, which inhibits urate synthesis (Ch. 26).

Probenecid inhibits the reabsorption of urate in the proximal tubule, increasing its excretion. It has the opposite effect on penicillin, inhibiting its secretion into the tubules and raising its plasma concentration. Given orally, probenecid is well absorbed in the gastrointestinal tract, maximal concentrations in the plasma occurring in about 3 h. Approximately 90% is bound to plasma albumin. Free drug passes into the glomerular filtrate but more is actively secreted into the proximal tubule, whence it may diffuse back because of its high lipid solubility (see also Ch. 9). Sulfinpyrazone acts similarly.

The main effect of uricosuric drugs is to block urate reabsorption and lower plasma urate concentration. Both probenecid and sulfinpyrazone inhibit the secretion as well as the reabsorption of urate and, if given in subtherapeutic doses, can actually increase plasma urate concentrations.

DRUGS USED IN RENAL FAILURE

Many drugs used in renal failure (e.g. antihypertensives, vitamin D preparations and **epoietin**) are covered in other chapters. Electrolyte disorders are particularly important in renal failure, notably *hyperphosphataemia* and *hyperkalaemia*, which may require drug treatment.

HYPERPHOSPHATAEMIA

Phosphate metabolism is closely linked with that of calcium and is discussed in Chapter 36.

The antacid **aluminium hydroxide** (Ch. 30) binds phosphate in the gastrointestinal tract, reducing its absorption, but may increase plasma aluminium in dialysis patients.[9] Calcium-based phosphate-binding agents (e.g. calcium carbonate) are widely used. They are contraindicated in hypercalcaemia or hypercalciuria but until recently have

---

[9]Before Kerr identified the cause in Newcastle, the use of alum to purify municipal water supplies led to a horrible and untreatable neurodegenerative condition known as 'dialysis dementia', and also to a particularly painful and refractory form of bone disease.

been believed to be otherwise safe. However, calcium salts may predispose to tissue calcification (including of artery walls), and calcium-containing phosphate binders may actually contribute to the very high death rates from cardiovascular disease in dialysis patients (Goldsmith et al., 2004).

An anion exchange resin, **sevelamer**, lowers plasma phosphate, and is less likely than calcium carbonate to cause arterial calcification (Tonelli et al., 2010). Sevelamer is not absorbed from the gut and has an additional effect in lowering low-density-lipoprotein cholesterol. It is given in gram doses by mouth three times a day with meals. Its adverse effects are gastrointestinal disturbance, and it is contraindicated in bowel obstruction.

HYPERKALAEMIA

Severe hyperkalaemia is life-threatening. Cardiac toxicity is counteracted directly by administering calcium gluconate intravenously (Table 21.1), and by measures that shift K^+ into the intracellular compartment, for example glucose plus insulin (Ch. 31). **Salbutamol (albuterol)**, administered intravenously or by inhalation, also causes cellular K^+ uptake and is used for this indication (e.g. Murdoch et al., 1991); it acts synergistically with insulin. Intravenous sodium bicarbonate is also often recommended, and moves potassium ions into cells in exchange for intracellular protons that emerge to buffer the extracellular fluid.

Removal of excessive potassium from the body can be achieved by cation exchange resins such as **sodium** or **calcium polystyrene sulfonate** administered by mouth (in combination with **sorbitol** to prevent constipation) or as an enema. Dialysis is often needed.

DRUGS USED IN URINARY TRACT DISORDERS

Bed wetting (enuresis) is normal in very young children and persists in around 5% of children aged 10. Disordered micturition is also extremely common in adults. However, it is not easy to prevent incontinence without causing urinary retention.

Nocturnal enuresis in children aged 10 or more may warrant **desmopressin** (an analogue of antidiuretic hormone, given by mouth or by nasal spray; Ch. 33) combined with restricting fluid intake.

Symptoms from benign prostatic hyperplasia may be improved by α_1-adrenoceptor antagonists, for example **doxazosin** or **tamsulosin** (Ch. 14), or by an inhibitor of androgen synthesis such as **finasteride** (Ch. 35).

Muscarinic receptor antagonists (Ch. 13) such as **oxybutinin** are used for neurogenic detrusor muscle instability, but the dose is limited by their adverse effects. A selective β_3 agonist (**mirabegron**) has recently been licensed for overactive bladder (Ch. 14).

REFERENCES AND FURTHER READING

Physiological aspects

Agre, P., 2004. Aquaporin water channels (Nobel lecture). Angew. Chem. Int. Ed. 43, 4278–4290.

Gamba, G., 2005. Molecular physiology and pathophysiology of electroneutral cation–chloride cotransporters. Physiol. Rev. 85, 423–493. (*Comprehensive review of the molecular biology, structure–function relationships, and physiological and pathophysiological roles of each co-transporter*)

Greger, R., 2000. Physiology of sodium transport. Am. J. Med. Sci. 319, 51–62. (*Outstanding article. Covers not only Na+ transport but also, briefly, that of K+, H+, Cl–, HCO3–, Ca2+, Mg2+ and some organic substances in each of the main parts of the nephron. Discusses regulatory factors, pathophysiological aspects and pharmacological principles*)

Lee, W., Kim, R.B., 2003. Transporters and renal drug elimination. Annu. Rev. Pharmacol. Toxicol. 44, 137–166. (*Review*).

Drugs and therapeutic aspects
Diuretics

Aung, K., Htay, T., 2011. Thiazide diuretics and the risk of hip fracture. Cochrane Database Syst. Rev. 10, Article Number: CD005185, doi:10.1002/14651858.CD005185.pub2.

Greger, R., Lang, F., Sebekova, K., Heidland, A., 2005. Action and clinical use of diuretics. In: Davison, A.M., Cameron, J.S., Grunfeld, J.P., et al. (Eds.), Oxford Textbook of Clinical Nephrology, third ed. Oxford University Press, Oxford, pp. 2619–2648. (*Succinct authoritative account of cellular mechanisms; strong on clinical uses*)

Shankar, S.S., Brater, D.C., 2003. Loop diuretics: from the Na–K–2Cl transporter to clinical use. Am. J. Physiol. Renal Physiol. 284, F11–F21. (*Reviews pharmacokinetics and pharmacodynamics of loop diuretics in health and in oedematous disorders; the authors hypothesise that altered expression or activity of the Na+/K+/2Cl– transporter possibly accounts for reduced diuretic responsiveness*)

Weinberger, M.H., 2004. Eplerenone – a new selective aldosterone receptor antagonist. Drugs Today 40, 481–485. (*Review*)

Ca^{2+}/PO_4^- (see also Diuretics section, above)

Cozzolino, M., Brancaccio, D., Gallieni, M., Slatopolsky, E., 2005. Pathogenesis of vascular calcification in chronic kidney disease. Kidney Int. 68, 429–436. (*Reviews hyperphosphataemia and hypercalcaemia as independent risk factors for higher incidence of cardiovascular events in patients with chronic kidney disease: '… hyperphosphatemia accelerates the*

progression of secondary hyperparathyroidism with the concomitant bone loss, possibly linked to vascular calcium-phosphate precipitation')

Goldsmith, D., Ritz, E., Covic, A., 2004. Vascular calcification: a stiff challenge for the nephrologist – does preventing bone disease cause arterial disease? Kidney Int. 66, 1315–1333. (*Potential danger of using calcium salts as phosphate binders in patients with chronic renal failure*)

Tonelli, M., Pannu, N., Manns, B., 2010. Drug therapy: oral phosphate binders in patients with kidney failure. N. Engl. J. Med. 362, 1312–1324.

Antihypertensives and renal protection

ALLHAT Officers and Coordinators for the ALLHAT Collaborative Research Group, 2002. Major outcomes in high-risk hypertensive patients randomized to angiotensin-converting enzyme inhibitor or calcium channel blocker vs diuretic: the Antihypertensive and Lipid-Lowering Treatment to Prevent Heart Attack Trial (ALLHAT). JAMA 288, 2981–2997. (*Massive trial; see also Appel, L.J. for editorial comment: 'The verdict from ALLHAT – thiazide diuretics are the preferred initial therapy for hypertension'. JAMA 288, 3039–3042*)

Nijenhuis, T., Vallon, V., van der Kemp, A.W., et al., 2005. Enhanced passive Ca^{2+} reabsorption and reduced Mg^{2+} channel abundance explains thiazide-induced hypocalciuria and hypomagnesemia. J. Clin. Invest. 115, 1651–1658. (*Micropuncture studies in mouse knockouts showing that enhanced passive Ca^{2+} transport in the proximal tubule rather than active Ca^{2+} transport in distal convolution explains thiazide-induced hypocalciuria*)

Sodium and potassium ion disorders

Coca, S.G., Perazella, M.A., Buller, G.K., 2005. The cardiovascular implications of hypokalemia. Am. J. Kidney Dis. 45, 233–247. (*The recent discovery that aldosterone antagonists decrease pathological injury of myocardium and endothelium has focused interest on their mechanism; this review addresses the relative benefits of modulating potassium balance versus non-renal effects of aldosterone blockade*)

Murdoch, I.A., Dos Anjos, R., Haycock, G.B., 1991. Treatment of hyperkalaemia with intravenous salbutamol. Arch. Dis. Child. 66, 527–528. (*First description of this approach in children*)

Drug utilisation in kidney disease

Carmichael, D.J.S., 2005. Handling of drugs in kidney disease. In: Davison, A.M., Cameron, J.S., Grunfeld, J.P., et al. (Eds.), Oxford Textbook of Clinical Nephrology, third ed. Oxford University Press, Oxford, pp. 2599–2618. (*Principles and practice of dose adjustment in patients with renal failure*)

The gastrointestinal tract

OVERVIEW

In addition to its main function of digestion and absorption of food, the gastrointestinal tract is one of the major endocrine systems in the body. It also has its own integrative neuronal network, the enteric nervous system (see Ch. 12), which contains almost the same number of neurons as the spinal cord. It is the site of many common pathologies, ranging from simple dyspepsia to complex autoimmune conditions such as Crohn's disease and medicines for treating gastrointestinal disorders comprise some 8% of all prescriptions. In this chapter, we briefly review the physiological control of gastrointestinal function and then discuss the pharmacological characteristics of drugs affecting gastric secretion and motility, and those used to treat intestinal inflammatory disease.

THE INNERVATION AND HORMONES OF THE GASTROINTESTINAL TRACT

The blood vessels and the glands (exocrine, endocrine and paracrine) of the gastrointestinal tract are under both neuronal and hormonal control.

NEURONAL CONTROL

There are two principal intramural plexuses in the tract: the *myenteric plexus* (*Auerbach's plexus*) lies between the outer, longitudinal and the middle, circular muscle layers, and the *submucous plexus* (*Meissner's plexus*) lies on the lumenal side of the circular muscle layer. These plexuses are interconnected and their ganglion cells receive preganglionic parasympathetic fibres from the vagus. These are mostly cholinergic and excitatory, although a few are inhibitory. Incoming sympathetic fibres are largely postganglionic. In addition to innervating blood vessels, smooth muscle and some glandular cells directly, some sympathetic fibres terminate in these plexuses, where they inhibit acetylcholine secretion (see Ch. 12).

The neurons within the plexuses constitute the *enteric nervous system* and secrete not only acetylcholine and noradrenaline (norepinephrine), but also 5-hydroxytryptamine (5-HT), purines, nitric oxide and a variety of pharmacologically active peptides (see Chs 12–20). The enteric plexus also contains sensory neurons, which respond to mechanical and chemical stimuli.

HORMONAL CONTROL

The hormones of the gastrointestinal tract include both endocrine and paracrine secretions. The endocrine secretions (i.e. substances released into the bloodstream) are mainly peptides synthesised by endocrine cells in the mucosa. Important examples include *gastrin* and *cholecystokinin*. The paracrine secretions include many regulatory peptides released from special cells found throughout the wall of the tract. These hormones act on nearby cells, and in the stomach the most important of these is *histamine*. Some of these paracrine factors also function as neurotransmitters.

Orally administered drugs are, of course, absorbed during their passage through the gastrointestinal tract (Ch. 8). Other functions of the gastrointestinal tract that are important from the viewpoint of pharmacological intervention are:

- gastric secretion
- vomiting (emesis) and nausea
- gut motility and defecation
- the formation and excretion of bile.

GASTRIC SECRETION

The stomach secretes about 2.5 litres of gastric juice daily. The principal exocrine components are proenzymes such as *prorennin* and *pepsinogen* elaborated by the *chief* or *peptic* cells, and *hydrochloric acid* (HCl) and *intrinsic factor* (see Ch. 25) secreted by the *parietal* or *oxyntic* cells. The production of acid is important for promoting proteolytic digestion of foodstuffs, iron absorption and killing pathogens. Mucus-secreting cells also abound in the gastric mucosa. Bicarbonate ions are secreted and trapped in the mucus, creating a gel-like protective barrier that maintains the mucosal surface at a pH of 6–7 in the face of a much more acidic environment (pH 1–2) in the lumen. Alcohol and bile can disrupt this protective layer. Locally produced 'cytoprotective' prostaglandins stimulate the secretion of both mucus and bicarbonate.

Disturbances in these secretory and protective mechanisms are thought to be involved in the pathogenesis of *peptic ulcer*, and indeed in other types of gastric damage such as *gastro-oesophageal reflux disease* (GORD)[1] and injury caused by non-steroidal anti-inflammatory drugs (NSAIDs).

THE REGULATION OF ACID SECERETION BY PARIETAL CELLS

Disturbances of acid secretion are important in the pathogenesis of peptic ulcer and constitute a particular target for drug action. The secretion of the parietal cells is an isotonic solution of HCl (150 mmol/l) with a pH less than 1, the concentration of hydrogen ions being more than a million times higher than that of the plasma. To produce this, Cl$^-$ is actively transported into *canaliculi* in the cells

---

[1] Or GERD in the USA, to reflect the different spelling of *esophageal*.

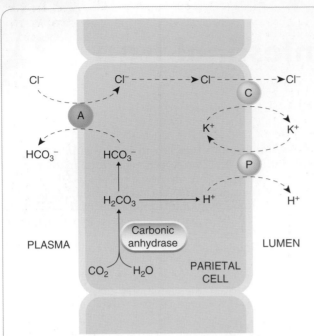

Fig. 30.1 A schematic illustration of the secretion of hydrochloric acid by the gastric parietal cell. Secretion involves a proton pump (P), which is an H^+-K^+-ATPase, a symport carrier (C) for K^+ and Cl^-, and an antiport (A), which exchanges Cl^- and HCO_3^-. An additional Na^+/H^+ antiport situated at the interface with the plasma may also have a role (not shown).

that communicate with the lumen of the gastric glands and thus with the stomach itself. This is accompanied by K^+ secretion, which is then exchanged for H^+ from within the cell by a K^+-H^+-ATPase (the 'proton pump', Fig. 30.1). Within the cell, carbonic anhydrase catalyses the combination of carbon dioxide and water to give carbonic acid, which dissociates into H^+ and bicarbonate ions. The latter exchanges across the basal membrane of the parietal cell for Cl^-. The principal mediators that directly – or indirectly – control parietal cell acid output are:

- histamine (a stimulatory local hormone)
- gastrin (a stimulatory peptide hormone)
- acetylcholine (a stimulatory neurotransmitter)
- prostaglandins E_2 and I_2 (local hormones that inhibit acid secretion)
- somatostatin (an inhibitory peptide hormone).

HISTAMINE

Histamine is discussed in Chapter 26, and only those aspects of its pharmacology relevant to gastric secretion will be dealt with here. Neuroendocrine cells abound in the stomach and the dominant type are the *ECL cells* (enterochromaffin-like cells). These are histamine-containing cells similar to mast cells, which lie close to the parietal cells. They sustain a steady basal release of histamine, which is further increased by gastrin and acetylcholine. Histamine acts in a paracrine fashion on parietal cell H_1 receptors, increasing intracellular cAMP. These cells are responsive to histamine concentrations that are below the threshold required for vascular H_2 receptor activation.

GASTRIN

Gastrin is a polypeptide of 34 residues but also exists in shorter forms. It is synthesised by *G cells* in the gastric antrum and secreted into the portal blood (i.e. it acts in an endocrine fashion). Its main action is stimulation of acid secretion by ECL cells through its action at gastrin/cholecystokinin $(CCK)_2$ receptors,[2] which elevate intracellular Ca^{2+}. Gastrin receptors also occur on the parietal cells but their significance in the control of physiological secretion is controversial. CCK_2 receptors are blocked by the experimental drug **proglumide** (Fig. 30.2), which weakly inhibits gastrin action.

Gastrin also stimulates histamine synthesis by ECL cells and indirectly increases pepsinogen secretion, stimulates blood flow and increases gastric motility. Release of this hormone is controlled by both neuronal transmitters and blood-borne mediators, as well as by the chemistry of the stomach contents. Amino acids and small peptides directly stimulate the gastrin-secreting cells, as do milk and solutions of calcium salts, explaining why it is inappropriate to use calcium-containing salts as antacids.

ACETYLCHOLINE

Acetylcholine (together with a battery of other neurotransmitters and peptides), released from postganglionic cholinergic neurons, stimulates specific muscarinic M_3 receptors on the surface of the parietal cells (see Ch. 13), thereby elevating intracellular Ca^{2+} and stimulating the release of protons. It also has complex effects on other cell types; by inhibiting somatostatin release from *D cells*, it potentiates its action on parietal cell acid secretion.

PROSTAGLANDINS

Most cells of the gastrointestinal tract produce prostaglandins (PGs; see Chs 6 and 17), the most important being PGE_2 and I_2. Prostaglandins exert 'cytoprotective' effects on many aspects of gastric function including increasing bicarbonate secretion ($EP_{1/2}$ receptors), increasing the release of protective mucin (EP_4 receptor), reducing gastric acid output probably by acting on $EP_{2/3}$ receptors on ECL cells and preventing the vasoconstriction (and thus damage to the mucosa) that follows injury or insult. The latter is probably an action mediated through $EP_{2/4}$ receptors. **Misoprostol** (see below) is a synthetic prostaglandin that probably exploits many of these effects to bring about its therapeutic action.

SOMATOSTATIN

This peptide hormone is released from *D cells* at several locations within the stomach. By acting at its somatostatin $(SST)_2$ receptor, it exerts paracrine inhibitory actions on gastrin release from G cells, histamine release from ECL cells, as well as directly on parietal cell acid output.

THE COORDINATION OF FACTORS REGULATING ACID SECRETION

The regulation of the parietal cell is complex and many local hormones probably play a role in the fine-tuning of the secretory response. The generally accepted model

[2]These two peptides share the same, biologically active, C-terminal pentapeptide sequence.

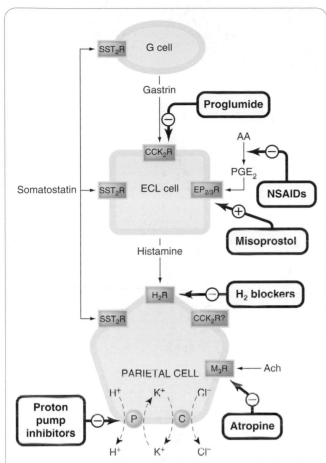

Fig. 30.2 Schematic diagram showing the regulation of the acid-secreting gastric parietal cell, illustrating the site of action of drugs influencing acid secretion. The initial step in controlling physiological secretion is the release of gastrin from G cells. This acts through its CCK$_2$ receptor on ECL cells to release histamine and may also have a secondary direct effect on parietal cells themselves, although this is not entirely clear. Histamine acts on parietal cell H$_2$ receptors to elevate cAMP that activates the secretion of acid by the proton pump. Direct vagal stimulation also provokes acid secretion and released acetylcholine directly stimulates M$_3$ receptors on parietal cells. Somatostatin probably exerts a tonic inhibitory influence on G cells, ECL cells and parietal cells, while local (or therapeutically administered) prostaglandins exert inhibitory effects predominately on ECL cell function. AA, arachidonic acid; ACh, acetylcholine; C, symport carrier for K$^+$ and Cl$^-$; CCK$_2$, gastrin/cholecystokinin receptor; ECL, mast cell-like histamine-secreting enterochromaffin cell; NSAIDs, non-steroidal anti-inflammatory drugs; P, proton pump (H$^+$-K$^+$-ATPase); PGE$_2$, prostaglandin E$_2$.

Direct vagal stimulation can also provoke acid secretion (the basis for 'stress ulcers') through a release of acetylcholine, which directly stimulates M$_3$ receptors on parietal cells. Somatostatin probably exerts a tonic inhibitory influence on G cells, ECL and parietal cells, and local (or therapeutically administered) prostaglandins, acting through EP$_{2/3}$ receptors, exert inhibitory effects predominantly on ECL cell function.

This control system is clearly complex but prolonged exposure of tissues to excess acid secretion is dangerous and must be tightly regulated (see Schubert & Peura, 2008).

Secretion of gastric acid, mucus and bicarbonate

The control of the gastrointestinal tract is through nervous and humoral mechanisms:

- acid is secreted from gastric parietal cells by a proton pump (K$^+$-H$^+$-ATPase)
- the three endogenous secretagogues for acid are histamine, acetylcholine and gastrin
- prostaglandins E$_2$ and I$_2$ inhibit acid, stimulate mucus and bicarbonate secretion, and dilate mucosal blood vessels
- somatostatin inhibits all phases of parietal cell activation.

The genesis of peptic ulcers involves:

- infection of the gastric mucosa with *Helicobacter pylori*
- an imbalance between the mucosal-damaging, (acid, pepsin) and the mucosal-protecting, agents (mucus, bicarbonate, prostaglandins E$_2$ and I$_2$, and nitric oxide).

DRUGS USED TO INHIBIT OR NEUTRALISE GASTRIC ACID SECRETION

The principal clinical indications for reducing acid secretion are *peptic ulceration* (both duodenal and gastric), *GORD* (in which gastric secretion causes damage to the oesophagus) and the *Zollinger–Ellison syndrome* (a rare hypersecretory condition caused by a gastrin-producing tumour). If untreated, GORD can cause a dysplasia of the oesophgeal epithelium which may progress to a potentially dangerous pre-cancerous condition called *Barrett's oesophagus*.

The reasons why peptic ulcers develop are not fully understood, although infection of the stomach mucosa with *Helicobacter pylori*[3] – a Gram-negative bacillus that causes chronic gastritis – is now generally considered to be a major cause (especially of duodenal ulcer) and, while there are some problems with this notion (see Axon, 2007), forms the usual basis for therapy. Treatment of *H. pylori* infection is discussed below.

Many non-specific NSAIDs (see Ch. 26) cause gastric bleeding and erosions by inhibiting cyclo-oxygenase-1, the enzyme responsible for synthesis of protective prostaglandins. More selective cyclo-oxygenase-2 inhibitors such as **celecoxib** appear to cause less stomach damage (but see Ch. 26 for a discussion of this issue).

today is that the *gastrin–ECL–parietal cell axis* is the dominant mechanism for controlling acid secretion. According to this idea (see Fig. 30.2), which is supported by the majority of transgenic 'knockout' mouse studies, the initial step in controlling physiological secretion is the release of gastrin from G cells. This acts through its CCK$_2$ receptor on ECL cells to release histamine and may also have a secondary direct effect on parietal cells themselves, although this has been disputed. Histamine acts on H$_2$ receptors on parietal cells to elevate cAMP and to activate the secretion of protons as described.

---

[3] *H. pylori* infection in the stomach has also been classified as a class 1 (definite) carcinogen for gastric cancer.

Therapy of peptic ulcer and reflux oesophagitis aims to decrease the secretion of gastric acid with H$_2$ receptor antagonists or proton pump inhibitors, and/or to neutralise secreted acid with antacids (see Huang & Hunt, 2001). These treatments are often coupled with measures to eradicate *H. pylori* (see Blaser, 1998, and Horn, 2000).

HISTAMINE H$_2$ RECEPTOR ANTAGONISTS

The discovery and development of histamine H$_2$-blocking drugs by Black and his colleagues in 1972 was a major breakthrough in the treatment of gastric ulcers – a condition that could hitherto only be treated by (sometimes rather heroic) surgery.[4] Indeed, the ability to distinguish between histamine receptor subtypes using pharmacological agents was, in itself, a major intellectual achievement. H$_2$ receptor antagonists competitively inhibit histamine actions at all H$_2$ receptors, but their main clinical use is as inhibitors of gastric acid secretion. They can inhibit histamine- and gastrin-stimulated acid secretion; pepsin secretion also falls with the reduction in volume of gastric juice. These agents not only decrease both basal and food-stimulated acid secretion by 90% or more, but numerous clinical trials indicate that they also promote healing of gastric and duodenal ulcers. However, relapses are likely to follow after cessation of treatment.

The main drugs used are **cimetidine**, **ranitidine** (sometimes in combination with **bismuth**), **nizatidine** and **famotidine**. There is little difference between them. The effect of cimetidine on gastric secretion in human subjects is shown in Figure 30.3. The clinical use of H$_2$ receptor antagonists is explained in the clinical box.

Pharmacokinetic aspects and unwanted effects

The drugs are generally given orally and are well absorbed, although preparations for intramuscular and intravenous use are also available (except famotidine). Dosage regimens vary depending on the condition under treatment. Low-dosage over-the-counter formulations of cimetidine, ranitidine and famotidine are available from pharmacies for short-term use, without prescription.

Unwanted effects are rare. Diarrhoea, dizziness, muscle pains, alopecia, transient rashes, confusion in the elderly and hypergastrinaemia have been reported. Cimetidine sometimes causes gynaecomastia in men and, rarely, a decrease in sexual function. This is probably caused by a modest affinity for androgen receptors. Cimetidine (but not other H$_2$ receptor antagonists) also inhibits cytochrome P450, and can retard the metabolism (and thus potentiate the action) of a range of drugs including oral anticoagulants and tricyclic antidepressants.

PROTON PUMP INHIBITORS

The first proton pump inhibitor was **omeprazole**, which irreversibly inhibits the H$^+$-K$^+$-ATPase (the proton pump), the terminal step in the acid secretory pathway (see Figs 30.1 and 30.2). Both basal and stimulated gastric acid secretion (Fig. 30.4) is reduced. The drug comprises a racemic mixture of two enantiomers. As a weak base, it accumulates in the acid environment of the canaliculi of the stimulated parietal cell where it is converted into an

---

[4]This era has been referred to as the 'BC' – before cimetidine – era of gastroenterology (Schubert & Peura, 2008)! It is an indication of the clinical importance of the development of this drug.

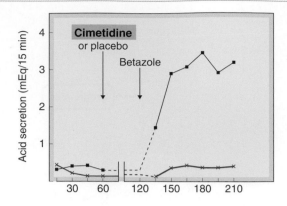

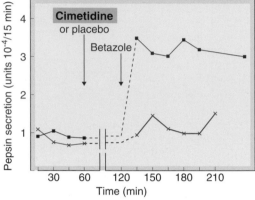

Fig. 30.3 **The effect of cimetidine on betazole-stimulated gastric acid and pepsin secretion in humans.** Either cimetidine or a placebo was given orally 60 min prior to a subcutaneous injection (1.5 mg/kg) of betazole, a relatively specific histamine H$_2$-receptor agonist that stimulates gastric acid secretion. *(Modified from Binder & Donaldson, 1978.)*

Clinical use of agents affecting gastric acidity

- Histamine H$_2$ receptor antagonists (e.g. **ranitidine**):
  - *peptic ulcer*
  - *reflux oesophagitis.*
- Proton pump inhibitors (e.g. **omeprazole**, **lansoprazole**):
  - *peptic ulcer*
  - *reflux oesophagitis*
  - as one component of therapy for *Helicobacter pylori* infection
  - *Zollinger–Ellison* syndrome (a rare condition caused by gastrin-secreting tumours).
- Antacids (e.g. **magnesium trisilicate**, **aluminium hydroxide**, **alginates**):
  - *dyspepsia*
  - symptomatic relief in *peptic ulcer* or (**alginate**) *oesophageal reflux.*
- **Bismuth chelate**:
  - as one component of therapy for *H. pylori* infection.

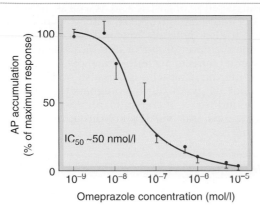

Fig. 30.4 The inhibitory action of omeprazole on acid secretion from isolated human gastric glands stimulated by 50 μmol/l histamine. Acid secretion was measured by the accumulation of a radiolabelled weak base, aminopyrine (AP), in the secretory channels. The data represent the mean and standard error of measurements from eight patients. *(Adapted from Lindberg P et al. 1987 Trends Pharmacol Sci 8, 399–402.)*

achiral form and is then able to react with, and inactivate, the ATPase. This preferential accumulation means that it has a specific effect on these cells. Other proton pump inhibitors (all of which have a similar mode of activation and pharmacology) include **esomeprazole** (the [S] isomer of omeprazole), **lansoprazole**, **pantoprazole** and **rabeprazole**. The clinical indication for these drugs is given in the clinical box (see above).

Pharmacokinetic aspects and unwanted effects

Oral administration is the most common route of administration, although some injectable preparations are available. Omeprazole is given orally, but as it degrades rapidly at low pH, it is administered as capsules containing enteric-coated granules. Following absorption in the small intestine, it passes from the blood into the parietal cells and then into the canaliculi where it exerts its effects. Increased doses give disproportionately higher increases in plasma concentration (possibly because its inhibitory effect on acid secretion improves its own bioavailability). Although its half-life is about 1 h, a single daily dose affects acid secretion for 2–3 days, partly because of the accumulation in the canaliculi and partly because it inhibits the H^+-K^+-ATPase irreversibly. With daily dosage, there is an increasing antisecretory effect for up to 5 days, after which a plateau is reached.

Unwanted effects of this class of drugs are uncommon. They may include headache, diarrhoea (both sometimes severe) and rashes. Dizziness, somnolence, mental confusion, impotence, gynaecomastia, and pain in muscles and joints have been reported. Proton pump inhibitors should be used with caution in patients with liver disease, or in women who are pregnant or breastfeeding. The use of these drugs may 'mask' the symptoms of gastric cancer.

ANTACIDS

Antacids are the simplest way to treat the symptoms of excessive gastric acid secretion. They directly neutralise acid and this also has the effect of inhibiting the activity of peptic enzymes, which practically ceases at pH 5. Given in sufficient quantity for long enough, they can produce healing of duodenal ulcers but are less effective for gastric ulcers.

Most antacids in common use are salts of magnesium and aluminium. Magnesium salts cause diarrhoea and aluminium salts, constipation – so mixtures of these two can, happily, be used to preserve normal bowel function. Preparations of these substances (e.g. **magnesium trisilicate** mixtures and some proprietary aluminium preparations) containing high concentrations of sodium should not be given to patients on a sodium-restricted diet. Numerous antacid preparations are available; a few of the more significant are given below.

Magnesium hydroxide is an insoluble powder that forms magnesium chloride in the stomach. It does not produce systemic alkalosis, because Mg^{2+} is poorly absorbed from the gut. Another salt, magnesium trisilicate, is an insoluble powder that reacts slowly with the gastric juice, forming magnesium chloride and colloidal silica. This agent has a prolonged antacid effect, and it also adsorbs pepsin. **Magnesium carbonate** is also used.

Aluminium hydroxide gel forms aluminium chloride in the stomach; when this reaches the intestine, the chloride is released and is reabsorbed. Aluminium hydroxide raises the pH of the gastric juice to about 4, and also adsorbs pepsin. Its action is gradual, and its effect continues for several hours.[5] Colloidal aluminium hydroxide combines with phosphates in the gastrointestinal tract and the increased excretion of phosphate in the faeces that occurs results in decreased excretion of phosphate via the kidney. This effect has been used in treating patients with chronic renal failure (see Ch. 29). Other preparations such as **hydrotalcite** contain mixtures of both aluminium and magnesium salts.

Alginates or **simeticone** are sometimes combined with antacids. Alginates are believed to increase the viscosity and adherence of mucus to the oesophageal mucosa, forming a protective barrier, whereas simeticone is an anti-foaming agent, intended to relieve bloating and flatulence.

TREATMENT OF *HELICOBACTER PYLORI* INFECTION

H. pylori infection has been implicated as a causative factor in the production of gastric and, more particularly, duodenal ulcers, as well as a risk factor for gastric cancer. Indeed, some would argue that infectious gastroduodenitis is actually the chief clinical entity associated with ulcers, and gastric cancer its prominent sequela. Certainly, eradication of *H. pylori* infection promotes rapid and long-term healing of ulcers, and it is routine practice to test for the organism in patients presenting with suggestive symptoms. If the test is positive, then the organism can generally be eradicated with a 1- or 2-week regimen of 'triple therapy', comprising a proton pump inhibitor in combination with the antibacterials **amoxicillin** and **metronidazole** or **clarithromycin** (see Ch. 51); other combinations are also used. Bismuth-containing preparations (see below) are sometimes added. While elimination of

---

[5]There was a suggestion – no longer widely believed – that aluminium could trigger Alzheimer's disease. In fact, aluminium is not absorbed to any significant extent following oral administration of aluminium hydroxide, although when introduced by other routes (e.g. during renal dialysis with aluminium-contaminated solutions) it is extremely toxic.

the bacillus can produce long-term remission of ulcers, reinfection with the organism can occur.

DRUGS THAT PROTECT THE MUCOSA

Some agents, termed *cytoprotective*, are said to enhance endogenous mucosal protection mechanisms and/or to provide a physical barrier over the surface of the ulcer.

Bismuth chelate

Bismuth chelate (tripotassium dicitratobismuthate) is sometimes used in combination regimens to treat *H. pylori*. It has toxic effects on the bacillus, and may also prevent its adherence to the mucosa or inhibit its bacterial proteolytic enzymes. It is also believed to have other mucosa-protecting actions, by mechanisms that are unclear, and is widely used as an over-the-counter remedy for mild gastrointestinal symptoms. Very little is absorbed, but if renal excretion is impaired, the raised plasma concentrations of bismuth can result in encephalopathy.

Unwanted effects include nausea and vomiting, and blackening of the tongue and faeces.

Sucralfate

Sucralfate is a complex of aluminium hydroxide and sulfated sucrose, which releases aluminium in the presence of acid. The residual complex carries a strong negative charge and binds to cationic groups in proteins, glycoproteins, etc. It can form complex gels with mucus, an action that is thought to decrease the degradation of mucus by pepsin and to limit the diffusion of H^+ ions. Sucralfate can also inhibit the action of pepsin and stimulate secretion of mucus, bicarbonate and prostaglandins from the gastric mucosa. All these actions contribute to its mucosa-protecting action.

Sucralfate is given orally and about 30% is still present in the stomach 3 h after administration. In the acid environment, the polymerised product forms a tenacious paste, which can sometimes produce an obstructive lump (known as a *bezoar*[6]) that gets stuck in the stomach. It reduces the absorption of a number of other drugs, including fluoroquinolone antibiotics, **theophylline**, **tetracycline**, **digoxin** and **amitriptyline**. Because it requires an acid environment for activation, antacids given concurrently or prior to its administration will reduce its efficacy.

Unwanted effects are few, the most common being constipation. Less common effects apart from bezoar formation, include dry mouth, nausea, vomiting, headache and rashes.

Misoprostol

Prostaglandins of the E and I series have a generally homeostatic protective action in the gastrointestinal tract, and a deficiency in endogenous production (after ingestion of a NSAID, for example) may contribute to ulcer formation. **Misoprostol** is a stable analogue of prostaglandin E_1. It is given orally and is used to promote the healing of ulcers or to prevent the gastric damage that can occur with chronic use of NSAIDs. It exerts a direct action on the ECL cell (and possibly parietal cell also; Fig. 30.2), inhibiting the basal secretion of gastric acid as well as the stimulation of production seen in response to food, pentagastrin and caffeine. It also increases mucosal blood flow and augments the secretion of mucus and bicarbonate.

Unwanted effects include diarrhoea and abdominal cramps; uterine contractions can also occur, so the drug should not be given during pregnancy (unless deliberately to induce a therapeutic abortion; see Ch. 35). Prostaglandins and NSAIDs are discussed more fully in Chs 6 and 26.

VOMITING

Nausea and vomiting are unwanted side effects of many clinically used drugs, notably those used for cancer chemotherapy but also opioids, general anaesthetics and digoxin. They also occur in motion sickness,[7] during early pregnancy and in numerous disease states (e.g. migraine) as well as bacterial and viral infections.

THE REFLEX MECHANISM OF VOMITING

Vomiting is a defensive response intended to rid the organism of toxic or irritating material. Poisonous compounds, bacterial toxins, many cytotoxic drugs (as well as mechanical distension) trigger the release, from enterochromaffin cells in the lining of the GI tract, of mediators such as 5-HT. These transmitters trigger signals in vagal afferent fibres. The physical act of vomiting is co-ordinated centrally by the *vomiting* (or *emetic*) *centre* in the medulla; see Figure 30.5. Actually, this is not a discrete anatomical location but a network of neural pathways that integrate signals arriving from other locations. One of these, in the *area postrema* is known as the *chemoreceptor trigger zone* (CTZ). The CTZ receives inputs from the labyrinth in the inner ear through the *vestibular nuclei* (which explains the mechanism of motion sickness) and vagal afferents arising from the GI tract. Toxic chemicals in the blood stream can also be detected directly by the CTZ because the blood–brain barrier is relatively permeable in this area. The CTZ is therefore a primary site of action of many emetic and antiemetic drugs (see Table 30.1).

The vomiting centre also receives signals directly from vagal afferents, as well as those relayed through the CTZ. In addition, it receives input from higher cortical centres, explaining why unpleasant or repulsive sights or smells, or strong emotional stimuli, can sometimes induce nausea and vomiting.

The main neurotransmitters involved in this neurocircuitry are acetylcholine, histamine, 5-HT, dopamine and substance P and receptors for these transmitters have been demonstrated in the relevant areas (see Chs 12–16 and 38). It has been hypothesised that enkephalins (see Ch. 42) are also implicated in the mediation of vomiting, acting possibly at δ (CTZ) or μ (vomiting centre) opioid receptors. Substance P (see Ch. 18) acting at neurokinin-1 receptors in the CTZ, and endocannabinoids (Ch. 19), may also be involved.

---

[6]From the Persian word meaning 'a cure for poisoning'. It refers to the belief that a concoction made from lumps of impacted rubbish retrieved from the stomach of goats would protect against poisoning by one's enemies.

[7]In fact, the word *nausea* is derived from the Greek word meaning 'boat', with the obvious implication of associated motion sickness. *Vomiting* is derived from the Latin and a *vomitorium* was the 'fast exit' passageway in ancient theatres. It has a certain resonance, as we think you will agree!

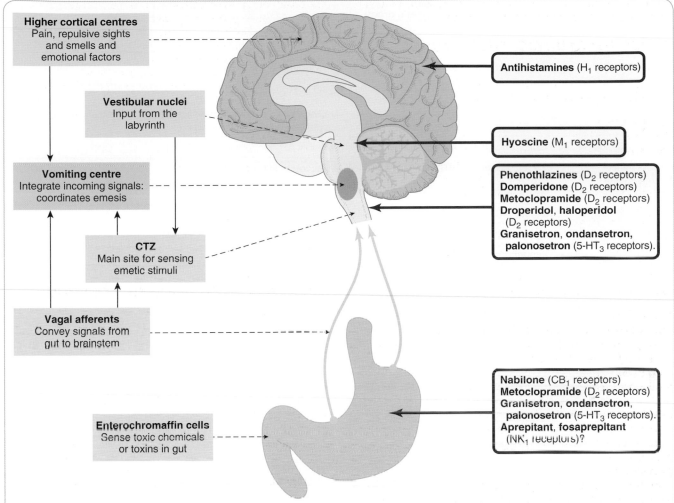

Fig. 30.5 Schematic diagram of the factors involved in the control of vomiting, with the probable sites of action of antiemetic drugs. There are three important centres located in the medulla. The chemoreceptor trigger zone (CTZ), the vomiting centre and the vestibular nuclei. The vomiting centre control receives inputs from the CTZ, the GI tract (through vagal afferent connections) and higher cortical centres and coordinates the physical act of emesis. Vagal afferents arising from the GI tract also feed into the CTZ directly as does input from the vestibular nuclei, which in turn, receive inputs from the labyrinth. *(Based partly on a diagram from Rojas & Slusher, 2012)*

The neurobiology of nausea is much less well understood. Nausea and vomiting may occur together or separately and may subserve different physiological functions (see Andrews & Horn, 2006). From the pharmacologist's viewpoint, it is easier to control vomiting than nausea, and many effective antiemetics (e.g. 5-HT$_3$ antagonists) are much less successful in this regard.

ANTIEMETIC DRUGS

Several antiemetic agents are available, and these are generally used for specific conditions, although there may be some overlap. Such drugs are of particular importance as an adjunct to cancer chemotherapy, where the nausea and vomiting produced by many cytotoxic drugs (see Ch. 56) can be almost unendurable.[8] In using drugs to treat the morning sickness of pregnancy, the problem of potential

damage to the fetus has always to be borne in mind. In general, all drugs should be avoided during the first 3 months of pregnancy, if possible. Details of the main categories of antiemetics are given below, and their main clinical uses are summarised in the box. The clinical box below and Table 30.1 give an overview of their likely sites of action and their clinical utility.

RECEPTOR ANTAGONISTS

Many H$_1$ (see Ch. 26), muscarinic (see Ch. 13), 5-HT$_3$ (see Ch. 15), dopamine (see Ch. 46) and NK$_1$ (see Ch. 15) receptor antagonists exhibit clinically useful antiemetic activity.

H$_1$ receptor antagonists

Cinnarizine, cyclizine and **promethazine** are the most commonly employed; they are effective against nausea and vomiting arising from many causes, including motion sickness and the presence of irritants in the stomach. None is very effective against substances that act directly on the CTZ. Promethazine is used for morning sickness of

---

[8]It was reported that a young, medically qualified patient being treated by combination chemotherapy for sarcoma stated that 'the severity of vomiting at times made the thought of death seem like a welcome relief'.

Table 30.1 Sites of action of common antiemetic drugs

Class	Drugs	Site of action	Comments
Antihistamines	Cinnarizine, cyclizine, promethazine	H_1 receptors in the CNS (causing sedation) and possibly anticholinergic actions in the vestibular apparatus	Widely effective regardless of cause of emesis
Antimuscarinics	Hyoscine	Anticholinergic actions in the vestibular apparatus and possibly elsewhere	Mainly MS
Cannabinoids	Nabilone	Probably CB_1 receptors in the GI tract	CINV
Dopamine antagonists	Phenothiazines: prochlorphenazine, perphenazine, trifluorphenazine, chlorpromazine	D_2 receptors in CTZ	CINV, PONV, NNV, RS
	Related drugs: droperidol, haloperidol	D_2 receptors in GI tract	CINV, PONV, RS
	Metoclopramide	D_2 receptors in the CTZ and GI tract	PONV, CINV
	Domperidone	D_2 receptors in CTZ	CINV
Glucocorticoids	Dexamethasone	Probably multiple sites of action, including the GI tract	CINV; often used in combination with other drugs
5-HT$_3$ antagonists	Granisteron, ondansetron, palonosetron	5-HT$_3$ receptors in CTZ and GI tract	PONV, CINV
Neurokinin-1 antagonists	Aprepitant, fosaprepitant	NK_1 receptors in CTZ, vomiting centre and possibly the GI tract	CINV; often given in combination with another drug

CINV, cytotoxic drug-induced vomiting; CNS, central nervous system; CTZ, chemoreceptor trigger zone; GI, gastrointestinal; PONV, postoperative nausea and vomiting; MS, motion sickness; RS, radiation sickness.

The reflex mechanism of vomiting

Emetic stimuli include:
- chemicals or drugs in the blood or intestine
- neuronal input from the gastrointestinal tract, labyrinth and central nervous system (CNS).

Pathways and mediators include:
- impulses from the chemoreceptor trigger zone and various other CNS centres relayed to the vomiting centre
- chemical transmitters such as histamine, acetylcholine, dopamine, 5-hydroxytryptamine and substance P, acting on H_1, muscarinic, D_2, 5-HT$_3$ and NK$_1$ receptors, respectively.

Antiemetic drugs include:
- H_1 receptor antagonists (e.g. **cinnarizine**)
- muscarinic antagonists (e.g. **hyoscine**)
- 5-HT$_3$ receptor antagonists (e.g. **ondansetron**)
- D_2 receptor antagonists (e.g. **metoclopramide**)
- cannabinoids (e.g. **nabilone**)
- neurokinin-1 antagonists (e.g. **aprepitant**, **fosaprepitant**).

Main side effects of principal antiemetics include:
- drowsiness and antiparasympathetic effects (**hyoscine**, **nabilone** > **cinnarizine**)
- dystonic reactions (**metoclopramide**)
- general CNS disturbances (**nabilone**)
- headache, gastrointestinal tract upsets (**ondansetron**).

Clinical use of antiemetic drugs

- Histamine H_1 receptor antagonists (see also clinical box in Ch. 26):
  - **cyclizine**: motion sickness
  - **cinnarizine**: motion sickness, vestibular disorders (e.g. Menière's disease)
  - **promethazine**: severe morning sickness of pregnancy.
- Muscarinic receptor antagonists:
  - **hyoscine**: motion sickness.
- Dopamine D_2 receptor antagonists:
  - phenothiazines (e.g. **prochlorperazine**): vomiting caused by uraemia, radiation, viral gastroenteritis, severe morning sickness of pregnancy
  - **metoclopramide**: vomiting caused by uraemia, radiation, gastrointestinal disorders, cytotoxic drugs
  - **domperidone** is less liable to cause CNS side effects as it penetrates the blood–brain barrier poorly.
- 5-Hydroxytryptamine 5-HT$_3$ receptor antagonists (e.g. **ondansetron**): cytotoxic drugs or radiation, postoperative vomiting.
- Cannabinoids (e.g. **nabilone**): cytotoxic drugs (see Ch. 19).

pregnancy (on the rare occasions when this is so severe that drug treatment is justified), and has been used by NASA to treat space motion sickness. Drowsiness and sedation, while possibly contributing to their clinical efficacy, are the chief unwanted effects.

Betahistine has complicated effects on histamine action, antagonising H_3 receptors but having a weak agonist activity on H_1 receptors. It is used to control the nausea and vertigo associated with *Menière's disease*.[9]

Muscarinic receptor antagonists

Hyoscine (scopolamine) is employed principally for prophylaxis and treatment of motion sickness, and may be administered orally or as a transdermal patch. Dry mouth and blurred vision are the most common unwanted effects. Drowsiness also occurs, but the drug has less sedative action than the antihistamines because of poor central nervous system penetration.

5-HT₃ receptor antagonists

Granisetron, **ondansetron** and **palonosetron** (see Ch. 15) are of particular value in preventing and treating the vomiting and, to a lesser extent the nausea, commonly encountered postoperatively as well as that caused by radiation therapy or administration of cytotoxic drugs such as **cisplatin**. The primary site of action of these drugs is the CTZ. They may be given orally or by injection (sometimes helpful if nausea is already present). Unwanted effects such as headache and gastrointestinal upsets are relatively uncommon.

Dopamine antagonists

Antipsychotic phenothiazines (see Ch. 45), such as **chlorpromazine**, **perphenazine**, **prochlorperazine** and **trifluoperazine**, are effective antiemetics commonly used for treating the more severe nausea and vomiting associated with cancer, radiation therapy, cytotoxic drugs, opioids, anaesthetics and other drugs. They can be administered orally, intravenously or by suppository. They act mainly as antagonists of the dopamine D_2 receptors in the CTZ (see Fig. 30.5) but they also block histamine and muscarinic receptors.

Unwanted effects are common and include sedation (especially chlorpromazine), hypotension and extrapyramidal symptoms including dystonias and tardive dyskinesia (Ch. 46).

Other antipsychotic drugs, such as **haloperidol**, the related compound **droperidol** and **levomepromazine** (Ch. 46), also act as D_2 antagonists in the CTZ and can be used for acute chemotherapy-induced emesis.

Metoclopramide and domperidone

Metoclopramide is a D_2 receptor antagonist (Fig. 30.5), closely related to the phenothiazine group, that acts centrally on the CTZ and also has a peripheral action on the gastrointestinal tract itself, increasing the motility of the oesophagus, stomach and intestine. This not only adds to the antiemetic effect, but explains its use in the treatment of gastro-oesophageal reflux and hepatic and biliary disorders. As metoclopramide also blocks dopamine receptors (see Ch. 44) elsewhere in the central nervous system, it produces a number of unwanted effects including disorders of movement (more common in children and young adults), fatigue, motor restlessness, spasmodic torticollis (involuntary twisting of the neck) and occulogyric crises (involuntary upward eye movements). It stimulates prolactin release (see Chs 33 and 35), causing galactorrhoea and disorders of menstruation.

Domperidone is a similar drug often used to treat vomiting due to cytotoxic therapy as well as gastrointestinal symptoms. Unlike metoclopramide, it does not readily penetrate the blood–brain barrier and is consequently less prone to producing central side effects. Both drugs are given orally, have plasma half-lives of 4–5 h and are excreted in the urine.

NK₁ receptor antagonists

Substance P causes vomiting when injected intravenously and is released by gastrointestinal vagal afferent nerves as well as in the vomiting centre itself. **Aprepitant** blocks substance P (NK_1) receptors (see Ch. 18) in the CTZ and vomiting centre. Aprepitant is given orally, and is effective in controlling the late phase of emesis caused by cytotoxic drugs, with few significant unwanted effects. **Fosaprepitant** is a prodrug of aprepitant, which is administered intravenously.

OTHER ANTIEMETIC DRUGS

Anecdotal evidence originally suggested the possibility of using cannabinoids (see Ch. 19) as antiemetics (see Pertwee, 2001) The synthetic cannabinol **nabilone** has been found to decrease vomiting caused by agents that stimulate the CTZ, and is sometimes effective where other drugs have failed. The antiemetic effect is antagonised by **naloxone**, which implies that opioid receptors may be important in the mechanism of action. Nabilone is given orally; it is well absorbed from the gastrointestinal tract and is metabolised in many tissues. Its plasma half-life is approximately 120 min, and its metabolites are excreted in the urine and faeces.

Unwanted effects are common, especially drowsiness, dizziness and dry mouth. Mood changes and postural hypotension are also fairly frequent. Some patients experience hallucinations and psychotic reactions, resembling the effect of other cannabinoids (see Ch. 19).

High-dose glucocorticoids (particularly **dexamethasone**; see Chs 26 and 33) can also control emesis, especially when this is caused by cytotoxic drugs. The mechanism of action is not clear. Dexamethasone can be used alone but is frequently deployed in combination with a phenothiazine, ondansetron or aprepitant.

THE MOTILITY OF THE GASTROINTESTINAL TRACT

Drugs that alter the motility of the gastrointestinal tract include:

- purgatives, which accelerate the passage of food through the intestine
- agents that increase the motility of the gastrointestinal smooth muscle without causing purgation
- antidiarrhoeal drugs, which decrease motility
- antispasmodic drugs, which decrease smooth muscle tone.

---

[9]A disabling condition named after the eponymous French physician who discovered that the nausea and vertigo that characterise this condition were associated with a disorder of the inner ear.

Clinical uses of drugs that affect the motility of the gastrointestinal tract are summarised in the clinical box below.

> ### Drugs and gastrointestinal tract motility
>
> - Purgatives include:
>   - bulk laxatives (e.g. **ispaghula husk**, first choice for slow action)
>   - osmotic laxatives (e.g. **lactulose**)
>   - faecal softeners (e.g. **docusate**)
>   - stimulant purgatives (e.g. **senna**).
> - Drugs that can increase motility without purgation:
>   - **domperidone**, used in disorders of gastric emptying.
> - Drugs used to treat diarrhoea:
>   - oral rehydration with isotonic solutions of NaCl plus glucose and starch-based cereal (important in infants)
>   - antimotility agents, e.g. **loperamide** (unwanted effects: drowsiness and nausea).

PURGATIVES

The transit of food through the intestine may be hastened by several different types of drugs, including laxatives, faecal softeners and stimulant purgatives. The latter agents may be used to relieve constipation or to clear the bowel prior to surgery or examination.

BULK AND OSMOTIC LAXATIVES

The *bulk laxatives* include **methylcellulose** and certain plant extracts such as **sterculia**, **agar**, **bran** and **ispaghula husk**. These agents are polysaccharide polymers that are not digested in the upper part of the gastrointestinal tract. They form a bulky hydrated mass in the gut lumen promoting peristalsis and improving faecal consistency. They may take several days to work but have no serious unwanted effects.

The *osmotic laxatives* consist of poorly absorbed solutes – the saline purgatives – and **lactulose**. The main salts in use are magnesium sulfate and magnesium hydroxide. By producing an osmotic load, these agents trap increased volumes of fluid in the lumen of the bowel, accelerating the transfer of the gut contents through the small intestine. This results in an abnormally large volume entering the colon, causing distension and purgation within about an hour. Abdominal cramps can occur. The amount of magnesium absorbed after an oral dose is usually too small to have adverse systemic effects, but these salts should be avoided in small children and in patients with poor renal function, in whom they can cause heart block, neuromuscular block or central nervous system depression. While isotonic or hypotonic solutions of saline purgatives cause purgation, hypertonic solutions can cause vomiting. Sometimes, other sodium salts of phosphate and citrate are given rectally, by suppository, to relieve constipation.

Lactulose is a semisynthetic disaccharide of fructose and galactose. It is poorly absorbed and produces an effect similar to that of the other osmotic laxatives. It takes 2–3 days to act. Unwanted effects, seen with high doses, include flatulence, cramps, diarrhoea and electrolyte disturbance. Tolerance can develop. Another agent, **macrogols**, which consists of inert ethylene glycol polymers, acts in the same way.

FAECAL SOFTENERS

Docusate sodium is a surface-active compound that acts in the gastrointestinal tract in a manner similar to a detergent and produces softer faeces. It is also a weak stimulant laxative. Other agents that achieve the same effect include **arachis oil**, which is given as an enema, and **liquid paraffin**, although this is now seldom used.

STIMULANT LAXATIVES

The stimulant laxative drugs act mainly by increasing electrolyte and hence water secretion by the mucosa, and also by increasing peristalsis – possibly by stimulating enteric nerves. Abdominal cramping may be experienced as a side effect with almost any of these drugs.

Bisacodyl may be given by mouth but is often given by suppository. In the latter case, it stimulates the rectal mucosa, inducing defecation in 15–30 min. Glycerol suppositories act in the same manner. **Sodium picosulfate** and docusate sodium have similar actions. The former is given orally and is often used in preparation for intestinal surgery or colonoscopy.

Senna and **dantron** are **anthroquinone** laxatives. The active principle (after hydrolysis of glycosidic linkages in the case of the plant extract, senna) directly stimulates the myenteric plexus, resulting in increased peristalsis and thus defecation. Dantron is similar. As this drug is a skin irritant and may be carcinogenic, it is generally used only in the terminally ill.

Laxatives of any type should not be used when there is obstruction of the bowel. Overuse can lead to an atonic colon where the natural propulsive activity is diminished. In these circumstances, the only way to achieve defecation is to take further amounts of laxatives, so a sort of dependency arises.

DRUGS THAT INCREASE GASTROINTESTINAL MOTILITY

Domperidone is primarily used as an antiemetic (as described above), but it also increases gastrointestinal motility (although the mechanism is unknown). Clinically, it increases lower oesophageal sphincter pressure (thus inhibiting gastro-oesophageal reflux), increases gastric emptying and enhances duodenal peristalsis. It is useful in disorders of gastric emptying and in chronic gastric reflux.

Metoclopramide (also an antiemetic) stimulates gastric motility, causing a marked acceleration of gastric emptying. It is useful in gastro-oesophageal reflux and in disorders of gastric emptying, but is ineffective in paralytic ileus.

Prucalopride is a selective 5-HT$_4$ receptor agonist that has marked prokinetic properties on the gut. It is generally only used when other types of laxative treatment have failed.

ANTIDIARRHOEAL AGENTS

There are numerous causes of diarrhoea, including underlying disease, infection, toxins and even anxiety. It may also arise as a side effect of drug or radiation therapy. The consequences range from mild discomfort and inconvenience to a medical emergency requiring hospitalisation, parenteral fluid and electrolyte replacement therapy. Globally, acute diarrhoeal disease is one of the principal causes of death in malnourished infants, especially in developing countries where medical care is less accessible and 1–2 million children die each year for want of simple counter-measures.

During an episode of diarrhoea, there is an increase in the motility of the gastrointestinal tract, accompanied by an increased secretion, coupled with a decreased absorption, of fluid. This leads to a loss of electrolytes (particularly Na⁺) and water. Cholera toxins and some other bacterial toxins produce a profound increase in electrolyte and fluid secretion by irreversibly activating the G proteins that couple the surface receptors of the mucosal cells to adenylyl cyclase (see Ch. 3).

There are three approaches to the treatment of severe acute diarrhoea:

- maintenance of fluid and electrolyte balance
- use of anti-infective agents
- use of spasmolytic or other antidiarrhoeal agents.

The maintenance of fluid and electrolyte balance by means of oral rehydration is the first priority. Wider application of this cheap and simple remedy could save the lives of many infants in the developing world. Indeed, many patients require no other treatment.

In the ileum, as in the nephron, there is co-transport of Na⁺ and glucose across the epithelial cell. The presence of glucose (and some amino acids) therefore enhances Na⁺ absorption and thus water uptake. Preparations of sodium chloride and glucose for oral rehydration are available in powder form, ready to be dissolved in water before use.

Many gastrointestinal infections are viral in origin. Those that are bacterial generally resolve fairly rapidly, so the use of anti-infective agents is usually neither necessary nor useful. Other cases may require more aggressive therapy, however. *Campylobacter* sp. is the commonest cause of bacterial gastroenteritis in the UK, and severe infections may require **ciprofloxacin**. The most common bacterial organisms encountered by travellers include *Escherichia coli*, *Salmonella* and *Shigella*, as well as protozoa such as *Giardia* and *Cryptosporidium* spp. Drug treatment (Chs 51 and 54) may be necessary in these and other more serious infections.

TRAVELLERS' DIARRHOEA

Millions of people cross international borders each year. Many travel hopefully, but many return with GI symptoms such as diarrhoea, having encountered enterotoxin-producing *E. coli* (the most common cause) or other organisms. Most infections are mild and self-limiting, requiring only oral replacement of fluid and salt, as detailed above. General principles for the drug treatment of travellers' diarrhoea are detailed by Gorbach (1987).[10]

Up-to-date information on the condition, including the prevalence of infectious organisms around the globe as well as recommended treatment guidelines, is issued in the UK by the National Travel Health Network and Centre (see Web links in the reference list).

ANTIMOTILITY AND SPASMOLYTIC AGENTS

The main pharmacological agents that decrease motility are opioids (Ch. 42) and muscarinic receptor antagonists (Ch. 13). Agents in this latter group are seldom employed as primary therapy for diarrhoea because of their actions on other systems, but small doses of **atropine** are sometimes used, combined with **diphenoxylate**. The action of **morphine**, the archetypal opiate, on the alimentary tract is complex; it increases the tone and rhythmic contractions of the intestine but diminishes propulsive activity. The pyloric, ileocolic and anal sphincters are contracted, and the tone of the large intestine is markedly increased. Its overall effect is constipating.

The main opioids used for the symptomatic relief of diarrhoea are **codeine** (a morphine congener), diphenoxylate and **loperamide** (both **pethidine** congeners that do not readily penetrate the blood–brain barrier and are used only for their actions in the gut). All may have unwanted effects, including constipation, abdominal cramps, drowsiness and dizziness. Complete loss of intestinal motility (paralytic ileus) can also occur. They should not be used in young (<4 years of age) children.

Loperamide is the drug of first choice for pharmacotherapy of travellers' diarrhoea and is a component of several proprietary antidiarrhoeal medicines. It has a relatively selective action on the gastrointestinal tract and undergoes significant enterohepatic cycling. It reduces the frequency of abdominal cramps, decreases the passage of faeces and shortens the duration of the illness.

Diphenoxylate also lacks morphine-like activity in the central nervous system, although large doses (25-fold higher) produce typical opioid effects. Preparations of diphenoxylate usually contain atropine as well. Codeine and loperamide have antisecretory actions in addition to their effects on intestinal motility.

'Endogenous opioids', enkephalins (Ch. 42), also play a role in regulation of intestinal secretion. **Racecadotril** is a prodrug of **thiorphan**, an inhibitor of enkephalinase. By preventing the breakdown of enkephalins, this drug reduces the excessive intestinal secretion seen during episodes of diarrhoea. It is used in combination with rehydration therapy.

Cannabinoid receptor agonists also reduce gut motility in animals, most probably by decreasing acetylcholine release from enteric nerves. There have been anecdotal reports of a beneficial effect of cannabis against dysentery and cholera.

Drugs that reduce gastrointestinal motility are also useful in irritable bowel syndrome and diverticular disease. Muscarinic receptor antagonists (Ch. 13) used for this purpose include atropine, hyoscine, **propantheline** and **dicycloverine**. The last named is thought to have some additional direct relaxant action on smooth muscle. All produce antimuscarinic side effects such as dry mouth, blurred vision and urinary retention. **Mebeverine**, a derivative of reserpine, has a direct relaxant action on gastrointestinal smooth muscle. Unwanted effects are few.

---

[10]Who flippantly (although accurately) observed that 'travel broadens the mind and loosens the bowels'.

ADSORBENTS

Adsorbent agents are used in the symptomatic treatment of some types of diarrhoea, although properly controlled trials proving efficacy have not been carried out. The main preparations used contain kaolin, pectin, chalk, charcoal, methylcellulose and activated attapulgite (magnesium aluminium silicate). It has been suggested that these agents may act by adsorbing microorganisms or toxins, by altering the intestinal flora or by coating and protecting the intestinal mucosa, but there is no hard evidence for this. Kaolin is sometimes given as a mixture with morphine (e.g. kaolin and morphine mixture BP).

DRUGS FOR CHRONIC BOWEL DISEASE

This category comprises *irritable bowel syndrome* (IBS) and *inflammatory bowel disease* (IBD). IBS is characterised by bouts of diarrhoea, constipation or abdominal pain. The aetiology of the disease is uncertain, but psychological factors may play a part. Treatment is symptomatic, with a high-residue diet plus loperamide or a laxative if needed.

Ulcerative colitis and *Crohn's disease* are forms of IBD, affecting the colon or ileum. They are autoimmune inflammatory disorders, which can be severe and progressive, requiring long-term drug treatment with anti-inflammatory and immunosuppressant drugs (see Ch. 26), and occasionally surgical resection. The following agents are commonly used.

GLUCOCORTICOIDS

Glucocorticoids are potent anti-inflammatory agents and are dealt with in Chapters 26 and 33. The drugs of choice are generally **prednisolone** or **budesonide** (although others can be used). They are administered orally or locally into the bowel by suppository or enema.

AMINOSALICYLATES

While glucocorticoids are useful for the acute attacks of inflammatory bowel diseases, they are not the ideal for the long-term treatment because of their side effects. Maintenance of remission in both ulcerative colitis and Crohn's disease is generally achieved with aminosalicylates, although they are less useful in the latter condition.

Sulfasalazine consists of the sulfonamide sulfapyridine linked to 5-aminosalicylic acid (5-ASA). The latter forms the active moiety when it is released in the colon. Its mechanism of action is obscure. It may reduce inflammation by scavenging free radicals, by inhibiting prostaglandin and leukotriene production, and/or by decreasing neutrophil chemotaxis and superoxide generation. Its unwanted effects include diarrhoea, salicylate sensitivity and interstitial nephritis. 5-ASA is not absorbed, but the sulfapyridine moiety, which seems to be therapeutically inert in this instance, is absorbed, and its unwanted effects are those associated with the sulfonamides (see Ch. 51).

Newer compounds in this class, which presumably share a similar mechanism of action, include **mesalazine** (5-ASA itself), **olsalazine** (a 5-ASA dimer linked by a bond that is hydrolysed by colonic bacteria) and **balsalazide** (a prodrug from which 5-ASA is also released following hydrolysis of a diazo linkage).

OTHER DRUGS

Methotrexate and the immunosuppressants **ciclosporin**, **azathioprine** and **6-mercaptopurine** (see Ch. 26) are also sometimes used in patients with severe inflammatory bowel disease. The biologics **infliximab** and **adalimumab**, monoclonal antibodies directed against tumour necrosis factor (TNF)-α, (see Ch. 26) have also been used with success. These drugs are expensive, and in the UK their use is restricted to moderate and severe Crohn's disease that is unresponsive to glucocorticoids or immunomodulators.

The antiallergy drug sodium **cromoglicate** (see Ch. 28) is sometimes used for treating gastrointestinal symptoms associated with food allergies.

DRUGS AFFECTING THE BILIARY SYSTEM

The commonest pathological condition of the biliary tract is *cholesterol cholelithiasis* – the formation of gallstones with high cholesterol content. Surgery is generally the preferred option, but there are orally active drugs that dissolve non-calcified 'radiolucent' cholesterol gallstones. The principal agent is **ursodeoxycholic acid**, a minor constituent of human bile (but the main bile acid in the bear, hence *urso-*). Diarrhoea is the main unwanted effect.

Biliary colic, the pain produced by the passage of gallstones through the bile duct, can be very intense, and immediate relief may be required. Morphine relieves the pain effectively, but it may have an undesirable local effect because it constricts the sphincter of Oddi and raises the pressure in the bile duct. **Buprenorphine** may be preferable. Pethidine has similar actions, although it relaxes other smooth muscle, for example that of the ureter. Atropine is commonly employed to relieve biliary spasm because it has antispasmodic action and may be used in conjunction with morphine. **Glyceryl trinitrate** (see Ch. 21) can produce a marked fall of intrabiliary pressure and may be used to relieve biliary spasm.

FUTURE DIRECTIONS

You might be forgiven for thinking that the widespread availability of several different types of safe antisecretory drug would have satisfied the current medical need for peptic ulcer treatment, but this is not so. Although the incidence of GI ulcers has dropped, thanks to the use of these drugs, other diseases associated with excess acid production (GORD, NSAID-induced damage) are on the increase, at least in the 'developed' countries. There are also many reasons why the existing drugs fail to perform adequately in some patients or become less active with longer duration treatments.

The quest for novel antisecretory drugs is therefore an ongoing task. Amongst the newer agents that are being actively considered are H_3 antagonists, gastrin receptor antagonists and potassium competitive acid-blocking drugs. The latter agents work because potassium ions are exchanged for protons by the proton pump (see Fig. 30.1) and so potassium antagonists would represent an alternative modality for inhibiting the secretion of acid. Unfortunately, the agents produced so far have been disappointing in clinical trial. An account of the unmet need in this area is given by Krznaric et al. (2011).

REFERENCES AND FURTHER READING

Innervation and hormones of the gastrointestinal tract

Hansen, M.B., 2003. The enteric nervous system II: gastrointestinal functions. Pharmacol. Toxicol. 92, 249–257. (*Small review on the role of the enteric nervous system in the control of gastrointestinal motility, secretory activity, blood flow and immune status; easy to read*)

Sanger, G.J., 2004. Neurokinin NK_1 and NK_3 receptors as targets for drugs to treat gastrointestinal motility disorders and pain. Br. J. Pharmacol. 141, 1303–1312. (*Useful review that deals with the present and potential future uses of neurokinin antagonists in gastrointestinal physiology and pathology*)

Spiller, R., 2002. Serotonergic modulating drugs for functional gastrointestinal diseases. Br. J. Clin. Pharmacol. 54, 11–20. (*An excellent and 'easily digestible' article describing the latest thinking on the use of 5-hydroxytryptamine agonists and antagonists in gastrointestinal function; useful diagrams*)

Gastric secretion

Binder, H.J., Donaldson, R.M. Jr., 1978. Effect of cimetidine on intrinsic factor and pepsin secretion in man. Gastroenterology 74, 371–375.

Chen, D., Friis-Hansen, L., Håkanson, R., Zhao, C.-M., 2005. Genetic dissection of the signaling pathways that control gastric acid secretion. Inflammopharmacology 13, 201–207. (*Describes experiments using receptor 'knock outs' to analyse the mechanisms that control gastric acid production*)

Cui, G., Waldum, H.L., 2007. Physiological and clinical significance of enterochromaffin-like cell activation in the regulation of gastric acid secretion. World J. Gastroenterol 13, 493–496. (*Short review on the central role of ECL cells in the regulation of gastric acid secretion. Easy to read*)

Horn, J., 2000. The proton-pump inhibitors: similarities and differences. Clin. Ther. 22, 266–280, discussion 265. (*Excellent overview*)

Huang, J.Q., Hunt, R.H., 2001. Pharmacological and pharmacodynamic essentials of H(2)-receptor antagonists and proton pump inhibitors for the practising physician. Best Pract. Res. Clin. Gastroenterol. 15, 355–370.

Krznaric, Z., Ljubas Kelecic, D., Rustemovic, N., et al., 2011. Pharmaceutical principles of acid inhibitors: unmet needs. Dig. Dis. 29, 469–475. (*A good account of the shortcomings of current anti-secretory drugs and the need for innovation in the field*)

Linberg, P., Brandstrom, A., Wallmark, B., 1987. Structure activity relationships of omeprazole analogues and their mechanism of action. Trends Pharmacol. Sci. 8, 399–402.

Schubert, M.L., Peura, D.A., 2008. Control of gastric acid secretion in health and disease. Gastroenterology 134, 1842–1860. (*Excellent review of the physiology and pharmacology of gastric acid secretion. Authoritative and well illustrated*)

Drugs in GI disorders

Axon, A.T., 2007. Relationship between *Helicobacter pylori* gastritis, gastric cancer and gastric acid secretion. Adv. Med. Sci. 52, 55–60. (*Takes a critical look at the epidemiological evidence for the relationship between* H. pylori *infection and gastric cancer*)

Black, J.W., Duncan, W.A.M., Durant, C.J., et al., 1972. Definition and antagonism of histamine H_2-receptors. Nature 236, 385–390. (*Seminal paper outlining the pharmacological approach to inhibition of acid secretion through antagonism at an alternative histamine receptor*)

Blaser, M.J., 1998. *Helicobacter pylori* and gastric diseases. BMJ 316, 1507–1510. (*Succinct review, emphasis on future developments*)

Klotz, U., 2000. The role of aminosalicylates at the beginning of the new millennium in the treatment of chronic inflammatory bowel disease. Eur. J. Clin. Pharmacol. 56, 353–362.

Mossner, J., Caca, K., 2005. Developments in the inhibition of gastric acid secretion. Eur. J. Clin. Invest. 35, 469–475. (*Useful overview of several new directions in gastrointestinal drug development*)

Pertwee, R.G., 2001. Cannabinoids and the gastrointestinal tract. Gut 48, 859–867.

Nausea and vomiting

Andrews, P.I., Horn, C.C., 2006. Signals for nausea and emesis: implications for models of upper gastrointestinal diseases. Auton. Neurosci. 125, 100–115.

Hesketh, P.J., 2001. Potential role of the NK_1 receptor antagonists in chemotherapy-induced nausea and vomiting. Support. Care Cancer 9, 350–354.

Hornby, P.J., 2001. Central neurocircuitry associated with emesis. Am. J. Med. 111, 106S–112S. (*Comprehensive review of central control of vomiting*)

Rojas, C., Slusher, B.S., 2012. Pharmacological mechanisms of 5-HT(3) and tachykinin NK(1) receptor antagonism to prevent chemotherapy-induced nausea and vomiting. Eur. J. Pharmacol. 684, 1–7.

Tramèr, M.R., Moore, R., Reynolds, D.J., McQuay, H.J., 1997. A quantitative systematic review of ondansetron in treatment of established postoperative nausea and vomiting. Br. Med. J. 314, 1088–1092.

Yates, B.J., Miller, A.D., Lucot, J.B., 1998. Physiological basis and pharmacology of motion sickness: an update. Brain Res. Bull. 5, 395–406. (*Good account of the mechanisms underlying motion sickness and its treatment*)

Motility of the gastrointestinal tract

De Las Casas, C., Adachi, J., Dupont, H., 1999. Travellers' diarrhoea. Aliment. Pharmacol. Ther. 13, 1373–1378. (*Review article*)

Gorbach, S.L., 1987. Bacterial diarrhoea and its treatment. Lancet ii, 1378–1382.

The biliary system

Bateson, M.C., 1997. Bile acid research and applications. Lancet 349, 5–6.

Useful Web resources

<www.nathnac.org> (*This is the site for the UK Health Protection Agency's National Travel Health Network and Centre. There are two components to the site, one for lay people and one for health professionals. Click on the latter and enter 'Travellers' diarrhoea' as a search term to retrieve current information and advice*)

31

The control of blood glucose and drug treatment of diabetes mellitus

OVERVIEW

In this chapter we describe the endocrine control of blood glucose by pancreatic hormones, especially *insulin* but also *glucagon* and *somatostatin*, and the gut hormones (*incretins*) *glucagon-like peptide-1* (GLP-1) and *gastric inhibitory peptide* (GIP, which is also known as glucose-dependent insulinotropic peptide). This underpins coverage of diabetes mellitus and its treatment with insulin preparations (including insulin analogues), and other hypoglycaemic agents – metformin, sulfonylureas, α-glucosidase inhibitors, glitazones, long-acting incretin mimetics such as exenatide, and gliptins, which potentiate incretins by blocking their degradation.

INTRODUCTION

Insulin is the main hormone controlling intermediary metabolism. Its most striking acute effect is to lower blood glucose. Reduced (or absent) secretion of insulin causes *diabetes mellitus*. It is often coupled with reduced sensitivity to its action, 'insulin resistance', which is closely related to obesity. Diabetes mellitus, recognised since ancient times, is named for the production of sugary urine in copious volumes (due to the osmotic diuretic action of the high urine glucose concentration). Diabetes is rapidly increasing to epidemic proportions (in step with obesity, Ch. 32), and its consequences are dire – especially accelerated atherosclerosis (myocardial and cerebral infarction, gangrene or limb amputation), kidney failure, neuropathy and blindness.

In this chapter, we first describe the control of blood sugar. The second part of the chapter is devoted to the different kinds of diabetes mellitus and the role of drugs in their treatment. Diabetes, along with obesity (Ch. 32), hypertension (Ch. 22) and dyslipidaemia (Ch. 23), comprise what is now termed 'metabolic syndrome', a common pathological cluster and a rapidly growing problem that is associated with many life-threatening conditions. New drugs, including several directed at controlling blood sugar, have been developed in recent years that act on some of the many mechanisms that become deranged in metabolic syndrome. Despite the effort and creativity that have gone into it, clinical success has so far been modest.

CONTROL OF BLOOD GLUCOSE

Glucose is the obligatory source of energy for the adult brain, and physiological control of blood glucose reflects the need to maintain adequate fuel supplies in the face of intermittent food intake and variable metabolic demands.

More fuel is made available by feeding than is required immediately, and excess calories are stored as glycogen or fat. During fasting, these energy stores need to be mobilised in a regulated manner. The most important regulatory hormone is *insulin*, the actions of which are described below. Increased blood glucose stimulates insulin secretion (Fig. 31.1), whereas reduced blood glucose reduces insulin secretion. The effect of glucose on insulin secretion depends on whether the glucose load is administered intravenously or by mouth. Glucose administered by mouth is more effective in stimulating insulin secretion because it stimulates release from the gut of incretin hormones which promote insulin secretion (Fig. 31.1). Glucose is less effective in stimulating insulin secretion in patients with diabetes (Fig. 31.2). *Hypoglycaemia*, caused by excessive exogenous insulin, not only reduces endogenous insulin secretion but also elicits secretion of an array of 'counter-regulatory' hormones, including *glucagon, adrenaline* (Ch. 14), *glucocorticoids* (Ch. 33) and *growth hormone* (Ch. 33), all of which increase blood glucose. Their main effects on glucose uptake and carbohydrate metabolism are summarised and contrasted with those of insulin in Table 31.1.

PANCREATIC ISLET HORMONES

The islets of Langerhans, the endocrine part of the pancreas, contain four main types of peptide-secreting cells: B (or β) cells secrete *insulin*, A (or α) cells secrete *glucagon*, D cells secrete *somatostatin,* and PP cells secrete *pancreatic polypeptide* (PP).

▼ PP is a 36 amino acid peptide closely related to neuropeptide Y (Ch. 14) and peptide YY (Ch. 32). It is released by eating a meal and is implicated in control of food intake (Ch. 32): PP acts on G protein-coupled receptors and also inhibits secretion of exocrine pancreatic secretions and contraction of intestinal and biliary smooth muscle.

The core of each islet contains mainly the predominant B cells surrounded by a mantle of A cells interspersed with D cells or PP cells (see Fig. 31.1). In addition to insulin, B cells secrete a peptide known as *islet amyloid polypeptide* or *amylin* which delays gastric emptying and opposes insulin by stimulating glycogen breakdown in striated muscle, and C-peptide (see p. 381). Glucagon opposes insulin, increasing blood glucose and stimulating protein breakdown in muscle. Somatostatin inhibits secretion of insulin and of glucagon. It is widely distributed outside the pancreas and is also released from the hypothalamus, inhibiting the release of growth hormone from the pituitary gland (Ch. 33).

INSULIN

Insulin was the first protein for which the amino acid sequence was determined (by Sanger's group in

Table 31.1   The effect of hormones on blood glucose

Hormone	Main actions	Main stimuli for secretion	Main effect
Main regulatory hormone			
Insulin	↑ Glucose uptake ↑ Glycogen synthesis ↓ Glycogenolysis ↓ Gluconeogenesis	Acute rise in blood glucoseIncretins (GIP and GLP-1)	↓ Blood glucose
Main counter-regulatory hormones			
Glucagon	↑ Glycogenolysis ↑ Glyconeogenesis		
Adrenaline (epinephrine)	↑ Glycogenolysis	Hypoglycaemia (i.e. blood glucose <3 mmol/l), (e.g. with exercise, stress, high protein meals), etc.	↑ Blood glucose
Glucocorticoids	↓ Glucose uptake ↑ Gluconeogenesis ↓ Glucose uptake and utilisation		
Growth hormone	↓ Glucose uptake		

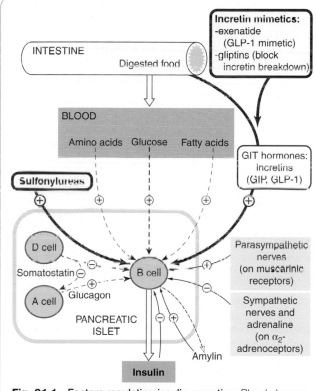

Fig. 31.1   Factors regulating insulin secretion. Blood glucose is the most important factor. Drugs used to stimulate insulin secretion are shown in red-bordered boxes. Glucagon potentiates insulin release but opposes some of its peripheral actions and increases blood glucose. GIP, gastric inhibitory peptide; GIT, gastrointestinal tract; GLP-1, glucagon-like peptide-1.

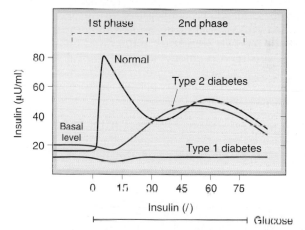

Fig. 31.2   Schematic diagram of the two-phase release of insulin in response to a constant glucose infusion. The first phase is missing in type 2 (non-insulin-dependent) diabetes mellitus, and both are missing in type 1 (insulin-dependent) diabetes mellitus. The first phase is also produced by amino acids, sulfonylureas, glucagon and gastrointestinal tract hormones. *(Data from Pfeifer MA, Halter JB, Porte D Jr 1981 Am J Med 70, 579–588.)*

Cambridge in 1955). It consists of two peptide chains (of 21 and 30 amino acid residues) linked by two disulfide bonds.

SYNTHESIS AND SECRETION

Like other peptide hormones (see Ch. 19), insulin is synthesised as a precursor (preproinsulin) in the rough endoplasmic reticulum. Preproinsulin is transported to the Golgi apparatus, where it undergoes proteolytic cleavage to proinsulin and then to insulin plus a fragment of uncertain function called C-peptide.[1] Insulin and C-peptide are stored in granules in B cells, and are normally co-secreted by exocytosis in equimolar amounts together with smaller and variable amounts of proinsulin.

The main factor controlling the synthesis and secretion of insulin is the blood glucose concentration (Fig. 31.1). B cells respond both to the absolute glucose concentration and to the rate of change of blood glucose. Other

---

[1]Not to be confused with C-reactive peptide, which is an acute-phase reactant used clinically as a marker of inflammation (Ch. 6).

Table 31.2 Effects of insulin on carbohydrate, fat and protein metabolism

Type of metabolism	Liver cells	Fat cells	Muscle
Carbohydrate metabolism	↓ Gluconeogenesis ↓ Glycogenolysis ↑ Glycolysis ↑ Glycogenesis	↑ Glucose uptake ↑ Glycerol synthesis	↑ Glucose uptake ↑ Glycolysis ↑ Glycogenesis
Fat metabolism	↑ Lipogenesis ↓ Lipolysis	↑ Synthesis of triglycerides ↑ Fatty acid synthesis ↓ Lipolysis	
Protein metabolism	↓ Protein breakdown	–	↑ Amino acid uptake ↑ Protein synthesis

physiological stimuli to insulin release include amino acids (particularly arginine and leucine), fatty acids, the parasympathetic nervous system and *incretins* (especially *GLP-1* and *GIP*, see p. 385). Pharmacologically, sulfonylurea drugs (see p. 388-389) act by releasing insulin.

There is a steady basal release of insulin and an increase in blood glucose stimulates an additional response. This response has two phases: an initial rapid phase reflecting release of stored hormone, and a slower, delayed phase reflecting continued release of stored hormone and new synthesis (Fig. 31.2). The response is abnormal in diabetes mellitus, as discussed later.

ATP-sensitive potassium channels (K_{ATP}; Ch. 4) determine the resting membrane potential in B cells. Glucose enters B cells via a surface membrane transporter called Glut-2, and its subsequent metabolism via glucokinase (which is the rate-limiting glycolytic enzyme in B cells) links insulin secretion to extracellular glucose. The consequent rise in ATP within B cells blocks K_{ATP} channels, causing membrane depolarisation. Depolarisation opens voltage-dependent calcium channels, leading to Ca^{2+} influx. This triggers insulin secretion in the presence of amplifying messengers including diacylglycerol, non-esterified arachidonic acid (which facilitates further Ca^{2+} entry), and 12-lipoxygenase products of arachidonic acid (mainly *12-S-hydroxyeicosatetraenoic acid* or 12-S-HETE; see Ch. 17). Phospholipases are commonly activated by Ca^{2+}, but free arachidonic acid is liberated in B cells by an ATP-sensitive Ca^{2+}-insensitive (ASCI) phospholipase A_2. Consequently, in B cells, Ca^{2+} entry and arachidonic acid production are both driven by ATP, linking cellular energy status to insulin secretion.

Insulin release is inhibited by the sympathetic nervous system (Fig. 31.1). Adrenaline (epinephrine) increases blood glucose by inhibiting insulin release (via α_2 adrenoceptors) and by promoting glycogenolysis via β_2 adrenoceptors in striated muscle and liver. Several peptides, including somatostatin, galanin (an endogenous K_{ATP} activator) and amylin, also inhibit insulin release.

About one-fifth of the insulin stored in the pancreas of the human adult is secreted daily. The plasma insulin concentration after an overnight fast is 20–50 pmol/l. Plasma insulin concentration is reduced in patients with type 1 (insulin-dependent) diabetes mellitus (see p. 386), and markedly increased in patients with *insulinomas* (uncommon functioning tumours of B cells), as is C-peptide, with which it is co-released.[2] It is also raised in obesity and other normoglycaemic insulin-resistant states.

ACTIONS

Insulin is the main hormone controlling intermediary metabolism, having its main actions on liver, fat and muscle (Table 31.2). It is an *anabolic hormone*: its overall effect is to conserve fuel by facilitating the uptake and storage of glucose, amino acids and fats after a meal. Acutely, it reduces blood glucose. Consequently, a fall in plasma insulin increases blood glucose. The biochemical pathways through which insulin exerts its effects are summarised in Figure 31.3, and molecular aspects of its mechanism are discussed below.

Insulin influences glucose metabolism in most tissues, especially the liver, where it inhibits glycogenolysis (glycogen breakdown) and gluconeogenesis (synthesis of glucose from non-carbohydrate sources) while stimulating glycogen synthesis. It also increases glucose utilisation by glycolysis, but the overall effect is to increase hepatic glycogen stores.

In muscle, unlike liver, uptake of glucose is slow and is the rate-limiting step in carbohydrate metabolism. Insulin causes a glucose transporter called Glut-4 which is sequestered in vesicles to be expressed within minutes on the surface membrane. This facilitates glucose uptake, and stimulates glycogen synthesis and glycolysis.

Insulin increases glucose uptake by Glut-4 in adipose tissue as well as in muscle. One of the main products of glucose metabolism in adipose tissue is glycerol, which is esterified with fatty acids to form triglycerides, thereby affecting fat metabolism (see Table 31.2).

Insulin increases synthesis of fatty acid and triglyceride in adipose tissue and in liver. It inhibits lipolysis, partly via dephosphorylation – and hence inactivation – of lipases (Table 31.2). It also inhibits the lipolytic actions of adrenaline, growth hormone and glucagon by opposing their actions on adenylyl cyclase.

---

[2]Insulin for injection does not contain C-peptide, which therefore provides a means of distinguishing endogenous from exogenous insulin. This is used to differentiate insulinoma (an insulin-secreting tumour causing high circulating insulin with high C-peptide) from surreptitious injection of insulin (high insulin with low C-peptide). Deliberate induction of hypoglycaemia by self-injection with insulin is a well-recognised, if unusual, manifestation of psychiatric disorder, especially in health professionals – it has also been used in murder.

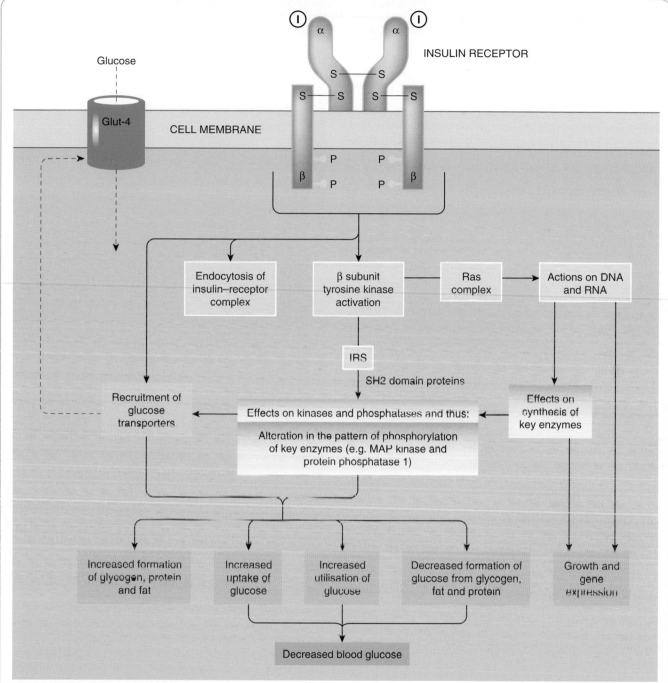

Fig. 31.3 **Insulin signalling pathways.** I, insulin; Glut-4, an insulin-sensitive glucose transporter present in muscle and fat cells; IRS, insulin receptor substrate (several forms: 1–4).

Insulin stimulates uptake of amino acids into muscle and increases protein synthesis. It also decreases protein catabolism and inhibits oxidation of amino acids in the liver.

Other metabolic effects of insulin include transport into cells of K^+, Ca^{2+}, nucleosides and inorganic phosphate.[3]

Long-term effects of insulin

In addition to rapid effects on metabolism, exerted via altered activity of enzymes and transport proteins, insulin has long-term actions via altered enzyme synthesis. It is an important anabolic hormone during fetal development. It stimulates cell proliferation and is implicated in somatic and visceral growth and development.

Mitogenic actions of insulin are of great concern in the development of insulin analogues; **insulin glargine** (one widely used analogue; see p. 387) is six- to eight-fold more

---

[3]The action on K^+ is exploited in the emergency treatment of hyperkalaemia by intravenous glucose with insulin (see Ch. 29).

mitogenic than human insulin, and cultured breast cancer cells proliferate in response to near-therapeutic concentrations of this analogue *in vitro*, but it is not known if there is any clinically significant parallel *in vivo*. Mammary tumours developed in rats given one long-acting insulin analogue.

Mechanism of action

Insulin binds to a specific receptor on the surface of its target cells. The receptor is a large transmembrane glycoprotein complex belonging to the tyrosine kinase-linked type 3 receptor superfamily (Ch. 3) and consisting of two α and two β subunits (Fig. 31.3). Occupied receptors aggregate into clusters, which are subsequently internalised in vesicles, resulting in downregulation. Internalised insulin is degraded in lysosomes, but the receptors are recycled to the plasma membrane.

▼ The signal transduction mechanisms that link receptor binding to the biological effects of insulin are complex. Receptor autophosphorylation – the first step in signal transduction – is a consequence of dimerisation, allowing each receptor to phosphorylate the other, as explained in Chapter 3.

Insulin receptor substrate (IRS) proteins undergo rapid tyrosine phosphorylation specifically in response to insulin and insulin-like growth factor-1 but not to other growth factors. The best-characterised substrate is IRS-1, which contains 22 tyrosine residues that are potential phosphorylation sites. It interacts with proteins that contain a so-called SH2 domain (see Ch. 3, Fig. 3.15), thereby passing on the insulin signal. Knockout mice lacking IRS-1 are hyporesponsive to insulin (insulin-resistant) but do not become diabetic, because of robust B-cell compensation with increased insulin secretion. By contrast, mice lacking IRS-2 fail to compensate and develop overt diabetes, implicating the IRS-2 gene as a candidate for human type 2 diabetes (IRS proteins are reviewed by Lee & White, 2004). Activation of phosphatidylinositol 3-kinase by interaction of its SH2 domain with phosphorylated IRS has several important effects, including recruitment of insulin-sensitive glucose transporters (Glut-4) from the Golgi apparatus to the plasma membrane in muscle and fat cells.

The longer-term actions of insulin entail effects on DNA and RNA, mediated partly at least by the Ras signalling complex. Ras is a protein that regulates cell growth and cycles between an active GTP-bound form and an inactive GDP-bound form (see Chs 3 and 56). Insulin shifts the equilibrium in favour of the active form, and initiates a phosphorylation cascade that results in activation of mitogen-activated protein kinase (MAP-kinase), which in turn activates several nuclear transcription factors, leading to the expression of genes that are involved with cell growth and with intermediary metabolism.

Insulin for treatment of diabetes mellitus is considered below.

GLUCAGON

SYNTHESIS AND SECRETION

Glucagon is a single-chain polypeptide of 21 amino acid residues synthesised mainly in the A cell of the islets, but also in the upper gastrointestinal tract. It has considerable structural homology with other gastrointestinal tract hormones, including secretin, vasoactive intestinal peptide and GIP (see Ch. 30).

Amino acids (especially L-arginine) stimulate glucagon secretion and ingestion of a high-protein meal increases glucagon secretion, but diurnal variation in plasma glucagon concentrations is less than for insulin. Glucagon secretion is stimulated by low and inhibited by high concentrations of glucose and fatty acids in the plasma. Sympathetic nerve activity and circulating adrenaline stimulate

glucagon release via β adrenoceptors. Parasympathetic nerve activity also increases secretion, whereas somatostatin, released from D cells adjacent to the glucagon-secreting A cells in the periphery of the islets, inhibits glucagon release.

> ### Endocrine pancreas and blood glucose
>
> - Islets of Langerhans secrete insulin from B (or β) cells, glucagon from A cells and somatostatin from D cells.
> - Many factors stimulate insulin secretion, but the main one is blood glucose. Incretins, especially GIP and GLP-1 secreted, respectively, by K and L cells in the gut are also important.
> - Insulin has essential metabolic actions as a fuel storage hormone and also affects cell growth and differentiation. It decreases blood glucose by:
>   - increasing glucose uptake into muscle and fat via Glut-4
>   - increasing glycogen synthesis
>   - decreasing gluconeogenesis
>   - decreasing glycogen breakdown.
> - Glucagon is a fuel-mobilising hormone, stimulating gluconeogenesis and glycogenolysis, also lipolysis and proteolysis. It increases blood sugar and also increases the force of contraction of the heart.
> - Diabetes mellitus is a chronic metabolic disorder in which there is hyperglycaemia. There are two main types:
>   - type 1 (insulin-dependent) diabetes, with an absolute deficiency of insulin
>   - type 2 (non-insulin-dependent) diabetes, with a relative deficiency of insulin associated with reduced sensitivity to its action (insulin resistance).

ACTIONS

Glucagon increases blood glucose and causes breakdown of fat and protein. It acts on specific G protein-coupled receptors to stimulate adenylyl cyclase, and its actions are somewhat similar to β-adrenoceptor-mediated actions of adrenaline. Unlike adrenaline, however, its metabolic effects are more pronounced than its cardiovascular actions. Glucagon is proportionately more active on liver, while the metabolic actions of adrenaline are more pronounced on muscle and fat. Glucagon stimulates glycogen breakdown and gluconeogenesis, and inhibits glycogen synthesis and glucose oxidation. Its metabolic actions on target tissues are thus the opposite of those of insulin. Glucagon increases the rate and force of contraction of the heart, although less markedly than adrenaline.

Clinical uses of glucagon are summarised in the clinical box.

SOMATOSTATIN

Somatostatin is secreted by the D cells of the islets. It is also generated in the hypothalamus, where it acts to inhibit the release of growth hormone (see Ch. 32). In the

Clinical uses of glucagon

- **Glucagon** can be given intramuscularly or subcutaneously as well as intravenously.
- Treatment of *hypoglycaemia* in unconscious patients (who cannot drink); unlike intravenous glucose, it can be administered by non-medical personnel (e.g. spouses or ambulance crew). It is useful if obtaining intravenous access is difficult.
- Treatment of *acute cardiac failure* precipitated by β-adrenoceptor antagonists.

islet, it inhibits release of insulin and of glucagon. **Octreotide** is a long-acting analogue of somatostatin. It inhibits release of a number of hormones, and is used clinically to relieve symptoms from several uncommon gastroenteropancreatic endocrine tumours, and for treatment of acromegaly[4] (the endocrine disorder caused by a functioning tumour of cells that secrete growth hormone from the anterior pituitary; see Ch. 33).

AMYLIN (ISLET AMYLOID POLYPEPTIDE)

▼ The term *amyloid* refers to amorphous protein deposits in different tissues that occur in a variety of diseases, including several neurodegenerative conditions (see Ch. 40). Amyloid deposits occur in the pancreas of patients with diabetes mellitus, although it is not known if this is functionally important. The major component of pancreatic amyloid is a 37-amino acid residue peptide known as islet amyloid polypeptide or amylin. This is stored with insulin in secretory granules in B cells and is co-secreted with insulin. Amylin delays gastric emptying. Supraphysiological concentrations stimulate the breakdown of glycogen to lactate in striated muscle. Amylin also inhibits insulin secretion (Fig. 31.1). It is structurally related to calcitonin (see Ch. 36) and has weak calcitonin-like actions on calcium metabolism and osteoclast activity. It is also about 50% identical with calcitonin gene-related peptide (CGRP; see Ch. 18), and large intravenous doses cause vasodilatation, presumably by an action on CGRP receptors.

Pramlintide, an amylin analogue with three proline substitutions that reduce its tendency to aggregate into insoluble fibrils, has been licensed since 2005 by the FDA for patients with type 1 diabetes and for type 2 diabetics who use insulin. It is injected subcutaneously before meals as an adjunct to insulin, and reduces insulin requirements. Unwanted effects include hypoglycaemia and nausea – it is contraindicated in patients with loss of gastric motility (gastroparesis), a complication of diabetic autonomic neuropathy (Younk et al., 2011).

INCRETINS

La Barre suggested in the 1930s that crude secretin contained two active principles: 'excretin', which stimulates the exocrine pancreas, and 'incretin', which stimulates insulin release. He proposed that incretin presented possibilities for the treatment of diabetes. 'Excretin' did not

catch on (perhaps not helped by an unfortunate association with other bodily functions – at least to an Anglo-Saxon ear), but 'incretin' has gone from strength to strength, and some 80 years later several incretin-based drugs are now licensed for clinical use (see below). Incretin action proved to be due to peptide hormones released from the gut, mainly *glucagon-like insulinotropic peptide* (GIP) and *glucagon like peptide-1* (GLP-1). These are both members of the glucagon peptide superfamily (Ch. 18). GIP is a 42-amino acid peptide stored in and secreted by enteroendocrine K cells in the duodenum and proximal jejunum. GLP-1 is secreted by L cells which are more widely distributed in the gut, including in the ileum and colon as well as more proximally. Two forms of GLP-1 are secreted after a meal: GLP-1(7-37) and GLP-1(7-36) amide; these are similarly potent. Most of the circulating activity is due to GLP-1(7-36) amide. Release of GIP and GLP-1 by ingested food provides an early stimulus to insulin secretion before absorbed glucose or other products of digestion reach the islet cells in the portal blood (Fig. 31.1). As well as stimulating insulin secretion, both these hormones inhibit pancreatic glucagon secretion and slow the rate of absorption of digested food by reducing gastric emptying. They are also implicated in control of food intake via appetite and satiety (see Ch. 32). The actions of GIP and GLP-1 are terminated rapidly by dipeptidyl peptidase-4 (DPP-4). This enzyme is a membrane glycoprotein with rather wide substrate specificity – it has been implicated in suppression of malignancy (e.g. Yu et al., 2010).

DIABETES MELLITUS

Diabetes mellitus is a chronic metabolic disorder characterised by a high blood glucose concentration – hyperglycaemia (fasting plasma glucose >7.0 mmol/l, or plasma glucose >11.1 mmol/l, 2 h after a meal) – caused by insulin deficiency, often combined with insulin resistance. Hyperglycaemia occurs because of uncontrolled hepatic glucose output and reduced uptake of glucose by skeletal muscle with reduced glycogen synthesis. When the renal threshold for glucose reabsorption is exceeded, glucose spills over into the urine (glycosuria) and causes an osmotic diuresis (polyuria) which, in turn, results in dehydration, thirst and increased drinking (polydipsia). Insulin deficiency causes muscle wasting through increased breakdown and reduced synthesis of proteins. Diabetic ketoacidosis is an acute emergency. It develops in the absence of insulin because of accelerated breakdown of fat to acetyl-CoA, which, in the absence of aerobic carbohydrate metabolism, is converted to acetoacetate and β-hydroxybutyrate (which cause acidosis) and acetone (a ketone).

Various complications develop as a consequence of the metabolic derangements in diabetes, often over several years. Many of these are the result of disease of blood vessels, either large (macrovascular disease) or small (microangiopathy). Dysfunction of vascular endothelium (see Ch. 22) is an early and critical event in the development of vascular complications. Oxygen-derived free radicals, protein kinase C and non-enzymic products of glucose and albumin called *advanced glycation end products* (AGE) have been implicated. Macrovascular disease consists of accelerated atheroma (Ch. 23) and its

[4]Octreotide is used either short term before surgery on the pituitary tumour, or while waiting for radiotherapy of the tumour to take effect, or if other treatments have been ineffective.

385

thrombotic complications (Ch. 24), which are commoner and more severe in diabetic patients. Microangiopathy is a distinctive feature of diabetes mellitus and particularly affects the retina, kidney and peripheral nerves. Diabetes mellitus is the commonest cause of chronic renal failure, a huge and rapidly increasing problem, and a major burden to society as well as to individual patients. Coexistent hypertension promotes progressive renal damage, and treatment of hypertension slows the progression of diabetic nephropathy and reduces the risk of myocardial infarction. Angiotensin-converting enzyme inhibitors or angiotensin receptor antagonists (Ch. 22) are more effective in preventing diabetic nephropathy than other antihypertensive drugs, perhaps because they prevent fibroproliferative actions of angiotensin II and aldosterone.

Diabetic neuropathy[5] is associated with accumulation of osmotically active metabolites of glucose, produced by the action of aldose reductase, but *aldose reductase inhibitors* have been disappointing as therapeutic drugs (see Farmer et al., 2012, for a review).

There are two main types of diabetes mellitus:

1. **Type 1 diabetes** (previously known as insulin-dependent diabetes mellitus – IDDM – or juvenile-onset diabetes).
2. **Type 2 diabetes** (previously known as non-insulin-dependent diabetes mellitus – NIDDM – or maturity-onset diabetes).

In type 1 diabetes, there is an absolute deficiency of insulin resulting from autoimmune destruction of pancreatic B cells. Without insulin treatment, such patients will sooner or later die with diabetic ketoacidosis.

▼ Type 1 diabetes can occur at any age, but patients are usually young (children or adolescents) and not obese when they first develop symptoms. There is an inherited predisposition, with a 10–15-fold increased incidence in first-degree relatives of an index case, and strong associations with particular histocompatibility antigens (HLA types). Identical twins are less than fully concordant, so environmental factors such as viral infection (e.g. with coxsackievirus or echovirus) are believed to be necessary for genetically predisposed individuals to express the disease. Viral infection may damage pancreatic B cells and expose antigens that initiate a self-perpetuating autoimmune process. The patient becomes overtly diabetic only when more than 90% of the B cells have been destroyed. This natural history provides a tantalising prospect of intervening in the prediabetic stage, and a variety of strategies have been mooted, including immunosuppression, early insulin therapy, antioxidants, nicotinamide and many others; so far these have disappointed, but this remains a very active field.

Type 2 diabetes is accompanied both by insulin resistance (which precedes overt disease) and by impaired insulin secretion, each of which are important in its pathogenesis. Such patients are often obese and usually present in adult life, the incidence rising progressively with age as B-cell function declines. Treatment is initially dietary, although oral hypoglycaemic drugs usually become necessary, and most patients ultimately benefit from exogenous insulin. Prospective studies have demonstrated a relentless deterioration in diabetic control[6] over the years.

Insulin secretion (basal, and in response to a meal) in a type 1 and a type 2 diabetic patient is contrasted schematically with that in a healthy control in Figure 31.2.

There are many other less common forms of diabetes mellitus in addition to the two main ones described above (for example, syndromes associated with autoantibodies directed against insulin receptors which cause severe insulin resistance, functional A-cell tumours, 'glucagonomas', and many other rarities), and hyperglycaemia can also be a clinically important adverse effect of several drugs, including glucocorticoids (Ch. 33), high doses of thiazide diuretics (Ch. 29) and several of the protease inhibitors used to treat HIV infection (Ch. 52).

TREATMENT OF DIABETES MELLITUS

Insulin is essential for the treatment of type 1 diabetes, and a valuable component of the treatment of many patients with type 2 disease.

▼ For many years it was assumed, as an act of faith, that normalising plasma glucose would prevent diabetic complications. The Diabetes Control and Complications Trial (American Diabetes Association, 1993) showed that this faith was well placed: type 1 diabetic patients were randomly allocated to intensive or conventional management. Mean fasting blood glucose concentration was 2.8 mmol/l lower in the intensively treated group, who had a substantial reduction in the occurrence and progression of retinopathy, nephropathy and neuropathy over a period of 4–9 years. Benefits, including reduced atheromatous as well as microvascular disease, were long-lasting and outweighed adverse effects, including a three-fold increase in severe hypoglycaemic attacks and modest excess weight gain.

The UK Prospective Diabetes Study showed that *lowering blood pressure* markedly improves outcome in type 2 diabetes. Normalisation of blood glucose was not achieved even in intensively treated patients. Better metabolic control did improve outcome, but (in contrast to lowering blood pressure) the magnitude of the benefit was disappointing and statistically significant only for microvascular complications. In long-term follow-up, patients from this study who had been allocated to intensive treatment continued to have better outcomes than patients treated with diet alone (despite diabetic control becoming similar in the two groups after the blinded treatment period had finished), suggesting that early diabetic control (within the first 12 years from diagnosis) is important (Holman et al., 2008). By contrast, studies of intensive control later in the course of the disease have been disappointing with harm from hypoglycaemia outweighing any benefit.

Realistic goals in type 2 diabetic patients are usually less ambitious than in younger type 1 patients. Dietary restriction leading to weight loss in overweight and obese patients is the cornerstone (albeit one with a tendency to crumble), combined with increased exercise. Oral agents are used to control symptoms from hyperglycaemia, as well as to limit microvascular complications, and are introduced early. Dietary measures and statins to prevent atheromatous disease (Ch. 24) are crucial. Details of dietary management and treatment for specific diabetic complications are beyond the scope of this book. Newer drugs (glitazones and drugs that mimic or potentiate incretins) have been shown to reduce glycated haemoglobin (typically by 0.5–1 percentage points) but their effects (if any) on clinical outcomes such as diabetic complications are unproven.

---

[5]Neuropathy ('disease of the nerves') causes dysfunction of peripheral nerve fibres, which can be motor, sensory or autonomic. Diabetic neuropathy often causes numbness in a 'stocking' distribution caused by damage to sensory fibres, and postural hypotension and erectile dysfunction due to autonomic neuropathy.

[6]Diabetic control is not easily estimated by determination of blood glucose, because this is so variable. Instead, glycated haemoglobin (haemoglobin A_{1C}) is measured. This provides an integrated measure of control over the lifespan of the red cell: approximately 120 days. In healthy individuals, 4–6% of haemoglobin is glycated; levels above 7% are indicative of diabetes.

INSULIN TREATMENT

The effects of insulin and its mechanism of action are described above. Here we describe pharmacokinetic aspects and adverse effects, both of which are central to its therapeutic use. Insulin for clinical use was once either porcine or bovine but is now almost entirely human (made by recombinant DNA technology). Animal insulins are liable to elicit an immune response; this is less of an issue with recombinant human insulins. Although recombinant insulin is more consistent in quality than insulins extracted from pancreases of freshly slaughtered animals, doses are still quantified in terms of units of activity (Ch. 7), with which doctors and patients are familiar, rather than of mass.

Pharmacokinetic aspects and insulin preparations

Insulin is destroyed in the gastrointestinal tract, and is ordinarily given by injection – usually subcutaneously, but intravenously or occasionally intramuscularly in emergencies. Intraperitoneal insulin can be used in diabetic patients with end-stage renal failure treated by ambulatory peritoneal dialysis. Pulmonary absorption of insulin occurs, but an aerosol formulation was withdrawn from therapeutic use. Other potential approaches include incorporation of insulin into biodegradable polymer microspheres as a slow-release formulation, and its encapsulation with a lectin in a glucose-permeable membrane.[7] Once absorbed, insulin has an elimination half-life of approximately 10 min. It is inactivated enzymatically in the liver and kidney, and 10% is excreted in the urine. Renal impairment reduces insulin requirement.

One of the main problems in using insulin is to avoid wide fluctuations in plasma concentration and thus in blood glucose. Different formulations vary in the timing of their peak effect and duration of action. *Soluble insulin* produces a rapid and short-lived effect. Longer-acting preparations are made by precipitating insulin with protamine or zinc, thus forming finely divided amorphous solid or relatively insoluble crystals, which are injected as a suspension from which insulin is slowly absorbed. These preparations include *isophane insulin* and amorphous or crystalline *insulin zinc suspensions*. Mixtures of different forms in fixed proportions are available. **Insulin lispro** is an insulin analogue in which a lysine and a proline residue are 'switched'. It acts more rapidly but for a shorter time than natural insulin, enabling patients to inject themselves immediately before the start of a meal. **Insulin glargine** is another modified insulin analogue, designed with the opposite intention, namely to provide a constant basal insulin supply and mimic physiological postabsorptive basal insulin secretion. Insulin glargine, which is a clear solution, forms a microprecipitate at the physiological pH of subcutaneous tissue, and absorption from the subcutaneous site of injection is prolonged. Used in conjunction with short-acting insulin, it lowers postabsorptive plasma glucose.

Various dosage regimens are used. Some type 1 patients inject a combination of short- and intermediate-acting insulins twice daily, before breakfast and before the evening meal. Improved control of blood glucose can be achieved with multiple daily injections of rapid-acting insulin analogues given with meals, and a basal insulin analogue injected once daily (often at night). Insulin pumps are used in hospital to control blood glucose acutely and sometimes, by specialists, in outpatients. The most sophisticated forms of pump regulate the dose by means of a sensor that continuously measures blood glucose, but these are not used routinely – this seemingly logical approach is limited by the complexity of insulin's effects on intermediary metabolism (see Table 31.2, Fig. 31.3) which are imperfectly captured by interstitial glucose concentration, and by risks of infection.

Unwanted effects

The main undesirable effect of insulin is hypoglycaemia. This is common and, if very severe, can cause brain damage or sudden cardiac death. In the Diabetes Control and Complications Trial mentioned above, intensive insulin therapy resulted in a three-fold increase in severe hypoglycaemic episodes compared with usual care. The treatment of hypoglycaemia is to take a sweet drink or snack or, if the patient is unconscious, to give intravenous glucose or intramuscular glucagon (see clinical box, p. 385). Rebound hyperglycaemia ('Somogyi effect') can follow insulin-induced hypoglycaemia, because of the release of counter-regulatory hormones (e.g. adrenaline, glucagon and glucocorticoids). This can cause hyperglycaemia before breakfast following an unrecognised hypoglycaemic attack during sleep in the early hours of the morning. It is essential to appreciate this possibility to avoid the mistake of increasing (rather than reducing) the evening dose of insulin in this situation.

Allergy to human insulin is unusual but can occur. It may take the form of local or systemic reactions. Insulin resistance as a consequence of antibody formation is rare. Theoretical concerns regarding mitogenic effects of insulin analogues are mentioned above (p. 383).

Clinical uses of insulin and other hypoglycaemic drugs for injection

- Patients with *type 1 diabetes* require long term **insulin**:
    - an intermediate-acting preparation (e.g. **isophane insulin**) or a long-acting analogue (e.g. **glargine**) is often combined with soluble insulin or a short-acting analogue (e.g. **lispro**) taken before meals.
- **Soluble insulin** is used (intravenously) in emergency treatment of hyperglycaemic emergencies (e.g. *diabetic ketoacidosis*).
- Approximately one-third of patients with *type 2 diabetes* ultimately benefit from **insulin**.
- Short-term treatment of patients with type 2 diabetes or impaired glucose tolerance during intercurrent events (e.g. *operations*, *infections*, *myocardial infarction*).
- During pregnancy, for *gestational diabetes* not controlled by diet alone.
- Emergency treatment of *hyperkalaemia*: **insulin** is given with glucose to lower extracellular K$^+$ via redistribution into cells.
- **Exenatide** for type 2 diabetes in addition to oral agents to improve control and lose weight.

---

[7]This could, in theory, provide variable release of insulin controlled by the prevailing glucose concentration, because glucose and glycated insulin compete for binding sites on the lectin.

OTHER HYPOGLYCAEMIC AGENTS

Biguanides

Metformin (present in French lilac, *Galega officinalis*, which was used to treat diabetes in traditional medicine for centuries) is the only biguanide used clinically to treat type 2 diabetes, for which it is now a drug of first choice.[8]

Actions and mechanism

The molecular target or targets through which biguanides act remains unclear, but their biochemical actions are well understood, and include:

- reduced hepatic glucose production (gluconeogenesis; gluconeogenesis is markedly increased in type 2 diabetes)
- increased glucose uptake and utilisation in skeletal muscle (i.e. they reduce insulin resistance)
- reduced carbohydrate absorption from the intestine
- increased fatty acid oxidation
- reduced circulating low-density and very-low-density lipoprotein (LDL and VLDL, respectively, see Ch. 23).

Reduced hepatic gluconeogenesis is especially important. The primary effect of metformin is to decrease hepatic glucose production by inhibiting the mitochondrial respiratory chain complex I (reviewed by Viollet et al., 2012). The resulting decrease in hepatic energy status activates AMPK (AMP-activated protein kinase) which is an important enzyme in metabolic control (Towler & Hardie, 2007). Activation of AMPK increases expression of a nuclear receptor that inhibits expression of genes that are important for gluconeogenesis in the liver (see Kim et al., 2008).

Metformin has a half-life of about 3 h and is excreted unchanged in the urine.

Unwanted effects

Metformin, while preventing hyperglycaemia, does *not* cause hypoglycaemia, and the commonest unwanted effects are dose-related gastrointestinal disturbances (e.g. anorexia, diarrhoea, nausea), which are usually but not always transient. Lactic acidosis is a rare but potentially fatal toxic effect, and metformin should not be given routinely to patients with renal or hepatic disease, hypoxic pulmonary disease or shock. Such patients are predisposed to lactic acidosis because of reduced drug elimination or reduced tissue oxygenation. Compensated heart failure is not a contraindication, and indeed metformin is associated with improved outcome in patients with diabetes and heart failure. It should be avoided in other situations that predispose to lactic acidosis including some forms of mitochondrial myopathy that are associated with diabetes. Long-term use may interfere with absorption of vitamin B_{12}.

Clinical use

Metformin is used to treat patients with type 2 diabetes. It does not stimulate appetite (rather the reverse; see above!) and is consequently the drug of first choice in the majority of type 2 patients who are obese, provided they have unimpaired renal and hepatic function. It can be combined with sulfonylureas, glitazones or insulin. Potential uses outside type 2 diabetes include other syndromes with accompanying insulin resistance including polycystic ovary syndrome, non-alcoholic fatty liver disease, gestational diabetes and some forms of premature puberty.

Sulfonylureas

The sulfonylureas were developed following the chance observation that a sulfonamide derivative (which was being used to treat typhoid) caused hypoglycaemia. Numerous sulfonylureas are available. The first used therapeutically were **tolbutamide** and **chlorpropamide**. Chlorpropamide has a long duration of action and a substantial fraction is excreted in the urine. Consequently, it can cause severe hypoglycaemia, especially in elderly patients in whom renal function declines inevitably but insidiously (Ch. 29). It causes flushing after alcohol because of a disulfiram-like effect (Ch. 49), and has an action like that of antidiuretic hormone on the distal nephron, giving rise to hyponatraemia and water intoxication. Williams (1994) comments that 'time honoured but idiosyncratic chlorpropamide should now be laid to rest' – a sentiment with which we concur. Tolbutamide, however, remains useful. So-called second-generation sulfonylureas (e.g. **glibenclamide**, **glipizide**; see Table 31.3) are more potent, but their maximum hypoglycaemic effect is no greater and control of blood glucose no better than with tolbutamide. These drugs all contain the sulfonylurea moiety and act in the same way, but different substitutions result in differences in pharmacokinetics and hence in duration of action (see Table 31.3).

Mechanism of action

The principal action of sulfonylureas is on B cells (Fig. 31.1), stimulating insulin secretion and thus reducing plasma glucose. High-affinity binding sites for sulfonylureas are present on the K_{ATP} channels (Ch. 4) in the surface membranes of B cells, and the binding of various sulfonylureas parallels their potency in stimulating insulin release. Block by sulfonylurea drugs of K_{ATP} channel activation causes depolarisation, Ca^{2+} entry and insulin secretion. (Compare this with the physiological control of insulin secretion, see Fig. 31.1.)

Pharmacokinetic aspects

Sulfonylureas are well absorbed after oral administration, and most reach peak plasma concentrations within 2–4 h. The duration of action varies (Table 31.3). All bind strongly to plasma albumin and are implicated in interactions with other drugs (e.g. salicylates and sulfonamides) that compete for these binding sites (see Ch. 8). Most sulfonylureas (or their active metabolites) are excreted in the urine, so their action is increased and prolonged in the elderly and in patients with renal disease.

Most sulfonylureas cross the placenta and enter breast milk and their use is contraindicated in pregnancy and in breastfeeding.

---

[8]Metformin had a very slow start. It was first synthesised in 1922, one of a large series of biguanides with many different pharmacological actions, which proved largely unsuitable for clinical use. Its glucose-lowering effect was noted early on, but was eclipsed by the discovery of insulin. It did not receive FDA approval until 1995. The only other biguanides in routine clinical use are the antimalarial antifolate drugs pyrimethamine and proguanil (Ch. 54).

Table 31.3 Oral hypoglycaemic sulfonylurea drugs

Drug	Relative potency[a]	Duration of action and (half-life) (hours)	Pharmacokinetic aspects[b]	General comments
Tolbutamide	1	6–12 (4)	Some converted in liver to weakly active hydroxytolbutamide; some carboxylated to inactive compound Renal excretion	A safe drug; least likely to cause hypoglycaemia May decrease iodide uptake by thyroid Contraindicated in liver failure
Glibenclamide[c]	150	18–24 (10)	Some is oxidised in the liver to moderately active products and is excreted in urine; 50% is excreted unchanged in the faeces	May cause hypoglycaemia The active metabolite accumulates in renal failure
Glipizide	100	16–24 (7)	Peak plasma levels in 1 h Most is metabolised in the liver to inactive products, which are excreted in urine; 12% is excreted in faeces	May cause hypoglycaemia Has diuretic action Only inactive products accumulate in renal failure

[a]Relative to tolbutamide.
[b]All are highly protein bound (90–95%).
[c]Termed gliburide in USA.

Unwanted effects

The sulfonylureas are usually well tolerated. Unwanted effects are specified in Table 31.3. The commonest adverse effect is hypoglycaemia, which can be severe and prolonged, the highest incidence occurring with long-acting chlorpropamide and glibenclamide and the lowest with tolbutamide. Long acting sulfonylureas are best avoided in the elderly and in patients with even mild renal impairment because of the risk of hypoglycaemia. Sulfonylureas stimulate appetite and often cause weight gain. This is a major concern in obese diabetic patients. About 3% of patients experience gastrointestinal upsets. Allergic skin rashes can occur, and bone marrow toxicity (Ch. 57), although rare, can be severe.

During and for a few days after acute myocardial infarction in diabetic patients, insulin must be substituted for sulfonylurea treatment. This is associated with a substantial reduction in short-term mortality, although it remains unclear if this is due to a beneficial effect specific to insulin or to a detrimental effect of sulfonylurea drugs in this setting, or both. Another vexing question is whether prolonged therapy with oral hypoglycaemic drugs has adverse effects on the cardiovascular system. Blockade of K_{ATP} in heart and vascular tissue could theoretically have adverse effects, and an observational study recorded an increased risk of death and cardiovascular disease during follow up for up to 8 years in newly diagnosed type 2 diabetic patients treated with sulfonylureas compared with those treated with metformin (Evans et al., 2006).

Drug interactions

Several drugs augment the hypoglycaemic effect of sulfonylureas. Non-steroidal anti-inflammatory drugs, warfarin, some uricosuric drugs (e.g. **sulfinpyrazone**), alcohol, monoamine oxidase inhibitors, some antibacterial drugs (including sulfonamides, **trimethoprim** and **chloramphenicol**) and some imidazole antifungal drugs have all been reported to produce severe hypoglycaemia when given

with a sulfonylurea. The probable basis of most of these interactions is competition for metabolising enzymes, but interference with plasma protein binding or with transport mechanisms facilitating excretion may play some part.

Agents that *decrease* the action of sulfonylureas on blood glucose include high doses of thiazide diuretics (Chs 22, 29) and glucocorticoids (pharmacodynamic interactions).

Clinical use

Sulfonylureas are used to treat type 2 diabetes in its early stages, but because they require functional B cells, they are not useful in type 1 or late stage type 2 diabetes. They can be combined with metformin or with thiazolidinediones.

OTHER DRUGS THAT STIMULATE INSULIN SECRETION

Several drugs that act, like the sulfonylureas, by blocking the sulfonylurea receptor on K_{ATP} channels in pancreatic B cells but lack the sulfonylurea moiety have recently been developed. These include **repaglinide** and **nateglinide** which, though much less potent than most sulfonylureas, have rapid onset and offset kinetics leading to short duration of action and a low risk of hypoglycaemia.[9] These drugs are administered shortly before a meal to reduce the postprandial rise in blood glucose in type 2 diabetic patients inadequately controlled with diet and exercise. They may cause less weight gain than conventional sulfonylureas. Later in the course of the disease, they can be combined with metformin or thiazolidinediones. Unlike glibenclamide, these drugs are relatively selective for K_{ATP} channels on B cells versus K_{ATP} channels in vascular smooth muscle.

[9]It is ironic that these aggressively marketed drugs share many of the properties of tolbutamide, the oldest, least expensive and least fashionable of the sulfonylureas.

Thiazolidinediones (glitazones): pioglitazone

The thiazolidinediones (or *glitazones*) were developed following the chance observation that a **clofibrate** analogue, **ciglitazone**, which was being screened for effects on lipids, unexpectedly lowered blood glucose. Ciglitazone caused liver toxicity, and this class of drugs (despite considerable commercial success) has been dogged by adverse effects (especially cardiovascular), regulatory withdrawals and controversy. No clinical trials of these agents have demonstrated a beneficial effect on mortality, and they were licensed on the basis of statistically significant effects on haemoglobin A1c (a surrogate marker of metabolic control) of uncertain clinical significance. **Pioglitazone** is the only drug of this class that remains in clinical use, its predecessors, rosiglitazone and troglitazone, having been withdrawn because of increased risk of heart attacks and liver damage, respectively – at the time, a *cause célèbre*, and very expensive for the companies involved.

Effects

The effect of thiazolidinediones on blood glucose is slow in onset, the maximum effect being achieved only after 1–2 months of treatment. They act by enhancing the effectiveness of endogenous insulin, thereby reducing hepatic glucose output, and increasing glucose uptake into muscle.

They reduce the amount of exogenous insulin needed to maintain a given level of blood glucose by approximately 30%. Reduced blood glucose concentration is accompanied by reduced insulin and free fatty acid concentrations. Triglycerides decline, while LDL and high-density lipoprotein (HDL) are unchanged or slightly increased. The proportion of small dense LDL particles (believed to be the most atherogenic; Ch. 23) is reduced. Weight gain of 1–4 kg is common, usually stabilising in 6–12 months. Some of this is attributable to fluid retention: there is an increase in plasma volume of up to 500 ml, with a concomitant reduction in haemoglobin concentration caused by haemodilution; there is also an increase in extravascular fluid, and increased deposition of subcutaneous (as opposed to visceral) fat.

Mechanism of action

Thiazolidinediones bind to a nuclear receptor called the *peroxisome proliferator-activated receptor-γ* (PPARγ), which is complexed with retinoid X receptor (RXR; see Ch. 3).[10] PPARγ occurs mainly in adipose tissue, but also in muscle and liver. It causes differentiation of adipocytes (this contributes to the unwanted effect of weight gain), increases lipogenesis and enhances uptake of fatty acids and glucose. It also promotes amiloride-sensitive sodium ion reabsorption in renal collecting ducts, explaining the adverse effect of fluid retention (Guan et al., 2005). Endogenous agonists of PPARγ include unsaturated fatty acids and various derivatives of these, including prostaglandin J₂. Thiazolidinediones are exogenous agonists, which cause the PPARγ–RXR complex to bind to DNA, promoting transcription of several genes with products that are important in insulin signalling. These include lipoprotein lipase, fatty acid transporter protein, adipocyte fatty acid-binding protein, Glut-4, phosphoenolpyruvate carboxykinase, malic enzyme and others. It remains something of a mystery that glucose homeostasis should be so responsive to drugs that bind to receptors found mainly in fat cells; it has been suggested that the explanation may lie in resetting of the glucose–fatty acid (Randle) cycle by the reduction in circulating free fatty acids.

Pharmacokinetic aspects

Pioglitazone is rapidly and nearly completely absorbed, with time to peak plasma concentration of less than 2 h. It is highly (>99%) bound to plasma proteins, and is subject to hepatic metabolism and has a short (<7 h) elimination half-life for the parent drug, but substantially longer (up to 24 h) for the metabolite. Pioglitazone is metabolised mainly by a CYP2C isozyme and CYP3A4 to active metabolites, which are eliminated mainly in bile.

Unwanted effects

Reports of liver dysfunction caused by pioglitazone have been rare; tests of liver function are recommended before treatment and periodically thereafter, especially if symptoms such as dark urine raise the possibility of liver disease. The commonest unwanted effects of pioglitazone are weight gain and fluid retention. Fluid retention is a substantial concern, because it can precipitate or worsen heart failure, which contraindicates its use. In addition to increased cardiovascular risk, both observational studies and meta-analysis of randomised controlled trials (Loke et al., 2009) indicate an increased risk (approximately a doubling of risk) of fractures with chronic use. Its use is associated with a small increased risk of bladder cancer. Non-specific symptoms, including headache, fatigue and gastrointestinal disturbances, have been reported. Pioglitazone is contraindicated in pregnant or breastfeeding women and in children. It is theoretically possible that these drugs could cause ovulation to resume in women who are anovulatory because of insulin resistance (e.g. with polycystic ovary syndrome).

Clinical use

Pioglitazone is additive with other oral hypoglycaemic drugs in terms of effect on blood glucose, and a combination tablet with metformin is marketed. It may lessen the progression of impaired glucose tolerance to diabetes, and may reduce the need for exogenous insulin in type 2 diabetic patients. Combination with insulin may increase the risk of heart disease.

α-Glucosidase inhibitors

Acarbose, an inhibitor of intestinal α-glucosidase, is used in type 2 diabetes inadequately controlled by diet with or without other agents. It delays carbohydrate absorption, reducing the postprandial increase in blood glucose. The commonest adverse effects are related to its main action and consist of flatulence, loose stools or diarrhoea, and abdominal pain and bloating. Like metformin, it may be particularly helpful in obese type 2 patients, and it can be co-administered with metformin.

Incretin mimetics and related drugs

Exenatide is a synthetic version of *exendin-4*, a peptide found in the saliva of the Gila monster (a lizard that presumably evolved this as means to disable its prey by rendering them hypoglycaemic).

Exenatide mimics the effects of GLP-1 (see above), but is longer acting. **Liraglutide** is an alternative injectable GLP-1 agonist. These drugs lower blood glucose after a

---

[10]Compare with fibrates (to which thiazolidinediones are structurally related), which bind to PPARα (see Ch. 23).

meal by increasing insulin secretion, suppressing glucagon secretion and slowing gastric emptying (see above). They reduce food intake (by an effect on satiety, see Ch. 32) and are associated with modest weight loss. They reduce hepatic fat accumulation.

Exenatide is not absorbed by the gut and is administered subcutaneously. It is much more stable than GLP-1, and is administered twice daily before the first and last meal of the day. A modified release formulation is available for once weekly injection and is used in combination with metformin and a sulfonylurea in poorly controlled obese patients. It can cause hypoglycaemia and a range of gastrointestinal effects. Pancreatitis is less common but potentially severe.

Exenatide or liraglutide are used in patients with type 2 diabetes in combination with other drugs (metformin with or without a sulfonylurea, pioglitazone, insulin); they are recommended in obese patients who have failed on dual therapy and it is recommended to continue them only if they cause a drop in haemoglobin A1c of ≥1 %-age point after 6 months together with a weight loss of at least 3%. As with the glitazones evidence of cardiovascular efficacy or effect on mortality is missing so risk benefit is arguable (see Cohen, 2013 for a popular account).

Gliptins

Gliptins (e.g. **sitagliptin**, **vildagliptin**, **saxagliptin**, **linagliptin**) are synthetic drugs that competitively inhibit dipeptidylpeptidase-4 (DPP-4), thereby lowering blood glucose by potentiating endogenous incretins (GLP-1 and GIP, see p. 385) which stimulate insulin secretion. They do not cause weight loss or weight gain.

They are absorbed from the gut and administered once (or, in the case of vildagliptin, twice) daily by mouth. They are eliminated partly by renal excretion and are also metabolised by hepatic CYP enzymes. They are usually well tolerated with a range of gastrointestinal adverse effects; occasional liver disease, worsening of heart failure and pancreatitis (incidence approximately 0.1–1%) are less common but potentially serious. There is also concern that they may act as tumour promoters (see Ch. 57). Gliptins are used for type 2 diabetes in addition to other oral hypoglycaemic drugs (see clinical box on uses of oral hypoglycaemic drugs, p. 392).

POTENTIAL NEW ANTIDIABETIC DRUGS

Several agents are currently being studied, including α_2-adrenoceptor antagonists, inhibitors of fatty acid oxidation and activators of glucokinase. Lipolysis in fat cells is controlled by adrenoceptors of the β_3 subtype (see Ch. 14). The possibility of using selective β_3 agonists, currently in development, in the treatment of obese patients with type 2 diabetes is being investigated (see Ch. 32).

Drugs used in diabetes mellitus

Insulin and other injectable drugs

- Human **insulin** is made by recombinant DNA technology. For routine use, it is given subcutaneously (by intravenous infusion in emergencies).
- Different formulations of **insulin** differ in their duration of action:
  - fast- and short-acting **soluble insulin**: peak action after subcutaneous dose 2–4 h and duration 6–8 h; it is the only formulation that can be given intravenously
  - intermediate-acting insulin (e.g. **isophane insulin**)
  - long-acting forms (e.g. **insulin zinc suspension**).
- The main unwanted effect is hypoglycaemia.
- Altering the amino acid sequence (insulin analogues, e.g. **lispro** and **glargine**) can usefully alter **insulin** kinetics.
- **Insulins** are used for all type 1 diabetic patients and approximately one-third of patients with type 2 diabetes.
- **Exenatide** and **liraglutide** are injectable GLP-1 agonists used as add-on treatment in certain inadequately controlled type 2 diabetic patients. Unlike **insulin** they cause weight loss.

Oral hypoglycaemic drugs

- These are used in type 2 diabetes.
- Biguanides (e.g. **metformin**):
  - have complex peripheral actions in the presence of residual insulin, increasing glucose uptake in striated muscle and inhibiting hepatic glucose output and intestinal glucose absorption
  - cause anorexia and encourage weight loss
  - can be combined with sulfonylureas.

- Sulfonylureas and other drugs that stimulate insulin secretion (e.g. **tolbutamide**, **glibenclamide**, **nateglinide**):
  - can cause hypoglycaemia (which stimulates appetite and leads to weight gain)
  - are effective only if B cells are functional
  block ATP-sensitive potassium channels in B cells
  - are well tolerated but promote weight gain and are associated with more cardiovascular disease than is **metformin**.
- Thiazolidinediones have been associated with serious hepatic and cardiac toxicity. **Pioglitazone** is the only one still marketed; it:
  - increases insulin sensitivity and lowers blood glucose in type 2 diabetes
  - can cause weight gain and oedema
  - increases osteoporotic fractures
  - is a peroxisome proliferator-activated receptor-γ (a nuclear receptor) agonist.
- Gliptins (e.g. **sitagliptin**):
  - potentiate endogenous incretins by blocking DPP-4
  - are added to other orally active drugs to improve control in patients with type 2 diabetes
  - are weight-neutral; they are usually well tolerated but pancreatitis is a concern.
- α-Glucosidase inhibitor, **acarbose**:
  - reduces carbohydrate absorption
  - causes flatulence and diarrhoea.

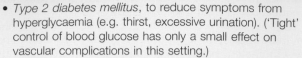

Clinical uses of oral hypoglycaemic drugs

- *Type 2 diabetes mellitus*, to reduce symptoms from hyperglycaemia (e.g. thirst, excessive urination). ('Tight' control of blood glucose has only a small effect on vascular complications in this setting.)
- **Metformin** is preferred, especially for obese patients unless contraindicated by factors that predispose to lactic acidosis (renal or liver failure, poorly compensated heart failure, hypoxaemia).
- **Acarbose** (α-glucosidase inhibitor) reduces carbohydrate absorption; it causes flatulence and diarrhoea.
- Drugs that act on the sulfonylurea receptor (e.g. **tolbutamide**, **glibenclamide**) are well tolerated but

often promote weight gain. They are associated with increased cardiovascular risk compared with **metformin**.
- **Pioglitazone** improves control (reduces haemoglobin A_{1c}) but increases weight, causes fluid retention and increases risk of fractures. GLP-1 agonists (**exenatide** or **liraglutide**) are injected once daily or (**extended release exenatide**) once weekly in obese patients inadequately controlled on two hypoglycaemic drugs.
- DPP4 inhibitors (gliptins, e.g. **sitagliptin**) improve control, are well tolerated and weight-neutral, but long-term experience is lacking, as is outcome evidence. Pancreatitis is a concern.

REFERENCES AND FURTHER READING

References

American Diabetes Association, 1993. Implications of the diabetes control and complications trial. Diabetes 42, 1555–1558. (*Landmark clinical trial*)

Cohen, D., 2013. Has pancreatic damage from GLP-1 based diabetes drugs been underplayed? Br. Med. J. 346, 16–21. (*Excellent journalistic account of current safety concerns*)

Evans, J.M.M., Ogston, S.A., Emslie-Smith, A., Morris, A.D., 2006. Risk of mortality and adverse cardiovascular outcomes in type 2 diabetes: a comparison of patients treated with sulfonylureas and metformin. Diabetologia 49, 930–936. (*Observational cohort study in 5700 newly treated type 2 patients, 1000 deaths in up to 8 years follow-up. Sulfonylurea use was associated with increased risk of death and of cardiovascular disease. Not proof but pretty suggestive!*)

Holman, R.R., Sanjoy, K.P., Bethel, M.A., et al., 2008. 10-year follow-up of intensive glucose control in type 2 diabetes. N. Engl. J. Med. 359, 1577–1589.

Kim, Y.D., Park, K.G., Lee, Y.S., et al., 2008. Metformin inhibits hepatic gluconeogenesis through AMP-activated protein kinase-dependent regulation of the orphan nuclear receptor SHP. Diabetes 57, 306–314.

Loke, Y.K., Singh, S., Furberg, C.D., et al., 2009. Long-term use of thiazolidinediones and fractures in type 2 diabetes: a meta-analysis. CMAJ 180, 32–39. (*Long-term thiazolidinedione use doubles the risk of fractures among women with type 2 diabetes, without a significant increase in risk of fractures among men with type 2 diabetes*)

Towler, M.C., Hardie, D.G., 2007. AMP-activated protein kinase in metabolic control and insulin signaling. Circ. Res. 100, 328–341.

Viollet, B., Guigas, B., Garcia, N.S., Leclerc, J., Foretz, M., Andreelli, F., 2012. Cellular and molecular mechanisms of metformin: an overview. Clin. Sci. 122, 253–270. (*Reviews mechanisms as a setting for novel therapeutic uses, for example in non-alcoholic fatty liver disease*)

Williams, G., 1994. Management of non-insulin dependent diabetes mellitus. Lancet 343, 95–100.

Yu, D.M.T., Yao, T.-W., Chowdhary, S., 2010. The dipeptidyl peptidase IV family in cancer and cell biology. FEBS J. 277, 1126–1144. (*Discusses current understanding of this unique family of enzymes*)

Further reading

Physiological and pathophysiological aspects

Lee, Y.H., White, M.F., 2004. Insulin receptor substrate proteins and diabetes. Arch. Pharm. Res. 27, 361–370. (*Reviews the discovery of IRS proteins and their role linking cell surface receptors to intracellular signalling cascades. 'Understanding the regulation and signaling by IRS1 and IRS2 in cell growth, metabolism and survival will reveal new strategies to prevent or cure diabetes and other metabolic diseases'*)

Withers, D.J., Gutierrez, J.S., Towery, H., et al., 1998. Disruption of IRS-2 causes type 2 diabetes in mice. Nature 391, 900–904.

(*Dysfunction of IRS-2 may 'contribute to the pathophysiology of human type 2 diabetes'; see also accompanying commentary by Avruch, J., A signal for β-cell failure, pp. 846–847*)

Zimmet, P., Alberti, K.G.M.M., Shaw, J., 2001. Global and societal implications of the diabetes epidemic. Nature 414, 782–787. (*Changes in human behaviour have resulted in a dramatic increase in type 2 diabetes worldwide*)

Insulins

Owens, D.R., Zinman, B., Bolli, G.B., 2001. Insulins today and beyond. Lancet 358, 739–746. (*Reviews the physiology of glucose homeostasis, genetically engineered 'designer' insulins and developments in insulin delivery and glucose sensing*)

Oral hypoglycaemic drugs

Gale, E.A.M., 2001. Lessons from the glitazones: a story of drug development. Lancet 357, 1870–1875. (*Fighting stuff: 'Troglitazone was voluntarily withdrawn in Europe, but went on to generate sales of over $2 billion in the USA and caused 90 cases of liver failure before being withdrawn. Rosiglitazone and pioglitazone reached the USA for use alone or in combination with other drugs whereas in Europe the same dossiers were used to apply for a limited licence as second-line agents. How should we use them? How did they achieve blockbuster status without any clear evidence of advantage over existing therapy?'*)

Guan, Y., Hao, C., Cha, D.R., et al., 2005. Thiazolidinediones expand body fluid volume through PPARγ stimulation of ENaC-mediated renal salt absorption. Nat. Med. 11, 861–865. (*Mechanism of fluid retention caused by thiazolidinediones and suggestion that amiloride may provide a specific therapy for this. Human studies will no doubt follow … See also News and Views article in the same issue: TZDs and diabetes: testing the waters, by A.F. Semenkovich, pp. 822–824*)

Other drugs for diabetes, and therapeutic aspects

Brenner, B.M., Cooper, M.E., de Zeeuw, D., et al., 2001. Effects of losartan on renal and cardiovascular outcomes in patients with type 2 diabetes and nephropathy. N. Engl. J. Med. 345, 861–869. (*Significant renal benefits from the AT₁ antagonist; see also two adjacent articles: Lewis, E.J., et al., pp. 851–860, and Parving, H.-H., et al., pp. 870–878, and an editorial on prevention of renal disease caused by type 2 diabetes by Hostetter, T.H., pp. 910–911*)

Farmer, K.L., Li, C.-Y., Dobrowsky, R.T., 2012. Diabetic neuropathy: should a chaperone accompany our therapeutic approach? Pharmacol. Rev. 64, 880–900. (*Currently no satisfactory therapy*)

Younk, L.M., Mikeladze, M., Davis, S.N., 2011. Pramlintide and the treatment of diabetes: a review of the data since its introduction. Expert Opin. Pharmacother. 12, 1439–1451. ('*Pramlintide significantly reduces hemoglobin A(1c) and body weight in patients with type 1 and type 2 diabetes mellitus. Newer research is focusing on weight loss effects of pramlintide and pramlintide plus metreleptin in nondiabetic obese individuals*')

Obesity 32

OVERVIEW

Obesity is a growing health issue around the world and is reaching epidemic proportions in some nations. The problem is not restricted to the inhabitants of the affluent countries, to the adult population or to any one socioeconomic class. Body fat represents stored energy and obesity occurs when the homeostatic mechanisms controlling energy balance become disordered or overwhelmed. In this chapter we first outline the endogenous regulation of appetite and body mass, and then consider the main health implications of obesity and its pathophysiology. We conclude with a discussion of the drugs currently licensed for the treatment of obesity and glance at the future of pharmacological treatment of this condition.

INTRODUCTION

Survival requires a continuous provision of energy to maintain homeostasis even when the supply of food is intermittent. Evolution has furnished a mechanism for storing excess energy latent in foodstuffs in adipose tissue as energy-dense triglycerides, such that these can be easily mobilised when food is scarce. This mechanism, controlled by the so-called thrifty genes, was an obvious asset to our hunter–gatherer ancestors. However, in many societies a combination of sedentary lifestyle, genetic susceptibility, cultural influences and unrestricted access to an ample supply of calorie-dense foods has lead to a global epidemic of obesity, or 'globesity' as it is sometimes called. Obesity is one component of a cluster of disorders described in other chapters, which often coexist in the same individual, comprising what is now described as 'metabolic syndrome', a rapidly growing public health problem.

DEFINITION OF OBESITY

'Obesity' may be defined as an illness where health (and hence life expectancy) is adversely affected by excess body fat.[1] But at what point does an individual become 'obese'? The generally accepted benchmark is the body mass index (BMI). The BMI is expressed as W/h^2, where W = body weight (in kg), h = height (in metres). Although it is not a perfect index (e.g. it does not distinguish between fat and lean mass), the BMI is generally well correlated with other measurements of body fat, and it is widely utilised as a convenient index. While there are problems in defining a 'healthy' weight for a particular population, the World Health Organization (WHO) classifies adults with a BMI of ≥25 as being overweight and those with a BMI of ≥30 as obese. Childhood obesity is more difficult to assess.

Since the BMI obviously depends on the overall energy balance, another operational definition of obesity would be that it is a multifactorial disorder of energy balance in which calorie intake over the long term exceeds energy output.

OBESITY AS A HEALTH PROBLEM

Obesity is a growing and costly global health problem. The WHO in 2008 estimated that there were already more than 1.4 billion overweight adults, approximately half of whom – amounting to more than 10% of the world's population – were obese according to the criteria outlined above. National obesity levels vary enormously, being less than 5% in China, Japan and parts of Africa, and a staggering 75% in parts of Samoa. Adult obesity levels in the USA, Europe and the UK (among others) have increased threefold since 1980, with figures of 35.9% being quoted for the USA (2010 figures; Xia & Grant, 2013) and about 25% for many other industrialised nations (Padwal et al., 2003). The disease is not confined to adults: some 40 million children under 5 years old are estimated to be overweight (2011 figures). In the USA, the number of overweight children has doubled and the number of overweight adolescents has trebled since 1980. Ironically, obesity often coexists with malnutrition in many developing countries. All socioeconomic classes are affected. In the poorest countries, it is the top socioeconomic classes in whom obesity is prevalent, but in the West it is usually the reverse.

Overall, more people die in the world from being overweight and obese than being underweight. The financial burden on the healthcare system is huge. The cost of treating obesity in the USA alone was $198 billion in 2010 (Xia & Grant, 2013).

▼ While obesity itself is rarely fatal, it often coexists with metabolic and other disorders (particularly hypertension, hypercholesterolaemia and type 2 diabetes), together comprising the *metabolic syndrome*. This carries a high risk of cardiovascular conditions, strokes, cancers (particularly hormone-dependent), respiratory disorders (particularly sleep apnoea) and digestive problems, as well as osteoarthritis. One commentator (Kopelman, 2000) has remarked that obesity 'is beginning to replace under-nutrition and infectious diseases as the most significant contributor to ill health'. Increasingly, social stigma is suffered by obese individuals, leading to a sense of psychological isolation.

The risk of developing type 2 diabetes (which represents 85% of all cases of the disease) rises sharply with increasing BMI. The WHO reports that 90% of those diagnosed with the disease are obese. In a study of the disease in women, the risk of developing diabetes was closely correlated with BMI, increasing five-fold when the BMI was 25 kg/m², to 93-fold when the BMI was 35 kg/m² or above (Colditz et al., 1995). Cardiovascular disease is also increased in the obese individual, and the increased thoracic and abdominal adipose tissue reduces lung volume and makes respiration difficult. Obese subjects also have an increased risk of colon, breast, prostate, gall bladder, ovarian and uterine cancer. Numerous other disorders are associated with excess body weight, including osteoarthritis, hyperuricaemia and male hypogonadism. 'Gross' obesity (BMI >40 kg/m²) is associated with a 12-fold increase in mortality in the group aged 25–35 years compared with those in this age group with a BMI of 20–25 kg/m².

---

[1]'Persons who are naturally very fat are apt to die earlier than those who are slender' observed Hippocrates.

HOMEOSTATIC MECHANISMS CONTROLLING ENERGY BALANCE

A common view, and one that is implicitly encouraged by authors of numerous books as well as the enormously lucrative dieting industry, is that obesity is simply the result of bad diet or willful overeating (hyperphagia). In truth, however, the situation is more complex. On its own, dieting seldom provides a lasting solution: the failure rate is high (probably 90%), and most dieters eventually return to their original starting weight. This suggests the operation of some intrinsic homeostatic system that operates to maintain a particular set weight. This mechanism is normally exceptionally precise, and is capable of regulating energy balance to 0.17% per decade (Weigle, 1994), a truly astonishing feat, considering the day-to-day variations in food intake.

When exposed to the same dietary choices some individuals will become obese whereas others will not. Studies of obesity in monozygotic and dizygotic twins have established a strong genetic influence on the susceptibility to the condition, and studies of rare mutations in mice (and more recently in humans) have led to the discovery and elucidation of the neuroendocrine pathways that match food intake with energy expenditure. These, in turn, have led to the concept that it is in fact disorders of these control systems that are largely responsible for the onset and maintenance of obesity.

THE ROLE OF GUT AND OTHER HORMONES IN BODY WEIGHT REGULATION

At the beginning of the 20th century it was observed that patients with damage to the hypothalamus tended to gain weight. In the 1940s it was also shown that discrete lesions in the hypothalamus of rodents caused them to become obese or exhibit unusual feeding behaviour. On the basis of experiments with rats, Kennedy proposed as early as 1953, that a hormone released from adipose tissue acted on the hypothalamus to regulate body fat and food intake. These seminal findings set the stage for future discoveries in this area.

It also was observed that mice could become obese as a result of mutations in certain genes. At least five of these have now been characterised, including the *Ob* (obesity), *Tub* (tubby), *Fat* and *Db* (diabetes) genes. Mice that are homozygous for mutant forms of these genes – *Ob/Ob* mice and *Db/Db* mice – eat excessively, have low energy expenditure, become grossly fat and have numerous metabolic and other abnormalities. Weight gain in an *Ob/Ob* mouse is suppressed if its circulation is linked to that of a normal mouse, implying that the obesity is caused by lack of a blood-borne factor.

An important conceptual breakthrough came in 1994, when Friedman and his colleagues (see Zhang et al., 1994) cloned the *Ob* gene and identified its protein product as leptin.[2] When recombinant leptin was administered systemically to *Ob/Ob* mice, it strikingly reduced food intake and body weight. It had a similar effect when injected directly into the lateral or the third ventricle, implying that it acted on the regions of the brain that control food intake and energy balance. Recombinant leptin has similar effects in humans (see Fig. 32.1).

Leptin mRNA is expressed in adipocytes; its synthesis is increased by glucocorticoids, insulin and oestrogens, and is reduced by β-adrenoceptor agonists. In normal human subjects, the release of leptin is pulsatile and varies according to the state of the fat stores and the BMI. Insulin (see Ch. 31) can also function in a similar manner.

Today, it is recognised that in addition to leptin and insulin, several other mediators originating mainly from the gastrointestinal (GI) tract as well as in the hypothalamus, play a crucial role in determining food intake, meal size and the feeling of satisfaction produced ('satiety').[3] Peptide hormones secreted by cells in the wall of the small intestine in response to the arrival of food (see Ch. 30) are important in this connection. Table 32.1 and Figure 32.2 summarise the chief characteristics of these mediators.

The majority of these factors are released either during, or in anticipation of, eating and most are inhibitory in nature, producing either satiety or satiation. Two exceptions are the gastric hormone, ghrelin, which promotes hunger, and leptin itself, which is controlled by the amount of adipose tissue and is thus more involved with the longer-term energy status of the individual. The main targets for these hormones are receptors on vagal afferent fibres or within the hypothalamus (or elsewhere in the central nervous system [CNS]). Here, they modulate the release of other neurotransmitters that exert a fine regulation over eating behaviour, energy expenditure and body weight. Other actions of these peptide hormones include the release of insulin by the *incretins* (see Ch. 31), which include glucagon-like peptide-1 (GLP-1) and gastric inhibitory peptide (GIP).

NEUROLOGICAL CIRCUITS THAT CONTROL BODY WEIGHT AND EATING BEHAVIOUR

CONTROL OF FOOD INTAKE

The manner in which all these hormonal signals are processed and integrated with other viscerosensory, gustatory or olfactory information within the CNS is complex. Many sites are involved in different aspects of the process and some 50 hormones and neurotransmitters are implicated. The account we present here is therefore necessarily an oversimplification: the Further Reading list should be consulted for a more complete picture.

As early lesioning studies predicted, the hypothalamus is the main brain centre that regulates appetite, feeding behaviour and energy status, although other sites in the brain such as the nucleus accumbens (NAc), the amygdala and especially the nucleus tractus solitarius (NTS) in the medulla, are also crucial. Within the hypothalamus, the arcuate nucleus (ARC), situated in the floor of the third ventricle, is a key site. It receives afferent signals originating from the GI tract and contains receptors for leptin and other significant hormones. It also has extensive reciprocal connections with other parts of the hypothalamus involved in monitoring energy status, in particular the paraventricular nuclei and the ventromedial hypothalamus. Figure 32.2 summarises in a simplified fashion some of the interactions that occur in the ARC.

Within the ARC are two groups of functionally distinct neurons that exert opposite effects on appetite. One group,

---

[2]The word is derived from the Greek *leptos*, meaning thin.

[3]The terminology can be confusing. 'Hunger' obviously refers to the desire to eat; 'satiation' is the feeling that you have eaten enough in the course of a meal. 'Satiety' refers to the feeling after a meal that you don't yet need another.

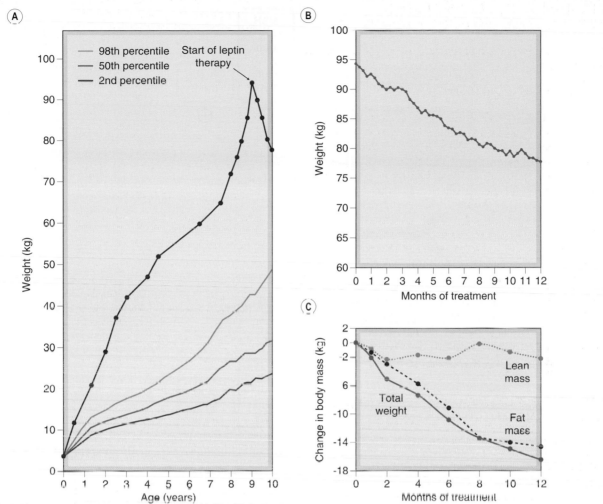

Fig. 32.1 The effect of recombinant leptin on body weight in a 9-year-old severely obese child with endogenous leptin deficiency because of a frame shift mutation in the leptin gene. Although of normal birth weight, the child began gaining weight at 4 months and was constantly demanding food. Prior to treatment, the child weighed 94.4 kg. Weight loss began after 2 weeks' treatment, and her eating pattern returned to normal. She had lost 15.6 kg of body fat after 1 year of treatment. (Data and figure adapted from Farooqi et al. 1999.)

Table 32.1 Some peripheral hormones that regulate eating behaviour

Hormone	Source	Stimulus to release	Target	Effect
CCK	GI tract	During feeding or just before	Vagal afferents	Limits size of meal
Amylin, insulin, glucagon	Pancreas	During feeding or just before	Vagal afferents	Limits size of meal
PYY3–36	Ileum, colon	After feeding	Brain stem, hypothalamus	Postpones need for next meal
GLP-1	Stomach	After feeding	Brain stem, hypothalamus	Postpones need for next meal
Oxcyntomodulin	Stomach	After feeding	Brain stem, hypothalamus	Postpones need for next meal
Leptin	Adipose tissue	Adiposity 'status'	Brain stem, arcuate nucleus	Longer-term regulation of food intake
Ghrelin	Stomach	Hunger, feeding	Vagus, hypothalamus	Increases food intake by increasing size and number of meals

CCK, cholecystokinin; GI, gastrointestinal; GLP-1, glucagon-like peptide-1; PYY3–36, peptide YY.

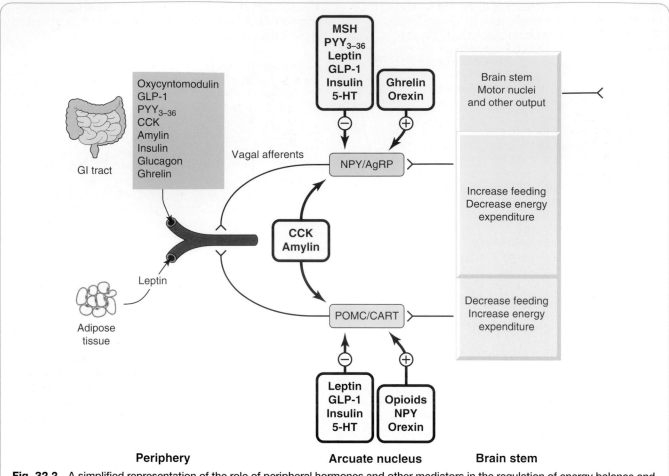

Fig. 32.2 A simplified representation of the role of peripheral hormones and other mediators in the regulation of energy balance and fat stores. The primary level of hypothalamic control is vested in two groups of neurons, with opposing actions, in the arcuate nucleus (ARC). In one group, the peptides neuropeptide Y (NPY) and agouti-related protein (AgRP) are co-localised; the other contains the polypeptides prepro-opiomelanocortin (POMC) and cocaine- and amphetamine-related transcript (CART), which release α-melanocyte-stimulating hormone (MSH). Blood-borne hormones arising from the gastrointestinal (GI) tract or adipose tissue are sensed by receptors on vagal and other afferents and are relayed through the nucleus tractus solitarius to modify the activity of these neuronal circuits. The influence of hormones on each neuronal group is indicated. Some (e.g. leptin) arise from the peripheral blood and influence the ARC neurons directly or indirectly through neuronal signals; while others (e.g. 5-hydroxytryptamine [5-HT], orexin) originate within the central nervous system itself. Activation of the NPY/AgRP group by, for example, a fall in leptin or an increase in ghrelin levels results in increased food intake and decreased energy expenditure. In the POMC/CART group of neurons, increased leptin or other hormone levels triggered by overfeeding produces a predominately inhibitory effect on feeding behaviour. A number of other hormones such as cholecystokinin (CCK) and amylin also alter the properties of the ARC neurons although the mechanism is not clear. GLP-1, glucagon-like peptide-1; PYY₃₋₃₆, peptide YY. (*Modified from Adan et al. 2008.*)

termed *anorexigenic* (appetite-suppressing), secrete pro-opiomelanocortin (POMC)-derived peptides (such as α-melanocyte-stimulating hormone; α-MSH) or cocaine- and amphetamine-regulated transcript (CART)[4]-derived peptides. The other group, termed *orexigenic* (appetite-promoting) neurons, secrete neuropeptide Y (NPY) or agouti-related peptide (AgRP). As these groups of neurons have opposing actions, energy homeostasis depends, in the first instance, on the balance between these actions whose final effects are transduced by the brain stem motor system and change feeding behaviour.

Monoamines such as noradrenaline, 5-hydroxy-tryptamine (5-HT) and dopamine also play a role in the modulation of satiety signals. Noradrenaline is co-localised with NPY in some neurons and greatly potentiates its hyperphagic action. Deficit of dopamine impairs feeding behaviour, as do agonists at the 5-HT₂C receptor; antagonists at this receptor have the reverse effect.

Many neural signals arising from the GI tract are integrated, and relayed on to the hypothalamus, by the NTS in the medulla. Some of these signals, including those of gustatory, olfactory, mechanical and viscerosensory signals, arise from vagal and other spinal afferents originating in the GI tract or liver. Endocrine signals have more complex signalling pathways. For example, cholecystokinin (CCK) is secreted by the duodenum in response to the process of eating and digestion of (especially fatty) foodstuffs. CCK acts locally on CCK_A receptors in the GI tract to stimulate vagal afferents and may also act on CCK_B receptors in the brain in order to function as a satiety factor. Ghrelin stimulates growth hormone release (Ch. 33) and also has a direct action on neurons in the ARC to

---

[4]So called because the administration of cocaine or amphetamine stimulates the transcription of this gene. Its expression in the hypothalamus is related to nutritional status implicating it in the control of appetite. Its receptor is unknown but it probably modulates the action of NPY and leptin.

modify feeding behaviour. Blood ghrelin levels normally fall after eating but not in obese individuals (English et al., 2002). Interestingly, polymorphisms in the ghrelin gene may be important in the pathogenesis of the *Prader–Willi syndrome*, a rare genetic childhood disorder that predisposes to life-threatening obesity.

Leptin also targets these neurons in the ARC. Falling leptin levels activate the orexigenic neurons, resulting in increased food intake and synthesis and storage of fat (anabolism), as well as decreased energy expenditure. Conversely, rising leptin levels activate the second group of neurons, producing the opposite anorexigenic and catabolic effect.

Inputs from other parts of the CNS also influence feeding behaviour. Of importance to us is the input from the NAc. This centre seems to regulate those aspects of eating that are driven by pleasure or reward – the so-called 'hedonic' aspects of eating (see also Ch. 49). The endocannabinoid system is important in this response. The hypothalamus contains large amounts of 2-arachidonyl glycerol and anandamide as well as the CB_1 receptor (Ch. 19). Administration of endogenous or exogenous (e.g. Δ9-THC) cannabinoids provokes a powerful feeding response.[5] This system in turn may be modulated by 'stress' and other factors in the environment.

CONTROL OF ENERGY EXPENDITURE

Balancing food intake is the energy expenditure required to maintain metabolism, physical activity and thermogenesis (heat production). The metabolic aspects include, among other things, cardiorespiratory work and the energy required by a multitude of enzymes. Physical activity increases all these, as well as increasing energy consumption by skeletal muscles. Exposure to cold also stimulates thermogenesis, and the reverse is also true. The, often dramatic (20–40% increase), thermogenic effect of feeding itself may provide a partial protection against developing obesity.

The sympathetic nervous system (sometimes in concert with thyroid hormone) plays a significant part in energy regulation in cardiovascular and skeletal muscle function during physical activity, as well as the thermogenic response of adipose tissue and the response to cold. Both 'white' and (especially) 'brown' fat cells (the colour is caused by the high density of mitochondria) play a major role in thermogenesis. Brown fat, which is densely innervated by the sympathetic nervous system, is abundant in rodents and human infants, although in human adults these cells are generally to be found more interspersed amongst white fat cells. Because of their abundant mitochondria, they are remarkable heat generators. The basis for this, as determined in mice, is the presence of mitochondrial uncoupling proteins (UCP). Three isoforms, UCP-1, -2 and -3, are known and have different distributions, although all are found in brown fat. These proteins 'uncouple' oxidative phosphorylation, so that mitochondria dissipate most energy as heat rather than producing ATP. As one might anticipate, exposure to cold or leptin administration increases both the activity and (after prolonged stimulation) the amount of UCP-1 in brown fat. Noradrenaline, acting on β adrenoceptors (mainly β_3) in brown fat, increases the activity of the peroxisome proliferator-activated receptor-γ (PPARγ) transcription factor,

which, in turn, activates the gene for UCP-1. The expression of β_3 adrenoceptors is decreased in genetically obese mice.

Energy balance

Energy balance depends on food intake, energy storage in fat and energy expenditure. In most individuals the process is tightly regulated by a homeostatic system that integrates inputs from a number of internal sensors and external factors. Important components of the system include the following:

- Hormones that signal the status of fat stores (e.g. leptin). Increasing fat storage promotes leptin release from adipocytes.
- Hormones released from the gut during feeding that convey sensations of hunger (e.g. ghrelin), satiety (e.g. CCK) or satiation (e.g. PYY3–36).
- This hormonal information together with neural, gustatory, olfactory and viscerosensory input is integrated in the hypothalamus. The arcuate nucleus is a key site.
- Two groups of opposing neurons in the arcuate nucleus sense hormonal and other signals. Those secreting POMC/CART products promote feeding while those secreting NPY/AgRP inhibit feeding. Many other CNS neurotransmitters (e.g. endocannabinoids) are involved.

The net output from this process is relayed to other sites in the brain stem motor nuclei that control feeding behaviour.

THE PATHOPHYSIOLOGY OF HUMAN OBESITY

In most adults, body fat and body weight remain more or less constant over many years, even decades, in the face of very large variations in food intake and energy expenditure amounting to about a million calories per year. The steady-state body weight and BMI of an individual, as explained, depends upon the integration of multiple interacting regulatory pathways. How, then, does obesity occur? Why is it so difficult for the obese to lose weight and maintain the lower weight?

The main determinant is manifestly a disturbance of the homeostatic mechanisms that control energy balance, and genetic endowment underlies this disturbance. Other factors, such as food availability and lack of physical activity, also contribute. Additionally, of course, there are overlaying social, cultural and psychological aspects. We discuss here the physiological and genetic mechanisms; the role of social, cultural and psychological aspects we will leave (with a profound sigh of relief) to the psychosociologists!

FOOD INTAKE AND OBESITY

As Spiegelman & Flier (1996) point out, 'one need not be a rocket scientist to notice that increased food intake tends to be associated with obesity'. A typical obese subject will usually gain 20 kg over a decade or so. This means that there has been a daily excess of energy input over energy requirement of 30–40 kcal initially, increasing gradually to maintain the increased body weight.

---

[5]This effect is responsible for the 'munchies', a common side effect of smoking cannabis.

The type of food eaten, as well as the quantity, can disturb energy homeostasis. Fat is an energy-dense foodstuff, and it may be that the satiety mechanisms regulating appetite, which react rapidly to carbohydrate and protein, react too slowly to stop an individual consuming excess fat.

However, when obese individuals reduce their calorie intake as part of a diet regime, they shift into negative energy balance. When they lose weight, the resting metabolic rate decreases, and there is a concomitant reduction in energy expenditure. Thus an individual who was previously obese and is now of normal weight generally needs fewer calories to maintain that weight than an individual who has never been obese. The decrease in energy expenditure appears to be largely caused by an alteration in the conversion efficiency of chemical energy to mechanical work in the skeletal muscles. This adaptation to the caloric reduction contributes to the difficulty of maintaining weight loss by diet.

PHYSICAL EXERCISE AND OBESITY

It used to be said that the only exercise effective in combating obesity was pushing one's chair back from the table. It is now recognised that physical activity – i.e. increased energy expenditure – has a much more positive role in reducing fat storage and adjusting energy balance in the obese, particularly if associated with modification of the diet. An inadvertent, natural population study provides an example. Many years ago, a tribe of Pima Indians split into two groups. One group in Mexico continued to live simply at subsistence level, eating frugally and spending most of the week in hard physical labour. They are generally lean and have a low incidence of type 2 diabetes. The other group settled in the USA – an environment with easy access to calorie-rich food and less need for hard physical work. They are, on average, 57 lb (26 kg) heavier than the Mexican group and have a high incidence of early-onset type 2 diabetes.

OBESITY AS A DISORDER OF THE HOMEOSTATIC CONTROL OF ENERGY BALANCE

Because the homeostatic control of energy balance is complex, it is not easy to determine exactly what goes wrong in obesity.[6] When the leptin story unfolded, it was thought that alterations in leptin kinetics might provide a simple explanation. There is a considerable interindividual variation in sensitivity to leptin, and some individuals seem to produce insufficient amounts of this hormone. Paradoxically, however, plasma leptin is often higher in obese compared with non-obese subjects, not lower as might be expected. The reason for this is that resistance to leptin, rather than insufficient hormone, is more prevalent in obesity. Such resistance could be caused by defects in leptin carriage in the circulation, transport into the CNS, in leptin receptors in the hypothalamus (as occurs in obese *Db/Db* mice) or in post-receptor signalling.

Mediators other than leptin are also implicated. For example, tumour necrosis factor (TNF)-α, a cytokine that can relay information from fat tissue to brain, is increased in the adipose tissue of insulin-resistant obese individuals. Reduced insulin sensitivity of muscle and fat also occurs, as well as decreased β_3 adrenoceptor function in brown adipose tissue; alternatively, the uncoupling protein UCP-2 in adipocytes, may be dysfunctional.

A further suggestion is that alterations in the function of specific nuclear receptors, such as PPARα, β and γ, may play a role in obesity. These receptors regulate gene expression of enzymes associated with lipid and glucose homeostasis, and they also promote the formation of adipose tissue. PPARγ is expressed preferentially in fat cells and synergises with another transcription factor, C/EBPα, to convert precursor cells to fat cells (see Spiegelman & Flier, 1996). The gene for UCP in white fat cells also has regulatory sites that respond to PPARα and C/EBPα. **Pioglitazone**, used to treat type 2 diabetes (see Ch. 31), activates PPARγ and causes weight gain. The pathophysiology of obesity could involve disturbance(s) in any of the multitude of other factors involved in energy balance.

GENETIC FACTORS AND OBESITY

Analyses of large-scale (>100 000) studies in human monozygotic and dizygotic twin pairs indicated that 50–90% of the variance of BMI can be attributed to genetic factors, and suggested a relatively minor role for environmental influences (Barsh et al., 2000). The prevailing view is that *susceptibility* to obesity is largely determined genetically, while environmental factors regulate the *expression* of the disease.

The discovery that spontaneous mutations arising in single genes (e.g. the *Ob/Ob* genotype) produced obese phenotypes in mice led to a search for equivalent genes in humans. A review (Pérusse et al., 2005) identified over 170 human obesity cases that could be traced to single gene mutations in 10 different genes. Leptin receptor or POMC mutations are sometimes observed, but melanocortin MC_4 receptor mutations seem to be more prevalent (3–5%) in obese patients (e.g. see Barsh et al., 2000), and MC_4 agonists are being explored as potential appetite suppressants (as well as potential treatments for erectile dysfunction – another hypothalamic function in which they are implicated).

Other genes that may be involved include the neurotransmitter receptors involved in the central processing of appetite/energy expenditure (e.g. the CB_1, D_2, 5-HT_{2C} receptors), the β_3 adrenoceptor and the glucocorticoid receptor. Decreased function of the β_3 adrenoceptor gene could be associated with impairment of lipolysis in white fat or with thermogenesis in brown fat. A mutation of this gene has been found to be associated with abdominal obesity, insulin resistance and early-onset type 2 diabetes in some subjects and a markedly increased propensity to gain weight in a separate group of morbidly obese subjects. Alterations in the function of the glucocorticoid receptor could be associated with obesity through the permissive effect of glucocorticoids on several aspects of fat metabolism and energy balance. The significance of polymorphisms in the ghrelin gene has already been mentioned.

Overall, some 600 genes, markers and chromosomal regions are under investigation for linkage to human obesity (Pérusse et al., 2005), and it is likely (see Xia & Grant, 2013), that obesity is probably a polygenic disorder

---

[6]Even the type of gut flora has come under scrutiny as a potential determining factor in obesity. The notion that this could be supplemented with 'probiotics' to modify the risk is attracting attention. 'Holy shit!' was the title of one magazine article on the subject (*The Economist*, 12 November 2009).

with many genes each having a small effect. And this is without taking into account any further contributions from epigenetic changes or alterations in copy number of genes that regulate obesity. Clearly it will be a while before we have a clear appreciation of all these issues.

Obesity

- Obesity is a multifactorial disorder of energy balance, in which long-term calorie intake exceeds energy output.
- A subject with a BMI (W/h^2) of 20–25 kg/m^2 is considered as having a healthy body weight, one with a BMI of 25–30 kg/m^2 as overweight, and one with a BMI >30 kg/m^2 as obese.
- Obesity is a growing problem in most rich nations; the incidence – at present approximately >30% in the USA and 15–20% in Europe – is increasing.
- A BMI > 30 kg/m^2 significantly increases the risk of type 2 diabetes, hypercholesterolaemia, hypertension, ischaemic heart disease, gallstones and some cancers.
- The causes of obesity include:
  - dietary, exercise, social, financial and cultural factors genetic susceptibility
  - deficiencies in the synthesis or action of leptin or other gut hormone signals
  - defects in the hypothalamic neuronal systems responding to any of these signals
  - defects in the systems controlling energy expenditure (e.g. reduced sympathetic activity), decreased metabolic expenditure of energy or decreased thermogenesis caused by a reduction in β_3 adrenoceptor-mediated tone and/or dysfunction of the proteins that uncouple oxidative phosphorylation.

PHARMACOLOGICAL APPROACHES TO THE PROBLEM OF OBESITY

The first weapons in the fight against obesity are diet and exercise. Unfortunately, these often fail or show only short-term efficacy, leaving surgical techniques (such as gastric stapling or bypass) or drug therapy as a viable alternative. *Bariatric* (weight loss) surgery is much more effective than currently licensed drugs, and is believed to work not by crudely limiting gastric capacity but by its demonstrated effects on gut hormone responses to feeding, acting for example to produce earlier satiety. It is thus potentially a 'proof-of-concept' for pharmacological measures designed to interrupt these messengers.

The attempt to control body weight with drugs has had a long and, regrettably, a largely undistinguished,[7] history. Many types of 'anorectic' (e.g. appetite suppressant) agents have been tested in the past, including the uncoupling agent dinitrophenol (DNP), amphetamines, **dexfenfluramine** and **fenfluramine**. All have been withdrawn from clinical use because of serious adverse effects. DNP, an industrial chemical, is advertised online for slimmers and body-builders as a weight loss and 'fat-burning agent', and has caused deaths among those who use it for this purpose. It blocks mitochondrial ATP production, diverting energy metabolism to generate heat instead of ATP and increasing the overall metabolic rate, which can cause life-threatening hyperthermia.[8]

CENTRALLY ACTING APPETITE SUPPRESSANTS

There have been many attempts to use centrally acting drugs to control appetite. Examples include **sibutramine** and **rimonobant** (both withdrawn in most countries) and **lorcaserin**, a 5-HT$_{2C}$ receptor agonist (see Ch. 39), recently approved as an appetite suppressant. In clinical trials it enhanced weight loss through dieting, but patients regained weight after stopping the drug.

▼ Sibutramine inhibits the reuptake of 5-HT and noradrenaline at the hypothalamic sites that regulate food intake.[9] Its main effects are to reduce food intake and cause dose-dependent weight loss (see Fig. 32.3), this being associated with a decrease in obesity-related risk factors. Sibutramine enhanced satiety and was reported to produce a reduction in waist circumference (i.e. a reduction in visceral fat), a decrease in plasma triglycerides and very-low-density lipoproteins, but an increase in high-density lipoproteins. In addition, beneficial effects on hyperinsulinaemia and glucose metabolism were reported. There is some evidence that the weight loss is associated with higher energy expenditure, possibly through an increase in thermogenesis mediated by the sympathetic nervous system. Like many similar drug regimes, sibutramine was much more effective when combined with lifestyle modification (Wadden et al., 2005).

Sibutramine was withdrawn in Europe because of concerns that its cardiovascular risks outweighed its benefits.

Another novel approach to centrally acting appetite suppressants originated from research in the cannabinoid field (see Ch. 19). As noted above, the endocannabinoid system is involved in the regulation of feeding behaviour and from this observation arose the idea that this could be a useful site of pharmacological intervention. Such a drug was the CB$_1$ receptor antagonist rimonabant that was originally developed for smoking cessation. This drug was introduced as an appetite suppressant following some encouraging clinical trials but was eventually withdrawn in 2008 because of adverse effects on mood seen in some patients. A similar fate overtook another promising CB$_1$ antagonist, **taranabant**.

ORLISTAT

The only drug currently (2013) licensed in the UK for the treatment of obesity is the lipase inhibitor **orlistat**, used with concomitant dietary and other therapy (e.g. exercise).

In the intestine, orlistat reacts with serine residues at the active sites of gastric and pancreatic lipases, irreversibly inhibiting these enzymes and thereby preventing the breakdown of dietary fat to fatty acids and glycerol. It therefore decreases absorption (and correspondingly causes faecal excretion) of some 30% of dietary fat. Given in conjunction with a low-calorie diet in obese

---

[7]As the showman Bynum said: 'there's a sucker born every minute … and one born to take him' … thyroxine (to increase metabolic rate, Ch. 34), swallowing parasites (intestinal worms compete for ingested food), amphetamines (Ch. 58), drugs that cause malabsorption (hence leaking fat per rectum (see later in this chapter) … really!

[8]DNP is reported to have been given to Russian soldiers in the Second World War, to keep them warm.
[9]Many antidepressant drugs act by the same mechanism (see Ch. 47), and also cause weight loss by reducing appetite. However, sibutramine does not have antidepressant properties. Furthermore, depressed patients are often obese, and antidepressant drugs are used to treat both conditions (see Appolinario et al., 2004).

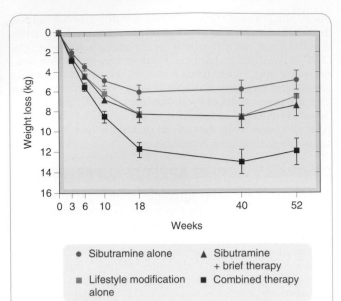

Fig. 32.3 **The effect of treatment with sibutramine alone or in combination with lifestyle modification.** In this study, 224 obese patient were given sibutramine alone, lifestyle modification counselling alone or sibutramine together with a 'brief' or more extensive programme of lifestyle counselling. The Y-axis shows the weight loss in kg (± SE) over time (X-axis). It is evident that sibutramine is far more effective as a weight-loss therapy when combined with lifestyle changes. This is a common experience when treating obesity. *(Modified from Wadden et al. 2005.)*

individuals, it produces a modest but consistent loss of weight compared with placebo-treated control subjects. In a meta-analysis of 11 long-term placebo-controlled trials encompassing more than 6000 patients, orlistat was found to produce a 2.9% greater reduction in body weight than in the control group, and 12% more patients lost 10% or more of their body weight compared with the controls (Padwal et al., 2003).

Orlistat is also reported to be effective in patients suffering from type 2 diabetes and other complications of obesity. It reduces leptin levels and blood pressure, protects against weight loss-induced changes in biliary secretion, delays gastric emptying and gastric secretion and improves several important metabolic parameters without interfering with the release or action of thyroid or other important hormones (Curran & Scott, 2004). It does not induce changes in energy expenditure.

PHARMACOKINETIC ASPECTS AND UNWANTED EFFECTS

Virtually all (97%) of orlistat is excreted in the faeces (83% unchanged), with only negligible amounts of the drug or its metabolites being absorbed.

Abdominal cramps, flatus with discharge and faecal incontinence can occur, as can intestinal borborygmi (rumbling) and oily spotting. Surprisingly, in view of the possibility of these antisocial effects occurring, the drug is well tolerated. Supplementary therapy with fat-soluble vitamins may be needed. The absorption of contraceptive pills and **ciclosporin** (see Ch. 26) may be decreased. The former is probably not clinically significant but the latter

is potentially more serious. Given its good safety record, orlistat has recently been licensed for inclusion in some over-the-counter medicines for weight loss.

Clinical uses of anti-obesity drugs

- The main treatment of obesity is a suitable diet and increased exercise.
- **Orlistat**, which causes fat malabsorption, is considered for severely obese individuals, especially with additional cardiovascular risk factors (e.g. diabetes mellitus, hypertension).
- Many centrally acting appetite suppressants have been withdrawn because of addiction, pulmonary hypertension or other serious adverse effects.

NEW APPROACHES TO OBESITY THERAPY

As might be imagined, the quest for further effective anti-obesity agents is the subject of a prodigious effort by the pharmaceutical industry.

Rare cases of leptin deficiency in patients have been successfully treated by long-term treatment with the hormone, but this is an unusual intervention and unlikely to be of more than limited use in the future. Many other approaches are being piloted (see Kang & Park, 2012). Some of these aim to exploit the action or production of neuroendocrine satiety signals such as CCK to produce appetite suppression. Many of these GI satiety hormones produce such effects when given systemically to humans or rodents, although these are not always useful; for example, CCK reduces meal size but increases meal frequency (West et al., 1984). Glucagon-like peptides such as **liraglutide**, which are used for treating type 2 diabetes (Ch. 31), also have anorexic actions and have shown promising activity in some trials (Astrup et al., 2009). Peptide YY (PYY, Fig. 32.2) is under investigation for human use. It reduces food intake by increasing satiety; a zinc conjugate (compare zinc insulins, Ch. 31) can be administered subcutaneously and acts as a depot.

Other strategies aim to alter the CNS levels of neurotransmitters such as NPY or melanocortins, which transduce changes in these hormonal signals (Halford, 2006). The tractability of the MC_4 receptor itself as a drug target, coupled with the observation that defects in MC_4 signalling are prevalent in obesity, has attracted much interest from the pharmaceutical industry.

Given the importance of the sympathetic nervous system in the control of energy regulation, one might predict that β_3-adrenoceptor agonists might be useful therapeutics. This field has been extensively researched (see Arch, 2008) but, disappointingly, has so far failed to produce an acceptable drug.

Kang and Park (2012) highlight the likely value of combination therapies that target the complex pathways involved in appetite regulation. Most drug therapies are much more effective when used in conjunction with lifestyle and other behavioural modification. The importance of this joint approach is reviewed by Vetter et al. (2010).

REFERENCES AND FURTHER READING

Body weight regulation

Adan, R.A., Vanderschuren, L.J., la Fleur, S.E., 2008. Anti-obesity drugs and neural circuits of feeding. Trends Pharmacol. Sci. 29, 208–217. (*Very accessible overview of the area. Recommended*)

Ahima, R.S., Flier, J.S., 2000. Leptin. Annu. Rev. Physiol. 62, 413–437. (*Comprehensive review of leptin: its expression, actions in hypothalamus, role in energy homeostasis and other actions*)

Ahima, R.S., Osei, S., 2001. Molecular regulation of eating behaviour: new insights and prospects for future strategies. Trends Mol. Med. 7, 205–213. (*Praiseworthy short review; excellent figures and useful tables of the mediators involved in stimulation and inhibition of feeding behaviour*)

English, P.J., Ghatei, M.A., Malik, I.A., et al., 2002. Food fails to suppress ghrelin levels in obese humans. J. Clin. Endocrinol. Metab. 87, 2984–2987.

Farooqi, I.S., Jebb, S.A., Langmack, G., et al., 1999. Effects of recombinant leptin therapy in a child with congenital leptin deficiency. N. Engl. J. Med. 341, 879–884. (*A classic clinical paper on the role of leptin in the control of feeding behaviour and weight control*)

Frühbeck, G., Gómez-Ambrosi, J., Muruzábal, F.J., Burrell, M.A., 2001. The adipocyte: a model for integration of endocrine and metabolic signalling in energy metabolism regulation. Am. J. Physiol. Endocrinol. Metab. 280, E827–E847. (*Detailed review covering receptors on and the factors secreted by the fat cell, and the role of these factors in energy homeostasis*)

Kennedy, G.C., 1953. The role of depot fat in the hypothalamic control of food intake in the rat. Proc. R. Soc. Lond. B. Biol Sci 140, 578–592. (*The paper that put forward the proposal, based on experiments on rats, that there was a hypothalamus-based homeostatic mechanism for controlling body fat*)

Schwartz, M.W., Woods, S.C., Porte, D.J., et al., 2000. Central nervous control of food intake. Nature 404, 661–671. (*Outlines a model that delineates the roles of hormones and neuropeptides in the control of food intake. Outstanding diagrams. Note that there are several other excellent articles in this Nature Insight supplement on obesity*)

Weigle, D.S., 1994. Appetite and the regulation of body composition. FASEB J. 8, 302–310.

Obesity

Barsh, G.S., Farooqi, I.S., O'Rahilly, S., 2000. Genetics of body weight regulation. Nature 404, 644–651.

Colditz, G.A., Willett, W.C., Rotnitzky, A., Manson, J.E., 1995. Weight gain as a risk factor for clinical diabetes mellitus in women. Ann. Intern. Med. 122, 481–486.

Kopelman, P.G., 2000. Obesity as a medical problem. Nature 404, 635–643.

Pérusse, C., Rankinen, T., Zuberi, A., et al., 2005. The human obesity gene map: the 2004 update. Obes. Res. 13, 381–490. (*Detailed review of the genes, markers and chromosomal regions that have been shown to be associated with human obesity*)

Spiegelman, B.M., Flier, J.S., 1996. Adipogenesis and obesity: rounding out the big picture. Cell 87, 377–389.

Spiegelman, B.M., Flier, J.S., 2001. Obesity regulation and energy balance. Cell 104, 531–543. (*Excellent review of the CNS control of energy intake/body weight, monogenic obesities, leptin physiology, central neural circuits, the melanocortin pathway, the role of insulin and adaptive thermogenesis*)

Xia, Q., Grant, S.F., 2013. The genetics of human obesity. Ann. N. Y. Acad. Sci. 1281, 178–190. (*A short and accessible paper dealing with this complex area*)

Zhang, Y., Proenca, R., Maffei, M., et al., 1994. Positional cloning of the mouse obese gene and its human homologue. Nature 372, 425–432.

Drugs in obesity

Appolinario, J.C., Bueno, J.R., Coutinho, W., 2004. Psychotropic drugs in the treatment of obesity: what promise? CNS Drugs 18, 629–651.

Chiesi, M., Huppertz, C., Hofbauer, K.G., 2001. Pharmacotherapy of obesity: targets and perspectives. Trends Pharmacol. Sci. 22, 247–254. (*Commendable, succinct review; table of the potential targets, and useful, simple figures of the central and peripheral pathways of energy regulation and of the regulation of thermogenesis*)

Clapham, J.C., Arch, J.R.S., Tadayyon, M., 2001. Anti-obesity drugs: a critical review of current therapies and future opportunities. Pharmacol. Ther. 89, 81–121. (*Comprehensive review covering, under energy intake; biogenic amines, cannabinoids, neuropeptides, leptin, gastrointestinal tract peptides and inhibitors of fat absorption; and under energy expenditure, β_3-adrenoceptor agonists and uncoupling proteins*)

Collins, P., Williams, G., 2001. Drug treatment of obesity: from past failures to future successes? Br. J. Clin. Pharmacol. 51, 13–25. (*Overview – from a clinical perspective – of currently available anti-obesity drugs and potential future drugs; well written*)

Crowley, V.E.F., Yeo, G.S.H., O'Rahilly, S., 2002. Obesity therapy: altering the energy intake-and-expenditure balance sheet. Nat. Rev. Drug Discov. 1, 276–286. (*Review stressing that pharmacological approaches to obesity therapy necessitate altering the balance between energy intake and expenditure and/or altering the partitioning of nutrients between lean tissue and fat*)

Curran, M.P., Scott, L.J., 2004. Orlistat: a review of its use in the management of patients with obesity. Drugs 64, 2845–2864.

Kang, J.G., Park, C.Y., 2012. Anti-obesity drugs: a review about their effects and safety. Diabetes Metab. J 36, 13–25. (*A brief and easy-to-read review dealing with prospective new drug therapies for obesity*)

Padwal, R., Li, S.K., Lau, D.C., 2003. Long-term pharmacotherapy for overweight and obesity: a systematic review and meta-analysis of randomized controlled trials. Int. J. Obes. Relat. Metab. Disord. 27, 1437–1446.

Wadden, T.A., Berkowitz, R.I., Womble, G., et al., 2005. Randomized trial of lifestyle modification and pharmacotherapy for obesity. N. Engl. J. Med. 353, 2111–2120.

Future drug treatments for obesity

Arch, J.R., 2008. The discovery of drugs for obesity, the metabolic effects of leptin and variable receptor pharmacology: perspectives from beta$_3$-adrenoceptor agonists. Naunyn Schmiedebergs Arch. Pharmacol. 378, 225–240 (*A comprehensive review that focuses on the quest for anti-obesity drugs that act through the β_3 adrenoceptor. Useful comments and insights into the field as a whole*)

Astrup, A., Rossner, S., Van Gaal, L., et al.; NN8022-1807 Study Group, 2009. Effects of liraglutide in the treatment of obesity: a randomised, double blind, placebo-controlled study. Lancet 374, 1606–1616.

Di Marzo, V., Matias, I., 2005. Endocannabinoid control of food intake and energy balance. Nat. Neurosci. 8, 585–589. (*A discussion of the putative role of endocannabinoids in this complex physiological mechanism; also considers therapeutic applications arising from this area*)

Fong, T.M., 2008. Development of anti-obesity agents: drugs that target neuropeptide and neurotransmitter systems. Expert Opin. Investig. Drugs 17, 321–325. (*Deals with drugs in late-stage development that target the regulatory neuropeptide pathways discussed in this chapter*)

Halford, J.C., 2006. Obesity drugs in clinical development. Curr. Opin. Invest. Drugs 7, 312–318.

Kaplan, L.M., 2005. Pharmacological therapies for obesity. Gastroenterol. Clin. North Am. 34, 91–104.

Vetter, M.L., Faulconbridge, L.F., Webb, V.L., Wadden, T.A., 2010. Behavioral and pharmacologic therapies for obesity. Nat. Rev. Endocrinol. 6, 578–588. (*This review stresses the importance of lifestyle changes in combination with drug therapy to combat obesity*)

West, D.B., Fey, D., Woods, S.C., 1984. Cholecystokinin persistently suppresses meal size but not food intake in free-feeding rats. Am. J. Physiol. 246, R776–R787.

Books

Wilding, J.P.H. (Ed.), 2008. Pharmacotherapy of obesity. In: Parnham, M.J., Bruinvels, J. (Eds.), Milestones in drug therapy. Birkhäuser, Basle. (*This book covers a wide variety of topics connected with obesity and its therapy. The contributors are experts in the field*)

Useful Web resource

<www.who.int> (*This is the World Health Organization Web page that carries data about the prevalence of 'globesity' and its distribution around the world; click on the 'Health Topics' link and navigate to 'Obesity' in the alphabetical list of topics for further information*)

33 The pituitary and the adrenal cortex

OVERVIEW

The pituitary gland and the adrenal cortex release hormones that regulate salt and water balance, energy expenditure, growth, sexual behaviour, immune function and many other vital mechanisms. The commander-in-chief of this impressive logistical exercise is the hypothalamus and the functioning unit is known as the *hypothalamo–pituitary–adrenal (HPA) axis*. In the first part of this chapter we examine the control of pituitary function by hypothalamic hormones and review the physiological roles and clinical uses of both anterior and posterior pituitary hormones. The second part of the chapter focuses on adrenal hormones and, in particular, the anti-inflammatory effect of glucocorticoids. This should be read in conjunction with the relevant sections of Chapters 3 and 26.

THE PITUITARY GLAND

The pituitary gland comprises three different structures arising from two different embryological precursors (see Fig. 33.1). The *anterior pituitary* and the *intermediate lobe* are derived from the endoderm of the buccal cavity, while the *posterior pituitary* is derived from neural ectoderm. The anterior and posterior lobes receive independent neuronal input from the hypothalamus, with which they have an intimate functional relationship.

THE ANTERIOR PITUITARY GLAND

The anterior pituitary gland (*adenohypophysis*) secretes a number of hormones crucial for normal physiological function. Within this tissue are specialised cells such as *corticotrophs*, *lactotrophs* (*mammotrophs*), *somatotrophs*, *thyrotrophs* and *gonadotrophs*, which secrete hormones that regulate different endocrine organs of the body (Table 33.1). Interspersed among these are other cell types, including *folliculostellate cells*, which exert a nurturing and regulatory influence on the hormone-secreting endocrine cells.

Secretion from the anterior pituitary is largely regulated by the release from the hypothalamus of 'factors' – in effect local hormones – that reach the pituitary through the bloodstream.[1] The blood supply to the hypothalamus divides to form a meshwork of capillaries, the *primary plexus*, which drains into the *hypophyseal portal vessels*. These pass through the pituitary stalk to feed a *secondary plexus* of capillaries in the anterior pituitary. Peptidergic neurons in the hypothalamus secrete a variety of releasing or inhibitory hormones directly into the capillaries of the

primary capillary plexus (Table 33.1 and Fig. 33.1). Most of these regulate the secretion of hormones from the anterior lobe, although the *melanocyte-stimulating hormones* (MSHs) are secreted mainly from the intermediate lobe.

The release of stimulatory hormones is regulated by negative feedback pathways between the hormones of the hypothalamus, the anterior pituitary and the peripheral endocrine glands. In *long negative feedback* pathways, hormones secreted from the peripheral glands exert regulatory actions on both the hypothalamus and the anterior pituitary. Anterior pituitary hormones acting directly on the hypothalamus comprise the *short negative feedback* pathway.

The peptidergic neurons in the hypothalamus are themselves influenced by other centres within the central nervous system (CNS) mediated through neural pathways that release dopamine, noradrenaline, 5-hydroxytryptamine and the opioid peptides (which are particularly abundant in the hypothalamus, see Ch. 15). Hypothalamic control of the anterior pituitary is also exerted through the *tuberohypophyseal dopaminergic pathway* (see Ch. 39), the neurons of which lie in close apposition to the primary capillary plexus. Dopamine secreted directly into the hypophyseal portal circulation reaches the anterior pituitary in the blood.

HYPOTHALAMIC HORMONES

The secretion of anterior pituitary hormones, then, is primarily regulated by the 'releasing factors' that originate in the hypothalamus. The most significant are described in more detail below. Somatostatin and gonadotrophin-releasing hormone are used therapeutically, the others being used mainly for diagnostic tests or as research tools. Some of these factors also function as neurotransmitters or neuromodulators elsewhere in the CNS (Ch. 39).

SOMATOSTATIN

Somatostatin is a peptide of 14 amino acid residues. It inhibits the release of growth hormone and thyroid-stimulating hormone (TSH, thyrotrophin) from the anterior pituitary (Fig. 33.2), and insulin and glucagon from the pancreas. It also decreases the release of most gastrointestinal hormones, and reduces gastric acid and pancreatic secretion.

Octreotide is a long-acting analogue of somatostatin. It is used for the treatment of *carcinoid* and other hormone-secreting tumours (Ch. 15). It also has a place in the therapy of *acromegaly* (a condition in which there is oversecretion of growth hormone in an adult). It also constricts splanchnic blood vessels, and is used to treat bleeding *oesophageal varices*. Octreotide is generally given subcutaneously. The peak action is at 2 h, and the suppressant effect lasts for up to 8 h.

Unwanted effects include pain at the injection site and gastrointestinal disturbances. Gallstones and postprandial

---

[1]The term 'factor' was originally coined at a time when their structure and function were not known. These are blood-borne messengers, and as such are clearly hormones. Nevertheless, the nomenclature, though irrational, lingers on.

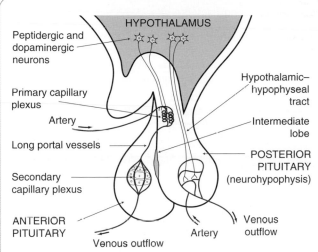

Fig. 33.1 Schematic diagram of vascular and neuronal relationships between the hypothalamus, the posterior pituitary and the anterior pituitary. The main portal vessels to the anterior pituitary lie in the pituitary stalk and arise from the primary plexus in the hypothalamus, but some (the short portal vessels) arise from the vascular bed in the posterior pituitary (not shown).

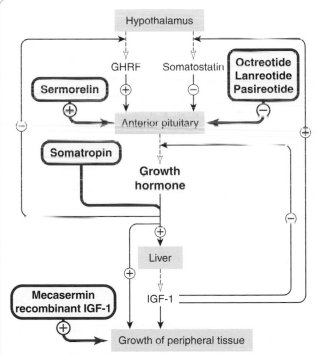

Fig. 33.2 Control of growth hormone secretion and its actions. Drugs are shown in red-bordered boxes. GHRF, growth hormone-releasing factor; IGF-1, insulin-like growth factor-1.

hyperglycaemia have also been reported, and acute hepatitis or pancreatitis has occurred in a few cases.

Lanreotide and **pasireotide** have similar effects. Lanreotide is also used in the treatment of thyroid tumours, while pasireotide, which is a particularly potent analogue, is used in the treatment of *Cushing's syndrome* when surgery is inappropriate or has been ineffective.

GONADOTROPHIN-RELEASING HORMONE

Gonadotrophin- (or luteinising hormone-) releasing hormone is a decapeptide that releases both *follicle-stimulating hormone* and *luteinising hormone* from gonadotrophs. **Gonadorelin**[2] and its analogues (**buserelin**, **goserelin**, **leuprorelin**, **nafarelin** and **triptorelin**) are used mainly in the treatment of infertility and some hormone-dependent tumours (see Ch. 35).

GROWTH HORMONE-RELEASING FACTOR (SOMATORELIN)

Growth hormone-releasing factor (GHRF) is a peptide with 44 amino acid residues. The main action of GHRF is summarised in Figure 33.2. An analogue, **sermorelin**, may be used as a diagnostic test for growth hormone secretion. Given intravenously, subcutaneously or intranasally, it causes secretion of growth hormone within minutes and peak concentrations in 1 h. The action is selective for the somatotrophs in the anterior pituitary, and no other pituitary hormones are affected. Unwanted effects are rare.

THYROTROPHIN-RELEASING HORMONE

Thyrotrophin-releasing hormone (TRH) from the hypothalamus releases TSH from the thyrotrophs.

▼ **Protirelin** is a synthetic TRH that has been used for the diagnosis of thyroid disorders (see Ch. 34). Given intravenously in normal subjects, it causes an increase in plasma TSH concentration, whereas in patients with hyperthyroidism there is a blunted response because the raised blood thyroxine concentration has a negative feedback effect on the anterior pituitary. The opposite occurs with hypothyroidism, where there is an intrinsic defect in the thyroid itself. Its use was recently discontinued in the UK.

CORTICOTROPHIN-RELEASING FACTOR

Corticotrophin-releasing factor (CRF) is a peptide that releases **adrenocorticotrophic hormone** (ACTH, corticotrophin) and β-endorphin from corticotrophs in the anterior pituitary gland. CRF acts synergistically with *antidiuretic hormone* (ADH; arginine-vasopressin), and both its action and release are inhibited by *glucocorticoids* (see Fig. 33.4). Synthetic preparations have been used to test the ability of the pituitary to secrete ACTH, and to assess whether ACTH deficiency is caused by a pituitary or a hypothalamic defect. It has also been used to evaluate hypothalamic pituitary function after therapy for Cushing's syndrome (see Fig. 33.7).

ANTERIOR PITUITARY HORMONES

The main hormones of the anterior pituitary are listed in Table 33.1. The gonadotrophins are dealt with in Chapter 35 and TSH in Chapter 34. The actions of the remainder are summarised below.

GROWTH HORMONE (SOMATOTROPHIN)

Growth hormone is secreted by the somatotroph cells and is the most abundant pituitary hormone. Secretion is high in the newborn, decreasing at 4 years to an intermediate level, which is then maintained until after puberty, after which there is a further decline. Recombinant

---

[2]In this context, the suffix '-relin' denotes peptides that stimulate hormone release.

Table 33.1 Hormones secreted by the hypothalamus and the anterior pituitary and related drugs.

Hypothalamic factor/hormone[a]	Effect on anterior pituitary	Main effects of anterior pituitary hormone
Corticotrophin-releasing factor (CRF)	Releases adrenocorticotrophic hormone (ACTH, corticotrophin) *Analogue*: tetracosactide	Stimulates secretion of adrenal cortical hormones (mainly glucocorticoids); maintains integrity of adrenal cortex
Thyrotrophin-releasing hormone (TRH) *Analogue*: protirelin	Releases thyroid-stimulating hormone (TSH; thyrotrophin)	Stimulates synthesis and secretion of thyroid hormones; maintains integrity of thyroid gland
Growth hormone-releasing factor (GHRF, somatorelin) *Analogue*: sermorelin	Releases growth hormone (GH; somatotrophin) *Analogue*: somatropin	Regulates growth, partly directly, partly through by releasing somatomedins from the liver and elsewhere; increases protein synthesis, increases blood glucose, stimulates lipolysis
Growth hormone release-inhibiting factor (somatostatin) *Analogues*: octreotide, lanreotide	Inhibits the release of GH	Prevents effects above as well as TSH release
Gonadotrophin (or luteinising hormone)-releasing hormone (GnRH) *Analogues*: 'gonadorelin analogues' – buserelin, goserelin, leuprorelin, naferelin, triptorelin	Releases follicle-stimulating hormone (FSH; see Ch. 35)	Stimulates the growth of the ovum and the Graafian follicle (female) and gametogenesis (male); with LH, stimulates the secretion of oestrogen throughout the menstrual cycle and progesterone in the second half
	Releases luteinising hormone (LH) or interstitial cell-stimulating hormone (see Ch. 35)	Stimulates ovulation and the development of the corpus luteum; with FSH, stimulates secretion of oestrogen and progesterone in the menstrual cycle; in male, regulates testosterone secretion
Prolactin-releasing factor (PRF)	Releases prolactin	Together with other hormones, prolactin promotes development of mammary tissue during pregnancy; stimulates milk production in the postpartum period
Prolactin release-inhibiting factor (probably dopamine)	Inhibits the release of prolactin	Prevents effects above
Melanocyte-stimulating hormone (MSH)-releasing factor	Releases α-, β- and γ-MSH	Promotes formation of melanin, which causes darkening of skin; MSH is anti-inflammatory and helps to regulate appetite/feeding
MSH release-inhibiting factor	Inhibits the release of α-, β- and γ-MSH	Prevents effects above

[a]These hormones are often spelled without the 'h' (e.g. corticotropin, thyrotropin, etc.) in contemporary texts. We have retained the original nomenclature in this edition.

human growth hormone, **somatropin**, is available for treating growth defects and other developmental problems.

Regulation of secretion

Secretion of growth hormone is regulated by the action of hypothalamic GHRF and modulated by somatostatin, as described above and outlined in Figure 33.2. A different peptide releaser of growth hormone ('ghrelin') is released from the stomach and pancreas and is implicated in the control of appetite and of body weight (Ch. 32). One of the mediators of growth hormone action, *insulin-like growth factor* (IGF)-1, which is released from the liver, has an inhibitory effect on growth hormone secretion by stimulating somatostatin release from the hypothalamus.

As with other anterior pituitary secretions, growth hormone release is pulsatile, and its plasma concentration may fluctuate 10- to 100-fold. These surges occur repeatedly during the day and night, and reflect the dynamics of hypothalamic control. Deep sleep is a potent stimulus to growth hormone secretion, particularly in children.

Actions

The main effect of growth hormone (and its analogues) is to stimulate normal growth. To do so, it acts in conjunction with other hormones secreted from the thyroid, the gonads and the adrenal cortex. It stimulates hepatic production of the IGFs – also termed *somatomedins* – which mediate most of its anabolic actions. IGF-1 (the principal mediator) mediates many of these anabolic effects and stimulates the uptake of amino acids and protein synthesis by skeletal muscle and the cartilage at the epiphyses of long bones, thus influencing bone growth. Receptors for IGF-1 exist on many other cell types, including liver cells and fat cells.

Disorders of production and clinical use

Deficiency of growth hormone (or failure of its action) results in *pituitary dwarfism*. In this condition, which may result from lack of GHRF or a lack of IGF generation or action, the normal proportions of the body are maintained. Growth hormone is used therapeutically in these patients (often children) as well as those suffering from the short stature associated with the chromosomal disorder known as *Turner's syndrome*. It may also be used to correct short stature caused by chronic renal insufficiency in children.

Humans are insensitive to growth hormone of other species, so human growth hormone (hGH) must be used clinically. This used to be obtained from human cadavers, but this led to the spread of *Creutzfeldt–Jakob disease*, a prion-mediated neurodegenerative disorder (Ch. 40). hGH is now prepared by recombinant DNA technology (somatropin), which avoids this risk. Satisfactory linear growth can be achieved by giving somatropin subcutaneously, six to seven times per week, and therapy is most successful when started early.

hGH is also used illicitly by athletes (see Ch. 58) to increase muscle mass. The large doses used have serious side effects, causing abnormal bone growth and cardiomegaly. It has also been tested as a means of combating the bodily changes in senescence; clinical trials have shown increases in body mass, but no functional improvement.

Human recombinant IGF-1 (**mecasermin**) is also available for the treatment of growth failure in children who lack adequate amounts of this hormone.

An excessive production of growth hormone in children results in *gigantism*. An excessive production in adults, which is usually the result of a benign pituitary tumour, results in acromegaly, in which there is enlargement mainly of the jaw and of the hands and feet. The dopamine agonist **bromocriptine** and octreotide may mitigate the condition. Another useful agent is **pegvisomant**, a modified analogue of growth hormone prepared by recombinant technology that is a highly selective antagonist of growth hormone actions.

PROLACTIN

Prolactin is secreted from the anterior pituitary gland by lactotroph (mammotroph) cells. These are abundant in the gland and increase in number during pregnancy, probably under the influence of oestrogen.

Regulation of secretion

Prolactin secretion is under tonic inhibitory control by dopamine (acting on D_2 receptors on the lactotrophs) released from the hypothalamus (Fig. 33.3 and Table 33.1). The main stimulus for release is suckling; in rats, both the smell and the sounds of hungry pups are also effective triggers. Neural reflexes from the breast may stimulate the secretion from the hypothalamus of prolactin-releasing factor(s), possible candidates for which include TRH and **oxytocin**. Oestrogens increase both prolactin secretion and the proliferation of lactotrophs through release, from a subset of lactotrophs, of the neuropeptide *galanin*. Dopamine antagonists (used mainly as antipsychotic drugs; see Ch. 46) are potent stimulants of prolactin release, whereas agonists such as **bromocriptine** (Chs 39 and 46) suppress prolactin release. Bromocriptine is also used in Parkinson's disease (Ch. 40).

Actions

The prolactin receptor is a single transmembrane domain receptor related to the cytokine receptors. Several different isoforms and splice variants are known. These are found not only in the mammary gland but are widely distributed throughout the body, including the brain, ovary, heart, lungs and immune system. The main

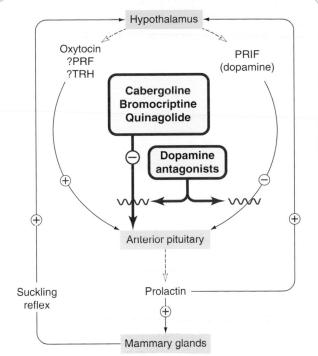

Fig. 33.3 **Control of prolactin secretion.** Drugs are shown in red-bordered boxes. PRF, prolactin-releasing factor(s); PRIF, prolactin release-inhibiting factor(s); TRH, thyrotrophin-releasing hormone.

function of prolactin in women is the control of milk production. At parturition the prolactin concentration rises and lactation is initiated. Maintenance of lactation depends on suckling (see above), which causes a 10- to 100-fold increase in blood hormone levels within 30 min.

Together with other hormones, prolactin is responsible for the proliferation and differentiation of mammary tissue during pregnancy. It also inhibits gonadotrophin release and/or the response of the ovaries to these trophic hormones. This is one of the reasons why ovulation does not usually occur during breastfeeding, and is believed to constitute a natural contraceptive mechanism.

▼ According to one rather appealing hypothesis, the high postpartum concentration of prolactin reflects its biological function as a 'parental' hormone. Certainly, broodiness and nest-building activity can be induced in birds, mice and rabbits by prolactin injections. Prolactin also exerts other, apparently unrelated, actions, including stimulating mitogenesis in lymphocytes. There is some evidence that it may play a part in regulating immune responses.

Modification of prolactin secretion

Prolactin itself is not used clinically. Bromocriptine, a dopamine receptor agonist, is used to decrease excessive prolactin secretion (*hyperprolactinaemia*). It is well absorbed orally, and peak concentrations occur after 2 h. Unwanted reactions include nausea and vomiting. Dizziness, constipation and postural hypotension may also occur. **Cabergoline** and **quinagolide** are similar.

ADRENOCORTICOTROPHIC HORMONE

Adrenocorticotrophic hormone (ACTH, corticotrophin) is the anterior pituitary secretion that controls the synthesis and release of the glucocorticoids of the adrenal cortex (see Table 33.1). It is a 39-residue peptide derived from

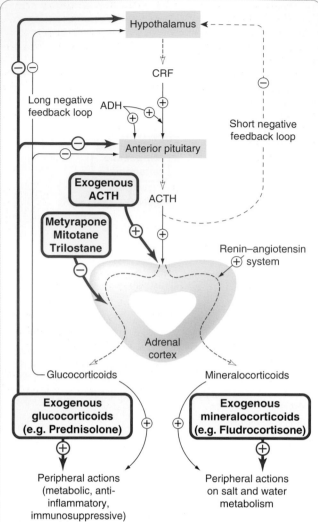

Fig. 33.4 Regulation of synthesis and secretion of adrenal corticosteroids. The long negative feedback loop is more important than the short loop (dashed lines). Adrenocorticotrophic hormone (ACTH, corticotrophin) has only a minimal effect on mineralocorticoid production. Drugs are shown in red-bordered boxes. ADH, antidiuretic hormone (vasopressin); CRF, corticotrophin-releasing factor.

Clinical uses of bromocriptine

- To prevent lactation.
- To treat galactorrhoea (i.e. non-puerperal lactation in either sex), owing to excessive prolactin secretion.
- To treat prolactin-secreting pituitary tumours (prolactinomas).
- In the treatment of Parkinson's disease (Ch. 40) and of acromegaly.

the precursor *pro-opiomelanocortin* (POMC) by sequential proteolytic processing. Failure of ACTH action because of defects in its receptor or intracellular signalling pathways can lead to severe glucocorticoid deficiency (Chan et al., 2008). Details of the regulation of ACTH secretion are shown in Figure 33.4.

▼ This hormone occupies (together with cortisone) an important place in the history of inflammation therapy because of the work of Hench and his colleagues in the 1940s, who first observed that both substances had anti-inflammatory effects in patients with rheumatoid disease. The effect of ACTH was thought to be secondary to stimulation of the adrenal cortex but, interestingly, the hormone also has anti-inflammatory actions in its own right, through activation of macrophage (melanocortin) MC_3 receptors (Getting et al., 2002).

Adrenocorticotrophic hormone itself is not often used in therapy today, because its action is less predictable than that of the corticosteroids and it may provoke antibody formation. **Tetracosactide (tetracosactrin)**, a synthetic polypeptide that consists of the first 24 N-terminal residues of human ACTH, has the same drawbacks but is now widely used in its stead for assessing the competency of the adrenal cortex.

The concentration of ACTH in the blood is reduced by glucocorticoids, forming the basis of the *dexamethasone suppression test*.

Actions

Acting through MC_2 receptors, tetracosactide and ACTH have two actions on the adrenal cortex:

- Stimulation of the synthesis and release of glucocorticoids. This action occurs within minutes of injection, and the ensuing biological actions are those of the steroids released.
- A trophic action on adrenal cortical cells, and regulation of the levels of key mitochondrial steroidogenic enzymes. The loss of this effect accounts for the adrenal atrophy that results from chronic glucocorticoid administration, which suppresses ACTH secretion.

The main use of tetracosactide is in the diagnosis of adrenal cortical insufficiency. The drug is given intramuscularly or intravenously, and the concentration of hydrocortisone in the plasma is measured by radioimmunoassay.

MELANOCYTE-STIMULATING HORMONE (MSH)

α-, β- and γ-MSH are peptide hormones with structural similarity to ACTH and are derived from the same precursor. Together, these peptides are referred to as *melanocortins*, because their first recognised action was to stimulate the production of melanin by specialised skin cells called *melanocytes*. As such, they play an important part in determining hair coloration, skin colour and reaction to ultraviolet light.

Melanocyte-stimulating hormone acts on melanocortin receptors, of which five (MC_{1-5}) have been cloned. These are G protein-coupled receptors (GPCRs) that activate cAMP synthesis. Melanin formation is controlled by the MC_1 receptor. Excessive α-MSH production can provoke abnormal proliferation of melanocytes and may predispose to melanoma.

▼ Melanocortins exhibit numerous other biological effects. For example, α-MSH inhibits the release of interleukin (IL)-1β and tumour necrosis factor (TNF)-α, reduces neutrophil infiltration, and exhibits anti-inflammatory and antipyretic activity. Levels of α-MSH are increased in synovial fluid of patients with rheumatoid arthritis. MC_1 and MC_3 receptors mediate the immunomodulatory effect of MSH. Agonists at these receptors with potential anti-inflammatory activity are being sought. Central injection of α-MSH also causes changes in animal behaviour, such as increased grooming and sexual activity as well as reduced feeding through actions on MC_4 receptors, and MC_4 agonists are under investigation as potential treatments for obesity and for erectile impotence.

Intracerebroventricular or intravenous injection of γ-MSH increases blood pressure, heart rate and cerebral blood flow. These effects are also likely to be mediated by the MC_4 receptor.

Two naturally occurring ligands for melanocortin receptors (*agouti-signalling protein* and *agouti-related peptide*, together called the *agouti*) have been discovered in human tissues. These are proteins that competitively antagonise the effect of MSH at melanocortin receptors.

The anterior pituitary gland and hypothalamus

- The anterior pituitary gland secretes hormones that regulate:
  - the release of *glucocorticoids* from the adrenal cortex
  - the release of *thyroid hormones*
  - the release of *sex hormones*: *ovulation* in the female and *spermatogenesis* in the male
  - *growth*
  - *mammary gland* structure and function.
- Each anterior pituitary hormone is regulated by a specific hypothalamic releasing factor. Feedback mechanisms govern the release of these factors. Substances available for clinical use include:
  - *growth hormone-releasing factor* (**sermorelin**) and analogues of growth hormone (**somatrophin**)
  - *thyrotrophin-releasing factor* (**protirelin**) and thyroid-stimulating hormone (thyrotrophin; used to test thyroid function)
  - **octreotide** and **lanreotide**, analogues of **somatostatin**, which inhibit growth hormone release
  - *corticotrophin-releasing factor*, used in diagnosis
  - *gonadotrophin-releasing factor*, **gonadorelin** and analogues. Used to treat infertility and some carcinomas.

Adrenocorticotrophic hormone and the adrenal steroids

- Adrenocorticotrophic hormone (ACTH; **tetracosactrin**, **tetracosactide**) stimulates synthesis and release of glucocorticoids (e.g. **hydrocortisone**), and also some androgens, from the adrenal cortex.
- Corticotrophin-releasing factor (CRF) from the hypothalamus regulates ACTH release, and is regulated in turn by neural factors and negative feedback effects of plasma glucocorticoids.
- Mineralocorticoid (e.g. aldosterone) release from the adrenal cortex is controlled by the renin–angiotensin system.

POSTERIOR PITUITARY GLAND

The posterior pituitary gland (neurohypophysis) consists largely of the terminals of nerve cells that lie in the *supraoptic* and *paraventricular nuclei* of the hypothalamus. Their axons form the *hypothalamic–hypophyseal tract*, and the fibres terminate in dilated nerve endings in close associa-

---

tion with capillaries in the posterior pituitary gland (Fig. 33.1). Peptides, synthesised in the hypothalamic nuclei, pass down these axons into the posterior pituitary, where they are stored and eventually secreted into the bloodstream.

The two main hormones of the posterior pituitary are **oxytocin** (which contracts the smooth muscle of the uterus; for details see Ch. 35) and **vasopressin** (antidiuretic hormone ADH; see Chs 22 and 29). They are highly homologous cyclic nonapeptides. Several analogues have been synthesised that vary in their antidiuretic, vasopressor and oxytocic (uterine stimulant) properties.

The posterior pituitary gland

- The posterior pituitary gland secretes:
  - oxytocin (see Ch. 35)
  - antidiuretic hormone (**vasopressin**), which acts on V_2 receptors in the distal kidney tubule to increase water reabsorption and, in higher concentrations, on V_{1A} receptors to cause vasoconstriction. It also stimulates adrenocorticotrophic hormone secretion.
- Substances available for clinical use are **vasopressin** and the analogues **desmopressin**, **felypressin** and **terlipressin**.

Clinical uses of antidiuretic hormone (vasopressin) and analogues

- Diabetes insipidus: **felypressin**, **desmopressin**.
- Initial treatment of bleeding oesophageal varices: **vasopressin**, **terlipressin**, **felypressin**. (Octreotide – a somatostatin analogue – is also used, but direct injection of sclerosant via an endoscope is the main treatment.)
- Prophylaxis against bleeding in haemophilia (e.g. before tooth extraction): **vasopressin**, **desmopressin** (by increasing the concentration of factor VIII).
- **Felypressin** is used as a vasoconstrictor with local anaesthetics (see Ch. 43)
- **Desmopressin** is used for persistent nocturnal enuresis in older children and adults.

VASOPRESSIN

Regulation of secretion and physiological role

Vasopressin released from the posterior pituitary has a crucial role in the control of the water content of the body through its action on the cells of the distal part of the nephron and the collecting tubules in the kidney (see Ch. 29). The hypothalamic nuclei that control fluid balance lie close to the nuclei that synthesise and secrete vasopressin.

One of the main stimuli for vasopressin release is an increase in plasma osmolarity (which produces a sensation of thirst). A decrease in circulating blood volume (*hypovolaemia*) is another, and here the stimuli arise from stretch receptors in the cardiovascular system or from angiotensin release. *Diabetes insipidus* is a condition in which large volumes of dilute urine are produced because vasopressin secretion is reduced or absent, or because of a reduced sensitivity of the kidney to the hormone.

Vasopressin receptors

There are three classes of receptor: V_{1A}, V_{1B} and V_2. All are GPCRs. V_2 receptors stimulate adenylyl cyclase, which mediates the main physiological actions of vasopressin in the kidney, whereas the V_{1A} and V_{1B} receptors are coupled to the phospholipase C/inositol trisphosphate system.

The receptor for oxytocin (OT receptor) is also a GPCR, which primarily signals through phospholipase C stimulation but has a secondary action on adenylyl cyclase. Vasopressin is a partial agonist at OT but its effects are limited by the distribution of the receptor, which, as might be inferred from its classic action on the pregnant uterus, is high in the myometrium, endometrium, mammary gland and ovary. The central actions of oxytocin (and vasopressin) have also attracted attention as they are apparently involved in 'pair bonding' and the other psychosocial interactions.[3]

Actions

Renal actions

Vasopressin binds to V_2 receptors in the basolateral membrane of the cells of the distal tubule and collecting ducts of the nephron. Its main effect in the collecting duct is to increase the rate of insertion of water channels (*aquaporins*) into the lumenal membrane, thus increasing the permeability of the membrane to water (see Ch. 29). It also activates urea transporters and transiently increases Na^+ absorption, particularly in the distal tubule.

Several drugs affect the action of vasopressin. Non-steroidal anti-inflammatory drugs and **carbamazepine** increase, and **lithium**, **colchicine** and **vinca alkaloids** decrease, vasopressin effects. The effects of the last two agents are secondary to their action on the microtubules required for translocation of water channels. The antagonists **demeclocycline** and **tolvaptan** counteract the action of vasopressin on the V_2 receptor in renal tubules and can be used to treat patients with water retention combined with urinary salt loss (and thus *hyponatraemia*) caused by excessive secretion of the hormone. This *syndrome of inappropriate ADH secretion* ('SIADH') is associated with lung or other malignancies or head injury. Specific V_2 receptor antagonists are also being investigated in the treatment of heart failure (Ch. 22).

Other non-renal actions

Vasopressin causes contraction of smooth muscle, particularly in the cardiovascular system, by acting on V_{1A} receptors (see Ch. 22). The affinity of vasopressin for these receptors is lower than that for V_2 receptors, and smooth muscle effects are seen only with doses larger than those affecting the kidney. Vasopressin also stimulates blood platelet aggregation and mobilisation of coagulation factors. When released into the pituitary portal circulation it promotes the release of ACTH from the anterior pituitary by an action on V_{1B} receptors (Fig. 33.4). In the CNS, vasopressin, like oxytocin, is believed to have a role in emotional and social behaviour.

Pharmacokinetic aspects

Vasopressin, as well as various peptide analogues, is used clinically either for the treatment of diabetes insipidus or as a vasoconstrictor. Several analogues have been developed to (a) increase the duration of action and (b) shift the relative potency between the V_1 and V_2 receptors.

The main substances used are:

- vasopressin itself; short duration of action, weak selectivity for V_2 receptors, given by subcutaneous or intramuscular injection, or by intravenous infusion;
- **desmopressin**; increased duration of action, V_2-selective and therefore fewer pressor effects, can be given by several routes including nasal spray;
- **terlipressin**; increased duration of action, low but protracted vasopressor action and minimal antidiuretic properties);
- **felypressin**; a short-acting vasoconstrictor that is injected with local anaesthetics such as **prilocaine** to prolong their action (see Ch. 43).

Vasopressin itself is rapidly eliminated, with a plasma half-life less than 10 min and a short duration of action. Metabolism is by tissue peptidases, and 33% is removed by the kidney. Desmopressin is less subject to degradation by peptidases, and its plasma half-life is 75 min.

Unwanted effects

There are few unwanted effects and they are mainly cardiovascular in nature: intravenous vasopressin may cause spasm of the coronary arteries with resultant angina, but this risk can be minimised if the antidiuretic peptides are administered intranasally.

THE ADRENAL CORTEX

The adrenal glands consist of two parts: the inner *medulla*, which secretes catecholamines (see Ch. 14), and the outer *cortex*, which secretes adrenal steroids. The cortex comprises three concentric zones: the *zona glomerulosa* (the outermost layer), which elaborates mineralocorticoids, the *zona fasciculate*, which elaborates glucocorticoids, and the innermost *zona reticularis*, which produces androgen precursors. The principal adrenal steroids are those with glucocorticoid and mineralocorticoid[4] activity. Androgen secretion (see Ch. 35) by the cortex is not considered further in this chapter.

The mineralocorticoids regulate water and electrolyte balance, and the main endogenous hormone is *aldosterone*. The glucocorticoids have widespread actions on intermediate metabolism, affecting carbohydrate and protein metabolism, as well as potent regulatory effects on host defence mechanisms (Chs 6 and 26). The adrenal gland secretes a mixture of glucocorticoids; in humans the main hormone is *hydrocortisone* (also, confusingly, known as *cortisol*), and in rodents, *corticosterone*. The mineralocorticoid and glucocorticoid actions are not completely

---

[3]Oxytocin is released during childbirth, lactation and orgasm and has been shown to promote trust and other prosocial behaviour. This has earned it the nickname, in the popular press and in the numerous Internet discussion groups that these findings have spawned, of the 'love hormone' or, even more nauseatingly, the 'cuddle hormone'.

[4]So named because early experimenters noticed that separate fractions of adrenal gland extracts caused changes in blood glucose or salt and water retention.

Table 33.2 Comparison of the main corticosteroid agents used for systemic therapy (using hydrocortisone as a standard)

Compound	Relative affinity for receptor[a]	Approximate relative potency in clinical use		Duration of action after oral dose[b]	Comments
		Anti-inflammatory	Sodium retaining		
Hydrocortisone	1	1	1	Short	Drug of choice for replacement therapy (cortisol)
Cortisone	Prodrug	0.8	0.8	Short	Cheap; inactive until converted to hydrocortisone; not used as anti-inflammatory because of mineralocorticoid effects
Deflazacort	Prodrug	3	?	Short	Converted by plasma esterases into active metabolite. Similar utility to prednisolone
Prednisolone	2.2	4	0.8	Intermediate	Drug of choice for systemic anti-inflammatory and immunosuppressive effects
Prednisone	Prodrug	4	0.8	Intermediate	Inactive until converted to prednisolone
Methylprednisolone	11.9	5	Minimal	Intermediate	Anti-inflammatory and immunosuppressive
Triamcinolone	1.9	5	None	Intermediate	Relatively more toxic than others
Dexamethasone	7.1	27	Minimal	Long	Anti-inflammatory and immunosuppressive, used especially where water retention is undesirable (e.g. cerebral oedema); drug of choice for suppression of ACTH production
Betamethasone	5.4	27	Negligible	Long	Anti-inflammatory and immunosuppressive, used especially when water retention is undesirable
Fludrocortisone	3.5	15	150	Short	Drug of choice for mineralocorticoid effects
Aldosterone	0.38	None	500	–	Endogenous mineralocorticoid

[a]Data obtained in human fetal lung cells.
[b]Duration of action (half lives in hours): short, 8–12; intermediate, 12–36, long, 36–72. Some drugs are inactive until converted to active compounds *in vivo* and therefore have negligible affinity for the glucocorticoid receptor.
(Data for relative affinity obtained from Baxter & Rousseau 1979)

separated in naturally occurring steroids and some glucocorticoids have quite substantial effects on water and electrolyte balance. In fact, hydrocortisone and aldosterone are equiactive on mineralocorticoid receptors but, in mineralocorticoid-sensitive tissues such as the kidney, the action of *11β-hydroxysteroid dehydrogenase* converts hydrocortisone to the inactive metabolite cortisone,[5] thereby preventing the tissue from responding to hydrocortisone.

With the exception of *replacement therapy*, glucocorticoids are most commonly employed for their anti-inflammatory and immunosuppressive properties (see Ch. 26). Under these circumstances, their metabolic and other actions are seen as unwanted side effects. Synthetic steroids have been developed in which it has been possible to separate, to some degree, the glucocorticoid from the mineralocorticoid actions (see Table 33.2), but it has not been possible to separate the anti-inflammatory from the other actions of the glucocorticoids completely.

---

[5]Oddly, it was cortisone that was originally demonstrated to have potent glucocorticoid anti-inflammatory activity in the classic studies of Hench and his colleagues in 1949. The reason for this apparent anomaly is that an isoform of 11 β-hydroxysteroid dehydrogenase present in some tissues can transform cortisone back to cortisol (i.e. hydrocortisone), thus restoring its biological activity.

▼ The adrenal gland is essential to life, and animals deprived of these glands are able to survive only under rigorously controlled conditions. In humans, a deficiency in corticosteroid production, termed *Addison's disease*, is characterised by muscular weakness, low blood pressure, depression, anorexia, loss of weight and hypoglycaemia. Addison's disease may have an autoimmune aetiology, or it may result from destruction of the gland by chronic inflammatory conditions such as tuberculosis.

When corticosteroids are produced in excess, the clinical picture depends on which species predominates. Excessive *glucocorticoid* activity results in *Cushing's syndrome*, the manifestations of which are outlined in Figure 33.7. This can be caused by hypersecretion from the adrenal glands or by prolonged therapeutic use of glucocorticoids. An excessive production of *mineralocorticoids* results in retention of Na$^+$ and loss of K$^+$. This may be caused by hyperactivity or tumours of the adrenals (*primary hyperaldosteronism*, or *Conn's syndrome*, an uncommon but important cause of hypertension; see Ch. 22), or by excessive activation of the renin–angiotensin system (such as occurs in some forms of kidney disease), cirrhosis of the liver or congestive cardiac failure (*secondary hyperaldosteronism*).

GLUCOCORTICOIDS

Synthesis and release

Glucocorticoids are not stored in the adrenal gland but are synthesised under the influence of circulating ACTH secreted from the anterior pituitary gland (Fig. 33.4) and released in a pulsatile fashion into the blood. While they are always present, there is a well-defined circadian rhythm in the secretion in healthy humans, with the net blood concentration being highest early in the morning, gradually diminishing throughout the day and reaching a low point in the evening or night. ACTH secretion itself (also pulsatile in nature) is regulated by CRF released from the hypothalamus, and by vasopressin released from the posterior pituitary gland. The release of both ACTH and CRF, in turn, is reflexly inhibited by the ensuing rising concentrations of glucocorticoids in the blood.

Opioid peptides also exercise a tonic inhibitory control on the secretion of CRF, and psychological factors, excessive heat or cold, injury or infections can also affect the release of both vasopressin and CRF. This is the principal mechanism whereby the HPA axis is activated in response to perceived threats in the external environment.

The precursor of glucocorticoids is cholesterol (Fig. 33.5). The initial conversion of cholesterol to *pregnenolone* is the rate-limiting step and is regulated by ACTH. Some biosynthetic reactions can be inhibited by drugs and these have a utility in treating Cushing's disease or adrenocortical carcinoma. **Metyrapone** prevents the β-hydroxylation at C11, and thus the formation of hydrocortisone and corticosterone. Synthesis is blocked at the 11-deoxycorticosteroid stage, leaving intermediates that have no effects on the hypothalamus and pituitary, so there is a marked increase in ACTH in the blood. Metyrapone can therefore be used to test ACTH production, and may also be used to treat patients with Cushing's syndrome. **Trilostane** (also of use in Cushing's syndrome and primary hyperaldosteronism) blocks an earlier enzyme in the pathway – the *3β-dehydrogenase*. **Aminoglutethimide** inhibits the initial step in the biosynthetic pathway and has the same overall effect as metyrapone.

Trilostane and aminoglutethamide are not currently used in the UK but **ketoconazole**, an antifungal agent (Ch. 53), also inhibits steroidogenesis and may be of value in the specialised treatment of Cushing's syndrome. **Mitotane** suppresses glucocorticoid synthesis by a direct (and unknown) mechanism on the adrenal gland. It is chiefly used to treat adrenocortical carcinomas.

Mechanism of glucocorticoid action

The glucocorticoid effects relevant to this discussion are initiated by interaction of the drugs with specific intracellular glucocorticoid receptors belonging to the nuclear receptor superfamily (although there may be other binding proteins or sites; see Norman et al., 2004). This superfamily (see Ch. 3) also includes the receptors for mineralocorticoids, the sex steroids, thyroid hormones, vitamin D_3 and retinoic acid. The actual mechanism of transcriptional control is complex, with at least four mechanisms operating within the nucleus. These are summarised diagrammatically in Figure 33.6.

When the nuclear actions of glucocorticoid receptors were first discovered it was thought that this mechanism could account for all the actions of the hormones, but a surprising discovery overturned this idea. Reichardt et al. (1998), using transgenic mice in which the glucocorticoid receptor was unable to dimerise, found that glucocorticoids were still able to exert a great many biological actions. This suggested that in addition to controlling gene expression within the nucleus, the liganded receptor itself, in either a monomeric or a dimeric form, could

Glucocorticoids

Common drugs used systemically include **hydrocortisone**, **prednisolone** and **dexamethasone**.

Metabolic actions

- *Carbohydrates*: decreased uptake and utilisation of glucose accompanied by increased gluconeogenesis; this causes a tendency to hyperglycaemia.
- *Proteins*: increased catabolism, reduced anabolism.
- *Lipids*: a permissive effect on lipolytic hormones and a redistribution of fat, as observed in Cushing's syndrome.

Regulatory actions

- *Hypothalamus and anterior pituitary gland*: a negative feedback action resulting in reduced release of endogenous glucocorticoids.
- *Cardiovascular system*: reduced vasodilatation, decreased fluid exudation.
- *Musculoskeletal*: decreased osteoblast and increased osteoclast activity.
- *Inflammation and immunity*:
  - acute inflammation: decreased influx and activity of leukocytes
  - chronic inflammation: decreased activity of mononuclear cells, decreased angiogenesis, less fibrosis
  - lymphoid tissues: decreased clonal expansion of T and B cells, and decreased action of cytokine-secreting T cells. Switch from Th1 to Th2 response.
- Mediators:
  - decreased production and action of many cytokines, including interleukins, tumour necrosis factor-α and granulocyte–macrophage colony-stimulating factor
  - reduced generation of eicosanoids
  - decreased generation of IgG
  - decrease in complement components in the blood
  - increased release of anti-inflammatory factors such as interleukin (IL)-10, IL-1ra and annexin 1.
- Overall effects: reduction in the activity of the innate and acquired immune systems, but also diminution in the protective aspects of the inflammatory response and sometimes decreased healing.

initiate important signal transduction events while still in the cytosolic compartment (there may even be a subpopulation of receptors that reside there permanently). One such effect seems to be interaction of the receptor with the regulatory complex, NF-κB (Ch. 3). Other important interactions may involve protein kinases/phosphatases that regulate glucocorticoid receptor behaviour and the time spent in the nuclear compartment. Some of these cytosolic actions are very rapid. For example, the glucocorticoid-induced phosphorylation by PKC and subsequent release of the protein *annexin-1*, which has potent inhibitory effects on leukocyte trafficking and other anti-inflammatory actions, occurs in minutes and could not be accounted for by changes in protein synthesis.

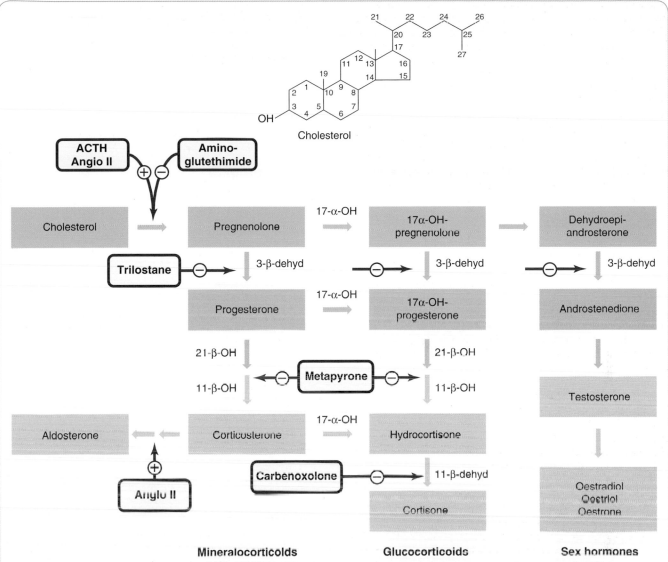

Fig. 33.5 **Biosynthesis of corticosteroids, mineralocorticoids and sex hormones.** All steroid hormones are synthesised from cholesterol. Successive steps of hydroxylation and dehydrogenation are important in the biosynthetic pathway and are targets for drugs. Intermediates are shown in green boxes; interconversions occur between the pathways. Blue boxes indicate circulating hormones. Drugs are shown in red-bordered boxes adjacent to their sites of action. Glucocorticoids are produced by cells of the zona fasciculata, and their synthesis is stimulated by adrenocorticotrophic hormone (ACTH); aldosterone is produced by cells of the zona glomerulosa, and its synthesis is stimulated by angiotensin II (angio II). Metyrapone inhibits glucocorticoid synthesis, aminoglutethimide and trilostane block synthesis of all three types of adrenal steroid (see text for details). Carbenoxolone inhibits the interconversion of hydrocortisone and cortisone in the kidney. Not shown is mitotane, which suppresses adrenal hormone synthesis through an unknown mechanism. Enzymes: 17-α-OH, 17-α-hydroxylase; 3-β-dehyd, 3-β-dehydrogenase; 21-β-OH, 21-β-hydroxylase; 11-β-OH, 11-β-hydroxylase; 11-β-dehyd, 11-β-hydroxysteroid dehydrogenase.

Actions

General metabolic and systemic effects

The main metabolic effects are on carbohydrate and protein metabolism. The glucocorticoids cause both a decrease in the uptake and utilisation of glucose and an increase in gluconeogenesis, resulting in a tendency to hyperglycaemia (see Ch. 31). There is a concomitant increase in glycogen storage, which may be a result of insulin secretion in response to the increase in blood sugar. Overall, there is decreased protein synthesis and increased protein breakdown, particularly in muscle, and this can lead to tissue wasting. Glucocorticoids also have a 'permissive' effect on the cAMP-dependent lipolytic response to catecholamines and other hormones. Such hormones cause lipase activation through a cAMP-dependent kinase, the synthesis of which requires the presence of glucocorticoids. Large doses of glucocorticoids given over a long period result in the redistribution of body fat characteristic of Cushing's syndrome (Fig. 33.7).

Glucocorticoids tend to produce a negative calcium balance by decreasing Ca^{2+} absorption in the gastrointestinal tract and increasing its excretion by the kidney. Together with increased breakdown of bone matrix

411

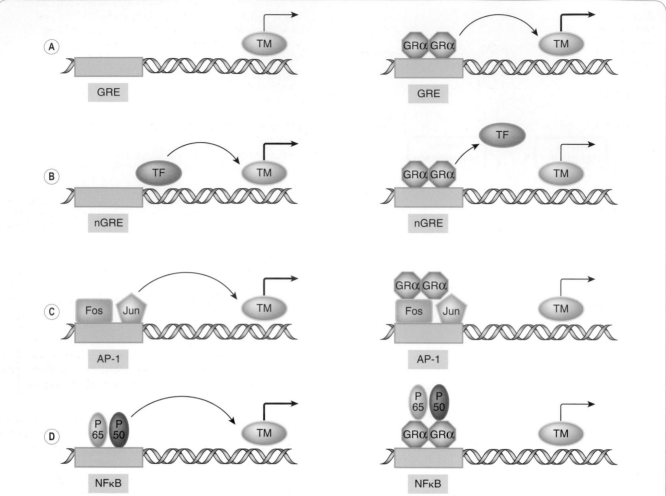

Fig. 33.6 Molecular mechanism of action of glucocorticoids. The schematic figure shows three possible ways by which the liganded glucocorticoid receptor can control gene expression following translocation to the nucleus. [**A**] Basic transactivation mechanism. Here, the transcriptional machinery (TM) is presumed to be operating at a low level. The liganded glucocorticoid receptor (GR) dimer binds to one or more 'positive' glucocorticoid response elements (GREs) within the promoter sequence (shaded zone) and upregulates transcription. [**B**] Basic transrepression mechanism. The transcriptional machinery is constitutively driven by transcription factors (TF). In binding to the 'negative' GRE (nGRE), the receptor complex displaces these factors and expression falls. [**C**] Fos/Jun mechanism. Transcription is driven at a high level by Fos/Jun transcription factors binding to their AP-1 regulatory site. This effect is reduced in the presence of the GR. [**D**] Nuclear factor (NF)κβ mechanism. The transcription factors P65 and P50 bind to the NF-κβ site, promoting gene expression. This is prevented by the presence of the GR, which binds the transcription factors, preventing their action (this may occur in the cytoplasm also). (For further details of the structure of the glucocorticoid receptor, see Ch. 3.) *(Modified from Oakley & Cidlowski 2001.)*

protein this may cause osteoporosis. In higher, non-physiological concentrations, the glucocorticoids have some mineralocorticoid actions, causing Na^+ retention and K^+ loss – possibly by swamping the protective 11β-hydroxysteroid dehydrogenase and acting at mineralocorticoid receptors.

Negative feedback effects on the anterior pituitary and hypothalamus

Both endogenous and exogenous glucocorticoids have a negative feedback effect on the secretion of CRF and ACTH (see Fig. 33.4), thus inhibiting the secretion of endogenous glucocorticoids and potentially causing atrophy of the adrenal cortex. If therapy is prolonged, it may take many months to return to normal function once the drugs are stopped.

Anti-inflammatory and immunosuppressive effects

Endogenous glucocorticoids maintain a low-level anti-inflammatory tone, and are secreted in response to inflammatory stimuli. Consequently, adrenalectomised animals show a heightened response to even mild inflammatory stimuli . On this basis, it has been suggested that a failure of appropriate secretion of glucocorticoids in response to injury or infection may underlie certain chronic inflammatory human pathologies.

Exogenous glucocorticoids are the anti-inflammatory drugs *par excellence*, and when given therapeutically inhibit the operation of both the innate and adaptive immune system. They reverse virtually all types of inflammatory reaction, whether caused by invading pathogens, by chemical or physical stimuli, or by inappropriately deployed immune responses such as are seen in hypersensitivity

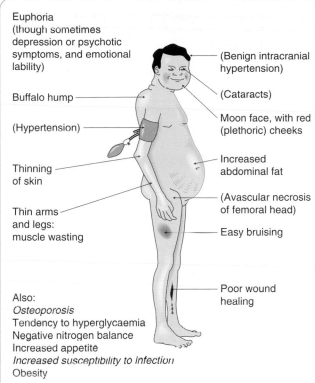

Euphoria
(though sometimes
depression or psychotic
symptoms, and emotional
lability)

Buffalo hump

(Hypertension)

Thinning
of skin

Thin arms
and legs:
muscle wasting

(Benign intracranial
hypertension)

(Cataracts)

Moon face, with red
(plethoric) cheeks

Increased
abdominal fat

(Avascular necrosis
of femoral head)

Easy bruising

Poor wound
healing

Also:
Osteoporosis
Tendency to hyperglycaemia
Negative nitrogen balance
Increased appetite
Increased susceptibility to infection
Obesity

Fig. 33.7 Cushing's syndrome. This is caused by excessive exposure to glucocorticoids, and may be caused by disease (e.g. an adrenocorticotrophic hormone-secreting tumour) or by prolonged administration of glucocorticoid drugs (iatrogenic Cushing's). Italicised effects are particularly common. Less frequent effects, related to dose and duration of therapy, are shown in parentheses. *(Adapted from Baxter & Rousseau 1979)*

or autoimmune disease. When used prophylactically to suppress graft rejection, glucocorticoids are more efficient in suppressing the initiation and generation of the immune response than they are in preventing the operation of an established response where clonal proliferation has already occurred.

Given that glucocorticoids modify the expression of so many genes, and that the extent and direction of regulation varies between tissues and even at different times during disease, you will not be surprised to learn that their anti-inflammatory effects are complex.

Actions on *inflammatory* cells include:

- decreased egress of neutrophils from blood vessels and reduced activation of neutrophils, macrophages and mast cells secondary to decreased transcription of the genes for cell adhesion factors and cytokines
- decreased overall activation of T-helper (Th) cells, reduced clonal proliferation of T cells, and a 'switch' from the Th1 to the Th2 immune response (see Ch. 6)
- decreased fibroblast function, less production of collagen and glycosaminoglycans, and, under some circumstances, reduced healing and repair.

Actions on the mediators of inflammatory and immune responses (Chs 17 and 18) include:

- decreased production of prostanoids through reduced expression of cyclo-oxygenase-2

- decreased generation of many cytokines, including IL-1, IL-2, IL-3, IL-4, IL-5, IL-6, IL-8, TNF-α, cell adhesion factors and granulocyte–macrophage colony-stimulating factor. These are largely secondary to inhibition of gene transcription
- reduction in the concentration of complement components in the plasma
- decreased generation of induced nitric oxide by nitric oxide synthase 2 (NOS2)
- decreased histamine release from basophils and mast cells
- decreased immunoglobulin G (IgG) production
- increased synthesis of anti-inflammatory factors such as IL-10, IL-1-soluble receptor and annexin-1.

Potent anti-inflammatory glucocorticoids circulate constantly in the blood and are increased during inflammatory episodes. It is suggested (see Munck et al., 1984), that the anti-inflammatory and immunosuppressive actions of endogenous glucocorticoids play a crucial counter-regulatory role, in that they prevent excessive activation of inflammation and other powerful defence reactions that might, if unchecked, themselves threaten homeostasis. Certainly, this view is borne out by experimental work. While these drugs are of great value in treating conditions characterised by hypersensitivity and unwanted inflammation, they carry the hazard that they are able to suppress the same defence reactions that provide protection from infection and other insults.

Unwanted effects

Low-dose glucocorticoid replacement therapy is usually without problems but serious unwanted effects occur with large doses or prolonged administration of glucocorticoids. The major effects are as follows:

- *Suppression of the response to infection or injury:* opportunistic infection can be potentially very serious unless quickly treated with antimicrobial agents along with an increase in the dose of steroid. Oral thrush (candidiasis, a fungal infection; see Ch. 53) frequently occurs when glucocorticoids are taken by inhalation, because of suppression of local anti-infective mechanisms. Wound healing is impaired, and peptic ulceration may also occur.
- *Cushing's syndrome* (see Fig. 33.7).
- *Osteoporosis*, with the attendant hazard of fractures, is one of the main limitations to long-term glucocorticoid therapy. These drugs influence bone density both by regulation of calcium and phosphate metabolism and through effects on collagen turnover. They reduce osteoblast function (which deposits bone matrix) and increase the activity of osteoclasts (which digest bone matrix). An effect on the blood supply to bone can result in avascular necrosis of the head of the femur (see Ch. 36).
- *Hyperglycaemia* produced by exogenous glucocorticoids may develop into actual diabetes.
- *Muscle wasting* and proximal muscle weakness.
- In children, *inhibition of growth*[6] if treatment is continued for more than 6 months.

---

[6]However, some of the diseases for which glucocorticoids are indicated themselves retard growth. In a classical trial, glucocorticoid treatment *increased* growth in adolescents with inflammatory bowel disease as the disease resolved (Whittington et al., 1977).

- *Central nervous system effects*: euphoria, depression and psychosis.
- *Other effects*: glaucoma (in genetically predisposed persons), raised intracranial pressure and an increased incidence of cataracts.

Sudden withdrawal of the drugs after prolonged therapy may result in acute adrenal insufficiency because of suppression of the patient's capacity to synthesise corticosteroids.[7] Careful procedures for phased withdrawal should be followed. Recovery of full adrenal function usually takes about 8 weeks, although it can take 18 months or more after prolonged high-dose treatment.

Mechanism of action of the glucocorticoids

- Glucocorticoids bind intracellular receptors that then dimerise, migrate to the nucleus and interact with DNA to modify gene transcription, inducing synthesis of some proteins and inhibiting synthesis of others.
- A substantial proportion of glucocorticoid actions are mediated by interactions of regulatory factors with the receptor in the cytosol. Some are very rapid.
- *Metabolic actions*: most mediator proteins are enzymes, for example cAMP-dependent kinase, but not all actions on genes are known.
- *Anti-inflammatory and immunosuppressive actions*. Known actions include:
  - inhibition of transcription of the genes for inducible cyclo-oxygenase-2 and inducible nitric oxide synthase, cytokines and interleukins, cell adhesion molecules
  - block of vitamin D_3-mediated induction of the osteocalcin gene in osteoblasts, and modification of transcription of the collagenase genes
  - increased synthesis and release of anti-inflammatory factors including annexin-1 in cells of the innate immune system. This has potent anti-inflammatory effects on cells and mediator release, and may also mediate negative feedback at the level of the hypothalamus and anterior pituitary gland.

Pharmacokinetic aspects

There are many glucocorticoid drugs in therapeutic use. Although **cortisol** (**hydrocortisone**), the endogenous hormone, is often used, synthetic derivatives are even more common. These have different physicochemical properties as well as varying potency and have been optimised for administration by different routes. They may be administered orally, systemically or intra-articularly; given by aerosol into the respiratory tract; administered as drops into the eye or sprayed into the nose; applied as creams or ointments to the skin (see Ch. 27); or as foam enemas to the gastrointestinal tract (Ch. 30). Topical administration diminishes the likelihood of systemic toxic effects unless large quantities are used. When prolonged use of systemic glucocorticoids is necessary, therapy on

Clinical uses of glucocorticoids

- Replacement therapy for patients with adrenal failure (*Addison's disease*).
- Anti-inflammatory/immunosuppressive therapy (see also Ch. 26):
  - in *asthma* (Ch. 28)
  - topically in various inflammatory conditions of skin, eye, ear or nose (e.g. *eczema, allergic conjunctivitis* or *rhinitis*; see Ch. 27)
  - *hypersensitivity states* (e.g. severe allergic reactions)
  - in miscellaneous diseases with autoimmune and inflammatory components (e.g. *rheumatoid arthritis* and other 'connective tissue' diseases, *inflammatory bowel diseases*, some forms of *haemolytic anaemia*, *idiopathic thrombocytopenic purpura*)
  - to prevent graft-versus-host disease following organ or bone marrow transplantation.
- In neoplastic disease (Ch. 56):
  - in combination with cytotoxic drugs in treatment of specific malignancies (e.g. *Hodgkin's disease, acute lymphocytic leukaemia*)
  - to reduce cerebral oedema in patients with metastatic or primary *brain tumours* (**dexamethasone**).

alternate days may decrease suppression of the HPA axis and other unwanted effects.

As small lipophilic molecules, glucocorticoids probably enter their target cells by simple diffusion. Hydrocortisone has a plasma half-life of 90 min, although its main biological effects have a latency of 2–8 h. Biological inactivation, which occurs in liver cells and elsewhere, is initiated by reduction of the C4–C5 double bond. Cortisone and **prednisone** are inactive until converted *in vivo* to hydrocortisone and **prednisolone**, respectively.

Endogenous glucocorticoids are transported in the plasma bound to *corticosteroid-binding globulin* (CBG) and to albumin. About 77% of plasma hydrocortisone is bound to CBG, but many synthetic glucocorticoids are not bound at all. Albumin has a lower affinity for hydrocortisone but binds both natural and synthetic steroids. Both CBG-bound and albumin-bound steroids are biologically inactive.

The clinical use of systemic glucocorticoids is given in the clinical box above. Dexamethasone has a special use: it is used to test HPA axis function. In the *dexamethasone suppression test* a relatively low dose of dexamethasone, usually given at night, would be expected to suppress the hypothalamus and pituitary, and result in reduced ACTH secretion and hydrocortisone output, as measured in the plasma about 9 h later. Failure of suppression implies hypersecretion of ACTH or of glucocorticoids (Cushing's syndrome).

MINERALOCORTICOIDS

The main endogenous mineralocorticoid is aldosterone. Its chief action is to increase Na^+ reabsorption by the distal tubules in the kidney, with a concomitant increase in excretion of K^+ and H^+ (see Ch. 29). An excessive secretion

---

[7]Patients on long-term glucocorticoid therapy are advised to carry a card stating, 'I am a patient on STEROID TREATMENT which must not be stopped abruptly'.

Pharmacokinetics and unwanted actions of the glucocorticoids

- Administration can be oral, topical or parenteral. Most naturally occurring glucocorticoids are transported in the blood by corticosteroid-binding globulin or albumen and enter cells by diffusion. They are metabolised in the liver.
- Unwanted effects are seen mainly after prolonged systemic use as anti-inflammatory or immunosuppressive agents but not usually following replacement therapy. The most important are:
  - suppression of response to infection
  - suppression of endogenous glucocorticoid synthesis
  - metabolic actions (see above)
  - osteoporosis
  - iatrogenic Cushing's syndrome (see Fig. 33.7).

of mineralocorticoids, as in *Conn's syndrome*, causes marked Na^+ and water retention, with increased extracellular fluid volume and sometimes hypokalaemia, alkalosis and hypertension. Decreased secretion, as in some patients with Addison's disease, causes Na^+ loss (desalinisation) and a marked decrease in extracellular fluid volume. There is a concomitant decrease in the excretion of K^+, resulting in hyperkalaemia.

Mineralocorticoids

Fludrocortisone is given orally to produce a mineralocorticoid effect. This drug:
- increases Na^+ reabsorption in distal tubules and increases K^+ and H^+ efflux into the tubules
- acts on intracellular receptors that modulate DNA transcription, causing synthesis of protein mediators
- is used together with a glucocorticoid in replacement therapy.

Regulation of aldosterone synthesis and release
The regulation of the synthesis and release of aldosterone depends mainly on the electrolyte composition of the plasma and on the angiotensin II system (Fig. 33.4; Chs 22 and 29). Low plasma Na^+ or high plasma K^+ concentrations affect the zona glomerulosa cells of the adrenal directly, stimulating aldosterone release. Depletion of body Na^+ also activates the renin–angiotensin system (see Ch. 22, Fig. 22.4). One of the effects of angiotensin II is to increase the synthesis and release of aldosterone (see Ch. 29, Fig. 29.5).

Mechanism of action
Like other steroid hormones, aldosterone acts through specific intracellular receptors of the nuclear receptor family. Unlike the glucocorticoid receptor, which is present in most cells, the *mineralocorticoid receptor* is restricted to a few tissues, such as the kidney and the transporting epithelia of the colon and bladder. Cells containing mineralocorticoid receptors also contain the 11β-hydroxysteroid

dehydrogenase type 2 enzyme, which converts hydrocortisone (cortisol) into inactive cortisone, but does not inactivate aldosterone. This ensures that the cells are appropriately affected only by the mineralocorticoid hormone itself. Interestingly, this enzyme is inhibited by **carbenoxolone,** a compound derived from liquorice (and previously used to treat gastric ulcers; see Ch. 30). If this inhibition is marked, cortisol accumulates and acts on the mineralocorticoid receptor, producing an effect similar to Conn's syndrome (*primary hyperaldosteronism*) except that the circulating aldosterone concentration is not raised.

As with the glucocorticoids, the interaction of aldosterone with its receptor initiates transcription and translation of specific proteins, resulting in an increase in the number of sodium channels in the apical membrane of the cell, and subsequently an increase in the number of Na^+-K^+-ATPase molecules in the basolateral membrane (see Fig. 29.5), causing increased K^+ excretion (see Ch. 29). In addition to the genomic effects, there is evidence for a rapid non-genomic effect of aldosterone on Na^+ influx, through an action on the Na^+-H^+ exchanger in the apical membrane.

Clinical use of mineralocorticoids and antagonists
The main clinical use of mineralocorticoids is in replacement therapy of patients with Addison's disease. The most commonly used drug is **fludrocortisone** (Table 33.2 and Fig. 33.4), which can be taken orally to supplement the necessary glucocorticoid replacement. **Spironolactone** is a competitive antagonist of aldosterone, and it also prevents the mineralocorticoid effects of other adrenal steroids on the renal tubule (Ch. 29). Side effects include gynaecomastia and impotence, because spironolactone also has some blocking action on androgen and progesterone receptors. It is used to treat primary or secondary hyperaldosteronism and, in conjunction with other drugs, in the treatment of resistant hypertension and of heart failure (Ch. 22) and oedema (Ch. 29). **Eplerenone** has a similar indication and mechanism of action, although fewer side effects as it has lower affinity for sex hormone receptors (Ch. 22).

NEW DIRECTIONS IN GLUCOCORTICOID THERAPY

Glucocorticoids are highly effective in controlling inflammation, but severely limited by their side effects. The ideal solution would be a glucocorticoid possessing the anti-inflammatory but not the unwanted metabolic or other effects.

Following the discovery of cortisol, the pharmaceutical industry pursued this ambitious goal by testing straightforward structural analogues of cortisol. While this yielded many new active and interesting compounds (several of which are in clinical use today), none achieved a true 'separation' of the glucocorticoid actions. Many considered that the possibilities afforded by this approach had been exhausted but recently there have been fresh attempts to accomplish this. The development of structural analogues at novel sites on the steroid template (e.g. Uings et al., 2013) has met with more success and the use of X-ray crystallography has even enabled the design of non-steroidal ligands that exploit unusual binding sites on the receptor (Biggadike et al., 2009).

Another idea has been to add other functional groups on to the steroid molecule. Fiorucci et al. (2002) attached a nitric oxide donating group to prednisolone, finding augmented efficacy and reduced unwanted effects. The compound is reported to be useful in the treatment of inflammatory bowel disease (see Schacke et al., 2007).

Many investigators in this area have been influenced by the 'transrepression hypothesis': this is the notion, based upon some experimental observations, that the therapeutic effects of glucocorticoids are generally caused by the *down*-regulation (*transrepression*) of genes such as those coding for cytokines, whilst the unwanted effects are usually caused by *up*-regulation (*transactivation*) of metabolic and other genes (e.g. tyrosine amino transferase and phosphoenol pyruvate carboxykinase). This could alter intermediate metabolism and lead to, for example, diabetes. Because transactivation and transrepression utilise different molecular pathways, researchers have sought **s**elective **g**lucocorticoid **r**eceptor **a**gonists (SEGRAs) that promote one set of actions without the other. The application of this idea has been reviewed by Schacke et al. (2007) and the development of one such compound to the clinical trial stage has been reported (Schacke et al., 2009). Clark and Belvisi (2012) have reviewed the evidence for this idea and, in particular, highlighted its shortcomings.

A related idea focuses upon the histone deacetylase enzymes that are responsible for facilitating the transcriptional regulation of genes following nuclear receptor binding to response elements (Hayashi et al., 2004). One current notion is that there may be a specific isoform of this enzyme that deals with gene upregulation, and that if this could be inhibited, it would lessen the possibility of those unwanted effects. Barnes (2011) has reviewed this approach particularly as it relates to the therapy of asthma. A more general review of the whole area with particular relevance to the treatment of rheumatic diseases has been provided by Strehl et al. (2011).

The quest for the glucocorticoid magic bullet continues.

REFERENCES AND FURTHER READING

The hypothalamus and pituitary

Chan, L.F., Clark, A.J., Metherell, L.A., 2008. Familial glucocorticoid deficiency: advances in the molecular understanding of ACTH action. Horm. Res. 69, 75–82. (*This paper and the one by the same group below (Clark et al.) discuss research into the role of the ACTH signalling system in familial glucocorticoid deficiency. An expert piece of scientific detective work. The second paper is more accessible*)

Chini, B., Manning, M., Guillon, G., 2008. Affinity and efficacy of selective agonists and antagonists for vasopressin and oxytocin receptors: an 'easy guide' to receptor pharmacology. Prog. Brain Res. 170, 513–517. (*The title is self-explanatory! Also deals with the prospects for new drugs in this area*)

Clark, A.J., Metherell, L.A., Cheetham, M.E., Huebner, A., 2005. Inherited ACTH insensitivity illuminates the mechanisms of ACTH action. Trends Endocrinol. Metab. 16, 451–457.

Drolet, G., Rivest, S., 2001. Corticotropin-releasing hormone and its receptors; an evaluation at the transcription level *in vivo*. Peptides 22, 761–767.

Freeman, M.E., Kanyicska, B., Lerant, A., Nagy, G., 2000. Prolactin: structure, function and regulation of secretion. Physiol. Res. 80, 1524–1585. (*Comprehensive review of prolactin and its receptors*)

Getting, S.J., Christian, H.C., Flower, R.J., Perretti, M., 2002. Activation of melanocortin type 3 receptor as a molecular mechanism for adrenocorticotropic hormone efficacy in gouty arthritis. Arthritis Rheum. 46, 2765–2775. (*Original paper that demonstrates that ACTH has intrinsic anti-inflammatory actions that are independent of the adrenals*)

Guillemin, R., 2005. Hypothalamic hormones a.k.a. hypothalamic releasing factors. J. Endocrinol. 184, 11–28. (*This little review focuses on the history of research in this area and covers the discovery and characterisation of the principal releasing factors. Something to read if you are drawn to this area*)

Lamberts, S.W.J., van der Lely, A.-J., de Herder, W.W., Hofland, L.J., 1996. Octreotide. N. Engl. J. Med. 334, 246–254. (*A review covering somatostatin receptors, somatostatin analogues and treatment of tumours expressing somatostatin receptors with octreotide*)

Maybauer, M.O., Maybauer, D.M., Enkhbaatar, P., Traber, D.L., 2008. Physiology of the vasopressin receptors. Best Pract. Res. Clin. Anaesthesiol. 22, 253–263. (*A small review written mainly from a clinical perspective. Discusses future therapeutic uses for receptor agonists*)

Okada, S., Kopchick, J.J., 2001. Biological effects of growth hormone and its antagonist. Trends Mol. Med. 7, 126–132.

Prakash, A., Goa, K.L., 1999. Sermorelin: a review of its use in the diagnosis and treatment of children with idiopathic growth hormone deficiency. Biodrugs 12, 139–157. (*Mainly a clinical appraisal of sermorelin utility in treating growth deficiency in contrast to growth hormone itself*)

Schneider, F., Tomek, W., Grundker, C., 2006. Gonadotropin-releasing hormone (GnRH) and its natural analogues: a review. Theriogenology 66, 691–709. (*Focuses mainly on the use of such agents in veterinary medicine*)

Thibonnier, M., Coles, P., Thibonnier, A., et al., 2001. The basic and clinical pharmacology of nonpeptide vasopressin receptor antagonists. Annu. Rev. Pharmacol. 41, 175–202. (*Authoritative account of ADH receptors and the search for new antagonists*)

Vance, M.L., 1994. Hypopituitarism. N. Engl. J. Med. 330, 1651–1662. (*Review of causes, clinical features and hormone replacement therapy of hypopituitarism*)

Wikberg, J.E.S., Muceniece, R., Mandrika, I., et al., 2000. New aspects on the melanocortins and their receptors. Pharmacol. Res. 42, 393–420. (*Detailed review of the varied biological roles of melanocortins and their receptors*)

Glucocorticoids

Adcock, I.M., 2003. Glucocorticoids: new mechanisms and future agents. Curr. Allergy Asthma Rep. 3, 249–257. (*Excellent review of advances in glucocorticoid pharmacology*)

Barnes, P.J., 2011. Glucocorticosteroids: current and future directions. Br. J. Pharmacol. 163 (1), 29–43. (*Useful and accessible review focusing on general mechanisms with especial reference to asthma*)

Baxter, J.D., Rousseau, G.G. (Eds.), 1979. Glucocorticoid hormone action. Monographs on Endocrinology. Springer-Verlag, Berlin, p. 12. (*Another very useful source of information although it is somewhat dated now*)

Biggadike, K., Bledsoe, R.K., Coe, D.M., et al., 2009. Design and x-ray crystal structures of high-potency nonsteroidal glucocorticoid agonists exploiting a novel binding site on the receptor. Proc. Natl Acad. Sci. U.S.A. 106, 18114–18119. (*Explores the design of new non-steroid drugs that bind to the glucocorticoid receptor*)

Borski, R.J., 2000. Nongenomic membrane actions of glucocorticoids in vertebrates. Trends Endocrinol. Metab. 11, 427–436. (*A thought-provoking account of the non-genomic effects of glucocorticoids*)

Buckingham, J.C., 1998. Stress and the hypothalamo–pituitary–immune axis. Int. J. Tissue React. 20, 23–34. (*Excellent review of the complexities of the effect of stress on HPA axis function*)

Clark, A.R., Belvisi, M.G., 2012. Maps and legends: the quest for dissociated ligands of the glucocorticoid receptor. Pharmacol. Ther. 134, 54–67. (*Very readable account of the 'transrepression' hypothesis and its shortcomings*)

D'Acquisto, F., Perretti, M., Flower, R.J., 2008. Annexin-A1: a pivotal regulator of the innate and adaptive immune systems. Br. J. Pharmacol. 155, 152–169. (*Reviews the role of the glucocorticoid-regulated protein annexin-A1 in mediating the anti-inflammatory action of glucocorticoid drugs*)

Falkenstein, E., Tillmann, H.C., Christ, M., et al., 2000. Multiple actions of steroid hormones – a focus on rapid, nongenomic effects. Pharmacol. Rev. 52, 513–556.

Fiorucci, S., Antonelli, E., Distrutti, E., et al., 2002. NCX-1015, a nitric-oxide derivative of prednisolone, enhances regulatory T cells in the lamina propria and protects against 2,4,6-trinitrobenzene sulfonic acid-induced colitis in mice. Proc. Natl Acad. Sci. U.S.A. 99, 15770–15775.

Hayashi, R., Wada, H., Ito, K., Adcock, I.M., 2004. Effects of glucocorticoids on gene transcription. Eur. J. Pharmacol. 500, 51–62. (*Good basic review of glucocorticoid action; easy to read*)

Kirwan, J., Power, L., 2007. Glucocorticoids: action and new therapeutic insights in rheumatoid arthritis. Curr. Opin. Rheumatol. 19, 233–237. (*Written mainly from the viewpoint of a practising rheumatologist, this review offers interesting insights into the use of these drugs to modify severe chronic arthritic disease*)

Munck, A., Guyre, P.M., Holbrook, N.J., 1984. Physiological functions of glucocorticoids in stress and their relation to pharmacological actions. Endocr. Rev. 5, 25–44. (*Seminal review suggesting that the anti-inflammatory/immunosuppressive actions of the glucocorticoids have a physiological function; required reading if you want to understand glucocorticoid physiology and pharmacology*)

Norman, A.W., Mizwicki, M.T., Norman, D.P., 2004. Steroid-hormone rapid actions, membrane receptors and a conformational ensemble model. Nat. Rev. Drug Discov. 3, 27–41. (*Fairly advanced reading but contains many useful tables and excellent diagrams; well worth the effort if this subject interests you*)

Oakley, R.H., Cidlowski, J.A., 2001. The glucocorticoid receptor: expression, function and regulation of glucocorticoid responsiveness. In: Goulding, N.J., Flower, R.J. (Eds.), Milestones in Drug Therapy: Glucocorticoids. Birkhäuser Verlag, Basle, pp. 55–80. (*The book is a useful source of information on all aspects of glucocorticoid biology and pharmacology, containing chapters by some of the leaders in the field*)

Reichardt, H.M., Kaestner, K.H., Tuckermann, J., et al., 1998. DNA binding of the glucocorticoid receptor is not essential for survival. Cell. 93, 531–541. (*An account of the work that changed the way we think about glucocorticoid receptor actions. A similar approach is employed in the following paper, with further discoveries*)

Reichardt, H.M., Tronche, F., Bauer, A., Schutz, G., 2000. Molecular genetic analysis of glucocorticoid signaling using the Cre/loxP system. Biol. Chem. 381, 961–964.

Schacke, H., Berger, M., Rehwinkel, H., Asadullah, K., 2007. Selective glucocorticoid receptor agonists (SEGRAs): novel ligands with an improved therapeutic index. Mol. Cell. Endocrinol. 275, 109–117. (*This paper and the next describe the ideas behind the 'SEGRA' concept and the drugs that have been produced as a result*)

Schacke, H., Zollner, T.M., Docke, W.D., et al., 2009. Characterization of ZK 245186, a novel, selective glucocorticoid receptor agonist for the topical treatment of inflammatory skin diseases. Br. J. Pharmacol. 158, 1088–1103.

Song, I.H., Gold, R., Straub, R.H., et al., 2005. New glucocorticoids on the horizon: repress, don't activate! J. Rheumatol. 32, 1199–1207. (*Good summary of the various approaches taken to circumvent glucocorticoid side effects*)

Strehl, C., Spies, C.M., Buttgereit, F., 2011. Pharmacodynamics of glucocorticoids. Clin. Exp. Rheumatol. 29, S13–S18. (*General review of glucocorticoid mechanisms with especial reference to the treatment of rheumatic disorders*)

Tak, P.P., Firestein, G.S., 2001. NF-kappaB: a key role in inflammatory diseases. J. Clin. Invest. 107, 7–11. (*Succinct and very readable account of the role of nuclear factor (NF)κβ in inflammation*)

Uings, I.J., Needham, D., Matthews, J., et al., 2013. Discovery of GW870086: a potent anti-inflammatory steroid with a unique pharmacological profile. Br. J. Pharmacol. 169, 1389–1403.

Whittington, P.F., Barnes, H.V., Bayless, T.M., 1977. Medical management of Crohn's disease in adolescence. Gastroenterology 72, 1338–1344.

Mineralocorticoids

Bastl, C., Hayslett, J.P., 1992. The cellular action of aldosterone in target epithelia. Kidney Int. 42, 250–264. (*A detailed review covering the aldosterone receptor and regulation of gene expression, aldosterone action on electrogenic and electroneutral Na^+ transport, and on K^+ and H^+ secretion*)

34 The thyroid

OVERVIEW

Diseases of the thyroid gland are common, and in this chapter we deal with drug therapy used to mitigate these disorders. We set the scene by briefly outlining the structure, regulation and physiology of the thyroid, and highlight the most common abnormalities of thyroid function. We then consider the drugs that can replace the thyroid hormones when these are deficient or cease to function adequately, and the drugs that decrease thyroid function when this is excessive.

SYNTHESIS, STORAGE AND SECRETION OF THYROID HORMONES

The thyroid gland secretes three main hormones: *thyroxine* (T_4), *tri-iodothyronine* (T_3) and *calcitonin*. T_4 and T_3 are critically important for normal growth and development and for controlling energy metabolism. Calcitonin is involved in the control of plasma [Ca^{2+}] and is used to treat osteoporosis and other metabolic bone diseases. It is dealt with in Chapter 36. The term 'thyroid hormones' will be used here solely to refer to T_4 and T_3.

The functional unit of the thyroid is the follicle or acinus. Each follicle consists of a single layer of epithelial cells around a cavity, the *follicle lumen*, which is filled with a thick colloid containing thyroglobulin. *Thyroglobulin* is a large glycoprotein, each molecule of which contains about 115 tyrosine residues. It is synthesised, glycosylated and then secreted into the lumen of the follicle, where iodination of the tyrosine residues occurs. Surrounding the follicles is a dense capillary network and the blood flow through the gland is very high in comparison with other tissues. The main steps in the synthesis, storage and secretion of thyroid hormone (Fig. 34.1) are:

- uptake of plasma iodide by the follicle cells
- oxidation of iodide and iodination of tyrosine residues of thyroglobulin
- secretion of thyroid hormone.

UPTAKE OF PLASMA IODIDE BY THE FOLLICLE CELLS

Iodide uptake must occur against a concentration gradient (normally about 25:1) so it is an energy-dependent process. Iodide is captured from the blood and moved to the lumen by two transporters: the Na^+/I^- symporter (NIS) located at the basolateral surface of the thyrocytes (the energy being provided by Na^+/K^+-ATPase), and *pendrin*[1] (PDS), an I^-/Cl^- porter in the apical membranes

[1]So called because it is implicated in the pathophysiology of *Pendred's syndrome*, named after the eponymous English physician who first described this autosomal recessive form of familial goitre in association with sensorineural deafness.

(Nilsson, 2001). Uptake is very rapid: labelled iodide (^{125}I) is found in the lumen within 40 s of intravenous injection. Numerous mutations have been discovered in the NIS and PDS genes and these contribute to thyroid disease in some patients.

OXIDATION OF IODIDE AND IODINATION OF TYROSINE RESIDUES

The oxidation of iodide and its incorporation into thyroglobulin (termed the *organification* of iodide) is catalysed by *thyroperoxidase*, an enzyme situated at the inner surface of the cell at the interface with the colloid. The reaction requires the presence of hydrogen peroxide (H_2O_2) as an oxidising agent. Iodination occurs after the tyrosine has been incorporated into thyroglobulin. The process is shown in Figure 34.2.

Tyrosine residues are iodinated first at position 3 on the ring, forming monoiodotyrosine (MIT) and then, in some molecules, at position 5 as well, forming di-iodotyrosine (DIT). While still incorporated into thyroglobulin, these molecules are then coupled in pairs, either MIT with DIT to form T_3, or two DIT molecules to form T_4. The mechanism for coupling is believed to involve a peroxidase system similar to that involved in iodination. About one-fifth of the tyrosine residues in thyroglobulin are iodinated in this way.

The iodinated thyroglobulin of the thyroid forms a large store of thyroid hormone within the gland, with a relatively slow turnover. This is in contrast to some other endocrine secretions (e.g. the hormones of the adrenal cortex), which are not stored but synthesised and released as required.

SECRETION OF THYROID HORMONE

The thyroglobulin molecule is taken up into the follicle cell by endocytosis (Fig. 34.1). The endocytotic vesicles then fuse with lysosomes, and proteolytic enzymes act on thyroglobulin, releasing T_4 and T_3 to be secreted into the plasma. The surplus MIT and DIT, which are released at the same time, are scavenged by the cell and the iodide is removed enzymatically and reused.

REGULATION OF THYROID FUNCTION

Thyrotrophin-releasing hormone (TRH), released from the hypothalamus in response to various stimuli, releases *thyroid-stimulating hormone* (TSH; thyrotrophin) from the anterior pituitary (Fig. 34.3), as does the synthetic tripeptide **protirelin** (pyroglutamyl-histidyl-proline amide), which is used in this way for diagnostic purposes. TSH acts on receptors on the membrane of thyroid follicle cells through a mechanism that involves cAMP and phosphatidylinositol 3-kinase. It has a trophic action on thyroid cells and controls all aspects of thyroid hormone synthesis, including:

- the uptake of iodide by follicle cells, by stimulating transcription of the iodide transporter genes; this is

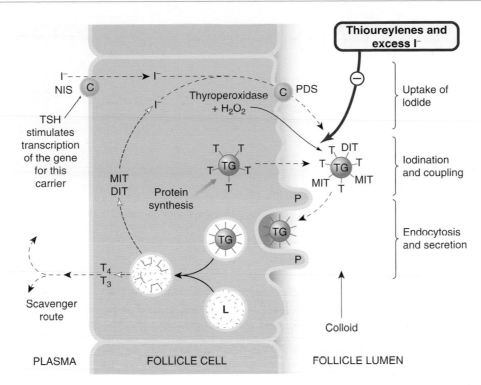

Fig. 34.1 Diagram of thyroid hormone synthesis and secretion, with the sites of action of some drugs used in the treatment of thyroid disorders. Iodide in the blood is transported by the carriers NIS and pendrin (PDS) through the follicular cell and into the colloid-rich lumen, where it is incorporated into thyroglobulin under the influence of the thyroperoxidase enzyme (see text for details). The hormones are produced by processing of the endocytosed thyroglobulin and exported into the blood. DIT, di-iodotyrosine; L, lysosome; MIT, monoiodotyrosine; P, pseudopod; T, tyrosine; T_3, tri-iodothyronine; T_4, thyroxine; TG, thyroglobulin; TSH, thyroid-stimulating hormone (thyrotrophin).

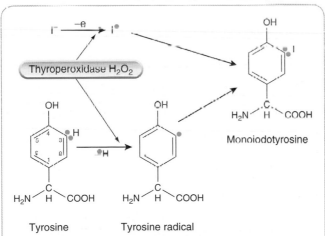

Fig. 34.2 Iodination of tyrosyl residues by the thyroperoxidase–H_2O_2 complex. This probably involves two sites on the enzyme, one of which removes an electron from iodide to give the free radical I•; another removes an electron from tyrosine to give the tyrosyl radical (shown by orange dot). Monoiodotyrosine results from the addition of the two radicals.

the main mechanism by which it regulates thyroid function and controls all aspects of thyroid hormone synthesis including:

- the synthesis and secretion of thyroglobulin
- the generation of H_2O_2 and the iodination of tyrosine

- the endocytosis and proteolysis of thyroglobulin
- the actual secretion of T_3 and T_4
- the blood flow through the gland.

The production of TSH is also regulated by a negative feedback effect of thyroid hormones on the anterior pituitary gland; T_3 is more active than T_4 in this respect. The peptide **somatostatin** also reduces basal TSH release. The control of the secretion of TSH thus depends on a balance between the actions of T_3/T_4 and TRH (and probably also somatostatin) on the pituitary.[2]

The other main factor influencing thyroid function is the plasma iodide concentration. About 100 nmol of T_4 is synthesised daily, necessitating uptake by the gland of approximately 500 nmol of iodide each day (equivalent to about 70 µg of iodine). A reduced iodine intake, with reduced plasma iodide concentration, will result in a decrease of hormone production and an increase in TSH secretion. An increased plasma iodide has the opposite effect, although this may be modified by other factors. The overall feedback mechanism responds to changes of iodide slowly over fairly long periods of days or weeks, because there is a large reserve capacity for the binding and uptake of iodide in the thyroid. The size and vascularity of the thyroid are reduced by an increase in plasma iodide and this is exploited therapeutically in preparing

---

[2]Other control systems may also operate under some circumstances. A 'long feedback' loop through which T_3/T_4 can act on the hypothalamus to reduce TSH has been demonstrated in some animals.

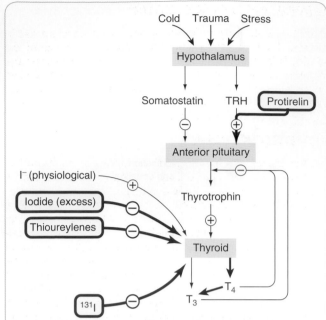

Fig. 34.3 Regulation of thyroid hormone secretion. Iodide (I⁻) is essential for thyroid hormone synthesis, but excess of endogenous or exogenous iodide (30 times the daily requirement of iodine) may be used to inhibit the increased thyroid hormone production of thyrotoxicosis. Protirelin as well as recombinant thyrotrophin-releasing hormone (TRH) is sometimes used to stimulate the system for diagnostic purposes. Larger amounts of this isotope are used for ablation of thyroid tissue (see text for details). T_3, tri-iodothyronine; T_4, thyroxine.

hyperthyroid patients for surgery to the gland. Diets deficient in iodine eventually result in a continuous excessive compensatory secretion of TSH, and eventually in an increase in vascularity and (sometimes gross) hypertrophy of the gland.[3]

ACTIONS OF THE THYROID HORMONES

The physiological actions of the thyroid hormones fall into two main categories: those affecting metabolism and those affecting growth and development.

EFFECTS ON METABOLISM

The thyroid hormones produce a general increase in the metabolism of carbohydrates, fats and proteins, and regulate these processes in most tissues, T_3 being three to five times more active than T_4 in this respect (Fig. 34.4). Although the thyroid hormones directly control the activity of some of the enzymes of carbohydrate metabolism, most effects are brought about in conjunction with other hormones, such as insulin, glucagon, the glucocorticoids and the catecholamines. There is an increase in oxygen consumption and heat production, which is manifested as an increase in the measured basal metabolic rate. This reflects the action of these hormones on tissues such as heart, kidney, liver and muscle, although not on others,

[3]'Derbyshire neck' was the name given to this condition in a part of the UK where sources of dietary iodine were once scarce.

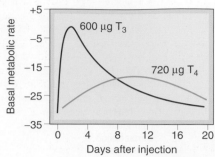

Fig. 34.4 The effect of equimolar doses of tri-iodothyronine (T_3) and thyroxine (T_4) on basal metabolic rate (BMR) in a hypothyroid subject. Note that this figure is meant only to illustrate overall differences in effect; thyroxine is not given clinically in a single bolus dose as here, but in regular daily doses so that the effect builds up to a plateau. The apparent differences in potency really represent differences in kinetics, reflecting the prehormone role of T_4. (*Modified from Blackburn et al., 1954.*)

such as the gonads, brain or spleen. The calorigenic action is important as part of the response to a cold environment. Administration of thyroid hormone results in augmented cardiac rate and output, and increased tendency to dysrhythmias such as atrial fibrillation.

EFFECTS ON GROWTH AND DEVELOPMENT

The thyroid hormones have a critical effect on growth, partly by a direct action on cells, and also indirectly by influencing growth hormone production and potentiating its effects on its target tissues. The hormones are important for a normal response to parathormone (Ch. 36) and calcitonin as well as for skeletal development; they are also essential for normal growth and maturation of the central nervous system.

MECHANISM OF ACTION

While there is some evidence for non-genomic actions (see Bassett et al., 2003), thyroid hormones act mainly through a specific nuclear receptor, TR (Ch. 3). Two distinct genes, TRα and TRβ, code for several receptor isoforms that have distinct functions. T_4 may be regarded as a prohormone, because when it enters the cell, it is converted to T_3, which then binds with high affinity to TR. This interaction is likely to take place in the nucleus, where TR isoforms generally act as a constitutive repressor of target genes. When T_3 is bound, these receptors change conformation, the co-repressor complex is released and a co-activator complex is recruited, which then activates transcription, resulting in generation of mRNA and protein synthesis.

TRANSPORT AND METABOLISM OF THYROID HORMONES

Both thyroid hormones are transported in the blood mainly bound to thyroxine-binding globulin (TBG). Plasma concentrations of these hormones can be measured by radioimmunoassay, and are approximately 1×10^{-7} mol/l (T_4) and 2×10^{-9} mol/l (T_3). Both are eventually metabolised in their target tissues by deiodination, deamination, decarboxylation and conjugation with glucuronic and sulfuric acids. The liver is a major site of metabolism and the free and conjugated forms are excreted partly in the bile and partly in the urine. The half-life of T_3 is a few hours, whereas that of T_4 varies between 3–4 days in hyperthyroidism, and 9–10 days in hypothyroidism.[4] Abnormalities in the metabolism of these hormones may occur naturally or be induced by drugs or heavy metals, and this may give rise to a variety of (uncommon) clinical conditions such as the 'low T_3 syndrome'.

ABNORMALITIES OF THYROID FUNCTION

Thyroid disorders are among the most common endocrine diseases, and subclinical thyroid disease is particularly prevalent in the middle-aged and elderly. They are accompanied by many extrathyroidal symptoms, particularly in the heart and skin. One (rare) cause of organ dysfunction is thyroid cancer. Many other thyroid disorders have an autoimmune basis. The reason for this is not clear, although it may be linked to polymorphisms in the PDS, tumour necrosis factor (TNF)-α or other genes. Regardless of causation, thyroid dysfunction is often associated with enlargement of the gland, known as *goitre*. Like other autoimmune diseases, such thyroid disorders are more common in women than men and occur with increased frequency during pregnancy (Cignini et al., 2012).

HYPERTHYROIDISM (THYROTOXICOSIS)

In thyrotoxicosis there is excessive secretion and activity of the thyroid hormones, resulting in a high metabolic rate, an increase in skin temperature and sweating, and heat intolerance. Nervousness, tremor, tachycardia and increased appetite associated with loss of weight occur. There are several types of hyperthyroidism, but only two are common: diffuse toxic goitre (also called *Graves' disease*[5] or exophthalmic goitre) and toxic nodular goitre.

Diffuse toxic goitre is an organ-specific autoimmune disease caused by autoantibodies to the TSH receptor which activate it, increasing thyroxine secretion. Constitutively active mutations of the TRH receptor may also be involved. As is indicated by the name, patients with exophthalmic goitre have protrusion of the eyeballs. The pathogenesis of this condition is not fully understood, but it is thought to be caused by the presence of TSH receptor-like proteins in orbital tissues. There is also an enhanced sensitivity to catecholamines. Toxic nodular goitre is caused by a benign neoplasm or adenoma, and may develop in patients with long-standing simple goitre. This condition does not usually have concomitant exophthalmos. The antidysrhythmic drug **amiodarone** (Ch. 21) is rich in iodine and can cause either hyperthyroidism or hypothyroidism. Some iodine-containing radiocontrast agents, such as **iopanoic acid** and its congeners, used as imaging agents to visualise the gall bladder, may also interfere with thyroid function. The chronic use of psychotropic agents may precipitate a variety of thyroid abnormalities (Bou Khalil & Richa, 2011).

SIMPLE, NON-TOXIC GOITRE

A dietary deficiency of iodine, if prolonged, causes a rise in plasma TRH and eventually an increase in the size of the gland. This condition is known as simple or non-toxic goitre. Another cause is ingestion of *goitrogens* (e.g. from cassava root). The enlarged thyroid usually manages to produce normal amounts of thyroid hormone, although if the iodine deficiency is very severe, hypothyroidism may supervene.

HYPOTHYROIDISM

A decreased activity of the thyroid results in hypothyroidism, and in severe cases *myxoedema*. Once again, this disease is immunological in origin, and the manifestations include low metabolic rate, slow speech, deep hoarse voice, lethargy, bradycardia, sensitivity to cold and mental impairment. Patients also develop a characteristic thickening of the skin (caused by the subcutaneous deposition of glycosaminoglycans), which gives myxoedema its name. *Hashimoto's thyroiditis*, a chronic autoimmune disease in which there is an immune reaction against thyroglobulin or some other component of thyroid tissue, can lead to both hypothyroidism and myxoedema. Genetic factors play an important role. Therapy of thyroid tumours with radioiodine is another cause of hypothyroidism.

Thyroid deficiency during development, which is the most prevalent endocrine disorder in the newborn (1 in 3000–4000 births) causes congenital hypothyroidism,[6] characterised by gross retardation of growth and mental deficiency.

DRUGS USED IN DISEASES OF THE THYROID

HYPERTHYROIDISM

Hyperthyroidism may be treated pharmacologically or surgically. In general, surgery is now used only when there are mechanical problems resulting from compression of the trachea by the thyroid. Under such circumstances it is usual to remove only part of the organ. Although the condition of hyperthyroidism can be controlled with antithyroid drugs, these drugs do not alter the underlying autoimmune mechanisms or improve the exophthalmos associated with Graves' disease.

RADIOIODINE

Radioiodine is a first-line treatment for hyperthyroidism (particularly in the USA). The isotope used is [131]I (usually as the sodium salt), and the dose generally 5–15 mCi. Given orally, it is taken up and processed by the thyroid in the same way as the stable form of iodide, eventually becoming incorporated into thyroglobulin. The isotope emits both β and γ radiation. The γ rays pass through the tissue without causing damage, but the β particles have a very short range; they are absorbed by the tissue and exert a powerful cytotoxic action that is restricted to the cells of the thyroid follicles, resulting in significant destruction of the tissue. [131]I has a half-life of 8 days, so by 2 months its radioactivity has effectively disappeared. It is given as one single dose, but its cytotoxic effect on the gland is delayed for 1–2 months and does not reach its maximum for a further 2 months.

---

[4]Correcting hypothyroidism by administration of T_4 therefore takes 2–3 weeks to reach equilibrium.
[5]After a Dublin physician who connected 'violent and long continued palpitations in females' with enlargement of the thyroid gland. Their complaints of fluttering hearts and lumps in their throats had previously been attributed to hysteria.

[6]An older term for this condition, *cretinism*, has been dropped.

The thyroid

- Thyroid hormones, tri-iodothyronine (T_3) and thyroxine (T_4), are synthesised by iodination of tyrosine residues on thyroglobulin within the lumen of the thyroid follicle.
- Hormone synthesis and secretion are regulated by thyroid-stimulating hormone (thyrotrophin) and influenced by plasma iodide.
- There is a large pool of T_4 in the body; it has a low turnover rate and is found mainly in the circulation.
- There is a small pool of T_3 in the body; it has a fast turnover rate and is found mainly intracellularly.
- Within target cells, the T_4 is converted to T_3, which interacts with a nuclear receptor to regulate gene transcription.
- T_3 and T_4 actions:
  - stimulation of metabolism, causing increased oxygen consumption and increased metabolic rate
  - regulation of growth and development.
- Abnormalities of thyroid function include:
  - hyperthyroidism (thyrotoxicosis); either diffuse toxic goitre or toxic nodular goitre
  - hypothyroidism; in adults this causes myxoedema, in infants, gross retardation of growth and mental deficiency
  - simple non-toxic goitre caused by dietary iodine deficiency, usually with normal thyroid function.

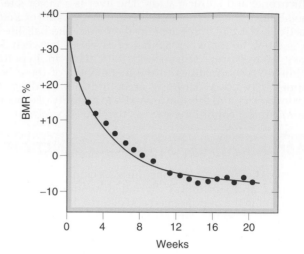

Fig. 34.5 Time course of fall of basal metabolic rate (BMR) during treatment with an antithyroid drug, **carbimazole.** The curve is exponential, corresponding to a daily decrease in BMR of 3.4%. *(Modified from Furth et al., 1963.)*

Hypothyroidism will eventually occur after treatment with radioiodine, particularly in patients with Graves' disease, but is easily managed by replacement therapy with T_4. Radioiodine is best avoided in children and also in pregnant patients because of potential damage to the fetus. There is theoretically an increased risk of thyroid cancer but this has not been seen following therapeutic treatment.

The uptake of ^{131}I and other isotopes of iodine is also used diagnostically as a test of thyroid function. A tracer dose of the isotope is given orally or intravenously and the amount accumulated by the thyroid is measured by a γ-scintillation counter placed over the gland. [131]I is also used for the treatment of thyroid cancer.

THIOUREYLENES

This group of drugs comprises **carbimazole**, **methimazole** and **propylthiouracil**. Chemically, they are related to thiourea, and the thiocarbamide (S–C–N) group is essential for antithyroid activity.

Mechanism of action

Thioureylenes decrease the output of thyroid hormones from the gland, and cause a gradual reduction in the signs and symptoms of thyrotoxicosis, the basal metabolic rate and pulse rate returning to normal over a period of 3–4 weeks. Their mode of action is not completely understood, but there is evidence that they inhibit the iodination of tyrosyl residues in thyroglobulin (see Figs 34.1 and 34.2). It is thought that they inhibit the thyroperoxidase-catalysed oxidation reactions by acting as substrates for the postulated peroxidase–iodinium complex, thus competitively inhibiting the interaction with tyrosine. Pro-

pylthiouracil has the additional effect of reducing the deiodination of T_4 to T_3 in peripheral tissues.

Pharmacokinetic aspects

Thioureylenes are given orally. Carbimazole is rapidly converted to its active metabolite methimazole, which is distributed throughout the body water and has a plasma half-life of 6–15 h. An average dose of carbimazole produces more than 90% inhibition of thyroid incorporation of iodine within 12 h. The full clinical response to this and other antithyroid drugs, however, may take several weeks (Fig. 34.5), partly because T_4 has a long half-life, and also because the thyroid may have large stores of hormone, which need to be depleted before the drug's action can be fully manifest. Propylthiouracil is thought to act somewhat more rapidly because of its additional effect as an inhibitor of the peripheral conversion of T_4 to T_3.

Both methimazole and propylthiouracil cross the placenta and also appear in the milk, but this effect is less pronounced with propylthiouracil, because it is more strongly bound to plasma protein. After degradation, the metabolites are excreted in the urine, propylthiouracil being excreted more rapidly than methimazole. The thioureylenes may be concentrated in the thyroid.

Unwanted effects

The most dangerous unwanted effect of thioureylene drugs is neutropenia and agranulocytosis (see Ch. 24). This is relatively rare, having an incidence of 0.1–1.2%, and is reversible on cessation of treatment. Patients must be warned to report symptoms (especially sore throat) immediately and have a blood count. Rashes (2–25%) and other symptoms including headaches, nausea, jaundice and pain in the joints, can also occur.

IODINE/IODIDE

Iodine is converted *in vivo* to iodide (I^-), which temporarily inhibits the release of thyroid hormones. When high doses of iodine are given to thyrotoxic patients, the symptoms subside within 1–2 days. There is inhibition of the secretion of thyroid hormones and, over a period of 10–14 days, a marked reduction in vascularity of the gland, which becomes smaller and firmer. Iodine is often given orally in a solution with potassium iodide ('*Lugol's iodine*'). With continuous administration, its effect reaches maximum within 10–15 days and then decreases. The mechanism of action is not entirely clear; it may inhibit iodination of thyroglobulin, possibly by reducing the H_2O_2 generation that is necessary for this process.

The main uses of iodine/iodide are for the preparation of hyperthyroid subjects for surgical resection of the gland, and as part of the treatment of severe thyrotoxic crisis (*thyroid storm*). It is also used following exposure to accidental leakage of radioactive iodine from nuclear reactors, to reduce uptake of the radioactive isotope in the thyroid. Allergic reactions can occur; these include angioedema, rashes and drug fever. Lacrimation, conjunctivitis, pain in the salivary glands and a cold-like syndrome are dose-related adverse effects connected to the concentration of iodide by transport mechanisms in tears and saliva.

OTHER DRUGS USED

The β-adrenoceptor antagonists, for example **propranolol** and **nadolol** (Ch. 14), are not antithyroid agents as such, but they are useful for decreasing many of the signs and symptoms of hyperthyroidism – the tachycardia, dysrhythmias, tremor and agitation. They are used during the preparation of thyrotoxic patients for surgery, as well as in most hyperthyroid patients during the initial treatment period while the thioureylenes or radioiodine take effect, or as part of the treatment of acute hyperthyroid crisis. Eye drops containing **guanethidine**, a noradrenergic-blocking agent (Ch. 14), are used to mitigate the exophthalmos of hyperthyroidism (which is not relieved by antithyroid drugs); it acts by relaxing the sympathetically innervated smooth muscle that causes eyelid retraction. Glucocorticoids (e.g. **prednisolone** or **hydrocortisone**) or surgical decompression may be needed to mitigate severe exophthalmia in Graves' disease. Some other drugs (e.g. cholecystographic agents or antiepileptic drugs) as well as environmental 'endocrine disruptors'[7] may interfere with the normal production of thyroid hormones.

HYPOTHYROIDISM

There are no drugs that specifically augment the synthesis or release of thyroid hormones. The only effective treatment for hypothyroidism, unless it is caused by iodine deficiency (which is treated with iodide), is to administer the thyroid hormones themselves as replacement therapy. Synthetic T_4 (official name: **levothyroxine**) and T_3 (official name: **liothyronine**), identical to the natural hormones, are given orally. Levothyroxine, as the sodium salt in doses of 50–100 µg/day, is the usual first-line drug of choice. Liothyronine has a faster onset but a shorter duration of action, and is generally reserved for acute emergencies such as the rare condition of myxoedema coma, where these properties are an advantage.

Unwanted effects may occur with overdose, and in addition to the signs and symptoms of hyperthyroidism

there is a risk of precipitating angina pectoris, cardiac dysrhythmias or even cardiac failure. The effects of less severe overdose are more insidious; the patient feels well but bone resorption is increased, leading to osteoporosis (Ch. 36).

The use of drugs to treat thyroid cancer (see Kojic et al., 2012) is a specialist subject and will not be covered here.

The use of drugs acting on the thyroid is summarised in the clinical box.

> ### Drugs in thyroid disease
>
>
> #### Drugs for hyperthyroidism
> - *Radioiodine* (^{131}I), given orally, is selectively taken up by thyroid and damages cells; it emits short-range β radiation, which affects only thyroid follicle cells. Hypothyroidism will eventually occur.
> - *Thioureylenes* (e.g. **carbimazole**, **propylthiouracil**) decrease the synthesis of thyroid hormones; the mechanism is through inhibition of thyroperoxidase, thus reducing iodination of thyroglobulin. They are given orally.
> - *Iodine*, given orally in high doses, transiently reduces thyroid hormone secretion and decreases vascularity of the gland.
>
> #### Drugs for hypothyroidism
> - **Levothyroxine** has all the actions of endogenous thyroxine; it is given orally.
> - **Liothyronine** has all the actions of endogenous tri-iodothyronine; it is given intravenously.

> ### Clinical use of drugs acting on the thyroid
>
> #### Radioiodine
> - Hyperthyroidism (Graves' disease, multinodular toxic goitre).
> - Relapse of hyperthyroidism after failed medical or surgical treatment.
>
> #### Carbimazole or propylthiouracil
> - Hyperthyroidism (diffuse toxic goitre); at least 1 year of treatment is needed.
> - Preliminary to surgery for toxic goitre.
> - Part of the treatment of thyroid storm (very severe hyperthyroidism); **propylthiouracil** is preferred. The β-adrenoceptor antagonists (e.g. **propranolol**) are also used.
>
> #### Thyroid hormones and iodine
> - **Levothyroxine** (T_4) is the standard replacement therapy for hypothyroidism.
> - **Liothyronine** (T_3) is the treatment of choice for myxoedema coma.
> - Iodine dissolved in aqueous potassium iodide (**'Lugol's iodine'**) is used short term to control thyrotoxicosis preoperatively. It reduces the vascularity of the gland.

---

[7]These are man-made chemicals such as pesticides or herbicides (e.g. polychlorinated biphenyls) that linger in the environment and are ingested in foodstuffs. The endocrine system is particularly sensitive to these, especially during development.

REFERENCES AND FURTHER READING

Bassett, J.H.D., Harvey, C.B., Williams, G.R., 2003. Mechanisms of thyroid hormone receptor-specific nuclear and extranuclear actions. Mol. Cell. Endocrinol. 213, 1–11. (*An excellent and comprehensive review dealing with the actions of thyroid hormones through the nuclear receptor mechanism as well as other actions through G protein-coupled receptors and other pathways*)

Blackburn, C.M., McConahey, W.M., Keating, F.R. Jr., Albert, A., 1954. Calorigenic effects of single intravenous doses of L-triiodothyronine and L-thyroxine in myxedematous persons. J. Clin. Invest. 33, 819–824.

Bou Khalil, R., Richa, S., 2011. Thyroid adverse effects of psychotropic drugs: a review. Clin. Neuropharmacol. 34, 248–255. (*Many patients taking psychotropic drugs present with thyroid problems. This review deals with the role played by antipsychotic drugs in this phenomenon*)

Braga, M., Cooper, D.S., 2001. Clinical review 129. Oral cholecystographic agents and the thyroid. J. Clin. Endocrinol. Metab. 86, 1853–1860. (*Discusses the deleterious effect of imaging agents on thyroid function*)

Cignini, P., Cafa, E.V., Giorlandino, C., Capriglione, S., Spata, A., Dugo, N., 2012. Thyroid physiology and common diseases in pregnancy: review of literature. J. Prenat. Med. 6, 64–71. (*Makes the point that increased rates of thyroid abnormalities are seen in pregnancy and that many go undiagnosed. Also deals with clinical management of these cases*)

Furth, E.D., Becker, D.V., Schwartz, M.S., 1963. Significance of rate of response of basal metabolic rate and serum cholesterol in hyperthyroid patients receiving neomercazole and other antithyroid agents. J. Clin. Endocrinol. Metab. 23, 1130–1140.

Hadj Kacem, H., Rebai, A., Kaffel, N., et al., 2003. PDS is a new susceptibility gene to autoimmune thyroid diseases: association and linkage study. J. Clin. Endocrinol. Metab. 88, 2274–2280. (*Interesting article on the PDS transporter protein and its contribution to disease susceptibility*)

Kahaly, G.J., Dillmann, W.H., 2005. Thyroid hormone action in the heart. Endocr. Rev. 26, 704–728. (*A very interesting review focusing on the cardiac actions of thyroid hormones; much historical detail*)

Kelly, G.S., 2000. Peripheral metabolism of thyroid hormones: a review. Altern. Med. Rev. 5, 306–333. (*This review focuses on the role of peripheral metabolism in thyroid hormone action*)

Kojic, K.L., Kojic, S.L., Wiseman, S.M., 2012. Differentiated thyroid cancers: a comprehensive review of novel targeted therapies. Exp. Rev. Anticancer Ther. 12, 345–357. (*A review dealing with the pharmacotherapy of the most common type of thyroid cancer, differentiated thyroid carcinoma*)

Lazarus, J.H., 1997. Hyperthyroidism. Lancet 349, 339–343. (*A 'seminar' covering aetiology, clinical features, pathophysiology, diagnosis and treatment*)

Lindsay, R.S., 1997. Hypothyroidism. Lancet 349, 413–417. (*A 'seminar' emphasising the management of hypothyroidism*)

Mastorakos, G., Karoutsou, E.I., Mizamtsidi, M., Creatsas, G., 2007. The menace of endocrine disruptors on thyroid hormone physiology and their impact on intrauterine development. Endocrine 3, 219–237. (*A review of endocrine disrupters and their effects on the thyroid. Not mainstream reading but an interesting topic*)

Nilsson, M., 2001. Iodide handling by the thyroid epithelial cell. Exp. Clin. Endocrinol. Diabetes 109, 13–17. (*Useful and readable review of iodide handling by the thyroid gland*)

Paschke, R., Ludgate, M., 1997. The thyrotropin receptor and its diseases. N. Engl. J. Med. 337, 1675–1679. (*Reviews aspects of TSH biology and disease*)

Roberts, C.G., Ladenson, P.W., 2004. Hypothyroidism. Lancet 363, 793–803. (*Authoritative and accessible review dealing with this thyroid pathology*)

Schmutzler, C., Kohrle, J., 1998. Implications of the molecular characterization of the sodium–iodide symporter (NIS). Exp. Clin. Endocrinol. Diabetes 106, S1–S10. (*Discusses the diagnostic and therapeutic implications of the information now available as a result of the cloning of NIS*)

Surks, M.I., Ortiz, E., Daniels, G.H., et al., 2004. Subclinical thyroid disease: scientific review and guidelines for diagnosis and management. JAMA 291, 228–238. (*Discusses and reviews the treatment of subclinical thyroid disease in detail; primarily of interest to clinical students*)

Yen, P.M., 2001. Physiological and molecular basis of thyroid hormone action. Physiol. Rev. 81, 1097–1142. (*Comprehensive review of thyroid hormone–receptor interaction and the effects of thyroid hormone on target tissues*)

Zhang, J., Lazar, M., 2000. The mechanism of action of thyroid hormones. Annu. Rev. Physiol. 62, 439–466. (*Detailed review of the molecular aspects of thyroid hormone–receptor interaction*)

The reproductive system

35

OVERVIEW

In this chapter, we describe the endocrine control of the female and male reproductive systems as the basis for understanding drug actions in sex hormone replacement, contraception, treatment of infertility, management of labour and treatment of erectile dysfunction.

INTRODUCTION

Drugs that affect reproduction (both by preventing conception and more recently for treating infertility) transformed society in the latter half of the last century. In this chapter, we briefly summarise salient points in reproductive endocrinology as a basis for understanding the numerous important drugs that work on the male and female reproductive systems. Such drugs are used for contraception, to treat infertility, as sex hormone replacement and in obstetric practice to influence labour. The principle of negative feedback is stressed and is central to understanding how hormones interact to control reproduction[1] – many drugs, including agents used to prevent or assist conception, work by influencing negative feedback mechanisms. The chapter concludes with a short section on erectile dysfunction.

ENDOCRINE CONTROL OF REPRODUCTION

Hormonal control of the reproductive systems in men and women involves sex steroids from the gonads, hypothalamic peptides and glycoprotein gonadotrophins from the anterior pituitary gland.

NEUROHORMONAL CONTROL OF THE FEMALE REPRODUCTIVE SYSTEM

Increased secretion of hypothalamic and anterior pituitary hormones occurs in girls at puberty and stimulates secretion of oestrogen from the ovaries. This causes maturation of the reproductive organs and development of secondary sexual characteristics, and also accelerated growth followed by closure of the epiphyses of the long bones. Sex steroids, *oestrogens* and *progesterone*, are thereafter involved in the menstrual cycle, and in pregnancy. A simplified outline is given in Figures 35.1 and 35.2.

The menstrual cycle begins with menstruation, which lasts for 3–6 days, during which the superficial layer of uterine endometrium is shed. The endometrium regenerates during the follicular phase of the cycle after menstrual flow has stopped. A releasing factor, *gonadotrophin-releasing hormone* (GnRH), is secreted from peptidergic neurons in the hypothalamus which discharge in a pulsatile fashion, approximately one burst per hour. GnRH stimulates the anterior pituitary to release gonadotrophic hormones (Fig. 35.1) – *follicle-stimulating hormone* (FSH) and *luteinising hormone* (LH). These act on the ovaries to promote development of small groups of follicles, each of which contains an ovum. One follicle develops faster than the others and forms the Graafian follicle (Figs 35.1 and 35.2E), which secretes oestrogens, and the rest degenerate. The ripening Graafian follicle consists of thecal and granulosa cells surrounding a fluid-filled centre, within which lies an ovum. Oestrogens are responsible for the proliferative phase of endometrial regeneration, which occurs from day 5 or 6 until mid-cycle (Fig. 35.2B,F). During this phase, the endometrium increases in thickness and vascularity, and at the peak of oestrogen secretion there is a prolific cervical secretion of mucus of pH 8–9, rich in protein and carbohydrate, which facilitates entry of spermatozoa. Oestrogen has a negative feedback effect on the anterior pituitary, decreasing gonadotrophin release during chronic administration of oestrogen as oral contraception (see p. 433-434). In contrast, the spike of endogenous oestrogen secretion just before mid-cycle sensitises LH-releasing cells of the pituitary to the action of the GnRH and causes the mid-cycle surge of LH secretion (Fig. 35.2C). This, in turn, causes rapid swelling and rupture of the Graafian follicle, resulting in ovulation. If fertilisation occurs, the fertilised ovum passes down the fallopian tubes to the uterus, starting to divide as it goes.

Stimulated by LH, cells of the ruptured follicle proliferate and develop into the *corpus luteum*, which secretes progesterone. Progesterone acts, in turn, on oestrogen-primed endometrium, stimulating the secretory phase of the cycle, which renders the endometrium suitable for the implantation of a fertilised ovum. During this phase, cervical mucus becomes more viscous, less alkaline, less copious and in general less welcoming for sperm. Progesterone exerts negative feedback on the hypothalamus and pituitary, decreasing the release of LH. It also has a thermogenic effect, causing a rise in body temperature of about 0.5 °C at ovulation, which is maintained until the end of the cycle.

If implantation of a fertilised ovum does not occur, progesterone secretion stops, triggering menstruation. If implantation does occur the corpus luteum continues to secrete progesterone which, by its effect on the hypothalamus and anterior pituitary, prevents further ovulation. The chorion (an antecedent of the placenta) secretes human chorionic gonadotrophin (HCG), which maintains the lining of the uterus during pregnancy. For reasons that are not physiologically obvious HCG has an additional pharmacological action, exploited therapeutically in treating infertility (see p. 433), of stimulating ovulation. As

---

[1]Recognition that negative feedback is central to endocrine control was a profound insight, made in 1930 by Dorothy Price, a laboratory assistant in the University of Chicago experimenting on effects of testosterone in rats. She referred to it as 'reciprocal influence' and it helps in understanding how many reproductive hormones seem, confusingly, to cause both an effect and its opposite if given in different doses or over different time courses.

425

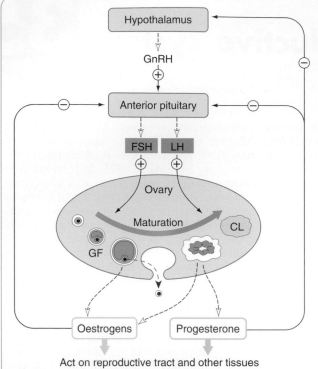

Fig. 35.1 Hormonal control of the female reproductive system. The Graafian follicle (GF) is shown developing on the left, then involuting to form the corpus luteum (CL) on the right, after the ovum (•) has been released. FSH, follicle-stimulating hormone; GnRH, gonadotrophin-releasing hormone; LH, luteinising hormone.

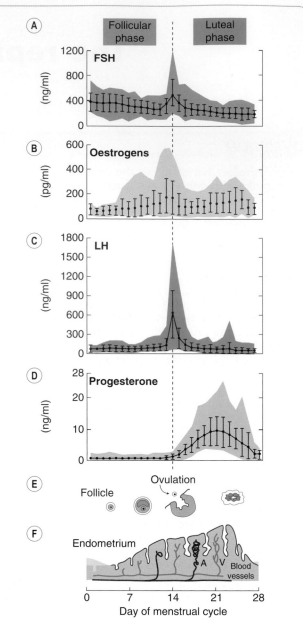

Fig. 35.2 Plasma concentrations of ovarian hormones and gonadotrophins in women during normal menstrual cycles. Values are the mean ± standard deviation of 40 women. The shaded areas indicate the entire range of observations. Day 1 is the onset of menstruation. E and F show diagrammatically the changes in the ovarian follicle and the endometrium during the cycle. Ovulation on day 14 of the menstrual cycle occurs with the mid-cycle peak of luteinising hormone (LH), represented by the vertical dashed line. A, arterioles; FSH, follicle-stimulating hormone; V, venules. *(After van de Wiele R L, Dyrenfurth I 1974 Pharmacol Rev 25, 189–217.)*

pregnancy proceeds, the placenta develops further hormonal functions and secretes a variety of hormones, including gonadotrophins, progesterone and oestrogens. Progesterone secreted during pregnancy controls the development of the secretory alveoli in the mammary gland, while oestrogen stimulates the lactiferous ducts. After parturition oestrogen, along with prolactin (see Ch. 33), is responsible for stimulating and maintaining lactation, whereas supraphysiological doses of oestrogen suppress lactation.

Oestrogens, progestogens (progesterone-like drugs), androgens and the gonadotrophins are described below – see Figure 35.3 for biosynthetic pathways.

NEUROHORMONAL CONTROL OF THE MALE REPRODUCTIVE SYSTEM

As in women, hypothalamic, anterior pituitary and gonadal hormones control the male reproductive system. A simplified outline is given in Figure 35.4. GnRH controls the secretion of gonadotrophins by the anterior pituitary. This secretion is not cyclical as in menstruating women, although it is pulsatile in both sexes, as with other anterior pituitary hormones (see Ch. 33). FSH is responsible for the integrity of the seminiferous tubules, and after puberty is important in gametogenesis through an action on Sertoli cells, which nourish and support developing spermatozoa. LH, which in the male is also called *interstitial cell-stimulating hormone* (ICSH), stimulates the interstitial cells (Leydig cells) to secrete androgens – in particular *testosterone*. LH/ICSH secretion begins at puberty, and the consequent secretion of testosterone causes maturation of the reproductive organs and development of secondary sexual characteristics. Thereafter, the primary function of testosterone is the maintenance of spermatogenesis and hence fertility – an action mediated by Sertoli cells. Testosterone is also important in the maturation of spermatozoa as they pass through the epididymis and vas deferens. A further action is a feedback effect on the anterior pituitary, modulating its sensitivity to GnRH and thus influencing secretion of LH/ICSH. Testosterone has marked anabolic effects, causing development of the musculature

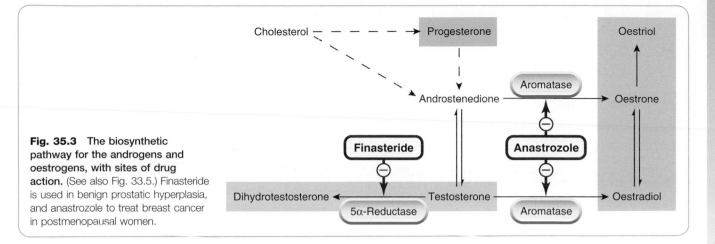

Fig. 35.3 The biosynthetic pathway for the androgens and oestrogens, with sites of drug action. (See also Fig. 33.5.) Finasteride is used in benign prostatic hyperplasia, and anastrozole to treat breast cancer in postmenopausal women.

Hormonal control of the female reproductive system

- The menstrual cycle starts with menstruation
- Gonadotrophin-releasing hormone, released from the hypothalamus, acts on the anterior pituitary to release follicle-stimulating hormone (FSH) and luteinising hormone (LH).
- FSH and LH stimulate follicle development in the ovary. FSH is the main hormone stimulating oestrogen release. LH stimulates ovulation at mid-cycle and is the main hormone controlling subsequent progesterone secretion from the corpus luteum.
- Oestrogen controls the proliferative phase of the endometrium and has negative feedback effects on the anterior pituitary. Progesterone controls the later secretory phase, and has negative feedback effects on both the hypothalamus and anterior pituitary.
- If a fertilised ovum is implanted, the corpus luteum continues to secrete progesterone.
- After implantation, human chorionic gonadotrophin (HCG) from the chorion becomes important, and later in pregnancy progesterone, HCG and other hormones are secreted by the placenta.

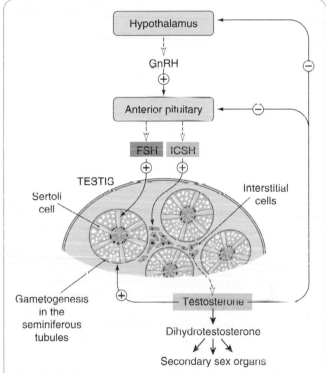

Fig. 35.4 Hormonal control of the male reproductive system. FSH, follicle-stimulating hormone; GnRH, gonadotrophin-releasing hormone; ICSH, interstitial cell-stimulating hormone.

and increased bone growth which results in the pubertal growth spurt, followed by closure of the epiphyses of the long bones.

Secretion of testosterone is mainly controlled by LH/ICSH, but FSH also plays a part, possibly by releasing a factor similar to GnRH from the Sertoli cells which are its primary target. The interstitial cells that synthesise testosterone also have receptors for prolactin, which may influence testosterone production by increasing the number of receptors for LH/ICSH.

BEHAVIOURAL EFFECTS OF SEX HORMONES

As well as controlling the menstrual cycle, sex steroids affect sexual behaviour. Two types of control are recognised: *organisational* and *activational*.

Organisational control refers to the fact that sexual differentiation of the brain can be permanently altered by the presence or absence of sex steroids at key stages in

development. In rats, administration of androgens to females within a few days of birth results in long-term virilisation of behaviour. Conversely, neonatal castration of male rats causes them to develop behaviourally as females. Brain development in the absence of sex steroids follows female lines, but is switched to the male pattern by exposure of the hypothalamus to androgen at a key stage of development. Similar but less complete behavioural virilisation of female offspring has been demonstrated following androgen administration in non-human primates, and probably also occurs in humans if pregnant women are exposed to excessive androgen.

The *activational* effect of sex steroids refers to their ability to modify sexual behaviour after brain development is complete. In general, oestrogens and androgens

427

increase sexual activity in the appropriate sex. **Oxytocin**, which is important during parturition (see p. 435), also has roles in mating and parenting behaviours, its action in the central nervous system being regulated by oestrogen (see Ch. 33).

DRUGS AFFECTING REPRODUCTIVE FUNCTION

OESTROGENS

Oestrogens are synthesised by the ovary and placenta, and in small amounts by the testis and adrenal cortex. The starting substance for synthesis of oestrogen (and other steroids) is cholesterol. The immediate precursors to the oestrogens are androgenic substances – androstenedione or testosterone (Fig. 35.3). There are three main endogenous oestrogens in humans: *oestradiol*, *oestrone* and *oestriol* (Fig. 35.3). Oestradiol is the most potent and is the principal oestrogen secreted by the ovary. At the beginning of the menstrual cycle, the plasma concentration is 0.2 nmol/l, rising to ~2.2 nmol/l in mid-cycle.

Actions

Oestrogen acts in concert with progesterone, and induces synthesis of progesterone receptors in uterus, vagina, anterior pituitary and hypothalamus. Conversely, progesterone decreases oestrogen receptor expression in the reproductive tract. *Prolactin* (see Ch. 33) also influences oestrogen action by increasing the numbers of oestrogen receptors in the mammary gland, but has no effect on oestrogen receptor expression in the uterus.

Effects of exogenous oestrogen depend on the state of sexual maturity when the oestrogen is administered:

- In primary hypogonadism: oestrogen stimulates development of secondary sexual characteristics and accelerates growth.
- In adults with primary amenorrhoea: oestrogen, given cyclically with a progestogen, induces an artificial cycle.
- In sexually mature women: oestrogen (with a progestogen) is contraceptive.
- At or after the menopause: oestrogen replacement prevents menopausal symptoms and bone loss.

Oestrogens have several metabolic actions, including mineralocorticoid (retention of salt and water) and mild anabolic actions. They increase plasma concentrations of high-density lipoproteins, a potentially beneficial effect (Ch. 23) that may contribute to the relatively low risk of atheromatous disease in premenopausal women compared with men of the same age. However, oestrogens also increase the coagulability of blood, and increase the risk of thromboembolism.

Mechanism of action

Oestrogen binds to nuclear receptors, as do other steroid hormones (Ch. 3). There are at least two types of oestrogen receptor, termed ERα and ERβ. Binding is followed by interaction of the resultant complexes with nuclear sites and subsequent genomic effects. In addition to these 'classic' intracellular receptors, some oestrogen effects, in particular its rapid vascular actions, are initiated by interaction with membrane receptors, including a G protein-coupled [o]estrogen receptor ('GPER', see review by Nilsson et al., 2011). Acute vasodilatation caused by 17-β-oestradiol is mediated by nitric oxide, and a plant-derived (phyto-) oestrogen called **genistein** (which is selective for ERβ, as well as having quite distinct effects due to inhibition of protein kinase C) is as potent as 17-β-oestradiol in this regard (Walker et al., 2001). Oestrogen receptor modulators (receptor-selective oestrogen agonists or antagonists) are mentioned below.

Preparations

Many preparations (oral, transdermal, intramuscular, implantable and topical) of oestrogens are available for a wide range of indications. These include natural (e.g. **oestradiol**, **oestriol**) and synthetic (e.g. **mestranol, ethinylestradiol, diethylstilbestrol**) oestrogens. Oestrogens are presented either as single agents or combined with progestogen.

Pharmacokinetic aspects

Natural and synthetic oestrogens are well absorbed in the gastrointestinal tract, but after absorption the natural oestrogens are rapidly metabolised in the liver, whereas synthetic oestrogens are degraded less rapidly. There is variable enterohepatic cycling. Most oestrogens are readily absorbed from skin and mucous membranes. They may be given as intravaginal creams or pessaries for local effect. In the plasma, natural oestrogens are bound to albumin and to a sex steroid-binding globulin. Natural oestrogens are excreted in the urine as glucuronides and sulfates.

Unwanted effects

Unwanted effects of oestrogens range from the common and tiresome to the life-threatening but rare: breast tenderness, nausea, vomiting, anorexia, retention of salt and water with resultant oedema, and increased risk of thromboembolism. More details of the unwanted effects of oral contraceptives are given below.

Used intermittently for postmenopausal replacement therapy, oestrogens cause menstruation-like bleeding. Oestrogen causes endometrial hyperplasia unless given cyclically with a progestogen. When administered to males, oestrogens result in feminisation.

Oestrogen administration to pregnant women can cause genital abnormalities in their offspring: carcinoma of the vagina was more common in young women whose mothers were given diethylstilbestrol in early pregnancy in a misguided attempt to prevent miscarriage (see Ch. 57).

The clinical uses of oestrogens and antioestrogens are summarised in the box (p. 429). In addition, see the section below on postmenopausal hormone replacement therapy (HRT).

OESTROGEN RECEPTOR MODULATORS

Raloxifene, a 'selective [o]estrogen receptor modulator' (SERM), has antioestrogenic effects on breast and uterus but oestrogenic effects on bone, lipid metabolism and blood coagulation. It is used for prevention and treatment of postmenopausal osteoporosis (Ch. 36) and reduces the incidence of oestrogen receptor-positive breast cancer similarly to **tamoxifen** but with fewer adverse events (Barret-Connor et al., 2006; Vogel et al., 2006). The US Food and Drug Administration has supported its use to reduce the risk of invasive breast cancer in postmenopausal women with osteoporosis and in postmenopausal women at high risk for invasive breast cancer. Unlike oestrogen, it does not prevent menopausal flushes.

Tamoxifen has an antioestrogenic action on mammary tissue but oestrogenic actions on plasma lipids, endometrium and bone. It produces mild oestrogen-like adverse effects consistent with partial agonist activity. The tamoxifen–oestrogen receptor complex does not readily dissociate, so there is interference with the recycling of receptors.

Tamoxifen upregulates transforming growth factor-β, a cytokine that retards the progression of malignancy, and that also has a role in controlling the balance between bone-producing osteoblasts and bone-resorbing osteoclasts (Ch. 36).

The use of tamoxifen to treat and prevent breast cancer is discussed further in Chapter 56.

ANTIOESTROGENS

Antioestrogens compete with natural oestrogens for receptors in target organs; in addition to SERMs (raloxifene, tamoxifen), which are partial agonists in some tissues and antagonists in others, there are drugs that are pure oestrogen-receptor antagonists.

Clomiphene inhibits oestrogen binding in the anterior pituitary, so preventing negative feedback and acutely increasing secretion of GnRH and gonadotrophins. This stimulates and enlarges the ovaries, increases oestrogen secretion and induces ovulation. It is used in treating infertility caused by lack of ovulation. Twins are common, but multiple pregnancy is unusual.

See the clinical box on oestrogens and antioestrogens for a summary of clinical uses.

PROGESTOGENS

The natural progestational hormone (progestogen) is *progesterone* (see Figs 35.2 and 35.3). This is secreted by the corpus luteum in the second part of the menstrual cycle, and by the placenta during pregnancy. Small amounts are also secreted by the testis and adrenal cortex.

Progestogens act, as do other steroid hormones, on nuclear receptors. The density of progesterone receptors is controlled by oestrogens (see p. 428).

Preparations
There are two main groups of progestogens:

1. The naturally occurring hormone and its derivatives (e.g. **hydroxyprogesterone**, **medroxyprogesterone**, **dydrogesterone**). Progesterone itself is virtually inactive orally, because of presystemic hepatic metabolism. Other derivatives are available for oral administration, intramuscular injection or administration via the vagina or rectum.
2. Testosterone derivatives (e.g. **norethisterone**, **norgestrel** and **ethynodiol**) can be given orally. The first two have some androgenic activity and are metabolised to give oestrogenic products. Newer progestogens used in contraception include **desogestrel** and **gestodene**; they may have fewer adverse effects on lipids than ethynodiol and may be considered for women who experience side effects such as acne, depression or breakthrough bleeding with the older drugs. However, these newer drugs have been associated with higher risks of venous thromboembolic disease (see below).

Oestrogens and antioestrogens

- The endogenous oestrogens are oestradiol (the most potent), oestrone and oestriol; there are numerous exogenous synthetic forms (e.g. **ethinylestradiol**).
- Mechanism of action involves interaction with nuclear receptors (ERα or ERβ) in target tissues, resulting in modification of gene transcription. Some of the rapid vascular effects of oestrogens are mediated by a G protein-coupled [o]estrogen receptor (GPER).
- Their pharmacological effects depend on the sexual maturity of the recipient:
  - before puberty, they stimulate development of secondary sexual characteristics
  - given cyclically in the female adult, they induce an artificial menstrual cycle and are used for contraception
  - given at or after the menopause, they prevent menopausal symptoms and protect against osteoporosis, but increase thromboembolism.
- Antioestrogens are competitive antagonists or partial agonists. **Tamoxifen** is used in oestrogen-dependent breast cancer. **Clomiphene** induces ovulation by inhibiting the negative feedback effects on the hypothalamus and anterior pituitary.
- Selective drugs that are oestrogen agonists in some tissues but antagonists in others are being developed. **Raloxifene** (one such drug) is used to treat and prevent osteoporosis.

Clinical uses of oestrogens and antioestrogens

Oestrogens
- Replacement therapy:
  - primary ovarian failure (e.g. Turner's syndrome)
  - secondary ovarian failure (menopause) for flushing, vaginal dryness and to preserve bone mass.
- Contraception.
- Prostate and breast cancer (these uses have largely been superseded by other hormonal manipulations; see Ch. 56).

Antioestrogens
- To treat oestrogen-sensitive breast cancer (**tamoxifen**).
- To induce ovulation (**clomiphene**) in treating infertility.

Actions
The pharmacological actions of the progestogens are in essence the same as the physiological actions of progesterone described above. Specific effects relevant to contraception are detailed below.

Pharmacokinetic aspects
Injected progesterone is bound to albumin, not to the sex steroid-binding globulin. Some is stored in adipose tissue. It is metabolised in the liver, and the products, pregnanolone and pregnanediol, are conjugated with glucuronic acid and excreted in the urine.

Unwanted effects

Unwanted effects of progestogens include weak androgenic actions. Other unwanted effects include acne, fluid retention, weight change, depression, change in libido, breast discomfort, premenstrual symptoms, irregular menstrual cycles and breakthrough bleeding. There is an increased incidence of thromboembolism.

Clinical uses of progestogens are summarised in the box below.

ANTIPROGESTOGENS

Mifepristone is a partial agonist at progesterone receptors. It sensitises the uterus to the action of prostaglandins. It is given orally and has a plasma half-life of 21 h. Mifepristone is used, in combination with a prostaglandin (e.g. **gemeprost**; see p. 436), as a medical alternative to surgical termination of pregnancy (see clinical box, opposite).

POSTMENOPAUSAL HORMONE REPLACEMENT THERAPY

At the menopause, whether natural or surgically induced, ovarian function decreases and oestrogen levels fall. There is a long history of disagreement regarding the pros and cons of hormone replacement therapy (HRT) in this context, with the prevailing wisdom undergoing several revisions over the years (see Davis et al., 2005). HRT normally involves the cyclic or continuous administration of low doses of one or more oestrogens, with or without a progestogen. Short-term HRT has some clear-cut benefits:

- improvement of symptoms caused by reduced oestrogen, for example hot flushes and vaginal dryness
- prevention and treatment of osteoporosis, but other drugs are usually preferable for this (Ch. 36).

Oestrogen replacement does not reduce the risk of coronary heart disease, despite earlier hopes, nor is there evidence that it reduces age-related decline in cognitive function. Drawbacks include:

- cyclical withdrawal bleeding
- adverse effects related to progestogen (see below)
- increased risk of endometrial cancer if oestrogen is given unopposed by progestogen
- increased risk of breast cancer, related to the duration of HRT use and disappearing within 5 years of stopping
- increased risk of venous thromboembolism (risk approximately doubled in women using combined HRT for 5 years).

See Web links in the reference list for best estimates of risks of cancer (breast, endometrium, ovary), venous thromboembolism, stroke and coronary artery disease in relation to age and duration of HRT use.

Oestrogens used in HRT can be given orally (conjugated oestrogens, oestradiol, oestriol), vaginally (oestriol), by transdermal patch (oestradiol) or by subcutaneous implant (oestradiol). **Tibolone** is marketed for the short-term treatment of symptoms of oestrogen deficiency. It has oestrogenic, progestogenic and weak androgenic activity, and can be used continuously without cyclical progesterone (avoiding the inconvenience of withdrawal bleeding).

Progestogens and antiprogestogens

- The endogenous hormone is progesterone. Examples of synthetic drugs are the progesterone derivative **medroxyprogesterone** and the testosterone derivative **norethisterone**.
- Mechanism of action involves intracellular receptor/altered gene expression, as for other steroid hormones. Oestrogen stimulates synthesis of progesterone receptors, whereas progesterone inhibits synthesis of oestrogen receptors.
- Main therapeutic uses are in oral contraception and oestrogen replacement regimens, and to treat endometriosis.
- The antiprogestogen **mifepristone**, in combination with prostaglandin analogues, is an effective medical alternative to surgical termination of early pregnancy.

Clinical uses of progestogens and antiprogestogens

Progestogens
- Contraception:
    - with **oestrogen** in *combined oral contraceptive pill*
    - as *progesterone-only contraceptive pill*
    - as *injectable* or *implantable* progesterone-only contraception
    - as part of an *intrauterine* contraceptive system.
- Combined with **oestrogen** for *oestrogen replacement therapy* in women with an intact uterus, to prevent endometrial hyperplasia and carcinoma.
- For *endometriosis*.
- In *endometrial carcinoma*; use in breast and renal cancer has declined.
- Poorly validated uses have included various menstrual disorders.

Antiprogestogens
- Medical termination of pregnancy: **mifepristone** (partial agonist) combined with a prostaglandin (e.g. **gemeprost**).

ANDROGENS

Testosterone is the main natural androgen. It is synthesised mainly by the interstitial cells of the testis, and in smaller amounts by the ovaries and adrenal cortex. Adrenal androgen production is influenced by adrenocorticotrophic hormone (ACTH, corticotrophin). As for other steroid hormones, cholesterol is the starting substance. Dehydroepiandrosterone and androstenedione are important intermediates. They are released from the gonads and the adrenal cortex, and converted to testosterone in the liver (see Fig. 35.3).

Actions

In general, the effects of exogenous androgens are the same as those of testosterone, and depend on the age and sex of the recipient. If given to prepubertal boys, the individuals concerned do not reach their full predicted height because of premature closure of the epiphyses of the long bones. In boys at the age of puberty, there is rapid development of secondary sexual characteristics (i.e. growth of facial, axillary and pubic hair, deepening of the voice), maturation of the reproductive organs and a marked increase in muscular strength. There is a growth spurt with an acceleration in the usual increase in height that occurs year on year in younger children, followed by cessation of linear growth. In adults, the anabolic effects can be accompanied by retention of salt and water. The skin thickens and may darken, and sebaceous glands become more active which can result in acne. Body weight and muscle mass increase, partly due to water retention. Androgens cause a feeling of well-being and an increase in physical vigour, and may increase libido. Whether they are responsible for sexual behaviour as such is controversial, as is their contribution to aggressive behaviour. Paradoxically, testosterone administration inhibits spermatogenesis, so reducing male fertility.

Administration of 'male' doses to women results in masculinisation, but lower doses (e.g. patches that release 300 mg of testosterone/day) restore plasma testosterone to normal female concentrations and improve sexual dysfunction in women following ovariectomy, without adverse effects (Braunstein et al., 2005).

Mechanism of action

In most target cells, testosterone works through an active metabolite, dihydrotestosterone, to which it is converted locally by a 5α-reductase enzyme. In contrast, testosterone itself causes virilisation of the genital tract in the male embryo and regulates LH/ICSH production in anterior pituitary cells. Testosterone and dihydrotestosterone modify gene transcription by interacting with nuclear receptors.

Preparations

Testosterone itself can be given by subcutaneous implantation or by transdermal patches (male replacement dose approximately 2.5 mg/day). Various esters (e.g. enanthate and proprionate) are given by intramuscular depot injection. Testosterone undecanoate and mesterolone can be given orally.

Pharmacokinetic aspects

If given orally, testosterone is rapidly metabolised in the liver. Virtually all testosterone in the circulation is bound to plasma protein – mainly to the sex steroid-binding globulin. Approximately 90% of endogenous testosterone is eliminated as metabolites. The elimination half-life of the free hormone is short (10–20 min). It is converted in the liver to androstenedione (see Fig. 35.3), which has weak androgenic activity. Synthetic androgens are less rapidly metabolised, and some are excreted in the urine unchanged.

Unwanted effects

Unwanted effects of androgens include decreased gonadotrophin release during continued use, with resultant infertility, and salt and water retention leading to oedema. Adenocarcinoma of the liver has been reported. Androgens impair growth in children (via premature fusion of epiphyses), cause acne and lead to masculinisation in girls. Adverse effects of testosterone replacement and monitoring for these are reviewed by Rhoden & Morgentaler (2004).

Androgens and the hormonal control of the male reproductive system

- Gonadotrophin-releasing hormone from the hypothalamus acts on the anterior pituitary to release both follicle-stimulating hormone, which stimulates gametogenesis, and luteinising hormone (also called interstitial cell-stimulating hormone), which stimulates androgen secretion.
- The endogenous hormone is testosterone; intramuscular depot injections of testosterone esters are used for replacement therapy.
- Mechanism of action is via intracellular receptors.
- Effects depend on age/sex, and include development of male secondary sexual characteristics in prepubertal boys and masculinisation in women.

Clinical uses of androgens and antiandrogens

- Androgens (**testosterone** preparations) as hormone replacement in:
  - male hypogonadism due to pituitary or testicular disease (e.g. 50–100 mg per day as gel applied to the skin)
  - female hyposexuality following ovariectomy (e.g. 300 µg/day patches).
- Antiandrogens (e.g. **flutamide**, **cyproterone**) are used as part of the treatment of prostatic cancer.
- 5α-Reductase inhibitors (e.g. **finasteride**) are used in benign prostatic hyperplasia.

The clinical uses of androgens are given in the clinical box above.

ANABOLIC STEROIDS

Androgens can be modified chemically to alter the balance of anabolic and other effects. 'Anabolic steroids' (e.g. **nandrolone**) increase protein synthesis and muscle development disproportionately, but clinical use (e.g. in debilitating disease) has been disappointing. They are used in the therapy of aplastic anaemia and (notoriously) abused by some athletes (Ch. 58), as is testosterone itself. Unwanted effects are described above, under Androgens. In addition, cholestatic jaundice, liver tumours and increased risk of coronary heart disease are recognised adverse effects of high-dose anabolic steroids.

ANTIANDROGENS

Both oestrogens and progestogens have antiandrogen activity, oestrogens mainly by inhibiting gonadotrophin secretion and progestogens by competing at androgen receptors in target organs. **Cyproterone** is a derivative of progesterone and has weak progestational activity. It is a partial agonist at androgen receptors, competing with dihydrotestosterone for receptors in androgen-sensitive target tissues. Through its effect in the hypothalamus, it

431

depresses the synthesis of gonadotrophins. It is used as an adjunct in the treatment of prostatic cancer during initiation of GnRH agonist treatment (see below). It is also used in the therapy of precocious puberty in males, and of masculinisation and acne in women. It also has a central nervous system effect, decreasing libido, and has been used to treat hypersexuality in male sexual offenders.[2]

Flutamide is a non-steroidal antiandrogen used with GnRH agonists in the treatment of prostate cancer.

Drugs can have antiandrogen action by inhibiting synthetic enzymes. **Finasteride** inhibits the enzyme (5α-reductase) that converts testosterone to dihydrotestosterone (Fig. 35.3). This active metabolite has greater affinity than testosterone for androgen receptors in the prostate gland. Finasteride is well absorbed after oral administration, has a half-life of about 7 h, and is excreted in the urine and faeces. It is used to treat benign prostatic hyperplasia, although α1-adrenoceptor antagonists, for example **terazosin** or **tamsulosin** (Chs 14 and 29), are more effective (working by the entirely different mechanism of relaxing smooth muscle in the capsule of the prostate gland and opposing α1-adrenoceptor-mediated prostatic growth). Surgery is another option.

GONADOTROPHIN-RELEASING HORMONE: AGONISTS AND ANTAGONISTS

Gonadotrophin-releasing hormone is a decapeptide that controls the secretion of FSH and LH by the anterior pituitary. Secretion of GnRH is controlled by neural input from other parts of the brain, and through negative feedback by the sex steroids (Figs 35.1 and 35.5). Exogenous androgens, oestrogens and progestogens all inhibit GnRH secretion, but only progestogens exert this effect at doses that do not have marked hormonal actions on peripheral tissues, presumably because progesterone receptors in the reproductive tract are sparse unless they have been induced by previous exposure to oestrogen. **Danazol** (see below) is a synthetic steroid that inhibits release of GnRH and, consequently, of gonadotrophins (FSH and LH). **Clomiphene** is an oestrogen antagonist that stimulates gonadotrophin release by inhibiting the negative feedback effects of endogenous oestrogen; it is used to treat infertility (see clinical box, p. 429, and Fig. 35.5).

Synthetic GnRH is termed **gonadorelin**. Numerous analogues of GnRH, both agonists and antagonists, have been synthesised. **Buserelin, leuprorelin, goserelin** and **nafarelin** are agonists, the last being 200 times more potent than endogenous GnRH.

Pharmacokinetics and clinical use

Gonadotrophin-releasing hormone agonists, given by subcutaneous infusion in pulses to mimic physiological secretion of GnRH, stimulate gonadotrophin release (Fig. 35.5) and induce ovulation. They are absorbed intact following nasal administration (Ch. 8). Continuous use, by nasal spray or as depot preparations, stimulates gonadotrophin release transiently, but then paradoxically inhibits gonadotrophin release (Fig. 35.5) because of downregulation (desensitisation) of GnRH receptors in the pituitary. GnRH analogues are given in this fashion to cause gonadal suppression in various sex hormone-dependent conditions, including prostate and breast cancers, endometriosis

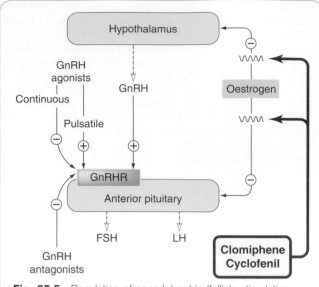

Fig. 35.5 Regulation of gonadotrophin (follicle-stimulating hormone, FSH; luteinising hormone, LH) release from the anterior pituitary. GnRHR, GnRH receptor.

(endometrial tissue outside the uterine cavity) and large uterine fibroids. Continuous, non-pulsatile administration inhibits spermatogenesis and ovulation. GnRH agonists are used by specialists in infertility treatment, not to stimulate ovulation (which is achieved using gonadotrophin preparations) but to suppress the pituitary before administration of FSH or HCG.

Unwanted effects of GnRH analogues

Unwanted effects of GnRH agonists in women, for example flushing, vaginal dryness and bone loss, result from hypo-oestrogenism. The initial stimulation of gonadotrophin secretion on starting treatment can cause transient worsening of pain from bone metastases in men with prostate cancer, so treatment is started only after the patient has received an androgen receptor antagonist such as **flutamide** (see above and Ch. 56).

DANAZOL

Actions and pharmacokinetics

Danazol inhibits gonadotrophin secretion (especially the mid-cycle surge), and consequently reduces oestrogen synthesis in the ovary (Fig. 35.5). In men, it reduces androgen synthesis and spermatogenesis. It has androgenic activity. It is orally active and metabolised in the liver.

Danazol is used in sex hormone-dependent conditions including endometriosis, breast dysplasia and gynaecomastia. An additional special use is to reduce attacks of swelling in hereditary angio-oedema (Ch. 28).

Unwanted effects are common, and include gastrointestinal disturbances, weight gain, fluid retention, dizziness, menopausal symptoms, muscle cramps and headache. Danazol is virilising in women.

GONADOTROPHINS AND ANALOGUES

Gonadotrophins (FSH, LH and HCG) are glycoproteins produced and secreted by the anterior pituitary (FSH and LH see Ch. 33) or chorion and placenta (HCG). Large amounts of gonadotrophins are present in the urine of

---

[2]Very different doses are used for these different conditions, for example 2 mg/day for acne, 100 mg/day for hypersexuality and 300 mg/day for prostatic cancer.

women following the menopause, in whom oestrogen no longer exerts feedback inhibition on the pituitary, which consequently secretes large amounts of FSH and LH.[3]

Preparations

Gonadotrophins are extracted from urine of pregnant (HCG) or postmenopausal women (human menopausal gonadotrophin, which contains a mixture of FSH and LH). Recombinant FSH (**follitropin**) and LH (**lutropin**) are also available.

Pharmacokinetics and clinical use

Gonadotrophin preparations are given by injection. They are used to treat infertility caused by lack of ovulation as a result of hypopituitarism, or following failure of treatment with **clomiphene**; they are also used by specialists to induce ovulation to enable eggs to be collected for in vitro fertilisation. For this use, gonadotrophin is usually administered after secretion of endogenous FSH and LH has been suppressed (see p. 432). Gonadotrophins are also sometimes used in men with infertility caused by a low sperm count as a result of hypogonadotrophic hypogonadism (a disorder that is sometimes accompanied by lifelong anosmia, i.e. lack of sense of smell). (Gonadotrophins do not, of course, work for patients whose low sperm count is the result of primary testicular failure.) HCG has been used to stimulate testosterone synthesis in boys with delayed puberty, but testosterone is usually preferred.

DRUGS USED FOR CONTRACEPTION

ORAL CONTRACEPTIVES

There are two main types of oral contraceptives:

1. Combinations of an oestrogen with a progestogen (the combined pill).
2. Progestogen alone (the progestogen-only pill).

THE COMBINED PILL

The combined oral contraceptive pill is extremely effective, at least in the absence of intercurrent illness and of treatment with potentially interacting drugs (see p. 434). The oestrogen in most combined preparations (second-generation pills)[4] is **ethinylestradiol**, although a few preparations contain **mestranol** instead. The progestogen may be **norethisterone**, **levonorgestrel**, **ethynodiol**, or – in 'third-generation' pills – **desogestrel** or **gestodene**, which are more potent, have less androgenic action and cause less change in lipoprotein metabolism, but which probably cause a greater risk of thromboembolism than do second-generation preparations. The oestrogen content is generally 20–50 μg of ethinylestradiol or its equivalent, and a preparation is chosen with the lowest oestrogen and progestogen content that is well tolerated and gives good cycle control in the individual woman. This combined pill is taken for 21 consecutive days followed by 7 pill-free days, which causes a withdrawal bleed. Normal cycles of

Gonadotrophin-releasing hormone and gonadotrophins

- Gonadotrophin-releasing hormone is a decapeptide; **gonadorelin** is the synthetic form. **Nafarelin** is a potent analogue.
- Given in pulsatile fashion, they stimulate gonadotrophin release; given continuously, they inhibit it.
- The gonadotrophins, follicle-stimulating hormone and luteinising hormone, are glycoproteins.
- Preparations of gonadotrophins (e.g. chorionic gonadotrophin) are used to treat infertility caused by lack of ovulation.
- **Danazol** is a modified progestogen that inhibits gonadotrophin production by an action on the hypothalamus and anterior pituitary.

menstruation usually commence fairly soon after discontinuing treatment, and permanent loss of fertility (which may be a result of early menopause rather than a long-term consequence of the contraceptive pill) is rare.

The mode of action is as follows:

- Oestrogen inhibits secretion of FSH via negative feedback on the anterior pituitary, and thus suppresses development of the ovarian follicle.
- Progestogen inhibits secretion of LH and thus prevents ovulation; it also makes the cervical mucus less suitable for the passage of sperm.
- Oestrogen and progestogen act in concert to alter the endometrium in such a way as to discourage implantation.

They may also interfere with the coordinated contractions of the cervix, uterus and fallopian tubes that facilitate fertilisation and implantation.

Hundreds of millions of women worldwide have used this method since the 1960s, and in general the combined pill constitutes a safe and effective method of contraception. There are distinct health benefits from taking the pill (see p. 434), and serious adverse effects are rare. However, minor unwanted effects constitute drawbacks to its use, and several important questions need to be considered.

Common adverse effects

The common adverse effects are:

- weight gain, owing to fluid retention or an anabolic effect, or both
- mild nausea, flushing, dizziness, depression or irritability
- skin changes (e.g. acne and/or an increase in pigmentation)
- amenorrhoea of variable duration on cessation of taking the pill.

Questions that need to be considered

Is there an increased risk of cardiovascular disease (venous thromboembolism, myocardial infarction, stroke)? With second-generation pills (oestrogen content less than 50 μg), the risk of thromboembolism is small (incidence approximately 15 per 100 000 users per year, compared with 5 per 100 000 non-pregnant non-users per year or 60 episodes of thromboembolism per

---

[3]This forms the basis for the standard blood test, estimation of plasma LH/FSH concentrations, to confirm whether a woman is postmenopausal.
[4]The first-generation pills, containing more than 50 μg of oestrogen, were shown in the 1970s to be associated with an increased risk of deep vein thrombosis and pulmonary embolism.

100000 pregnancies). The risk is greatest in subgroups with additional factors, such as smoking (which increases risk substantially) and long-continued use of the pill, especially in women over 35 years of age. The incidence of thromboembolic disease is approximately 25 per 100000 users per year in users of preparations containing **desogestrel** or **gestodene**, which is still a small absolute risk compared with the risk of thromboembolism in an unwanted pregnancy. In general, provided risk factors, e.g. smoking, hypertension and obesity, have been identified, combined oral contraceptives are safe for most women for most of their reproductive lives.

Is cancer risk affected? Ovarian and endometrial cancer risk is *reduced*.

Is blood pressure increased? A marked increase in arterial blood pressure occurs in a small percentage of women shortly after starting the combined oral contraceptive pill. This is associated with increased circulating angiotensinogen, and disappears when treatment is stopped. Blood pressure is therefore monitored carefully when oral contraceptive treatment is started, and an alternative contraceptive substituted if necessary.

Beneficial effects

Besides avoiding unwanted pregnancy, other desirable effects of the combined contraceptive pill include decreased menstrual symptoms such as irregular periods and intermenstrual bleeding. Iron deficiency anaemia and premenstrual tension are reduced, as are benign breast disease, uterine fibroids and functional cysts of the ovaries.

THE PROGESTOGEN-ONLY PILL

The drugs used in progestogen-only pills include **norethisterone**, **levonorgestrel** or **ethynodiol**. The pill is taken daily without interruption. The mode of action is primarily on the cervical mucus, which is made inhospitable to sperm. The progestogen probably also hinders implantation through its effect on the endometrium (Fig. 35.2) and on the motility and secretions of the fallopian tubes (see p. 433).

Potential beneficial and unwanted effects

Progestogen-only contraceptives offer a suitable alternative to the combined pill for some women in whom oestrogen is contraindicated, and are suitable for women whose blood pressure increases unacceptably during treatment with oestrogen. However, their contraceptive effect is less reliable than that of the combination pill, and missing a dose may result in conception. Disturbances of menstruation (especially irregular bleeding) are common. Only a small proportion of women use this form of contraception, so long-term safety data are less reliable than for the combined pill.

Pharmacokinetics of oral contraceptives: drug interactions

Combined and progestogen-only oral contraceptives are metabolised by hepatic cytochrome P450 enzymes. Because the minimum effective dose of oestrogen is used (in order to avoid excess risk of thromboembolism), any increase in its clearance may result in contraceptive failure, and indeed enzyme-inducing drugs can have this effect not only for combined but also for progesterone-only pills. Such drugs include **rifampicin** and **rifabutin**, as well as **carbamazepine**, **phenytoin** and others, including the herbal preparation St John's Wort (Ch. 47).

Oral contraceptives

The combined pill

- The combined pill contains an oestrogen and a progestogen. It is taken for 21 consecutive days out of 28.
- Mode of action: the oestrogen inhibits follicle-stimulating hormone release and therefore follicle development; the progestogen inhibits luteinising hormone release and therefore ovulation, and makes cervical mucus inhospitable for sperm; together, they render the endometrium unsuitable for implantation.
- Drawbacks: weight gain, nausea, mood changes and skin pigmentation can occur.
- Serious unwanted effects are rare. A small proportion of women develop reversible hypertension; there is a small increase in diagnosis of breast cancer, possibly attributable to earlier diagnosis, and of cervical cancer. There is an increased risk of thromboembolism with third-generation pills especially in women with additional risk factors (e.g. smoking) and with prolonged use.
- There are several beneficial effects, not least the avoidance of unwanted pregnancy, which itself carries risks to health.

The progestogen-only pill

- The progestogen-only pill is taken continuously. It differs from the combined pill in that the contraceptive effect is less reliable and is mainly a result of the alteration of cervical mucus. Irregular bleeding is common.

OTHER DRUG REGIMENS USED FOR CONTRACEPTION

POSTCOITAL (EMERGENCY) CONTRACEPTION

Oral administration of **levonorgestrel**, alone or combined with oestrogen, is effective if taken within 72 h of unprotected intercourse and repeated 12 h later. Nausea and vomiting are common (and the pills may then be lost: replacement tablets can be taken with an antiemetic such as **domperidone**). Insertion of an intrauterine device is more effective than hormonal methods, and works up to 5 days after intercourse.

LONG-ACTING PROGESTOGEN-ONLY CONTRACEPTION

Medroxyprogesterone can be given intramuscularly as a contraceptive. This is effective and safe. However, menstrual irregularities are common, and infertility may persist for many months after cessation of treatment.

Levonorgestrel implanted subcutaneously in non-biodegradable capsules is used by approximately 3 million women worldwide. This route of administration avoids first-pass metabolism. The capsules release their progestogen content slowly over 5 years. Irregular bleeding and headache are common.

A levonorgestrel-impregnated intrauterine system provides prolonged, reliable contraception and, in contrast to standard copper containing devices, *reduces* menstrual bleeding.

THE UTERUS

The physiological and pharmacological responses of the uterus vary at different stages of the menstrual cycle and during pregnancy.

THE MOTILITY OF THE UTERUS

Uterine muscle contracts rhythmically both *in vitro* and *in vivo*, contractions originating in the muscle itself. Myometrial cells in the fundus act as pacemakers and give rise to conducted action potentials. The electrophysiological activity of these pacemaker cells is regulated by the sex hormones.

The non-pregnant human uterus contracts spontaneously but weakly during the first part of the cycle, and more strongly during the luteal phase and during menstruation. Uterine movements are depressed in early pregnancy because oestrogen, potentiated by progesterone, hyperpolarises myometrial cells. This suppresses spontaneous contractions. Towards the end of gestation, however, contractions recommence; these increase in force and frequency, and become fully coordinated during parturition. The nerve supply to the uterus includes both excitatory and inhibitory sympathetic components: adrenaline, acting on β_2 adrenoceptors, inhibits uterine contraction, whereas noradrenaline, acting on α adrenoceptors, stimulates contraction.

DRUGS THAT STIMULATE THE UTERUS

Drugs that stimulate the pregnant uterus and are important in obstetrics include **oxytocin**, **ergometrine** and prostaglandins.

OXYTOCIN

The neurohypophyseal hormone oxytocin (an octapeptide) regulates myometrial activity, causing uterine contraction. Oxytocin release is stimulated by cervical dilatation, and by suckling; its role in parturition is incompletely understood but the fact that an antagonist (**atosiban**, see below) is effective in delaying the onset of labour implicates it in the physiology of parturition.

Oestrogen induces oxytocin receptor synthesis and, consequently, the uterus at term is highly sensitive to this hormone. Given by slow intravenous infusion to induce labour, oxytocin causes regular coordinated contractions that travel from fundus to cervix. Both amplitude and frequency of these contractions are related to dose, the uterus relaxing completely between contractions during low-dose infusion. Larger doses further increase the frequency of the contractions, and there is incomplete relaxation between them. Still higher doses cause sustained contractions that interfere with blood flow through the placenta and cause fetal distress or death.

Oxytocin contracts myoepithelial cells in the mammary gland, which causes 'milk let-down' – the expression of milk from the alveoli and ducts. It also has a vasodilator action. A weak antidiuretic action can result in water retention, which can be problematic in patients with cardiac or renal disease, or with pre-eclampsia.[5] Oxytocin

and oxytocin receptors are also found in the brain, particularly in the limbic system, and are believed to play a role in mating and parenting behaviour.

The clinical use of synthetic oxytocin is given in the box on p. 436.

Oxytocin can be given by intravenous injection or intramuscularly, but is most often given by intravenous infusion. It is inactivated in the liver and kidneys, and by circulating placental oxytocinase.

Unwanted effects of oxytocin include dose-related hypotension, due to vasodilatation, with associated reflex tachycardia. Its antidiuretic hormone-like effect on water excretion by the kidney causes water retention and, unless water intake is curtailed, consequent hyponatraemia.

ERGOMETRINE

Ergot (*Claviceps purpurea*) is a fungus that grows on rye and contains a surprising variety of pharmacologically active substances (see Ch. 15). Ergot poisoning, which was once common, was often associated with abortion. In 1935, **ergometrine** was isolated and was recognised as the oxytocic principle in ergot.

Ergometrine contracts the human uterus. This action depends partly on the contractile state of the organ. On a contracted uterus (the normal state following delivery), ergometrine has relatively little effect. However, if the uterus is inappropriately relaxed, ergometrine initiates strong contraction and reduces bleeding from the placental bed (the raw surface from which the placenta has detached). Ergometrine also has a moderate vasoconstrictor action.

The mechanism of action of ergometrine on smooth muscle is not understood. It is possible that it acts partly on α adrenoceptors, like the related alkaloid ergotamine (see Ch. 14), and partly on 5-hydroxytryptamine receptors.

The clinical use of ergometrine is given in the box on p. 436.

Ergometrine can be given orally, intramuscularly or intravenously. It has a very rapid onset of action and its effect lasts for 3–6 h.

Ergometrine can produce vomiting, probably by an effect on dopamine D_2 receptors in the chemoreceptor trigger zone (see Ch. 30, Fig. 30.5). Vasoconstriction with an increase in blood pressure associated with nausea, blurred vision and headache can occur, as can vasospasm of the coronary arteries, resulting in angina.

PROSTAGLANDINS

Prostaglandins are discussed in detail in Chapter 17. The endometrium and myometrium have substantial prostaglandin-synthesising capacity, particularly in the second, proliferative phase of the menstrual cycle. Prostaglandin $(PG)F_{2\alpha}$ is generated in large amounts, and has been implicated in the ischaemic necrosis of the endometrium that precedes menstruation (although it has relatively little vasoconstrictor action on many human blood vessels, in contrast to some other mammalian species). Vasodilator prostaglandins, PGE_2 and PGI_2 (prostacyclin), are also generated by the uterus.

In addition to their vasoactive properties, the E and F prostaglandins contract uterine smooth muscle whose sensitivity to these prostaglandins increases during gestation. Their role in parturition is not fully understood, but

---

[5]Eclampsia is a pathological condition (involving, among other things, high blood pressure, swelling and seizures) that occurs in pregnant women.

as cyclo-oxygenase inhibitors can delay labour (see below), they probably play some part in this.

Prostaglandins also play a part in two of the main disorders of menstruation: dysmenorrhoea (painful menstruation) and menorrhagia (excessive blood loss). Dysmenorrhoea is associated with increased production of PGE_2 and $PGF_{2\alpha}$; non-steroidal anti-inflammatory drugs, which inhibit prostaglandin biosynthesis (see Ch. 26), are used to treat dysmenorrhoea. Menorrhagia, in the absence of uterine pathology, may be caused by a combination of increased vasodilatation and reduced haemostasis. Increased generation by the uterus of PGI_2 (which inhibits platelet aggregation) could impair haemostasis as well as causing vasodilatation. Non-steroidal anti-inflammatory drugs (e.g. **mefenamic acid**) are used to treat menorrhagia as well as dysmenorrhoea.

Prostaglandin preparations

Prostaglandins of the E and F series promote coordinated contractions of the body of the pregnant uterus, while relaxing the cervix. E and F prostaglandins reliably cause abortion in early and middle pregnancy, unlike oxytocin which generally does not cause expulsion of the uterine contents at this stage. The prostaglandins used in obstetrics are **dinoprostone** (PGE_2), **carboprost** (15-methyl $PGF_{2\alpha}$) and **gemeprost** or **misoprostol** (PGE_1 analogues). Dinoprostone can be given intravaginally as a gel or as tablets. Carboprost is given by deep intramuscular injection. Gemeprost or misoprostol are given intravaginally.

Unwanted effects

Unwanted effects include uterine pain, nausea and vomiting, and diarrhoea. Dinoprost can cause hypotension. When combined with mifepristone, a progestogen antagonist that sensitises the uterus to prostaglandins, lower doses of the prostaglandins (e.g. misoprostol) can be used to terminate pregnancy and side effects are reduced.

See the clinical box for the clinical uses of prostaglandins (see Ch. 17).

DRUGS THAT INHIBIT UTERINE CONTRACTION

Selective β_2-adrenoceptor agonists, such as **ritodrine** or **salbutamol**, inhibit spontaneous or oxytocin-induced contractions of the pregnant uterus. These uterine relaxants are used in selected patients to prevent premature labour occurring between 22 and 33 weeks of gestation in otherwise uncomplicated pregnancies. They can delay delivery by 48 h, time that can be used to administer glucocorticoid therapy to the mother so as to mature the lungs of the baby and reduce neonatal respiratory distress. It has been difficult to demonstrate that any of the drugs used to delay labour improve the outcome for the baby. Risks to the mother, especially pulmonary oedema, increase after 48 h, and myometrial response is reduced, so prolonged treatment is avoided. Cyclo-oxygenase inhibitors (e.g. **indometacin**) inhibit labour, but their use could cause problems in the baby, including renal dysfunction and delayed closure of the ductus arteriosus, both of which are influenced by endogenous prostaglandins.

An oxytocin receptor antagonist, **atosiban**, provides an alternative to a β_2-adrenoceptor agonist. It is given as an intravenous bolus followed by an intravenous infusion for not more than 48 h. Adverse effects include vasodilatation, nausea, vomiting and hyperglycaemia.

> ### Clinical uses of drugs acting on the uterus
>
> **Myometrial stimulants (oxytocics)**
> - **Oxytocin** is used to *induce or augment labour* when the uterine muscle is not functioning adequately. It can also be used to treat *postpartum haemorrhage*.
> - **Ergometrine** can be used to treat *postpartum haemorrhage*. **Carboprost** can be used if patients do not respond to **ergometrine**.
> - A preparation containing both **oxytocin** and **ergometrine** is used for the management of the third stage of labour; the two agents together can also be used, prior to surgery, to control bleeding due to incomplete abortion.
> - **Gemeprost** (intravaginally) or **misoprostol** (intravaginally or by mouth) are used in *therapeutic abortion* and **misoprostol** (unlicensed use) in *induction of labour*.
> - **Gemeprost**, given as vaginal pessary following **mifepristone**, is used as a medical alternative to surgical *termination of pregnancy* (up to 63 days of gestation).
>
> **Myometrial relaxants**
> - The β-adrenoceptor agonists (e.g. **ritodrine**) are used to delay *preterm labour*.
> - **Atosiban** (oxytocin antagonist) also delays preterm labour.

> ### Drugs acting on the uterus
>
> - At parturition, **oxytocin** causes regular coordinated uterine contractions, each followed by relaxation; **ergometrine**, an ergot alkaloid, causes uterine contractions with an increase in basal tone. **Atosiban**, an antagonist of oxytocin, delays labour.
> - Prostaglandin (PG) analogues, for example **dinoprostone** (PGE_2) and **dinoprost** ($PGF_{2\alpha}$), contract the pregnant uterus but relax the cervix. Cyclo-oxygenase inhibitors inhibit PG synthesis and delay labour. They also alleviate symptoms of dysmenorrhoea and menorrhagia.
> - The β_2-adrenoceptor agonists (e.g. **ritodrine**) inhibit spontaneous and oxytocin-induced contractions of the pregnant uterus.

ERECTILE DYSFUNCTION

Erectile function depends on complex interactions between physiological and psychological factors. Erection is caused by vasorelaxation in the arteries and arterioles supplying the erectile tissue. This increases penile blood flow; the consequent increase in sinusoidal filling compresses the venules, occluding venous outflow and causing erection. During sexual intercourse, reflex contraction of the ischiocavernosus muscles compresses the base of the corpora cavernosa, and the intracavernosal pressure can reach several hundred millimetres of mercury during this phase of rigid erection. Innervation of the penis includes autonomic and somatic nerves. Nitric oxide is probably the main mediator of erection and is released both from nitrergic nerves and from endothelium (Ch. 20; Fig. 20.6).

Erectile function is adversely affected by several therapeutic drugs (including many antipsychotic, antidepressant and antihypertensive agents), and psychiatric and vascular disease (especially in association with endothelial dysfunction) can themselves cause erectile dysfunction, which is common in middle-aged and older men, even if they have no psychiatric or cardiovascular problems.[6] There are several organic causes, including hypogonadism (see clinical box, p. 431), hyperprolactinaemia (see Ch. 33), arterial disease and various causes of neuropathy (most commonly diabetes), but often no organic cause is identified.

Over the centuries, there has been a huge trade in parts of various creatures that have the misfortune to bear some fancied resemblance to human genitalia, in the pathetic belief that consuming these will restore virility or act as an aphrodisiac (i.e. a drug that stimulates libido). Alcohol (Ch. 49) 'provokes the desire but takes away the performance', and cannabis (Ch. 19) can also release inhibitions and probably does the same. **Yohimbine** (an α_2-adrenoceptor antagonist; Ch. 14) may have some positive effect in this regard, but trials have proved inconclusive. **Apomorphine** (a dopamine agonist; Ch. 40) causes erections in humans as well as in rodents when injected subcutaneously, but it is a powerful emetic, a disadvantage in this context. The picture picked up somewhat when it was found that injecting vasodilator drugs directly into the corpora cavernosa causes penile erection. **Papaverine** (Ch. 22), if necessary with the addition of **phentolamine**, was used in this way. The route of administration is not acceptable to most men, but diabetics in particular are often not needle-shy, and this approach was a real boon to many such patients. **PGE₁** (alprostadil) is often combined with other vasodilators when given intracavernosally. It can also be given transurethrally as an alternative (albeit still a somewhat unromantic one) to injection. Adverse effects of all these drugs include priapism (prolonged and painful erection with risk of permanent tissue damage), which is no joke. Treatment consists of aspiration of blood (using sterile technique) and, if necessary, cautious intracavernosal administration of a vasoconstrictor such as **phenylephrine**. Intracavernosal and transurethral preparations are still available, but orally active phosphodiesterase inhibitors are now generally the drugs of choice.

PHOSPHODIESTERASE TYPE V INHIBITORS

Sildenafil, the first selective phosphodiesterase type V inhibitor (see also Chs 20 and 22), was found accidentally to influence erectile function.[7] **Tadalafil** and **vardenafil** are also phosphodiesterase type V inhibitors licensed to treat erectile dysfunction. Tadalafil is longer acting than sildenafil. In contrast to intracavernosal vasodilators, phosphodiesterase type V inhibitors do not cause erection

independent of sexual desire, but enhance the erectile response to sexual stimulation. They have transformed the treatment of erectile dysfunction.

Mechanism of action

Phosphodiesterase V is the isoform that inactivates cGMP. Nitrergic nerves release nitric oxide (or a related nitrosothiol) which diffuses into smooth muscle cells, where it activates guanylyl cyclase. The resulting increase in cytoplasmic cGMP mediates vasodilatation via activation of protein kinase G (Ch. 4, Fig. 4.10). Consequently, inhibition of phosphodiesterase V potentiates the effect on penile vascular smooth muscle of endothelium-derived nitric oxide and of nitrergic nerves that are activated by sexual stimulation (Fig. 35.6). Other vascular beds are also affected, suggesting other possible uses, notably in pulmonary hypertension (Ch. 22).

Pharmacokinetic aspects and drug interactions

Peak plasma concentrations of sildenafil occur approximately 30–120 min after an oral dose and are delayed by eating, so it is taken an hour or more before sexual activity. It is given as a single dose as needed. It is metabolised by CYP3A4, which is induced by **carbamazepine**, **rifampicin** and **barbiturates**, and inhibited by **cimetidine**, macrolide antibiotics, antifungal imidazolines and some antiviral drugs (such as **ritonavir**). These drugs can

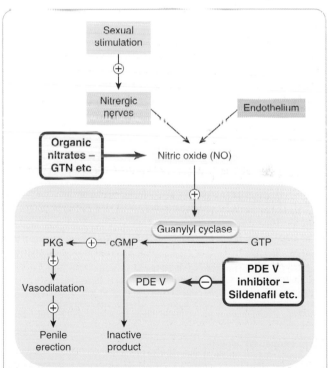

Fig. 35.6 Mechanism of phosphodiesterase V (PDE V) inhibitors on penile erection, and of the interaction of PDE V inhibitors with organic nitrates. The large grey rectangle denotes a vascular smooth muscle cell in the corpora cavernosa. Sexual stimulation releases nitric oxide (NO) from nitrergic nerves and this activates guanylyl cyclase, increasing cGMP production and hence activating protein kinase G (PKG), causing vasodilatation and penile erection. cGMP is inactivated by PDE V, so PDE V inhibitors (e.g. sildenafil) potentiate NO and promote penile erection. NO from organic nitrates such as glyceryl trinitrate (GTN) is also potentiated leading to generalised vasodilatation and hypotension.

---

[6]In randomised controlled trials, an appreciable proportion of men who discontinued treatment because of erectile dysfunction had been receiving placebo.

[7]Sildenafil was originally intended to treat angina, but volunteers in early phase trials reported an effect on affairs of the heart in a quite different anatomical region from the precordium.

interact with sildenafil. Tadalafil has a longer half-life than sildenafil, so can be taken longer before sexual activity. A clinically important pharmacodynamic interaction of all phosphodiesterase V inhibitors occurs with all organic nitrates, which work through increasing cGMP (Ch. 20) and are therefore markedly potentiated by sildenafil (Ch. 35, Fig. 35.6). Consequently, concurrent nitrate use, including use of **nicorandil**, contraindicates the use of any phosphodiesterase type V inhibitor.[8]

---

[8]This is important not only for sufferers from angina who take nitrates such as glyceryl trinitrate or isosorbide mononitrate therapeutically or prophylactically and are at risk of hypotension because of coronary artery disease, but also asymptomatic individuals who take amyl nitrate recreationally ('poppers') because of its effect on pelvic musculature.

Unwanted effects

Many of the unwanted effects of phosphodiesterase type V inhibitors are caused by vasodilatation in other vascular beds; these effects include hypotension, flushing and headache. Visual disturbances have occasionally been reported and are of concern because sildenafil has some action on phosphodiesterase VI, which is present in the retina and important in vision. The manufacturers advise that sildenafil should not be used in patients with hereditary retinal degenerative diseases (such as retinitis pigmentosa) because of the theoretical risk posed by this. Vardenafil is more selective for the type V isozyme than is sildenafil (reviewed by Doggrell, 2005), but is also contraindicated in patients with hereditary retinal disorders.

REFERENCES AND FURTHER READING

Sex hormones and their control

Barrett-Connor, E., Mosca, L., Collins, P., et al., 2006. Effects of raloxifene on cardiovascular events and breast cancer in postmenopausal women. N. Engl. J. Med. 355, 125–137. (*Reduced breast cancer*)

Chen, Z., Yuhanna, I.S., Galcheva-Gargova, Z., et al., 1999. Estrogen receptor-alpha mediates the nongenomic activation of endothelial nitric oxide synthase by estrogen. J. Clin. Invest. 103, 401–406. (*Acute vasodilator action of oestrogen may involve membrane ER rather than the classic intracellular receptor pathway*)

Gruber, C.J., Tschugguel, W., Schneeberger, C., Huber, J.C., 2002. Production and actions of estrogens. N. Engl. J. Med. 346, 340–352. (*Review focusing on the new biochemical aspects of the action of oestrogen – including phyto-oestrogens and selective oestrogen receptor modulators – as well as physiological and clinical aspects*)

Nilsson, B.L., Olde, G., Leeb-Lundberg, L.M.F., 2011. G protein-coupled oestrogen receptor 1 (GPER1)/GPR30: a new player in cardiovascular and metabolic oestrogenic signalling. Br. J. Pharmacol. 163, 1131–1139.

Rhoden, E.L., Morgentaler, A., 2004. Risks of testosterone-replacement therapy and recommendations for monitoring. N. Engl. J. Med. 350, 482–492. (*Review*)

Vogel, V., Constantino, J., Wickerman, L., et al., 2006. Effects of tamoxifen vs. raloxifene on the risk of developing invasive breast cancer and other disease outcomes. JAMA 295, 2727–2741. (*Raloxifene had similar efficacy as tamoxifen with fewer thrombotic events*)

Walker, H.A., Dean, T.S., Sanders, T.A.B., 2001. The phytoestrogen genistein produces acute nitric oxide-dependent dilation of human forearm vasculature with similar potency to 17 beta-estradiol. Circulation 103, 258–262.

Contraceptives

Djerassi, C., 2001. This Man's Pill: Reflections on the 50th Birthday of the Pill. Oxford University Press, New York. (*Scientific and autobiographical memoir by polymath steroid chemist who worked on 'the pill' at its inception under Syntex in Mexico, and has continued thinking about human reproduction in a broad biological and biosocial sense ever since*)

Postmenopausal aspects

Braunstein, G.D., Sundwall, D.A., Katz, M., et al., 2005. Safety and efficacy of a testosterone patch for the treatment of hypoactive sexual desire disorder in surgically menopausal women: a randomized, placebo-controlled trial. Arch. Intern. Med. 165, 1582–1589. (*A 300 mg/day testosterone patch increased sexual desire and frequency of satisfying sexual activity and was well tolerated in women who developed hypoactive sexual desire disorder after surgical menopause*)

Davis, S.R., Dinatale, I., Rivera-Woll, L., Davison, S., 2005. Postmenopausal hormone therapy: from monkey glands to transdermal patches. J. Endocrinol. 185, 207–222. (*Reviews the history of knowledge of the menopause and the development of hormonal therapy for climacteric complaints, and summarises current evidence for specific benefits and risks of hormone treatment*)

Hulley, S., Grady, D., Bush, T., et al., 1998. Randomized trial of estrogen plus progestin for secondary prevention of coronary heart disease in postmenopausal women. JAMA 280, 605–613. (*Study showing that incidence of fatal myocardial infarction was similar in the two groups, despite favourable changes in low- and high-density-lipoprotein cholesterol in the HRT group. Venous thromboembolism was increased by a factor of 2.89 in the active group*)

The uterus

Norwitz, E.R., Robinson, J.N., Challis, J.R., 1999. The control of labor. N. Engl. J. Med. 341, 660–666. (*Review*)

Thornton, S., Vatish, M., Slater, D., 2001. Oxytocin antagonists: clinical and scientific considerations. Exp. Physiol. 86, 297–302. (*Reviews rationale for uterine relaxants in preterm labour; evidence for administering atosiban and the role of oxytocin, vasopressin and their receptors in the onset of labour*)

Erectile dysfunction

Doggrell, S.A., 2005. Comparison of clinical trials with sildenafil, vardenafil and tadalafil in erectile dysfunction. Expert Opin. Pharmacother. 6, 75–84. (*Vardenafil is similarly effective to sildenafil. Its only advantage is that it does not inhibit phosphodiesterase VI to alter colour perception, a rare side effect that sometimes occurs with sildenafil. Tadalafil has a longer duration of action*)

Useful Web resource

www.mhra.gov.uk/home/groups/pl-p/documents/websiteresources/con2032228.pdf (*Risks of cancer [breast, endometrium, ovary], venous thromboembolism, stroke and coronary artery disease in relation to age and duration of HRT use*)

Bone metabolism

OVERVIEW

In this chapter we consider first the cellular and biochemical processes involved in bone remodelling, and the various mediators that regulate these processes. We then describe the drugs used to treat disorders of bone, including new agents.

INTRODUCTION

The human skeleton undergoes a continuous process of remodelling throughout life – some bone being resorbed and new bone being laid down continuously – resulting in the complete skeleton being replaced every 10 years. Structural deterioration and decreased bone mass (osteoporosis) occur with advancing age and constitute a worldwide health problem. Other conditions that lead to treatable pathological changes in bone include nutritional deficiencies and malignancy. There have recently been significant advances in the understanding of bone biology, which have led in turn to several valuable new drugs.

BONE STRUCTURE AND COMPOSITION

The human skeleton consists of 80% cortical bone and 20% trabecular bone. Cortical bone is the dense, compact outer part and trabecular bone, the inner meshwork. The former predominates in the shafts of long bones, the latter in the vertebrae, the epiphyses of long bones and the iliac crest. Trabecular bone, having a large surface area, is metabolically more active and more affected by factors that lead to bone loss (see opposite).

The main minerals in bone are calcium and phosphates. More than 99% of the calcium in the body is in the skeleton, mostly as crystalline hydroxyapatite but some as non-crystalline phosphates and carbonates; together, these make up half the bone mass.

The main bone cells are *osteoblasts*, *osteoclasts* and *osteocytes*.

- Osteoblasts are bone-forming cells derived from precursor cells in the bone marrow and the periosteum: they secrete important components (particularly collagen) of the extracellular matrix of bone – which is known as *osteoid*. They also have a role in the activation of osteoclasts (see Figs 36.1 and 36.2).
- Osteoclasts are multinucleated bone-resorbing cells derived from precursor cells of the macrophage/monocyte lineage.
- Osteocytes are derived from osteoblasts which, during the formation of new bone, become embedded in the bony matrix and differentiate into osteocytes. These cells form a connected cellular network that, along with nerve fibres located in bone, influences the response to mechanical loading. Osteocytes sense mechanical strain, and respond by triggering bone remodelling and secreting *sclerostin*, a mediator that reduces bone formation (Khosla et al., 2008).
- Other important cells in bone include monocytes/macrophages, lymphocytes and vascular endothelial cells; these secrete cytokines and other mediators implicated in bone remodelling.

Osteoid is the organic matrix of bone and its principal component is collagen. Other components such as *proteoglycans*, *osteocalcin* and various phosphoproteins are also important; one of these, *osteonectin*, binds to both calcium and collagen and thus links these two major constituents of bone matrix.

Calcium phosphate crystals are deposited as hydroxyapatite $[Ca_{10}(PO_4)_6(OH)_2]$ in the osteoid, converting it into hard bone matrix.

In addition to its structural function, bone plays a major role in calcium homeostasis.

BONE REMODELLING

There has been substantial progress in our understanding of bone remodelling (see reviews by Boyce & Xing, 2008; Gallagher, 2008; Deal, 2009; Wright et al., 2009.)

The process of remodelling involves:

- activity of osteoblasts and osteoclasts (Fig. 36.1)
- actions of various cytokines (Figs 36.1 and 36.2)
- turnover of bone minerals – particularly calcium and phosphate
- actions of several hormones: parathyroid hormone (PTH), the vitamin D family, oestrogens, growth hormone, steroids, calcitonin and various cytokines.

Diet, drugs and physical factors (exercise, loading) also affect remodelling. Bone loss – of 0.5–1% per year – starts aged 35–40 in both sexes, and accelerates by as much as 10-fold during the menopause in women or with castration in men, and then gradually settles at 1–3% per year. The loss during the menopause is due to increased osteoclast activity and affects mainly trabecular bone; the later loss in both sexes with increasing age is due to decreased osteoblast numbers and affects mainly cortical bone.

THE ACTION OF CELLS AND CYTOKINES

A cycle of remodelling starts with recruitment of osteoclast precursors followed by cytokine-induced differentiation of these to mature multinucleated osteoclasts (Fig. 36.1). The osteoclasts adhere to an area of trabecular bone, developing a ruffled border at the attachment site. They move along the bone, digging a pit by secreting hydrogen ions and proteolytic enzymes, mainly *cathepsin*

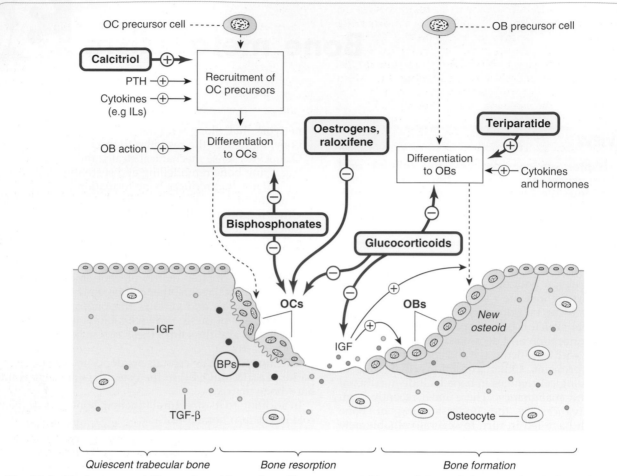

Fig. 36.1 The bone-remodelling cycle and the action of hormones, cytokines and drugs. *Quiescent trabecular bone:* Cytokines such as insulin-like growth factor (IGF) and transforming growth factor (TGF)-β, shown as dots, are embedded in the bone matrix. *Bone resorption* and *bone formation* are illustrated. Embedded bisphosphonates (BPs), are ingested by osteoclasts (OCs) when bone is resorbed (not shown); IL, interleukin; PTH, parathyroid hormone.

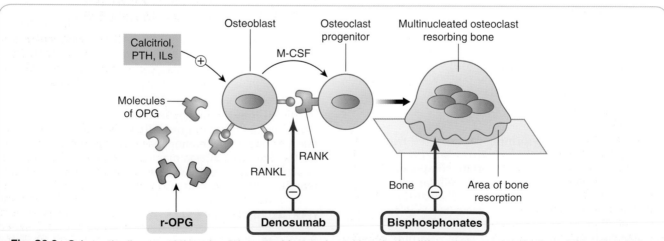

Fig. 36.2 Schematic diagram of the role of the osteoblast and cytokines in the differentiation and activation of the osteoclast and the action of drugs thereon. The osteoblast is stimulated to express a surface ligand, the RANK ligand (RANKL). RANKL interacts with a receptor on the osteoclast – an osteoclast differentiation and activation receptor termed RANK (receptor activator of nuclear factor kappa B), which causes differentiation and activation of the osteoclast progenitors to form mature osteoclasts. Bisphosphonates inhibit bone resorption by osteoclasts. Anti-RANKL antibodies (e.g. denosumab) bind RANKL and prevent the RANK–RANKL interaction. Drugs used clinically are in red-bordered boxes.

K. This process gradually liberates cytokines such as insulin-like growth factor (IGF)-1 and transforming growth factor (TGF)-β, which have been embedded in the osteoid (Fig. 36.1); these in turn recruit and activate successive teams of osteoblasts that have been stimulated to develop from precursor cells and are awaiting the call to duty (see Fig. 36.1). The osteoblasts invade the site, synthesising and secreting osteoid and secreting IGF-1 and TGF-β (which become embedded in the osteoid; see above). Some osteoblasts become embedded in the osteoid, forming osteocytes; others interact with and activate osteoclast precursors – and we are back to the beginning of the cycle.

Cytokines other than IGF-1 and TGF-β involved in bone remodelling include other members of the TGF-β family, including *bone morphogenic proteins* (BMPs), several interleukins, various hormones and members of the tumour necrosis factor (TNF) family. A member of this last family – a ligand for a receptor on the osteoclast precursor cell – is of particular importance. The receptor is termed (wait for it – biological terminology has fallen over its own feet here) *RANK*, which stands for *receptor activator of nuclear factor kappa B* (NFκB), NFκB being the principal transcription factor involved in osteoclast differentiation and activation. And the ligand is termed, unsurprisingly, RANK ligand (RANKL).

▼ Osteoblasts synthesise and release *osteoprotegerin* (OPG) which is identical with RANK and functions as a decoy receptor. In a sibling-undermining process by osteoblast and osteoclast precursor cells, OPG can bind to RANKL[1] (generated by the very same cells as OPG) and inhibit RANKL's binding to the functional receptor, RANK, on the osteoclast precursor cell (Fig. 36.2). The ratio of RANKL to OPG is critical in the formation and activity of osteoclasts and the RANK, RANKL, OPG system is fundamental to bone remodelling (reviewed by Boyce & Xing, 2008; Wright et al., 2009).

THE TURNOVER OF BONE MINERALS

The main bone minerals are calcium and phosphates.

CALCIUM METABOLISM

The daily turnover of bone minerals during remodelling involves about 700 mg of calcium. Calcium has numerous roles in physiological functioning. Intracellular Ca^{2+} is part of the signal transduction mechanism of many cells (see Ch. 4), so the concentration of Ca^{2+} in the extracellular fluid and the plasma, normally about 2.5 mmol/l, needs to be controlled with great precision. The plasma Ca^{2+} concentration is regulated by interactions between PTH and various forms of vitamin D (Figs 36.3 and 36.4); calcitonin also plays a part.

Calcium absorption in the intestine involves a Ca^{2+}-binding protein whose synthesis is regulated by calcitriol (see Fig. 36.3). It is probable that the overall calcium content of the body is regulated largely by this absorption mechanism, because urinary Ca^{2+} excretion normally remains more or less constant. However, with high blood Ca^{2+} concentrations urinary excretion increases, and with low blood concentrations urinary excretion can be reduced by PTH and calcitriol, both of which enhance Ca^{2+} reabsorption in the renal tubules (Fig. 36.3).

PHOSPHATE METABOLISM

Phosphates are important constituents of bone, and are also critically important in the structure and function of all the cells of the body. They are constituents of nucleic acids, provide energy in the form of ATP, and control – through phosphorylation – the activity of many functional proteins. They also have roles as intracellular buffers and in the excretion of hydrogen ions in the kidney.

Phosphate absorption is an energy-requiring process regulated by *calcitriol*. Phosphate deposition in bone, as hydroxyapatite, depends on the plasma concentration of PTH, which, with calcitriol, mobilises both Ca^{2+} and phosphate from the bone matrix. Phosphate is excreted by the kidney; here PTH inhibits reabsorption and thus increases excretion.

Bone remodelling

- Bone is continuously remodelled throughout life. The events of the remodelling cycle are as follows:
  - osteoclasts, having been activated by osteoblasts, resorb bone by digging pits in trabecular bone. Into these pits the bone-forming osteoblasts secrete osteoid (bone matrix), which consists mainly of collagen but also contains osteocalcin, osteonectin, phosphoproteins and the cytokines insulin growth factor (IGF) and transforming growth factor (TGF)-β
  - the osteoid is then mineralised, i.e. complex calcium phosphate crystals (hydroxyapatites) are deposited.
- Bone metabolism and mineralisation involve the action of parathyroid hormone, the vitamin D family, and various cytokines (e.g. IGF, the TGF-β family and interleukins). Declining physiological levels of oestrogens and therapeutic levels of glucocorticoids can result in bone resorption not balanced by bone formation – leading to osteoporosis.

HORMONES INVOLVED IN BONE METABOLISM AND REMODELLING

The main hormones involved in bone metabolism and remodelling are parathyroid hormone (PTH), members of the vitamin D family, oestrogens and calcitonin. Glucocorticoids and thyroid hormone also affect bone.

PARATHYROID HORMONE

Parathyroid hormone, which consists of a single-chain polypeptide of 84 amino acids, is an important physiological regulator of Ca^{2+} metabolism. It acts on PTH receptors in various tissues (bone, kidney, gastrointestinal tract) to maintain the plasma Ca^{2+} concentration. It mobilises Ca^{2+} from bone, promotes its reabsorption by the kidney and stimulates the synthesis of calcitriol, which in turn increases Ca^{2+} absorption from the intestine and synergises with PTH in mobilising bone Ca^{2+} (Figs 36.3 and 36.4). PTH promotes phosphate excretion, and thus its net effect is to increase the concentration of Ca^{2+} in the plasma and lower that of phosphate.

The mobilisation of Ca^{2+} from bone by PTH is mediated, at least in part, by stimulation of the recruitment and activation of osteoclasts. Pathological oversecretion of

---

[1]RANKL is also sometimes confusingly termed OPG ligand.

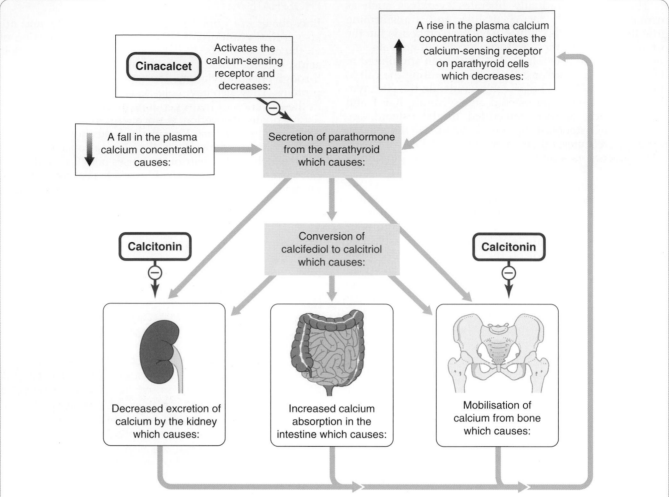

Fig. 36.3 **The main factors involved in maintaining the concentration of Ca^{2+} in the plasma and the action of drugs.** The calcium receptor on the parathyroid cell is a G protein-coupled receptor. Calcifediol and calcitriol are metabolites of vitamin D$_3$ and constitute the 'hormones' 25-hydroxy-vitamin D$_3$ and 1,25-dihydroxy-vitamin D$_3$, respectively. Endogenous calcitonin, secreted by the thyroid, inhibits Ca^{2+} mobilisation from bone and decreases its reabsorption in the kidney, thus reducing blood Ca^{2+}. Calcitonin is also used therapeutically in osteoporosis.

PTH (hyperparathyroidism) inhibits osteoblast activity (not shown in Fig. 36.1). But given therapeutically in a low intermittent dose, PTH and fragments of PTH paradoxically stimulate osteoblast activity and enhance bone formation.

Parathyroid hormone is synthesised in the cells of the parathyroid glands and stored in vesicles. The principal factor controlling secretion is the concentration of ionised calcium in the plasma, low plasma Ca^{2+} stimulating secretion, high plasma Ca^{2+} decreasing it by binding to and activating a Ca^{2+}-sensing G protein-coupled surface receptor (see Ch. 3 and Fig. 36.3). (For reviews, see Stewart, 2004; Deal, 2009.)

VITAMIN D

Vitamin D (calciferol) consists of a group of lipophilic precursors that are converted in the body into biologically active metabolites that function as true hormones, circulating in the blood and regulating the activities of various cell types (see Reichel et al., 1989). Their main action, mediated by nuclear receptors of the steroid receptor superfamily (see Ch. 3), is the maintenance of plasma Ca^{2+} by increasing Ca^{2+} absorption in the intestine, mobilising Ca^{2+} from bone and decreasing its renal excretion (see Fig. 36.3). In humans, there are two important forms of vitamin D, termed D$_2$ and D$_3$:

1. Dietary *ergocalciferol* (D$_2$), derived from ergosterol in plants.
2. *Cholecalciferol* (D$_3$), generated in the skin from 7-dehydrocholesterol by the action of ultraviolet irradiation during sun exposure, or formed from cholesterol in the wall of the intestine.

Cholecalciferol is converted to *calcifediol* (25-hydroxy-vitamin D$_3$) in the liver, and this is converted to a series of other metabolites of varying activity in the kidney, the most potent of which is *calcitriol* (1,25-dihydroxy-vitamin D$_3$); see Figure 36.4.

The synthesis of calcitriol from calcifediol is regulated by PTH, and is also influenced by the phosphate concentration in the plasma and by the calcitriol concentration itself through a negative feedback mechanism (Fig. 36.4).

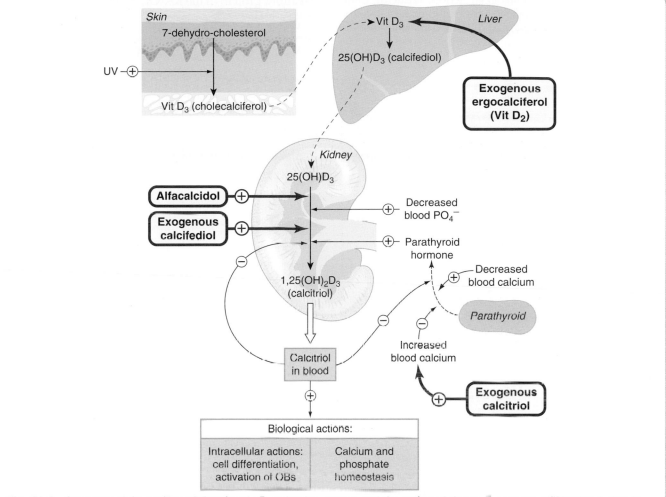

Fig. 36.4 **Summary of the actions of the vitamin D endocrine system and the action of drugs.** Exogenous ergocalciferol, vitamin (Vit) D_2 (formed in plants by ultraviolet [UV] light), is converted to the corresponding D_2 metabolites in liver and kidney, as is the D_2 analogue dihydrotachysterol (not shown). Alfacalcidol (1α-hydroxycholecalciferol) is 25-hydroxylated to calcitriol in the liver. OB, osteoblast.

Receptors for calcitriol are ubiquitous, and calcitriol is important in the functioning of many cell types.

The main actions of calcitriol are the stimulation of absorption of Ca^{2+} and phosphate in the intestine, and the mobilisation of Ca^{2+} from bone, but it also increases Ca^{2+} reabsorption in the kidney tubules (Fig. 36.3). Its effect on bone involves promotion of maturation of osteoclasts and indirect stimulation of their activity (Figs 36.1 and 36.3). It decreases collagen synthesis by osteoblasts. However, the effect on bone is complex and not confined to mobilising Ca^{2+}, because in clinical vitamin D deficiency (see p. 444), in which the mineralisation of bone is impaired, administration of vitamin D restores bone formation. One explanation may lie in the fact that calcitriol stimulates synthesis of *osteocalcin*, the Ca^{2+}-binding protein of bone matrix.

OESTROGENS

Oestrogens have an important role in maintaining bone integrity in adult women, acting on osteoblasts and osteoclasts. Oestrogen inhibits the cytokines that recruit osteoclasts and opposes the bone-resorbing, Ca^{2+}-mobilising action of PTH. It increases osteoblast proliferation, augments production of TGF-β and bone morphogenic proteins, and inhibits apoptosis (see Ch. 5). Withdrawal of oestrogen, as happens physiologically at the menopause, frequently leads to osteoporosis.

CALCITONIN

Calcitonin is a peptide hormone secreted by 'C' cells found in the thyroid follicles (see Ch. 34).

The main action of calcitonin is on bone; it inhibits bone resorption by binding to an inhibitory receptor on osteoclasts. In the kidney, it decreases the reabsorption of Ca^{2+} and phosphate in the proximal tubules. Its overall effect is to decrease the plasma Ca^{2+} concentration (Fig. 36.3).

Secretion is determined mainly by the plasma Ca^{2+} concentration.

OTHER HORMONES

Physiological concentrations of glucocorticoids are required for osteoblast differentiation. Higher concentrations inhibit bone formation by inhibiting osteoblast differentiation and activity, and may stimulate osteoclast action – leading to osteoporosis, which is a feature of Cushing's syndrome (Fig. 33.7) and an important adverse effect of glucocorticoid administration (Ch. 33).

Thyroxine stimulates osteoclast action, reducing bone density and liberating Ca^{2+}. Osteoporosis occurs in association with thyrotoxicosis, and it is important not to use excessive thyroxine for treating hypothyroidism (see Ch. 34).

> ## Parathyroid hormone, vitamin D and bone mineral homeostasis
>
> - The vitamin D family give rise to true hormones; precursors are converted to calcifediol in the liver, then to the main hormone, calcitriol, in the kidney.
> - Calcitriol increases plasma Ca^{2+} by mobilising it from bone, increasing its absorption in the intestine and decreasing its excretion by the kidney.
> - Parathyroid hormone (PTH) increases blood Ca^{2+} by increasing calcitriol synthesis, mobilising Ca^{2+} from bone and reducing renal Ca^{2+} excretion. Paradoxically, small doses of PTH given intermittently *increase* bone formation through an anabolic effect.
> - Calcitonin (secreted from the thyroid) reduces Ca^{2+} resorption from bone by inhibiting osteoclast activity.

DISORDERS OF BONE

The reduction of bone mass with distortion of the microarchitecture is termed *osteoporosis*; a reduction in the mineral content is termed *osteopenia*. Dual-energy X-ray absorptiometry (DXA) and quantitative computed tomography are the standard methods for assessing osteoporosis severity and monitoring the effect of treatment (Riggs et al., 2012). Osteoporotic bone fractures easily after minimal trauma. The commonest causes of osteoporosis are postmenopausal deficiency of oestrogen and age-related deterioration in bone homeostasis. It is estimated that 50% of women and 20% of men over the age of 50 will have a fracture due to osteoporosis. With increasing life expectancy, osteoporosis has increased to epidemic proportions and is an important public health problem, affecting about 75 million people in the USA, Japan and Europe. Other predisposing factors include catabolic hormones that favour protein breakdown such as excessive thyroxine or glucocorticoid administration. Other preventable or treatable diseases of bone include *osteomalacia* and *rickets* (the juvenile form of osteomalacia), in which there are defects in bone mineralisation due to vitamin D deficiency, either due to dietary deficiency of vitamin D and lack of sunlight, or to renal disease resulting in reduced synthesis of the active calcitriol hormone (Ch. 29) and *Paget's disease*, in which there is distortion of the processes of bone resorption and remodelling as a consequence of mutation in the gene that codes for a ubiquitin-binding protein[2] called sequestosome 1 (Rea et al., 2013) which is

a scaffold protein in the RANK/NFκB signalling pathway (see p. 441).

DRUGS USED IN BONE DISORDERS

Two types of agent are currently used for treatment of osteoporosis:

1. *Antiresorptive drugs* that decrease bone loss, e.g. bisphosphonates, calcitonin, selective [o]estrogen receptor modulators (SERMs), **denusomab**, calcium.
2. *Anabolic agents* that increase bone formation, e.g. PTH, **teriparatide**.

Strontium has both actions.

Rickets and osteomalacia are treated with vitamin D preparations.

Paget's disease is common but only a small percentage of patients are symptomatic; if medical treatment is needed, bisphosphonates such as **pamidronate** or **zoledronate** (see below) are very effective and much more convenient than frequent injections of **salmon calcitonin**, previously the only effective medical treatment. A single intravenous dose of zoledronate (5 mg) can suppress the elevated plasma alkaline phosphatase that signals disease activity in Paget's disease for more than 2 years.

BISPHOSPHONATES

Bisphosphonates (Fig. 36.5) are enzyme-resistant analogues of pyrophosphate, a normal constituent of tissue fluids that accumulates in bone, and has a role in regulating bone resorption. Bisphosphonates inhibit bone resorption by an action mainly on the osteoclasts. They form tight complexes with calcium in the bone matrix, and are

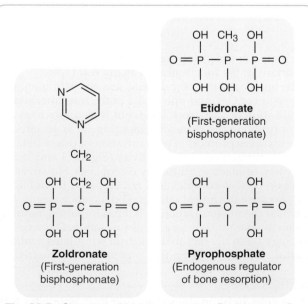

Fig. 36.5 **Structure of bisphosphonates.** Replacement of the oxygen atom in pyrophosphate renders the compounds enzyme-resistant. Addition of an N-containing side chain alters the mechanism of action (see text) and greatly increases potency.

---

[2]Ubiquitin (Ch. 5) is a small regulatory protein present in almost all cells of the body ('ubiquitous'). It directs proteins to compartments in the cell, including the proteasome which destroys and recycles proteins. Ubiquitin-binding proteins interact with ubiquitinated targets and regulate diverse biological processes, including endocytosis, signal transduction, transcription and DNA repair.

released slowly as bone is resorbed by the osteoclasts, which are thus exposed to high local bisphosphonate concentrations.

Mechanism of action

Bisphosphonates reduce the rate of bone turnover. They can be grouped into two classes:

1. Simple compounds that are very similar to pyrophosphate (e.g. **etidronate**). These are incorporated into ATP analogues that accumulate within the osteoclasts and promote their apoptosis.
2. Potent, amino-bisphosphonates (e.g. **pamidronate**, **alendronate**, **risedronate**, **ibandronate**, **zoledronate**). These prevent bone resorption by interfering with the anchoring of cell surface proteins to the osteoclast membrane by prenylation, thereby preventing osteoclast attachment to bone (see Strewler, 2005).

Pharmacokinetic aspects

Bisphosphonates are given orally on an empty stomach with plenty of water in a sitting or standing position at least 30 minutes before breakfast because of their propensity to cause severe oesophageal problems or, in the case of pamidronate, ibandronate and of zoledronate, intravenously. They are poorly absorbed from the gut. About 50% of absorbed drug accumulates at sites of bone mineralisation, where it remains adsorbed onto hydroxyapatite crystals, potentially for months or years, until the bone is resorbed. The free drug is excreted unchanged by the kidney.

Absorption is impaired by food, particularly milk, so the drugs must be taken on an empty stomach.

Unwanted effects include gastrointestinal disturbances including peptic ulcers and oesophagitis (sometimes with erosions or stricture formation). Bone pain occurs occasionally. Atypical femoral fractures are described during long-term treatment, especially of osteoporosis, and the need for continued use should be re-evaluated periodically (e.g. after 5 years). Given intravenously, some bisphosphonates (in particular zoledronate) can lead to osteonecrosis (literally 'death of bone') of the jaw, especially in patients with malignant disease; a dental check is needed before treatment (followed by any indicated remedial work). After zoledronate infusion supplemental calcium and vitamin D are administered for at least ten days.

Clinical use

Alendronate and risedronate are given orally for prophylaxis and treatment of osteoporosis. Etidronate is an alternative. Clodronate is used in patients with malignant disease involving bone and pamidronate is given by intravenous infusion to treat hypercalcaemia of malignancy or to treat Paget's disease. Ibandronate is given intravenously every 3–4 weeks in patients with breast cancer metastatic to bone, or every 3 months to treat postmenopausal osteoporosis. Zoledronate, which is given as an intravenous infusion, is used for advanced malignancy involving bone, for Paget's disease and for selected cases of osteoporosis (postmenopausal or in men) when it is administered once a year or even less frequently (see clinical box below).

Bisphosphonates

- Orally active, stable analogues of pyrophosphate, which are incorporated into remodelling bone and remain there for months to years.
- Released when osteoclast-mediated bone resorption occurs, exposing osteoclasts to their effects.
- First-generation compounds (e.g. **etidronate**) act by promoting apoptosis of osteoclasts.
- Second-generation compounds (e.g. **risedronate**) with N-containing side chains are much more potent, and prevent osteoclast action by inhibiting prenylation reactions required for membrane anchoring of functional proteins.
- Used long term for prevention and treatment of osteoporosis, and for symptomatic Paget's disease.
- Main unwanted effect is gastrointestinal (especially oesophageal) disturbance; a rare but serious adverse effect of the most potent drugs (notably **zoledronate**) is osteonecrosis of the jaw.

Clinical uses of bisphosphonates

- *Osteoporosis*:
  - 'primary' prevention of fractures in high-risk individuals (e.g. with established osteoporosis, several risk factors for osteoporosis, chronic treatment with systemic glucocorticoids)
  - 'secondary' prevention after an osteoporotic fracture
  - **alendronate** by mouth, given daily or once weekly in addition to calcium with vitamin D₃. **Risedronate** or **etidronate** are alternatives; **zoledronate** is given annually or even less often by intravenous infusion; it is the most potent bisphosphonate and more likely to cause osteonecrosis of the jaw – dental check and remedial dental work are prerequisites of treatment.
- *Malignant disease* involving bone (e.g. metastatic breast cancer, multiple myeloma):
  - to reduce bone damage, pain and hypercalcaemia (e.g. **clodronate**, **ibandronate**, **zoledronate**).
- *Paget's disease* of bone (e.g. **etidronate**, **pamidronate**) administered intermittently and with monitoring of serum phosphate, alkaline phosphatase and urinary hydroxyproline (a marker of collagen turnover).

OESTROGENS AND RELATED COMPOUNDS

The decline in endogenous oestrogen is a major factor in postmenopausal osteoporosis, and there is evidence that giving oestrogen as hormone replacement therapy (HRT; see Ch. 35) can ameliorate this. But HRT has actions on many systems, and newer agents (e.g. **raloxifene**, see Ch. 35) have been developed that exhibit agonist actions on some tissues and antagonist actions on others. These are termed *selective oestrogen receptor modulators* (SERMs).

RALOXIFENE

Raloxifene is a SERM that stimulates osteoblasts and inhibits osteoclasts. It also has agonist actions on the cardiovascular system, and antagonist activity on mammary tissue and the uterus.

It is well absorbed in the gastrointestinal tract, and undergoes extensive first-pass metabolism in the liver to give the glucuronide, which undergoes enterohepatic recycling. Overall bioavailability is only about 2%. Despite the low plasma concentration, raloxifene is concentrated in tissues, and is converted to an active metabolite in liver, lungs, bone, spleen, uterus and kidney. Its half-life averages 32 h. It is excreted mainly in the faeces.

Unwanted effects include hot flushes, leg cramps, flu-like symptoms and peripheral oedema. Less common are thrombophlebitis and thromboembolism. Other rarer adverse effects are thrombocytopenia, gastrointestinal disturbances, rashes, raised blood pressure and arterial thromboembolism. Raloxifene is not recommended for primary prevention of osteoporotic fractures, but is one alternative to a bisphosphonate for secondary prevention in postmenopausal women who cannot tolerate a bisphosphonate.

PARATHYROID HORMONE AND TERIPARATIDE

PTH and fragments of PTH given in small doses paradoxically *stimulate* osteoblast activity and *enhance* bone formation, and are used by specialists to treat selected male or female patients with osteoporosis, especially those with severe disease. The main compound currently used is **teriparatide** – the peptide fragment (1–34) of recombinant PTH. Another peptide analogue (**ostabolin,** cyclic PTH1–35, which it is hoped will increase bone mass with less effect on bone resorption and hence on plasma calcium concentration than PTH or teriparatide) is in development.

Teriparatide reverses osteoporosis by stimulating new bone formation (Yasothan & Santwana, 2008). It increases bone mass, structural integrity and bone strength by increasing the number of osteoblasts and by activating those osteoblasts already in bone. It also reduces osteoblast apoptosis.

It acts on PTH_1 and PTH_2, G protein-coupled receptors in the cell membranes of target cells, and its effects are mediated through activation of adenylyl cyclase and phospholipases A, C and D, and consequent increases in cyclic AMP and intracellular Ca^{2+} (see Deal, 2009).

Teriparatide is given subcutaneously once daily. It is well tolerated, and serious adverse effects are few. Nausea, dizziness, headache and arthralgias can occur. Mild hypercalcaemia, transient orthostatic hypotension and leg cramps have been reported.

STRONTIUM

Strontium (a Scottish element discovered in the tin mines around Strontian and given as the ranelate salt) inhibits bone resorption and also stimulates bone formation. It prevents vertebral and non-vertebral fractures in older women (see Fogelman & Blake, 2005). However, like barium it blocks potassium channels responsible for basal vasodilator tone, and is associated with an increased risk of cardiovascular disease, including myocardial infarction. It can also cause severe allergic reactions, and its use is restricted to specialists treating severe forms of osteoporosis.

The precise mechanism is not clear. Like calcium, strontium is absorbed from the intestine, incorporated into bone and excreted via the kidney. Strontium ions stimulate the calcium-sensing receptor causing pre-osteoblasts to differentiate into osteoblasts, which increase bone formation and secrete osteoprotegerin. Strontium inhibits osteoclasts so decreasing bone resorption. Strontium atoms are adsorbed onto the hydroxyapatite crystals, but eventually exchange for calcium in the bone minerals and remain in bone for many years.

The drug is well tolerated; a low incidence of nausea and diarrhoea is reported.

VITAMIN D PREPARATIONS

Vitamin D preparations are used in the treatment of vitamin D deficiencies, bone problems associated with renal failure ('renal osteodystrophy') and hypoparathyroidism – acute hypoparathyroidism is treated with intravenous calcium and injectable vitamin D preparations.

The main vitamin D preparation used clinically is **ergocalciferol**. Other preparations are **alfacalcidol** and **calcitriol**. All can be given orally and are well absorbed unless there is obstructive liver disease (vitamin D is fat soluble, and bile salts are necessary for absorption). **Paricalcitol,** a synthetic vitamin D analogue with less potential to cause hypercalcaemia, is used to treat and prevent the secondary hyperparathyroidism that occurs in patients with chronic renal failure because of associated hyperphosphataemia (Salusky, 2005).

Given orally, vitamin D is bound to a specific α-globulin in the blood and exogenous vitamin D can be found in fat for many months after dosing. The main route of elimination is in the faeces.

The clinical uses of vitamin D preparations are given in the box.

Excessive intake of vitamin D causes hypercalcaemia. If hypercalcaemia persists, especially in the presence of elevated phosphate concentrations, calcium salts are deposited in the kidney and urine, causing renal failure and kidney stones.

Clinical uses of vitamin D

- Deficiency states: prevention and treatment of *rickets*, *osteomalacia* and vitamin D deficiency owing to *malabsorption* and *liver disease* (**ergocalciferol**).
- Hypocalcaemia caused by *hypoparathyroidism* (**ergocalciferol**).
- *Osteodystrophy* of *chronic renal failure*, which is the consequence of decreased calcitriol generation (**calcitriol** or **alphacalcidol**).
  Plasma Ca^{2+} levels should be monitored during therapy with vitamin D.

BIOLOGICALS

Denosumab is a recombinant human monoclonal antibody that inhibits RANKL, the primary signal for bone resorption (see p. 441). It was approved by the US Food and Drug Administration in 2010 for use in postmenopausal women at risk of osteoporosis, and to prevent skeleton-related events in patients with bone metastases from solid tumours. Trials in other indications are ongoing. It is especially useful when bisphosphonates are not appropriate. Calcium and vitamin D deficiencies need to be corrected and necessary dental work needs to be undertaken before treatment with denosumab to reduce the risk of osteonecrosis of the jaw (as with potent bisphosphonates, see clinical box, p. 445). It is administered as subcutaneous injections (60 mg) every 6 months for women with postmenopausal osteoporosis or men with prostate cancer at increased risk of osteoporosis because of hormone ablation, or more frequently (monthly) in patients with bone metastases. Adverse effects include altered bowel habit (diarrhoea or constipation), dyspnoea, hypocalcaemia, hypophosphataemia, infection (including respiratory, ear, cellulitis) or rash as well as (rarely) osteonecrosis of the jaw.

CALCITONIN

The main preparation available for clinical use (see the clinical box) is **salcatonin** (synthetic salmon calcitonin). Synthetic human calcitonin is also available. Calcitonin is given by subcutaneous or intramuscular injection, and there may be a local inflammatory action at the injection site. It can also be given intranasally, which is more convenient but less effective. Its plasma half-life is 4–12 min, but its action lasts for several hours.

Unwanted effects include nausea and vomiting. Facial flushing may occur, as may a tingling sensation in the hands and an unpleasant taste in the mouth.

> ### Clinical uses of calcitonin/salcatonin
>
>
> These agents are now less used.
> - *Hypercalcaemia* (e.g. associated with neoplasia).
> - *Paget's disease* of bone (to relieve pain and reduce neurological complications) – but it is much less convenient than an injected high potency bisphosphonate.
> - Postmenopausal and corticosteroid-induced *osteoporosis* (with other agents).

CALCIUM SALTS

Calcium salts used therapeutically include **calcium gluconate** and **calcium lactate**, given orally. Calcium gluconate is also used for intravenous injection in emergency treatment of hyperkalaemia (Ch. 29); intramuscular injection is not used because it causes local necrosis.

Calcium carbonate, an antacid and phosphate binder (Ch. 29), is usually very little absorbed from the gut (an advantage since an effect within the stomach or intestine is the desired outcome for a drug intended to buffer gastric acid and to reduce ileal phosphate absorption), but there is concern that low level systemic absorption has the potential to cause arterial calcification in patients with renal failure, especially if complicated by hyperphosphataemia (the product of calcium and phosphate ion concentrations is sometimes used clinically to estimate the risk of tissue deposition of insoluble calcium phosphate).

Unwanted effects: oral calcium salts can cause gastrointestinal disturbance. Intravenous administration in emergency treatment of hyperkalaemia requires care, especially in patients receiving cardiac glycosides, the toxicity of which is influenced by extracellular calcium ion concentration (see Ch. 21).

The clinical uses of calcium salts are given in the clinical box.

> ### Clinical uses of calcium salts
>
>
> - Dietary deficiency.
> - Hypocalcaemia caused by *hypoparathyroidism* or *malabsorption* (intravenous for acute tetany).
> - Calcium carbonate is an antacid; it is poorly absorbed and binds phosphate in the gut. It is used to treat *hyperphosphataemia* (Ch. 29).
> - Prevention and treatment of *osteoporosis* (often with oestrogen or SERM in women, bisphosphonate, vitamin D).
> - Cardiac dysrhythmias caused by severe *hyperkalaemia* (intravenous; see Ch. 21).

CALCIMIMETIC COMPOUNDS

Calcimimetics enhance the sensitivity of the parathyroid Ca^{2+}-sensing receptor to the concentration of blood Ca^{2+}, with a consequent decrease in secretion of PTH and reduction in serum Ca^{2+} concentration. There are two types of calcimimetics:

1. Type I are agonists, and include various inorganic and organic cations; Sr^{2+} is an example (see p. 446).
2. Type II are allosteric activators (see Ch. 3) that activate the receptor indirectly. **Cinacalcet**, which is used for the treatment of hyperparathyroidism (Fig. 36.3; Peacock et al., 2005) is an example.

POTENTIAL NEW THERAPIES

Improved understanding of bone remodelling (Yasothan & Kar, 2008; Deal, 2009) has opened several therapeutic approaches that will hopefully yield useful new drugs in the foreseeable future. These include cathepsin K inhibitors (e.g. **odanacatib** – which may be submitted for regulatory review in 2014). Other promising targets are discussed by Deal (2009).

REFERENCES AND FURTHER READING

Bone disorders and bone remodelling

Boyce, B.F., Xing, L., 2008. Functions of RANKL/RANK/OPG in bone modeling and remodeling. Arch. Biochem. Biophys. 473, 139–146. (*Good review of the role of the RANK/RANKL/OPG in osteoclast formation and the transcription factors involved*)

Deal, C., 2009. Potential new drug targets for osteoporosis. Nat. Clin. Pract. Rheumatol. 5, 174–180. (*Outstanding review; good diagrams*)

Deftos, L.J., 2005. Treatment of Paget's disease – taming the wild osteoclast. N. Engl. J. Med. 353, 872–875. (*Editorial covering the use of OPG and zoledronic acid for Paget's disease. See also article by Cundy et al. in the same issue, pp. 918–923*)

Gallagher, J.C., 2008. Advances in bone biology and new treatments for bone loss. Maturitas 20, 65–69. (*Article on preventing bone loss by targeting the RANK/RANKL/OPG system with denosumab*)

Imai, Y., Youn, M.-Y., Inoue, K., 2013. Nuclear receptors in bone physiology and diseases. Physiol. Rev. 93, 481–523. (*Reviews roles of various nuclear receptor-mediated signalling pathways in bone physiology and disease*)

Khosla, S., Westendorf, J.J., Oursler, M.J., 2008. Building bone to reverse osteoporosis and repair fractures. J. Clin. Invest. 118, 421–428. (*Good review; covers the role of Wnt signalling and sclerostin secretion*)

Rea, S.L., Walsh, J.P., Layfield, R., Ratajczak, T., Xu, J., 2013. New insights into the role of sequestosome 1/p62 mutant proteins in the pathogenesis of Paget's disease of bone. Endocrine Rev. 34, 501-524. (*Outlines recent advances in understanding of the multiple pathophysiological roles of SQSTM1/p62 protein, with particular emphasis on their relationship to Paget's disease of bone*)

Reichel, H., Koeftler, H.P., Norman, A.W., 1989. The role of the vitamin D endocrine system in health and disease. N. Engl. J. Med. 320, 980–991. (*Classic*)

Reid, R., 2008. Anti-resorptive therapies for osteoporosis. Semin. Cell Dev. Biol. 19, 5473–5478. (*Excellent review of the actions of current and novel anti-resorptive drugs*)

Riggs, B.L., Khosla, S., Melton, L.J., 2012. Better tools for assessing osteoporosis. J. Clin. Invest. 122, 4323–4324. (*Describes the current gold standard methods of dual-energy X-ray absorptiometry (DXA) and quantitative computed tomography*)

Stewart, J.F., 2004. Translational implications of the parathyroid calcium receptor. N. Engl. J. Med. 351, 324–326. (*Succinct article with useful diagrams*)

Wright, H.L., McCarthy, H.S., Middleton, J., Marshall, M.J., 2009. RANK, RANKL and osteoprotegerin in bone biology and disease. Curr. Rev. Musculoskelet. Med. 2, 56–64. (*Synopsis of the structures of RANK, RANKL and OPG, and the intracellular RANK/RANKL signalling pathways with a review of diseases linked to their malfunction*)

Drugs used to treat bone disorders

Brennan, T.C., Rybchyn, M.S., Green, W., et al., 2009. Osteoblasts play key roles in the mechanisms of action of strontium ranelate. Br. J. Pharmacol. 57, 1291–1300. (*A study in human cells showing that strontium ranelate acts at least in part by activating the calcium-sensing receptor*)

Clemett, D., Spenser, C.M., 2000. Raloxifene: a review of its use in postmenopausal osteoporosis. Drugs 60, 379–411. (*Comprehensive review covering the mechanism of action, pharmacology, pharmacokinetic aspects, therapeutic use and adverse effects of raloxifene*)

Cummings, S.R., San Martin, J., McClung, M.R., et al., 2009. Denosumab for prevention of fractures in postmenopausal women with osteoporosis. N. Engl. J. Med. 361, 818–820. ('*Freedom Trial' with 239 collaborators. Denosumab was effective in reducing fracture risk in women with osteoporosis*)

Fogelman, I., Blake, G.M., 2005. Strontium ranelate for the treatment of osteoporosis. Br. Med. J. 330, 1400–1401. (*Crisp editorial analysis*)

Khosla, K., 2009. Increasing options for the treatment of osteoporosis. N. Engl. J. Med. 361, 818–820. (*Editorial*)

Nemeth, E.F., Heaton, W.H., Miller, M., et al., 2004. Pharmacodynamics of the type II calcimimetic compound cinacalcet HCl. J. Pharmacol. Exp. Ther. 398, 627–635. (*Detailed study of pharmacokinetic aspects and the pharmacological action of cinacalcet hydrochloride*)

Peacock, M., Bilezikian, J.P., Klassen, P.S., et al., 2005. Cinacalcet hydrochloride maintains long-term normocalcaemia in patients with primary hyperparathyroidism. J. Clin. Endocrinol. Metab. 90, 135–141.

Reginster, J.Y., Deroisy, R., Neuprez, A., et al., 2009. Strontium ranelate: new data on fracture prevention and mechanisms of action. Curr. Osteoporos. Rep. 7, 96–102. (*Stresses that in 5-year studies this drug has proved efficacious in both decreasing bone reabsorption and stimulating bone formation, and has a positive risk–benefit ratio*)

Rogers, M.J., 2003. New insights into the mechanisms of action of the bisphosphonates. Curr. Pharm. Des. 9, 2643–2658. (*Covers the different mechanisms of action of the simple bisphosphonates and the nitrogen-containing bisphosphonates*)

Salusky, I.B., 2005. Are new vitamin D analogues in renal bone disease superior to calcitriol? Pediatr. Nephrol. 20, 393–398.

Strewler, G.J., 2005. Decimal point – osteoporosis therapy at the 10-year mark. N. Engl. J. Med. 350, 1172–1174. (*Crisp article concentrating mainly on bisphosphonates*)

Whyte, M.P., 2006. The long and the short of bone therapy. N. Engl. J. Med. 354, 860–863. (*Present status of and future possibilities for bone therapy.*)

Yasothan, U., Kar, S., 2008. Osteoporosis: overview and pipeline. Nat. Rev. Drug Discov. 7, 725–726.

Yasothan, U., Santwana, K., 2008. From the analyst's couch. Osteoporosis: overview and pipeline. Nat. Rev. Drug Discov. 7, 725–726. (*Crisp outline of current antiosteoporosis drugs with table of new drugs in phase I and phase II development*)

Chemical transmission and drug action in the central nervous system

37

OVERVIEW

Brain function is the single most important aspect of physiology that defines the difference between humans and other species. Disorders of brain function, whether primary or secondary to malfunction of other systems, are a major concern of human society, and a field in which pharmacological intervention plays a key role. In this chapter we introduce some basic principles of neuropharmacology that underlie much of the material in the rest of this section.

INTRODUCTION

There are two reasons why understanding the action of drugs on the central nervous system (CNS) presents a particularly challenging problem. The first is that centrally acting drugs are of special significance to humankind. Not only are they of major therapeutic importance,[1] but they are also the drugs that humans most commonly administer to themselves for non medical reasons (e.g. alcohol, tea and coffee, cannabis, nicotine, opioids, amphetamines and so on). The second reason is that the CNS is functionally far more complex than any other system in the body, and this makes the understanding of drug effects very much more difficult. The relationship between the behaviour of individual cells and that of the organ as a whole is far less direct in the brain than in other organs. Currently, the links between a drug's action at the biochemical and cellular level and its effects on brain function remain largely mysterious. Functional brain imaging is beginning to reveal relationships between brain activity in specific regions and mental function, and this tool is being used increasingly to probe drug effects. Despite sustained progress in understanding the cellular and biochemical effects produced by centrally acting drugs, and the increasing use of brain imaging to study brain function and drug effects, the gulf between our understanding of drug action at the cellular level and at the functional and behavioural level remains, for the most part, very wide.

In some instances, our understanding of brain function and how drugs alter it is more advanced. Thus, the relationship between dopaminergic pathways in the extrapyramidal system and the effects of drugs in alleviating or exacerbating the symptoms of Parkinson's disease (see Ch. 40) is clear cut. Many CNS drugs are used to treat psychiatric disorders that are defined according to their symptomatology rather than on the basis of

causative factors or clinical signs and investigations. What is called 'schizophrenia' or 'depression' on the basis of particular symptoms is likely to consist of several distinct disorders caused by different mechanisms and responding to drugs in different ways. Much effort is going into pinning down the biological basis of psychiatric disorders – a necessary step to improve the design of better drugs for clinical use – but the task is daunting and progress is slow.

In this chapter we outline the general principles governing the action of drugs on the CNS. Most neuroactive drugs work by interfering with the chemical signals that underlie brain function, and the next two chapters discuss the major CNS transmitter systems and the ways in which drugs affect them. In Chapter 40, we focus on neurodegenerative diseases, and the remaining chapters in this section deal with the main classes of neuroactive drugs that are currently in use.

Background information will be found in neurobiology and neuropharmacology textbooks such as Kandel et al. (2013), Nestler et al. (2008) and Iversen et al. (2009).

CHEMICAL SIGNALLING IN THE NERVOUS SYSTEM

The brain (like every other organ in the body!) is basically a chemical machine; it controls the main functions of a higher animal across timescales ranging from milliseconds (e.g. returning a 100 mph tennis serve) to years (e.g. remembering how to ride a bicycle).[2] The chemical signalling mechanisms cover a correspondingly wide dynamic range, as summarised, in a very general way, in Figure 37.1. Currently, we understand much about drug effects on events at the fast end of the spectrum – synaptic transmission and neuromodulation – but much less about long-term adaptive processes, although it is quite evident that the latter are of great importance for the neurological and psychiatric disorders that are susceptible to drug treatment.

The original concept of neurotransmission envisaged a substance released by one neuron and acting rapidly, briefly and at short range on the membrane of an adjacent (postsynaptic) neuron, causing excitation or inhibition. The principles outlined in Chapter 12 apply to the central as well as the peripheral nervous system. It is now clear that chemical mediators within the brain can produce slow and long-lasting effects; that they can act rather diffusely, at a considerable distance from their site of release (e.g. GABA acting at extrasynaptic $GABA_A$ receptors, see Ch. 38); and that they can also produce other diverse effects, for example on transmitter synthesis, on the

---

[1]In Britain in 2008/2009, 145 million prescriptions (about 20% of all prescriptions), costing £1.7 billion, were for CNS drugs as defined by the *British National Formulary*. This amounted to over two per person across the whole population.

[2]Memory of drug names and the basic facts of pharmacology seems to come somewhere in the middle of this range (skewed towards the short end).

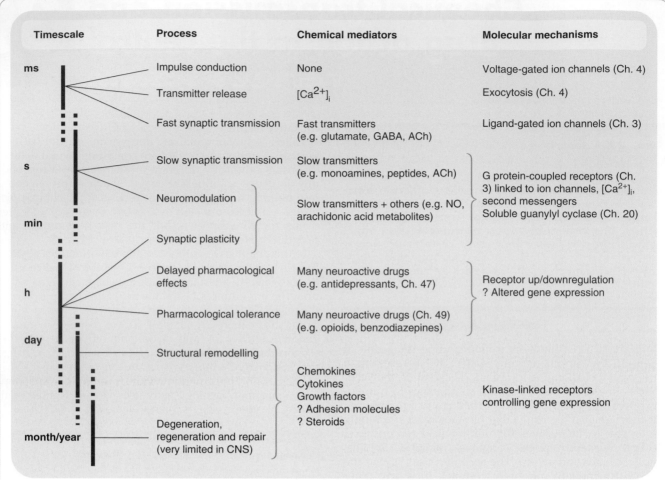

Fig. 37.1 **Chemical signalling in the nervous system.** Knowledge of the mediators and mechanisms becomes sparser as we move from the rapid events of synaptic transmission to the slower ones involving remodelling and alterations of gene expression. ACh, acetylcholine; CNS, central nervous system; NO, nitric oxide.

expression of neurotransmitter receptors and on neuronal morphology, in addition to affecting the ionic conductance of the postsynaptic cell membrane. The term *neuromodulator* is often used to denote a mediator, the actions of which do not conform to the original neurotransmitter concept. The term is not clearly defined, and it covers not only the diffusely acting neuropeptide mediators, but also mediators such as nitric oxide (NO, Ch. 20) and arachidonic acid metabolites (Ch. 17), which are not stored and released like conventional neurotransmitters, and may come from non-neuronal cells, particularly glia, as well as neurons. In general, *neuromodulation* relates to synaptic plasticity, including short-term physiological events such as the regulation of presynaptic transmitter release or postsynaptic excitability. Longer-term *neurotrophic* effects are involved in regulating the growth and morphology of neurons, as well as their functional properties. Table 37.1 summarises the types of chemical mediator that operate in the CNS.

Glial cells, particularly astrocytes, which are the main non-neuronal cells in the CNS and outnumber neurons by 10 to 1, also play an important signalling role. Once thought of mainly as housekeeping cells, whose function was merely to look after the fastidious neurons, they are increasingly seen as 'inexcitable neurons' with a major communications role (see Matsas & Tsacopolous, 2013),

albeit on a slower timescale than that of neuronal communication. These cells express a range of receptors and transporters, and also release a wide variety of mediators, including glutamate, D-serine, ATP, lipid mediators and growth factors. They respond to chemical signals from neurons, and also from neighbouring astrocytes and microglial cells (the CNS equivalent of macrophages, which function much like inflammatory cells in peripheral tissues). Electrical coupling between astrocytes causes them often to respond in concert in a particular brain region, thus controlling the chemical environment in which the neurons operate. Although they do not conduct action potentials, and do not send signals to other parts of the body, astrocytes are otherwise very similar to neurons and play a crucial communication role within the brain. Because they are difficult to study in situ, however, our knowledge of how they function, and how they respond to drugs, is still fragmentary. It is an area to watch closely.

TARGETS FOR DRUG ACTION

▼ To recapitulate what was discussed in Chapters 2 and 3, neuroactive drugs act on one of four types of target proteins, namely ion channels, receptors, enzymes and transport proteins. Of the four main receptor families – ionotropic receptors, G protein-coupled

Table 37.1 Types of chemical mediators in the central nervous system

Mediator type[a]	Examples	Targets	Main functional role
Conventional small-molecule mediators	Glutamate, GABA, acetylcholine, dopamine, 5-hydroxytryptamine, etc.	Ligand-gated ion channels G protein-coupled receptors	Fast and slow synaptic neurotransmission Neuromodulation
Neuropeptides	Substance P, neuropeptide Y, endorphins, corticotrophin-releasing factor, etc.	G protein-coupled receptors	Neuromodulation
Lipid mediators	Prostaglandins, endocannabinoids	G protein-coupled receptors	Neuromodulation
'Gaseous' mediators	Nitric oxide Carbon monoxide	Guanylyl cyclase	Neuromodulation
Neurotrophins, cytokines	Nerve growth factor, brain-derived neurotrophic factor, interleukin-1	Kinase-linked receptors	Neuronal growth, survival and functional plasticity
Steroids	Androgens, oestrogens	Nuclear and membrane receptors	Functional plasticity

[a]Most central nervous system pharmacology is currently centred on small-molecule mediators and, less commonly, neuropeptides. Other mediator types are now being targeted for therapeutic purposes.

Chemical transmission in the central nervous system

- The basic processes of synaptic transmission in the central nervous system are essentially similar to those operating in the periphery (Ch. 12).
- Glial cells, particularly astrocytes, participate actively in chemical signalling, functioning essentially as 'inexcitable neurons'.
- The terms *neurotransmitter*, *neuromodulator* and *neurotrophic factor* refer to chemical mediators that operate over different timescales. In general:
  - *neurotransmitters* are released by presynaptic terminals and produce rapid excitatory or inhibitory responses in postsynaptic neurons
  - fast neurotransmitters (e.g. glutamate, GABA) operate through ligand-gated ion channels
  - slow neurotransmitters and neuromodulators (e.g. dopamine, neuropeptides, prostanoids) operate mainly through G protein-coupled receptors

  - *neuromodulators* are released by neurons and by astrocytes, and produce slower pre- or postsynaptic responses
  - *neurotrophic factors* are released mainly by non-neuronal cells and act on tyrosine kinase-linked receptors that regulate gene expression and control neuronal growth and phenotypic characteristics.
- The same agent (e.g. glutamate, 5-hydroxytryptamine, acetylcholine) may act through both ligand-gated channels and G protein-coupled receptors, and function as both neurotransmitter and neuromodulator.
- Many chemical mediators, including glutamate, nitric oxide and arachidonic acid metabolites, are produced by glia as well as neurons.
- Many mediators (e.g. cytokines, chemokines, growth factors and steroids) control long-term changes in the brain (e.g. synaptic plasticity and remodelling), mainly by affecting gene transcription.

receptors, kinase-linked receptors and nuclear receptors – current neuroactive drugs target mainly the first two.

In the last three decades, knowledge about these targets in the CNS has accumulated rapidly, particularly as follows:

- As well as 40 or more small-molecule and peptide mediators, the importance of other 'non-classical' mediators – nitric oxide, eicosanoids, growth factors, etc. – has become apparent.
- Considerable molecular diversity of known receptor molecules and ion channels (see Ch. 3) has been revealed.
- The receptors and channels are each expressed in several subtypes, with characteristic distributions in different brain areas. In most cases, we are only beginning to discover what this diversity means at a functional level, mainly through the study of transgenic animals. The molecular diversity of such targets raises the possibility of developing drugs with improved selectivity of action, e.g. interacting with one kind of GABA$_A$ receptor without affecting others (see Ch. 44). The potential of these new approaches in terms of improved drugs for neurological and psychiatric diseases is large but as yet unrealised.

- The pathophysiology of neurodegeneration is beginning to be understood (see Ch. 40), and progress is being made in understanding the mechanisms underlying drug dependence (see Ch. 49), suggesting new strategies for treating these disabling conditions. The neurobiology of epilepsy, schizophrenia and depressive illnesses is also advancing.
- Cognitive dysfunction in CNS disorders such as schizophrenia, depressive illness and drug addiction is a potential target for drug therapy.

DRUG ACTION IN THE CENTRAL NERVOUS SYSTEM

As already emphasised, the molecular and cellular mechanisms underlying drug action in the CNS and in the periphery have much in common. Understanding how drugs affect brain function is, however, problematic. One difficulty is the complexity of neuronal interconnections in the brain – the wiring diagram. Figure 37.2 illustrates in a schematic way the kind of interconnections that typically exist for, say, a noradrenergic neuron in the *locus coeruleus* (see Ch. 39), shown as **neuron 1** in the diagram, releasing **transmitter *a*** at its terminals. Release of *a* affects **neuron 2** (which releases **transmitter *b***), and also affects neuron 1 by direct feedback and, indirectly, by affecting presynaptic inputs impinging on neuron 1. The firing pattern of neuron 2 also affects the system, partly through interneuronal connections (**neuron 3**, releasing **transmitter *c***). Even at this grossly oversimplified level, the effects on the system of blocking or enhancing the release or actions of one or other of the transmitters are difficult to predict, and will depend greatly on the relative strength of the various excitatory and inhibitory synaptic connections, and on external inputs (*x* and *y* in the diagram). Added to this complexity is the influence of glial cells, mentioned above.

A further important complicating factor is that a range of secondary, adaptive responses is generally set in train by any drug-induced perturbation of the system. Typically, an increase in transmitter release, or interference with transmitter reuptake, is countered by inhibition of transmitter synthesis, enhanced transporter expression or decreased receptor expression. These changes, which involve altered gene expression, generally take time (hours, days or weeks) to develop and are not evident in acute pharmacological experiments.

In the clinical situation, the effects of psychotropic drugs often take weeks to develop, so it is likely that they reflect adaptive responses and slowly developing changes in perception rather than the immediate pharmacodynamic effects of the drug. This is well documented for antipsychotic and antidepressant drugs (Chs 46 and 47). The development of dependence on opioids, benzodiazepines and psychostimulants is similarly gradual in onset (Ch. 49). Thus, one has to take into account not only the primary interaction of the drug with its target, but also the secondary response of the brain to this primary effect; it is often the secondary response, rather than the primary effect, which leads to clinical benefit.

BLOOD–BRAIN BARRIER

▼ A key factor in CNS pharmacology is the blood–brain barrier (see Ch. 8), penetration of which requires molecules to traverse the vascular endothelial cells rather than going between them. Inflammation can disrupt the integrity of the blood–brain barrier, allowing previously impermeable drugs such as **penicillin** to cross. In

general, only small non-polar molecules can diffuse passively across cell membranes. Some neuroactive drugs penetrate the blood–brain barrier in this way, but many do so via transporters, which either facilitate entry into the brain or diminish it by pumping the compound from the endothelial cell interior back into the bloodstream. Drugs that gain entry in this way include **levodopa** (Ch. 40), **valproate** (Ch. 45) and various sedative histamine antagonists (Ch. 17). Active extrusion of drugs from the brain occurs via P-glycoprotein, an ATP-driven drug efflux transporter, and related transporter proteins (see Ch. 8). Many antibacterial and anticancer drugs are excluded from the brain while some CNS-acting drugs – including certain opioid, antidepressant, antipsychotic and antiepileptic drugs – are actively extruded from the brain see (Linnet & Ejsing, 2008). Variation in the activity of efflux transporters between individuals is an important consideration (Chs 8 and 11).

THE CLASSIFICATION OF PSYCHOTROPIC DRUGS

Psychotropic drugs are defined as those that affect mood and behaviour. Because these indices of brain function are difficult to define and measure, there is no consistent basis for classifying psychotropic drugs. Instead, we find a confusing mêlée of terms relating to chemical structure (*benzodiazepines, butyrophenones*, etc.), biochemical target (*monoamine oxidase inhibitors, serotonin reuptake inhibitors*, etc.), behavioural effect (*hallucinogens, psychomotor stimulants*) or clinical use (*antidepressants, antipsychotic agents, antiepileptic drugs*, etc.), together with a number of indefinable rogue categories (*atypical antipsychotic drugs, nootropic drugs*) thrown in for good measure.

Some drugs defy classification in this scheme, for example **lithium** (see Ch. 47), which is used in the treatment of manic depressive psychosis, and **ketamine** (see Ch. 41), which is classed as a dissociative anaesthetic but produces psychotropic effects rather similar to those produced by phencyclidine.

In practice, the use of drugs in psychiatric illness frequently cuts across specific therapeutic categories. For example, it is common for antipsychotic drugs to be used as 'tranquillisers' to control extremely anxious or unruly patients, or to treat bipolar depression (Ch. 47). Antidepressant drugs are often used to treat anxiety (Ch. 44) and neuropathic pain (Ch. 42), and certain psychostimulants are of proven efficacy for treating hyperactive children (Ch. 48). Here we will adhere to the conventional pharmacological categories, but it needs to be emphasised that in clinical use these distinctions are often disregarded.

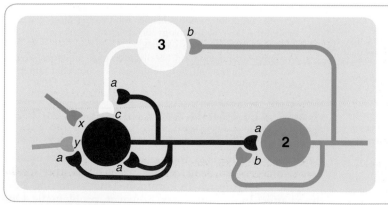

Fig. 37.2 **Simplified scheme of neuronal interconnections in the central nervous system.** Neurons 1, 2 and 3 are shown releasing transmitters *a*, *b* and *c*, respectively, which may be excitatory or inhibitory. Boutons of neuron 1 terminate on neuron 2, but also on neuron 1 itself, and on presynaptic terminals of other neurons that make synaptic connections with neuron 1. Neuron 2 also feeds back on neuron 1 via interneuron 3. Transmitters (*x* and *y*) released by other neurons are also shown impinging on neuron 1. Even with such a simple network, the effects of drug-induced interference with specific transmitter systems can be difficult to predict.

Table 37.2 General classification of drugs acting on the central nervous system

Class	Definition	Examples	See Chapter
General anaesthetic agents	Drugs used to produce surgical anaesthesia	Isoflurane, desflurane, propofol, etomidate	41
Analgesic drugs	Drugs used clinically for controlling pain	Opiates Neuropathic pain – carbamazepine, gabapentin, amitriptyline, duloxetine	42
Anxiolytics and sedatives	Drugs that reduce anxiety and cause sleep	Benzodiazepines (e.g. diazepam, chlordiazepoxide, flurazepam, clonazepam)	44
Antiepileptic drugs Synonym: anticonvulsants	Drugs used to reduce seizures	Carbamazepine, valproate, lamotrigine	45
Antipsychotic drugs Synonym: antischizophrenic drugs	Drugs used to relieve the symptoms of schizophrenic illness	Clozapine, haloperidol, risperidone	46
Antidepressant drugs	Drugs that alleviate the symptoms of depressive illness	Selective serotonin reuptake inhibitors, tricyclic antidepressants, monoamine oxidase inhibitors	47
Psychomotor stimulants Synonym: psychostimulants	Drugs that cause wakefulness and euphoria	Amphetamine, cocaine, methylphenidate, caffeine	48
Psychotomimetic drugs Synonym: hallucinogens	Drugs that cause disturbance of perception (particularly visual hallucinations) and of behaviour in ways that cannot be simply characterised as sedative or stimulant effects	Lysergic acid diethylamide, mescaline, MDMA (ecstasy)	48
Cognition enhancers Synonym: nootropic drugs	Drugs that improve memory and cognitive performance	Acetylcholinesterase inhibitors: donepezil, galantamine, rivastigmine	40
		NMDA receptor antagonists: memantine	37
		Others: piracetam, modafinil	

Drug action in the central nervous system

- The basic types of drug target (ion channels, receptors, enzymes and transporter proteins) described in Chapter 3 apply in the central nervous system, as elsewhere.
- Most of these targets occur in several different molecular isoforms, giving rise to subtle differences in function and pharmacology.
- Many of the currently available neuroactive drugs are relatively non-specific, affecting several different targets,

the principal ones being receptors, ion channels and transporters.
- The relationship between the pharmacological profile and the therapeutic effect of neuroactive drugs is often unclear.
- Slowly developing secondary responses to the primary interaction of the drug with its target are often important (e.g. the delayed efficacy of antidepressant drugs, and tolerance and dependence with opioids).

REFERENCES AND FURTHER READING

Iversen, L.L., Iversen, S.D., Bloom, F.E., Roth, R.H., 2009. Introduction to Neuropsychopharmacology. Oxford University Press, New York. (*Excellent and readable account focusing on basic rather than clinical aspects*)

Kandel, E., Schwartz, J.H., Jessell, T.M., 2013. Principles of Neural Science, fifth ed. Elsevier, New York. (*Excellent and detailed standard text on neurobiology – little emphasis on pharmacology*)

Linnet, K., Ejsing, T.B., 2008. A review on the impact of P-glycoprotein on the penetration of drugs into the brain. Focus on psychotropic

drugs. Eur. Neuropsychopharmacol. 18, 157–169. (*Review of how P-glycoprotein can limit the brain concentration of antidepressant and antipsychotic drugs*)

Matsas, R., Tsacopolous, M., 2013. The functional roles of glial cells in health and disease: dialogue between glia and neurons. Adv. Exp. Biol. Med. 468. (*This volume contains a number of chapters on the emerging view of glial cell function*)

Nestler, E.J., Hyman, S.E., Malenka, R.C., 2008. Molecular neuropharmacology, second ed. McGraw-Hill, New York. (*Good textbook*)

38 Amino acid transmitters

OVERVIEW

In this chapter we discuss the major neurotransmitters in the central nervous system (CNS), namely the excitatory transmitter, glutamate, and the inhibitory transmitters, GABA and glycine. It is an area in which scientific interest has been intense in recent years. Unravelling the complexities of amino acid receptors and signalling mechanisms has thrown considerable light on their role in brain function and their likely involvement in CNS disease. Drugs that target specific receptors and transporters have been developed, but translating this knowledge into drugs for therapeutic use is only now beginning to happen. Here, we present the pharmacological principles and include recent references for those seeking more detail.

EXCITATORY AMINO ACIDS

EXCITATORY AMINO ACIDS AS CNS TRANSMITTERS

L-Glutamate is the principal and ubiquitous excitatory transmitter in the central nervous system. **Aspartate** plays a similar role in certain brain regions, and possibly also **homocysteate**, but this is controversial.

▼ The realisation of glutamate's importance came slowly (see Watkins & Jane, 2006). By the 1950s, work on the peripheral nervous system had highlighted the transmitter roles of acetylcholine and catecholamines and, as the brain also contained these substances, there seemed little reason to look further. The presence of **γ-aminobutyric acid** (GABA; see p. 462) in the brain, and its powerful inhibitory effect on neurons, were discovered in the 1950s, and its transmitter role was postulated. At the same time, work by Curtis's group in Canberra showed that glutamate and various other acidic amino acids produced a strong excitatory effect, but it seemed inconceivable that such workaday metabolites could actually be transmitters. Through the 1960s, GABA and excitatory amino acids (EAAs) were thought, even by their discoverers, to be mere pharmacological curiosities. In the 1970s, the humblest amino acid, glycine, was established as an inhibitory transmitter in the spinal cord, giving the lie to the idea that transmitters had to be exotic molecules, too beautiful for any role but to sink into the arms of a receptor. Once glycine had been accepted, the rest quickly followed. A major advance was the discovery of EAA antagonists, based on the work of Watkins in Bristol, which enabled the physiological role of glutamate to be established unequivocally, and also led to the realisation that EAA receptors are heterogeneous.

To do justice to the wealth of discovery in this field in the past 25 years is beyond the range of this book; for more detail see Traynelis et al. (2010) and Nicoletti et al. (2011). Here we concentrate on pharmacological aspects. With regard to novel drug development, many promising new compounds interacting with EAAs commenced development for the treatment of a wide range of neurological and psychiatric disorders but have failed because of lack of efficacy or adverse effects and only a few drugs[1] have made it into clinical use. The field has yet to make a major impact on therapeutics. The major problem has been that EAA-mediated neurotransmission is ubiquitous in the brain and so agonist and antagonist drugs exert effects at many sites, giving rise not only to therapeutically beneficial effects, but also to other, unwanted, harmful effects.

METABOLISM AND RELEASE OF EXCITATORY AMINO ACIDS

Glutamate is widely and fairly uniformly distributed in the CNS, where its concentration is much higher than in other tissues. It has an important metabolic role, the metabolic and neurotransmitter pools being linked by transaminase enzymes that catalyse the interconversion of glutamate and α-oxoglutarate (Fig. 38.1). Glutamate in the CNS comes mainly from either glucose, via the Krebs cycle, or glutamine, which is synthesised by glial cells and taken up by the neurons; very little comes from the periphery. The interconnection between the pathways for the synthesis of EAAs and inhibitory amino acids (GABA and glycine), shown in Figure 38.1, makes it difficult to use experimental manipulations of transmitter synthesis to study the functional role of individual amino acids, because disturbance of any one step will affect both excitatory and inhibitory mediators.

In common with other fast neurotransmitters, glutamate is stored in synaptic vesicles and released by Ca^{2+}-dependent exocytosis; specific transporter proteins account for its uptake by neurons and other cells, and for its accumulation by synaptic vesicles (see Ch. 12). Released glutamate is taken up into nerve terminals and neighbouring astrocytes (Fig. 38.2) by $Na^+/H^+/K^+$ dependent transporters (cf. monoamine transporters – Chs 12 and 14), and transported into synaptic vesicles, by a different transporter driven by the proton gradient across the vesicle membrane. Several EAA transporters have been cloned and characterised in detail (see Beart & O'Shea, 2007). Glutamate transport can, under some circumstances (e.g. depolarisation by increased extracellular $[K^+]$), operate in reverse and constitute a source of glutamate release, a process that may occur under pathological conditions such as brain ischaemia (see Ch. 40). Glutamate taken up by astrocytes is converted to glutamine and recycled, via transporters, back to the neurons, which convert the glutamine back to glutamate (Fig. 38.2). Glutamine, which lacks the pharmacological activity of glutamate, thus

---

[1]**Perampanel**, a non-competitive AMPA receptor antagonist, has recently been approved for the treatment of epilepsy (Ch. 45). **Memantine**, an N-methyl-D-aspartate (NMDA) antagonist, licensed for the treatment of moderate to severe Alzheimer's disease (Ch. 40), has been used for some time, as has the dissociative anaesthetic **ketamine**, an NMDA channel blocker (Ch. 41).

in clinical use) are known that interfere specifically with glutamate metabolism.

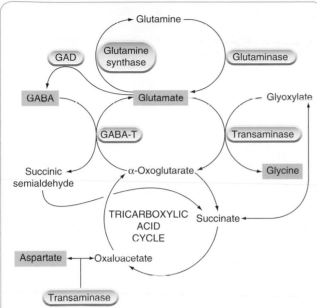

Fig. 38.1 Metabolism of transmitter amino acids in the brain. Transmitter substances are marked with green boxes. GABA-T, GABA transaminase; GAD, glutamic acid decarboxylase.

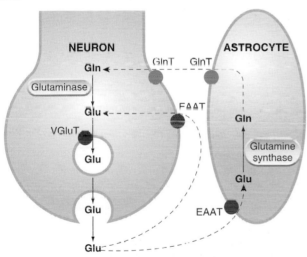

Fig. 38.2 Transport of glutamate (Glu) and glutamine (Gln) by neurons and astrocytes. Released glutamate is captured partly by neurons and partly by astrocytes, which convert most of it to glutamine. EAAT, excitatory amino acid transporter; GlnT, glutamine transporter; VGluT, vesicular glutamate transporter.

serves as a pool of inactive transmitter under the regulatory control of the astrocytes, which act as ball boys, returning the ammunition in harmless form in order to rearm the neurons.

There may be value in developing enhancers and inhibitors of glutamate uptake (see Bunch et al., 2009) for the treatment of CNS disorders in which the level of extracellular glutamate may be abnormal, e.g. neurodegeneration (see Ch. 40), schizophrenia (see Ch. 46) and depression (see Ch. 47). In contrast to the situation with monoamine synthesis and transport (Chs 14 and 39), few drugs (none

GLUTAMATE

GLUTAMATE RECEPTOR SUBTYPES

Glutamate and related excitatory amino acids activate both ionotropic (ligand-gated cation channels) and metabotropic (G protein-coupled) receptors (see Ch. 3 for a general description of ionotropic and metabotropic receptors).

IONOTROPIC GLUTAMATE RECEPTORS

On the basis of studies with selective agonists and antagonists (Fig. 38.3), three main subtypes of ionotropic receptors for glutamate can be distinguished: **NMDA**, **AMPA** and **kainate**[2] receptors, named originally according to their specific agonists (Table 38.1). These ligand-gated channels can be homomeric or heteromeric assemblies of four subunits, each with the 'pore loop' structure shown in Figure 3.18 (Ch. 3). There are some 16 different receptor subunits and their nomenclature has, until recently, been somewhat confusing.[3] Here, in this brief, general description, we use the new International Union of Basic and Clinical Pharmacology (IUPHAR) recommended terminology because it simplifies the subject considerably, but beware confusion when reading older papers. NMDA receptors are assembled from seven types of subunit (GluN1, GluN2A, GluN2B, GluN2C, GluN2D, GluN3A, GluN3B). The subunits comprising AMPA receptors (GluA1–4)[4] and kainate receptors (GluK1–5) are closely related to, but distinct from, GluN subunits. Receptors comprising different subunits can have different pharmacological and physiological characteristics, e.g. AMPA receptors lacking the GluA2 subunit have much higher permeability to Ca^{2+} than the others, which has important functional consequences (see Ch. 4).

AMPA receptors, and in certain brain regions kainate receptors, serve to mediate fast excitatory synaptic transmission in the CNS – absolutely essential for our brains to function. NMDA receptors (which often coexist with AMPA receptors) contribute a slow component to the excitatory synaptic potential (Fig. 38.4B), the magnitude of which varies in different pathways. Kainate and NMDA receptors are also expressed on nerve terminals where they can enhance or reduce transmitter release (see Corlew et al., 2008; Jane et al., 2009).[5] AMPA receptors occur on astrocytes as well as on neurons, and these cells play an important role in communication in the brain.

[2]In the past, AMPA and kainate receptors were often lumped together as AMPA/kainate or non-NMDA receptors, but nowadays it is realised that they each have distinct subunit compositions and should not be grouped together.
[3]An international committee has sought to bring order to the area but, despite the logic of their recommendations, how generally accepted they will be remains to be seen (see Collingridge et al., 2009 and www.guidetopharmacology.org). Scientists can get very stuck in their ways.
[4]AMPA receptor subunits are also subject to other kinds of variation, namely alternative splicing, giving rise to the engagingly named *flip* and *flop* variants, and RNA editing at the single amino acid level, both of which contribute yet more functional diversity to this diverse family.
[5]In the CNS, presynaptic ligand-gated ion channels such as kainate and NMDA receptors as well as nicotinic and P2X receptors (see Ch. 39) control neurotransmitter release. An explanation of how this control can be either facilitatory or inhibitory is given in Khakh & Henderson (2000).

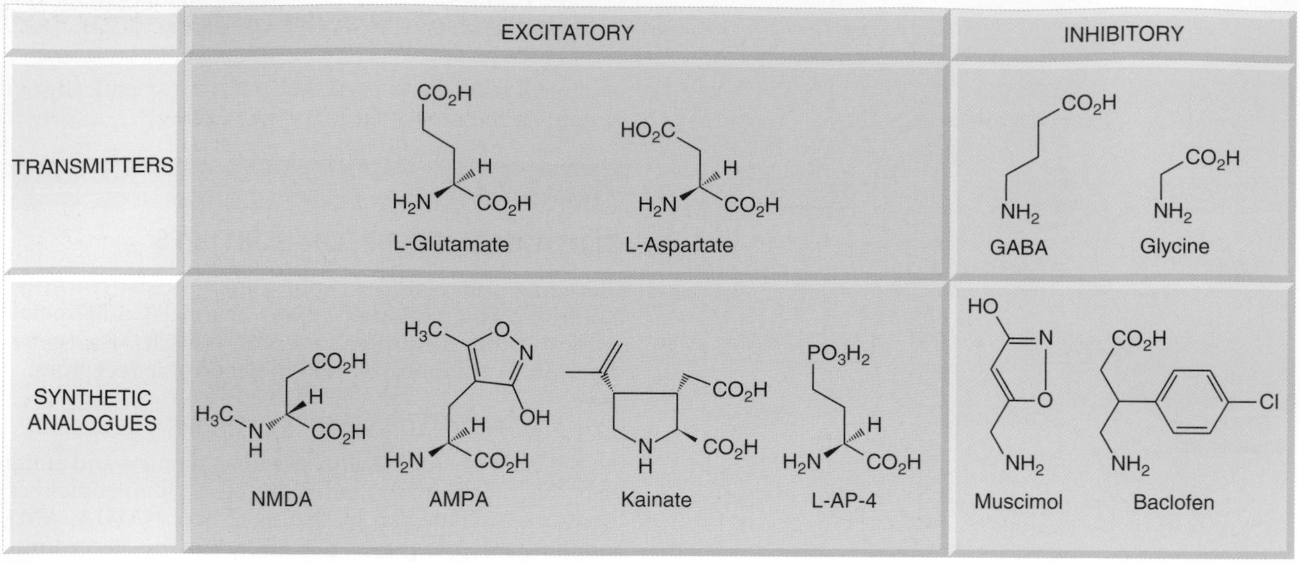

Fig. 38.3 Structures of agonists acting on glutamate, GABA and glycine receptors. The receptor specificity of these compounds is shown in Tables 38.1 and 38.2. AMPA, (S)-α-amino-3-hydroxy-5-methylisoxazole-4-propionic acid; L-AP4, L-2-amino-4-phosphonopentanoic acid; NMDA, N-methyl-D-aspartic acid.

Table 38.1 Properties of ionotropic glutamate receptors

	NMDA		AMPA	Kainate
Subunit composition	Tetramers consisting of GluN1–3 subunits		Tetramers consisting of GluA1–4 subunits (variants splicing and RNA editing)	Tetramers consisting of GluK1–5 subunits
	Receptor site	*Modulatory site (glycine)*		
Endogenous agonist(s)	Glutamate Aspartate	Glycine D-Serine	Glutamate	Glutamate
Other agonist(s)[a]	NMDA	Cycloserine	AMPA Quisqualate	Kainate Domoate[b]
Antagonist(s)[a]	AP5, CPP	7-Chloro-kynurenic acid, HA-966	NBQX	NBQX ACET
Other modulators	Polyamines (e.g. spermine, spermidine) Mg^{2+}, Zn^{2+}		Cyclothiazide Perampanel Piracetam CX-516	–
Channel blockers	Dizocilpine (MK801) Phencyclidine, ketamine Remacemide Memantine Mg^{2+}		–	–
Effector mechanism	Ligand-gated cation channel (slow kinetics, high Ca^{2+} permeability)		Ligand-gated cation channel (fast kinetics; channels possessing GluA2 subunits show low Ca^{2+} permeability)	Ligand-gated cation channel (fast kinetics, low Ca^{2+} permeability)
Location	Postsynaptic (some presynaptic, also glial) Wide distribution		Postsynaptic (also glial)	Pre- and postsynaptic
Function	Slow epsp Synaptic plasticity (long-term potentiation, long-term depression) Excitotoxicity		Fast epsp Wide distribution	Fast epsp Presynaptic inhibition Limited distribution

[a]Structures of experimental compounds can be found in Brauner-Osborne et al. (2002).
[b]A neurotoxin from mussels (see Ch. 40).
ACET, -(S)-1-(2-amino-2-carboxyethyl)-3-(2-carboxy-5-phenylthiophene-3-yl-methyl)-5-methylpyrimidine-2,4-dione; AP5, 2-amino-5-phosphonopentanoic acid; CPP, 3-(2-carboxypiperazin-4-yl)-propyl-1-phosphonic acid; CX-516, 1-(quinoxalin-6-ylcarbonyl)-piperidine; epsp, excitatory postsynaptic potential; NBQX, 2,3-dihydro-6-nitro-7-sulfamoyl-benzoquinoxaline. (Other structures are shown in Figure 38.3.)

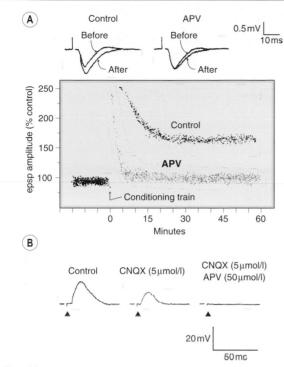

Fig. 38.4 Effects of excitatory amino acid receptor antagonists on synaptic transmission. **[A]** AP5 (NMDA antagonist) prevents long-term potentiation (LTP) in the rat hippocampus without affecting the fast excitatory postsynaptic potential (epsp). Top records show the extracellularly recorded fast epsp (downward deflection) before, and 50 min after, a conditioning train of stimuli (100 Hz for 2 s). The presence of LTP in the control preparation is indicated by the increase in epsp amplitude. In the presence of AP5 (50 μmol/l), the normal epsp is unchanged, but LTP does not occur. Lower trace shows epsp amplitude as a function of time. The conditioning train produces a short-lasting increase in epsp amplitude, which still occurs in the presence of AP5, but the long-lasting effect is prevented. **[B]** Block of fast and slow components of epsp by CNQX (6-cyano-7-nitroquinoxaline-2,3-dione; AMPA receptor antagonist) and AP5 (NMDA receptor antagonist). The epsp (upward deflection) in a hippocampal neuron recorded with intracellular electrode is partly blocked by CNQX (5 μmol/l), leaving behind a slow component, which is blocked by AP5 (50 μmol/l). *(Panel [A] from Malinow R, Madison D, Tsien R W 1988 Nature 335, 821; panel [B] from Andreasen M, Lambert J D, Jensen M S 1989 J Physiol 414, 317–336.)*

Binding studies show that ionotropic glutamate receptors are most abundant in the cortex, basal ganglia and sensory pathways. NMDA and AMPA receptors are generally co-localised, but kainate receptors have a much more restricted distribution. Expression of the many different receptor subtypes in the brain also shows distinct regional differences, but we have hardly begun to understand the significance of this extreme organisational complexity.

Special features of NMDA receptors

NMDA receptors and their associated channels have been studied in more detail than the other types and show special pharmacological properties, summarised in Fig. 38.5, that are postulated to play a role in pathophysiological mechanisms.

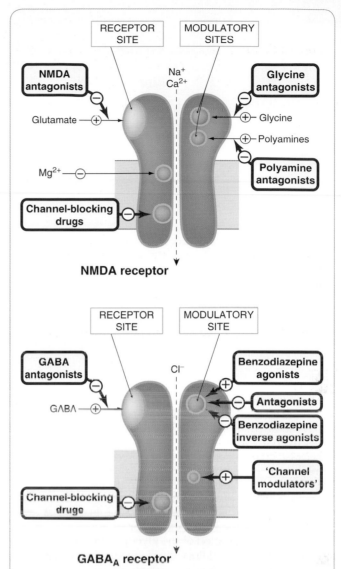

Fig. 38.5 Main sites of drug action on NMDA and GABA$_A$ receptors. Both receptors are multimeric ligand-gated ion channels. Drugs can act as agonists or antagonists at the neurotransmitter receptor site or at modulatory sites associated with the receptor. They can also act to block the ion channel at one or more distinct sites. In the case of the GABA$_A$ receptor, the mechanism by which 'channel modulators' (e.g. ethanol, anaesthetic agents, neurosteroids) facilitate channel opening is uncertain; they may affect both ligand binding and channel sites. The location of the different binding sites shown in the figure is largely imaginary, although study of mutated receptors is beginning to reveal where they actually reside. Examples of the different drug classes are given in Tables 38.1 and 38.3.

- They are highly permeable to Ca^{2+}, as well as to other cations, so activation of NMDA receptors is particularly effective in promoting Ca^{2+} entry.
- They are readily blocked by Mg^{2+}, and this block shows marked voltage dependence. It occurs at physiological Mg^{2+} concentrations when the cell is normally polarised, but disappears if the cell is depolarised.
- Activation of NMDA receptors requires glycine as well as glutamate (Fig. 38.6). The binding site for

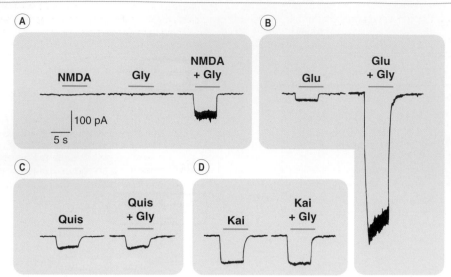

Fig. 38.6   Facilitation of NMDA by glycine. Recordings from mouse brain neurons in culture (whole-cell patch clamp technique). Downward deflections represent inward current through excitatory amino acid-activated ion channels. **[A]** NMDA (10 μmol/l) or glycine (1 μmol/l) applied separately had little or no effect, but together produced a response. **[B]** The response to glutamate (Glu, 10 μmol/l) was strongly potentiated by glycine (Gly, 1 μmol/l). **[C]** and **[D]** Responses of AMPA and kainate receptors to quisqualate (Quis) and kainate (Kai) were unaffected by glycine. *(From Johnson JW, Ascher P 1987 Glycine potentiates the NMDA response in cultured mouse brain neurons. Nature 325, 529–531.)*

glycine is distinct from the glutamate binding site, i.e. glycine is an allosteric modulator (see Ch. 2), and both have to be occupied for the channel to open. This discovery by Johnson and Ascher caused a stir, because glycine had hitherto been recognised as an inhibitory transmitter (see p. 465), so to find it facilitating excitation ran counter to the prevailing doctrine. The concentration of glycine required depends on the subunit composition of the NMDA receptor: for some NMDA receptor subtypes, physiological variation of the glycine concentration may serve as a regulatory mechanism, whereas others are fully activated at all physiological glycine concentrations. Competitive antagonists at the glycine site (see Table 38.1) indirectly inhibit the action of glutamate. **D-serine**, somewhat surprisingly,[6] has been found to activate the NMDA receptor via the glycine site and to be released from astrocytes.

- Some endogenous polyamines (e.g. **spermine**, **spermidine**) act at an allosteric site distinct from that of glycine to facilitate channel opening. The experimental drugs **ifenprodil** and **eliprodil** block their action.
- Recently other allosteric sites have been identified on the NMDA receptor and positive and negative allosteric modulators with novel patterns of GluN2 subunit selectivity have been discovered (Monaghan et al., 2012).
- Some well-known anaesthetic and psychotomimetic agents, such as **ketamine** (Ch. 41) and **phencyclidine** (Ch. 48), are selective blocking agents for NMDA-operated channels. The experimental compound **dizocilpine** shares this property.

METABOTROPIC GLUTAMATE RECEPTORS

There are eight different metabotropic glutamate receptors (mGlu$_{1-8}$) which are unusual in showing no sequence homology with other G protein-coupled receptors (Ferraguti & Shigemoto, 2006). They function as homo- and heterodimers[7] (see Ch. 3) cross-linked by a disulfide bridge across the extracellular domain of each protein (see Goudet et al., 2009). They are members of class C G protein-coupled receptors, possessing a large extracellular N-terminus domain that forms a venus fly trap-like structure into which glutamate binds. They can be divided into three groups on the basis of their sequence homology, G protein coupling and pharmacology (see Table 38.2). Alternatively, spliced receptor variants have been reported.

mGlu receptors are widely distributed throughout the central nervous system (see Ferraguti & Shigemoto, 2006) on neurons, where they regulate cell excitability and synaptic transmission, and on glia. Neuronal group 1 mGlu receptors are located postsynaptically and are largely excitatory. By raising intracellular [Ca^{2+}], they modify responses through ionotropic glutamate receptors (see Fig. 38.7). Group 2 and 3 mGlu receptors are mostly presynaptic receptors and their activation tends to reduce synaptic transmission and neuronal excitability. They can be autoreceptors, involved in reducing glutamate release or heteroreceptors, e.g. when present on GABA-containing terminals.

SYNAPTIC PLASTICITY AND LONG-TERM POTENTIATION

▼ In general, it appears that NMDA and mGlu receptors play a particular role in long-term adaptive and pathological changes in the

[6]Surprising, because it is the 'wrong' enantiomer for amino acids of higher organisms. Nevertheless, vertebrates possess specific enzymes and transporters for this D-amino acid, which is abundant in the brain.

[7]It has been suggested that mGlu receptors may form heterodimers with non mGlu receptors such as the 5-HT$_{2A}$ receptor (Gonzalez-Maeso et al., 2008).

Table 38.2 Metabotropic glutamate receptors

	Group 1	Group 2	Group 3
Members	mGlu$_1$, mGlu$_5$	mGlu$_2$, mGlu$_3$	mGlu$_4$, mGlu$_6$,[a] mGlu$_7$, mGlu$_8$
G protein coupling	G$_q$	G$_i$/G$_o$	G$_i$/G$_o$
Agonist	DHPG CHPG[b]	LY354740	L-AP4 (S)-3,4-DCPG[c]
Antagonist	LY367385[d] S-4-CPG	LY341495	CPPG
Neuronal location	Somatodendritic	Somatodendritic and nerve terminals	Nerve terminals

[a]mGlu$_6$ is found only in the retina.
[b]mGlu$_5$ selective.
[c]mGlu$_8$ selective.
[d]mGlu$_1$ selective.
CHPG, (RS)-2-chloro-5-hydroxyphenylglycine; CPPG, (RS)-α-cyclopropyl 4 phosphonophenylglycine; DHPG, 3,5-dihydroxyphenylglycine; L-AP4, 2-amino-4-phosphonobutyrate; (S)-3,4-DCPG, (S)-3,4-dicarboxyphenylglycine; S-4-CPG, (S)-4-carboxyphenylglycine.

brain, and are of particular interest as potential drug targets. AMPA receptors, on the other hand, are mainly responsible for fast excitatory transmission. They too are involved in synaptic plasticity.

Two aspects of glutamate receptor function are of particular pathophysiological importance, namely *synaptic plasticity*, discussed here, and *excitotoxicity* (discussed in Ch. 40).

Synaptic plasticity is a general term used to describe long-term changes in synaptic connectivity and efficacy, either following physiological alterations in neuronal activity (as in learning and memory), or resulting from pathological disturbances (as in epilepsy, chronic pain or drug dependence). Synaptic plasticity underlies much of what we call 'brain function'. Needless to say, no single mechanism is responsible; however, one significant and much-studied component is *long-term potentiation* (LTP), a phenomenon in which AMPA and NMDA receptors play a central role.

Long-term potentiation (LTP; see Bear et al., 2006; Bliss & Cooke, 2011) is a prolonged (hours *in vitro*, days or weeks *in vivo*) enhancement of synaptic transmission that occurs at various CNS synapses following a short (conditioning) burst of high-frequency presynaptic stimulation. Its counterpart is *long-term depression* (LTD), which is produced at some synapses by a longer train of stimuli at lower frequency (see Massey & Bashir, 2007; Bliss & Cooke, 2011). These phenomena have been studied at various synapses in the CNS, most especially in the hippocampus, which plays a central role in learning and memory (Fig. 38.4). It has been argued that 'learning', in the synaptic sense, can occur if synaptic strength is enhanced following simultaneous activity in both pre- and postsynaptic neurons. LTP shows this characteristic; it does not occur if presynaptic activity fails to excite the postsynaptic neuron, or if the latter is activated independently, for instance by a different presynaptic input. The mechanisms underlying both LTP and LTD differ somewhat at different synapses in the brain (see Bear et al., 2006). Here only a brief, generic view of the underlying events is given. LTP initiation may involve both presynaptic and postsynaptic components, and results from

enhanced activation of postsynaptic AMPA receptors at EAA synapses and (probably) to enhanced glutamate release (although the argument rumbles on about whether increased transmitter release does or does not occur in LTP; see Kullman, 2012). The response of postsynaptic AMPA receptors to glutamate is increased due to phosphorylation of the AMPA receptor subunits by kinases such as Ca^{2+}/calmodulin-dependent protein kinase (CaMKII) and protein kinase C (PKC), thus enhancing their conductance, as well as to increased expression and trafficking of AMPA receptors to synaptic sites. LTD, on the other hand, results from modest Ca^{2+} entry into the cell through AMPA receptors (NMDA receptors remain blocked by Mg^{2+}) activating phosphatases that reduce AMPA receptor phosphorylation and enhance AMPA receptor internalisation.

LTP is reduced by agents that block the synthesis or effects of nitric oxide or arachidonic acid. These mediators (see Chs 17 and 20) may act as retrograde messengers through which events in the postsynaptic cell are able to influence the presynaptic nerve terminal. Endogenous cannabinoids released by the postsynaptic cell, may also act as retrograde messengers to enhance glutamate release (see Chs 19 and 39).

Two special properties of the NMDA receptor underlie its involvement in LTP, namely voltage-dependent channel block by Mg^{2+} and its high Ca^{2+} permeability. At normal membrane potentials, the NMDA channel is blocked by Mg^{2+}; a sustained postsynaptic depolarisation produced by glutamate acting repeatedly on AMPA receptors, however, removes the Mg^{2+} block, and NMDA receptor activation then allows Ca^{2+} to enter the cell. Activation of group 1 mGlu receptors also contributes to the increase in [Ca^{2+}]$_i$. This rise in [Ca^{2+}]$_i$ in the postsynaptic cell activates protein kinases, phospholipases and nitric oxide synthase, which act jointly with other cellular processes (by mechanisms that are not yet fully understood) to facilitate transmission via AMPA receptors. Initially, during the induction phase of LTP, phosphorylation of AMPA receptors increases their responsiveness to glutamate. Later, during the maintenance phase, more AMPA receptors are recruited to the membrane of postsynaptic dendritic spines as a result of altered receptor trafficking; later still, various other mediators and signalling pathways are activated, causing structural changes and leading to a permanent increase in the number of synaptic contacts.

The general description of LTP given above is intended to provide the uninitiated reader with an overview of the topic. There are subtle differences in its forms and in the mechanisms underlying it at different synapses in the CNS. How LTP, in all of its guises, relates to different forms of memory is slowly being worked out (see Bear et al., 2006; Kessels & Malinow, 2009). Thus there is hope that drugs capable of enhancing LTP may improve learning and memory.

DRUGS ACTING ON GLUTAMATE RECEPTORS

ANTAGONISTS AND NEGATIVE MODULATORS

Inotropic glutamate receptor antagonists

The main types and examples of ionotropic glutamate antagonists are shown in Table 38.1. They are selective for the main receptor types but generally not for specific subtypes. Many of these compounds, although very useful as experimental tools *in vitro*, are unable to penetrate the blood–brain barrier, so they are not effective when given systemically.

NMDA receptors, as discussed above, require glycine as well as NMDA to activate them, so blocking the glycine site is an alternative way to produce antagonism. **Kynurenic acid** and the more potent analogue **7-chlorokynurenic acid** act in this way. Another site of block is the channel itself, where substances such as ketamine, phencyclidine and **memantine** act. These agents are lipid-soluble and thus able to cross the blood–brain barrier.

The potential therapeutic interest in ionotropic glutamate receptor antagonists lies mainly in the reduction of brain damage following strokes and head injury (Ch. 40), as well as in the treatment of epilepsy (Ch. 45) and Alzheimer's disease (Ch. 40). They have also been considered for indications such as drug dependence (Ch. 49),

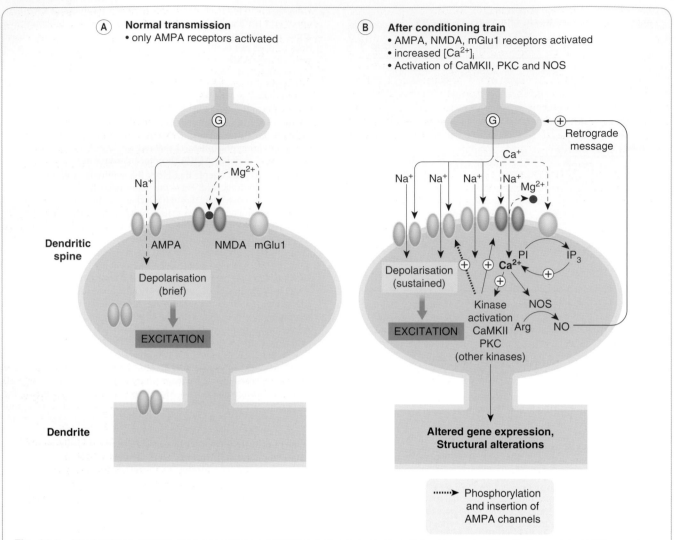

Fig. 38.7 **Mechanisms of long-term potentiation.** [**A**] With infrequent synaptic activity, glutamate (G) activates mainly AMPA receptors. There is insufficient glutamate to activate metabotropic receptors, and NMDA receptor channels are blocked by Mg^{2+}. [**B**] After a conditioning train of stimuli, enough glutamate is released to activate metabotropic receptors, and NMDA channels are unblocked by the sustained depolarisation. The resulting increase in $[Ca^{2+}]_i$ activates various enzymes, including the following:

- Ca^{2+}/calmodulin-dependent protein kinase (CaMKII) and protein kinase C (PKC) phosphorylate various proteins, including AMPA receptors (causing them to be trafficked to areas of synaptic contact on dendritic spines and facilitation of transmitter action) and other signal transduction molecules controlling gene transcription (not shown) in the postsynaptic cell.
- Nitric oxide synthase (NOS); release of nitric oxide (NO) facilitates glutamate release (retrograde signalling, otherwise known as NO turning back).
- Phospholipase A_2 (not shown) catalyses the formation of arachidonic acid (Ch. 17), a retrograde messenger that increases presynaptic glutamate release.
- A phospholipase (NAPE-PLD, not shown) that catalyses production of the endocannabinoids (Ch. 19) that act as retrograde messengers to enhance glutamate release.
- The neurotrophic factor BDNF released from nerve terminals and postsynaptic structures (not shown) plays a multimodal role in the early and later stages of LTP.

Arg, arginine; IP_3, inositol (1,4,5) trisphosphate; NO, nitric oxide; PI, phosphatidylinositol.

schizophrenia (Ch. 46) and depression (Ch. 47). Trials with NMDA antagonists and channel blockers have so far proved disappointing, and a serious drawback of these agents is their tendency to cause hallucinatory and other disturbances (also a feature of phencyclidine; Ch. 48). Only two NMDA receptor antagonists, **ketamine** (anaesthesia, analgesia and depression; see Chs 41, 42 and 47) and **memantine** (Alzheimer's disease; Ch. 40), are in clinical use. It is possible that antagonists selective for NMDA receptors containing the GluN2B subunit, which is highly Ca^{2+} permeable, may be effective for treating neurodegeneration and have fewer CNS side effects. The noncompetitive AMPA receptor antagonist **perampanel** has been introduced as an antiepileptic drug. The prospects for kainate receptor antagonists appear promising – antagonists for GluK1 have shown potential for the treatment of pain, migraine, epilepsy, stroke and anxiety (see Jane et al., 2009).

Overall, the promise foreseen for ionotropic glutamate receptor antagonists in the clinic has been less successful than was hoped. The problem may be that glutamate is such a ubiquitous and multifunctional mediator – involved, it seems, in almost every aspect of brain function – that attempting to improve a specific malfunction by flooding the brain with a compound that affects the glutamate system in some way is just too crude a strategy. The new hope is that subunit selective negative allosteric modulators may have fewer side effects than previous generations of orthosteric antagonists.

Metabotropic glutamate receptor antagonists

While antagonists that discriminate between the different groups of mGlu receptors are available (see Table 38.2), it has proven more difficult to develop selective antagonists for the subtypes within the groups. mGlu receptors, like many G protein-coupled receptors, possess allosteric modulatory sites, which can be either inhibitory or facilitatory (see Ch. 3). Antagonists or negative allosteric modulators acting at group 1 mGlu receptors have potential for the treatment of fragile X syndrome,[8] various pain states, Parkinson's disease (including the control of **levodopa**-induced dyskinesias, see Ch. 40), neuroprotection, epilepsy and drug abuse; whereas antagonists or negative allosteric modulators of group 2 mGlu receptors have potential as cognition enhancers (see Nicoletti et al., 2011).

AGONISTS AND POSITIVE MODULATORS

Ionotropic glutamate receptors

Various agonists at ionotropic glutamate receptors that are used experimentally are shown in Table 38.1. From the clinical perspective, interest centres on the theory that positive AMPA receptor modulators may improve memory and cognitive performance. Early examples include **cyclothiazide**, **piracetam** and CX-516 (**Ampalex**). These positive allosteric modulators, known as *ampakines*, can act in subtly different ways to increase response amplitude, slow deactivation and attenuate desensitisation of AMPA receptor-mediated currents. They therefore increase AMPA-mediated synaptic responses and enhance long-term potentiation as well as upregulating the production of nerve growth factors such as *brain-derived neurotrophic factor* (BDNF). Originally ampakines were thought to have therapeutic potential as cognition enhancers and for the treatment of schizophrenia, depression, attention deficit hyperactivity disorder (ADHD) and Parkinson's disease (see Lynch, 2006) but so far clinical trials have been disappointing. A more recently developed ampakine, CX1739, is in Phase II clinical trial for the treatment of drug-induced respiratory depression. Inhibition of the glycine transporter GlyT1 leads to an elevation of extracellular glycine levels throughout the brain and, through potentiation of NMDA receptor-mediated responses, could be beneficial in the treatment of various neurological disorders (see Harvey & Yee, 2013).

Metabotropic glutamate receptors

Developing selective agonists of mGlu receptors has proven to be quite difficult; recently, selective positive allosteric modulators have been developed (see Nicoletti et al., 2011). Group 2 and 3 mGlu receptors are located presynaptically on nerve terminals and agonists at these receptors decrease glutamate release. Group 2 mGlu agonists and positive allosteric modulators were therefore thought to have therapeutic potential to decrease neuronal cell death in stroke and in the treatment of epilepsy, but to date clinical trials have been disappointing. Agonists and positive allosteric modulators may be useful in treating anxiety as well as in controlling the positive symptoms of schizophrenia. Group 3 mGlu receptor positive allosteric modulators may be useful in treating anxiety and Parkinson's disease.

Excitatory amino acids

- Excitatory amino acids (EAAs), namely glutamate and aspartate, are the main fast excitatory transmitters in the central nervous system.
- Glutamate is formed mainly from the Krebs cycle intermediate α-oxoglutarate by the action of GABA transaminase.
- There are three main ionotropic glutamate receptors and eight metabotropic receptors.
- NMDA, AMPA and kainate receptors are ionotropic receptors regulating cation channels.
- The channels controlled by NMDA receptors are highly permeable to Ca^{2+} and are blocked by Mg^{2+}.
- AMPA and kainate receptors are involved in fast excitatory transmission; NMDA receptors mediate slower excitatory responses and, through their effect in controlling Ca^{2+} entry, play a more complex role in controlling synaptic plasticity (e.g. long-term potentiation).
- Competitive NMDA receptor antagonists include **AP5** (2-amino-5-phosphonopentanoic acid) and **CPP** (3-(2-carboxypirazin-4-yl)-propyl-1-phosphonic acid); the NMDA-operated ion channel is blocked by **ketamine** and **phencyclidine**.
- **NBQX** (2,3-dihydro-6-nitro-7-sulfamoyl-benzoquinoxaline) is an AMPA and kainate receptor antagonist.
- NMDA receptors require low concentrations of glycine as a co-agonist, in addition to glutamate; **7-chlorokynurenic acid** blocks this action of glycine.
- NMDA receptor activation is increased by endogenous polyamines, such as **spermine**, acting on a modulatory site that is blocked by **ifenprodil**.
- The entry of excessive amounts of Ca^{2+} produced by NMDA receptor activation can result in cell death – excitotoxicity (see Ch. 40).
- Metabotropic glutamate receptors ($mGlu_{1-8}$) are dimeric G protein-coupled receptors. $mGlu_1$ and $mGlu_5$ receptors couple through G_q to inositol trisphosphate formation and intracellular Ca^{2+} release. They play a part in glutamate-mediated synaptic plasticity and excitotoxicity. The other mGlu receptors couple to G_i/G_o and inhibit neurotransmitter release, most importantly glutamate release.
- Some specific metabotropic glutamate receptor agonists and antagonists are available, as are positive and negative allosteric modulators.

---

[8]Fragile X syndrome is caused by mutation of a single gene on the X chromosome. It affects about 1:4000 children of either sex, causing mental retardation, autism and motor disturbances.

γ-AMINOBUTYRIC ACID (GABA)

GABA is the main inhibitory transmitter in the brain. In the spinal cord and brain stem, glycine is also important (see p. 465).

SYNTHESIS, STORAGE AND FUNCTION

GABA occurs in brain tissue but not in other mammalian tissues, except in trace amounts. It is particularly abundant (about 10 μmol/g tissue) in the nigrostriatal system, but occurs at lower concentrations (2–5 μmol/g) throughout the grey matter.

GABA is formed from glutamate (Fig. 38.1) by the action of glutamic acid decarboxylase (GAD), an enzyme found only in GABA-synthesising neurons in the brain. Immunohistochemical labelling of GAD is used to map the GABA pathways in the brain. GABAergic neurons and astrocytes take up GABA via specific transporters, thus removing GABA after it has been released. GAT1 is the predominant GABA transporter in the brain and is located primarily on GABAergic nerve terminals where it recycles GABA. GAT3 is located predominantly on astrocytes around the GABAergic synapse. GABA transport is inhibited by **guvacine**, **nipecotic acid** and **tiagabine**. Tiagabine is used to treat epilepsy (Ch. 45). In astrocytes GABA can be destroyed by a transamination reaction in which the amino group is transferred to α-oxoglutaric acid (to yield glutamate), with the production of succinic semialdehyde and then succinic acid. This reaction is catalysed by GABA transaminase, an enzyme located primarily in astrocytes. It is inhibited by **vigabatrine**, another compound used to treat epilepsy (Ch. 45).

GABA functions as an inhibitory transmitter in many different CNS pathways. About 20% of CNS neurons are GABAergic; most are short interneurons, but there are some long GABAergic tracts, e.g. from the striatum to the substantia nigra and globus pallidus (see Ch. 40 and Fig. 40.4). The widespread distribution of GABA – GABA serves as a transmitter at about 30% of all the synapses in the CNS – and the fact that virtually all neurons are sensitive to its inhibitory effect suggests that its function is ubiquitous in the brain. That antagonists such as **bicuculline** induce seizures illustrates the important, ongoing inhibitory role of GABA in the brain.

GABA RECEPTORS: STRUCTURE AND PHARMACOLOGY

GABA acts on two distinct types of receptor: GABA$_A$ receptors are ligand-gated ion channels whereas GABA$_B$ receptors are G protein-coupled.

GABA$_A$ RECEPTORS

GABA$_A$ receptors[9] are members of the *cys-loop* family of receptors that also includes the glycine, nicotinic and 5-HT$_3$ receptors (see Ch. 3, Fig. 3.18). The GABA$_A$ receptors are pentamers made up of different subunits. The reader

should not despair when informed that 19 GABA$_A$ receptor subunits have been cloned (α1–6, β1–3, γ1–3, δ, ε, θ, π and ρ1–3) and that splice variants of some subunits also exist. Although the number of possible combinations is large, only a few dozen have been shown to exist. The most common are α1β2γ2 (by far the most abundant), α2β3γ2 and α3β3γ2 subunits. To make up the pentamer, each receptor contains two α, two β and one γ subunit arranged in a circle in the sequence α–β–α–β–γ around the pore when viewed from the extracellular side of the membrane. GABA binds at each of the interfaces between the α and β subunits whereas benzodiazepines (see Ch. 44) bind at the α/γ interface. A novel benzodiazepine binding site at the α/β interface has recently been described but its function is unclear at present. Receptors containing different α and γ subunits exhibit differential sensitivity to benzodiazepines and mediate different behavioural responses to these drugs. This raises the tantalising prospect of developing new agents with greater selectivity and potentially fewer side effects. The GABA$_A$ receptor should therefore be thought of as a group of receptors exhibiting subtle differences in their physiological and pharmacological properties.

GABA$_A$ receptors are primarily located postsynaptically and mediate both fast and tonic postsynaptic inhibition. The GABA$_A$ channel is selectively permeable to Cl$^-$ and because the equilibrium membrane potential for Cl$^-$ is usually negative to the resting potential, increasing Cl$^-$ permeability hyperpolarises the cell as Cl$^-$ ions enter, thereby reducing its excitability.[10] In the postsynaptic cell GABA$_A$ receptors are located both at areas of synaptic contact and extrasynaptically (see Fig 38.8 and Farrant & Nusser, 2005). Thus GABA produces inhibition by acting both as a fast 'point-to-point' transmitter and as an 'action-at-a-distance' neuromodulator, as the extrasynaptic GABA$_A$ receptors can be tonically activated by GABA that has diffused away from its site of release. Extrasynaptic GABA$_A$ receptors contain α4 and α6 subunits as well as the δ subunit, and are highly sensitive to general anaesthetic agents (see Ch. 41) and ethanol (see Ch. 49), have higher affinities for GABA and show less desensitisation. **Gaboxadol** (previously known as THIP from its chemical structure) is a selective GABA$_A$ receptor agonist with a preference for δ subunit-containing GABA$_A$ receptors.

GABA$_B$ RECEPTORS

GABA$_B$ receptors (see Bettler et al., 2004) are located pre- and postsynaptically. They are class C G protein-coupled receptors that couple through G_i/G_o to inhibit voltage-gated Ca^{2+} channels (thus reducing transmitter release), to open potassium channels (thus reducing postsynaptic excitability) and to inhibit adenylyl cyclase.

▼ For GABA$_B$ receptors, the functional receptor is a dimer (see Ch. 3) consisting of two different seven-transmembrane subunits, B1 and B2, held together by a coil/coil interaction between their C-terminal tails. In the absence of B2, the B1 subunit does not traffic to the plasma membrane as it possesses an endoplasmic reticulum retention signal. Interaction of B1 with B2 masks the retention signal and facilitates trafficking to the membrane. Activation of the dimer results from GABA binding to the extracellular, 'venus fly trap' domain of B1 (even although the B2 subunit possesses a similar domain) whereas it is the B2 subunit that interacts with and activates the G protein (Fig. 38.9).

---

[9]The IUPHAR Nomenclature Committee has recommended (see Olsen & Sieghart, 2008) that the receptors previously referred to as 'GABA$_C$' receptors, because they were insensitive to bicuculline, benzodiazepines and baclofen, should be subtypes of the GABA$_A$ receptor family as they are pentameric Cl$^-$-permeable ligand-gated channels comprising homo- or heteromeric assemblies of ρ subunits. Their functional significance is slowly being worked out (see Chebib, 2004).

[10]During early brain development (in which GABA plays an important role), and also in some regions of the adult brain, GABA has an excitatory rather than an inhibitory effect, because the intracellular Cl$^-$ concentration is relatively high, so that the equilibrium potential is positive to the resting membrane potential.

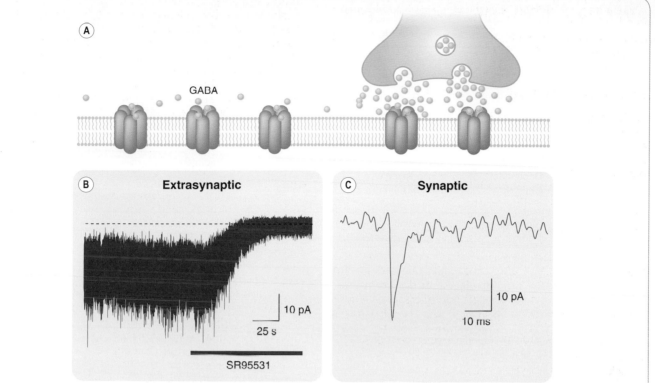

Fig. 38.8 Synaptic and extrasynaptic GABA$_A$ receptors. [A] Diagram depicting GABA$_A$ receptors at synaptic and extrasynaptic sites in the plasma membrane. The blue dots represent GABA molecules. [B] Tonic activation of extrasynaptic GABA$_A$ receptors gives rise to a steady state inward current (distance from the baseline indicated by the dashed line) and increased 'noise' on the trace. The current is blocked on application of the GABA$_A$ receptor antagonist SR95531. [C] Phasic release of GABA from the presynaptic terminal evokes a fast synaptic current (rapid downward deflection). Note the different timescales in [B] and [C]. *(Figure courtesy of M Usowicz.)*

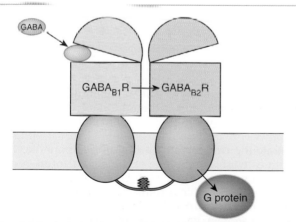

Fig 38.9 Dimeric structure of the GABA$_B$ receptor. The receptor is made up of two seven-transmembrane domain subunits held together by a coil/coil interaction between their C-terminal tails. Activation of the receptor occurs when GABA binds to the extracellular domain of the B1 subunit (known as the venus fly trap, because it snaps shut when GABA binds). This produces an allosteric change in the B2 subunit which is coupled to the G protein. *(Adapted from Kubo Y, Tateyama M 2005 Towards a view of functioning dimeric metabotropic receptors. Curr Opin Neurobiol 15, 289–295.)*

DRUGS ACTING ON GABA RECEPTORS

GABA$_A$ RECEPTORS

GABA$_A$ receptors resemble NMDA receptors in that drugs may act at several different sites (Fig. 38.5). These include:

* the GABA-binding site
* several modulatory sites
* the ion channel.

There is growing evidence that the different receptor subtypes differ in their pharmacological properties.

GABA$_A$ receptors are the target for several important centrally acting drugs, notably benzodiazepines (see Ch. 44), alcohol (see Ch. 49), barbiturates, neurosteroids (see p. 464, Table 38.3) and many general anaesthetics (see Ch. 41). The main agonists, antagonists and modulatory substances that act on GABA receptors are shown in Table 38.3.

Muscimol, derived from a hallucinogenic mushroom, resembles GABA chemically (see Fig. 38.3) and is a powerful GABA$_A$ receptor agonist. A synthetic analogue, **gaboxadol** is a partial agonist that was developed as a hypnotic drug (Ch. 44) but has now been withdrawn. **Bicuculline**, a naturally occurring convulsant compound, is a specific antagonist that blocks the fast inhibitory synaptic potential in most CNS synapses. **Gabazine**, a synthetic GABA analogue, is similar. These compounds are useful experimental tools but have no therapeutic uses.

Benzodiazepines, which have powerful sedative, anxiolytic and anticonvulsant effects (see Ch. 44), selectively potentiate the effects of GABA on some GABA$_A$ receptors

Table 38.3 Properties of inhibitory amino acid receptors

| | GABA_A | | | GABA_B | Glycine |
	Receptor site	Modulatory site (benzodiazepine)	Modulatory site (others)		
Endogenous agonists	GABA	Unknown, several postulated (see text)	Various neurosteroids (e.g. progesterone metabolites)	GABA	Glycine β-Alanine Taurine
Other agonist(s)	Muscimol Gaboxadol (THIP,[a] a partial agonist)	Anxiolytic benzodiazepines (e.g. diazepam)	Barbiturates Steroid anaesthetics (e.g. alphaxalone)	Baclofen	–
Antagonist(s)	Bicuculline Gabazine	Flumazenil (inverse agonist?)	–	2-Hydroxy-saclofen CGP 35348 and others	Strychnine
Channel blocker	Picrotoxin[b]			Not applicable	–
Effector mechanism(s)	Ligand-gated chloride channel			G protein-coupled receptor; inhibition of Ca^{2+} channels, activation of K^+ channels, inhibition of adenylyl cyclase	Ligand-gated chloride channel
Location	Widespread; primarily postsynaptic			Pre- and postsynaptic Widespread	Postsynaptic Mainly in brain stem and spinal cord
Function	Postsynaptic inhibition (fast ipsp and tonic inhibition)			Presynaptic inhibition (decreased Ca^{2+} entry) Postsynaptic inhibition (increased K^+ permeability)	Postsynaptic inhibition (fast ipsp)

[a]THIP is an abbreviation of the chemical name of gaboxadol. It is reported to have preference for δ subunit-containing extrasynaptic GABA_A receptors.
[b]Picrotoxin also blocks glycine receptors.
ipsp, inhibitory postsynaptic potential.

depending upon the subunit composition of the receptor. They bind with high affinity to an accessory site (the 'benzodiazepine receptor') on the GABA_A receptor, in such a way that the binding of GABA is facilitated and its agonist effect is enhanced. Conversely, inverse agonists at the benzodiazepine receptor (e.g. Ro15-4513) reduce GABA binding and are anxiogenic and proconvulsant – they are unlikely to be therapeutically useful!

Modulators that also enhance the action of GABA, but whose site of action is less well defined than that of benzodiazepines (shown as 'channel modulators' in Fig. 38.5), include other CNS depressants such as barbiturates (Ch. 44), anaesthetic agents (Ch. 41) and neurosteroids. Neurosteroids (see Lambert et al., 2009) are compounds that are related to steroid hormones but that act to enhance activation of GABA_A receptors – those containing δ subunits appear most sensitive. Interestingly, they include metabolites of progesterone and androgens that are formed in the nervous system, and are believed to have a physiological role. Synthetic neurosteroids include **alphaxalone**, developed as an anaesthetic agent (Ch. 41).

Picrotoxin, a plant product, is a convulsant that acts by blocking the GABA_A receptor chloride channel, thus blocking the postsynaptic inhibitory effect of GABA. It also blocks glycine receptors. It has no therapeutic uses.

GABA_B RECEPTORS

When the importance of GABA as an inhibitory transmitter was recognised, it was thought that a GABA-like substance might prove to be effective in controlling epilepsy and other convulsive states; because GABA itself fails to penetrate the blood–brain barrier, more lipophilic GABA analogues were sought, one of which, **baclofen** (see Fig. 38.3), was introduced in 1972. Unlike GABA, its actions are not blocked by bicuculline. These findings led to the recognition of the GABA_B receptor, for which baclofen is a selective agonist. Baclofen is used to treat spasticity and related motor disorders (Ch. 45) and may also be useful in the treatment of drug dependence (see Ch. 49).

Competitive antagonists for the GABA_B receptor include a number of experimental compounds (e.g. **2-hydroxy-saclofen** and more potent compounds with improved brain penetration, such as CGP 35348). Tests in animals showed that these compounds produce only slight effects on CNS function (in contrast to the powerful convulsant effects of GABA_A antagonists). The main effect observed, paradoxically, was an antiepileptic action, specifically in an animal model of absence seizures (see Ch. 45), together with enhanced cognitive performance. However, as in many areas of pharmacology, such preclinical promise has not resulted in the development of a new therapeutic drug.

γ-HYDROXYBUTYRATE

γ-Hydroxybutyrate (**sodium oxybate** or GHB; see Wong et al., 2004) occurs naturally in the brain as a side product of GABA synthesis. As a synthetic drug it can be used to treat narcolepsy and alcoholism. In addition it has found favour with bodybuilders, based on its ability to evoke the release of growth hormone, and with party-goers, based on its euphoric and disinhibitory effects. It is also used as an intoxicant and date rape drug. In common with many abused drugs (see Ch. 49), it activates 'reward pathways' in the brain, and its use is now illegal in most countries. GHB is an agonist at $GABA_A$ receptors containing α4 and δ subunits, a weak partial agonist at $GABA_B$ receptors and an agonist at an 'orphan' G protein-coupled receptor, GPR172A.

GLYCINE

Glycine is an important inhibitory neurotransmitter in the spinal cord and brain stem. It is present in particularly high concentration (5 μmol/g) in the grey matter of the spinal cord. Applied ionophoretically to motor neurons or interneurons, it produces an inhibitory hyperpolarisation that is indistinguishable from the inhibitory synaptic response. **Strychnine**, a convulsant poison that acts mainly on the spinal cord, blocks both the synaptic inhibitory response and the response to glycine. This, together with direct measurements of glycine release in response to nerve stimulation, provides strong evidence for its physiological transmitter role. **β-Alanine** has pharmacological effects and a pattern of distribution very similar to those of glycine, but its action is not blocked by strychnine.

The inhibitory effect of glycine is quite distinct from its role in facilitating activation of NMDA receptors (see p. 457–458).

▼ The glycine receptor (see Dutertre et al., 2012) resembles the $GABA_A$ receptor in that it is a cys-loop, pentameric ligand-gated chloride channel. There are no specific metabotropic receptors for glycine. Five glycine receptor subunits have been cloned (α1–4, β) and it appears that in the adult brain the main forms of glycine receptor are homomers of α subunits or a heteromeric complex of α and β subunits, probably with a stoichiometry of 2α and 3β. Receptors made up only of α subunits are sensitive to glycine and strychnine, indicating that the binding site for these drugs is on the α subunit. The situation for glycine is therefore much simpler than for GABA (see p. 462). Glycine receptors are involved in the regulation of respiratory rhythms, motor control and muscle tone as well as in the processing of pain signals. Mutations of the receptor have been identified in some inherited neurological disorders associated with muscle spasm and reflex hyperexcitability. There are as yet no therapeutic drugs that act specifically by modifying glycine receptors.

Tetanus toxin, a bacterial toxin resembling **botulinum toxin** (Ch. 13), acts selectively to prevent glycine release from inhibitory interneurons in the spinal cord, causing excessive reflex hyperexcitability and violent muscle spasms (lockjaw).

Glycine is removed from the extracellular space by two transporters GlyT1 and GlyT2 (Eulenburg et al., 2005). GlyT1 is located primarily on astrocytes and expressed throughout most regions of the CNS. GlyT2 on the other hand is expressed on glycinergic neurons in the spinal cord, brain stem and cerebellum. GlyT2 inhibitors may have potential as analgesics.

Inhibitory amino acids: GABA and glycine

- GABA is the main inhibitory transmitter in the brain.
- It is present fairly uniformly throughout the brain; there is very little in peripheral tissues.
- GABA is formed from glutamate by the action of glutamic acid decarboxylase. Its action is terminated mainly by reuptake, but also by deamination, catalysed by GABA transaminase.
- There are two main types of GABA receptor: $GABA_A$ and $GABA_B$.
- $GABA_A$ receptors, which occur mainly postsynaptically, are directly coupled to chloride channels, the opening of which reduces membrane excitability.
- **Muscimol** is a specific $GABA_A$ agonist, and the convulsant **bicuculline** is an antagonist.
- Other drugs that interact with $GABA_A$ receptors and channels include:
  - benzodiazepines, which act at an accessory binding site to facilitate the action of GABA
  - convulsants such as **picrotoxin**, which block the anion channel
  - neurosteroids, including endogenous progesterone metabolites
  - CNS depressants, such as barbiturates and many general anaesthetic agents, which facilitate the action of GABA.
- $GABA_B$ receptors are heterodimeric G protein-coupled receptors. They cause pre- and postsynaptic inhibition by inhibiting Ca^{2+} channel opening and increasing K^+ conductance. **Baclofen** is a $GABA_B$ receptor agonist used to treat spasticity. $GABA_B$ antagonists are not in clinical use.
- Glycine is an inhibitory transmitter mainly in the spinal cord, acting on its own receptor, structurally and functionally similar to the $GABA_A$ receptor.
- The convulsant drug **strychnine** is a competitive glycine antagonist. Tetanus toxin acts mainly by interfering with glycine release.

CONCLUDING REMARKS

The study of amino acids and their receptors in the brain has been one of the most active fields of research in the past 25 years, and the amount of information available is prodigious. These signalling systems have been speculatively implicated in almost every kind of neurological and psychiatric disorder, and the pharmaceutical industry has put a great deal of effort into identifying specific ligands – agonists, antagonists, modulators, enzyme inhibitors, transport inhibitors – designed to influence them. However, while a large number of pharmacologically unimpeachable compounds have emerged, and many clinical trials have been undertaken, there have been few therapeutic breakthroughs. The optimistic view is that a better understanding of the particular functions of the many molecular subtypes of these targets, and the design of more subtype-specific ligands, will lead to future breakthroughs. Expectations have, however, undoubtedly dimmed in recent years.

REFERENCES AND FURTHER READING

Excitatory amino acids

Beart, P.M., O'Shea, R.D., 2007. Transporters for L-glutamate: an update on their molecular pharmacology and pathological involvement. Br. J. Pharmacol. 150, 5–17.

Bräuner-Osborne, H., Egebjerg, J., Nielsen, E.Ø., Madsen, U., Krogsgaard-Larsen, P., 2000. Ligands for glutamate receptors: design and therapeutic prospects. J. Med. Chem. 43, 2609–2645.

Bunch, L., Enrichsen, M.N., Jensen, A.A., 2009. Excitatory amino acid transporters as potential drug targets. Expert Opin. Ther. Targets 13, 719–731.

Collingridge, G.L., Olsen, R.W., Peters, J., Spedding, M., 2009. A nomenclature for ligand-gated ion channels. Neuropharmacology 56, 2–5.

Corlew, R., Brasier, D.J., Feldman, D.E., Philpot, B.D., 2008. Presynaptic NMDA receptors: newly appreciated roles in cortical synaptic function and plasticity. Neuroscientist 14, 609–625.

Ferraguti, F., Shigemoto, R., 2006. Metabotropic glutamate receptors. Cell Tissue Res. 326, 483–504.

González-Maeso, J., Ang, R.L., Yuen, T., et al., 2008. Identification of a serotonin/glutamate receptor complex implicated in psychosis. Nature 452, 93–99.

Goudet, C., Magnaghi, V., Landry, M., et al., 2009. Metabotropic receptors for glutamate and GABA in pain. Brain Res. Rev. 60, 43–56.

Harvey, R.J., Yee, B.K., 2013. Glycine transporters as novel therapeutic targets in schizophrenia, alcohol dependence and pain. Nature Rev. Drug Discov. 12, 866–885.

Jane, D.E., Lodge, D., Collingridge, G.L., 2009. Kainate receptors: pharmacology, function and therapeutic potential. Neuropharmacology 56, 90–113.

Lynch, G., 2006. Glutamate-based therapeutic approaches: ampakines. Curr. Opin. Pharmacol. 6, 82–88.

Monaghan, D.T., Irvine, M.W., Costa, B.M., Fang, G., Jane, D.E., 2012. Pharmacological modulation of NMDA receptor activity and the advent of negative and positive allosteric modulators. Neurochem. Int. 61, 581–592. (*Report of new allosteric sites on NMDA receptors*)

Nicoletti, F., Bockaert, J., Collingridge, G.L., et al., 2011. Metabotropic glutamate receptors: from the workbench to the bedside. Neuropharmacology 60, 1017–1041. (*Extensive review of the scientific developments in this field and their potential clinical significance in relation to the development of new drugs*)

Traynelis, S.F., Wollmuth, L.P., McBain, C.J., et al., 2010. Glutamate receptor ion channels: structure, regulation and function. Pharmacol. Rev. 62, 405–496.

Watkins, J.C., Jane, D.E., 2006. The glutamate story. Br. J. Pharmacol. 147 (Suppl. 1), S100–S108. (*A brief and engaging history by one of the pioneers in the discovery of glutamate as a CNS transmitter*)

Inhibitory amino acids

Bettler, B., Kaupmann, K., Mosbacher, J., Gassmann, M., 2004. Molecular structure and function of $GABA_B$ receptors. Physiol. Rev. 84, 835–867. (*Comprehensive review article by the team that first cloned the $GABA_B$ receptor and discovered its unusual heterodimeric structure*)

Chebib, M., 2004. $GABA_C$ receptor ion channels. Clin. Exp. Pharmacol. Physiol. 31, 800–804.

Dutertre, S., Becker, C.M., Betz, H., 2012. Inhibitory glycine receptors: an update. J. Biol. Chem. 287, 40216–40223.

Eulenburg, V., Armsen, W., Betz, H., Gomez, J., 2005. Glycine transporters: essential regulators of neurotransmission. Trends Biochem. Sci. 30, 325–333.

Farrant, M., Nusser, Z., 2005. Variations on an inhibitory theme: phasic and tonic activation of $GABA_A$ receptors. Nat. Rev. Neurosci. 6, 215–229.

Lambert, J.J., Cooper, M.A., Simmons, R.D., Weir, C.J., Belelli, D., 2009. Neurosteroids: endogenous allosteric modulators of GABA(A) receptors. Psychoneuroendocrinology 34 (Suppl. 1), S48–S58.

Olsen, R.W., Sieghart, W., 2008. International Union of Pharmacology. LXX. Subtypes of γ-aminobutyric acid$_A$ receptors: classification on the basis of subunit composition, pharmacology, and function. Update. Pharmacol. Rev. 60, 243–260. (*IUPHAR Nomenclature Subcommittee report containing an extensive discussion of the subtypes of $GABA_A$ receptor depending upon subunit composition. It also contains the recommendation that $GABA_C$ receptors should be considered as subtypes of the $GABA_A$ receptor*)

Wong, C.G.T., Gibson, K.M., Snead, O.C., 2004. From street to brain: neurobiology of the recreational drug gamma-hydroxybutyric acid. Trends Pharmacol. Sci. 25, 29–34. (*Short review article*)

Physiological aspects

Bear, M.F., Connors, B.W., Paradiso, M.A., 2006. Neuroscience: exploring the brain, third ed. Lippincott, Williams & Wilkins, Baltimore. (*Major neuroscience textbook that discusses in detail long-term potentiation and memory mechanisms*)

Bliss, T.V., Cooke, S.F., 2011. Long-term potentiation and long-term depression: a clinical perspective. Clinics (São Paulo) 66 (Suppl. 1), 3–17.

Kessels, H.W., Malinow, R., 2009. Synaptic AMPA receptor plasticity and behavior. Neuron 61, 340–350.

Khakh, B.S., Henderson, G., 2000. Modulation of fast synaptic transmission by presynaptic ligand-gated cation channels. J. Auton. Nerv. Syst. 81, 110–121. (*Describes how activation of presynaptic ligand-gated cation channels can either enhance or inhibit neurotransmitter release*)

Kullmann, D.M., 2012. The Mother of All Battles 20 years on: is LTP expressed pre- or postsynaptically? J. Physiol. 590, 2213–2216.

Massey, P.V., Bashir, Z.I., 2007. Long-term depression: multiple forms and implications for brain function. Trends Neurosci. 30, 176–184.

Other transmitters and modulators 39

OVERVIEW

The principal 'amine' transmitters in the central nervous system (CNS), namely noradrenaline, dopamine, 5-hydroxytryptamine (5-HT, serotonin) and acetylcholine (ACh), are described in this chapter, with briefer coverage of other mediators, including histamine, melatonin and purines. The monoamines were the first CNS transmitters to be identified, and during the 1960s a combination of neurochemistry and neuropharmacology led to many important discoveries about their role, and about the ability of drugs to influence these systems. Amine mediators differ from the amino acid transmitters discussed in Chapter 38 in being localised to small populations of neurons with cell bodies in the brain stem and basal forebrain, which project diffusely both rostrally to cortical and other areas, and in some cases caudally to the spinal cord. These amine-containing neurons are broadly associated with high-level behaviours (e.g. emotion, cognition and awareness), rather than with localised synaptic excitation or inhibition.[1] More recently, some 'atypical' chemical mediators, such as nitric oxide (NO; Ch. 20) and endocannabinoids (Ch. 19) have come on the scene, and they are discussed at the end of the chapter. The other major class of CNS mediators, the neuropeptides, are described in Chapter 18, and information on specific neuropeptides (e.g. endorphins, neurokinins and orexins) appears in later chapters in this section.

INTRODUCTION

Although we know much about the many different mediators, their cognate receptors and signalling mechanisms at the cellular level, when describing their effects on brain function and behaviour we fall back on relatively crude terms – psychopharmacologists will be at our throats for so under-rating the sophistication of their measurements – such as 'motor coordination', 'arousal', 'cognitive impairment' and 'exploratory behaviour'. The gap between these two levels of understanding still frustrates the best efforts to link drug action at the molecular level to drug action at the therapeutic level. Modern approaches, such as the use of transgenic animal technology (see Ch. 7) and non-invasive imaging techniques, are helping to forge links, but there is still a long way to go.

More detail on the content of this chapter can be found in Nestler et al. (2008) and Iversen et al. (2009).

[1]They are, if you like, voices from the nether regions, which make you happy or sad, sleepy or alert, cautious or adventurous, energetic or lazy, although you do not quite know why – very much the stuff of mental illness.

NORADRENALINE

The basic processes responsible for the synthesis, storage and release of noradrenaline are the same in the CNS as in the periphery (Ch. 14). In the CNS, inactivation of released noradrenaline is by neuronal reuptake or by metabolism, largely through the *monamine oxidase, aldehyde reductase* and *catechol-O-methyl transferase* mediated pathway to 3-hydroxy-4-methoxyphenylglycol (MHPG) (see Fig. 14.4).

NORADRENERGIC PATHWAYS IN THE CNS

Although the transmitter role of noradrenaline in the brain was suspected in the 1950s, detailed analysis of its neuronal distribution became possible only when a technique, based on the formation of fluorescent catecholamine derivatives when tissues are exposed to formaldehyde, was devised by Falck and Hillarp. Detailed maps of the pathway of noradrenergic, dopaminergic and serotonergic neurons in laboratory animals were produced and later confirmed in human brains. The cell bodies of noradrenergic neurons occur in small clusters in the *pons* and *medulla*, and they send extensively branching axons to many other parts of the brain and spinal cord (Fig. 39.1). The most prominent cluster is the locus coeruleus (LC), located in the pons. Although it contains only about 10 000 neurons in humans, the axons, running in a discrete *medial forebrain bundle*, give rise to many millions of noradrenergic nerve terminals throughout the cortex, hippocampus, thalamus, hypothalamus and cerebellum. These nerve terminals do not form distinct synaptic contacts but appear to release transmitter somewhat diffusely. The LC also projects to the spinal cord and is involved in the descending control of pain (Ch. 42).

Other noradrenergic neurons lie close to the LC in the pons and project to the amygdala, hypothalamus, hippocampus and other parts of the forebrain, as well as to the spinal cord. A small cluster of adrenergic neurons, which release adrenaline rather than noradrenaline, lies more ventrally in the brain stem. These cells contain phenylethanolamine *N*-methyl transferase, the enzyme that converts noradrenaline to adrenaline (see Ch. 14), and project mainly to the pons, medulla and hypothalamus. Rather little is known about them, but they are believed to be important in cardiovascular control.

FUNCTIONAL ASPECTS

With the exception of the β_3 adrenoceptor, all of the adrenoceptors (α_{1A}, α_{1B}, α_{1C}, α_{2A}, α_{2B}, α_{2C}, β_1 and β_2) are expressed in the CNS (see Bylund, 2007). They are G protein-coupled receptors that interact with a variety of effector mechanisms (see Table 14.1). The role of α_1 receptors in the CNS is poorly understood. They are widely

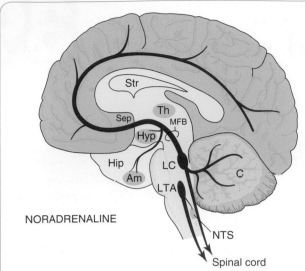

Fig. 39.1 Simplified diagram of the noradrenaline pathways in the brain. The location of the main groups of cell bodies and fibre tracts is in solid colour. Light-shaded areas show the location of noradrenergic terminals. Am, amygdaloid nucleus; C, cerebellum; Hip, hippocampus; Hyp, hypothalamus; LC, locus coeruleus; LTA, lateral tegmental area, part of the reticular formation; MFB, medial forebrain bundle; NTS, nucleus of the tractus solitarius (vagal sensory nucleus); Sep, septum; Str, corpus striatum; Th, thalamus.

distributed, located both on postsynaptic neurons and on glial cells, and may be involved in motor control, cognition and fear. α_2 Adrenoceptors are located on noradrenergic neurons (in both somatodendritic and nerve terminal regions where they function as inhibitory autoreceptors) as well as on postsynaptic non-noradrenergic neurons. They are involved in blood pressure control (see below), sedation (α_2 agonists such as **medetomidine** are used as anaesthetics in veterinary practice) and analgesia. β_1 Receptors are found in the cortex, striatum and hippocampus whereas β_2 receptors are largely found in the cerebellum. They have been implicated in the long-term effects of antidepressant drugs but quite how remains a mystery (see Ch. 47).

Research on the α_2-adrenoceptor antagonist **idazoxan** has led to the identification of other putative 'imidazoline receptors' (see Head & Mayorov, 2006). These are the I_1 receptor, which plays a role in the central control of blood pressure (see Ch. 22); the I_2 receptor, an allosteric binding site on monoamine oxidase, and the I_3 receptor, present in the pancreas with a role in regulating insulin secretion.

Arousal and mood

Attention has focused mainly on the LC, which is the source of most of the noradrenaline released in the brain, and from which neuronal activity can be measured by implanted electrodes. LC neurons are silent during sleep, and their activity increases with behavioural arousal. 'Wake-up' stimuli of an unfamiliar or threatening kind excite these neurons much more effectively than familiar stimuli. Amphetamine-like drugs, which release catecholamines in the brain, increase wakefulness, alertness and exploratory activity (although, in this case, firing of LC

neurons is actually reduced by feedback mechanisms; see Ch. 48).

There is a close relationship between mood and state of arousal; depressed individuals are usually lethargic and unresponsive to external stimuli. The catecholamine hypothesis of depression (see Ch. 47) suggested that it results from a functional deficiency of noradrenaline in certain parts of the brain, while mania results from an excess. This remains controversial, and subsequent findings suggest that 5-HT may be more important than noradrenaline in relation to mood.

Blood pressure regulation

The role of central, as well as peripheral, noradrenergic synapses in blood pressure control is shown by the action of hypotensive drugs such as **clonidine** and **methyldopa** (see Chs 14 and 22), which decrease the discharge of sympathetic nerves emerging from the CNS. They cause hypotension when injected locally into the medulla or fourth ventricle, in much smaller amounts than are required when the drugs are given systemically. Noradrenaline and other α_2-adrenoceptor agonists have the same effect when injected locally. Noradrenergic synapses in the medulla probably form part of the baroreceptor reflex pathway, because stimulation or antagonism of α_2 adrenoceptors in this part of the brain has a powerful effect on the activity of baroreceptor reflexes.

Ascending noradrenergic fibres run to the hypothalamus, and descending fibres run to the lateral horn region of the spinal cord, acting to increase sympathetic discharge in the periphery. It has been suggested that these regulatory neurons may release adrenaline rather than noradrenaline as inhibition of phenylethanolamine *N*-methyl transferase, the enzyme that converts noradrenaline to adrenaline, interferes with the baroreceptor reflex.

Moxonidine, reported to be an I_1-receptor agonist with less activity at α_2 adrenoceptors, acts centrally to reduce peripheral sympathetic activity, thus decreasing peripheral vascular resistance.

DOPAMINE

Dopamine is particularly important in relation to neuropharmacology, because it is involved in several common disorders of brain function, notably Parkinson's disease, schizophrenia and attention deficit disorder, as well as in drug dependence and certain endocrine disorders. Many of the drugs used clinically to treat these conditions work by influencing dopamine transmission.

The distribution of dopamine in the brain is more restricted than that of noradrenaline. Dopamine is most abundant in the *corpus striatum*, a part of the extrapyramidal motor system concerned with the coordination of movement (see Ch. 40), and high concentrations also occur in certain parts of the frontal cortex, limbic system and hypothalamus (where its release into the pituitary blood supply inhibits secretion of prolactin; Ch. 33).

The synthesis of dopamine follows the same route as that of noradrenaline (see Fig. 14.2), namely conversion of tyrosine to dopa (the rate-limiting step), followed by decarboxylation to form dopamine. Dopaminergic neurons lack dopamine β-hydroxylase, and thus do not convert dopamine to noradrenaline.

Dopamine is largely recaptured, following its release from nerve terminals, by a specific dopamine transporter,

Noradrenaline in the CNS

- Mechanisms for synthesis, storage, release and reuptake of noradrenaline in the central nervous system (CNS) are essentially the same as in the periphery, as are the receptors (Ch. 14).
- Noradrenergic cell bodies occur in discrete clusters, mainly in the pons and medulla, one important such cell group being the locus coeruleus.
- Noradrenergic pathways, running mainly in the medial forebrain bundle and descending spinal tracts, terminate diffusely in the cortex, hippocampus, hypothalamus, cerebellum and spinal cord.
- The actions of noradrenaline are mediated through α_1, α_2, β_1 and β_2 receptors.
- Noradrenergic transmission is believed to be important in:
  - the 'arousal' system, controlling wakefulness and alertness
  - blood pressure regulation
  - control of mood (functional deficiency contributing to depression).
- Psychotropic drugs that act partly or mainly on noradrenergic transmission in the CNS include antidepressants, **cocaine** and **amphetamine**. Some antihypertensive drugs (e.g. **clonidine**, **methyldopa**) act mainly on noradrenergic transmission in the CNS.

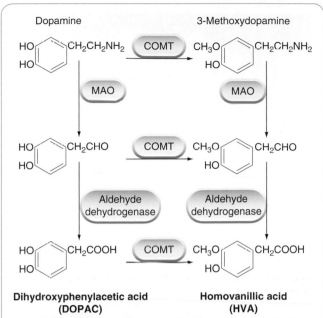

Fig. 39.2 The main pathways for dopamine metabolism in the brain. COMT, catechol-O-methyl transferase; MAO, monoamine oxidase.

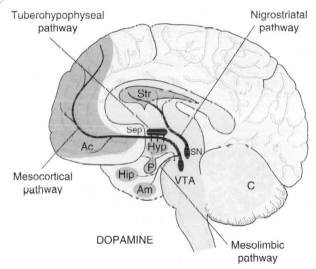

Fig. 39.3 Simplified diagram of the dopamine pathways in the brain, drawn as in Figure 39.1. The pituitary gland (P) is shown, innervated with dopaminergic fibres from the hypothalamus. Ac, nucleus accumbens; SN, substantia nigra; VTA, ventral tegmental area; other abbreviations as in Figure 39.1.

one of the large family of monoamine transporters (see Ch. 14). It is metabolised by monoamine oxidase and catechol-O-methyl transferase (Fig. 39.2), the main products being *dihydroxyphenylacetic acid* (DOPAC) and *homovanillic acid* (HVA), the methoxy derivative of DOPAC. The brain content of HVA is often used in animal experiments as an index of dopamine turnover. Drugs that cause the release of dopamine increase HVA, often without changing the concentration of dopamine. DOPAC and HVA, and their sulfate conjugates, are excreted in the urine, which provides an index of dopamine release in human subjects.

6-Hydroxydopamine, which selectively destroys dopaminergic nerve terminals, is commonly used as a research tool. It is taken up by the dopamine transporter and converted to a reactive metabolite that causes oxidative cytotoxicity.

DOPAMINERGIC PATHWAYS IN THE CNS

There are four main dopaminergic pathways in the brain (Fig. 39.3):

1. The **nigrostriatal pathway**, accounting for about 75% of the dopamine in the brain, consists of cell bodies largely in the substantia nigra whose axons terminate in the corpus striatum. These fibres run in the medial forebrain bundle along with other monoamine-containing fibres. The abundance of dopamine-containing neurons in the human striatum can be appreciated from the image shown in Figure 39.4, which was obtained by injecting a dopa derivative containing radioactive fluorine, and scanning for

radioactivity 3 h later by positron emission tomography.

2. The **mesolimbic pathway**, whose cell bodies occur in the midbrain ventral tegmental area (VTA), adjacent to the substantia nigra, and whose fibres project via the medial forebrain bundle to parts of the limbic system, especially the *nucleus accumbens* and the *amygdaloid nucleus*.

3. The **mesocortical pathway**, whose cell bodies also lie in the VTA and which project via the medial forebrain bundle to the frontal cortex.

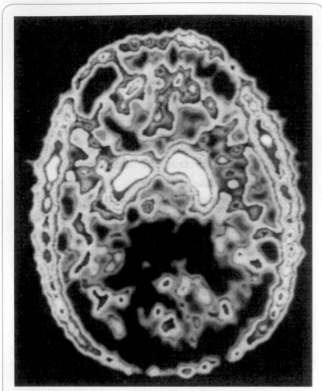

Fig. 39.4 Dopamine in the basal ganglia of a human subject. The subject was injected with 5-fluoro-dopa labelled with the positron-emitting isotope ^{18}F, which was localised 3 h later by the technique of positron emission tomography. The isotope is accumulated (white areas) by the dopa uptake system of the neurons of the basal ganglia, and to a smaller extent in the frontal cortex. It is also seen in the scalp and temporalis muscles. *(From Garnett ES, Firnau G, Nahmias C 1983 Nature 305, 137–138.)*

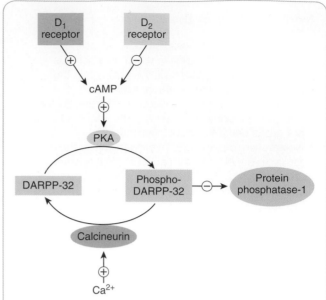

Fig. 39.5 The role of the neuron-specific phosphoprotein DARPP-32 in signalling by dopamine receptors (see text). PKA, protein kinase A.

calcium channels and adenylyl cyclase. In addition, they can also affect other cellular second messenger cascades (see Ch. 3). An interesting component in the dopamine signal transduction pathway is the protein DARPP-32 (*32-kDa dopamine- and cAMP-regulated phosphoprotein* also known as *protein phosphatase 1 regulatory subunit 1B*; see Girault & Greengard, 2004), which is highly expressed in dopamine-sensitive neurons. When intracellular cAMP is increased through activation of D_1 receptors, activating protein kinase A, DARPP-32 is phosphorylated (Fig. 39.5). Phosphorylated DARPP-32 acts as an inhibitor of protein phosphatase-1, thus acting in concert with protein kinases and favouring protein phosphorylation – effectively an amplifying mechanism. In general, activation of D_2 receptors opposes the effects of D_1 receptor activation.

Dopamine receptors are expressed in the brain in distinct but overlapping areas. D_1 receptors are the most abundant and widespread in areas receiving a dopaminergic innervation (namely the striatum, limbic system, thalamus and hypothalamus; Fig. 39.3), as are D_2 receptors, which also occur in the pituitary gland. D_2 receptors are found not only on dopaminergic neurons (cell bodies, dendrites and nerve terminals), where they function as inhibitory autoreceptors, but also on non-dopaminergic neurons (see De Mei et al., 2009). D_3 receptors occur in the limbic system but not in the striatum. The D_4 receptor is much more weakly expressed, mainly in the cortex and limbic systems.

Dopamine, like many other transmitters and modulators, acts presynaptically as well as postsynaptically. Presynaptic D_2 receptors act as autoreceptors on dopaminergic neurons, for example those in the striatum and limbic system, where they act to inhibit dopamine synthesis and release. Dopamine antagonists, by blocking these receptors, increase dopamine synthesis and release, and cause accumulation of dopamine metabolites in these parts of the brain. They also cause an increase in the rate of firing of dopaminergic neurons, probably by blocking feedback at the somatodendritic level mediated by locally released dopamine. Inhibitory D_2 receptors are also located on glutamatergic, GABAergic and cholinergic nerve terminals.

4. The **tuberohypophyseal** (or **tuberoinfundibular**) system is a group of short neurons running from the ventral hypothalamus to the median eminence and pituitary gland, the secretions of which they regulate.

There are also dopaminergic neurons in other brain regions and in the retina. For a more complete description, see Björklund & Dunnett (2007). The functions of the main dopaminergic pathways are discussed below.

DOPAMINE RECEPTORS

Two types of receptor, D_1 and D_2, were originally distinguished on pharmacological and biochemical grounds. Gene cloning revealed further subgroups, D_1 to D_5. The original D_1 family now includes D_1 and D_5, while the D_2 family consists of D_2, D_3 and D_4 (see Table 39.1). Splice variants, leading to long and short forms of D_2, and genetic polymorphisms, particularly of D_4, have subsequently been identified.

▼ All belong to the family of G protein-coupled transmembrane receptors described in Chapter 3. D_1 and D_5 receptors link through G_s to stimulate adenylyl cyclase and activation of protein kinase A (PKA). PKA mediates many of the effects of D_1 and D_5 receptors by phosphorylating a wide array of proteins, including voltage-activated sodium, potassium and calcium channels as well as ionotropic glutamate and GABA receptors. D_2, D_3, and D_4 receptors link through G_i/G_o and activate potassium channels as well as inhibiting

Table 39.1 Dopamine receptors

Functional role	D₁ type		D₂ type		
	D_1	D_5	D_2	D_3	D_4
Distribution					
Cortex — Arousal, mood	+++	–	++	–	+
Limbic system — Emotion, stereotypic behaviour	+++	+	++	+	+
Striatum — Prolactin secretion	+++	+	++	+	+
Ventral hypothalamus and anterior pituitary — Prolactin secretion	–	–	++	+	–
Agonists					
Dopamine	+ (Low potency)		+ (High potency)		
Apomorphine	PA (Low potency)		+ (High potency)		
Bromocriptine	PA (Low potency)		+ (High potency)		
Quinpirole	Inactive		Active		
Antagonists					
Chlorpromazine	++	++	++	++	++
Haloperidol	++	+	+++	++	+++
Spiperone	++	+	+++	+++	+++
Sulpiride	–	–	++	++	+
Clozapine	+	+	+	+	++
Aripiprazole	–	–	+++ (PA)	–	++
Raclopride	–	–	+++	++	+
Signal transduction	G_s coupled – activates adenylyl cyclase		G_i/G_o coupled – inhibits adenylyl cyclase, activates K⁺ channels, inhibits Ca²⁺ channels, may also activate phospholipase C		
Effect	Mainly postsynaptic inhibition		Pre- and postsynaptic inhibition Stimulation/inhibition of hormone release		

PA, partial agonist.

Affinity data based on data contained in the IUPHAR/BPS Guide to Pharmacology database (www.guidetopharmacology.org)

Dopamine receptors also mediate various effects in the periphery (mediated by D_1 receptors), notably renal vasodilatation and increased myocardial contractility (dopamine itself has been used clinically in the treatment of circulatory shock; see Ch. 22).

FUNCTIONAL ASPECTS

The functions of dopaminergic pathways divide broadly into:

- motor control (nigrostriatal system)
- behavioural effects (mesolimbic and mesocortical systems)
- endocrine control (tuberohypophyseal system).

Dopamine and motor systems

Ungerstedt showed, in 1968, that bilateral ablation of the substantia nigra in rats, which destroys the nigrostriatal neurons, causes profound catalepsy, the animals becoming so inactive that they die of starvation unless artificially fed. Parkinson's disease (Ch. 40) is a disorder of motor control, associated with a deficiency of dopamine in the nigrostriatal pathway.

In treating CNS disorders, it is often desired that a certain receptor type be activated or inhibited only in one part of the brain but the problem is that drugs are rarely brain region selective and will affect a given receptor type throughout the brain. For example, many antipsychotic drugs (see Ch. 46) are D_2 receptor antagonists, exerting a beneficial effect by blocking D_2 receptors in the mesolimbic pathway. However, their D_2 antagonist property also gives rise to their major side effect, which is to cause movement disorders, by simultaneously blocking D_2 receptors in the nigrostriatal pathway.

Behavioural effects

Administration of **amphetamine** to rats, which releases both dopamine and noradrenaline, causes a cessation of normal 'ratty' behaviour (exploration and grooming), and the appearance of repeated 'stereotyped' behaviour (rearing, gnawing and so on) unrelated to external stimuli. These amphetamine-induced motor disturbances in rats probably reflect hyperactivity in the nigrostriatal dopaminergic system, and are prevented by dopamine antagonists and by destruction of dopamine-containing cell bodies in the midbrain, but not by drugs that inhibit the noradrenergic system.

Amphetamine and **cocaine** (which act by inhibiting the dopamine transporter) and also other drugs of abuse (Ch. 49) activate mesolimbic dopaminergic 'reward' pathways to produce feelings of euphoria in humans. The main receptor involved appears to be D_1, and transgenic mice lacking D_1 receptors behave as though generally demotivated, with reduced food intake and insensitivity to amphetamine and cocaine.

Neuroendocrine function

The tuberohypophyseal dopaminergic pathway (see Fig. 39.3) is involved in the control of prolactin secretion. The hypothalamus secretes various mediators (mostly small peptides; see Ch. 33), which control the secretion of different hormones from the pituitary gland. One of these mediators, which has an inhibitory effect on prolactin release, is dopamine. This system is of clinical importance. Many antipsychotic drugs (see Ch. 46), by blocking D_2 receptors, increase prolactin secretion and can cause breast development and lactation, even in males. **Bromocriptine**, a dopamine receptor agonist derived from ergot, is used clinically to suppress prolactin secretion by tumours of the pituitary gland.

Growth hormone production is increased in normal subjects by dopamine, but bromocriptine paradoxically inhibits the excessive secretion responsible for acromegaly (probably because it desensitises dopamine receptors, in contrast to the physiological release of dopamine, which is pulsatile) and has a useful therapeutic effect, provided it is given before excessive growth has taken place. It is now rarely used, as other agents are more effective (see Ch. 33). Bromocriptine and other dopamine agonists, such as **cabergoline**, enhance libido and sexual performance.

Vomiting

Pharmacological evidence strongly suggests that dopaminergic neurons have a role in the production of nausea and vomiting. Thus nearly all dopamine receptor agonists (e.g. bromocriptine) and other drugs that increase dopamine release in the brain (e.g. **levodopa**; Ch. 40) cause nausea and vomiting as side effects, while many dopamine antagonists (e.g. phenothiazines, **metoclopramide**; Ch. 30) have antiemetic activity. D_2 receptors occur in the area of the medulla (chemoreceptor trigger zone) associated with the initiation of vomiting (Ch. 30), and are assumed to mediate this effect.

5-HYDROXYTRYPTAMINE

The occurrence and functions of 5-HT (serotonin) in the periphery are described in Chapter 15. Interest in 5-HT as a possible CNS transmitter dates from 1953, when Gaddum found that **lysergic acid diethylamide** (LSD), a drug known to be a powerful hallucinogen (see Ch. 48), acted as a 5-HT antagonist on peripheral tissues, and suggested that its central effects might also be related to this action. The presence of 5-HT in the brain was demonstrated a few years later. Even though brain 5-HT accounts for only about 1% of the total body content, 5-HT is an important CNS transmitter (see Iversen et al., 2009; Muller & Jacobs, 2009). 5-HT is involved in various physiological processes, including sleep, appetite, thermoregulation and pain perception as well as in disorders such as migraine, depression, mania, anxiety, obsessive–compulsive disorders, schizophrenia, autism and drug abuse.

In its formation, storage and release, 5-HT resembles noradrenaline. Its precursor is tryptophan, an amino acid

Dopamine in the CNS

- Dopamine is a neurotransmitter as well as being the precursor for noradrenaline. It is degraded in a similar fashion to noradrenaline, giving rise mainly to dihydroxyphenylacetic acid and homovanillic acid, which are excreted in the urine.
- There are four main dopaminergic pathways:
  - nigrostriatal pathway, important in motor control
  - mesolimbic pathway, running from groups of cells in the midbrain to parts of the limbic system, especially the nucleus accumbens, involved in emotion and drug-induced reward
  - mesocortical pathway, running from the midbrain to the cortex, involved in emotion
  - tuberohypophyseal neurons, running from the hypothalamus to the pituitary gland, whose secretions they regulate.
- There are five dopamine receptor subtypes. D_1 and D_5 receptors are linked to stimulation of adenylyl cyclase. D_2, D_3 and D_4 receptors are linked to activation of K^+ channels and inhibition of Ca^{2+} channels as well as to inhibition of adenylyl cyclase.
- D_2 receptors may be implicated in the positive symptoms and D_1 receptors in the negative symptoms of schizophrenia.
- Parkinson's disease is associated with a deficiency of nigrostriatal dopaminergic neurons.
- Hormone release from the anterior pituitary gland is regulated by dopamine, especially prolactin release (inhibited) and growth hormone release (stimulated).
- Dopamine acts on the chemoreceptor trigger zone to cause nausea and vomiting.

derived from dietary protein, the plasma content of which varies considerably according to food intake and time of day. 5-HT does not cross the blood–brain barrier and is synthesised in the CNS. Tryptophan is actively taken up into neurons, converted by tryptophan hydroxylase to 5-hydroxytryptophan (see Fig. 15.1), and then decarboxylated by a non-specific amino acid decarboxylase to form 5-HT. Tryptophan hydroxylase can be selectively and irreversibly inhibited by *p*-chlorophenylalanine (PCPA). Availability of tryptophan and the activity of tryptophan hydroxylase are thought to be the main factors that regulate 5-HT synthesis. The decarboxylase is very similar, if not identical, to dopa decarboxylase, and does not play any role in regulating 5-HT synthesis. Following release, 5-HT is largely recovered by neuronal uptake, through a specific transporter (see Ch. 3) similar to, but not identical with, those that take up noradrenaline and dopamine. 5-HT reuptake is specifically inhibited by *selective serotonin reuptake inhibitors* (SSRIs) such as **fluoxetine** and by many of the drugs that inhibit catecholamine uptake (e.g. *tricyclic antidepressants*). SSRIs (see Chs 44 and Ch. 47) constitute an important group of antidepressant and antianxiety drugs. 5-HT is degraded almost entirely by monoamine oxidase (Fig. 15.1), which converts it to 5-hydroxyindole acetaldehyde, most of which is then dehydrogenated to form 5-hydroxyindole acetic acid (5-HIAA) and excreted in the urine.

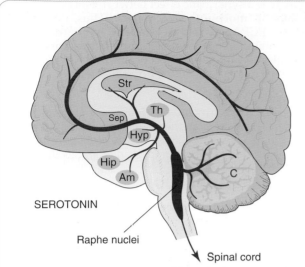

Fig. 39.6 Simplified diagram of the 5-hydroxytryptamine pathways in the brain, drawn as in **Figure 39.1**. Abbreviations as in Figure 39.1.

5-HT PATHWAYS IN THE CNS

The distribution of 5-HT-containing neurons (Fig. 39.6) resembles that of noradrenergic neurons. The cell bodies are grouped in the pons and upper medulla, close to the midline (raphe), and are often referred to as raphe nuclei. The rostrally situated nuclei project, via the medial forebrain bundle, to many parts of the cortex, hippocampus, basal ganglia, limbic system and hypothalamus. The caudally situated cells project to the cerebellum, medulla and spinal cord.

5-HT RECEPTORS IN THE CNS

The main 5-HT receptor types are shown in Table 15.1. All are G protein-coupled receptors except for 5-HT₃, which is a ligand-gated cation channel (see below). All are expressed in the CNS, and their functional roles have been extensively analysed. With some 14 identified subtypes plus numerous splice variants, and a large number of pharmacological tools of relatively low specificity, assigning clear-cut functions to 5-HT receptors is not simple. Detailed accounts of our present state of knowledge are given by Filip & Bader (2009).

Certain generalisations can be made:

- 5-HT$_1$ receptors (5-HT$_{1A}$, 5-HT$_{1B}$, 5-HT$_{1D}$, 5-HT$_{1E}$, 5-HT$_{1F}$)[2] are predominantly inhibitory in their effects. 5-HT$_{1A}$ receptors are expressed as somatodendritic autoreceptors by the 5-HT neurons in the raphe nuclei, and their autoinhibitory effect tends to limit the rate of firing of these cells. They are also widely distributed in the limbic system, and are believed to be a major target for drugs used to treat anxiety and depression (see Chs 44 and 47). 5-HT$_{1B}$ and 5-HT$_{1D}$ receptors are found mainly as presynaptic inhibitory receptors on both 5-HT-containing and other nerve terminals in the basal ganglia and cortex. Agonists acting on 5-HT$_{1B}$

and 5-HT$_{1D}$ receptors such as **sumatriptan** are used to treat migraine (see Ch. 15).
- 5-HT$_2$ receptors (5-HT$_{2A}$, 5-HT$_{2B}$ and 5-HT$_{2C}$) are abundant in the cortex and limbic system, where they are located at both pre- and postsynaptic sites. They can exert excitatory or inhibitory effects by enhancing the release of glutamate and GABA. They are believed to be the target of some antidepressants (see Ch. 47) and antipsychotic drugs (see Ch. 46) as well as various hallucinogenic drugs (see Ch. 48). **Lorcaserin**, a 5-HT$_{2C}$ agonist is an anti obesity drug (see Ch 32). The use of 5-HT$_2$ receptor antagonists such as **methysergide** in treating migraine is discussed in Chapter 15.
- 5-HT$_3$ receptors are pentameric ligand-gated cation channels that can be either homomeric or heteromeric complexes of different 5-HT$_3$ receptor subunits (see Peters et al., 2005). While 5-HT3A and 5-HT3B subunits are the most extensively studied, the roles of other subunits remain to be fully investigated (see Jensen et al., 2008). In the brain, 5-HT$_3$ receptors are found in the *area postrema* (a region of the medulla involved in vomiting; see Ch. 30) and other parts of the brain stem, extending to the dorsal horn of the spinal cord. They are also present in certain parts of the cortex, as well as in the peripheral nervous system. They are excitatory ionotropic receptors, and specific antagonists (e.g. **granisetron** and **ondansetron**; see Chs 15 and 30) are used to treat nausea and vomiting.
- 5-HT$_4$ receptors are important in the gastrointestinal tract (see Chs 15 and 30), and are also expressed in the brain, particularly in the limbic system, basal ganglia, hippocampus and substantia nigra. They are located at both pre- and postsynaptic sites. They exert a presynaptic facilitatory effect, particularly on ACh release, thus enhancing cognitive performance (see Ch. 40). Activation of medullary 5-HT$_4$ receptors opposes the respiratory depressant actions of opioids (see Ch. 42).
- There are two 5-HT$_5$ receptors, 5-HT$_{5A}$ and 5-HT$_{5B}$. In the human only 5-HT$_{5A}$ is functional. Antagonists may have anxiolytic, antidepressant and antipsychotic activity.
- 5-HT$_6$ receptors occur primarily in the CNS, particularly in the hippocampus, cortex and limbic system. Blockade of 5-HT$_6$ receptors increases glutamate and Ach release and 5HT$_6$-antagonists are considered potential drugs to improve cognition or relieve symptoms of schizophrenia.
- 5-HT$_7$ receptors occur in the hippocampus, cortex, amygdala, thalamus and hypothalamus. They are found on the soma and axon terminals of GABAergic neurons. They are also expressed in blood vessels and the gastrointestinal tract. Likely CNS functions include thermoregulation and endocrine regulation, as well as suspected involvement in mood, cognitive function and sleep. Selective antagonists are being developed for clinical use in a variety of potential indications.

FUNCTIONAL ASPECTS

The precise localisation of 5-HT neurons in the brain stem has allowed their electrical activity to be studied in detail and correlated with behavioural and other effects

---

[2]There is no 5-HT$_{1C}$ receptor. The original 5-HT$_{1C}$ receptor has been reclassified as 5-HT$_{2C}$.

produced by drugs thought to affect 5-HT-mediated transmission. 5-HT cells show an unusual, highly regular, slow discharge pattern, and are strongly inhibited by 5-HT$_1$ receptor agonists, suggesting a local inhibitory feedback mechanism.

In vertebrates, certain physiological and behavioural functions relate particularly to 5-HT pathways namely:

- hallucinations and behavioural changes
- sleep, wakefulness and mood
- feeding behaviour
- control of sensory transmission (especially pain pathways; see Ch. 42).

Hallucinatory effects

Many hallucinogenic drugs (e.g. LSD; Ch. 48) are agonists at 5-HT$_{2A}$ receptors. It is suggested that a loss of cortical inhibition underlies the hallucinogenic effect, as well as certain behavioural effects in experimental animals, such as the 'wet dog shakes' that occur in rats when the 5-HT precursor 5-hydroxytryptophan is administered. Many antipsychotic drugs (Ch. 46) are antagonists at 5-HT$_{2A}$ receptors in addition to blocking dopamine D$_2$ receptors. The psychostimulant properties of MDMA ('ecstasy'; see Ch. 48) are due partly to its ability to release 5-HT. MDMA is taken up by the serotonin transporter, causing it to displace 5-HT from storage vesicles – a mechanism analogous to the action of amphetamine on noradrenergic nerve terminals (Ch. 14).

Sleep, wakefulness and mood

Lesions of the raphe nuclei, or depletion of 5-HT by PCPA administration, abolish sleep in experimental animals, whereas microinjection of 5-HT at specific points in the brain stem induces sleep. 5-HT$_7$ receptor antagonists inhibit 'rapid-eye-movement' (REM) sleep and increase the latency to onset of REM sleep. Attempts to cure insomnia in humans by giving 5-HT precursors (tryptophan or 5-hydroxytryptophan) have, however, proved unsuccessful. There is strong evidence that 5-HT, as well as noradrenaline, may be involved in the control of mood (see Ch. 47), and the use of tryptophan to enhance 5-HT synthesis has been tried in depression, with equivocal results.

Feeding and appetite

In experimental animals, 5-HT$_{1A}$ agonists such as 8-hydroxy-2-(di-n-propylamino)tetralin (8-OH-DPAT) cause hyperphagia, leading to obesity. Antagonists acting on 5-HT$_2$ receptors, including several antipsychotic drugs used clinically, also increase appetite and cause weight gain. On the other hand, antidepressant drugs that inhibit 5-HT uptake (see Ch. 47) cause loss of appetite, as does the 5-HT$_{2C}$ receptor agonist **lorcaserin**.

Sensory transmission

After lesions of the raphe nuclei or administration of PCPA, animals show exaggerated responses to many forms of sensory stimulus. They are startled much more easily, and also quickly develop avoidance responses to stimuli that would not normally bother them. It appears that the normal ability to disregard irrelevant forms of sensory input requires intact 5-HT pathways. The 'sensory enhancement' produced by hallucinogenic drugs may be partly due to loss of this gatekeeper function of 5-HT. 5-HT also exerts an inhibitory effect on transmission in the pain pathway, both in the spinal cord and in the brain,

and there is a synergistic effect between 5-HT and analgesics such as **morphine** (see Ch. 42). Thus, depletion of 5-HT by PCPA, or selective lesions to the descending 5-HT-containing neurons that run to the dorsal horn, antagonise the analgesic effect of morphine, while inhibitors of 5-HT uptake have the opposite effect.

Other roles

Other roles of 5-HT include various autonomic and endocrine functions, such as the regulation of body temperature, blood pressure and sexual function. Further information can be found in Iversen et al. (2009).

CLINICALLY USED DRUGS

Several classes of drugs used clinically influence 5-HT-mediated transmission. They include:

- 5-HT reuptake inhibitors, such as fluoxetine, used as antidepressants (Ch. 47) and anxiolytic agents (Ch. 44)
- 5-HT$_{1D}$ receptor agonists, such as sumatriptan, used to treat migraine (Ch. 15)
- buspirone, a 5-HT$_{1A}$ receptor agonist used in treating anxiety (Ch. 44)
- 5-HT$_3$ receptor antagonists, such as ondansetron, used as antiemetic agents (see Ch. 30)
- antipsychotic drugs (e.g. clozapine, Ch. 46), which owe their efficacy partly to an action on 5-HT receptors.

ACETYLCHOLINE

There are numerous cholinergic neurons in the CNS, and the basic processes by which ACh is synthesised, stored and released are the same as in the periphery (see Ch. 13). Various biochemical markers have been used to locate cholinergic neurons in the brain, the most useful being choline acetyltransferase, the enzyme responsible for ACh synthesis, and the transporters that capture choline and package ACh, which can be labelled by immunofluorescence. Biochemical studies on ACh precursors and metabolites are generally more difficult than corresponding studies on other amine transmitters, because the relevant substances, choline and acetate, are involved in many processes other than ACh metabolism.

CHOLINERGIC PATHWAYS IN THE CNS

Acetylcholine is very widely distributed in the brain, occurring in all parts of the forebrain (including the cortex), midbrain and brain stem, although there is little in the cerebellum. Cholinergic neurons in the forebrain and brain stem send diffuse projections to many parts of the brain (see Fig. 39.7). Cholinergic neurons in the forebrain lie in a discrete area, forming the magnocellular forebrain nuclei (so called because the cell bodies are conspicuously large). Degeneration of one of these, the *nucleus basalis of Meynert*, which projects mainly to the cortex, is associated with Alzheimer's disease (Ch. 40). Another cluster, the *septohippocampal nucleus*, provides the main cholinergic input to the hippocampus, and is involved in memory. In addition, there are – in contrast to the monoamine pathways – many local cholinergic interneurons, particularly in the corpus striatum, these being

5-Hydroxytryptamine in the CNS

- The processes of synthesis, storage, release, reuptake and degradation of 5-hydroxytryptamine (5-HT) in the brain are very similar to events in the periphery (Ch. 15).
- Availability of tryptophan is the main factor regulating synthesis.
- Urinary excretion of 5-hydroxyindole acetic acid provides a measure of 5-HT turnover.
- 5-HT neurons are concentrated in the midline raphe nuclei in the brain stem projecting diffusely to the cortex, limbic system, hypothalamus and spinal cord, similar to the noradrenergic projections.
- Functions associated with 5-HT pathways include:
  - various behavioural responses (e.g. hallucinatory behaviour, 'wet dog shakes')
  - feeding behaviour
  - control of mood and emotion
  - control of sleep/wakefulness
  - control of sensory pathways, including nociception
  - control of body temperature
  - vomiting.
- 5-HT can exert inhibitory or excitatory effects on individual neurons, acting either presynaptically or postsynaptically.
- The main receptor subtypes (see Table 15.1) in the CNS are 5-HT$_{1A}$, 5-HT$_{1B}$, 5-HT$_{1D}$, 5-HT$_{2A}$, 5-HT$_{2C}$ and 5-HT$_3$. Associations of behavioural and physiological functions with these receptors have been partly worked out. Other receptor types (5-HT$_{4-7}$) also occur in the central nervous system, but less is known about their function.
- Drugs acting selectively on 5-HT receptors or transporters include:
  - **buspirone**, 5-HT$_{1A}$ receptor agonist used to treat anxiety (see Ch. 44)
  - 'triptans' (e.g. **sumatriptan**), 5-HT$_{1D}$ agonists used to treat migraine (see Ch. 15)
  - 5-HT$_2$ antagonists (e.g. **pizotifen**) used for migraine prophylaxis (see Ch. 15)
  - selective serotonin uptake inhibitors (e.g. **fluoxetine**) used to treat depression (see Ch. 47)
  - **ondansetron**, a 5-HT$_3$ antagonist, used to treat chemotherapy-induced emesis (see Chs 15 and 30)
  - **MDMA** (ecstasy), a substrate for the 5-HT transporter. It then displaces 5-HT from nerve terminals onto 5-HT receptors to produce its mood-altering effects (see Ch. 48).

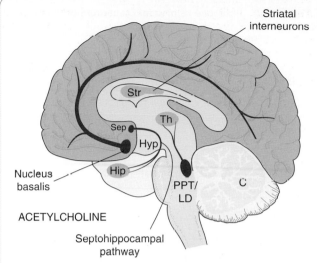

Fig. 39.7 Simplified diagram of the acetylcholine pathways in the brain, drawn as in Figure 39.1. PPT/LD, pedunculopontine and laterodorsal tegmental nuclei; other abbreviations as in Figure 39.1.

important in relation to Parkinson's disease and Huntington's chorea (Ch. 40).

ACETYLCHOLINE RECEPTORS

Acetylcholine acts on both muscarinic (G protein-coupled) and nicotinic (ionotropic) receptors in the CNS (see Ch. 13).

The muscarinic ACh receptors (mAChRs) in the brain are predominantly of the G$_q$-coupled M$_1$ class (i.e. M$_1$, M$_3$ and M$_5$ subtypes; see Ch. 13). Activation of these receptors can result in excitation through blockade of M-type (KCNQ/Kv7) K$^+$ channels (see Delmas & Brown, 2005) G$_i$/G$_o$-coupled M$_2$ and M$_4$ receptors, on the other hand, are inhibitory through activation of inwardly rectifying K$^+$ channels and inhibition of voltage-sensitive Ca^{2+} channels. mAChRs on cholinergic terminals function to inhibit ACh release, and muscarinic antagonists, by blocking this inhibition, markedly increase ACh release. Many of the behavioural effects associated with cholinergic pathways seem to be produced by ACh acting on mAChRs.

Nicotinic ACh receptors (nAChRs) are ligand-gated cation channels permeable to Na$^+$, K$^+$ and Ca^{2+} ions (see Ch. 13). They are pentamers and can be formed as homomeric or heteromeric combinations of α (α2–7) and β (β2–4) subunits (Ch. 3; see Gotti et al., 2008) distributed widely throughout the brain (see Table 39.2). The heteromeric α4β2 and the homomeric α7 subtypes are the most extensively characterised. The lack of subtype-specific ligands and the fact that some neurons express multiple subtypes has made the elucidation of the functions of each receptor subtype extremely difficult. Nicotine (see Ch. 49) exerts its central effects by agonist action on nAChRs.

In large part, nAChRs are located presynaptically and act usually to facilitate the release of other transmitters such as glutamate, dopamine and GABA.[3] In some situations, they function postsynaptically to mediate fast excitatory transmission, as in the periphery.

Many of the drugs that block nAChRs (e.g. **tubocurarine**; see Ch. 13) do not cross the blood–brain barrier, and even those that do (e.g. **mecamylamine**) produce only modest CNS effects. Various nAChR knockout mouse strains have been produced and studied. Deletion of the various CNS-specific nAChR subtypes generally has rather little effect, although some cognitive impairment can be detected. Mutations in nAChRs may be the cause of some forms of epilepsy and changes in nAChR expression may occur in disorders such as schizophrenia,

Table 39.2 Presence of nicotinic receptors of different subunit composition in selected regions of the central nervous system

Brain region	Nicotinic receptors						
	α7	α3β2	α3β4	α4β2	α4α5β	α6β2β3	α6α4β2β3
Cortex	+			+	+		
Hippocampus	+		+	+	+		
Striatum				+	+	+	+
Amygdala	+			+			
Thalamus				+			
Hypothalamus	+			+			
Substantia nigra	+		+	+	+	+	
Cerebellum	+	+	+	+			
Spinal cord	+	+		+			

nAChRs comprising α2β2 and α3β3β4 are found in some other areas of the brain.
Data taken from Gotti et al. 2006.

attention deficit hyperactivity disorder, depression and anxiety, as well as following neurodegeneration in Alzheimer's and Parkinson's diseases.

FUNCTIONAL ASPECTS

The main functions ascribed to cholinergic pathways are related to arousal, reward, learning and memory, and motor control. The cholinergic projection from the ventral forebrain to the cortex is thought to mediate arousal, whereas the septohippocampal pathway is involved in learning and short-term memory (see Hasselmo, 2006). Cholinergic interneurons in the striatum are involved in motor control (see Ch. 40).

Muscarinic agonists have been shown to restore partially learning and memory deficits induced in experimental animals by lesions of the septohippocampal cholinergic pathway. **Hyoscine**, a muscarinic antagonist, impairs memory in human subjects and causes amnesia when used as preanaesthetic medication. M_1 receptor knockout mice, however, show only slight impairment of learning and memory (see Wess, 2004).

Nicotine increases alertness and also enhances learning and memory, as do various synthetic agonists at neuronal nAChRs. Conversely, CNS-active nAChR antagonists such as mecamylamine cause detectable, although slight, impairment of learning and memory. Transgenic mice with disruption of brain nAChRs are only slightly impaired in spatial learning tasks. In the dopaminergic VTA to accumbens 'reward' pathway, nicotine affects neuronal firing at the level of the cell soma in the VTA and modulates dopamine release from terminals in the nucleus accumbens to modify dopamine release in this reward pathway (see Ch. 49).

In conclusion, both nAChRs and mAChRs may play a role in learning and memory, while nAChRs also mediate behavioural arousal. Receptor knockout mice are surprisingly little affected, suggesting that alternative mechanisms may be able to compensate for the loss of ACh receptor signalling.

The importance of cholinergic neurons in neurodegenerative conditions such as dementia and Parkinson's disease is discussed in Chapter 40. The role of nAChRs in addiction to nicotine is described in Chapter 49 and their role in modulating pain transmission in the CNS is described in Chapter 41.

PURINES

Both adenosine and ATP act as transmitters and/or modulators in the CNS (for review, see Fredholm et al., 2005; Khakh & North, 2012) as they do in the periphery (Ch. 16). Mapping the pathways is difficult, because purinergic neurons are not easily identifiable histochemically. It is likely that adenosine and ATP serve as neuromodulators.

Adenosine is produced intracellularly from ATP. It is not packaged into vesicles but is released mainly by carrier-mediated transport. Because the intracellular concentration of ATP (several mmol/l) greatly exceeds that of adenosine, conversion of a small proportion of ATP results in a large increase in adenosine. ATP is packaged into vesicles and released by exocytosis as a conventional transmitter, but can also leak out of cells in large amounts under conditions of tissue damage. In high concentrations, ATP can act as an excitotoxin (like glutamate; see Ch. 40) and cause further neuronal damage. It is also quickly converted to adenosine, which exerts a protective effect. These special characteristics of adenosine metabolism suggest that it serves mainly as a safety

---

[3]See Khakh & Henderson (2000) for a description of how presynaptic cation-selective ligand-gated channels can, under different circumstances, facilitate or enhance neurotransmitter release.

Acetylcholine in the CNS

- Synthesis, storage and release of acetylcholine (ACh) in the central nervous system (CNS) are essentially the same as in the periphery (Ch. 13).
- ACh is widely distributed in the CNS, important pathways being:
  - basal forebrain (magnocellular) nuclei, which send a diffuse projection to most forebrain structures, including the cortex
  - septohippocampal projection
  - short interneurons in the striatum and nucleus accumbens.
- Certain neurodegenerative diseases, especially dementia and Parkinson's disease (see Ch. 40), are associated with abnormalities in cholinergic pathways.
- Both nicotinic and muscarinic (predominantly M_1) ACh receptors occur in the CNS. The former mediate the central effects of nicotine. Nicotinic receptors are mainly located presynaptically; there are few examples of transmission mediated by postsynaptic nicotinic receptors.
- Muscarinic receptors appear to mediate the main behavioural effects associated with ACh, namely effects on arousal, and on learning and short-term memory.
- Muscarinic antagonists (e.g. **hyoscine**) cause amnesia.

mechanism, protecting the neurons from damage when their viability is threatened, for example by ischaemia or seizure activity.

Adenosine produces its effects through G protein-coupled adenosine A receptors (see Ch. 16). There are four adenosine receptors – A_1, A_{2A}, A_{2B} and A_3 – distributed throughout the CNS. The overall effect of adenosine, or of various adenosine receptor agonists, is inhibitory, leading to effects such as drowsiness and sedation, motor incoordination, analgesia and anticonvulsant activity. Xanthines, such as **caffeine** (Ch. 48), which are antagonists at A_2 receptors, produce arousal and alertness.

For ATP there are two forms of receptor – P2X and P2Y receptors (see Ch. 16 also). P2X receptor subunits (P2X1-7) are trimeric ligand-gated cation channels that can be homomeric or heteromeric in composition. The evidence in favour of ATP acting on postsynaptic P2X receptors mediating fast synaptic transmission in the brain remains weak. P2X receptors are located on the postsynaptic cell membrane away from sites of synaptic contact, on nerve terminals and on astrocytes. Like acetylcholine at nicotinic receptors (see p. 475), ATP acting on P2X receptors appears to play a neuromodulatory role. There are eight P2Y receptors,[4] all are G protein coupled (see Table 16.1).

While there is little doubt that purinergic signalling plays a significant role in CNS function, our understanding is still very limited. There is optimism that purinergic receptor ligands – both agonists and antagonists – will prove useful in a wide range of CNS disorders (see Burnstock, 2008; Chen et al., 2013).

HISTAMINE

▼ Histamine is present in the brain in much smaller amounts than in other tissues, such as skin and lung, but undoubtedly serves a neurotransmitter role (see Brown et al., 2001). The cell bodies of histaminergic neurons, which also synthesise and release a variety of other transmitters, are restricted to a small part of the hypothalamus, and their axons run to virtually all parts of the brain. Unusually, no uptake mechanism for histamine is present, its action being terminated instead by enzymic methylation.

Histamine acts on four types of receptor (H_{1-4}; Ch. 17) in the brain H_1–H_3 occur in most brain regions, H_4 has a more restricted distribution. All are G protein coupled – H_1 receptors to G_q, H_2 to G_s and H_3 and H_4 to G_i/G_o. H_3 receptors are inhibitory receptors on histamine-releasing neurons as well as on terminals releasing other neurotransmitters.

Like other monoamine transmitters, histamine is involved in many different CNS functions. Histamine release follows a distinct circadian pattern, the neurons being active by day and silent by night. H_1 receptors in the cortex and reticular activating system contribute to arousal and wakefulness, and H_1 receptor antagonists produce sedation (see Ch. 43). Antihistamines are widely used to control nausea and vomiting, for example in motion sickness and middle ear disorders, as well as to induce sleep. Recent pharmaceutical industry activity has centred on the development of selective H_3 receptor antagonists as they may have potential for the treatment of cognitive impairment associated with Alzheimer's disease (see Ch. 40), schizophrenia (see Ch. 46), attention deficit hyperactivity disorder (see Ch. 48) and Parkinson's disease (see Ch. 40) as well as for the treatment of narcolepsy, obesity and pain states (Leurs et al., 2011).

OTHER CNS MEDIATORS

We now move from the familiar neuropharmacological territory of the 'classic' monoamines to some of the frontier towns, bordering on the Wild West. Useful drugs are still few and far between in this area, and if applied pharmacology is your main concern, you can safely skip the next part and wait a few years for law and order to be established.

MELATONIN

▼ Melatonin (N-acetyl-5-methoxytryptamine) (reviewed by Dubocovich et al., 2003) is synthesised exclusively in the pineal, an endocrine gland that plays a role in establishing circadian rhythms. The gland contains two enzymes, not found elsewhere, which convert 5-HT by acetylation and O-methylation to melatonin, its hormonal product.

There are two well-defined melatonin receptors (MT_1 and MT_2) which are G protein-coupled receptors – both coupling to G_i/G_o – found mainly in the brain and retina but also in peripheral

---

[4]Unfortunately the nomenclature for P2Y receptors has developed in a rather haphazard manner. There is compelling evidence for the existence of $P2Y_{1,2,4,6,11,12,13}$ and $_{14}$ receptors but not for others.

tissues (see Jockers et al., 2008). Another type (termed MT$_3$) has been suggested to be the enzyme quinone reductase 2 (QR2). The function of the interaction between melatonin and QR2 is still unclear.

Melatonin secretion (in all animals, whether diurnal or nocturnal in their habits) is high at night and low by day. This rhythm is controlled by input from the retina via a noradrenergic retinohypothalamic tract that terminates in the suprachiasmatic nucleus (SCN) in the hypothalamus, a structure often termed the 'biological clock', which generates the circadian rhythm. Activation of MT$_1$ receptors inhibits neuronal firing in the SCN and prolactin secretion from the pituitary. Activation of MT$_2$ receptors phase shifts circadian rhythms generated within the SCN. Melatonin has antioxidant properties and may be neuroprotective in Alzheimer's disease and Parkinson's disease (see Ch. 40).

Given orally, melatonin is well absorbed but quickly metabolised, its plasma half-life being a few minutes. It has been promoted as a means of controlling jet lag, or of improving the performance of night-shift workers, based on its ability to reset the circadian clock but detailed analysis does not support this view (Buscemi et al., 2006). It may be useful for the treatment of insomnia in the elderly and in autistic children with disturbed sleep. **Ramelteon**, an agonist at MT$_1$ and MT$_2$ receptors, is used to treat insomnia (see Ch. 44) and **agomelatine**, which has agonist actions at MT$_1$ and MT$_2$ receptors as well as antagonist actions at 5-HT$_{2C}$ receptors, is a novel antidepressant drug (see Ch. 47).

NITRIC OXIDE

Nitric oxide (NO) as a peripheral mediator is discussed in Chapter 20. Its significance as an important chemical mediator in the nervous system has demanded a considerable readjustment of our views about neurotransmission and neuromodulation (for review, see Garthwaite, 2008). The main defining criteria for transmitter substances – namely that neurons should possess machinery for synthesising and storing the substance, that it should be released from neurons by exocytosis, that it should interact with specific membrane receptors and that there should be mechanisms for its inactivation – do not apply to NO. Moreover, it is an inorganic gas, not at all like the kind of molecule we are used to. The mediator function of NO is now well established (Zhou & Zhu, 2009). NO diffuses rapidly through cell membranes, and its action is not highly localised. Its half-life depends greatly on the chemical environment, ranging from seconds in blood to several minutes in normal tissues. The rate of inactivation of NO (see Ch. 20, reaction 20.1) increases disproportionately with NO concentration, so low levels of NO are relatively stable. The presence of superoxide, with which NO reacts (see below), shortens its half-life considerably.

Nitric oxide in the nervous system is produced mainly by the constitutive neuronal form of *nitric oxide synthase* (nNOS; see Ch. 20), which can be detected either histochemically or by immunolabelling. This enzyme is present in roughly 2% of neurons, both short interneurons and long-tract neurons, in virtually all brain areas, with particular concentrations in the cerebellum and hippocampus. It occurs in cell bodies and dendrites, as well as in axon terminals, suggesting that NO may be produced both pre- and postsynaptically. nNOS is calmodulin-dependent and is activated by a rise in intracellular Ca^{2+} concentration, which can occur by many mechanisms, including action potential conduction and neurotransmitter action, especially by glutamate activation of Ca^{2+}-permeable NMDA receptors. NO is not stored, but

released as it is made. Many studies have shown that NO production is increased by activation of synaptic pathways, or by other events, such as brain ischaemia (see Ch. 40).

Nitric oxide exerts pre- and postsynaptic actions on neurons as well as acting on glial cells (Garthwaite, 2008). It produces its effects in two main ways:

1. By activation of soluble guanylyl cyclase, leading to the production of cGMP, which itself or through activation of protein kinase G can affect membrane ion channels (Steinert et al., 2010). This 'physiological' control mechanism operates at low NO concentrations of about 0.1 μmol/l.
2. By reacting with the superoxide free radical to generate peroxynitrite, a highly toxic anion that acts by oxidising various intracellular proteins. This requires concentrations of 1–10 μmol/l, which are achieved in brain ischaemia.

There is good evidence that NO plays a role in synaptic plasticity (see Ch. 38), because long-term potentiation and depression are reduced or prevented by NOS inhibitors and are absent in transgenic mice in which the *nNOS* gene has been disrupted.

Based on the same kind of evidence, NO is also believed to play an important part in the mechanisms by which ischaemia causes neuronal death (see Ch. 40). There is also evidence that it may be involved in other processes, including neurodegeneration in Parkinson's disease, senile dementia and amyotrophic lateral sclerosis, and the local control of blood flow linked to neuronal activity.

▼ **Carbon monoxide** (CO) is best known as a poisonous gas present in vehicle exhaust, which binds strongly to haemoglobin, causing tissue anoxia. However, it is also formed endogenously and has many features in common with NO. Neurons and other cells contain a CO-generating enzyme, haem oxygenase, and CO, like NO, activates guanylyl cyclase.

The role of CO as a CNS mediator is not well established, but there is some evidence that it plays a role in memory mechanisms in the hippocampus (see Cutajar & Edwards, 2007).

LIPID MEDIATORS

▼ The formation of arachidonic acid, and its conversion to eicosanoids (mainly prostaglandins, leukotrienes and hydroxyeicosatetraenoic acids (HETEs); see Ch. 17) and to endocannabinoids, anandamide and 2-arachidonoylglycerol (see Ch. 19), also take place in the CNS (for review see Pertwee, 2008).

Phospholipid cleavage, leading to arachidonic acid production, occurs in neurons in response to receptor activation by many different mediators, including neurotransmitters. The arachidonic acid so formed can act directly as an intracellular messenger, controlling both ion channels and various parts of the protein kinase cascade (see Ch. 3), producing both rapid and delayed effects on neuronal function. Both arachidonic acid itself and its products escape readily from the cell of origin and can affect neighbouring structures, including presynaptic terminals (retrograde signalling) and adjacent cells (paracrine signalling), by acting on receptors or by acting directly as intracellular messengers. Figure 39.8 shows a schematic view of the variety of different roles these agents can play at the synapse.

Arachidonic acid can be metabolised to eicosanoids, some of which (principally the HETEs) can also act as intracellular messengers acting in the same cell. Eicosanoids can also exert an autocrine effect via membrane receptors expressed by the cell (see Ch. 17). The eicosanoids play important roles in neural function including pain,

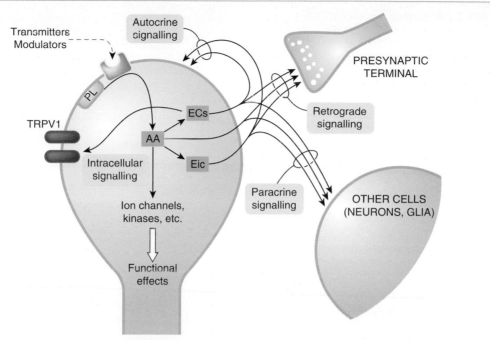

Fig. 39.8 **Postulated modes of signalling by lipid mediators.** Arachidonic acid (AA) is formed by receptor-mediated cleavage of membrane phospholipid. It can act directly as an intracellular messenger on ion channels or components of different kinase cascades, producing various long- and short-term effects. It can also be converted to eicosanoids (prostaglandins, leukotrienes or hydroxyeicosatetraenoic acids [HETEs]) or to the endocannabinoids (ECs), anandamide and 2-arachidonoylglycerol. Endocannabinoids can also act as intracellular messengers to activate TRPV1 channels. HETEs can also act directly as intracellular messengers. All these mediators also diffuse out of the cell, and exert effects on presynaptic terminals and neighbouring cells, acting either on extracellular receptors or intracellularly. There are examples of most of these modes of signalling but only limited information about their functional significance in the nervous system. Eic, eicosanoids; PL, membrane phospholipid.

temperature regulation, sleep induction, synaptic plasticity and spatial learning.

It is now generally accepted that the endocannabinoids act as retrograde synaptic messengers. They are synthesised and secreted in response to a rise in intracellular Ca^{2+} and activate presynaptic CB_1 receptors resulting in an inhibition of the release of neurotransmitters such as glutamate and GABA and the production of both long-term and short-term depression (see Castillo et al., 2012). CB_1 receptors are widely distributed in the brain and spinal cord whereas CB_2 receptor expression is much less. Agonists at CB_1 receptors have therapeutic potential for the treatment of vomiting, pain (CB_2 receptor agonists may also be effective in some pain states), muscle spasms as occur in conditions such as multiple sclerosis and anxiety, as well as in other brain disorders including Alzheimer's disease and tardive dyskinesias (see Pertwee, 2008). Endocannabinoids such as anandamide are metabolised by fatty acid amyl hydrolase (FAAH; see Ch. 19). Inhibitors of FAAH potentiate the effects of endocannabinoids and are effective analgesics in animal models of pain (Roques et al., 2012). The CB_1-receptor antagonist **rimonabant** was introduced as an antiobesity agent but subsequently had to be withdrawn because of negative effects on mood (see Ch. 19). One surprise in this field has been the discovery that endocannabinoids, besides being agonists at cannabinoid receptors, also activate TRPV1 channels (see Fig. 39.8 and Ch. 42), which are involved in the response of peripheral sensory nerve terminals to painful stimuli.

A FINAL MESSAGE

In the last two chapters we have taken a long and tortuous tour through the brain and its chemistry, with two questions at the back of our minds. What mediators and what receptors play a key role in what brain functions? How does the information relate to existing and future drugs that aim to correct malfunctions? Through the efforts of a huge army of researchers deploying an arsenal of powerful new techniques, the answers to these questions are slowly being produced. The array of potential CNS targets – comprising multiple receptor subtypes, many with the added complexity of heteromeric assemblies, splice variants, etc., along with regulatory mechanisms that control their expression and localisation – continues to grow in complexity. Speculation about the best target to aim at in order to ameliorate the effect of a particular brain malfunction, such as stroke or schizophrenia, has become less focused, even if better informed, than it was two decades ago. In the ensuing chapters in this section we shall find that most of the therapeutic successes have come from chance discoveries that were followed up empirically; few have followed a logical, mechanism-based route to success. The optimistic view is that this is changing, and that future therapeutic discoveries will depend less on luck and more on molecular logic. But the revolution is slow in coming. One of the key problems, perhaps, is that the brain puts cells, organelles and molecules exactly where they are needed, and uses the same molecules to perform different functions in different locations. Drug discovery scientists are getting quite good at devising molecule-specific ligands (see Ch. 60), but we lack delivery systems able to target them anatomically even to macroscopic brain regions, let alone to specific cells and subcellular structures.

Other transmitters and modulators

Purines

- ATP functions as a neurotransmitter, being stored in vesicles and released by exocytosis. It acts via ionotropic P2X receptors and metabotropic P2Y receptors.
- Cytosolic ATP is present at relatively high concentration and can be released directly if neuronal viability is compromised (e.g. in stroke). Excessive release may be neurotoxic.
- Released ATP is rapidly converted to ADP, AMP and adenosine.
- Adenosine is not stored in vesicles but is released by carrier mechanisms or generated from released ATP, mainly under pathological conditions.
- Adenosine exerts mainly inhibitory effects, through A_1 and A_2 receptors, resulting in sedative, anticonvulsant and neuroprotective effects, and acting as a safety mechanism.
- Methylxanthines (e.g. **caffeine**) are antagonists at A_2 receptors and increase wakefulness.

Histamine

- Histamine fulfils the criteria for a neurotransmitter. Histaminergic neurons originate in a small area of the hypothalamus and have a widespread distribution.
- H_1, H_2 and H_3 receptors are widespread in the brain.
- The functions of histamine are not well understood, the main clues being that histaminergic neurons are active during waking hours, and H_1 receptor antagonists are strongly sedative.
- H_1 receptor antagonists are antiemetic.

Melatonin

- Melatonin is synthesised from 5-hydroxytryptamine, mainly in the pineal gland, from which it is released as a circulating hormone.
- Secretion is controlled by light intensity, being low by day and high by night. Fibres from the retina run to the suprachiasmatic nucleus ('biological clock'), which controls the pineal gland via its sympathetic innervation.
- Melatonin acts on MT_1 and MT_2 receptors in the brain.
- Agonists at melatonin receptors induce sleep and have antidepressant properties.

Nitric oxide (see Ch. 20)

- Neuronal nitric oxide synthase (nNOS) is present in many central nervous system neurons, and nitric oxide (NO) production is increased by mechanisms (e.g. transmitter action) that raise intracellular Ca^{2+}.
- NO affects neuronal function by increasing cGMP formation, producing both inhibitory and excitatory effects on neurons.
- In larger amounts, NO forms peroxynitrite, which contributes to neurotoxicity.
- Inhibition of nNOS reduces long-term potentiation and long-term depression, probably because NO functions as a retrograde messenger. Inhibition of nNOS also protects against ischaemic brain damage in animal models.
- Carbon monoxide shares many properties with NO and may also be a neural mediator.

Lipid mediators

- Arachidonic acid is produced in neurons by receptor-mediated hydrolysis of phospholipid. It is converted to various eicosanoids and endocannabinoids.
- Arachidonic acid itself, as well as its active products, can produce rapid and slow effects by regulation of ion channels and protein kinase cascades. Such effects can occur in the donor cell or in adjacent cells and nerve terminals.
- Anandamide and 2-arachidonoylglycerol are endogenous activators of cannabinoid CB_1 and CB_2 receptors (Ch. 19) and also of the TRPV1 receptor (Ch. 42).

REFERENCES AND FURTHER READING

General references

Iversen, L.L., Iversen, S.D., Bloom, F.E., Roth, R.H., 2009. Introduction to Neuropsychopharmacology. Oxford University Press, New York. (*Clear and well-written textbook giving more detailed information on many topics covered in this chapter*)

Nestler, E.J., Hyman, S.E., Malenka, R.C., 2008. Molecular Neuropharmacology: A Foundation for Clinical Neuroscience, second ed. McGraw-Hill, New York. (*Good textbook*)

Noradrenaline

Bylund, D.B., 2007. Receptors for norepinephrine and signal transduction pathways. In: Ordway, G.A., Schwartz, M.A., Frazer, A. (Eds.), Brain Norepinephrine. Cambridge University Press, London.

Head, G.A., Mayorov, D.N., 2006. Imidazoline receptors, novel agents and therapeutic potential. Cardiovasc. Hematol. Agents Med. Chem. 4, 17–32. (*Provides an update on the elusive imidazoline receptors*)

Dopamine

Björklund, A., Dunnett, S.B., 2007. Dopamine neuron systems in the brain: an update. Trends Neurosci. 30, 194–202. (*Short review of the anatomy of dopaminergic neurons in the central nervous system*)

De Mei, C., Ramos, M., Iitaka, C., Borrelli, E., 2009. Getting specialized: presynaptic and postsynaptic dopamine D_2 receptors. Curr. Opin. Pharmacol. 9, 53–58.

Girault, J.-A., Greengard, P., 2004. The neurobiology of dopamine signalling. Arch. Neurol. 61, 641–644. (*Short review article*)

5-Hydroxytryptamine

Filip, M., Bader, M., 2009. Overview of 5-HT receptors and their role in physiology and pathology of the central nervous system. Pharm. Rep. 61, 761–777.

Jensen, A.A., Davies, P.A., Bräuner-Osborne, H., Krzywkowski, K., 2008. 3B but which 3B? And that's just one of the questions: the heterogeneity of human $5-HT_3$ receptors. Trends Pharmacol. Sci. 29, 437–444. (*Discusses the potential complexity of $5-HT_3$ receptors now that new subunits have been discovered*)

Muller, C., Jacobs, B., 2009. Handbook of Behavioral Neurobiology of Serotonin, vol. 18, (Handbook of Behavioral Neuroscience). Academic Press, Oxford. (*Extensive coverage of the role of 5-HT in the brain*)

Peters, J.A., Hales, T.G., Lambert, J.J., 2005. Molecular determinants of single-channel conductance and ion selectivity in the Cys-loop family:

insights from the 5-HT$_3$ receptor. Trends Pharmacol. Sci. 26, 587–594. (*For those who thought ligand-gated ion channels were just simple pores opened by neurotransmitters, this review will contain a few surprises!*)

Acetylcholine

Delmas, P., Brown, D.A., 2005. Pathways modulating neural KCNQ/M (Kv7) potassium channels. Nat. Rev. Neurosci. 6, 850–862. (*Gives information on the functional significance of the 'M-current' and the therapeutic potential of drugs that modify it*)

Gotti, C., Zoli, M., Clementi, F., 2008. Brain nicotinic acetylcholine receptors: native subtypes and their relevance. Trends Pharmacol. Sci. 27, 482–491.

Hasselmo, M.E., 2006. The role of acetylcholine in learning and memory. Curr. Opin. Neurobiol. 16, 710–715.

Khakh, B.S., Henderson, G., 2000. Modulation of fast synaptic transmission by presynaptic ligand-gated cation channels. J. Auton. Nerv. Syst. 81, 110–121. (*Describes how activation of presynaptic ligand-gated cation channels can either enhance or inhibit neurotransmitter release*)

Wess, J., 2004. Muscarinic acetylcholine receptor knockout mice: novel phenotypes and clinical implications. Annu. Rev. Pharmacol. Toxicol. 44, 423–450. (*Description of functional effects of deleting various peripheral and central mAChR isoforms*)

Other messengers

Brown, R.E., Stevens, D.R., Haas, H.L., 2001. The physiology of brain histamine. Prog. Neurobiol. 63, 637–672. (*Useful review article*)

Burnstock, G., 2008. Purinergic signalling and disorders of the central nervous system. Nat. Rev. Drug Discov. 7, 575–590. (*Extensive discussion of the therapeutic potential of drugs acting at purinergic receptors*)

Buscemi, N., Vandermeer, B., Hooton, N., et al., 2006. Efficacy and safety of exogenous melatonin for secondary sleep disorders and sleep disorders accompanying sleep restriction: meta-analysis. BMJ 332, 385–393.

Castillo, P.E., Younts, T.J., Chávez, A.E., Hashimotodani, Y., 2012. Endocannabinoid signaling and synaptic function. Neuron 76, 70–81.

Chen, J.F., Eltzschig, H.K., Fredholm, B.B., 2013. Adenosine receptors as drug targets – what are the challenges? Nat. Rev. Drug Discov. 12, 265–286.

Cutajar, M.C., Edwards, T.M., 2007. Evidence for the role of endogenous carbon monoxide in memory processing. J. Cogn. Neurosci. 19, 557–562.

Dubocovich, M.L., Rivera-Bermudez, M.A., Gerdin, M.J., Masana, M.I., 2003. Molecular pharmacology, regulation and function of mammalian melatonin receptors. Front. Biosci. 8, 1093–1108.

Fredholm, B.B., Chen, J.F., Masino, S.A., Vaugeois, J.M., 2005. Actions of adenosine at its receptors in the CNS: insights from knockouts and from drugs. Annu. Rev. Pharmacol. Toxicol. 45, 395–412.

Garthwaite, J., 2008. Concepts of neural nitric oxide-mediated transmission. Eur. J. Neurosci. 27, 2783–2802.

Jockers, R., Maurice, P., Boutin, J.A., Delagrange, P., 2008. Melatonin receptors, heterodimerization, signal transduction and binding sites: what's new? Br. J. Pharmacol. 154, 1182–1195.

Khakh, B.S., North, R.A., 2012. Neuromodulation by extracellular ATP and P2X receptors in the CNS. Neuron 76, 51–69.

Leurs, R., Vischer, H.F., Wijtmans, M., de Esch, I.J., 2011. En route to new blockbuster anti-histamines: surveying the offspring of the expanding histamine receptor family. Trends Pharmacol. Sci. 32, 250–257.

Pertwee, R.G., 2008. Ligands that target cannabinoid receptors in the brain: from THC to anandamide and beyond. Addict. Biol. 13, 147–159.

Roques, B.P., Fournié-Zaluski, M.-C., Wurm, M., 2012. Inhibiting the breakdown of endogenous opioids and cannabinoids to alleviate pain. Nat. Rev. Drug Discov. 11, 292–310. (*Interesting review of potential for such inhibitors to reduce pain*)

Steinert, J.R., Chernova, T., Forsythe, I.D., 2010. Nitric oxide signaling in brain function, dysfunction, and dementia. Neuroscientist 16, 435–452.

Zhou, L., Zhu, D.-Y., 2009. Neuronal nitric oxide synthase: structure, subcellular localization, regulation and clinical implications. Nitric Oxide 20, 223–230.

40 Neurodegenerative diseases

OVERVIEW

As a rule, dead neurons in the adult central nervous system (CNS) are not replaced,[1] nor can their terminals regenerate when their axons are interrupted. Therefore any pathological process causing neuronal death generally has irreversible consequences. At first sight, this appears to be very unpromising territory for pharmacological intervention, and indeed drug therapy is currently very limited, except in the case of Parkinson's disease (PD; see p. 491). Nevertheless, the incidence and social impact of neurodegenerative brain disorders in ageing populations has resulted in a massive research effort in recent years.

In this chapter, we focus mainly on three common neurodegenerative conditions: Alzheimer's disease (AD), PD and ischaemic brain damage (stroke). AD and PD are the commonest examples of a group of chronic, slowly developing conditions that include various prion diseases (e.g. Creutzfeldt–Jakob disease, CJD). They have a common aetiology in that they are caused by the aggregation of misfolded variants of normal physiological proteins. The high hopes that new pathophysiological understanding would lead to significant therapeutic progress in this important area remain largely unrealised, and to date the available therapeutic interventions are aimed at compensating for, rather than preventing or reversing, the neuronal loss. Stroke, which is a common disorder of enormous socioeconomic importance, results from acute ischaemic brain damage, quite different from the aetiology of chronic neurodegenerative diseases, requiring different but equally challenging therapeutic approaches.

Looking into the future, the hope is that stem cell therapies will be developed for these disorders. The main topics discussed in this chapter are:

- mechanisms responsible for neuronal death, focusing on protein aggregation (e.g. amyloidosis), excitotoxicity, oxidative stress and apoptosis
- pharmacological approaches to neuroprotection, based on the above mechanisms
- pharmacological approaches to compensation for neuronal loss (applicable mainly to AD and PD).

---

[1]It is recognised that new neurons are formed from progenitor cells (*neurogenesis*) in certain regions of the adult brain and can become functionally integrated, even in primates (see Rakic, 2002; Zhao et al., 2008). Neurogenesis in the hippocampus is thought to play a role in learning and memory, but plays little if any role in brain repair. However, learning how to harness the inherent ability of neuronal progenitors (stem cells) to form new neurons is seen as an obvious approach to treating neurodegenerative disorders.

PROTEIN MISFOLDING AND AGGREGATION IN CHRONIC NEURODEGENERATIVE DISEASES

Protein misfolding and aggregation is the first step in many neurodegenerative diseases (see Peden & Ironside, 2012). Misfolding means the adoption of abnormal conformations, by certain normally expressed proteins, such that they tend to form large insoluble aggregates (Fig. 40.1). The conversion of the linear amino acid chain produced by the ribosome into a functional protein requires it to be folded correctly into a compact conformation with specific amino acids correctly located on its surface. This complicated stepwise sequence can easily go wrong and lead to misfolded variants that are unable to find a way back to the correct 'native' conformation. The misfolded molecules lack the normal function of the protein, but can nonetheless make mischief within the cell. The misfolding often means that hydrophobic residues that would normally be buried in the core of the protein are exposed on its surface, which gives the molecules a strong tendency to stick to cell membranes and aggregate, initially as oligomers and then as insoluble microscopic aggregates (Fig. 40.1), leading to the death of neurons. The tendency to adopt such conformations may be favoured by specific mutations of the protein in question, or by infection with prions.

Misfolded conformations can be generated spontaneously at a low rate throughout life, so that aggregates accumulate gradually with age. In the nervous system, the aggregates often form distinct structures, generally known as *amyloid deposits*, that are visible under the microscope and are characteristic of neurodegenerative disease. Although the mechanisms are not clear, such aggregates, or the misfolded protein precursors, lead to neuronal death. Examples of neurodegenerative diseases that are caused by such protein misfolding and aggregation are shown in Table 40.1.

The brain possesses a variety of protective mechanisms that limit the accumulation of such protein aggregates. The main ones involve the production of 'chaperone' proteins, which bind to newly synthesised or misfolded proteins and encourage them to fold correctly, and the 'ubiquitination' reaction, which prepares proteins for destruction within the cell. Accumulation of protein deposits occurs when these protective mechanisms are unable to cope.

MECHANISMS OF NEURONAL DEATH

Acute injury to cells causes them to undergo *necrosis*, recognised pathologically by cell swelling, vacuolisation and lysis, and associated with Ca^{2+} overload of the cells and

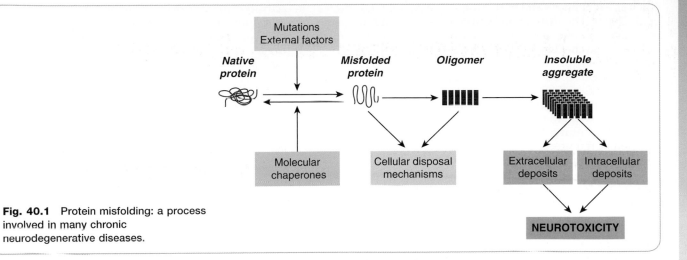

Fig. 40.1 Protein misfolding: a process involved in many chronic neurodegenerative diseases.

Table 40.1 Examples of neurodegenerative diseases associated with protein misfolding and aggregation[a]

Disease	Protein	Characteristic pathology	Notes
Alzheimer's disease	β-Amyloid (Aβ)	Amyloid plaques	Aβ mutations occur in rare familial forms of Alzheimer's disease
	Tau	Neurofibrillary tangles	Implicated in other pathologies ('tauopathies') as well as Alzheimer's disease
Parkinson's disease	α-Synuclein	Lewy bodies	α-Synuclein mutations occur in some types of familial Parkinson's disease
Creutzfeldt–Jakob disease	Prion protein	Insoluble aggregates of prion protein	Transmitted by infection with prion protein in its misfolded state
Huntington's disease	Huntingtin	No gross lesions	One of several genetic 'polyglutamine repeat' disorders
Amyotrophic lateral sclerosis (motor neuron disease)	Superoxide dismutase	Loss of motor neurons	Mutated superoxide dismutase tends to form aggregates; loss of enzyme function increases susceptibility to oxidative stress

[a]Protein aggregation disorders are often collectively known as amyloidoses and commonly affect organs other than the brain.

Protein misfolding

- Many chronic neurodegenerative diseases involve the misfolding of normal or mutated forms of physiological proteins. Examples include Alzheimer's disease, Parkinson's disease, amyotrophic lateral sclerosis and many less common diseases.
- Misfolded proteins are normally removed by intracellular degradation pathways, which may be altered in neurodegenerative disorders.
- Misfolded proteins tend to aggregate, initially as soluble oligomers, later as large insoluble aggregates that accumulate intracellularly or extracellularly as microscopic deposits, which are stable and resistant to proteolysis.
- Misfolded proteins often present hydrophobic surface residues that promote aggregation and association with membranes.
- The mechanisms responsible for neuronal death are unclear, but there is evidence that both the soluble aggregates and the microscopic deposits may be neurotoxic.

membrane damage (see p. 484). Necrotic cells typically spill their contents into the surrounding tissue, evoking an inflammatory response. Chronic inflammation is a feature of most neurodegenerative disorders (see Schwab & McGeer, 2008), and a possible target for therapeutic intervention.

Cells can also die by *apoptosis* or programmed cell death (see Ch. 5), a mechanism that is essential for many processes throughout life, including development, immune regulation and tissue remodelling. Apoptosis, as well as necrosis, occurs in both acute neurodegenerative disorders (such as stroke and head injury) and chronic ones (such as Alzheimer's and Parkinson's disease; see Okouchi et al., 2007). The distinction between necrosis and apoptosis as processes leading to neurodegeneration is not absolute, for challenges such as excitotoxicity and oxidative stress may be enough to kill cells directly by necrosis or, if less intense, may induce them to undergo apoptosis. Both processes therefore represent possible targets for putative neuroprotective drug therapy. Pharmacological interference with the apoptotic pathway may become possible in the future, but for the present most efforts are directed at the processes involved in cell necrosis, and at compensating pharmacologically for the neuronal loss.

EXCITOTOXICITY

Despite its ubiquitous role as a neurotransmitter, **glutamate** is highly toxic to neurons, a phenomenon dubbed *excitotoxicity* (see Ch. 38). A low concentration of glutamate applied to neurons in culture kills the cells, and the finding in the 1970s that glutamate given orally produces neurodegeneration *in vivo* caused considerable alarm because of the widespread use of glutamate as a 'taste-enhancing' food additive. The 'Chinese restaurant syndrome' – an acute attack of neck stiffness and chest pain – is well known, but so far the possibility of more serious neurotoxicity is only hypothetical.

Local injection of the glutamate receptor agonist *kainic acid* is used experimentally to produce neurotoxic lesions. It acts by excitation of local glutamate-releasing neurons, and the release of glutamate, acting on NMDA receptors, and also metabotropic receptors (Ch. 38), leads to neuronal death.

Calcium overload is the essential factor in excitotoxicity. The mechanisms by which this occurs and leads to cell death are as follows (Fig. 40.2):

- Glutamate activates NMDA, AMPA and metabotropic receptors (sites 1, 2 and 3). Activation of AMPA receptors depolarises the cell, which removes the Mg^{2+} block of NMDA channels (see Ch. 38), permitting Ca^{2+} entry. Depolarisation also opens voltage-dependent calcium channels (site 4). Metabotropic receptors cause the release of intracellular Ca^{2+} from the endoplasmic reticulum. Na^+ entry further contributes to Ca^{2+} entry by stimulating Ca^{2+}/Na^+ exchange (site 5). Depolarisation inhibits or reverses glutamate uptake (site 6), thus increasing the extracellular glutamate concentration.
- The mechanisms that normally operate to counteract the rise in cytosolic free Ca^{2+} concentration, $[Ca^{2+}]_i$, include the Ca^{2+} efflux pump (site 7) and, indirectly, the Na^+ pump (site 8).
- The mitochondria and endoplasmic reticulum act as capacious sinks for Ca^{2+} and normally keep $[Ca^{2+}]_i$ under control. Loading of the mitochondrial stores beyond a certain point, however, disrupts mitochondrial function, reducing ATP synthesis, thus reducing the energy available for the membrane pumps and for Ca^{2+} accumulation by the endoplasmic reticulum. Formation of reactive oxygen species is also enhanced. This represents the danger point at which positive feedback exaggerates the process.
- Raised $[Ca^{2+}]_i$ affects many processes, the chief ones relevant to neurotoxicity being:
  – increased glutamate release from nerve terminals
  – activation of proteases (calpains) and lipases, causing membrane damage

– activation of nitric oxide synthase; while low concentrations of nitric oxide are neuroprotective, high concentrations in the presence of reactive oxygen species generate peroxynitrite and hydroxyl free radicals, which damage many important biomolecules, including membrane lipids, proteins and DNA
– increased arachidonic acid release, which increases free radical and inflammatory mediator production and also inhibits glutamate uptake (site 6).

Glutamate and Ca^{2+} are arguably the two most ubiquitous chemical signals, extracellular and intracellular, respectively, underlying brain function, so it is disconcerting that such cytotoxic mayhem can be unleashed when they get out of control. Both are stored in dangerous amounts in subcellular organelles, like hand grenades in an ammunition store. Defence against excitotoxicity is clearly essential if our brains are to have any chance of staying alive. Mitochondrial energy metabolism provides one line of defence (see p. 486), and impaired mitochondrial function, by rendering neurons vulnerable to excitotoxic damage, may be a factor in various neurodegenerative conditions, including PD. Furthermore, impaired mitochondrial function can cause release of cytochrome c, which is an important initiator of apoptosis.

The role of excitotoxicity in ischaemic brain damage is well established (see p. 486), and it is also believed to be a factor in other neurodegenerative diseases, such as those discussed below.

▼ There are several examples of neurodegenerative conditions caused by environmental toxins acting as agonists on glutamate receptors. *Domoic acid* is a glutamate analogue produced by mussels, which was identified as the cause of an epidemic of severe mental and neurological deterioration in a group of Newfoundlanders in 1987. On the island of Guam, a syndrome combining the features of dementia, paralysis and PD was traced to an excitotoxic amino acid, β-methylamino-alanine, in the seeds of a local plant. Discouraging the consumption of these seeds has largely eliminated the disease.

Disappointingly, intense effort, based on the mechanisms described above, to find effective drugs for a range of neurodegenerative disorders in which excitotoxicity is believed to play a part has had very limited success. **Riluzole** retards to some degree the deterioration of patients with amyotrophic lateral sclerosis. Its precise mechanism of action is unclear. **Memantine**, a compound first described 40 years ago, is a weak NMDA receptor antagonist that produces slight improvement in moderate-to-severe cases of AD.

APOPTOSIS

Apoptosis can be initiated by various cell surface signals (see Ch. 5). The cell is systematically dismantled, and the shrunken remnants are removed by macrophages without causing inflammation. Apoptotic cells can be identified by a staining technique that detects the characteristic DNA breaks. Many different signalling pathways can result in apoptosis, but in all cases the final pathway resulting in cell death is the activation of a family of proteases (caspases), which inactivate various intracellular proteins. Neural apoptosis is normally prevented by neuronal growth factors, including *nerve growth factor* and *brain-derived neurotrophic factor*, secreted proteins that are required for the survival of different populations of neurons in the CNS. These growth factors regulate the expression of the two gene products Bax and Bcl-2, Bax

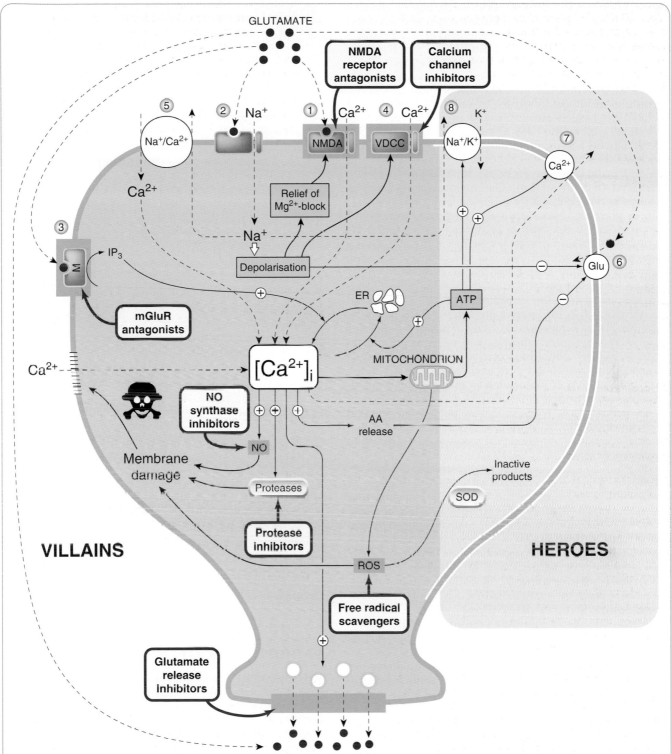

Fig. 40.2 **Mechanisms of excitotoxicity.** Membrane receptors, ion channels and transporters, identified by numbers 1–8, are discussed in the text. Possible sites of action of neuroprotective drugs (not yet of proven clinical value) are highlighted. Mechanisms on the left (villains) are those that favour cell death, while those on the right (heroes) are protective. See text for details. AA, arachidonic acid; ER, endoplasmic reticulum; Glu, glutamate uptake; IP$_3$, inositol trisphosphate; M, mGluR, metabotropic glutamate receptor; NO, nitric oxide; ROS, reactive oxygen species; SOD, superoxide dismutase; VDCC, voltage-dependent calcium channel.

being proapoptotic and Bcl-2 being antiapoptotic (see Ch. 5). Blocking apoptosis by interfering at specific points on these pathways represents an attractive strategy for developing neuroprotective drugs, but one that has yet to bear fruit.

OXIDATIVE STRESS

The brain has high energy needs, which are met almost entirely by mitochondrial oxidative phosphorylation, generating ATP at the same time as reducing molecular

O_2 to H_2O. Under certain conditions, highly reactive oxygen species (ROS), for example oxygen and hydroxyl free radicals and H_2O_2, may be generated as side products of this process (see Coyle & Puttfarken, 1993; Barnham et al., 2004). Oxidative stress is the result of excessive production of these reactive species. They can also be produced as a byproduct of other biochemical pathways, including nitric oxide synthesis and arachidonic acid metabolism (which are implicated in excitotoxicity; see p. 484), as well as the P450 mono-oxygenase system (see Ch. 9). Unchecked, reactive oxygen radicals attack many key molecules, including enzymes, membrane lipids and DNA. During periods of tissue reperfusion following ischaemia (e.g. in stroke), delinquent leukocytes may exacerbate this problem by releasing their own cytotoxic oxygen products. Not surprisingly, defence mechanisms are provided, in the form of enzymes such as *superoxide dismutase* (SOD) and *catalase*, as well as antioxidants such as ascorbic acid, glutathione and α-tocopherol (vitamin E), which normally keep these reactive species in check. Some cytokines, especially tumour necrosis factor (TNF)-α, which is produced in conditions of brain ischaemia or inflammation (Ch.18), exert a protective effect, partly by increasing the expression of SOD. Transgenic animals lacking TNF receptors show enhanced susceptibility to brain ischaemia. Mutations of the gene encoding SOD (Fig. 40.2) are associated with *amyotrophic lateral sclerosis* (ALS, also known as motor neuron disease), a fatal paralytic disease resulting from progressive degeneration of motor neurons, and transgenic mice expressing mutated SOD develop a similar condition.[2] Accumulation of aggregates of misfolded mutated SOD may also contribute to neurodegeneration.

Mitochondria play a central role in energy metabolism, failure of which leads to oxidative stress. Damage to mitochondria, leading to the release of cytochrome c into the cytosol, also initiates apoptosis. Mitochondrial integrity is therefore essential for neuronal survival, and mitochondrial dysfunction is seen as a major factor in many neurodegenerative disorders (see Itoh et al., 2013). It is possible that accumulated or inherited mutations in enzymes such as those of the mitochondrial respiratory chain lead to a congenital or age-related increase in susceptibility to oxidative stress, which is manifest in different kinds of inherited neurodegenerative disorders (such as Huntington's disease), and in age-related neurodegeneration.

Oxidative stress is both a cause and consequence of inflammation (Ch. 6), which is a general feature of neurodegenerative disease and is thought to contribute to neuronal damage (see Schwab & McGeer, 2008).

Several possible targets for therapeutic intervention with neuroprotective drugs are shown in Figure 40.2.

ISCHAEMIC BRAIN DAMAGE

After heart disease and cancer, strokes are the commonest cause of death in Europe and North America, and the 70% that are non-fatal are the commonest cause of disability. Approximately 85% of strokes are *ischaemic*, usually due to

---

Excitotoxicity and oxidative stress

- Excitatory amino acids, especially glutamate, can cause neuronal death.
- Excitotoxicity is associated mainly with activation of NMDA receptors, but other types of excitatory amino acid receptors also contribute.
- Excitotoxicity results from a sustained rise in intracellular Ca^{2+} concentration (Ca^{2+} overload).
- Excitotoxicity can occur under pathological conditions (e.g. cerebral ischaemia, epilepsy) in which excessive glutamate release occurs. It can also occur when chemicals such as **kainic acid** are administered.
- Raised intracellular Ca^{2+} causes cell death by various mechanisms, including activation of proteases, formation of free radicals and lipid peroxidation. Formation of nitric oxide and arachidonic acid are also involved.
- Various mechanisms act normally to protect neurons against excitotoxicity, the main ones being Ca^{2+} transport systems, mitochondrial function and the production of free radical scavengers.
- Oxidative stress refers to conditions (e.g. hypoxia) in which the protective mechanisms are compromised, reactive oxygen species accumulate and neurons become more susceptible to excitotoxic damage.
- Excitotoxicity due to environmental chemicals may contribute to some neurodegenerative disorders.
- Measures designed to reduce excitotoxicity include the use of glutamate antagonists, calcium channel-blocking drugs and free radical scavengers; none is yet proven for clinical use.
- Mitochondrial dysfunction, associated with ageing, environmental toxins and genetic abnormalities, leads to oxidative stress and is a common feature of neurodegenerative diseases.

---

thrombosis of a major cerebral artery. The remainder are *haemorrhagic*, due to rupture of a cerebral artery. Atherosclerosis is the usual underlying cause of both types.

PATHOPHYSIOLOGY

Interruption of blood supply to the brain initiates the cascade of neuronal events shown in Figure 40.2, which lead in turn to later consequences, including cerebral oedema and inflammation, which can also contribute to brain damage. Further damage can occur following reperfusion,[3] because of the production of reactive oxygen species when the oxygenation is restored. Reperfusion injury may be an important component in stroke patients. These secondary processes often take hours to develop, providing a window of opportunity for therapeutic intervention. The lesion produced by occlusion of a major cerebral artery consists of a central core in which the neurons quickly undergo irreversible necrosis, surrounded by a penumbra of compromised tissue in which inflammation

---

[2]Surprisingly, some SOD mutations associated with ALS are more, rather than less, active than the normal enzyme. The mechanism responsible for neurodegeneration probably involves abnormal accumulation of the enzyme in mitochondria.

[3]Nevertheless, early reperfusion (within 3 h of the thrombosis) is clearly beneficial, based on clinical evidence with fibrinolytic drugs.

and apoptotic cell death develop over a period of several hours. It is assumed that neuroprotective therapies, given within a few hours, might inhibit this secondary penumbral damage.

Glutamate excitotoxicity plays a critical role in brain ischaemia. Ischaemia causes depolarisation of neurons, and the release of large amounts of glutamate. Ca^{2+} accumulation occurs, partly as a result of glutamate acting on NMDA receptors, as both Ca^{2+} entry and cell death following cerebral ischaemia are inhibited by drugs that block NMDA receptors or channels (see Ch. 38). Nitric oxide is also produced in amounts much greater than result from normal neuronal activity (i.e. to levels that are toxic rather than modulatory).

THERAPEUTIC APPROACHES

The only drug currently approved for treating strokes is a recombinant tissue plasminogen activator, **alteplase**, given intravenously, which helps to restore blood flow by dispersing the thrombus (see Ch. 24). A controlled trial showed that it did not reduce mortality (about 8%), but gave significant functional benefit to patients who survive. To be effective, it must be given within about 3 h of the thrombotic episode. Also, it must not be given in the 15% of cases where the cause is haemorrhage rather than thrombosis, so preliminary computerised tomography (CT) scanning is essential. These stringent requirements seriously limit the use of fibrinolytic agents for treating stroke, except where specialised rapid response facilities are available. The use of early surgical procedures to remove clots, in combination with alteplase, is increasing in specialised acute stroke treatment centres.

A preferable approach would be to use neuroprotective agents aimed at rescuing cells in the penumbral region of the lesion, which are otherwise likely to die. In animal models involving cerebral artery occlusion, many drugs targeted at the mechanisms shown in Figure 40.2 (not to mention many others that have been tested on the basis of more far-flung theories) act in this way to reduce the size of the infarct. These include glutamate antagonists, calcium and sodium channel inhibitors, free radical scavengers, anti-inflammatory drugs, protease inhibitors and others (see Green, 2008). It seems that almost anything works in these animal models. However, of the many drugs that have been tested in over 100 clinical trials, none was effective. The dispiriting list of failures includes calcium- and sodium-channel blockers (e.g. **nimodipine**, **fosphenytoin**), NMDA-receptor antagonists (**selfotel**, **eliprodil**, **dextromethorphan**), drugs that inhibit glutamate release (adenosine analogues, **lobeluzole**), drugs that enhance GABA effects (e.g. **chlormethiazole**), 5-HT antagonists, metal chelators and various free radical scavengers (e.g. **tirilazad**). There is still hope that mGlu1-receptor antagonists or negative allosteric modulators might be effective in the treatment of ischemic brain damage.

Controlled clinical trials on stroke patients are problematic and very expensive, partly because of the large variability of outcome in terms of functional recovery, which means that large groups of patients (typically thousands) need to be observed for several months. The need to start therapy within hours of the attack is an additional problem.

One area of promise is the use of subanaesthetic doses of **xenon**, which has NMDA receptor antagonist properties (Ch. 41), in combination with hypothermia to treat hypoxia-induced brain damage in neonates (Esencan et al., 2013).

Stroke treatment is certainly not – so far at least – one of pharmacology's success stories, and medical hopes rest more on prevention (e.g. by controlling blood pressure, taking aspirin and preventing atherosclerosis) than on treatment.[4]

> ### Stroke
>
> - Associated with intracerebral thrombosis or haemorrhage (less common), resulting in rapid death of neurons by necrosis in the centre of the lesion, followed by more gradual (hours) degeneration of cells in the penumbra due to excitotoxicity and inflammation.
> - Spontaneous functional recovery occurs to a highly variable degree.
> - Although many types of drug that interfere with excitotoxicity are able to reduce infarct size in experimental animals, none of these has so far proved efficacious in humans.
> - Recombinant tissue plasminogen activator (**alteplase**), which disperses blood clots, is beneficial if it is given within 3 h; haemorrhagic stroke must be excluded by imaging before its administration.

ALZHEIMER'S DISEASE

Loss of cognitive ability with age is considered to be a normal process whose rate and extent is very variable. AD was originally defined as presenile dementia, but it now appears that the same pathology underlies the dementia[5] irrespective of the age of onset. AD refers to dementia that does not have an antecedent cause, such as stroke, brain trauma or alcohol. Its prevalence rises sharply with age, from about 5% at 65 to 90% or more at 95. Until recently, age-related dementia was considered to result from the steady loss of neurons that normally goes on throughout life, possibly accelerated by a failing blood supply associated with atherosclerosis. Studies over the past three decades have, however, revealed specific genetic and molecular mechanisms underlying AD (see Querfurth & LaFerla, 2010). These advances have raised hopes of more effective treatments, but success has proved elusive.

PATHOGENESIS OF ALZHEIMER'S DISEASE

Alzheimer's disease is associated with brain shrinkage and localised loss of neurons, mainly in the hippocampus and basal forebrain. The loss of cholinergic neurons in the hippocampus and frontal cortex is a feature of the disease, and is thought to underlie the cognitive

---

[4]Eating dark chocolate is believed to reduce the risk of stroke. Flavonoids in the chocolate may be protective due to antioxidant, anti-clotting and anti-inflammatory properties. However, this is not a reason to over indulge.
[5]The term *dementia* is used to describe progressive loss of cognitive function rather than being 'demented', i.e. behaving irrationally due to anger.

deficit and loss of short-term memory that occur in AD. Two microscopic features are characteristic of the disease, namely extracellular *amyloid plaques*, consisting of amorphous extracellular deposits of β-amyloid protein (known as Aβ), and intraneuronal *neurofibrillary tangles*, comprising filaments of a phosphorylated form of a microtubule-associated protein (Tau). Both of these deposits are protein aggregates that result from misfolding of native proteins, as discussed above. They appear also in normal brains, although in smaller numbers. The early appearance of amyloid deposits presages the development of AD, although symptoms may not develop for many years. Altered processing of amyloid protein from its precursor (*amyloid precursor protein*, APP) is now recognised as the key to the pathogenesis of AD. This conclusion is based on several lines of evidence, particularly the genetic analysis of certain, relatively rare, types of familial AD, in which mutations of the APP gene, or of other genes (e.g. for presenilins and sortilin-related receptor 1) that

control amyloid processing, have been discovered. The APP gene resides on chromosome 21, of which an extra copy is the cause of Down's syndrome, in which early AD-like dementia occurs in association with overexpression of APP.

▼ Amyloid deposits consist of aggregates of Aβ (Fig. 40.3), a 40- or 42-residue segment of APP, generated by the action of specific proteases (*secretases*). Aβ40 is produced normally in small amounts, whereas Aβ42 is overproduced as a result of the genetic mutations mentioned above. Both proteins aggregate to form *amyloid plaques*, but Aβ42 shows a stronger tendency than Aβ40 to do so, and appears to be the main culprit in amyloid formation. APP is a 770-amino acid membrane protein normally expressed by many cells, including CNS neurons. Cleavage by α-secretase releases the large extracellular domain as *soluble APP*, which is believed to serve a physiological trophic function. Formation of Aβ involves cleavage at two different points, including one in the intramembrane domain of APP, by β- and γ-secretases (Fig. 40.3). γ-Secretase is a clumsy enzyme – actually a large intramembrane complex of several proteins – that lacks precision and cuts APP at different points in the

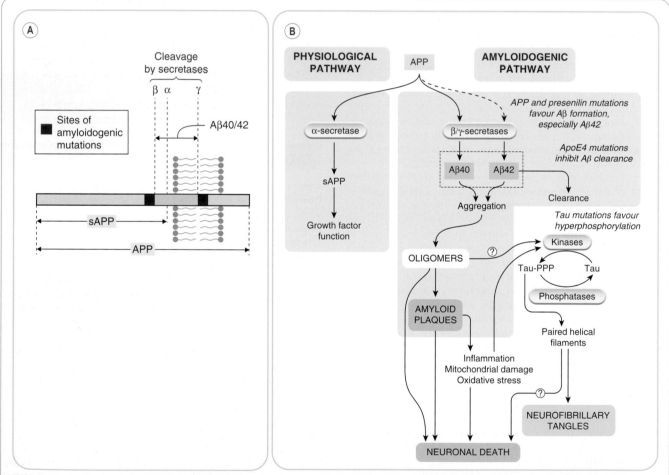

Fig. 40.3 **Pathogenesis of Alzheimer's disease.** [**A**] Structure of amyloid precursor protein (APP), showing origin of secreted APP (sAPP) and Aβ amyloid protein. The regions involved in amyloidogenic mutations discovered in some cases of familial Alzheimer's disease are shown flanking the Aβ sequence. APP cleavage involves three proteases: secretases α, β and γ. α-Secretase produces soluble APP, whereas β- and γ-secretases generate Aβ amyloid protein. γ-Secretase can cut at different points, generating Aβ peptides of varying lengths, including Aβ40 and Aβ42, the latter having a high tendency to aggregate as amyloid plaques. [**B**] Processing of APP. The main 'physiological' pathway gives rise to sAPP, which exerts a number of trophic functions. Cleavage of APP at different sites gives rise to Aβ, the predominant form normally being Aβ40, which is weakly amyloidogenic. Mutations in APP or presenilins increase the proportion of APP, which is degraded via the amyloidogenic pathway, and also increase the proportion converted to the much more strongly amyloidogenic form Aβ42. Clearance of Aβ is impaired by mutations in the apoE4 gene. Hyperphosphorylated Tau results in dissociation of Tau from microtubules, misfolding and aggregation to form paired helical filaments, which enhance Aβ toxicity.

transmembrane domain, generating Aβ fragments of different lengths, including Aβ40 and 42. Mutations in this region of the APP gene affect the preferred cleavage point, tending to favour formation of Aβ42. Mutations of the unrelated presenilin genes result in increased activity of γ-secretase, because the presenilin proteins form part of the γ-secretase complex. These different AD-related mutations increase the ratio of Aβ42:Aβ40, which can be detected in plasma, serving as a marker for familial AD. Mutations in another gene, that for the lipid transport protein ApoE4 which facilitates the clearance of Aβ oligomers, also predispose to AD, probably because the mutant form of ApoE4 proteins are less effective in this function.

It is uncertain exactly how Aβ accumulation causes neurodegeneration, and whether the damage is done by soluble Aβ monomers or oligomers or by amyloid plaques. There is evidence that the cells die by apoptosis, although an inflammatory response is also evident. Expression of Alzheimer mutations in transgenic animals (see Götz & Ittner, 2008) causes plaque formation and neurodegeneration, and also increases the susceptibility of CNS neurons to other challenges, such as ischaemia, excitotoxicity and oxidative stress, and this increased vulnerability may be the cause of the progressive neurodegeneration in AD. These transgenic models are potentially of great value in testing drug therapies aimed at retarding the neurodegenerative process.

The other main player on the biochemical stage is *Tau*, the protein of which the neurofibrillary tangles are composed (Fig. 40.3). Its role in neurodegeneration is unclear, although similar 'tauopathies' occur in many neurodegenerative conditions (see Brunden et al., 2009; Hanger et al., 2009). Tau is a normal constituent of neurons, being associated with the intracellular microtubules that serve as tracks for transporting materials along nerve axons. In AD and other tauopathies, Tau is abnormally phosphorylated by the action of various kinases, including glycogen synthase kinase-3β (GSK-3β) and cyclin-dependent kinase 5 (CDK5), and dissociates from microtubules to be deposited intracellularly as *paired helical filaments* with a characteristic microscopic appearance. When the cells die, these filaments aggregate as extracellular *neurofibrillary tangles*. Tau phosphorylation is enhanced by the presence of Aβ, possibly by activation of kinases. Conversely, hyperphosphorylated Tau favours the formation of amyloid deposits. Whether hyperphosphorylation and intracellular deposition of Tau directly harms the cell is not certain, although it is known that it impairs fast axonal transport, a process that depends on microtubules.

Loss of cholinergic neurons

Although changes in many transmitter systems have been observed, mainly from measurements on postmortem AD brain tissue, a relatively selective loss of cholinergic neurons in the basal forebrain nuclei (Ch. 39) is characteristic. This discovery, made in 1976, implied that pharmacological approaches to restoring cholinergic function might be feasible, leading to the use of cholinesterase inhibitors to treat AD (see below).

Choline acetyl transferase activity, acetylcholine content and acetylcholinesterase and choline transport in the cortex and hippocampus are all reduced considerably in AD but not in other disorders, such as depression or schizophrenia. Muscarinic receptor density, determined by binding studies, is not affected, but nicotinic receptors, particularly in the cortex, are reduced. The reason for the selective loss of cholinergic neurons resulting from Aβ formation is not known.

THERAPEUTIC APPROACHES

Unravelling the mechanism of neurodegeneration in AD has yet to result in therapies able to retard it. Currently, cholinesterase inhibitors (see Ch. 13) and **memantine** are the only drugs approved for treating AD. Many

Alzheimer's disease

- Alzheimer's disease (AD) is a common age-related dementia distinct from vascular dementia associated with brain infarction.
- The main pathological features of AD comprise amyloid plaques, neurofibrillary tangles and a loss of neurons (particularly cholinergic neurons of the basal forebrain).
- Amyloid plaques consist of aggregates of the Aβ fragment of amyloid precursor protein (APP), a normal neuronal membrane protein, produced by the action of β- and γ-secretases. AD is associated with excessive Aβ formation, resulting in neurotoxicity.
- Familial AD (rare) results from mutations in the APP gene, or in presenilin genes (involved in γ-secretase function), both of which cause increased Aβ formation.
- Mutations in the lipoprotein ApoE4 increase the risk of developing AD, probably by interfering with Aβ clearance.
- Neurofibrillary tangles comprise intracellular aggregates of a highly phosphorylated form of a normal neuronal protein (Tau). Hyperphosphorylated Tau and Aβ act synergistically to cause neurodegeneration.
- Loss of cholinergic neurons is believed to account for much of the learning and memory deficit in AD.

other approaches have been explored, based on the amyloid hypothesis as well as other ideas for neuroprotection (see Spencer et al., 2007), so far without success in clinical trials.[6]

CHOLINESTERASE INHIBITORS

Tacrine, the first drug approved for treating AD, was investigated on the basis that enhancement of cholinergic transmission might compensate for the cholinergic deficit. Trials showed modest improvements in tests of memory and cognition in about 40% of AD patients, but no improvement in other functional measures that affect quality of life. Tacrine has to be given four times daily and produces cholinergic side effects such as nausea and abdominal cramps, as well as hepatotoxicity in some patients, so it is far from an ideal drug. Later compounds, which also have limited efficacy but are more effective than tacrine in improving quality of life, include **donepezil**, **rivastigmine** and **galantamine** (Table 40.2). These drugs produce a measurable, although slight, improvement of cognitive function in AD patients, but this may be too small to be significant in terms of everyday life.

There is some evidence from laboratory studies that cholinesterase inhibitors may act somehow to reduce the formation or neurotoxicity of Aβ, and therefore retard the progression of AD as well as producing symptomatic

---

[6]The authors admit to disappointment that, despite intense research efforts, no new drugs worthy of mention have emerged since the last edition of this book.

Table 40.2 Cholinesterase inhibitors used in the treatment of Alzheimer's disease[a]

Drug	Type of inhibition	Duration of action and dosage	Main side effects	Notes
Tacrine	Affects both AChE and BuChE Not CNS selective	~6 h 2–3 times daily oral dosage	Cholinergic side effects (abdominal pain, nausea, diarrhoea), hepatotoxicity	The first anticholinesterase shown to be efficacious in AD Monitoring for hepatotoxicity needed
Donepezil	CNS, AChE selective	~24 h Once-daily oral dosage	Slight cholinergic side effects	–
Rivastigmine	CNS selective	~8 h Twice-daily oral dosage	Cholinergic side effects that tend to subside with continuing treatment	Gradual dose escalation to minimise side effects
Galantamine	Affects both AChE and BuChE Also enhances nicotinic ACh receptor activation by allosteric action	~8 h Twice-daily oral dosage	Slight cholinergic side effects	–

[a]Similar level of limited clinical benefit for all drugs. No clinical evidence for retardation of disease process, although animal tests suggest diminution of Aβ and plaque formation by a mechanism not related to cholinesterase inhibition.
AChE, acetylcholinesterase; BuChE, butyryl cholinesterase.

benefit. Clinical trials, however, have shown only a small improvement in cognitive function, with no effect on disease progression.

Other drugs aimed at improving cholinergic function that are being investigated include other cholinesterase inhibitors and a variety of muscarinic and nicotinic receptor agonists. To date the lack of selectivity of muscarinic orthosteric agonists has hindered their use to treat CNS disorders due to the incidence of side effects, but the hope is that positive allosteric modulators (see Ch. 3) that are selective (e.g. for the M_1 receptor) will be developed.

MEMANTINE

The other drug currently approved for the treatment of AD is **memantine**, an orally active weak antagonist at NMDA receptors. It was originally introduced as an antiviral drug, and resurrected as a potential inhibitor of excitotoxicity. It produces – surprisingly – a modest cognitive improvement in moderate or severe AD, but does not appear to be neuroprotective. It may work by selectively inhibiting excessive, pathological NMDA receptor activation while preserving more physiological activation. It has a long plasma half-life, and its adverse effects include headache, dizziness, drowsiness, constipation, shortness of breath and hypertension as well as a raft of less common problems. The potential for other drugs acting as agonists or allosteric modulators at NMDA receptors to enhance cognition is discussed by Collingridge et al. (2013).

Inhibiting neurodegeneration

▼ For most of the disorders discussed in this chapter, including AD, the Holy Grail, which so far eludes us, would be a drug that retards neurodegeneration. Although several well-characterised targets were identified, such as Aβ formation by the β- and γ-secretases, and

Clinical use of drugs in dementia

- Acetylcholinesterase inhibitors and NMDA antagonists detectably improve cognitive impairment in clinical trials but have significant adverse effects and are of limited use clinically. They have not been shown to retard neurodegeneration.
- Efficacy is monitored periodically in individual patients, and administration continued only if the drugs are believed to be working and their effect in slowing functional and behavioural deterioration is judged to outweigh adverse effects.

Acetylcholinesterase inhibitors:
- **Donepezil, galantamine, rivastigmine. Tacrine** is also effective, but may cause liver damage. Unwanted cholinergic effects may be troublesome.
- Used in mild to moderate Alzheimer's disease.

NMDA receptor antagonists:
- For example, **memantine** (see Ch. 38).
- Used in moderate to severe Alzheimer's disease.

Aβ neurotoxicity, together with a range of transgenic animal models of AD on which compounds can be tested, subsequent clinical trials of drugs targeting these processes have been disappointing (Corbett et al., 2012). Inhibitors of β- and γ-secretase were identified. Though they are effective in reducing Aβ formation, they appear to make cognition impairment worse. Several proved toxic to the immune system and gastrointestinal tract, and development has been halted. Kinase inhibitors aimed at preventing Tau phosphorylation were also investigated (see Brunden et al., 2009). The large number of phosphorylation sites and different kinases make this a difficult approach.

An ingenious approach was taken by Schenk et al. (1999), who immunised AD transgenic mice with Aβ protein, and found that this not only prevented but also reversed plaque formation. Initial trials in humans had to be terminated because of neuroinflammatory complications. More recent clinical trials with monoclonal Aβ antibodies have been disappointing but it is possible that the antibody treatments were given too late in the progression of the disease and that earlier intervention might reveal therapeutic benefit.

Epidemiological studies suggested that some non-steroidal anti-inflammatory drugs (NSAIDs; see Ch. 26) used routinely to treat arthritis reduced the likelihood of developing AD. This idea has been supported by numerous animal studies in which genetic mouse models lacking specific prostaglandin receptor subtypes have proved resistant to experimental models of neurodegenerative disease. Unfortunately, clinical trials with various NSAIDs have so far failed to show evidence of consistent benefit (Breitner et al., 2011). Indeed, NSAIDs can have adverse effects in later stages of AD, but in asymptomatic individuals **naproxen** can reduce the long-term incidence of AD.

Aβ plaques bind copper and zinc, and removal of these metal ions promotes dissolution of the plaques. The amoebicidal drug **clioquinol** is a metal-chelating agent that causes regression of amyloid deposits in animal models of AD, and showed some benefit in initial clinical trials. Clioquinol itself has known toxic effects in humans, which preclude its routine clinical use, but less toxic metal-chelating agents are under investigation.

Shortage of growth factors (particularly nerve growth factor) may contribute to the loss of forebrain cholinergic neurons in AD. Administering growth factors into the brain is not realistic for routine therapy, but alternative approaches, such as implanting cells engineered to secrete nerve growth factor, are under investigation.

Other approaches. These include the development of new drugs as well as the use of established drugs already in use to treat other unrelated conditions (see Corbett et al., 2012).

New potent and selective histamine H_3 antagonists may improve cognition in AD (see Brioni et al., 2011). They also increase wakefulness and may be used to treat narcolepsy (see Ch. 48).

Levetiracetam, an anticonvulsant with a novel mechanism of action, may slow the development of AD.

Longitudinal cohort studies suggest that antihypertensive therapy may be correlated with a reduction in the incidence of AD (see Corbett et al., 2012). The reasons for this are unclear but could relate to a reduction in inflammatory processes in the brain.

Caprylidene (caprylic triglyceride) is formulated from coconut oil.[7] It is broken down in the body to release ketones which provide an alternative energy source to glucose. There is some evidence that in AD glucose utilisation is impaired. It may be useful in mild to moderate AD to improve memory and cognitive function but it does not reverse neuronal degeneration.

Latrepirdine is in clinical trials for the treatment of AD. It has a complex pharmacology and which of its actions are responsible for any therapeutic benefit still needs to be determined.

Observational studies suggested that statins might prevent dementia, but this has not been prospectively confirmed in clinical trials.

PARKINSON'S DISEASE

FEATURES OF PARKINSON'S DISEASE

Parkinson's disease (see review by Schapira, 2009) is a progressive disorder of movement that occurs mainly in the elderly. The chief symptoms are:

- suppression of voluntary movements (*bradykinesia*), due partly to muscle rigidity and partly to an

inherent inertia of the motor system, which means that motor activity is difficult to stop as well as to initiate
- tremor at rest, usually starting in the hands ('pill-rolling' tremor), which tends to diminish during voluntary activity
- muscle rigidity, detectable as an increased resistance in passive limb movement
- a variable degree of cognitive impairment.

Parkinsonian patients walk with a characteristic shuffling gait. They find it hard to start, and once in progress they cannot quickly stop or change direction. PD is commonly associated with dementia, depression and autonomic dysfunction, because the degenerative process is not confined to the basal ganglia but also affects other parts of the brain. Non-motor symptoms may appear before motor symptoms and often predominate in the later stages of the disease.

Parkinson's disease often occurs with no obvious underlying cause, but it may be the result of cerebral ischaemia, viral encephalitis or other types of pathological damage. The symptoms can also be drug-induced, the main drugs involved being those that reduce the amount of dopamine in the brain (e.g. **reserpine**; see Ch. 14) or block dopamine receptors (e.g. antipsychotic drugs such as **chlorpromazine**; see Ch. 46). There are rare instances of familial early-onset PD, and several gene mutations have been identified, including those encoding *synuclein* and *parkin* (see p. 492). Mutations in the gene encoding leucine-rich repeat kinase 2 (LRRK2) have also been associated with PD. Study of gene mutations has given some clues about the mechanism underlying the neurodegenerative process.

Neurochemical changes

Parkinson's disease affects the basal ganglia, and its neurochemical origin was discovered in 1960 by Hornykiewicz, who showed that the dopamine content of the substantia nigra and corpus striatum (see Ch. 39) in post-mortem brains of PD patients was extremely low (usually less than 10% of normal), associated with a loss of dopaminergic neurons in the substantia nigra and degeneration of nerve terminals in the striatum.[8] Neurons containing other monoamines such as noradrenaline and 5-hydroxytryptamine are also affected. Gradual loss of dopamine occurs over several years, with symptoms of PD appearing only when the striatal dopamine content has fallen to 20–40% of normal. Lesions of the nigrostriatal tract or chemically induced depletion of dopamine in experimental animals also produce symptoms of PD. The symptom most clearly related to dopamine deficiency is *bradykinesia*, which occurs immediately and invariably in lesioned animals. Rigidity and tremor involve more complex neurochemical disturbances of other transmitters (particularly acetylcholine, noradrenaline, 5-hydroxytryptamine and GABA) as well as dopamine. In experimental lesions, two secondary consequences follow damage to the nigrostriatal tract, namely a hyperactivity of the remaining dopaminergic neurons, which show an increased rate of transmitter turnover, and

---

[7]It is sometimes referred to as a 'medical food'.

[8]It is emerging that other types of neuron are also affected. Here we concentrate on the dopaminergic nigrostriatal pathway as it is the most important in relation to current therapies.

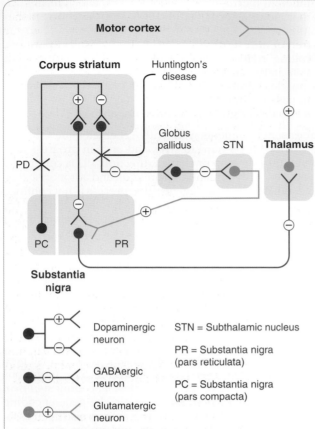

Fig. 40.4 Simplified diagram of the organisation of the extrapyramidal motor system and the defects that occur in Parkinson's disease (PD) and Huntington's disease. Normally, activity in nigrostriatal dopamine neurons causes excitation of striatonigral neurons and inhibition of striatal neurons that project to the globus pallidus. Because of the different pathways involved, the activity of GABAergic neurons in the substantia nigra is suppressed, releasing the restraint on the thalamus and cortex, causing motor stimulation. In PD, the dopaminergic pathway from the substantia nigra (pars compacta) to the striatum is impaired. In Huntington's disease, the GABAergic striatopallidal pathway is impaired, producing effects opposite to the changes in PD.

In the figure legend:
- Dopaminergic neuron
- GABAergic neuron
- Glutamatergic neuron
- STN = Subthalamic nucleus
- PR = Substantia nigra (pars reticulata)
- PC = Substantia nigra (pars compacta)

an increase in the number of dopamine receptors, which produces a state of denervation hypersensitivity (see Ch. 12). The striatum expresses mainly D_1 (excitatory) and D_2 (inhibitory) receptors (see Ch. 39), but fewer D_3 and D_4 receptors. A simplified diagram of the neuronal circuitry involved, and the pathways primarily affected in PD and Huntington's disease, is shown in Figure 40.4.

Cholinergic interneurons of the corpus striatum (not shown in Fig. 40.4) are also involved in PD and Huntington's disease. Acetylcholine release from the striatum is strongly inhibited by dopamine, and it is suggested that hyperactivity of these cholinergic neurons contributes to the symptoms of PD. The opposite happens in Huntington's disease, and in both conditions therapies aimed at redressing the balance between the dopaminergic and cholinergic neurons are, up to a point, beneficial.

PATHOGENESIS OF PARKINSON'S DISEASE

As with other neurodegenerative disorders, the neuronal damage in PD is caused by protein misfolding and aggregation, aided and abetted by other familiar villains, namely excitotoxicity, mitochondrial dysfunction, oxidative stress, inflammation and apoptosis. Aspects of the pathogenesis and animal models of PD are described by Duty & Jenner (2011).

Neurotoxins

New light was thrown on the possible aetiology of PD by a chance event. In 1982, a group of young drug addicts in California suddenly developed an exceptionally severe form of PD (known as the 'frozen addict' syndrome), and the cause was traced to the compound 1-methyl-4-phenyl-1,2,3,6-tetrahydropyridine (MPTP), which was a contaminant in the illegal preparation of a heroin substitute (see Langston, 1985). MPTP causes irreversible destruction of nigrostriatal dopaminergic neurons in various species, and produces a PD-like state in primates. MPTP acts by being converted to a toxic metabolite, MPP^+, by the enzyme monoamine oxidase (MAO, specifically by the MAO-B subtype that is located in glial cells; see Chs 14 and 47). MPP^+ is then taken up by the dopamine transport system, and thus acts selectively on dopaminergic neurons; it inhibits mitochondrial oxidation reactions, producing oxidative stress. MPTP appears to be selective in destroying nigrostriatal neurons and does not affect dopaminergic neurons elsewhere – the reason for this is unknown. It is also less effective in rats than in primates, yet mice show some susceptibility. **Selegiline**, a selective MAO-B inhibitor, prevents MPTP-induced neurotoxicity by blocking its conversion to MPP^+. Selegiline is also used in treating PD (see p. 495); as well as inhibiting dopamine breakdown, it might also work by blocking the metabolic activation of a putative endogenous, or environmental, MPTP-like substance, which is involved in the causation of PD. It is possible that dopamine itself could be the culprit, because oxidation of dopamine gives rise to potentially toxic metabolites. Whether or not the action of MPTP reflects the natural pathogenesis of PD, the MPTP model is a very useful experimental tool for testing possible therapies.

Impaired mitochondrial function is a feature of the disease in humans. Various herbicides, such as **rotenone**, that selectively inhibit mitochondrial function cause a PD-like syndrome in animals. PD in humans is more common in agricultural areas than in cities, suggesting that environmental toxins could be a factor in its causation.

Molecular aspects

▼ Parkinson's disease, as well as several other neurodegenerative disorders, is associated with the development of intracellular protein aggregates known as *Lewy bodies* in various parts of the brain. They consist largely of α-synuclein, a synaptic protein, present in large amounts in normal brains. Recent evidence suggests that α-synuclein may act as a prion-like protein (see p. 496) and that PD is in fact a prion-like disease (Poewe et al., 2012). α-Synuclein normally exists in an α-helical conformation. However, under certain circumstances, such as genetic duplication or triplication or genetic mutation it can undergo a conformational change to a β-sheet-rich structure that polymerises to form toxic aggregates and amyloid plaques. Mutations occur in rare types of hereditary PD (see p. 493). It is believed that misfolding and aggregation renders the protein resistant to degradation within cells, causing it to pile up in Lewy bodies. In parkinsonian patients who received fetal dopaminergic neuron grafts (see p. 495) over time the grafted neurons developed Lewy bodies. Misfolded α-synuclein is thought to have migrated from the native tissue to the grafted tissue.

It is possible (see Lotharius & Brundin, 2002) that the normal function of α-synuclein is related to synaptic vesicle recycling, and that the misfolded form loses this functionality, with the result that vesicular storage of dopamine is impaired. This may lead to an increase in cytosolic dopamine, degradation of which produces reactive oxygen species and hence neurotoxicity. Consistent with the α-synuclein hypothesis, another mutation associated with PD (*parkin*) also involves a protein that participates in the intracellular degradation of rogue proteins.

▼ Other gene mutations that have been identified as risk factors for early-onset PD code for proteins involved in mitochondrial function, making cells more susceptible to oxidative stress. Thus, a picture similar to AD pathogenesis is slowly emerging. Misfolded α-synuclein, facilitated by overexpression, genetic mutations or possibly by environmental factors, builds up in the cell as a result of impaired protein degradation (resulting from defective parkin) in the form of Lewy bodies, which, by unknown mechanisms, compromise cell survival. If oxidative stress is increased, as a result of ischaemia, mitochondrial poisons or mutations of certin mitochondrial proteins, the result is cell death.

Parkinson's disease

- Degenerative disease of the basal ganglia causing hypokinesia, tremor at rest and muscle rigidity, often with dementia and autonomic dysfunction.
- Associated with aggregation of α-synuclein (a protein normally involved in vesicle recycling) in the form of characteristic Lewy bodies.
- Often idiopathic but may follow stroke or virus infection; can be drug-induced (antipsychotic drugs). Rare familial forms also occur, associated with various gene mutations, including α-synuclein.
- Associated with degeneration of dopaminergic nigrostriatal neurons that gives rise to the motor symptoms, as well as more general neurodegeneration resulting in dementia and depression.
- Can be induced by 1-methyl-4-phenyl-1,2,3,6-tetrahydropyridine (**MPTP**), a neurotoxin affecting dopamine neurons. Similar environmental neurotoxins, as well as genetic factors, may be involved in human Parkinson's disease.

DRUG TREATMENT OF PARKINSON'S DISEASE

Currently, the main drugs used (see Fig. 40.5) are:

- **levodopa** (often in combination with **carbidopa** and **entacapone**)
- dopamine agonists (e.g. **pramipexole, ropinirole, bromocriptine**)
- monoamine oxidase-B (MAO-B) inhibitors (e.g. **selegiline, rasagiline**)
- muscarinic ACh receptor antagonists (e.g. **orphenadrine, procyclidine** and **trihexyphenidyl**) are occasionally used.

None of the drugs used to treat PD affects the progression of the disease. For general reviews of current and future approaches, see Schapira (2009) and Poewe et al. (2012).

LEVODOPA

Levodopa is the first-line treatment for PD and is combined with a peripherally acting dopa decarboxylase inhibitor, such as **carbidopa** or **benserazide**, which reduces the dose needed by about 10-fold and diminishes the peripheral side effects. It is well absorbed from the small intestine, a process that relies on active transport, although much of it is inactivated by MAO in the wall of the intestine. The plasma half-life is short (about 2 h). Oral and subcutaneous slow release preparations have been developed. Conversion to dopamine in the periphery, which would otherwise account for about 95% of the levodopa dose and cause troublesome side effects, is largely prevented by the decarboxylase inhibitor. Decarboxylation occurs rapidly within the brain, because the decarboxylase inhibitors do not penetrate the blood–brain barrier. It is not certain whether the effect depends on an increased release of dopamine from the few surviving dopaminergic neurons or on a 'flooding' of the synapse with dopamine formed elsewhere. Because synthetic dopamine agonists (see p. 494) are equally effective, the latter explanation is more likely, and animal studies suggest that levodopa can act even when no dopaminergic nerve terminals are present. On the other hand, the therapeutic effectiveness of levodopa decreases as the disease advances, so part of its action may rely on the presence of functional dopaminergic neurons. Combination of levodopa plus a dopa decarboxylase inhibitor with a catechol-O-methyl transferase (COMT) inhibitor (e.g. **entacapone** or **tolcapone**, see Ch. 14) to inhibit its degradation, is used in patients troubled by 'end of dose' motor fluctuations.

Therapeutic effectiveness

About 80% of patients show initial improvement with levodopa, particularly of rigidity and bradykinesia, and about 20% are restored virtually to normal motor function. As time progresses, the effectiveness of levodopa gradually declines (Fig. 40.6). In a typical study of 100 patients treated with levodopa for 5 years, only 34 were better than they had been at the beginning of the trial, 32 patients having died and 21 having withdrawn from the trial. It is likely that the loss of effectiveness of levodopa mainly reflects the natural progression of the disease, but receptor downregulation and other compensatory mechanisms may also contribute. There is no evidence that levodopa can actually accelerate the neurodegenerative process through overproduction of dopamine, as was suspected on theoretical grounds. Overall, levodopa increases the life expectancy of PD patients, probably as a result of improved motor function, although some symptoms (e.g. dysphagia, cognitive decline) are not improved.

Unwanted effects

There are two main types of unwanted effect:

1. Involuntary movements (dyskinesia), which do not appear initially but develop in the majority of patients within 2 years of starting levodopa therapy. These movements usually affect the face and limbs, and can become very severe. They occur at the time of the peak therapeutic effect, and the margin between the beneficial and the dyskinetic effect becomes progressively narrower. Levodopa is short acting, and the fluctuating plasma concentration of the drug may favour the development of dyskinesias, as longer-acting dopamine agonists are less problematic in this regard.
2. Rapid fluctuations in clinical state, where bradykinesia and rigidity may suddenly worsen for

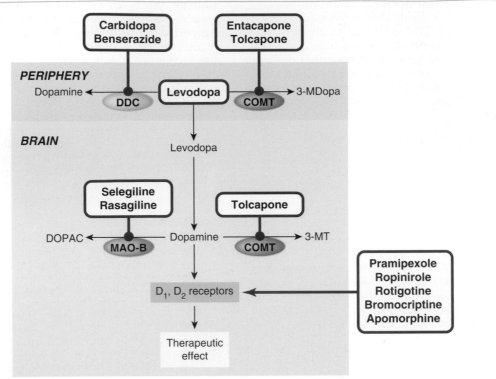

Fig. 40.5 **Sites of action of drugs used to treat Parkinson's disease.** Levodopa enters the brain and is converted to dopamine (the deficient neurotransmitter). Inactivation of levodopa in the periphery is prevented by inhibitors of DDC and COMT. Inactivation in the brain is prevented by inhibitors of COMT and MAO-B. Dopamine agonists act directly on striatal dopamine receptors. 3-MDopa, 3-methoxydopa; 3-MT, 3-methoxytyrosine; COMT, catechol-*O*-methyl transferase; DDC, DOPA decarboxylase; DOPAC, dihydroxyphenylacetic acid; MAO-B, monoamine oxidase B.

anything from a few minutes to a few hours, and then improve again. This 'on–off effect' is not seen in untreated PD patients or with other anti-PD drugs. The 'off effect' can be so sudden that the patient stops while walking and feels rooted to the spot, or is unable to rise from a chair, having sat down normally a few moments earlier. As with the dyskinesias, the problem seems to reflect the fluctuating plasma concentration of levodopa, and it is suggested that as the disease advances, the ability of neurons to store dopamine is lost, so the therapeutic benefit of levodopa depends increasingly on the continuous formation of extraneuronal dopamine, which requires a continuous supply of levodopa. The use of sustained-release preparations, or co-administration of COMT inhibitors such as **entacapone**, may be used to counteract the fluctuations in plasma concentration of levodopa.

In addition to these slowly developing side effects, levodopa produces several acute effects, which are experienced by most patients at first but tend to disappear after a few weeks. The main ones are as follow:

- Nausea and anorexia. **Domperidone**, a dopamine antagonist that works in the chemoreceptor trigger zone (where the blood–brain barrier is leaky) but does not gain access to the basal ganglia, may be useful in preventing this effect.
- Hypotension. Postural hypotension is a problem in a few patients.

- Psychological effects. Levodopa, by increasing dopamine activity in the brain, can produce a schizophrenia-like syndrome (see Ch. 46) with delusions and hallucinations. More commonly, in about 20% of patients, it causes confusion, disorientation, insomnia or nightmares.

DOPAMINE AGONISTS

Bromocriptine, **pergolide** and **cabergoline** exhibit slight selectivity for $D_{2/3}$ over D_1 receptors (see Ch. 39). Bromocriptine, which inhibits the release of prolactin from the anterior pituitary gland, was first introduced for the treatment of galactorrhoea and gynaecomastia (Ch. 33). Though effective in controlling the symptoms of PD, their usefulness is limited by side effects, such as nausea and vomiting, and somnolence and a risk of fibrotic reactions in the lungs, retroperitoneum and pericardium. These disadvantages have led to the replacement of these drugs by **pramipexole** and **ropinirole**, which are $D_{2/3}$ selective and better tolerated, and do not show the fluctuations in efficacy associated with levodopa. They do, however, cause somnolence and sometimes hallucinations, and recent evidence suggests that they may predispose to compulsive behaviours, such as excessive gambling,[9]

[9]In 2008 a plaintiff was awarded $8.2m damages by a US court, having become a compulsive gambler (and losing a lot of money) after taking pramipexole for PD – a side effect of which the pharmaceutical company had been aware.

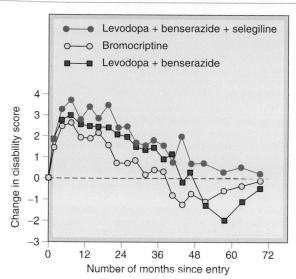

Fig. 40.6 Comparison of levodopa/benserazide, levodopa/benserazide/selegiline and bromocriptine on progression of Parkinson's disease symptoms. Patients (249–271 in each treatment group) were assessed on a standard disability rating score. Before treatment, the average rate of decline was 0.7 units/year. All three treatments produced improvement over the initial rating for 2–3 years, but the effect declined, either because of refractoriness to the drugs or disease progression. Bromocriptine appeared slightly less effective than levodopa regimens, and there was a higher drop-out rate due to side effects in this group. *(From Parkinson's Disease Research Group 1993 Br Med J 307, 469–472.)*

over-eating and sexual excess, related to the 'reward' functions of dopamine (see Ch. 49).

A disadvantage of current dopamine agonists is their short plasma half-life (6–8 h), requiring three-times daily dosage, though slow-release once-daily formulations are now available.

Rotigotine is a newer agent, delivered as a transdermal patch, with similar efficacy and side effects.

Apomorphine, given by injection, is sometimes used to control the 'off effect' with levodopa. Because of its powerful emetic action, it must be combined with an oral antiemetic drug. It has other serious adverse effects (mood and behavioural changes, cardiac dysrhythmias, hypotension) and is a last resort if other drugs fail.

MAO-B INHIBITORS

Selegiline is a selective MAO-B[10] inhibitor, which lacks the unwanted peripheral effects of non-selective MAO inhibitors used to treat depression (Ch. 47) and, in contrast to them, does not provoke the 'cheese reaction' or interact so frequently with other drugs. Inhibition of MAO-B protects dopamine from extraneuronal degradation and was initially used as an adjunct to levodopa. Long-term trials showed that the combination of selegiline and levodopa was more effective than levodopa alone in relieving symptoms and prolonging life. Recogni-

tion of the role of MAO-B in neurotoxicity (see p. 492) suggested that selegiline might be neuroprotective rather than merely enhancing the action of levodopa, but clinical studies do not support this. A large-scale trial (Fig. 40.6) showed no difference when selegiline was added to levodopa/benserazide treatment. Selegiline is metabolised to amphetamine, and sometimes causes excitement, anxiety and insomnia. **Rasagiline**, a very similar drug, does not have this unwanted effect, and may somewhat retard disease progression, as well alleviating symptoms (Olanow et al., 2009). **Safinamide**, undergoing clinical trials, is a new drug that inhibits both MAO-B and dopamine reuptake.

OTHER DRUGS USED IN PARKINSON'S DISEASE

Amantadine

▼ Amantadine was introduced as an antiviral drug and discovered by accident in 1969 to be beneficial in PD. Many possible mechanisms for its action have been suggested based on neurochemical evidence of increased dopamine release, inhibition of amine uptake or a direct action on dopamine receptors. More recently block of NMDA receptors by stabilising closed states of the channel has been described and this may be a novel target for antiparkinsonian drugs.

Amantadine is less effective than levodopa or bromocriptine in treating PD is but it is effective in reducing the dyskinesias induced by prolonged levodopa treatment (see p. 493).

Acetylcholine antagonists

▼ For more than a century, until levodopa was discovered, atropine and related drugs were the main form of treatment for PD. Muscarinic acetylcholine receptors exert an inhibitory effect on dopaminergic nerve terminals, suppression of which compensates for a lack of dopamine. The side effects of muscarinic antagonists – dry mouth, constipation, impaired vision, urinary retention – are troublesome, and they are now rarely used, except to treat parkinsonian symptoms in patients receiving antipsychotic drugs (which are dopamine antagonists and thus nullify the effect of levodopa; see Ch. 46).

NEW PHARMACOLOGICAL APPROACHES

▼ Potential new treatments for PD include adenosine A_{2A} receptor antagonists (e.g. **istradefylline** and **preladenant**), 5-HT$_{1A}$ antagonists (e.g. **sarizotan**) and glutamate receptor antagonists or negative allosteric modulators (acting at mGluR5, AMPA or NMDA receptors) as well as new, improved COMT inhibitors. For further information see Poewe et al. (2012).

NEURAL TRANSPLANTATION, GENE THERAPY AND BRAIN STIMULATION

▼ Parkinson's disease is the first neurodegenerative disease for which neural transplantation was attempted in 1982, amid much publicity. Various transplantation approaches have been tried, based on the injection of dissociated fetal cells (neuroblasts) directly into the striatum. Trials in patients with PD (Barker et al., 2013) have mainly involved injection of midbrain cells from aborted human fetuses. Although such transplants have been shown to survive and establish functional dopaminergic connections this approach has fallen out of favour recently. Some patients have gone on to develop serious dyskinesias, possibly due to dopamine overproduction. The use of fetal material is, of course, fraught with difficulties (usually cells from five or more fetuses are needed for one transplant), and hopes for the future rest mainly on the possibility of developing stem cell transplants (see Lindvall & Kokaia, 2009; Nishimura & Takahashi, 2013).

Gene therapy (see Ch. 59) for PD is aimed at increasing the synthesis of neurotransmitters and neurotrophic factors such as:

---

[10]MAO-B in the brain is located mainly in glial cells, and also in 5-HT neurons (though, surprisingly, it does not appear to be expressed in dopamine neurons).

Drugs used in Parkinson's disease

- Drugs act by counteracting deficiency of dopamine in basal ganglia or by blocking muscarinic receptors. None of the available drugs affect the underlying neurodegeneration.
- Drugs include:
  - **levodopa** (dopamine precursor; Ch. 14), given with an inhibitor of peripheral dopa decarboxylase (e.g. **carbidopa**) to minimise side effects; sometimes a catechol-*O*-methyl transferase inhibitor (e.g. **entacapone**) is also given, especially to patients with 'end of dose' motor fluctuations
  - dopamine receptor agonists (**pramipexole, ropinirole, rotigotine, bromocriptine**); **rotigotine** is available as a transdermal patch
  - monoamine oxidase B inhibitors (**selegiline, rasagiline**)
  - **amantadine** (which may enhance dopamine release)
  - **orphenadrine** (muscarinic receptor antagonist used for parkinsonism caused by antipsychotic drugs).
- Neurotransplantation, still in an experimental phase, may be effective but results are variable, and slowly developing dyskinesias may occur.

- dopamine in the striatum – by expressing tyrosine hydroxylase or dopa decarboxylase
- GABA in the subthalamic nucleus – by overexpression of glutamic acid decarboxylase (to reduce the excitatory input to the substantia nigra (see Fig. 40.4)
- neurotrophic factors such as neurturin, a glial-derived neurotrophic factor (GDNF) analogue.

Electrical stimulation of the subthalamic nuclei with implanted electrodes (which inhibits ongoing neural activity, equivalent to reversible ablation) is used in severe cases, and can improve motor dysfunction in PD, but does not improve cognitive and other symptoms and does not stop the neurodegenerative process (see Okun, 2012).

HUNTINGTON'S DISEASE

▼ Huntington's disease (HD) is an inherited (autosomal dominant) disorder resulting in progressive brain degeneration, starting in adulthood and causing rapid deterioration and death. As well as dementia, it causes severe motor symptoms in the form of choreiform (i.e. rapid, jerky involuntary) movements, especially of fingers, face or tongue. It is the commonest of a group of so-called *trinucleotide repeat* neurodegenerative diseases, associated with the expansion of the number of repeats of the CAG sequence in specific genes, and hence the number (50 or more) of consecutive glutamine residues at the N-terminal of the expressed protein (see Walker, 2007). The larger the number of repeats, the earlier the appearance of symptoms. The protein coded by the HD gene, *huntingtin*, which normally possesses a chain of fewer than 30 glutamine residues, is a soluble cytosolic protein of unknown function found in all cells. HD develops when the mutant protein contains 40 or more repeats. The long poly-Gln chains reduce the solubility of huntingtin, and favour the formation of aggregates, which are formed from proteolytic N-terminal fragments that include the poly-Gln region. As with AD and PD, aggregation is probably responsible for the neuronal loss, which affects mainly the cortex and the striatum, resulting in progressive dementia and severe involuntary choreiform movements. Studies on postmortem brains showed that the dopamine content of the striatum was normal or slightly increased, while there was a 75% reduction in the activity of glutamic acid decarboxylase, the enzyme responsible for GABA synthesis (Ch. 38). It is believed that the loss of GABA-mediated inhibition in the basal ganglia produces a hyperactivity of dopaminergic synapses, so the syndrome is in some senses a mirror image of PD (Fig. 40.4).

The effects of drugs that influence dopaminergic transmission are correspondingly the opposite of those that are observed in PD, dopamine antagonists being effective in reducing the involuntary movements, while drugs such as levodopa and bromocriptine make them worse. Drugs used to alleviate the motor symptoms include **tetrabenazine** (an inhibitor of the vesicular monoamine transporter (see Ch. 14) that reduces dopamine storage, dopamine antagonists such as **chlorpromazine** (Ch. 46) and the GABA agonist **baclofen** (Ch. 38). Other drug treatments include antidepressants, mood stabilisers (see Ch. 47) and benzodiazepines (see Ch. 44) to reduce the depression, mood swings and anxiety associated with the disorder. None of these drugs affects dementia or retards the course of the disease. It is possible that drugs that inhibit excitotoxicity, antisense to reduce mutant huntingtin expression, or possibly neural transplantation procedures when these become available, may prove useful.

NEURODEGENERATIVE PRION DISEASES

▼ A group of human and animal diseases associated with a characteristic type of neurodegeneration, known as *spongiform encephalopathy* because of the vacuolated appearance of the affected brain, has been the focus of intense research activity (see Collinge, 2001; Prusiner, 2001). A key feature of these diseases is that they are transmissible through an infective agent, although not, in general, across species. The recent upsurge of interest has been spurred mainly by the discovery that the bovine form of the disease, bovine spongiform encephalopathy (BSE), is transmissible to humans. Different human forms of spongiform encephalopathy include Creutzfeld–Jakob disease (CJD) which is unrelated to BSE, and the new variant form (vCJD), which results from eating, or close contact with, infected beef or human tissue. Another human form is *kuru*, a neurodegenerative disease affecting cannibalistic tribes in Papua New Guinea. These diseases cause a progressive, and sometimes rapid, dementia and loss of motor coordination, for which no therapies currently exist. *Scrapie*, a common disease of domestic sheep, is another example, and it may have been the practice of feeding sheep offal to domestic cattle that initiated an epidemic of BSE in Britain during the 1980s, leading to the appearance of vCJD in humans in the mid-1990s. Although the BSE epidemic has been controlled, there is concern that more human cases may develop in its wake, because the incubation period – known to be long – is uncertain.

Prion diseases are examples of protein misfolding diseases (see p. 482) in which the prion protein adopts a misfolded conformation that forms insoluble aggregates. The infectious agent responsible for transmissible spongiform encephalopathies such as vCJD is, unusually, a protein, known as a prion. The protein involved (PrP^C) is a normal cytosolic constituent of the brain and other tissues, whose functions are not known. As a result of altered glycosylation, the protein can become misfolded, forming the insoluble PrP^{Sc} form, which has the ability to recruit normal PrP^C molecules to the misfolded PrP^{Sc}, thus starting a chain reaction. PrP^{Sc} – the infective agent – accumulates and aggregates as insoluble fibrils, and is responsible for the progressive neurodegeneration. In support of this unusual form of infectivity, it has been shown that injection of PrP^{Sc} into normal mice causes spongiform encephalopathy, whereas PrP knockout mice, which are otherwise fairly normal, are resistant because they lack the substrate for the autocatalytic generation of PrP^{Sc}. Fortunately, the infection does not easily cross between species, because there are differences between the *PrP* genes of different species. It is possible that a mutation of the *PrP* gene in either sheep or cattle produced the variant form that became infective in humans.

This chain of events bears some similarity to that of AD, in that the brain accumulates an abnormal form of a normally expressed protein. There is as yet no known treatment for this type of encephalopathy. There was hope that **quinacrine** (an antimalarial drug), **chlorpromazine** or **pentosan polyphosphate** might inhibit disease progression, but clinical trials have proven negative. Interest has now turned to anti-prion antibodies and these are being investigated. Opioid drugs (see Ch. 42) are used to relieve pain, while clonazepam and sodium valproate (see Ch. 45) may help to relieve involuntary muscle jerks.

REFERENCES AND FURTHER READING

General mechanisms of neurodegeneration

Barnham, K.J., Masters, C.L., Bush, A.I., 2004. Neurodegenerative diseases and oxidative stress. Nat. Rev. Drug Discov. 3, 205–214. (*Update on the oxidative stress model of neurodegeneration, including evidence based on various transgenic animal models*)

Brunden, K., Trojanowski, J.O., Lee, V.M.-Y., 2009. Advances in Tau-focused drug discovery for Alzheimer's disease and related tauopathies. Nat. Rev. Drug Discov. 8, 783–793. (*Good detailed review of the current status of Tau-directed drug discovery efforts, with a realistic assessment of the problems that have to be overcome*)

Coyle, J.T., Puttfarken, P., 1993. Oxidative stress, glutamate and neurodegenerative disorders. Science 262, 689–695. (*Good review article*)

Hanger, D.P., Anderton, B.H., Noble, W., 2009. Tau phosphorylation: the therapeutic challenge for neurodegenerative disease. Trends Mol. Med. 15, 112–119.

Itoh, K., Nakamura, K., Iijima, M., Sesaki, H., 2013. Mitochondrial dynamics in neurodegeneration. Trends Cell Biol. 23, 64–71. (*Summarises evidence for the involvement of mitochondrial dysfunction in several neurodegenerative diseases*)

Okouchi, M., Ekshyyan, O., Maracine, M., Aw, T.Y., 2007. Neuronal apoptosis in neurodegeneration. Antioxid. Redox Signal. 9, 1059–1096. (*Detailed review describing the role of apoptosis, the factors that induce it and possible therapeutic strategies aimed at preventing it, in various neurodegenerative disorders*)

Peden, A.H., Ironside, J.W., 2012. Molecular pathology in neurodegenerative diseases. Curr. Drug Targets 13, 1548–1559. (*Compares the molecular pathology of neurodegenerative and prion-mediated disorders*)

Zhao, C., Deng, W., Gage, F.H., 2008. Mechanisms and functional implications of adult neurogenesis. Cell 132, 645–660. (*Review by one of the pioneers in this controversial field. Neurogenesis probably contributes to learning, but evidence for involvement in neural repair is weak*)

Alzheimer's disease

Breitner, J.C., Baker, L.D., Montine, T.J., et al., 2011. Extended results of the Alzheimer's disease anti-inflammatory prevention trial. Alzheimers Dement. 7, 402–411. (*Reports on a long-term trial of NSAIDs in AD*)

Brioni, J.D., Esbenshade, T.A., Garrison, T.R., 2011. Discovery of histamine H$_3$ antagonists for the treatment of cognitive disorders and Alzheimer's disease. J. Pharmacol. Exp. Ther. 336, 38–46. (*Reviews preclinical and clinical data on the effectiveness of H$_3$ antagonists to treat a variety of CNS disorders*)

Collingridge, G.L., Volianskis, A., Bannister, N., et al., 2013. The NMDA receptor as a target for cognitive enhancement. Neuropharmacology 64, 13–26. (*Reviews the preclinical evidence that various types of drug acting at the NMDA receptor might improve cognition*)

Corbett, A., Pickett, J., Burns, A., et al., 2012. Drug repositioning for Alzheimer's disease. Nat. Rev. Drug Discov. 11, 833–846. (*Describes recent failures in drug development and discusses how drugs currently used for other conditions might be effective in treating AD*)

Götz, J., Ittner, L.M., 2008. Animal models of Alzheimer's disease and frontotemporal dementia. Nat. Rev. Neurosci. 9, 532–544. (*Detailed review focusing on transgenic models*)

Querfurth, H.W., LaFerla, F.M., 2010. Mechanisms of disease: Alzheimer's disease. N. Engl. J. Med. 362, 329–344.

Rakic, P., 2002. Neurogenesis in the primate cortex: an evaluation of the evidence. Nat. Rev. Neurosci. 3, 65–71.

Schenk, D., Barbour, R., Dunn, W., et al., 1999. Immunization with amyloid-beta attenuates Alzheimer-disease-like pathology in the PDAPP mouse. Nature 400, 173–177. (*Report of an ingenious experiment that could have implications for AD treatment in humans*)

Schwab, C., McGeer, P.L., 2008. Inflammatory aspects of Alzheimer disease and other neurodegenerative disorders. J. Alzheimer Dis. 13, 359–369. (*Discusses the role of inflammation in neurodegeneration and repair*)

Spencer, B., Rockenstein, E., Crews, L., et al., 2007. Novel strategies for Alzheimer's disease treatment. Exp. Opin. Biol. Ther. 7, 1853–1867. (*Focus on potential applications of gene therapy and other biological approaches*)

Weggen, S., Rogers, M., Eriksen, J., 2007. NSAIDs: small molecules for prevention of Alzheimer's disease or precursors for future drug development. Trends Pharmacol. Sci. 28, 536–543. (*Summarises data relating to effects of NSAIDs on AD and concludes that mechanisms other than cyclo-oxygenase inhibition may be relevant in the search for new anti-AD drugs*)

Parkinson's disease

Barker, R.A., Barrett, J., Mason, S.L., Björklund, A., 2013. Fetal dopaminergic transplantation trials and the future of neural grafting in Parkinson's disease. Lancet Neurol. 12, 84–91. (*Recent update by pioneers in the field*)

Duty, S., Jenner, P., 2011. Animal models of Parkinson's disease: a source of novel treatments and clues to the cause of the disease. Br. J. Pharmacol. 164, 1357–1391. (*Describes the value of various animal models in the search for new therapies for PD*)

Langston, W.J., 1985. MPTP and Parkinson's disease. Trends Neurosci. 8, 79–83. (*Readable account of the MPTP story by its discoverer*)

Lindvall, O., Kokaia, Z., 2009. Prospects of stem cell therapy for replacing dopamine neurons in Parkinson's disease. Trends Pharmacol. Sci. 30, 260–267. (*Suggests the way ahead for neurotransplantation for treating PD*)

Lotharius, J., Brundin, P., 2002. Pathogenesis of Parkinson's disease: dopamine, vesicles and α-synuclein. Nat. Rev. Neurosci. 3, 833–842. (*Review of PD pathogenesis, emphasising the possible role of dopamine itself as a likely source of neurotoxic metabolites*)

Nishimura, K., Takahashi, J., 2013. Therapeutic application of stem cell technology toward the treatment of Parkinson's disease. Biol. Pharm. Bull. 36, 171–175.

Okun, M.S., 2012. Deep-brain stimulation for Parkinson's disease. N. Engl. J. Med. 367, 1529–1538. (*Review of the clinical use of deep brain stimulation to treat Parkinson's disease*)

Olanow, C.W., Brundin, P., 2013. Parkinson's disease and alpha synuclein: is Parkinson's disease a prion-like disorder? Mov. Disord. 28, 31–40.

Olanow, C.W., Rascol, O., Hauser, R., et al., 2009. A double-blind, delayed-start trial of rasagiline in Parkinson's disease. N. Engl. J. Med. 139, 1268–1278. (*Well-conducted trial showing that rasagiline can significantly retard disease progression in patients with early PD*)

Poewe, W., Mahlknecht, P., Jankovic, J., 2012. Emerging therapies for Parkinson's disease. Curr. Opin. Neurol. 25, 448–459.

Schapira, A.H.V., 2009. Neurobiology and treatment of Parkinson's disease. Trends Pharmacol. Sci. 30, 41–47. (*Short review of pathophysiology and treatment of PD, including summary of recent trials*)

Stroke

Esencan, E., Yuksel, S., Tosun, Y.B., Robinot, A., Solaroglu, I., Zhang, J.H., 2013. Xenon in medical area: emphasis on neuroprotection in hypoxia and anesthesia. Med. Gas Res. 3, 4. (*Outlines the potential for xenon as a neuroprotective agent*)

Green, A.R., 2008. Pharmacological approaches to acute ischaemic stroke: reperfusion, neuroprotection possibly. Br. J. Pharmacol. 153 (Suppl. 1), S325–S338. (*Update on efforts – largely unsuccessful so far – to develop neuroprotective agents*)

Huntington's disease

Walker, F.O., 2007. Huntington's disease. Lancet 369, 218–228. (*General review of genetics, pathogenesis and treatment of HD*)

Prion diseases

Collinge, J., 2001. Prion diseases of humans and animals: their causes and molecular basis. Annu. Rev. Neurosci. 24, 519–550. (*Useful review article*)

Prusiner, S.B., 2001. Neurodegenerative disease and prions. N. Engl. J. Med. 344, 1544–1551. (*General review article by the discoverer of prions*)

41

General anaesthetic agents

OVERVIEW

General anaesthesia aims to provide balanced anaesthesia meeting the requirements of amnesia, analgesia and relaxation tailored for the intended medical procedure. Different general anaesthetic agents provide varying amounts of the components of balanced anaesthesia but they are rarely used nowadays in isolation. Neuromuscular blocking drugs (Ch. 13), sedative and anxiolytic drugs (Ch. 44), and analgesic drugs (Ch. 42) are frequently co-administered. General anaesthetics are given systemically and exert their main effects on the central nervous system (CNS), in contrast to local anaesthetics (Ch. 43). Although we now take them for granted, general anaesthetics are the drugs that paved the way for modern surgery. Without them, much of modern medicine would be impossible.

In this chapter we first describe the pharmacology of the main agents in current use, which fall into two groups: intravenous agents and inhalation agents (gases and volatile liquids). The use of anaesthetics in combination with other drugs to produce balanced anaesthesia is discussed at the end of the chapter. Detailed information on the clinical pharmacology and use of anaesthetic agents can be found in specialised textbooks (e.g. Aitkenhead et al., 2013).

INTRODUCTION

It was only when inhalation anaesthetics were first discovered, in 1846, that most surgical operations became a practical possibility. Until that time, surgeons relied on being able to operate on struggling patients at lightning speed, and most operations were amputations.

▼ The use of **nitrous oxide** to relieve the pain of surgery was suggested by Humphrey Davy in 1800. He was the first person to make nitrous oxide, and he tested its effects on several people, including himself and the Prime Minister, noting that it caused euphoria, analgesia and loss of consciousness. The use of nitrous oxide, billed as 'laughing gas', became a popular fairground entertainment and came to the notice of an American dentist, Horace Wells, who had a tooth extracted under its influence, while he himself squeezed the inhalation bag. Ether also first gained publicity in a disreputable way, through the spread of 'ether frolics', at which it was used to produce euphoria among the guests. William Morton, also a dentist and a student at Harvard Medical School, used it successfully to extract a tooth in 1846 and then suggested to Warren, the illustrious chief surgeon at Massachusetts General Hospital, that he should administer it for one of Warren's operations. Warren grudgingly agreed, and on 16 October 1846 a large audience was gathered in the main operating theatre;[1] after some preliminary fumbling, Morton's demonstration was a spectacular success. 'Gentlemen, this is no humbug', was the most gracious comment that Warren could bring himself to make to the assembled audience.

In the same year, James Simpson, Professor of Midwifery at Edinburgh University, used chloroform to relieve the pain of childbirth, bringing on himself fierce denunciation from the clergy, one of whom wrote: 'Chloroform is a decoy of Satan, apparently offering itself to bless women; but in the end it will harden society and rob God of the deep, earnest cries which arise in time of trouble, for help.' Opposition was effectively silenced in 1853, when Queen Victoria gave birth to her seventh child under the influence of chloroform, and the procedure became known as *anaesthésie à la reine*.

MECHANISM OF ACTION OF ANAESTHETIC DRUGS

Unlike most drugs, anaesthetics, which include substances as diverse as simple gases (e.g. **nitrous oxide** and **xenon**), halogenated hydrocarbons (e.g. **isoflurane**), barbiturates (e.g. **thiopental**) and steroids (e.g. **alphaxalone**), belong to no recognisable chemical class. At one time it appeared that the shape and electronic configuration of the molecule were relatively unimportant, and the pharmacological action required only that the molecule had certain physicochemical properties. We now know much more about how different anaesthetics interact with neuronal membrane proteins and have come to realise that there are multiple mechanisms by which anaesthesia can be produced and that different anaesthetics work by different mechanisms.

As the concentration of an anaesthetic is increased, the switch from being conscious to unconscious occurs over a very narrow concentration range (approximately 0.2 of a log unit). This is a much steeper concentration–response curve than that seen with drugs that interact as agonists or antagonists at classical receptors (see Ch. 2).

LIPID SOLUBILITY

Overton and Meyer, at the turn of the 20th century, showed a close correlation between anaesthetic potency and lipid solubility in a diverse group of simple and unreactive organic compounds that were tested for their ability to immobilise tadpoles. This led to a bold theory, formulated by Meyer in 1937: 'Narcosis commences when any chemically indifferent substance has attained a certain molar concentration in the lipids of the cell.'

The relationship between anaesthetic activity and lipid solubility has been repeatedly confirmed for a diverse array of agents. Anaesthetic potency in humans is usually expressed as the minimal alveolar concentration (MAC) required to abolish the response to surgical incision in 50% of subjects. Figure 41.1 shows the correlation between MAC (inversely proportional to potency) and lipid solubility, expressed as oil:gas partition coefficient, for a wide range of inhalation anaesthetics. The Overton–Meyer studies did not suggest any particular mechanism, but revealed an impressive correlation, for which any theory of anaesthesia needs to account. Oil:gas partition was assumed to predict partition into membrane lipids,

---

[1]Now preserved as the Ether Dome, a museum piece at Massachusetts General Hospital.

consistent with the suggestion that anaesthesia results from an alteration of membrane function.

How the simple introduction of inert foreign molecules into the lipid bilayer could cause a functional disturbance was not explained. Two possible mechanisms, namely volume expansion and increased membrane fluidity, have been suggested and tested experimentally, but both are now largely discredited and attention has swung from lipids to proteins, the correlation of potency with lipid solubility being explained by molecules of anaesthetic binding to hydrophobic pockets within specific membrane protein targets.

EFFECTS ON ION CHANNELS

Following early studies that showed that anaesthetics can bind to various proteins as well as lipids, it was found that anaesthetics affect several different types of ion channels (see Rudolph & Antkowiak, 2004; Franks, 2008). For most anaesthetics, there are no known competitive antagonists, so this approach to identify sites of action is denied. Therefore the main criterion for identifying putative mechanisms of action of general anaesthetics is that, for an effect to be relevant to the anaesthetic or analgesic actions of these agents, it must occur at therapeutically relevant concentrations.

Cys-loop ligand-gated ion channels. Almost all anaesthetics (with the exceptions of **cyclopropane**, **ketamine** and **xenon**[2]) potentiate the action of GABA at GABA$_A$ receptors (Olsen & Li, 2011). As described in detail in Chapter 37, GABA$_A$ receptors are ligand-gated Cl$^-$ channels made up of five subunits (generally comprising two α, two β and one γ or δ subunit). Anaesthetics can bind to hydrophobic pockets within different GABA$_A$ receptor subunits (see Fig. 41.2).

Specific mutations of the amino acid sequence of the α subunit inhibit the actions of volatile anaesthetics but not those of intravenous anaesthetics, whereas mutations of the β subunit inhibit both volatile and intravenous anaesthetics (see Franks, 2008). This suggest that volatile anaesthetics may bind at the interface between α and β subunits (analogous to benzodiazepines that bind at the interface between α and γ/δ subunits, see Ch. 38), whereas the

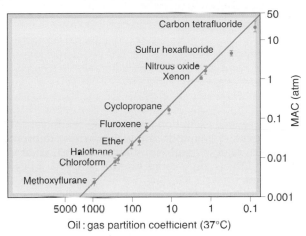

Fig. 41.1 Correlation of anaesthetic potency with oil:gas partition coefficient. Anaesthetic potency in humans is expressed as minimum alveolar partial pressure (MAC) required to produce surgical anaesthesia. There is a close correlation with lipid solubility, expressed as the oil:gas partition coefficient. *(From Halsey MJ 1989. Physicochemical properties of inhalation anaesthetics. In: Nunn JF, Utting JE, Brown BR (eds) General Anaesthesia. Butterworth, London.)*

---

[2]There is some controversy about whether or not xenon potentiates GABA$_A$ responses but at present the weight of evidence suggests it does not.

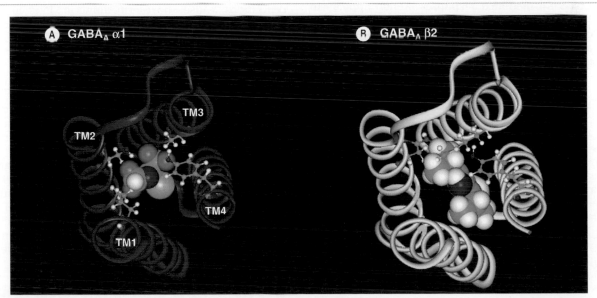

Fig. 41.2 Putative anaesthetic binding sites on GABA$_A$ receptor subunits. [A] A model of the α1 subunit of the GABA$_A$ receptor with a molecule of isoflurane shown sitting in a putative binding site. The transmembrane α-helices (TM) are numbered 1–4. [B] A model of the β2 subunit of the GABA$_A$ receptor with a molecule of propofol shown sitting in the putative binding site. *(Adapted from Hemmings HC et al. 2005 Trends Pharmacol Sci 26, 503–510.)*

intravenous anaesthetics may bind only on the β subunit. However, photoaffinity labelling experiments suggest that **etomidate** may bind to amino acid residues on both the α and β subunits. A further level of complexity arises because there are different subtypes of each subunit (see Ch. 38). Different subunit compositions give rise to subtly different subtypes of GABA$_A$ receptor and these may be involved in different aspects of anaesthetic action. GABA$_A$ receptors clustered at the synapse have different pharmacological and kinetic properties from those that are distributed elsewhere across the cell (extrasynaptic receptors; see Ch. 38). Extrasynaptic GABA$_A$ receptors contain α4 and α6 subunits as well as the δ subunit, and anaesthetics appear to have a greater potentiating effect on these extrasynaptic GABA$_A$ receptors.

General anaesthetics also affect other neuronal cys-loop ligand-gated channels such as those activated by glycine (Ch. 38), acetylcholine and 5-hydroxytryptamine (Ch. 39). Their actions on these channels are similar to those on GABA$_A$ receptors but the relative importance of such actions to general anaesthesia is still to be determined.

Two-pore domain K$^+$ channels. These belong to a family of 'background' K$^+$ channels that modulate neuronal excitability. They are homomeric or heteromeric assemblies of a family of structurally related subunits (Bayliss & Barrett, 2008). Channels made up of TREK1, TREK2, TASK1, TASK3 or TRESK (see Ch 4, Table 4.2) subunits can be directly activated by low concentrations of volatile and gaseous anaesthetics, thus reducing membrane excitability (see Franks, 2008). This may contribute to the analgesic, hypnotic and immobilising effects of these agents. Two-pore domain K$^+$ channels do not appear to be affected by intravenous anaesthetics.

NMDA receptors. **Glutamate**, the major excitatory neurotransmitter in the CNS, activates three main classes of ionotropic receptor – AMPA, kainate and NMDA receptors (see Ch. 38). NMDA receptors are an important site of action for anaesthetics such as **nitrous oxide**, **xenon** and **ketamine** which act, in different ways, to reduce NMDA receptor-mediated responses. Xenon appears to inhibit NMDA receptors by competing with glycine for its regulatory site on this receptor whereas ketamine blocks the pore of the channel (see Ch. 38). Other inhalation anaesthetics may also exert effects on the NMDA receptor in addition to their effects on other proteins such as the GABA$_A$ receptor.

Other ion channels. Anaesthetics may also exert actions at cyclic nucleotide-gated K$^+$ channels and K$_{ATP}$ channels. Some general anaesthetics inhibit certain subtypes of voltage-gated Na$^+$ channels. Inhibition of presynaptic Na$^+$ channels may give rise to the inhibition of transmitter release at excitatory synapses.

It may be overly simplistic to think of each anaesthetic as having only one mechanism of action: individual anaesthetics differ in their actions and affect cellular function in several different ways, so a single mechanism is unlikely to be sufficient.

Comprehensive reviews of the molecular and cellular actions of general anaesthetics can be found in Schüttler & Schwilden (2008).

EFFECTS ON THE NERVOUS SYSTEM

At the cellular level, the effects of anaesthetics are to enhance tonic inhibition (through enhancing the actions

Theories of anaesthesia

- Many simple, unreactive compounds produce general anaesthesia, the extreme example being the inert gas **xenon**.
- Anaesthetic potency is closely correlated with lipid solubility (Overton–Meyer correlation), not with chemical structure.
- Earlier theories of anaesthesia postulated interaction with the lipid membrane bilayer. Recent work favours interaction with membrane ion channels.
- Most anaesthetics enhance the activity of inhibitory GABA$_A$ receptors and other cys-loop ligand-gated ion channels. Other important effects are the activation of a subfamily of potassium channels (the two-pore domain K$^+$ channels) and inhibition of excitatory NMDA receptors.

of GABA), reduce excitation (opening K$^+$ channels) and to inhibit excitatory synaptic transmission (by depressing transmitter release and inhibiting ligand-gated ion channels). Effects on axonal conduction are relatively unimportant.

The anaesthetised state comprises several components, including *unconsciousness*, loss of reflexes (*muscle relaxation*) and *analgesia*. Much effort has gone into identifying the brain regions on which anaesthetics act to produce these effects. The most sensitive regions appear to be the midbrain reticular formation, thalamic sensory relay nuclei and, to a lesser extent, parts of the cortex. Inhibition of these regions results in unconsciousness and analgesia. Some anaesthetics – particularly volatile anaesthetics – cause inhibition at the spinal level, producing a loss of reflex responses to painful stimuli, although, in practice, neuromuscular-blocking drugs (Ch. 13) are used as an adjunct to produce muscle relaxation rather than relying on the anaesthetic alone. Anaesthetics, even in low concentrations, cause short-term amnesia. It is likely that interference with hippocampal function produces this effect, because the hippocampus is involved in short-term memory, and certain hippocampal synapses are highly susceptible to inhibition by anaesthetics.

As the anaesthetic concentration is increased, all brain functions are progressively affected, including motor control and reflex activity, respiration and autonomic regulation. Therefore it is not possible to identify a critical 'target site' in the brain responsible for all the phenomena of anaesthesia.

High concentrations of any general anaesthetic affect all parts of the CNS, causing profound inhibition which, in the absence of artificial respiration, leads to death from respiratory failure. The margin between surgical anaesthesia and potentially fatal respiratory and circulatory depression is quite narrow, requiring careful monitoring by the anaesthetist and adjustment of the level of anaesthesia.

EFFECTS ON THE CARDIOVASCULAR AND RESPIRATORY SYSTEMS

Most anaesthetics decrease cardiac contractility, but their effects on cardiac output and blood pressure vary because of concomitant actions on the sympathetic nervous system and vascular smooth muscle. **Isoflurane** and other halogenated anaesthetics inhibit sympathetic outflow, reduce arterial and venous tone and thus decrease arterial pressure and venous pressure. By contrast, **nitrous oxide** and **ketamine** increase sympathetic discharge and plasma noradrenaline concentration and, if used alone, increase heart rate and maintain blood pressure.

Many anaesthetics, especially **halothane**, cause ventricular extrasystoles. The mechanism involves sensitisation to adrenaline. Electrocardiogram monitoring shows that extrasystolic beats occur commonly in patients under anaesthesia, with no harm coming to the patient. If catecholamine secretion is excessive, however (*par excellence* in phaeochromocytoma, a neuroendocrine tumour that secretes catecholamines into the circulation; see Ch. 14), there is a risk of precipitating ventricular fibrillation.

With the exception of **nitrous oxide, ketamine** and **xenon**, all anaesthetics depress respiration markedly and increase arterial $P\text{CO}_2$. Nitrous oxide has much less effect, in part because its low potency prevents very deep anaesthesia from being produced with this drug. Some inhalation anaesthetics are pungent, particularly **desflurane**, which is liable to cause coughing, laryngospasm and bronchospasm, so desflurane is not used for induction of anaesthesia but only for maintenance.

INTRAVENOUS ANAESTHETIC AGENTS

Even the fastest-acting inhalation anaesthetics take a few minutes to act and cause a period of excitement before anaesthesia is induced. Intravenous anaesthetics act more rapidly, producing unconsciousness in about 20 s, as soon as the drug reaches the brain from its site of injection. These drugs (e.g. **propofol**, **thiopental** and **etomidate**) are normally used for induction of anaesthesia. They are preferred by many patients because injection generally lacks the menacing quality associated with a face mask in an apprehensive individual. With propofol, recovery is also fast due to rapid metabolism.

Although many intravenous anaesthetics are not suitable for maintaining anaesthesia because their elimination from the body is relatively slow compared with that of inhalation agents, propofol can be used as a continuous infusion, and the duration of action of ketamine is sufficient that it can be administered as a single bolus for short operations without the need for an inhalation agent. Under these circumstances a short-acting opioid such as **alfentanil** or **remifentanil** (Ch. 42) may be co-administered to provide analgesia.

The properties of the main intravenous anaesthetics are summarised in Table 41.1.[3]

PROPOFOL

Propofol, introduced in 1983, has now largely replaced thiopental as an induction agent. It has a rapid onset of action (approximately 30 s) and a rapid rate of redistribution ($t_{1/2}$ 2–4 min), which makes it short acting. Because of its low water solubility, it is administered as an

---

[3]**Propanidid** and **alphaxalone** were withdrawn because of allergic reactions including hypotension and bronchoconstriction – probably attributable to the solvent Cremophor – but a new formulation of alphaxalone has been reintroduced to veterinary medicine and is thought to be less allergenic.

Pharmacological effects of anaesthetic agents

- Anaesthesia involves three main neurophysiological changes: unconsciousness, loss of response to painful stimulation and loss of reflexes (motor and autonomic).
- At supra-anaesthetic doses, all anaesthetic agents can cause death by loss of cardiovascular reflexes and respiratory paralysis.
- At the cellular level, anaesthetic agents affect synaptic transmission and neuronal excitability rather than axonal conduction. GABA-mediated inhibitory transmission is enhanced by most anaesthetics. The release of excitatory transmitters and the response of the postsynaptic receptors are also inhibited.
- Although all parts of the nervous system are affected by anaesthetic agents, the main targets appear to be the cortex, thalamus, hippocampus, midbrain reticular formation and spinal cord.
- Most anaesthetic agents (with the exception of **ketamine**, **nitrous oxide** and **xenon**) produce similar neurophysiological effects and differ mainly in respect of their pharmacokinetic properties and toxicity.
- Most anaesthetic agents cause cardiovascular depression by effects on the myocardium and blood vessels, as well as on the nervous system. Halogenated anaesthetic agents are likely to cause cardiac dysrhythmias, accentuated by circulating catecholamines.

oil-in-water emulsion, which can cause pain on injection, and supports microbial growth. **Fospropofol** is a recently developed water-soluble derivative that is less painful on injection and rapidly converted by alkaline phosphatases to propofol in the body. Propofol metabolism to inactive conjugates and quinols follows first-order kinetics, in contrast to thiopental (see below), resulting in more rapid recovery and less hangover effect than occurs with thiopental. It has a cardiovascular depressant effect that may lead to hypotension and bradycardia. Respiratory depression may also occur. It is particularly useful for day-case surgery, especially as it causes less nausea and vomiting than do inhalation anaesthetics.

There have been reports of a propofol infusion syndrome occurring in approximately 1 in 300 patients when it has been given for a prolonged period to maintain sedation, particularly to sick patients – especially children in whom it is contraindicated in this setting – in intensive care units. This is characterised by severe metabolic acidosis, skeletal muscle necrosis (rhabdomyolysis), hyperkalaemia, lipaemia, hepatomegaly, renal failure, arrhythmia and cardiovascular collapse.

THIOPENTAL

Thiopental is the only remaining barbiturate in common use. It has very high lipid solubility, and this accounts for the speed of onset and transience of its effect when it is injected intravenously. The free acid is insoluble in water, so thiopental is given as the sodium salt. On intravenous injection, thiopental causes unconsciousness within about

Table 41.1 Properties of intravenous anaesthetic agents

Drug	Speed of induction and recovery	Main unwanted effect(s)	Notes
Propofol	Fast onset, very fast recovery	Cardiovascular and respiratory depression	Rapidly metabolised Possible to use as continuous infusion Causes pain at injection site
Thiopental	Fast (accumulation occurs, giving slow recovery) 'Hangover'	Cardiovascular and respiratory depression	Largely replaced by propofol Causes pain at injection site Risk of precipitating porphyria in susceptible patients
Etomidate	Fast onset, fairly fast recovery	Excitatory effects during induction and recovery Adrenocortical suppression	Less cardiovascular and respiratory depression than with thiopental Causes pain at injection site
Ketamine	Slow onset, after effects common during recovery	Psychotomimetic effects following recovery Postoperative nausea, vomiting and salivation Raised intracranial pressure	Produces good analgesia and amnesia with little respiratory depression
Midazolam	Slower than other agents	–	Little respiratory or cardiovascular depression

20 s, lasting for 5–10 min. The anaesthetic effect closely parallels the concentration of thiopental in the blood reaching the brain, because its high lipid solubility allows it to cross the blood–brain barrier without noticeable delay.

The blood concentration of thiopental declines rapidly, by about 80% within 1–2 min, following the initial peak after intravenous injection, because the drug is redistributed, first to tissues with a large blood flow (liver, kidneys, brain, etc.) and more slowly to muscle. Uptake into body fat, although favoured by the high lipid solubility of thiopental, occurs only slowly, because of the low blood flow to this tissue. After several hours, however, most of the thiopental present in the body will have accumulated in body fat, the rest having been metabolised. Recovery from the anaesthetic effect of a bolus dose occurs within about 5 min, governed entirely by redistribution of the drug to well-perfused tissues; very little is metabolised in this time. After the initial rapid decline, the blood concentration drops more slowly, over several hours, as the drug is taken up by body fat and metabolised. Consequently, thiopental produces a long-lasting hangover. Thiopental metabolism shows saturation kinetics (Ch. 10). Because of this, large doses or repeated intravenous doses cause progressively longer periods of anaesthesia, as the plateau in blood concentration becomes progressively more elevated as more drug accumulates in the body and metabolism saturates. For this reason, thiopental is not used to maintain surgical anaesthesia but only as an induction agent. It is also still used to terminate status epilepticus (see Ch. 45) or (in patients with a secured airway) to lower intracranial pressure.

Thiopental binds to plasma albumin (roughly 85% of the blood content normally being bound). The fraction bound is less in states of malnutrition, liver disease or renal disease, which affect the concentration and drug-binding properties of plasma albumin, and this can appreciably reduce the dose needed for induction of anaesthesia.

If thiopental – a strongly alkaline solution – is accidentally injected around rather than into a vein, or into an artery, this can cause pain, local tissue necrosis and ulceration or severe arterial spasm that can result in gangrene.

The actions of thiopental on the nervous system are very similar to those of inhalation anaesthetics, although it has little analgesic effect and can cause profound respiratory depression even in amounts that fail to abolish reflex responses to painful stimuli. Its long after-effect, associated with a slowly declining plasma concentration, means that drowsiness and some degree of respiratory depression persist for some hours.

ETOMIDATE

Etomidate has gained favour over thiopental on account of the larger margin between the anaesthetic dose and the dose needed to produce cardiovascular depression. It is more rapidly metabolised than thiopental, and thus less likely to cause a prolonged hangover. It causes less hypotension than propofol or thiopental. In other respects, etomidate is very similar to thiopental, although involuntary movements during induction, postoperative nausea and vomiting, and pain at the injection site are problems with its use. Etomidate suppresses the production of adrenal steroids, an effect that has been associated with an increase in mortality in severely ill patients. It should be avoided in patients at risk of having adrenal insufficiency, e.g. in sepsis. It is preferable to thiopental in patients at risk of circulatory failure.

OTHER INTRAVENOUS AGENTS

KETAMINE

▼ **Ketamine** closely resembles, both chemically and pharmacologically, **phencyclidine**. Both are used recreationally for their pronounced effects on sensory perception (see Ch. 48). Both drugs are believed to act by blocking activation of the NMDA receptor (see Ch. 38). They produce a similar anaesthesia-like state and profound analgesia, but ketamine produces less euphoria and sensory distortion than phencyclidine and is thus more useful in anaesthesia. Ketamine can be used in lower doses as an analgesic (Ch. 42) and as an acute treatment for depression (Ch. 47).

Intravenous anaesthetic agents

- Most commonly used for induction of anaesthesia, followed by inhalation agent. **Propofol** can also be used to maintain anaesthesia during surgery.
- **Propofol, thiopental** and **etomidate** are most commonly used; all act within 20–30 s if given intravenously.
- **Propofol**:
  - potent
  - rapid onset and distribution
  - rapidly metabolised
  - very rapid recovery; limited cumulative effect
  - useful for day-case surgery
  - low incidence of nausea and vomiting
  - risk of bradycardia
  - may induce an adverse 'propofol infusion syndrome' when administered at high doses for prolonged periods of time.
- **Thiopental**:
  - barbiturate with very high lipid solubility
  - rapid action due to rapid transfer across blood–brain barrier; short duration (about 5 min) due to redistribution, mainly to muscle
  - reduces intracranial pressure
  - slowly metabolised and liable to accumulate in body fat, therefore may cause prolonged effect if given repeatedly

- narrow margin between anaesthetic dose and dose causing cardiovascular depression
- risk of tissue damage if accidentally injected extravascularly or into an artery
- can precipitate an attack of porphyria in susceptible individuals (see Ch. 11).
- **Etomidate**:
  - similar to thiopental but more quickly metabolised
  - less risk of cardiovascular depression
  - may cause involuntary movements during induction and high incidence of nausea
  - possible risk of adrenocortical suppression.
- **Ketamine**:
  - analogue of **phencyclidine**, with similar properties
  - action differs from other agents, probably related to inhibition of NMDA-type glutamate receptors
  - onset of effect is relatively slow (1–2 min)
  - powerful analgesic
  - produces 'dissociative' anaesthesia, in which the patient may remain conscious although amnesic and insensitive to pain
  - high incidence of dysphoria, hallucinations, etc. during recovery; used mainly for minor procedures in children
  - can raise intracranial pressure.

Given intravenously, ketamine takes effect more slowly (1–2 min) than thiopental, and produces a different effect, known as 'dissociative anaesthesia', in which there is a marked sensory loss and analgesia, as well as amnesia, without complete loss of consciousness. During induction and recovery, involuntary movements and peculiar sensory experiences often occur. Ketamine does not act simply as a CNS depressant, and it produces cardiovascular and respiratory effects quite different from those of most anaesthetics. Blood pressure and heart rate are usually increased, and respiration is unaffected by effective anaesthetic doses. This makes it relatively safe to use in low-technology healthcare situations or in accident and emergency situations where it can be administered intramuscularly if intravenous administration is not possible.[4] However, ketamine, unlike other intravenous anaesthetic drugs, can increase intracranial pressure, so it should not be given to patients with raised intracranial pressure or at risk of cerebral ischaemia. The other main drawback of ketamine is that hallucinations, and sometimes delirium and irrational behaviour, are common during recovery. These after-effects limit the usefulness of ketamine but are said to be less marked in children,[5] and ketamine, often in conjunction with a benzodiazepine, is sometimes still used for minor procedures in paediatrics.

MIDAZOLAM

Midazolam, a benzodiazepine (Ch. 44), is slower in onset and offset than the drugs discussed above but, like ketamine, causes less respiratory or cardiovascular depression. Midazolam (or **diazepam**) is often used as a preoperative sedative and during procedures such as endoscopy, where full anaesthesia is not required. It can be administered in combination with an analgesic such as **alfentanil**. In the event of overdose it can be reversed by **flumazenil** (see Ch. 44).

INHALATION ANAESTHETICS

Many inhalation anaesthetics that were once widely used, such as ether, chloroform, trichloroethylene, cyclopropane, methoxyflurane and enflurane, have now been replaced in clinical practice, particularly by **isoflurane**, **sevoflurane** and **desflurane**, which have improved pharmacokinetic properties, fewer side effects and are non-flammable. Of the older agents, nitrous oxide is still used widely (especially in obstetric practice), and halothane now only occasionally.

PHARMACOKINETIC ASPECTS

An important characteristic of an inhalation anaesthetic is the speed at which the arterial blood concentration, which governs the pharmacological effect in the brain, follows changes in the partial pressure of the drug in the inspired gas mixture. Ideally, the blood concentration should follow as quickly as possible, so that the depth of anaesthesia can be controlled rapidly. In particular, the blood concentration should fall to a subanaesthetic level rapidly when administration is stopped, so that the patient recovers consciousness with minimal delay. A prolonged semi-comatose state, in which respiratory reflexes are weak or absent, is particularly hazardous.

---

[4]An anaesthetist colleague tells of coming across a motorway accident where most of a victim was hidden under a mass of distorted metal but enough of a limb was available for an injection of ketamine to be given.
[5]A cautionary note: many adverse effects are claimed to be less marked in children, perhaps because they cannot verbalise their experiences. At one time, muscle relaxants alone were used without anaesthesia during cardiac surgery in neonates. The babies did not complain of pain, but their circulating catecholamines reached extreme levels.

The lungs are the only quantitatively important route by which inhalation anaesthetics enter and leave the body. For modern inhalation anaesthetics, metabolic degradation is generally insignificant in determining their duration of action. Inhalation anaesthetics are all small, lipid-soluble molecules that readily cross alveolar membranes. It is therefore the rates of delivery of drug to and from the lungs, via (respectively) the inspired air and bloodstream, which determine the overall kinetic behaviour of an anaesthetic. The reason that anaesthetics vary in their kinetic behaviour is that their relative solubilities in blood, and in body fat, vary between one drug and another.

The main factors that determine the speed of induction and recovery can be summarised as follows:

- Properties of the anaesthetic:
  - blood : gas partition coefficient (i.e. solubility in blood)
  - oil : gas partition coefficient (i.e. solubility in fat).
- Physiological factors:
  - alveolar ventilation rate
  - cardiac output.

SOLUBILITY OF INHALATION ANAESTHETICS

Inhalation anaesthetics can be regarded physicochemically as ideal gases: their solubility in different media is expressed as *partition coefficients*, defined as the ratio of the concentration of the agent in two phases at equilibrium.

The *blood:gas partition coefficient* is the main factor that determines the rate of induction and recovery of an inhalation anaesthetic, and the lower the blood:gas partition coefficient, the faster is induction and recovery (Table 41.2). This is because it is the partial pressure of the gas in the alveolar space that governs the concentration in the blood. The lower the blood:gas partition coefficient, the more rapidly the partial pressure of the gas in the alveolar space will equal that being administered in the inspired air (see below).

The *oil:gas partition coefficient*, a measure of fat solubility, determines the potency of an anaesthetic (as already discussed) and also influences the kinetics of its distribution in the body, the main effect being that high lipid solubility delays recovery from anaesthesia. Values of blood:gas and oil:gas partition coefficients for some anaesthetics are given in Table 41.2.

INDUCTION AND RECOVERY

Cerebral blood flow is a substantial fraction of cardiac output (~15%), and the blood–brain barrier is freely permeable to anaesthetics, so the concentration of anaesthetic in the brain closely tracks that in the arterial blood. The kinetics of transfer of anaesthetic between the inspired air and the arterial blood therefore determine the kinetics of the pharmacological effect.

When a volatile anaesthetic is first administered, the initial breaths are diluted into the residual gas volume in the lungs resulting in a reduction in the alveolar partial pressure of the anaesthetic as compared with the inspired gas mixture. With subsequent breaths, the alveolar partial pressure rises towards equilibrium. For an anaesthetic with a low blood:gas partition coefficient, the absorption into the blood will be slower, so with repeated breaths the partial pressure in the alveolar space will rise faster than

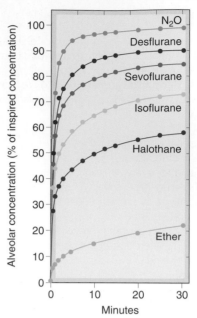

Fig. 41.3 Rate of equilibration of inhalation anaesthetics in humans. The curves show alveolar concentration (which closely reflects arterial blood concentration) as a function of time during induction. The initial rate of equilibration reflects solubility in blood. There is also a slow phase of equilibration, most marked with highly lipid-soluble drugs (ether and halothane), owing to the slow transfer between blood and fat (Fig. 41.4). *(Adapted from Yasuda N, Lockhart SH, Eger El II, et al. 1991 Comparison of kinetics of sevoflurane and isoflurane in humans. Anesth Analg 72, 316–324.)*

with an agent of high blood:gas partition coefficient. Thus a smaller number of breaths (i.e. a shorter time) will be needed to reach equilibrium. Therefore, contrary to what one might intuitively suppose, the *lower* the solubility in blood, the *faster* is the process of equilibration. Figure 41.3 shows the much faster equilibration for **nitrous oxide**, a low-solubility agent, than for **ether**, a high-solubility agent.

The rate of absorption into the blood can be enhanced by administering a volatile anaesthetic along with nitrous oxide. The rapid movement of nitrous oxide from the alveoli into the blood concentrates the volatile anaesthetic in the alveoli which will increase its movement into the blood – referred to as the *concentration effect*. Furthermore, replacement of the gas taken up into the blood by an increase in inspired ventilation augments the amount of volatile anaesthetic present in the alveoli – referred to as the *second gas effect*.

The transfer of anaesthetic between blood and tissues also affects the kinetics of equilibration. Figure 41.4 shows a very simple model of the circulation, in which two tissue compartments are included. Body fat has a low blood flow but has a high capacity to take up anaesthetics, and constitutes about 20% of the volume of a representative man. Therefore, for a drug such as **halothane**, which is about 100 times more soluble in fat than in water, the amount present in fat after complete equilibration would be roughly 95% of the total amount in the body. Because of the low blood flow to adipose tissue, it takes many hours for the drug to enter and leave the fat, which results in a pronounced slow phase of equilibration following the

Table 41.2 Characteristics of inhalation anaesthetics

Drug	Partition coefficient Blood:gas	Oil:gas	Minimum alveolar concentration (% v/v)	Induction/ recovery	Main adverse effect(s) and disadvantage(s)	Notes
Nitrous oxide	0.5	1.4	100[a]	Fast	Few adverse effects Risk of anaemia (with prolonged or repeated use) Accumulation in gaseous cavities	Good analgesic effect Low potency precludes use as sole anaesthetic agent – normally combined with other inhalation agents
Isoflurane	1.4	91	1.2	Medium	Few adverse effects Possible risk of coronary ischemia in susceptible patients	Widely used Has replaced halothane
Desflurane	0.4	23	6.1	Fast	Respiratory tract irritation, cough, bronchospasm	Used for day-case surgery because of fast onset and recovery (comparable with nitrous oxide)
Sevoflurane	0.6	53	2.1	Fast	Few reported Theoretical risk of renal toxicity owing to fluoride	Similar to desflurane
Halothane	2.4	220	0.8	Medium	Hypotension Cardiac arrhythmias Hepatotoxicity (with repeated use) Malignant hyperthermia (rare)	Little used nowadays Significant metabolism to trifluoracetate
Enflurane	1.9	98	1.7	Medium	Risk of convulsions (slight) Malignant hyperthermia (rare)	Has declined in use May induce seizures
Ether	12.0	65	1.9	Slow	Respiratory irritation Nausea and vomiting Explosion risk	Now obsolete, except where modern facilities are lacking

[a]Theoretical value based on experiments under hyperbaric conditions.

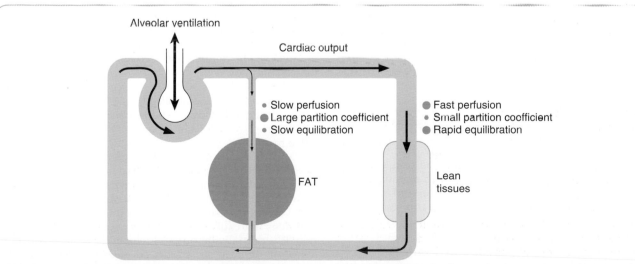

Fig. 41.4 Factors affecting the rate of equilibration of inhalation anaesthetics in the body. The body is represented as two compartments. Lean tissues, including the brain, have a large blood flow and low partition coefficient for anaesthetics, and therefore equilibrate rapidly with the blood. Fat tissues have a small blood flow and large partition coefficient, and therefore equilibrate slowly, acting as a reservoir of drug during the recovery phase.

rapid phase associated with the blood–gas exchanges (Fig. 41.3). The more fat-soluble the anaesthetic and the fatter the patient, the more pronounced this slow phase becomes and recovery will also be delayed.

Of the physiological factors affecting the rate of equilibration of inhalation anaesthetics, alveolar ventilation is the most important. The greater the minute volume (respiration rate × tidal volume), the faster is equilibration, particularly for drugs that have high blood:gas partition coefficients. Respiratory depressant drugs such as **morphine** (see Ch. 42) can thus retard recovery from anaesthesia. The effect of changes in cardiac output on the rate of equilibration is more complex. By reducing alveolar perfusion, a reduction of cardiac output reduces alveolar absorption of the anaesthetic, and thus speeds up induction, but this is partially offset by a reduction of cerebral blood flow slowing down delivery to the brain.

Recovery from anaesthesia involves the same processes as induction but in reverse, the rapid phase of recovery being followed by a slow 'hangover'. Because of these kinetic factors, the search for improved inhalation anaesthetics has focused on agents with low blood and tissue solubility. Newer drugs, which show kinetic properties similar to those of nitrous oxide but have higher potency, include **sevoflurane** and **desflurane** (Table 41.2 and Fig. 41.3).

METABOLISM AND TOXICITY

Metabolism, although not quantitatively important as a route of elimination of inhalation anaesthetics, can generate toxic metabolites (Ch. 57).[6] This is the main reason that agents that are now obsolete or obsolescent, such as chloroform, methoxyflurane and halothane, have been replaced by the less toxic alternatives described below.

Malignant hyperthermia is an important but rare *idiosyncratic reaction* (see Ch. 57), caused by heat production in skeletal muscle, due to excessive release of Ca^{2+} from the sarcoplasmic reticulum. The result is muscle contracture, acidosis, increased metabolism and an associated dramatic rise in body temperature that can be fatal unless treated promptly. Triggers include halogenated anaesthetics and depolarising neuromuscular-blocking drugs (see Ch. 13). Susceptibility has a genetic basis, being associated with mutations in the gene encoding the ryanodine receptor, which controls Ca^{2+} release from the sarcoplasmic reticulum (Ch. 4). Malignant hyperthermia is treated with **dantrolene**, a muscle relaxant drug that blocks these calcium-release channels.

INDIVIDUAL INHALATION ANAESTHETICS

The main inhalation anaesthetics currently used in developed countries are **isoflurane**, **desflurane** and **sevoflurane**, sometimes used in combination with **nitrous oxide**. Due to its relatively rapid onset of action and pleasant smell sevoflurane is used, under some circumstances, on its own to induce anaesthesia, e.g. in paediatrics or in adults frightened by the prospect of venous cannulation. **Xenon**, an inert gas shown many years ago to have

---

[6]The problem of toxicity of low concentrations of anaesthetics inhaled over long periods by operating theatre staff has been a cause for concern. Strict measures are now used to minimise the escape of anaesthetics into the air of operating theatres.

Pharmacokinetic properties of inhalation anaesthetics

- Rapid induction and recovery are important properties of an anaesthetic agent, allowing flexible control over the depth of anaesthesia.
- Speed of induction and recovery are determined by two properties of the anaesthetic: solubility in blood (blood:gas partition coefficient) and solubility in fat (lipid solubility).
- Agents with low blood:gas partition coefficients produce rapid induction and recovery (e.g. **nitrous oxide**, **desflurane**); agents with high blood:gas partition coefficients show slow induction and recovery.
- Agents with high lipid solubility accumulate gradually in body fat and may produce a prolonged 'hangover' if used for a long operation.
- Some halogenated anaesthetics (especially **halothane** and **methoxyflurane**) are metabolised. This is not very important in determining their duration of action, but contributes to toxicity (e.g. renal toxicity associated with fluoride production with **methoxyflurane** – no longer used).

---

anaesthetic properties, is making something of a comeback in the clinic because – not surprisingly for an inert gas – it lacks toxicity, but its relatively low potency and high cost are disadvantages. It may also be neuroprotective in neonatal hypoxia (see Ch. 40).

ISOFLURANE, DESFLURANE, SEVOFLURANE, ENFLURANE AND HALOTHANE

Isoflurane is now the most widely used volatile anaesthetic. It is not appreciably metabolised and lacks the proconvulsive property of enflurane. It can cause hypotension and is a powerful coronary vasodilator. This can exacerbate cardiac ischaemia in patients with coronary disease, because of the 'steal' phenomenon (see Ch. 21).

Desflurane is chemically similar to isoflurane, but its lower solubility in blood and fat means that adjustment of anaesthetic depth and recovery are faster, so it is increasingly used as an anaesthetic in obese patients undergoing bariatric surgery and for day-case surgery. It is not appreciably metabolised. It is less potent than the drugs described above. At the concentrations used for induction of anaesthesia (about 10%), desflurane causes some respiratory tract irritation, which can lead to coughing and bronchospasm. Rapid increases in the depth of desflurane anaesthesia can be associated with a striking increase in sympathetic activity, which is undesirable in patients with ischaemic heart disease.

Sevoflurane resembles desflurane but is more potent and does not cause the same degree of respiratory irritation. It is partially (about 3%) metabolised, and detectable levels of fluoride are produced, although this does not appear to be sufficient to cause toxicity.

Enflurane has a moderate speed of induction but is little used nowadays. It was originally introduced as an alternative to methoxyflurane. It can cause seizures, either during induction or following recovery from anaesthesia, especially in patients suffering from epilepsy. In this connection, it is interesting that a related substance, the fluorine-substituted diethyl-ether hexafluoroether, is a powerful convulsant agent, although the mechanism is not understood.

Halothane was an important drug in the development of volatile inhalation anaesthetics, but its use has declined in favour of isoflurane due to the potential for accumulation of toxic metabolites. Halothane has a marked relaxant effect on the uterus which can cause postpartum bleeding and limits its usefulness for obstetric purposes.

NITROUS OXIDE

Nitrous oxide (N_2O, not to be confused with nitric oxide, NO) is an odourless gas with many advantageous features for anaesthesia. It is rapid in onset of action because of its low blood:gas partition coefficient (Table 41.2), and is an effective analgesic in concentrations too low to cause unconsciousness. Its potency is low. It is used as a 50:50 mixture with O_2 to reduce pain during childbirth. It must never be given as 100% of the inspired gas as patients do need to breathe oxygen! Even at 80% in the inspired gas mixture, nitrous oxide does not produce surgical anaesthesia. It is not therefore used on its own as an anaesthetic, but is used (as 70% nitrous oxide in oxygen) as an adjunct to volatile anaesthetics to speed up induction – see description of the second gas effect (p. 504). During recovery from nitrous oxide anaesthesia, the transfer of the gas from the blood into the alveoli can be sufficient to reduce, by dilution, the alveolar partial pressure of oxygen, producing transient hypoxia (known as *diffusional hypoxia*). This is important for patients with respiratory disease.

Nitrous oxide tends to enter gaseous cavities in the body causing them to expand. This can be dangerous if a pneumothorax or vascular air embolus is present, or if the intestine is obstructed.

Given for brief periods, nitrous oxide is devoid of any serious toxic effects, but prolonged exposure (>6 h) causes inactivation of methionine synthase, an enzyme required for DNA and protein synthesis, resulting in bone marrow depression that may cause anaemia and leucopenia, so its use should be avoided in patients with anaemia related to vitamin B_{12} deficiency. Bone marrow depression does not occur with brief exposure to nitrous oxide, but prolonged or repeated use (for example, in intermittently painful conditions such as sickle cell anaemia) should be avoided. Nitrous oxide 'sniffers' are subject to this danger.

BALANCED ANAESTHESIA

Only in simple, short surgical procedures would a single anaesthetic be used on its own. In complex surgery, an array of drugs will be given at various times throughout the procedure. These may include a sedative or anxiolytic premedication (e.g. a benzodiazepine, see Ch. 44), an intravenous anaesthetic for rapid induction (e.g. **propofol**), a perioperative opioid analgesic (e.g. **alfentanil** or **remifentanil**, see Ch. 42), an inhalation anaesthetic to maintain anaesthesia during surgery (e.g. **nitrous oxide** and **isoflurane**), a neuromuscular blocking agent to produce adequate muscle relaxation (e.g. **vecuronium**, see Ch. 13) for access to the abdominal cavity for example, an antiemetic agent (e.g. **ondansetron**, see Ch. 30) and a muscarinic antagonist to prevent or treat bradycardia or to reduce bronchial and salivary secretions (e.g. **atropine** or **glycopyrrolate**,

Individual inhalation anaesthetics

- The main agents in current use in developed countries are **isoflurane**, **desflurane** and **sevoflurane**, sometimes supplemented with **nitrous oxide**.
- As a rare but serious hazard, inhalation anaesthetics can cause malignant hyperthermia.
- **Nitrous oxide**:
  - low potency, therefore must be combined with other agents
  - rapid induction and recovery
  - good analgesic properties
  - risk of bone marrow depression with prolonged administration
  - accumulates in gaseous cavities.
- **Isoflurane**:
  - similar to **enflurane** but lacks epileptogenic property
  - may precipitate myocardial ischaemia in patients with coronary disease
  - irritant to respiratory tract.
- **Desflurane**:
  - similar to **isoflurane** but with faster onset and recovery
  - respiratory irritant, so liable to cause coughing and laryngospasm
  - useful for day-case surgery.
- **Sevoflurane**:
  - similar to **desflurane**, with lack of respiratory irritation.

Clinical uses of general anaesthetics

- *Intravenous anaesthetics* are used for:
  - induction of anaesthesia (e.g. **propofol** or **thiopental**)
  - maintenance of anaesthesia throughout surgery ('total intravenous anaesthesia', e.g. **propofol** sometimes in combination with muscle relaxants and analgesics).
- *Inhalational anaesthetics* (gases or volatile liquids) are used for maintenance of anaesthesia. Points to note are that:
  - volatile anaesthetics (e.g. **isoflurane**, **sevoflurane**) are delivered in air, oxygen or oxygen–nitrous oxide mixtures as the carrier gas
  - **nitrous oxide** must always be given with oxygen
  - because of its potential for inducing hepatotoxicity, **halothane** has largely been replaced by newer volatile anaesthetics such as **isoflurane**
  - all inhalational anaesthetics can trigger *malignant hyperthermia* in susceptible individuals.

see Ch. 13) and, towards the end of the procedure, an anticholinesterase agent (e.g. **neostigmine**, see Ch. 13) to reverse the neuromuscular blockade and an analgesic for postoperative pain relief (e.g. an opioid such as **morphine** and/or a non-steroidal anti-inflammatory drug, see Ch. 42).

507

Such combinations of drugs result in much faster induction and recovery, avoiding long (and potentially hazardous) periods of semiconsciousness, good analgesia and muscle relaxation and it enables surgery to be carried out with less undesirable cardiorespiratory depression.

Low doses of general anaesthetics may be used to provide sedation where a local anaesthetic (Ch. 43) administered intrathecally, is used to provide analgesia and relaxation needed to perform surgery to the lower parts of the body.

REFERENCES AND FURTHER READING

Aitkenhead, A.R., Moppett, I., Thompson, J., 2013. Textbook of Anaesthesia. Churchill Livingstone/Elsevier, Edinburgh. (*Major textbook of anaesthesia*)

Bayliss, D.A., Barrett, P.Q., 2008. Emerging roles for two-pore-domain potassium channels and their potential therapeutic impact. Trends Pharmacol. Sci. 29, 566–575.

Franks, N.P., 2008. General anaesthesia: from molecular targets to neuronal pathways of sleep and arousal. Nat. Rev. Neurosci. 9, 370–386. (*Detailed discussion of the sites of action of general anaesthetics on specific ion channels*)

Olsen, R.W., Li, G.D., 2011. GABA$_A$ receptors as molecular targets of general anesthetics: identification of binding sites provides clues to allosteric modulation. Can. J. Anaesth. 58, 206–215. (*Useful update on the interaction of general anaesthetics with the GABA$_A$ receptor*)

Rudolph, U., Antkowiak, B., 2004. Molecular and neuronal substrates for general anaesthetics. Nat. Rev. Neurosci. 5, 709–720. (*Useful review article covering both the interaction of general anaesthetic agents with different ion channels, and the neuronal pathways that are affected*)

Schüttler, J., Schwilden, H., 2008. Modern anesthetics. Handb. Exp. Pharmacol. 182. (*Entire volume given over to multiauthor reviews of the mechanisms of action of general anaesthetics*)

Analgesic drugs 42

OVERVIEW

Pain is a disabling accompaniment of many medical conditions, and pain control is one of the most important therapeutic priorities.

In this chapter, we discuss the neural mechanisms responsible for different types of pain, and the various drugs that are used to reduce it. The 'classic' analgesic drugs, notably opioids and non-steroidal anti-inflammatory drugs (NSAIDs; described in Ch. 26), have their origins in natural products that have been used for centuries. The original compounds, typified by morphine and aspirin, are still in widespread use, but many synthetic compounds that act by the same mechanisms have been developed. Opioid analgesics are described in this chapter. Next, we consider various other drug classes, such as antidepressants and antiepileptic drugs, which clinical experience has shown to be effective in certain types of pain. Finally, looking into the future, many potential new drug targets have emerged as our knowledge of the neural mechanisms underlying pain has advanced. We describe briefly some of these new approaches at the end of the chapter.

NEURAL MECHANISMS OF PAIN

Pain is a subjective experience, hard to define exactly, even though we all know what we mean by it. Typically, it is a direct response to an untoward event associated with tissue damage, such as injury, inflammation or cancer, but severe pain can arise independently of any obvious predisposing cause (e.g. trigeminal neuralgia), or persist long after the precipitating injury has healed (e.g. phantom limb pain). It can also occur as a consequence of brain or nerve injury (e.g. following a stroke or herpes infection). Painful conditions of the latter kind, not directly linked to tissue injury, are often described as 'neuropathic pains'. They are very common and a major cause of disability and distress, and in general they respond less well to conventional analgesic drugs than do conditions where the immediate cause is clear. In these cases, we need to think of pain in terms of disordered neural function rather than simply as a 'normal' response to tissue injury.

The perception of noxious stimuli (termed *nociception* by Sherrington) is not the same thing as pain, which is a subjective experience and includes a strong emotional (affective) component. The amount of pain that a particular stimulus produces depends on many factors other than the stimulus itself. It is recognised clinically that many analgesics, particularly those of the morphine type, can greatly reduce the distress associated with pain. The affective component may be at least as significant as the antinociceptive component in the action of these drugs.

Good accounts of the neural basis of pain can be found in McMahon & Koltzenburg (2006).

NOCICEPTIVE AFFERENT NEURONS

Under normal conditions, pain is associated with impulse activity in small-diameter (C and Aδ) primary afferent fibres of peripheral nerves. These nerves have sensory endings in peripheral tissues and are activated by stimuli of various kinds (mechanical, thermal, chemical). The majority of unmyelinated (C) fibres are associated with *polymodal nociceptive* endings and convey a dull, diffuse, burning pain, whereas myelinated (Aδ) fibres convey a sensation of sharp, well-localised pain. C and Aδ fibres convey nociceptive information from muscle and viscera as well as from the skin.

With many pathological conditions, tissue injury is the immediate cause of the pain and results in the local release of a variety of chemicals that act on the nerve terminals, either activating them directly or enhancing their sensitivity to other forms of stimulation (Fig. 42.1). The pharmacological properties of nociceptive nerve terminals are discussed in more detail below.

The cell bodies of spinal nociceptive afferent fibres lie in dorsal root ganglia; fibres enter the spinal cord via the dorsal roots, ending in the grey matter of the dorsal horn. Most of the nociceptive afferents terminate in the superficial region of the dorsal horn, the C fibres and some Aδ fibres innervating cell bodies in laminae I and II (also known as the *substantia gelatinosa*), while other A fibres penetrate deeper into the dorsal horn (lamina V). The substantia gelatinosa is rich in both endogenous opioid peptides and opioid receptors, and may be an important site of action for morphine-like drugs (see p. 513, Fig. 42.4).

Cells in laminae I and V give rise to the main projection pathways from the dorsal horn to the thalamus. For a more detailed account of dorsal horn circuitry, see Fields et al. (2006).

The nociceptive afferent neurons release glutamate and possibly ATP as the fast neurotransmitters at their central synapses in the dorsal horn. Glutamate acting on AMPA receptors is responsible for fast synaptic transmission at the first synapse in the dorsal horn. There is also a slower NMDA receptor-mediated response, which is important in relation to the phenomenon of 'wind-up' (see Fig. 42.2). The nociceptive afferent neurons also contain several neuropeptides (see Ch. 18), particularly substance P, calcitonin gene-related peptide (CGRP) and galanin. These are released as mediators at both the central and the peripheral terminals, and play an important role in the pathology of pain. In the periphery, substance P and CGRP produce some of the features of neurogenic inflammation whereas galanin is anti-inflammatory. CGRP antagonists have potential for the treatment of migraine (see Ch. 15) but have not proved effective for other pain states. In animal models, substance P acting on NK_1 receptors was shown to be involved in wind-up and central sensitisation in the dorsal horn (see Fig 42.2). Surprisingly, however, antagonists of substance P at NK_1 receptors turned out to be ineffective as analgesics in humans, although they do have antiemetic activity (Ch. 30).

509

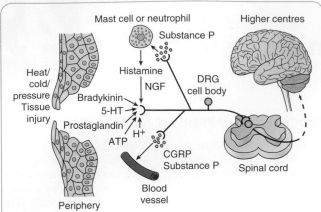

Fig. 42.1 Activation of nociceptive neurons. Various stimuli (physical and chemical) can initiate or enhance the rate of action potential firing in nociceptive primary afferent neurons (i.e. induce pain). These afferent fibres project to the dorsal horn of the spinal cord where they synapse on neurons projecting to higher centres. 5-HT, 5-hydroxytryptamine; ATP, adenosine triphosphate; CGRP, calcitonin gene-related peptide; DRG, dorsal root ganglion; NGF, nerve growth factor. *(Adapted from Julius D, Basbaum A I 2001 Nature 413, 203–210.)*

MODULATION IN THE NOCICEPTIVE PATHWAY

Acute pain is generally well accounted for in terms of nociception – an excessive noxious stimulus giving rise to an intense and unpleasant sensation. In contrast, most chronic pain states[1] are associated with aberrations of the normal physiological pathway, giving rise to *hyperalgesia* (an increased amount of pain associated with a mild noxious stimulus), *allodynia* (pain evoked by a non-noxious stimulus) or spontaneous pain without any precipitating stimulus. Some of the main mechanisms are summarised in Figure 42.3.

HYPERALGESIA AND ALLODYNIA

▼ Anyone who has suffered a burn or sprained ankle has experienced hyperalgesia and allodynia. Hyperalgesia involves both sensitisation of peripheral nociceptive nerve terminals and central facilitation of transmission at the level of the dorsal horn and thalamus. The peripheral component is due to the action of mediators such as bradykinin and prostaglandins acting on the nerve terminals. The central component reflects facilitation of synaptic transmission in the dorsal horn of the spinal cord (see Yaksh, 1999). The synaptic responses of dorsal horn neurons to nociceptive inputs display the phenomenon of 'wind-up' – i.e. the synaptic potentials steadily increase in amplitude with each stimulus – when repeated stimuli are delivered at physiological frequencies. This activity-dependent facilitation of transmission has features in common with the phenomenon of long-term potentiation, described in Chapter 38, and the chemical mechanisms underlying it may also be similar. In the dorsal horn, the facilitation is blocked by NMDA-receptor antagonists and also in part by antagonists of substance P and by inhibitors of nitric oxide (NO) synthesis (see Figs 42.2 and 42.3).

---

[1]Defined as pain that outlasts the precipitating tissue injury. Many clinical pain states fall into this category. The dissociation of pain from noxious input is most evident in 'phantom limb' pain, which occurs after amputations and may be very severe. At the other extreme, noxious input with no pain, there are many well-documented reports of mystics and showmen who subject themselves to horrifying ordeals with knives, burning embers, nails and hooks (undoubtedly causing massive afferent input) without apparently suffering pain.

Substance P and CGRP released from primary afferent neurons (see Fig. 42.1) also act in the periphery, promoting inflammation by their effects on blood vessels and cells of the immune system (Ch. 18). This mechanism, known as neurogenic inflammation, amplifies and sustains the inflammatory reaction and the accompanying activation of nociceptive afferent fibres.

Central facilitation is an important component of pathological hyperalgesia (e.g. that associated with inflammatory responses). The mediators responsible for central facilitation include substance P, CGRP, brain-derived neurotrophic factor (BDNF) and NO as well as many others. For example, nerve growth factor (NGF), a cytokine-like mediator produced by peripheral tissues, particularly in inflammation, acts on a kinase-linked receptor (known as TrkA) on nociceptive afferent neurons, increasing their electrical excitability, chemosensitivity and peptide content, and also promoting the formation of synaptic contacts. Increased NGF production may be an important mechanism by which nociceptive transmission becomes facilitated by tissue damage, leading to hyperalgesia (see Mantyh et al., 2011). Increased gene expression in sensory neurons is induced by NGF and other inflammatory mediators; the upregulated genes include those for neuropeptides and neuromodulators (e.g. CGRP, substance P and BDNF) as well as for receptors (e.g. transient receptor potential TRPV1 and P2X) and sodium channels, and have the overall effect of facilitating transmission at the first synaptic relay in the dorsal horn. BDNF released from primary afferent nerve terminals activates the kinase-linked TrkB receptor on postsynaptic dorsal horn neurons leading to phosphorylation of the NMDA subunit GluN1 and thus sensitisation of these glutamate receptors, resulting in synaptic facilitation, in the dorsal horn.

Excitation of nociceptive sensory neurons depends, as in other neurons (see Ch. 4), on voltage-gated sodium channels. Individuals who express non-functional mutations of $Na_v1.7$ are unable to experience pain. The expression of certain sodium-channel subtypes (e.g. $Na_v1.3$, $Na_v1.7$ and $Na_v1.8$ channels) is increased in sensory neurons in various pathological pain states and their enhanced activity underlies the sensitisation to external stimuli that occurs in inflammatory pain and hyperalgesia (see Ch. 4 for more detail on voltage-activated sodium channels). Consistent with this hypothesis is the fact that many antiepileptic and antidysrhythmic drugs, which act by blocking sodium channels (see Chs 21 and 45), also find clinical application as analgesics.

TRANSMISSION OF PAIN TO HIGHER CENTRES

From the dorsal horn, ascending nerve axons travel in the contralateral spinothalamic tracts, and synapse on neurons in the ventral and medial parts of the thalamus, from which there are further projections to the somatosensory cortex. In the medial thalamus in particular, many cells respond specifically to noxious stimuli in the periphery, and lesions in this area cause analgesia. Functional brain imaging studies in conscious subjects have been performed to localise regions involved in pain processing. These include sensory, discriminatory areas such as primary and secondary somatosensory cortex, thalamus and posterior parts of insula as well as affective, cognitive areas such as the anterior parts of insula, anterior cingulate cortex and prefrontal cortex (see Tracey, 2008).

DESCENDING INHIBITORY CONTROLS

Descending pathways (Fig. 42.4) control impulse transmission in the dorsal horn. A key part of this descending system is the *periaqueductal grey* (PAG) area of the midbrain, a small area of grey matter surrounding the central canal. In 1969, Reynolds found that electrical stimulation of this brain area in the rat caused analgesia sufficiently intense that abdominal surgery could be performed without anaesthesia and without eliciting any marked response. Non-painful sensations were unaffected. The

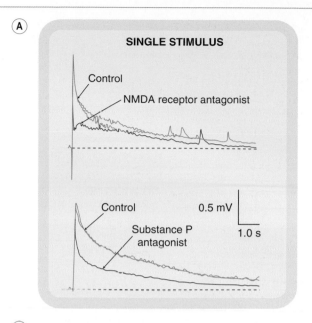

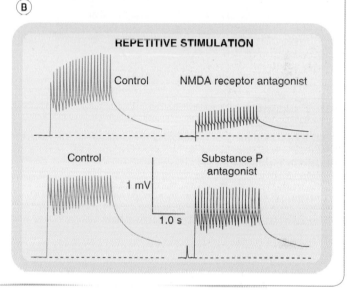

Fig. 42.2 Effect of glutamate and substance P antagonists on nociceptive transmission in the rat spinal cord. The rat paw was inflamed by ultraviolet irradiation 2 days before the experiment, a procedure that induces hyperalgesia and spinal cord facilitation. The synaptic response was recorded from the ventral root, in response to stimulation of C fibres in the dorsal root with [**A**] single stimuli or [**B**] repetitive stimuli. The effects of the NMDA receptor antagonist D-AP-5 (see Ch. 38) and the substance P antagonist RP 67580 (selective for neurokinin type 2, (NK$_2$) receptors) are shown. The slow component of the synaptic response is reduced by both antagonists [**A**] as in the 'wind-up' in response to repetitive stimulation [**B**]. These effects are much less pronounced in the normal animal. Thus both glutamate, acting on NMDA receptors, and substance P, acting on NK$_2$ receptors, are involved in nociceptive transmission, and their contribution increases as a result of inflammatory hyperalgesia. (Records kindly provided by L Urban and SW Thompson.)

PAG receives inputs from many other brain regions, including the hypothalamus, amygdala and cortex, and is the main pathway through which cortical and other inputs act to control the nociceptive 'gate' in the dorsal horn.

The PAG projects first to the rostroventral medulla (RVM) and thence via the dorsolateral funiculus of the spinal cord to the dorsal horn. Two important transmitters in this pathway are 5-hydroxytryptamine (5-HT; serotonin) and the enkephalins, which act directly or via interneurons to inhibit the discharge of spinothalamic neurons (Fig. 42.4).

The descending inhibitory pathway is probably an important site of action for opioid analgesics. Both PAG and substantia gelatinosa (SG) are particularly rich in enkephalin-containing neurons, and opioid antagonists such as naloxone (see p. 526) can prevent electrically induced analgesia, which would suggest that endogenous opioid peptides may function as transmitters in this system. The physiological role of opioid peptides in regulating pain transmission has been controversial, mainly because under normal conditions naloxone has relatively little effect on pain threshold. Under pathological conditions, however, when stress is present, naloxone causes hyperalgesia, implying that the opioid system is active.

GABA (see Ch. 38) is contained in interneurons in the dorsal horn. Activation of these interneurons releases GABA, which inhibits transmitter release from primary afferent terminals.

There is also a noradrenergic pathway from the *locus coeruleus* (LC; see Ch. 39), which has a similar inhibitory effect on transmission in the dorsal horn. Surprisingly, opioids inhibit rather than activate this pathway. The use of tricyclic antidepressants to control pain probably depends on potentiating this pathway.

It is thought that descending inhibitory purinergic pathways may release adenosine on to A$_1$ receptors on dorsal horn neurons to produce analgesia.

NEUROPATHIC PAIN

Neurological disease affecting the sensory pathway can produce severe chronic pain – termed *neuropathic pain*

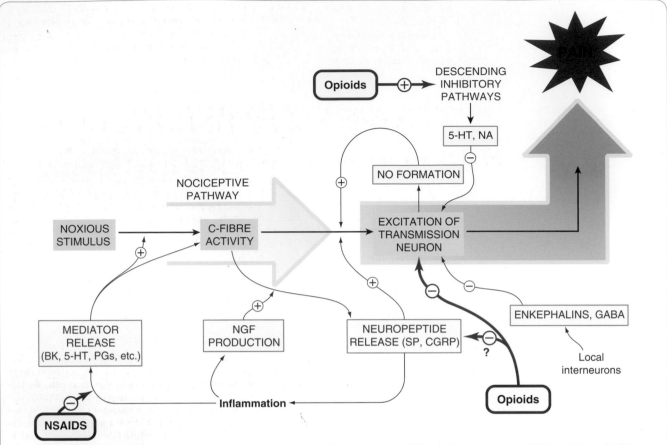

Fig. 42.3 Summary of modulatory mechanisms in the nociceptive pathway. 5-HT, 5-hydroxytryptamine; BK, bradykinin; CGRP, calcitonin gene-related peptide; NA, noradrenaline; NGF, nerve growth factor; NO, nitric oxide; NSAID, non-steroidal anti-inflammatory drug; PG, prostaglandin; SP, substance P.

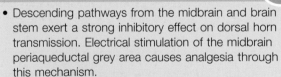

Modulation of pain transmission

- Descending pathways from the midbrain and brain stem exert a strong inhibitory effect on dorsal horn transmission. Electrical stimulation of the midbrain periaqueductal grey area causes analgesia through this mechanism.
- The descending inhibition is mediated mainly by endogenous opioid peptides, 5-hydroxytryptamine (serotonin), noradrenaline and adenosine. Opioids cause analgesia partly by activating these descending pathways, partly by inhibiting transmission in the dorsal horn and partly by inhibiting excitation of sensory nerve terminals in the periphery.
- Repetitive C-fibre activity facilitates transmission through the dorsal horn ('wind-up') by mechanisms involving activation of NMDA and substance P receptors.

– unrelated to any peripheral tissue injury. This occurs with central nervous system (CNS) disorders such as stroke and multiple sclerosis, or with conditions associated with peripheral nerve damage, such as mechanical injury, diabetic neuropathy or herpes zoster infection (shingles). The pathophysiological mechanisms underlying this kind of pain are poorly understood, although spontaneous activity in damaged sensory neurons, due to overexpression or

redistribution of voltage-gated sodium channels, is thought to be a factor. In addition, central sensitisation occurs. The sympathetic nervous system also plays a part, because damaged sensory neurons can express α adrenoceptors and develop a sensitivity to noradrenaline that they do not possess under normal conditions. Thus, physiological stimuli that evoke sympathetic responses can produce severe pain, a phenomenon described clinically as sympathetically mediated pain. Neuropathic pain, which appears to be a component of many types of clinical pain (including common conditions such as back pain and cancer pain, as well as amputation pain), responds poorly to conventional analgesic drugs but can be relieved by some antidepressant and antiepileptic agents (see p. 527). Potential new targets are discussed at the end of this chapter.

CHEMICAL SIGNALLING IN THE NOCICEPTIVE PATHWAY

CHEMOSENSITIVITY OF NOCICEPTIVE NERVE ENDINGS

In most cases, stimulation of nociceptive endings in the periphery is chemical in origin. Excessive mechanical or thermal stimuli can obviously cause acute pain, but the persistence of such pain after the stimulus has been removed, or the pain resulting from inflammatory or ischaemic changes in tissues, generally reflects an altered chemical environment of the pain afferents. The current state of knowledge is summarised in Figure 42.5.

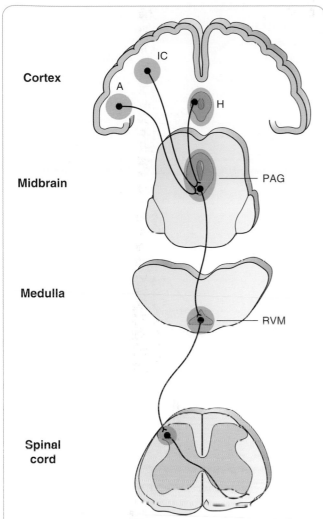

Fig. 42.4 The descending pain control system and sites of action of opioids to relieve pain. Opioids induce analgesia when microinjected into the insular cortex (IC), amygdala (A), hypothalamus (H), periaqueductal grey (PAG) region and rostroventral medulla (RVM) as well as into the dorsal horn of the spinal cord. The PAG receives input from higher centres and is the main output centre of the limbic system. It projects to the RVM. From the RVM, descending inhibitory fibres, some of which contain 5-hydroxytryptamine, project to the dorsal horn of the spinal cord. Pink shaded areas indicate regions expressing μ opioid receptors. The pathways shown in this diagram represent a considerable oversimplification. (*Adapted from Fields H 2001 Prog Brain Res 122, 245–253. For a fuller account of the descending pain modulating pathways, see Fields, 2004.*)

TRP channels – thermal sensation and pain

The *transient receptor potential* (TRP) channel family comprises some 27 or more structurally related ion channels that serve a wide variety of physiological functions (see Flockerzi & Nilius, 2007). Within this family are a group of channels present on sensory neurons that are activated both by thermal stimuli across a wide range of temperatures and by chemical agents (Table 42.1). With respect to pain, the most important channels are TRPV1, TRPM8 and TRPA1.

▼ **Capsaicin**, the substance in chilli peppers that gives them their pungency, selectively excites nociceptive nerve terminals, causing intense pain if injected into the skin or applied to sensitive structures

such as the cornea.[2] It produces this effect by activating TRPV1.[3] Agonists such as capsaicin open the channel, which is permeable to Na^+, Ca^{2+} and other cations, causing depolarisation and initiation of action potentials. The large influx of Ca^{2+} into peripheral nerve terminals also results in peptide release (mainly substance P and CGRP), causing intense vascular and other physiological responses. The Ca^{2+} influx may be enough to cause nerve terminal degeneration, which takes days or weeks to recover. Attempts to use topically applied capsaicin to relieve painful skin conditions have had some success, but the initial strong irritant effect is a major disadvantage. Capsaicin applied to the bladder causes degeneration of primary afferent nerve terminals, and has been used to treat incontinence associated with bladder hyper-reactivity in stroke or spinal injury patients. C-fibre afferents in the bladder serve a local reflex function, which promotes emptying when the bladder is distended, the reflex being exaggerated when central control is lost.

TRPV1 responds not only to capsaicin-like agonists but also to other stimuli (see Table 42.1), including temperatures in excess of about 42°C (the threshold for pain) and proton concentrations in the micromolar range (pH 5.5 and below), which also cause pain. The receptor thus has unusual 'polymodal' characteristics and is believed to play a central role in nociception. TRPV1 is, like many other ionotropic receptors, modulated by phosphorylation, and several of the pain-producing substances that act through G protein-coupled receptors (e.g. bradykinin) work by sensitising TRPV1. A search for endogenous ligands for TRPV1 revealed, surprisingly, that **anandamide** (a lipid mediator previously identified as an agonist at cannabinoid receptors; see Ch. 19) is also a TRPV1 agonist, although less potent than capsaicin. TRPV1 knockout mice show reduced responsiveness to noxious heat and also fail to show thermal hyperalgesia in response to inflammation. The latter observation is interesting, because TRPV1 expression is known to be increased by inflammation and this may be a key mechanism by which hyperalgesia is produced. A number of pharmaceutical companies have been developing TRPV1 agonists – to act as desensitising agents – and antagonists as analgesic agents. However, TRPV1 agonists were found to induce hypothermia, associated with activation of hypothalamic thermosensitive neurons, and TRPV1 antagonists were found to induce hyperthermia, consistent with a role of TRPV1 in body temperature control as well as nociception.

TRPM8 and TRPA1 respond to cold rather than heat (Table 42.1). TRPM8 is important in cold hypersensitivity, which is often a feature of neuropathic pain. TRPA1 is activated in some experimental settings by noxious cold temperatures, calcium, pain-producing substances and inflammatory mediators; it can therefore also be considered to be a polymodal sensor. It may be important for the analgesic action of paracetamol (see p. 526).

Kinins

When applied to sensory nerve endings, *bradykinin* and *kallidin* (see Ch. 18) induce intense pain. These two closely related peptides are produced under conditions of tissue injury by the proteolytic cleavage of the active kinins from a precursor protein contained in the plasma. Bradykinin acts partly by release of prostaglandins, which strongly enhance the direct action of bradykinin on the nerve terminals (Fig. 42.6). Bradykinin acts on B_2 receptors (see Ch. 18) on nociceptive neurons. B_2 receptors are coupled to activation of a specific isoform of protein kinase C (PKCε), which phosphorylates TRPV1 and facilitates opening of the TRPV1 channel.

▼ Bradykinin is converted in tissues by removal of a terminal arginine residue to *des-Arg9 bradykinin*, which acts selectively on B_1 receptors. B_1 receptors are normally expressed at very low levels, but their expression is strongly upregulated in inflamed tissues.

---

[2]Anyone who has rubbed their eyes after cutting up chilli peppers will know this.
[3]The receptor was originally known as the vanilloid receptor because many capsaicin-like compounds are based on the structure of vanillic acid.

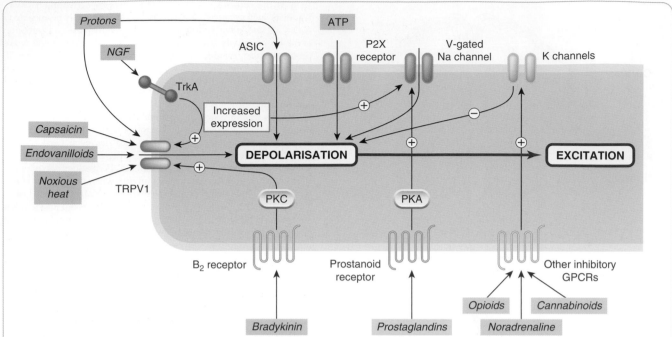

Fig. 42.5 Channels, receptors and transduction mechanisms of nociceptive afferent terminals. Only the main channels and receptors are shown. Ligand-gated channels include acid-sensitive ion channels (ASICs), ATP-sensitive channels (P2X receptors) and the capsaicin-sensitive channel (TRPV1), which is also sensitive to protons and to temperature. Various facilitatory and inhibitory G protein-coupled receptors (GPCRs) are shown, which regulate channel function through various second messenger systems. Growth factors such as nerve growth factor (NGF) act via kinase-linked receptors (TrkA) to control ion channel function and gene expression. B_2 receptor, bradykinin type 2 receptor; PKA, protein kinase A; PKC, protein kinase C.

Table 42.1 Thermosensitive TRP channels expressed on sensory neurons

Channel type	TRPA1	TRPM8	TRPV4	TRPV3	TRPV1	TRPV2
Activation temperature (°C)	<17	8–28	>27	>33	>42	>52
Chemical activators	Icilin Wintergreen oil Mustard oil	Menthol Icilin Eucalyptol Geraniol	4αPDD	Camphor Menthol Eugenol	Capsaicin Protons Anandamide Camphor Resiniferatoxin Eugenol	Δ^9-THC

4αPDD, 4 alpha-phorbol 12,13-didecanoate; Δ^9-THC, Δ^9-tetrahydrocannabinol.

Transgenic knockout animals lacking either type of receptor show reduced inflammatory hyperalgesia. Specific competitive antagonists for both B_1 and B_2 receptors are known, including peptides such as the B_2 antagonist **icatibant** (Ch. 18), as well as non-peptides. These show analgesic and anti-inflammatory properties, but are not yet developed for clinical use.

Prostaglandins
Prostaglandins do not themselves cause pain, but they strongly enhance the pain-producing effect of other agents such as 5-hydroxytryptamine or bradykinin (Fig. 42.6). Prostaglandins of the E and F series are released in inflammation (Ch. 17) and also during tissue ischaemia. Antagonists at EP_1 receptors decrease inflammatory hyperalgesia in animal models. Prostaglandins sensitise nerve terminals to other agents, partly by inhibiting potassium channels and partly by facilitating – through second messenger-mediated phosphorylation reactions (see Ch. 3) – the cation channels opened by noxious agents. It is of interest that bradykinin itself causes prostaglandin release, and thus has a powerful 'self-sensitising' effect on nociceptive afferents. Other eicosanoids, including prostacyclin, leukotrienes and the unstable hydroxyeicosatetraenoic acid (HETE) derivatives (Ch. 17), may also be important. The analgesic effects of NSAIDs (Ch. 26) result from inhibition of prostaglandin synthesis.

Other peripheral mediators
Various metabolites and substances are released from damaged or ischaemic cells, or inflamed tissues, including ATP, protons (produced by lactic acid), 5-HT, histamine and K^+, many of which affect nociceptive nerve terminals.

ATP excites nociceptive nerve terminals by acting on homomeric $P2X_3$ receptors or heteromeric $P2X_2/P2X_3$ receptors (see Ch. 16), ligand-gated ion channels that are selectively expressed by these neurons. Downregulation

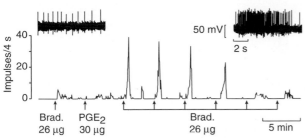

Fig. 42.6 Response of a nociceptive afferent neuron to bradykinin (Brad.) and prostaglandin. Recordings were made from a nociceptive afferent fibre supplying a muscle, and drugs were injected into the arterial supply. Upper records: single-fibre recordings showing discharge caused by bradykinin alone (left), and by bradykinin following injection of prostaglandin (right). Lower trace: ratemeter recording of single-fibre discharge, showing long-lasting enhancement of response to bradykinin after an injection of prostaglandin E₂ (PGE₂). Prostaglandin itself did not evoke a discharge. *(From Mense S 1981 Brain Res 225, 95.)*

Mechanisms of pain and nociception

- Nociception is the mechanism whereby noxious peripheral stimuli are transmitted to the central nervous system. Pain is a subjective experience not always associated with nociception.
- Polymodal nociceptors (PMNs) are the main type of peripheral sensory neuron that responds to noxious stimuli. The majority are non-myelinated C fibres whose endings respond to thermal, mechanical and chemical stimuli.
- Chemical stimuli acting on PMNs to cause pain include bradykinin, protons, ATP and vanilloids (e.g. **capsaicin**). PMNs are sensitised by prostaglandins, which explains the analgesic effect of **aspirin**-like drugs, particularly in the presence of inflammation.
- The TRPV1 receptor responds to noxious heat as well as to **capsaicin**-like agonists. The lipid mediator **anandamide** is an agonist at TRPV1 receptors, as well as being an endogenous cannabinoid-receptor agonist.
- Nociceptive fibres terminate in the superficial layers of the dorsal horn, forming synaptic connections with transmission neurons running to the thalamus.
- PMN neurons release glutamate (fast transmitter) and various peptides that act as slow transmitters. Peptides are also released peripherally and contribute to neurogenic inflammation.
- Neuropathic pain, associated with damage to neurons of the nociceptive pathway rather than an excessive peripheral stimulus, is frequently a component of chronic pain states and may respond poorly to opioid analgesics.

of P2X₃ receptors, by antisense DNA, reduces inflammatory pain.[4] Antagonists at this receptor are analgesic in animal models and may be developed for clinical use. They may also be effective in treating cough. Other P2X receptors (P2X₄ and P2X₇) are expressed on microglia in the spinal cord; activation results in the release of cytokines and chemokines that then act on neighbouring neurons to promote hypersensitivity. ATP and other purine mediators, such as adenosine, also play a role in the dorsal horn, and other types of purinoceptor may also be targeted by analgesic drugs in the future. In the periphery adenosine exerts dual effects – acting on A₁ receptors it causes analgesia but on A₂ receptors it does the opposite.

Low pH excites nociceptive afferent neurons partly by opening proton-activated cation channels (acid-sensitive ion channels) and partly by facilitation of TRPV1 (see p. 513).

5-Hydroxytryptamine causes excitation, but studies with antagonists suggest that it plays at most a minor role. Histamine is also active but causes itching rather than pain. Both these substances are released locally in inflammation (see Chs 15 and 17).

In summary, pain endings can be activated or sensitised by a wide variety of endogenous mediators, the receptors for which are often up- or downregulated under pathophysiological conditions.

ANALGESIC DRUGS

OPIOID DRUGS

Opium is an extract of the juice of the poppy *Papaver somniferum* that contains **morphine** and other related alkaloids. It has been used for social and medicinal purposes for thousands of years as an agent to produce euphoria, analgesia and sleep, and to prevent diarrhoea. It was introduced in Britain at the end of the 17th century, usually taken orally as 'tincture of laudanum', addiction to which acquired a certain social cachet during the next 200 years. The situation changed when the hypodermic

syringe and needle were invented in the mid 19th century, and opioid dependence began to take on a more sinister significance (see Ch. 49).

The history of opioid research is reviewed by Corbett et al. (2006).

CHEMICAL ASPECTS

The structure of morphine (Fig. 42.7) was determined in 1902, and since then many semisynthetic compounds (produced by chemical modification of morphine) and fully synthetic opioids have been studied. Important members of each chemical class are shown in Figure 42.7, with chemical structures drawn in a style that highlights their similarity to morphine.

Morphine is a phenanthrene derivative with two planar rings and two aliphatic ring structures, which occupy a plane roughly at right-angles to the rest of the molecule (Fig. 42.7). The most important parts of the molecule for opioid activity are the free hydroxyl on the benzene ring that is linked by two carbon atoms to a nitrogen atom. Variants of the morphine molecule have been produced by substitution at one or both of the hydroxyls (e.g. **diamorphine**[5]

---

[4]P2X₃ knockout mice are, in contrast, fairly normal in this respect, presumably because other mechanisms take over.

[5]While 'diamorphine' is the recommended International Nonproprietary Name (rINN), this drug is widely known as heroin.

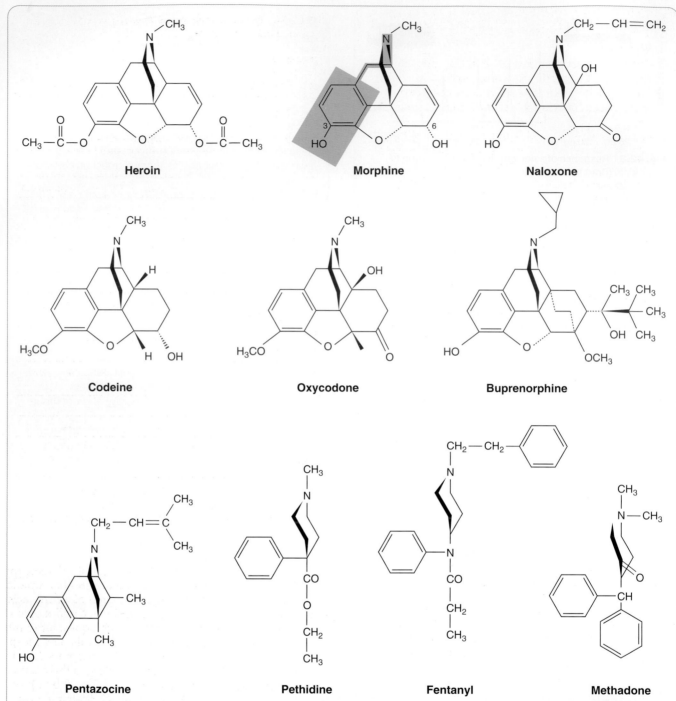

Fig. 42.7 Structures of some opioid analgesics. The red shaded area indicates the part of the morphine molecule that is structurally similar to tyrosine, the N-terminal amino acid in the endorphins. Carbon atoms 3 and 6 in the morphine structure are indicated. Diamorphine (heroin) is 3,6-diacetylmorphine and morphine is metabolised by addition of a glucuronide moiety at either position 3 or position 6.

3,6-diacetylmorphine, **codeine** 3-methoxymorphine and **oxycodone**). **Pethidine** and **fentanyl** represent more dramatic changes to the basic morphine structure. Pethidine was originally investigated as a new antimuscarinic agent but was found to have opioid analgesic activity. Although the structure of **methadone** bears no obvious chemical relationship to that of morphine, it is thought to assume a similar conformation in solution. Substitution of a bulky substituent on the nitrogen atom of morphine introduces antagonist activity to the molecule (e.g. **naloxone**).

OPIOID RECEPTORS

The proposal that opioids produce analgesia and their other effects by interacting with specific receptors first arose in the 1950s, based on the strict structural and stereochemical requirements essential for activity. It was, however, only with the development of molecules with antagonist activity (e.g. naloxone) that the notion of a specific receptor became accepted. Martin and co-workers then provided pharmacological evidence for multiple types of opioid receptors. They proposed three

Opioid analgesics

- Terminology:
  - *opioid*: any substance, whether endogenous or synthetic, that produces **morphine**-like effects that are blocked by antagonists such as **naloxone**
  - *opiate*: compounds such as **morphine** and **codeine** that are found in the opium poppy
  - *narcotic analgesic*: old term for opioids; *narcotic* refers to their ability to induce sleep. Unfortunately, the term narcotic has subsequently been hijacked and used inappropriately by some to refer generically to drugs of abuse (see Ch. 49).
- Important morphine-like agonists include **diamorphine**, **oxycodone** and **codeine**.
- The main groups of synthetic analogues are the piperidines (e.g. **pethidine** and **fentanyl**), the **methadone**-like drugs, the benzomorphans (e.g. **pentazocine**) and the thebaine derivatives (e.g. **buprenorphine**).
- Opioid analgesics may be given orally, by injection or intrathecally to produce analgesia.

Table 42.2 Functional effects associated with the main types of opioid receptor

Receptor (classical terminology)	μ	δ	κ	ORL$_1$
Receptor (recommended new terminology)	MOPr	DOPr	KOPr	NOPr
Analgesia				
Supraspinal	+++	–?	–	Anti-opioid[a]
Spinal	++	++	+	++
Peripheral	++	–	++	–
Respiratory depression	+++	++	–	–
Pupil constriction	++	–	+	–
Reduced gastrointestinal motility	++	++	+	–
Euphoria	+++	–	–	–
Dysphoria and hallucinations	–	–	+++	–
Sedation	++		++	
Catatonia	–	–	–	++
Physical dependence	+++	–	–	–

[a]ORL$_1$ agonists were originally thought to produce nociception or hyperalgesia but it was later shown that they reverse the supraspinal analgesic effects of endogenous and exogenous μ-opioid-receptor agonists.

different types of receptor, called μ, κ and σ.[6] Subsequently, in the early 1970s, radioligand binding (see Ch. 2) was used to demonstrate the presence of μ receptors in the brain.

Why are there specific receptors in the brain for morphine, a drug that is present in the opium poppy? Hughes and Kosterlitz argued that there must be an endogenous substance or substances in the brain that activated these receptors.[7] In 1975 they reported the isolation and characterisation of the first endogenous ligands, the *enkephalins*. We now know that the enkephalins are only two members of a larger family of endogenous opioid peptides known collectively as the *endorphins*, all of which possess a tyrosine residue at their N-terminus. The chemical structure of tyrosine includes an amine group separated from a phenol ring by two carbon atoms. This same structure (phenol-2 carbon atom chain-amine) is also contained within the morphine structure (Fig. 42.7). It is probably just chance (good or bad luck depending on one's viewpoint) that the opium poppy synthesises a semi-rigid alkaloid molecule, morphine, part of which structurally resembles the tyrosine residue in the endogenous opioid peptides.

Following on from the discovery of the enkephalins, pharmacological and ligand-binding studies revealed

another receptor, δ, and the three recognised receptor types (μ, δ and κ) were cloned. Later, another opioid receptor (ORL$_1$) that had a high a degree of amino acid sequence homology (>60%) towards the μ, δ and κ opioid receptors was identified by cloning techniques, although the antagonist, naloxone, did not bind to this new receptor. The terminology used for opioid receptors has in recent years been through several revisions; in this chapter we shall use the classical terminology. The four opioid receptors, μ, δ, κ and ORL$_1$ are all G protein-coupled receptors (see Ch. 3).[8] The main behavioural effects resulting from their activation are summarised in Table 42.2. The interaction of various endogenous opioid peptides with the various receptor types is summarised in Table 42.3. Some agents that are used as experimental tools for distinguishing the different receptor types are also shown.

[6]The σ 'receptor' is no longer considered to be an opioid receptor. It was postulated in order to account for the dysphoric effects (anxiety, hallucinations, bad dreams, etc.) produced by some opioids. It is now accepted that these effects result from drug-induced block of the NMDA receptor channel pore, an effect that is also produced by agents such as ketamine (see Ch. 41). Subsequently, the term σ receptor has also been used to describe other, non-NMDA receptor sites and a subdivision into σ$_1$ and σ$_2$ subtypes proposed. These proteins may be novel drug targets for psychiatric disorders.

[7]It may seem obvious today that if there is a receptor then there is likely also to be an endogenous ligand for that receptor but it was the search for, and subsequent discovery of, the enkephalins that gave credence to this idea. There are, however, exceptions to this rule. For example, although several endogenous ligands for the benzodiazepine 'receptor' or binding site on the GABA$_A$ receptor have been suggested, none so far has achieved universal acceptance (see Ch. 44).

[8]The opioid receptors are unusual among G protein-coupled receptors. First, in that there are many (20 or more) opioid peptides but only four receptors. In contrast, 5-hydroxytryptamine (5-HT), for example, is a single mediator interacting with many (about 14) receptors, which is the more common pattern. Second, all four receptors couple to the same types of G protein (G$_i$/G$_o$) and therefore activate the same spectrum of cellular effector mechanisms. In contrast, other receptor families (e.g. muscarinic receptors) couple to different types of G proteins and therefore give rise to different cellular responses (see Ch. 13).

Table 42.3 Endogenous opioid peptides and receptor-selective drugs

	μ	δ	κ	ORL₁
Endogenous peptides				
β-Endorphin	+++	+++	+	–
Leu-enkephalin	(++)	+++	+	–
Met-enkephalin	++	+++	+	–
Dynorphin	+	+	+++	–
Orphanin FQ/nociceptin[a]	–	–	–	+++
Research tools				
AGONISTS				
DAMGO[b]	+++	–	–	–
DPDPE[b]	–	++	–	–
Enadoline	–	–	+++	–
Ro64-6198	–	–	–	+++
ANTAGONISTS				
CTOP[b]	+++	–	–	–
Naltrindole	–	+++	+	–
Nor-binaltorphimine	+	+	+++	–
SB 612111	–	–	–	+++

Note: + symbols represent agonists activity; partial agonists in parentheses; – symbols represent weak or no activity.
[a]The endogenous ligand for the ORL₁ receptor is referred to in the literature both as orphanin FQ and as nociceptin.
[b]DAMGO, DPDPE and CTOP are synthetic peptides.

Opioid receptors

- μ Receptors are responsible for most of the analgesic effects of opioids, and for some major unwanted effects (e.g. respiratory depression, constipation, euphoria, sedation and dependence).
- δ Receptor activation results in analgesia but also can be proconvulsant.
- κ Receptors contribute to analgesia at the spinal level and may elicit sedation, dysphoria and hallucinations. Some analgesics are mixed κ agonists/μ antagonists.
- ORL₁ receptors are also members of the opioid receptor family. Activation results in an antiopioid effect (supraspinal), analgesia (spinal), immobility and impairment of learning.
- σ Receptors are not true opioid receptors but are the site of action of certain psychotomimetic drugs, with which some opioids also interact.
- All opioid receptors are linked through Gᵢ/Gₒ proteins and thus open potassium channels (causing hyperpolarisation) and inhibit the opening of calcium channels (inhibiting transmitter release). In addition they inhibit adenylyl cyclase and activate the MAP kinase (ERK) pathway.
- Functional heteromers, formed by combination of different types of opioid receptor or with other types of G protein-coupled receptor, may occur and give rise to further pharmacological diversity.

The development of transgenic mouse strains lacking each of the three main opioid receptor types has revealed that the major pharmacological effects of morphine, including analgesia, are mediated by the μ receptor.

All four opioid receptors appear to form homomeric as well as heteromeric receptor complexes. Opioid receptors are, in fact, quite promiscuous and can form heteromers with non-opioid receptors. Heteromerisation between opioid receptors has been shown to result in pharmacological characteristics distinct from those observed with the monomeric receptors and may explain some of the subtypes of each receptor that have been proposed. Another level of complexity may reflect 'bias' (see Ch. 3), whereby different ligands acting on the same opioid receptor can elicit different cellular responses and differential receptor trafficking (see Kelly, 2013).

AGONISTS AND ANTAGONISTS

Opioids vary not only in their receptor specificity but also in their efficacy at the different types of receptor. Thus, some agents act as agonists or partial agonists on one type of receptor, and antagonists or partial agonists at another, producing a very complicated pharmacological picture.

Morphine is in fact a partial agonist at the μ opioid receptor. This may surprise some clinicians because it is a powerful analgesic that can, at high doses, induce death

due to severe respiratory depression. However, when considering receptor activation, it has lower intrinsic efficacy than full agonists (see Ch. 2). Other opioid drugs, notably **codeine** and **dextropropoxyphene**, are sometimes referred to as weak agonists because their maximal effects, both analgesic and unwanted, are less than those of morphine. **Buprenorphine** is a partial agonist that dissociates slowly from opioid receptors. It induces less respiratory depression than other opioids. It is a very potent drug that can also antagonise the effect of other opioids by virtue of its high affinity and low efficacy. **Pentazocine** combines a degree of κ agonist and μ antagonist (or weak partial agonist) activity. Drugs with κ agonist tend to cause dysphoria rather than euphoria. Antagonists such as **naloxone** and **naltrexone** produce very little effect when given on their own to healthy subjects, while worsening chronic pain and blocking the effects of opioids.

MECHANISM OF ACTION OF OPIOIDS

The opioids have probably been studied more intensively than any other group of drugs in the effort to understand their powerful effects in molecular, cellular and physiological terms, and to use this understanding to develop new drugs as analgesics with significant advantages over morphine. Even so, morphine – described by Osler as 'God's own medicine' – remains the standard against which any new analgesic is assessed.

Cellular actions

All four types of opioid receptor belong to the family of Gᵢ/Gₒ protein-coupled receptors. Opioids thus exert powerful effects on ion channels on neuronal membranes through a direct G protein coupling to the channel. Opioids promote the opening of potassium channels (see Ch. 4) and inhibit the opening of voltage-gated calcium channels. These membrane effects decrease neuronal excitability (because the increased K^+ conductance causes hyperpolarisation of the membrane making the cell less likely to fire action potentials) and reduce transmitter release (due to inhibition of Ca^{2+} entry). The overall effect is therefore inhibitory at the cellular level. Nonetheless, opioids do increase activity in some neuronal pathways (see p. 513, Fig. 42.4). They do this by a process of *disinhibition* whereby they cause excitation of projection neurons by suppressing the activity of inhibitory interneurons that tonically inhibit the projection neurons (see Ch. 37, Fig. 37.2).

At the biochemical level, all four receptor types inhibit adenylyl cyclase and cause MAP kinase (ERK) activation (see Ch. 3). These cellular responses are likely to be important in mediating the long-term adaptive changes that occur in response to prolonged receptor activation and which, for μ-receptor agonists, may underlie the phenomenon of physical dependence (see Ch. 49).

At the cellular level, therefore, all four types of opioid receptor mediate very similar effects. It is their heterogeneous anatomical distributions across the CNS that give rise to the different behavioural responses seen with selective agonists for each type of receptor.

Sites of action of opioids to produce analgesia

Opioid receptors are widely distributed in the brain and spinal cord. Opioids are effective as analgesics when injected in minute doses into a number of specific brain nuclei (such as the insular cortex, amygdala, hypothalamus, PAG region and RVM) as well as into the dorsal horn of the spinal cord (see Fig. 42.4). There is evidence to suggest that supraspinal opioid analgesia involves endogenous opioid peptide release both at supraspinal and spinal sites and that at the spinal level there is also a component of the analgesia that results from the release of serotonin (5-HT) from descending inhibitory fibres. Surgical interruption of the descending pathway from the RVM to the spinal cord reduces analgesia induced by morphine that has been given systemically or microinjected into supraspinal sites, implying that a combination of effects at supraspinal and spinal sites contribute to the analgesic response.

At the spinal level, morphine inhibits transmission of nociceptive impulses through the dorsal horn and suppresses nociceptive spinal reflexes, even in patients with spinal cord transection. It can act presynaptically to inhibit release of various neurotransmitters from primary afferent terminals in the dorsal horn as well as acting postsynaptically to reduce the excitability of dorsal horn neurons.

There is also evidence (see Sawynok, 2003) that opioids inhibit the discharge of nociceptive afferent terminals in the periphery, particularly under conditions of inflammation, in which the expression of opioid receptors by sensory neurons is increased. Injection of morphine into the knee joint following surgery to the joint provides effective analgesia, undermining the age-old belief that opioid analgesia is exclusively a central phenomenon.

PHARMACOLOGICAL ACTIONS

Morphine is typical of many opioid analgesics and will be taken as the reference compound.

The most important effects of morphine are on the CNS and the gastrointestinal tract, although numerous effects of lesser significance on many other systems have been described.

Effects on the central nervous system
Analgesia
Morphine is effective in most kinds of acute and chronic pain, although opioids in general are less effective in neuropathic pain than in pain associated with tissue injury, inflammation or tumour growth.

As well as being antinociceptive, morphine also reduces the affective component of pain. This reflects its supraspinal action, possibly at the level of the limbic system, which is probably involved in the euphoria-producing effect. Drugs such as pentazocine share the antinociceptive actions of morphine but have much less effect on the psychological response to pain.

Hyperalgesia
In both animal studies and in patients receiving opioids for pain relief, prolonged exposure to opioids may paradoxically induce a state of hyperalgesia in which pain sensitisation or allodynia occurs (see Lee et al., 2011). This can appear as a reduced analgesic response to a given dose of opioid but should not be confused with tolerance, which is a reduced responsiveness due in large part to μ receptor desensitisation (see p. 521) and occurs with other opioid-induced behaviours in addition to analgesia. Hyperalgesia appears to have peripheral, spinal and supraspinal components. At the neuronal level, the mechanisms underlying this phenomenon are still unclear but appear to involve PKC and NMDA receptor activation. In addition, $P2X_4$ receptor expression in microglia is upregulated resulting in BDNF release, TrkB signalling and downregulation of the K^+/Cl^- co-transporter KCC2. In mice in which BDNF has been deleted from microglia hyperalgesia to morphine does not occur, whereas antinociception and tolerance are unaffected. Opioid-induced hyperalgesia can be reduced by ketamine, an NMDA antagonist, propofol, α_2-adrenoceptor agonists and COX-2 inhibitors. Switching to another opioid can also reduce hyperalgesia; in this regard, methadone may be a good choice as it is a weak NMDA receptor antagonist.

Euphoria
Morphine causes a powerful sense of contentment and well-being (see also Ch. 49). This is an important component of its analgesic effect, because the agitation and anxiety associated with a painful illness or injury are thereby reduced. If morphine or diamorphine (heroin) is given intravenously, the result is a sudden 'rush' likened to an 'abdominal orgasm'. The euphoria produced by morphine depends considerably on the circumstances. In patients who are distressed, it is pronounced, but in patients who become accustomed to chronic pain, morphine causes analgesia with little or no euphoria. Some patients report restlessness rather than euphoria under these circumstances.

Euphoria is mediated through μ receptors, whereas κ-receptor activation produces dysphoria and hallucinations (see Table 42.2). Thus, different opioid drugs vary greatly in the amount of euphoria that they produce. It does not occur with codeine or with pentazocine to any marked extent. There is evidence that antagonists at the κ receptor have antidepressant properties which may indicate that release of endogenous κ agonists may occur in depression.

Respiratory depression

Respiratory depression, resulting in increased arterial P_{CO_2}, occurs with a normal analgesic dose of morphine or related compounds, although in patients in severe pain the degree of respiratory depression produced may be less than anticipated. Respiratory depression is mediated by μ receptors. The depressant effect is associated with a decrease in the sensitivity of the respiratory centres to arterial P_{CO_2} and an inhibition of respiratory rhythm generation. Changes in P_{CO_2} are detected by chemosensitive neurons in a number of brain stem and medullary nuclei. Increased arterial CO_2 (hypercapnia) thus normally results in a compensatory increase in minute ventilation rate (V_E). In some of the chemosensitive regions, opioids exert a depressant effect on the hypercapnic response, making the increase in V_E insufficient to counteract the increased CO_2. Respiratory movements originate from activity of a rhythm generator (the *pre-Bötzinger complex*) within the ventral respiratory column of the medulla. μ Opioid receptors are located in this region, and local injection of opioid agonists decreases respiratory frequency.

Respiratory depression by opioids is not accompanied by depression of the medullary centres controlling cardiovascular function (in contrast to the action of general anaesthetics and other CNS depressants). This means that respiratory depression produced by opioids is much better tolerated than a similar degree of depression caused by, say, a barbiturate. Nonetheless, respiratory depression is a dangerous unwanted effect of these drugs and, unlike that due to general CNS depressant drugs, it occurs at therapeutic doses. It is the commonest cause of death in acute opioid poisoning.

Depression of cough reflex

Cough suppression (antitussive effect; see also Ch. 28), surprisingly, does not correlate closely with the analgesic and respiratory depressant actions of opioids, and its mechanism at the receptor level is unclear. In general, increasing substitution on the phenolic hydroxyl group of morphine increases antitussive relative to analgesic activity. **Codeine** and **pholcodine** suppress cough in subanalgesic doses but they cause constipation as an unwanted effect.

▼ **Dextromethorphan**, the dextro-isomer of the opioid analgesic **levorphanol**, has no affinity for opioid receptors and its cough suppression is not antagonised by naloxone. It is an uncompetitive NMDA receptor antagonist – this might explain why at high doses it evokes CNS effects similar to ketamine – and has putative actions at σ receptors. It is believed to work at various sites in the brain stem and medulla to suppress cough. In addition to its antitussive action, dextromethorphan is neuroprotective (see Ch. 40) and has an analgesic action in neuropathic pain (see p. 527-528).

Nausea and vomiting

Nausea and vomiting occur in up to 40% of patients to whom morphine is given, and do not seem to be separable from the analgesic effect among a range of opioid analgesics. The site of action is the *area postrema* (chemoreceptor trigger zone), a region of the medulla where chemical stimuli of many kinds may initiate vomiting (see Ch. 30).[9]

Nausea and vomiting following morphine injection are usually transient and disappear with repeated administration, although in some individuals they persist and can limit patient compliance.

Pupillary constriction

Pupillary constriction is caused by μ and κ receptor-mediated stimulation of the oculomotor nucleus. Pinpoint pupils are an important diagnostic feature in opioid poisoning,[10] because most other causes of coma and respiratory depression produce pupillary dilatation. Tolerance does not develop to the pupillary constriction induced by opioids and therefore can be observed in opioid-dependent drug users who may have been taking opioids for a considerable time.

Effects on the gastrointestinal tract

Opioids increase tone and reduce motility in many parts of the gastrointestinal system, resulting in constipation, which may be severe and very troublesome to the patient.[11] The resulting delay in gastric emptying can considerably retard the absorption of other drugs. Pressure in the biliary tract increases because of contraction of the gall bladder and constriction of the biliary sphincter. Opioids should be avoided in patients suffering from biliary colic due to gallstones, in whom pain may be increased rather than relieved. The rise in intrabiliary pressure can cause a transient increase in the concentration of amylase and lipase in the plasma.

The action of morphine on visceral smooth muscle is probably mediated mainly through the intramural nerve plexuses, because the increase in tone is reduced or abolished by atropine. It is also partly mediated by a central action, because intracerebroventricular injection of morphine inhibits propulsive gastrointestinal movements. **Methylnaltrexone bromide** (see also Ch. 8) and **alvimopan** are opioid antagonists that do not cross the blood–brain barrier. They have been developed to reduce unwanted peripheral side effects of opioids such as constipation without significantly reducing analgesia or precipitating withdrawal in dependent individuals.

Other actions of opioids

Morphine releases histamine from mast cells by an action unrelated to opioid receptors. Pethidine and fentanyl do not produce this effect. The release of histamine can cause local effects, such as urticaria and itching at the site of the injection, or systemic effects, namely bronchoconstriction and hypotension. The bronchoconstrictor effect can have serious consequences for asthmatic patients, to whom morphine should not be given.

Hypotension and bradycardia occur with large doses of most opioids, due to an action on the medulla. With morphine and similar drugs, histamine release may contribute to the hypotension.

Effects on smooth muscle other than that of the gastrointestinal tract and bronchi are slight, although spasms of the ureters, bladder and uterus sometimes occur. Opioids also exert complex immunosuppressant effects, which may be important as a link between the nervous

---

[9]The chemically related compound apomorphine is more strongly emetic than morphine, through its action as a dopamine agonist; despite its name, it is inactive on opioid receptors.

[10]The exception is pethidine, which causes pupillary dilatation because it blocks muscarinic receptors.

[11]In treating pain, constipation is considered as an undesirable side effect. However, opioids such as codeine and morphine can be used to treat diarrhoea.

system and immune function. The pharmacological significance of this is not yet clear, but there is evidence in humans that the immune system is depressed by long-term opioid use, and that in addicts suffering from AIDS the use of opioids may exacerbated the immune deficiency.

Actions of morphine

- The main pharmacological effects are:
  - analgesia
  - euphoria and sedation
  - respiratory depression
  - suppression of cough
  - nausea and vomiting
  - pupillary constriction
  - reduced gastrointestinal motility, causing constipation
  - histamine release, causing itch, bronchoconstriction and hypotension.
- The most troublesome unwanted effects are nausea and vomiting, constipation and respiratory depression.
- Acute overdosage with **morphine** produces coma and respiratory depression.
- **Diamorphine** is inactive at opioid receptors but is rapidly cleaved in the brain to 6-acetylmorphine and **morphine**
- **Codeine** is also converted to **morphine** but more slowly by liver metabolism.

TOLERANCE AND DEPENDENCE

Tolerance to many of the actions of opioids (i.e. an increase in the dose needed to produce a given pharmacological effect) develops within a few days during repeated administration. There is some controversy over whether significant tolerance develops to the analgesic effects of morphine, especially in palliative care patients with severe cancer pain (see McQuay, 1999; Ballantyne & Mao, 2003). Drug rotation (changing from one opioid to another) is frequently used clinically to overcome loss of effectiveness. As tolerance is likely to depend upon the level of receptor occupancy, the degree of tolerance observed may reflect the response being assessed, the intrinsic efficacy of the drug and the dose being administered.

Physical dependence refers to a state in which withdrawal of the drug causes adverse physiological effects, i.e. the abstinence syndrome.

Different adaptive cellular mechanisms underlie tolerance and dependence (see Williams et al., 2013; see also Chs 2 and 49). These phenomena occur to some degree whenever opioids are administered for more than a few days. They must not be confused with addiction (see Ch. 49), in which physical dependence is much more pronounced and psychological dependence (or 'craving') is the main driving force.

Tolerance

In animal experiments, tolerance can be detected even with a single dose of morphine. Tolerance extends to most of the pharmacological effects of morphine, including analgesia, emesis, euphoria and respiratory depression, but affects the constipating and pupil-constricting actions much less. Therefore, addicts may take 50 times the normal analgesic dose of morphine with relatively little

respiratory depression but marked constipation and pupillary constriction.

The cellular mechanisms responsible for tolerance are discussed in Chapter 2. Tolerance results in part from desensitisation of the μ opioid receptors (i.e. at the level of the drug target) as well as from long-term adaptive changes at the cellular, synaptic and network levels (see Williams et al., 2013). Tolerance is a general phenomenon of opioid-receptor ligands, irrespective of which type of receptor they act on. Cross-tolerance occurs between drugs acting at the same receptor, but not between opioids that act on different receptors. In clinical settings, the opioid dose required for effective pain relief may increase as a result of developing tolerance, but it does not constitute a major problem.

Physical dependence

Physical dependence is characterised by a clear-cut abstinence syndrome. In experimental animals (e.g. rats), abrupt withdrawal of morphine after repeated administration for a few days, or the administration of an antagonist such as naloxone, causes an increased irritability, diarrhoea, loss of weight and a variety of abnormal behaviour patterns, such as body shakes, writhing, jumping and signs of aggression. These reactions decrease after a few days, but abnormal irritability and aggression persist for many weeks. The signs of physical dependence are much less intense if the opioid is withdrawn gradually. Humans often experience an abstinence syndrome when opioids are withdrawn after being used for pain relief over days or weeks, with symptoms of restlessness, runny nose, diarrhoea, shivering and piloerection.[12]

Many physiological changes have been described in relation to the abstinence syndrome. For example, spinal reflex hyperexcitability occurs in morphine-dependent animals and can be produced by chronic intrathecal as well as systemic administration of morphine. The noradrenergic pathways emanating from the LC (see Ch. 39) may also play an important role in causing the abstinence syndrome and the α2-adrenoceptor agonist clonidine (Ch. 14) can be used to alleviate it. The rate of firing of LC neurons is reduced by opioids and increased during the abstinence syndrome. In animal models, and also in humans, the abstinence syndrome is reduced by giving NMDA receptor antagonists (e.g. ketamine).

PHARMACOKINETIC ASPECTS

Table 42.4 summarises the pharmacokinetic properties of the main opioid analgesics. The absorption of morphine congeners by mouth is variable. Morphine itself is slowly and erratically absorbed, and is commonly given by intravenous injection to treat acute severe pain; oral morphine is, however, often used in treating chronic pain, and slow-release preparations are available to increase its duration of action. Oxycodone is also available as a slow-release oral preparation. Codeine is well absorbed and normally given by mouth. Most morphine-like drugs undergo considerable first-pass metabolism, and are therefore markedly less potent when taken orally than when injected.

The plasma half-life of most morphine analogues is 3–6 h. Hepatic metabolism is the main mode of inactivation, usually by conjugation with glucuronide. This occurs

---

[12]Causing goose pimples. This is the origin of the phrase 'cold turkey' used to describe the effect of morphine withdrawal.

Table 42.4 Characteristics of the main opioid analgesic drugs

Drug	Use(s)	Route(s) of administration	Pharmacokinetic aspects	Main adverse effects	Notes
Morphine	Widely used for acute and chronic pain	Oral, including sustained-release form Injection[a] Intrathecal	Half-life 3–4 h Converted to active metabolite (morphine-6-glucuronide)	Sedation Respiratory depression Constipation Nausea and vomiting Itching (histamine release) Tolerance and dependence Euphoria	Tolerance and withdrawal effects not common when used for analgesia
Diamorphine (heroin)	Acute and chronic pain	Oral Injection	Acts more rapidly than morphine because of rapid brain penetration.	As morphine	Not available in all countries Metabolised to morphine and other active metabolites
Hydromorphone	Acute and chronic pain	Oral Injection	Half-life 2–4 h No active metabolites	As morphine but allegedly less sedative	Levorphanol is similar, with longer duration of action
Oxycodone	Acute and chronic pain	Oral, including sustained-release form Injection	Half-life 3–4.5 h	As morphine	Claims for less abuse potential are unfounded
Methadone	Chronic pain Maintenance of addicts	Oral Injection	Long half-life (>24 h) Slow onset	As morphine but less euphoric effect Accumulation may occur	Slow recovery results in attenuated withdrawal syndrome because of long half-life
Pethidine	Acute pain	Oral Intramuscular injection	Half-life 2–4 h Active metabolite (norpethidine) may account for stimulant effects	As morphine Anticholinergic effects Risk of excitement and convulsions	Known as meperidine in USA Interacts with monoamine oxidase inhibitors (Ch. 47)
Buprenorphine	Acute and chronic pain Maintenance of addicts	Sublingual Injection Intrathecal	Half-life about 12 h Slow onset Inactive orally because of first-pass metabolism	As morphine but less pronounced Respiratory depression not reversed by naloxone (therefore not suitable for obstetric use) May precipitate opioid withdrawal (partial agonist)	Useful in chronic pain with patient-controlled injection systems

Drug	Use	Route	Pharmacokinetics	Unwanted effects	Notes
Pentazocine	Mainly acute pain	Oral Injection	Half-life 2–4 h	Psychotomimetic effects (dysphoria) Irritation at injection site May precipitate opioid withdrawal (μ antagonist effect)	Nalbuphine is similar
Dipipenone	Moderate to severe pain	Oral	Half-life 3.5 h (although there are longer values quoted)	In addition to effects similar to morphine it produces psychosis	Marketed in combination with cyclizine (Diconal) and became a popular IV drug of abuse
Fentanyl	Acute pain Anaesthesia	Intravenous Epidermal Transdermal patch	Half-life 1–2 h	As morphine	High potency allows transdermal administration Sufentanil is similar
Remifentanil	Anaesthesia	Intravenous infusion	Half-life 5 min	Respiratory depression	Very rapid onset and recovery
Codeine	Mild pain	Oral	Acts as prodrug Metabolised to morphine and other active metabolites	Mainly constipation No dependence liability	Effective only in mild pain Also used to suppress cough Dihydrocodeine is similar
Dextropropoxyphene	Mild pain	Mainly oral	Half-life ~4 h Active metabolite (norpropoxyphene) with half-life ~24 h	Respiratory depression May cause convulsions (possibly by action of norpropoxyphene)	Similar to codeine No longer recommended
Tramadol	Acute (mainly postoperative) and chronic pain	Oral Intravenous	Well absorbed Half-life 4–6 h	Dizziness May cause convulsions No respiratory depression	Mechanism of action uncertain Weak agonist at opioid receptors Also inhibits monoamine uptake. Tapentadol is similar

aInjections may by given intravenously, intramuscularly or subcutaneously for most drugs.

Tolerance and dependence

- Tolerance develops rapidly.
- The mechanism of tolerance involves receptor desensitisation. It is not pharmacokinetic in origin.
- Dependence comprises two components:
  - physical dependence, associated with the withdrawal syndrome and lasting for a few days
  - psychological dependence, associated with craving and lasting for months or years; it rarely occurs in patients being given opioids as analgesics.
- Physical dependence, characterised by a withdrawal syndrome on cessation of drug administration, occurs with μ-receptor agonists.
- The withdrawal syndrome is precipitated by μ-receptor antagonists.
- Long-acting μ-receptor agonists such as **methadone** and **buprenorphine** may be used to relieve withdrawal symptoms.
- Certain opioid analgesics, such as **codeine**, **pentazocine**, **buprenorphine** and **tramadol**, are much less likely to cause physical or psychological dependence.

at the 3- and 6-OH groups (see Fig 42.7), and these glucuronides constitute a considerable fraction of the drug in the bloodstream. Morphine-6-glucuronide is more active as an analgesic than morphine itself, and contributes substantially to the pharmacological effect. Morphine-3-glucuronide has been claimed to antagonise the analgesic effect of morphine, but the significance of this experimental finding is uncertain as this metabolite has little or no affinity for opioid receptors. Morphine glucuronides are excreted in the urine, so the dose needs to be reduced in cases of renal failure. Glucuronides also reach the gut via biliary excretion, where they are hydrolysed, most of the morphine being reabsorbed (enterohepatic circulation). Because of low conjugating capacity in neonates, morphine-like drugs have a much longer duration of action; because even a small degree of respiratory depression can be hazardous, morphine congeners should not be used in the neonatal period, nor used as analgesics during childbirth. Pethidine (see p. 525) is a safer alternative for this purpose.

Analogues that have no free hydroxyl group in the 3 position (i.e. diamorphine, codeine) are converted to morphine, which accounts for all or part of their pharmacological activity. With heroin the conversion occurs rapidly in aqueous solution and in the brain but with codeine the effect is slower and occurs by metabolism in the liver. Morphine produces very effective analgesia when administered intrathecally, and is often used in this way by anaesthetists, the advantage being that the sedative and respiratory depressant effects are reduced, although not completely avoided. **Remifentanil** is rapidly hydrolysed and eliminated with a half life of 3–4 min. The advantage of this is that when given by intravenous infusion during general anaesthesia, the level of the drug can be manipulated rapidly when required (see Ch. 10 for a description of how, for intravenous infusion, both the rate of rise and

the rate of decay of the plasma concentration are determined by the half-time of elimination).

For the treatment of chronic or postoperative pain, opioids are often given 'on demand' (patient-controlled analgesia). The patients are provided with an infusion pump that they control, the maximum possible rate of administration being limited to avoid acute toxicity. Patients show little tendency to use excessively large doses and become dependent; instead, the dose is adjusted to achieve analgesia without excessive sedation, and is reduced as the pain subsides. Being in control of their own analgesia, the patients' anxiety and distress are reduced, and analgesic consumption actually tends to decrease. In chronic pain, especially that associated with cancer, patients often experience sudden, sharp increases in the level of pain they are experiencing. This is referred to as breakthrough pain. To combat this, there is a therapeutic need to be able to increase rapidly the amount of opioid being administered. This has led to the development of touch-sensitive transdermal patches containing potent opioids such as fentanyl that rapidly release drug into the bloodstream.

The opioid antagonist, naloxone, has a shorter biological half-life than most opioid agonists. In the treatment of opioid overdose, it must be given repeatedly to avoid the respiratory depressant effect of the agonist reoccurring once the naloxone has been eliminated. Naltrexone has a longer biological half-life.

UNWANTED EFFECTS

The main unwanted effects of morphine and related drugs are listed in Table 42.4.

Acute overdosage with morphine results in coma and respiratory depression, with characteristically constricted pupils. It is treated by giving naloxone intravenously. This also serves as a diagnostic test, for failure to respond to naloxone suggests a cause other than opioid poisoning for the comatose state.[13] There is a danger of precipitating a severe withdrawal syndrome with naloxone, because opioid poisoning occurs mainly in addicts.

Individual variability

▼ Individuals vary by as much as 10-fold in their sensitivity to opioid analgesics. This can be due to altered metabolism or altered sensitivity of the receptors (for extensive review, see Rollason et al., 2008). For morphine, reduced responsiveness may result from mutations in a number of genes including that for the drug transporter, P-glycoprotein (see Chs 9 and 11), for glucuronyltransferase that metabolises morphine and for the μ receptor itself. Mutations of various cytochrome P450 (CYP) enzymes influence the metabolism of codeine, oxycodone, methadone, tramadol and dextromethorphan. Genotyping could in principle be used to identify opioid-resistant individuals, but first the contribution of genotype to clinical outcome must be confirmed in the population at large.

OTHER OPIOID ANALGESICS

Diamorphine (heroin) is 3,6-diacetylmorphine; it can be considered as a prodrug as its high analgesic potency is attributable to rapid conversion to 6-monoacetylmorphine and morphine. Its effects are indistinguishable from those of morphine following oral administration. However, because of its greater lipid solubility, it crosses the blood–brain barrier more rapidly than morphine and gives a

---

[13]Naloxone is less effective in reversing the effects of buprenorphine as this agonist dissociates very slowly from the receptors.

greater 'buzz' when injected intravenously. It is said to be less emetic than morphine, but the evidence for this is slight. It is still available in Britain for use as an analgesic, although it is banned in many countries. Its only advantage over morphine is its greater solubility, which allows smaller volumes to be given orally, subcutaneously or intrathecally. It exerts the same respiratory depressant effect as morphine and, if given intravenously, is more likely to cause dependence.

Codeine (3-methoxymorphine) is more reliably absorbed by mouth than morphine, but has only 20% or less of the analgesic potency. Its analgesic effect does not increase appreciably at higher dose levels. It is therefore used mainly as an oral analgesic for mild types of pain (headache, backache, etc.). It is metabolised to morphine as well as undergoing glucuronidation in the liver. About 10% of the population is resistant to the analgesic effect of codeine, because they lack the demethylating enzyme that converts it to morphine. Unlike morphine, it causes little or no euphoria and is rarely addictive. It is often combined with **paracetamol** in proprietary analgesic preparations (see later section on combined use of opioids and NSAIDs). In relation to its analgesic effect, codeine produces the same degree of respiratory depression as morphine, but the limited response even at high doses means that it is seldom a problem in practice. It does, however, cause constipation. Codeine has marked antitussive activity and is often used in cough mixtures (see Ch. 28). **Dihydrocodeine** is pharmacologically very similar, having no substantial advantages or disadvantages over codeine.

Oxycodone is used in the treatment of acute and chronic pain. The suggestion that it acts on a subtype of κ opioid receptor is not generally accepted. Claims that it has less euphoric effect and less abuse potential appear unfounded. It is available as a slow release oral preparation but diversion to the street where addicts grind up the tablets that contain large amounts of drug has resulted in it becoming a major drug of abuse (see Ch. 49), sometimes referred to as 'hillbilly heroin'.

Fentanyl, alfentanil, sufentanil and **remifentanil** are highly potent phenylpiperidine derivatives, with actions similar to those of morphine but with a more rapid onset and shorter duration of action, particularly remifentanil. They are used extensively in anaesthesia, and they may be given intrathecally. Fentanyl, alfentanil and sufentanil are also used in patient-controlled infusion systems and in severe chronic pain, when they are administered via patches applied to the skin. The rapid onset is advantageous in breakthrough pain.

Methadone is orally active and pharmacologically similar to morphine, the main difference being that its duration of action is considerably longer (plasma half-life >24 h). The increased duration seems to occur because the drug is bound in the extravascular compartment and slowly released. On withdrawal, the physical abstinence syndrome is less acute than with morphine, although the psychological dependence is no less pronounced. Methadone is widely used as a means of treating heroin addiction (see Ch. 49). It is possible to wean addicts from heroin by giving regular oral doses of methadone – an improvement if not a cure.[14] Methadone has actions at other sites in the CNS, including block of potassium channels,

NMDA receptors and 5-HT receptors that may explain its CNS side effect profile. There is also interindividual variation in the response to methadone, probably due to genetic variability between individuals in its metabolism.

Pethidine (meperidine) is very similar to morphine in its pharmacological effects, except that it tends to cause restlessness rather than sedation, and it has an additional antimuscarinic action that may cause dry mouth and blurring of vision as side effects. It produces a very similar euphoric effect and is equally liable to cause dependence. Its duration of action is the same or slightly shorter than that of morphine, but the route of metabolic degradation is different. Pethidine is partly N-demethylated in the liver to norpethidine, which has hallucinogenic and convulsant effects. These become significant with large oral doses of pethidine, producing an overdose syndrome rather different from that of morphine. Pethidine is preferred to morphine for analgesia during labour, because it does not reduce the force of uterine contraction. Pethidine is only slowly eliminated in the neonate, and naloxone may be needed to reverse respiratory depression in the baby. (Morphine is even more problematic in this regard, because the conjugation reactions on which the excretion of morphine, but not of pethidine, depends are deficient in the newborn.) Severe reactions, consisting of excitement, hyperthermia and convulsions, have been reported when pethidine is given to patients receiving monoamine oxidase inhibitors. This seems to be due to inhibition of an alternative metabolic pathway, leading to increased norpethidine formation, but the details are not known.

Etorphine is a morphine analogue of remarkable potency, more than 1000 times that of morphine, but otherwise very similar in its actions. Its high potency confers no particular human clinical advantage, but it is used in veterinary practice, especially in large animals. It can be used in conjunction with sedative agents (neuroleptanalgesia) to immobilise wild animals for trapping.[15]

Buprenorphine is a partial agonist on μ receptors that produces strong analgesia but there is a ceiling to its respiratory depressant effect. Because of its antagonist actions, it can produce mild withdrawal symptoms in patients dependent on other opioids. It has a long duration of action and can be difficult to reverse with naloxone. It has abuse liability but, like methadone, it is also used in the treatment of heroin addiction. When heroin is injected 'on top' of buprenorphine, less euphoria is obtained because buprenorphine is a partial agonist. It is marketed as a sublingual preparation combined with naloxone for the management of opioid dependence; when administered as intended the naloxone is not absorbed and does not influence the effect of the buprenorphine, but if it is administered parenterally the effects of the buprenorphine are hopefully reduced by the naloxone, discouraging such abuse. How effective this is in practice has been questioned.

Meptazinol is an opioid of unusual chemical structure. It can be given orally or by injection and has a duration of action shorter than that of morphine. It seems to be relatively free of morphine-like side effects, causing neither euphoria nor dysphoria, nor severe respiratory depression. It does, however, produce nausea, sedation

---

[14]The benefits come mainly from removing the risks of self-injection and the need to finance the drug habit through crime.

[15]The required dose of etorphine, even for an elephant, is small enough to be incorporated into a dart or pellet.

and dizziness, and has atropine-like actions. Because of its short duration of action and lack of respiratory depression, it may have advantages for obstetric analgesia.

Tramadol is widely used as an analgesic for postoperative pain. It is a weak agonist at µ opioid receptors and also a weak inhibitor of monoamine reuptake. It is effective as an analgesic and appears to have a better side effect profile than most opioids, although psychiatric reactions have been reported. It is given by mouth or by intramuscular or intravenous injection for moderate to severe pain. **Tapentadol** acts similarly and is effective in acute and chronic pain, including the pain associated with diabetic neuropathy (see p. 527).

Pentazocine is a mixed κ agonist/µ antagonist with analgesic properties similar to those of morphine. However, it causes marked dysphoria, with nightmares and hallucinations, rather than euphoria, and is now rarely used.

Loperamide is an opioid that is effectively extruded from the brain by P-glycoprotein and therefore lacks analgesic activity. It inhibits peristalsis, and is used to control diarrhoea (see Ch. 30).

OPIOID ANTAGONISTS

Naloxone was the first pure opioid antagonist, with affinity for all three classic opioid receptors (µ > κ ≥ δ). It blocks the actions of endogenous opioid peptides as well as those of morphine-like drugs, and has been extensively used as an experimental tool to determine the physiological role of these peptides, particularly in pain transmission.

Given on its own, naloxone produces very little effect in normal subjects but produces a rapid reversal of the effects of morphine and other opioids. It has little effect on pain threshold under normal conditions but causes hyperalgesia under conditions of stress or inflammation, when endogenous opioids are produced. This occurs, for example, in patients undergoing dental surgery, or in animals subjected to physical stress. Naloxone also inhibits acupuncture analgesia, which is known to be associated with the release of endogenous opioid peptides. Analgesia produced by PAG stimulation is also prevented.

The main clinical uses of naloxone are to treat respiratory depression caused by opioid overdosage, and occasionally to reverse the effect of opioid analgesics, used during labour, on the respiration of the newborn baby. It is usually given intravenously, and its effects are produced immediately. It is rapidly metabolised by the liver, and its effect lasts only 2–4 h, which is considerably shorter than that of most morphine-like drugs and therefore it may have to be given repeatedly.

Naloxone has no important unwanted effects of its own but precipitates withdrawal symptoms in addicts. It can be used to detect opioid addiction.

Naltrexone is very similar to naloxone but with the advantage of a much longer duration of action (half-life about 10 h). It may be of value in addicts who have been 'detoxified', because it nullifies the effect of a dose of opioid should the patient's resolve fail. For this purpose, it is available in a slow-release subcutaneous implant formulation. It is also effective in reducing alcohol consumption in heavy drinkers (see Ch. 49), the rationale being that part of the high from alcohol comes from the release of endogenous opioid peptides. It may also have beneficial effects in septic shock. It is effective in treating chronic itching (pruritus), as occurs in chronic liver disease. Again,

this may indicate the involvement of endogenous opioid peptides in the pathophysiology of such itch conditions.

Methylnaltrexone bromide and **alvimopan** are µ opioid-receptor antagonists that do not cross the blood–brain barrier. They can be used in combination with opioid agonists to block unwanted effects, most notably reduced gastrointestinal motility, nausea and vomiting.

Specific antagonists at µ, δ and κ receptors are available for experimental use (Table 42.3) but they are not used clinically.

> ## Opioid antagonists
>
> - Pure antagonists include **naloxone** (short acting) and **naltrexone** (longer acting). They block µ, δ and κ receptors. Selective antagonists are available as experimental tools.
> - **Alvimopan** is a µ-receptor antagonist that does not cross the blood–brain barrier. It blocks opioid-induced constipation, nausea and vomiting.
> - Some drugs, such as **pentazocine**, produce a mixture of κ agonist and µ antagonist effects.
> - **Naloxone** does not affect pain threshold normally but blocks stress-induced analgesia and can exacerbate clinical pain.
> - **Naloxone** rapidly reverses opioid-induced analgesia and respiratory depression, and is used mainly to treat opioid overdose or to improve breathing in newborn babies affected by opioids given to the mother.
> - **Naloxone** precipitates withdrawal symptoms in **morphine**-dependent patients or animals. **Pentazocine** may also do this.

PARACETAMOL

Non-steroidal anti-inflammatory drugs (NSAIDs, covered in detail in Ch. 26) are widely used to treat painful inflammatory conditions and to reduce fever. **Paracetamol** (known as **acetaminophen** in the USA) deserves special mention. It was first synthesised more than a century ago, and since the 1950s has (alongside aspirin and ibuprofen) been the most widely used over-the-counter remedy for minor aches and pains. Paracetamol differs from other NSAIDs in producing analgesic and antipyretic effects while lacking anti-inflammatory effects. It also lacks the tendency of other NSAIDs to cause gastric ulceration and bleeding. The reason for the difference between paracetamol and other NSAIDs is unclear. Biochemical tests showed it to be only a weak cyclo-oxygenase (COX) inhibitor, with some selectivity for brain COX. It remains contentious whether paracetamol relieves pain centrally by inhibiting COX-3 (not a separate gene product but a splice variant of COX-1) or by inhibiting COX-2 at low rates of enzyme activity. Interestingly, the antinociceptive effects of paracetamol are absent in mice lacking the TRPA1 receptor (see p. 513). The antinociceptive effect appears to be mediated by metabolites (i.e. *N*-acetyl-*p*-benzoquinoneimine and *p*-benzoquinone), not by paracetamol itself. These activate TRPA1 and thus reduce voltage-gated calcium and sodium currents in primary sensory neurons.

Paracetamol is well absorbed by mouth, and its plasma half-life is about 3 h. It is metabolised by hydroxylation, conjugated mainly as glucuronide, and excreted in the urine. In therapeutic doses, it has few adverse effects. However, in overdose, paracetamol causes severe liver damage, which is commonly fatal (see Chs 26 and 57), and the drug is often used in attempted suicide.

USE OF OPIOIDS AND NSAIDS IN COMBINATION

The rationale behind co-administration of two drugs that produce analgesia by different mechanisms is that, if the effects are additive, less of each drug can therefore be given but the same degree of analgesia produced. This has the effect of reducing the intensity of the unwanted side effects produced by each drug. In the case of opioids (e.g. codeine) in combination with paracetamol or aspirin, the combination appears to produce synergy rather than simple additivity. The combination of dextropropoxyphene and paracetamol has been withdrawn in the UK due to concerns about overdosing.

TREATMENT OF NEUROPATHIC PAIN

Neuropathic pain is the severe, debilitating, chronic pain that occurs in conditions such as trigeminal neuralgia, diabetic neuropathy, postherpetic neuralgia and phantom limb pain, affecting millions of people worldwide. It is often stated that neuropathic pain is opioid-resistant. However, clinical studies have shown opioids such as morphine, oxycodone, levorphanol, tramadol and tapentadol to be effective in the treatment of neuropathic pain, provided an adequate dose can be reached that provides analgesia without excessive side effects. The monamine uptake inhibiting properties of tramadol and tapentadol may contribute to their effectiveness.

Several non-opioid drugs that are also used clinically for effects other than analgesia have been found to be effective in neuropathic pain (see Dworkin et al., 2010), largely as a result of serendipitous observations rather than a rational programme of drug discovery.

Tricyclic antidepressants, particularly **amitriptyline**, **nortriptyline** and **desipramine** (Ch. 47) are widely used. These drugs act centrally by inhibiting noradrenaline reuptake and are highly effective in relieving neuropathic pain in some, but not all, cases. Their action is independent of their antidepressant effects. Drugs such as **duloxetine** and **venlafaxine**, which inhibit serotonin and noradrenaline uptake, are also effective and have a different side effect profile, but selective serotonin reuptake inhibitors show little or no benefit.

Gabapentin and its congener, **pregabalin**, are antiepileptic drugs (Ch. 45) that are also effective in the treatment of neuropathic pain. They reduce the expression of $\alpha 2\delta$ subunits of voltage-activated calcium channels on the nerve membrane (see Ch. 4) and reduce neurotransmitter release. The $\alpha 2\delta$ subunits are upregulated in damaged sensory neurons, thus explaining why these agents are more effective across a range of pain states associated with nerve damage than in other forms of pain.

Carbamazepine, another type of antiepileptic drug, is effective in trigeminal neuralgia but evidence for effectiveness against other neuropathic pains is lacking. Carbamazepine blocks voltage-gated sodium channels (see Ch. 4) being slightly more potent in blocking $Na_v1.8$ than $Na_v1.7$ and $Na_v1.3$ channels; all of these channel subtypes are thought to be upregulated by nerve damage and contribute to the sensation of pain. At higher concentrations,

it inhibits voltage-activated calcium channels. **Phenytoin** administered intravenously is sometimes used in a crisis.

Other antiepileptic agents such as **valproic acid**, **lamotrogine**, **oxcarbazepine** and **topiramate**, may have efficacy in some neuropathic pain states.

Lidocaine (lignocaine), a local anaesthetic drug (Ch. 43), can be used topically to relieve neuropathic pain. It probably acts by blocking spontaneous discharges from damaged sensory nerve terminals. Some antidysrhythmic drugs (e.g. **mexiletine**, **tocainide**, **flecainide**; see Ch. 21) are effective orally.

Other analgesic drugs

- **Paracetamol** resembles non-steroidal anti-inflammatory drugs and is effective as an analgesic, but it lacks anti-inflammatory activity. It may act by inhibiting cyclo-oxygenase (COX) 3, a splice variant of COX-1, but probably has other effects as well. In overdose, it causes hepatotoxicity.
- **Nefopam** is an amine uptake inhibitor that can be used to treat opioid-resistant pain.
- Various antidepressants (e.g. **amitriptyline**), as well as antiepileptic drugs (e.g. **carbamazepine**, **gabapentin**), are used mainly to treat neuropathic pain.
- The NMDA-receptor antagonist **ketamine** is occasionally used.

Drugs used to treat neuropathic pain

- Opioids may be effective at higher doses if side effects can be tolerated.
- Various antidepressants (e.g. **amitriptyline**, **duloxetine**) provide therapeutic benefit.
- **Gabapentin** and **pregabalin** are now used more to relieve neuropathic pain than as antiepileptic agents.
- **Carbamazepine**, as well as some other antiepileptic agents that block sodium channels, can be effective in treating trigeminal neuralgia.
- **Lidocaine** may provide relief when applied topically.

TREATMENT OF FIBROMYALGIA

Fibromyalgia is a chronic disorder characterised by widespread musculoskeletal pain, fatigue and insomnia. Its cause is unknown, with no obvious characteristic pathology being apparent. It is associated with allodynia. As with neuropathic pain, classical analgesics (i.e NSAIDs and opioids), while bringing some relief, are not very effective in treating this disorder. Various antidepressant drugs (e.g. amitriptyline, **citalopram**, **milnacipram**, duloxetine, venlafaxine; see Ch. 47), antiepileptic agents (e.g. gabapentin, pregabalin; see Ch. 45), benzodiazepines (e.g. **clonazepam**, **zopiclone**; see Ch. 44) are currently used for this disorder – this long list reflecting their uncertain efficacy.

OTHER PAIN-RELIEVING DRUGS

Nefopam, an inhibitor of amine uptake with some sodium channel blocking properties is used in the treatment of persistent pain unresponsive to non-opioid drugs. It does not depress respiration but does produce sympathomimetic and antimuscarinic side effects.

Ketamine, a dissociative anaesthetic (Ch. 41), **memantine** and **dextromethorphan** work by blocking NMDA receptor channels, and probably reduce the wind-up phenomenon in the dorsal horn (Fig. 42.2). Given intrathecally, ketamine's effects on memory and cognitive function are largely avoided.

Ziconotide, a synthetic analogue of the N-type calcium-channel blocking peptide ω-conotoxin MVIIA, is effective when administered by the intrathecal route. It is used in patients whose pain does not respond to other analgesic agents. Blockers of low-voltage-activated T-type calcium channels may also be effective analgesics in some pain states.

Cannabinoids acting at CB₁ receptors are effective pain-relieving agents in animal pain models, including models of acute, antinociceptive, inflammatory and neuropathic pain. Although in clinical trials on neuropathic pain these drugs are able to reduce pain perception, the effect is generally weak and clinical relevance remains under evaluation (see Hosking & Zajicek, 2008). The strongest evidence of their benefit is for central neuropathic pain in multiple sclerosis. **Sativex** is an extract of the cannabis plant containing Δ9-tetrahydrocannabinol (THC) and cannabidiol that has been suggested to have improved therapeutic efficacy. CB₂-receptor agonists may also be potential analgesic agents.

In addition, cannabinoids and related drugs that lack agonist action at CB₁ receptors have been observed to induce analgesia by potentiating the actions of the inhibitory amino acid glycine at the ionotropic glycine receptor (see Ch. 38) in the spinal cord. This may lead to the development of new therapeutic agents lacking the unwanted effects of CB₁ agonism.

Botulinum toxin injections are effective in relieving back pain and the pain associated with spasticity. This effect is due mainly to a relief of muscle spasm (Ch. 13).

Ropinirole, **pramipexole** and **rotigotine**, dopamine-receptor agonists (see Ch. 39) are used to treat restless leg syndrome, which can be painful in some individuals.

Clinical uses of analgesic drugs (1)

- Analgesics are used to treat and prevent pain, for example:
  - pre- and postoperatively
  - common painful conditions including headache, dysmenorrhoea, labour, trauma and burns
  - many medical and surgical emergencies (e.g. myocardial infarction and renal colic)
  - terminal disease (especially metastatic cancer).
- Opioid analgesics are used in some non-painful conditions, for example acute heart failure (because of their haemodynamic effects) and terminal chronic heart failure (to relieve distress).
- The choice and route of administration of analgesic drugs depends on the nature and duration of the pain.
- A progressive approach is often used, starting with non-steroidal anti-inflammatory drugs (NSAIDs), supplemented first by weak opioid analgesics and then by strong opioids.
- In general, severe acute pain is treated with strong opioids (e.g. **morphine**, **fentanyl**) given by injection. Mild inflammatory pain (e.g. sprains, mild arthralgia) is treated with NSAIDs (e.g. **ibuprofen**) or by **paracetamol** supplemented by weak opioids (e.g. **codeine**). Severe pain (e.g. cancer pain) is treated with strong opioids given orally, intrathecally, epidurally or by subcutaneous injection. Patient-controlled infusion systems are useful postoperatively.
- Chronic neuropathic pain is less responsive to opioids and can be treated with tricyclic antidepressants (e.g. **amitriptyline**) or anticonvulsants (e.g. **carbamazepine**, **gabapentin**).

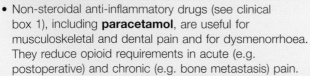

Clinical uses of analgesic drugs (2)

- Non-steroidal anti-inflammatory drugs (see clinical box 1), including **paracetamol**, are useful for musculoskeletal and dental pain and for dysmenorrhoea. They reduce opioid requirements in acute (e.g. postoperative) and chronic (e.g. bone metastasis) pain.
- Weak opioids (e.g. **codeine**) combined with **paracetamol** are useful in moderately severe pain if non-opioids are not sufficient. **Tramadol** (a weak opioid with additional action on 5-hydroxytryptamine and noradrenaline uptake) is an alternative.
- Strong opioids (e.g. **morphine**) are used for severe pain, particularly of visceral origin.
- Note that:
  - the intravenous route provides rapid relief from pain and distress
  - the intravenous dose is much lower than the oral dose because of presystemic metabolism

- **morphine** is given orally as a solution or as 'immediate-release' tablets every 4 h
- dose is titrated; when the daily requirement is apparent, the preparation is changed to a modified-release formulation to allow once- or twice-daily dosing
- **morphine** and **oxycodone** can be given orally in slow-release tablet form
- transdermal administration (e.g. patches of **fentanyl**) is an alternative, rapid means of pain relief
- adverse effects (nausea, constipation) are anticipated and treated pre-emptively
- addiction is not an issue in the setting of terminal care.
- Subanaesthetic doses of **nitrous oxide** (Ch. 41) are analgesic, and self-administration of a mixture of **nitrous oxide** with oxygen is widely used during labour or for painful dressing changes.

NEW APPROACHES

▼ As in other fields of neuropharmacology, increasing knowledge of the various chemical mediators and signalling pathways responsible for pain sensation suggests many new approaches to the control of pain. Pain treatment is currently far from perfect, and novel approaches are being explored.

- *Nerve growth factor* (NGF) is a major mediator of both inflammatory and neuropathic pain (Mantyh et al., 2011). It is therefore an important therapeutic target. It has proved difficult to design small-molecule, selective antagonists of NGF. Current alternative options being explored include the development of monoclonal antibodies to NGF or its receptor TrkA and the sequestration of NGF using a soluble decoy receptor protein that binds NGF with picomolar affinity.
- *TRP channel ligands*. It was hoped that TRPV1 antagonists would be effective analgesics but despite promising results in animal models, none has yet been developed for human use, mainly because they cause hyperthermia, and may suppress thermosensitivity and thus predispose to burn injury. TRPV1 agonists induce receptor desensitisation or a reversible sensory nerve terminal degeneration due to prolonged cation influx. Topical high-dose **capsaicin** is efficacious in a number of neuropathic pain conditions, but causes burning pain initially.
- *Other TRP channels* have been suggested to be involved in pain particularly when sensitised by some pathophysiological changes. Agonists and antagonists for TRPA1 and TRPM8 are in development. TRPM8 may also be a target for anticancer drugs.

- It had been hoped that *sodium channel blockers* especially those with selectivity at channels upregulated in chronic pain states would be effective pain relieving drugs. Clinical trials with **lacosamide** (antiepileptic) and **ralfinamide** in chronic pain have been disappointing.
- **Retigabine**, a K_v7 (M-current) *opener* (see Ch. 45) inhibits C-fibre- and Aδ-fibre-mediated nociceptive responses in dorsal horn neurons in both naive and neuropathic rats. It is chemically related to **flupirtine** which is used as an analgesic agent in some countries.
- Agonists at *nicotinic acetylcholine receptors*, based on **epibatidine** (an alkaloid from frog skin, which is a potent nicotinic agonist) show – unexpectedly – potent analgesic effects in animal models. Derivatives with fewer side effects are under investigation.
- Various *neuropeptides*, such as **somatostatin** (see Ch. 34) and **calcitonin** (see Ch. 36), produce powerful analgesia when applied intrathecally, and there are clinical reports suggesting that they may have similar effects when used systemically to treat endocrine disorders.
- *Glutamate antagonists* acting on NMDA or AMPA receptors show analgesic activity in animal models, but it has not yet been possible – with the exception of ketamine – to obtain this effect in humans without unacceptable side effects. To circumvent this, attempts are being made to develop antagonists selective for channels of different subunit compositions (see Ch. 38) or antagonists at the glycine site on the NMDA receptor. Paradoxically inhibitors of glycine reuptake may also be analgesic. Antagonists of metabotropic glutamate receptors, mGluR1 and mGluR5, are currently in development and may have fewer side effects.

REFERENCES AND FURTHER READING

General

Fields, H.L., Basbaum, A.I., Heinricher, M.M., 2006. Central nervous system mechanisms of pain modulation. In: McMahon, S.B., Koltzenburg, M. (Eds.), Wall & Melzack's Textbook of Pain, fifth ed. Elsevier, Edinburgh, pp. 125–142. (*Detailed account of central pathways that inhibit or enhance transmission in the dorsal horn*)

McMahon, S.B., Koltzenburg, M. (Eds.), 2006. Wall & Melzack's Textbook of Pain, fifth ed. Elsevier, Edinburgh. (*Large multiauthor reference book*)

Tracey, I., 2008. Imaging pain. Br. J. Anaesth. 101, 32–39. (*Description of brain imaging studies on which parts of the brain process pain information*)

Yaksh, T.L., 1999. Spinal systems and pain processing: development of novel analgesic drugs with mechanistically defined models. Trends Pharmacol. Sci. 20, 329–337. (*Good general review article on spinal cord mechanisms – more general than its title suggests*)

TRP channels

Flockerzi, V., Nilius, B. (Eds.), 2007. Transient receptor potential (TRP) channels. Handb. Exp. Pharmacol. 179. (*An entire volume given over to this topic, with individual chapters written by experts in the field*)

BDNF and TrkA

Mantyh, P.W., Koltzenburg, M., Mendell, L.M., Tive, L., Shelton, D.L., 2011. Antagonism of nerve growth factor-TrkA signaling and the relief of pain. Anesthesiology 115, 189–204.

Opioids

Ballantyne, J.C., Mao, J., 2003. Opioid therapy for chronic pain. N. Engl. J. Med. 349, 1943–1953. (*Considers whether or not tolerance is a problem when opioids are used to treat chronic pain*)

Corbett, A.D., Henderson, G., McKnight, A.T., et al., 2006. 75 years of opioid research: the exciting but vain search for the holy grail. Br. J. Pharmacol. 147, S153–S162. (*Comprehensive historical review of opioid research*)

Fields, H., 2004. State-dependent opioid control of pain. Nat. Rev. Neurosci. 5, 565–575.

Hashimoto, K., Ishiwata, K., 2006. Sigma receptor ligands: possible application as therapeutic drugs and as radiopharmaceuticals. Curr. Pharm. Des. 12, 3857–3876.

Kelly, E., 2013. Efficacy and ligand bias at the μ-opioid receptor. Br. J. Pharmacol. 169, 1430–1446.

Lee, M., Silverman, S.M., Hansen, H., Patel, V.B., Manchikanti, L., 2011. A comprehensive review of opioid-induced hyperalgesia. Pain Physician 14, 145–161.

McQuay, H., 1999. Opioids in pain management. Lancet 353, 2229–2232. (*Discusses whether or not tolerance occurs to opioids in clinical situations*)

Rollason, V., Samer, C., Piquet, V., et al., 2008. Pharmacogenetics of analgesics: towards the personalization of prescription. Pharmacogenomics 9, 905–933.

Sawynok, J., 2003. Topical and peripherally acting analgesics. Pharmacol. Rev. 55, 1–20. (*Review of the numerous mechanisms by which drugs interfere with nociceptive mechanisms in the periphery*)

Williams, J.T., Ingram, S.L., Henderson, G., et al., 2013. Regulation of μ-opioid receptors: desensitization, phosphorylation, internalization, and tolerance. Pharmacol. Rev. 65, 223–254. (*Very comprehensive review of the molecular and cellular mechanisms underlying opioid tolerance*)

Neuropathic pain and new drug targets

Dworkin, R.H., O'Connor, A.B., Audette, J., et al., 2010. Recommendations for the pharmacological management of neuropathic pain: an overview and literature update. Mayo Clin. Proc. 85 (3 Suppl), S3–S14. (*An evaluation of the clinical effectiveness of current drugs used to treat neuropathic pain*)

Hosking, R.D., Zajicek, J.P., 2008. Therapeutic potential of cannabis in pain medicine. Br. J. Anaesth. 101, 59–68.

43 Local anaesthetics and other drugs affecting sodium channels

OVERVIEW

As described in Chapter 4, the property of electrical excitability is what enables the membranes of nerve and muscle cells to generate propagated action potentials, which are essential for communication in the nervous system and for the initiation of mechanical activity in striated muscle. Initiation of the action potential depends on voltage-gated sodium channels, which open transiently when the membrane is depolarised. Here we discuss local anaesthetics, which act mainly by blocking sodium channels, and mention briefly other drugs that affect sodium-channel function.

There are, broadly speaking, two ways in which channel function may be modified, namely block of the channels and modification of gating behaviour. Blocking sodium channels reduces excitability. On the other hand, different types of drugs can either facilitate channel opening and thus increase excitability, or inhibit channel opening and reduce excitability.

LOCAL ANAESTHETICS

Although many drugs can, at high concentrations, block voltage-sensitive sodium channels and inhibit the generation of the action potential, the only drugs used clinically for this effect are the local anaesthetics, various antiepileptic and analgesic drugs (see Chs 42 and 45) and class I antidysrhythmic drugs (see Ch. 21).

HISTORY

Coca leaves have been chewed for their psychotropic effects for thousands of years (see Ch. 48) by South American Indians, who knew about the numbing effect they produced on the mouth and tongue. **Cocaine** was isolated in 1860 and proposed as a local anaesthetic for surgical procedures. Sigmund Freud, who tried unsuccessfully to make use of its 'psychic energising' power, gave some cocaine to his ophthalmologist friend in Vienna, Carl Köller, who reported in 1884 that reversible corneal anaesthesia could be produced by dropping cocaine into the eye. The idea was rapidly taken up, and within a few years cocaine anaesthesia was introduced into dentistry and general surgery. A synthetic substitute, **procaine**, was discovered in 1905, and many other useful compounds were later developed.

CHEMICAL ASPECTS

Local anaesthetic molecules consist of an aromatic part linked by an ester or amide bond to a basic side-chain (Fig. 43.1). They are weak bases, with pK_a values mainly in the range 8–9, so that they are mainly, but not completely, ionised at physiological pH (see Ch. 8 for an explanation of how pH influences the ionisation of weak bases). This is important in relation to their ability to penetrate the nerve sheath and axon membrane; quaternary derivatives such as QX-314, which are fully ionised irrespective of pH, are ineffective as local anaesthetics but have important experimental uses. **Benzocaine**, an atypical local anaesthetic, has no basic group.

The presence of the ester or amide bond in local anaesthetic molecules is important because of its susceptibility to metabolic hydrolysis. The ester-containing compounds are fairly rapidly inactivated in the plasma and tissues (mainly liver) by non-specific esterases. Amides are more stable, and these anaesthetics generally have longer plasma half-lives.

MECHANISM OF ACTION

Local anaesthetics block the initiation and propagation of action potentials by preventing the voltage-dependent increase in Na^+ conductance (see Ch. 4) (see Strichartz & Ritchie, 1987; Hille, 2001). At low concentrations they decrease the rate of rise of the action potential, increasing its duration, and increase the refractory period thus reducing the firing rate. At higher concentrations they prevent action potential firing. Currently available local anaesthetic agents do not by and large distinguish between different sodium channel subtypes although their potencies vary (see Ch. 4). They block sodium channels, by physically plugging the transmembrane pore, interacting with various amino acid residues of the S6 transmembrane helical domain of the channel protein (see Ragsdale et al., 1994).

▼ Local anaesthetic activity is strongly pH-dependent, being increased at alkaline extracellular pH (i.e. when the proportion of ionised molecules is low) and reduced at acid pH. This is because the compound needs to penetrate the nerve sheath and the axon membrane to reach the inner end of the sodium channel (where the local anaesthetic-binding site resides). Because the ionised form is not membrane-permeant, penetration is very poor at acid pH. Once inside the axon, it is primarily the ionised form of the local anaesthetic molecule that binds to the channel and blocks it (Fig. 43.2), the unionised form having only weak channel-blocking activity. This pH dependence can be clinically important, because the extracellular fluid of inflamed tissues is often relatively acidic and such tissues are thus somewhat resistant to local anaesthetic agents.

Further analysis of local anaesthetic action (see Strichartz & Ritchie, 1987) has shown that many drugs exhibit the property of 'use-dependent' block of sodium channels, as well as affecting, to some extent, the gating of the channels. Use-dependence means that the more the channels are opened, the greater the block becomes. It is a prominent feature of the action of many class I antidysrhythmic drugs (Ch. 21) and antiepileptic drugs (Ch. 45), and occurs because the blocking molecule enters the channel much more readily when the channel is open than when it is closed. Furthermore, for local anaesthetics that rapidly dissociate from the channel, block only occurs at high frequencies of action potential firing when the time between action potentials is too short for drug dissociation from the channel to occur. The channel can exist in three functional states: resting, open and inactivated (see Ch. 4). Many local anaesthetics

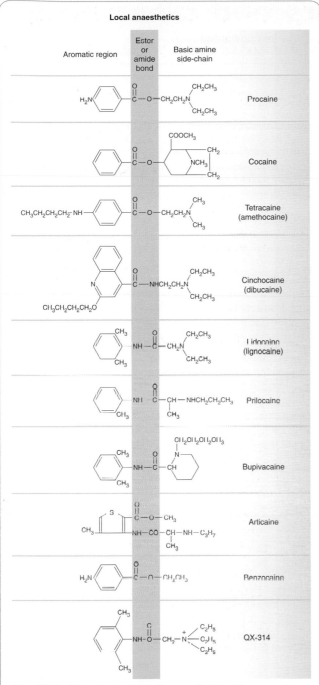

Fig. 43.1   Structures of local anaesthetics. The general structure of local anaesthetic molecules consists of an aromatic group (left), ester or amide group (shaded blue) and amine group (right).

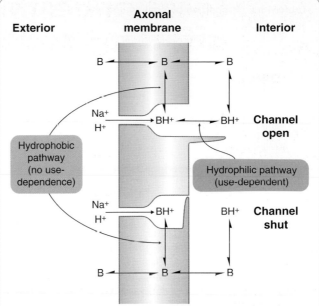

Fig. 43.2   Interaction of local anaesthetics with sodium channels. The blocking site within the channel can be reached via the open channel gate on the inner surface of the membrane by the charged species BH⁺ (hydrophilic pathway), or directly from the membrane by the uncharged species B (hydrophilic pathway).

use-dependence, which explains in part why pain transmission may be blocked more effectively than other sensory modalities.

Quaternary amine local anaesthetics only work when applied to the inside of the membrane and the channels must be cycled through their open state a few times before the blocking effect appears. With tertiary amine local anaesthetics, block can develop even if the channels are not open, and it is likely that the blocking molecule (uncharged) can reach the channel either directly from the membrane phase or via the open gate (Fig. 43.2). The relative importance of these two blocking pathways – the hydrophobic pathway via the membrane and the hydrophilic pathway via the inner mouth of the channel – varies according to the lipid solubility of the drug.

Local anaesthetics exert a number of effects on other ion channels as well as on membrane and intracellular signalling proteins. The importance of these actions to local anaesthetic action is as yet unclear (see Yanagidate & Stricharz, 2007).

In general, local anaesthetics block conduction in small-diameter nerve fibres more readily than in large fibres. Because nociceptive impulses are carried by Aδ and C fibres (Ch. 42), pain sensation is blocked more readily than other sensory modalities (touch, proprioception, etc.). Motor axons, being large in diameter, are also relatively resistant. The differences in sensitivity among different nerve fibres, although easily measured experimentally, are not of much practical importance, and it is not possible to block pain sensation without affecting other sensory modalities.

Local anaesthetics, as their name implies, are mainly used to produce local nerve block. At low concentrations, they are also able to suppress the spontaneous action potential discharge in sensory neurons that occurs in neuropathic pain. The properties of individual local anaesthetic drugs are summarised in Table 43.1.

bind most strongly to the inactivated state of the channel. Therefore, at any given membrane potential, the equilibrium between resting and inactivated channels will, in the presence of a local anaesthetic, be shifted in favour of the inactivated state, and this factor contributes to the overall blocking effect by reducing the number of channels available for opening, and by prolonging the refractory period following an action potential. The passage of a train of action potentials, for example when a painful stimulus is applied to a sensory nerve, causes the channels to cycle through the open and inactivated states, both of which are more likely to bind local anaesthetic molecules than the resting state; thus both mechanisms contribute to

Table 43.1 Properties of local anaesthetics

Drug	Onset	Duration	Tissue penetration	Plasma half-life (h)	Main unwanted effects	Notes
Cocaine	Medium	Medium	Good	~1	Cardiovascular and CNS effects owing to block of amine uptake	Rarely used, only as spray for upper respiratory tract
Procaine	Medium	Short	Poor	<1	CNS: restlessness, shivering, anxiety, occasionally convulsions followed by respiratory depression Cardiovascular system: bradycardia and decreased cardiac output; vasodilatation, which can cause cardiovascular collapse	The first synthetic agent No longer used
Lidocaine (lignocaine)	Rapid	Medium	Good	~2	As procaine but less tendency to cause CNS effects	Widely used for local anaesthesia Also used intravenously for treating ventricular dysrhythmias though no longer as first choice (Ch. 21)
Mepivacaine	Rapid	Medium	Good	~2	As procaine	Less vasodilatation (may be administered without a vasoconstrictor)
Tetracaine (amethocaine)	Very slow	Long	Moderate	~1	As lidocaine	Used mainly for spinal and corneal anaesthesia
Bupivacaine	Slow	Long	Moderate	~2	As lidocaine but greater cardiotoxicity	Widely used because of long duration of action Ropivacaine is similar, with less cardiotoxicity Levobupivacaine causes less cardiotoxicity and CNS depression than the racemate, bupivacaine
Prilocaine	Medium	Medium	Moderate	~2	No vasodilator activity Can cause methaemoglobinaemia	Widely used; not for obstetric analgesia because of risk of neonatal methaemoglobinaemia
Articaine	Rapid	Short	Good	0.5	As lidocaine	Used in dentistry While its chemical structure contains an amide linkage it also has an ester group on a side chain (Fig 43.1). Hydrolysis of the side chain inactivates the drug

CNS, central nervous system.

UNWANTED EFFECTS

When used clinically as local anaesthetics, the main unwanted effects involve the central nervous system (CNS) and the cardiovascular system (Table 43.1). Their action on the heart can also be of use in treating cardiac arrhythmias (see Ch. 21). Although local anaesthetics are usually administered in such a way as to minimise their spread to other parts of the body, they are ultimately absorbed into the systemic circulation. They may also be injected into veins or arterioles by accident.

Most local anaesthetics produce a mixture of depressant and stimulant effects on the CNS. Depressant effects predominate at low plasma concentrations, giving way to stimulation at higher concentrations, resulting in restlessness, tremor and sometimes convulsions, accompanied by subjective effects ranging from confusion to extreme

Actions of local anaesthetics

- Local anaesthetics block action potential generation by blocking sodium channels.
- Local anaesthetics are amphiphilic molecules with a hydrophobic aromatic group and a basic amine group.
- Local anaesthetics are weak bases that act in their cationic form but must reach their site of action by penetrating the nerve sheath and axonal membrane as un-ionised species.
- Many local anaesthetics show use-dependence (depth of block increases with action potential frequency). This arises:
  - because anaesthetic molecules gain access to the channel more readily when the channel is open
  - because anaesthetic molecules have higher affinity for inactivated than for resting channels.
- Use-dependence is mainly of importance in relation to antidysrhythmic and antiepileptic effects of sodium channel blockers.
- Local anaesthetics block conduction in peripheral nerves in the following order: small myelinated axons, non-myelinated axons, large myelinated axons. Nociceptive and sympathetic transmission is thus blocked first.
- Sodium-channel block in cardiac muscle and in CNS neurons is exploited in the therapy of cardiac dysrhythmias (Ch. 21) and epilepsy (Ch. 45).

agitation. Further increasing the dose produces profound CNS depression and death due to respiratory depression. The only local anaesthetic with markedly different CNS effects is **cocaine** (see Ch. 48), which produces euphoria at doses well below those that cause other CNS effects. This relates to its specific effect on monoamine uptake, an effect not shared by other local anaesthetics. **Procaine** is particularly liable to produce unwanted central effects, and has been superseded in clinical use by agents such as **lidocaine** and **prilocaine**. Studies with **bupivacaine**, a widely used long-acting local anaesthetic prepared as a racemic mixture of two optical isomers, suggested that its CNS and cardiac effects were mainly due to the $S(+)$ isomer. The $R(-)$ isomer (**levobupivacaine**) has a better margin of safety.

The adverse cardiovascular effects of local anaesthetics are due mainly to myocardial depression, conduction block and vasodilatation. Reduction of myocardial contractility probably results indirectly from an inhibition of the Na^+ current in cardiac muscle (see Ch. 21). The resulting decrease of $[Na^+]_i$ in turn reduces intracellular Ca^{2+} stores (see Ch. 4), and this reduces the force of contraction. Interference with atrioventricular conduction can result in partial or complete heart block, as well as other types of dysrhythmia. **Ropivacaine** has less cardiotoxicity than bupivacaine.

Vasodilatation, mainly affecting arterioles, is due partly to a direct effect on vascular smooth muscle, and partly to inhibition of the sympathetic nervous system. This leads to a fall in blood pressure, which may be sudden and life-threatening. Cocaine is an exception in respect of its cardiovascular effects, because of its ability to inhibit noradrenaline reuptake (see Chs 14 and 48). This enhances sympathetic activity, leading to tachycardia, increased cardiac output, vasoconstriction and increased arterial pressure.

Hypersensitivity reactions sometimes occur with local anaesthetics, usually in the form of allergic dermatitis but rarely as an acute anaphylactic reaction. Other unwanted effects that are specific to particular drugs include mucosal irritation (cocaine) and methaemoglobinaemia (which occurs after large doses of prilocaine, because of the production of a toxic metabolite).

PHARMACOKINETIC ASPECTS

Local anaesthetics vary a good deal in the rapidity with which they penetrate tissues, and this affects the rate at which they cause nerve block when injected into tissues, and the rate of onset of, and recovery from, anaesthesia (Table 43.1; see Becker & Reed, 2012). It also affects their usefulness as surface anaesthetics for application to mucous membranes.

Most of the ester-linked local anaesthetics (e.g. **tetracaine**) are rapidly hydrolysed by plasma cholinesterase, so their plasma half-life is short. Procaine – now rarely used – is hydrolysed to p-aminobenzoic acid, a folate precursor that interferes with the antibacterial effect of sulfonamides (see Ch. 51). The amide-linked drugs (e.g. lidocaine and prilocaine) are metabolised mainly in the liver, usually by N-dealkylation rather than cleavage of the amide bond, and the metabolites are often pharmacologically active.

Benzocaine is an unusual local anaesthetic of very low solubility, which is used as a dry powder to dress painful skin ulcers, or as throat lozenges. The drug is slowly released and produces long-lasting surface anaesthesia.[1]

The routes of administration, uses and main adverse effects of local anaesthetics are summarised in Table 43.2.

Most local anaesthetics have a direct vasodilator action, which increases the rate at which they are absorbed into the systemic circulation, thus increasing their potential toxicity and reducing their local anaesthetic action. **Adrenaline** (**epinephrine**) or **felypressin**, a short-acting vasopressin analogue (see Ch. 33), may be added to local anaesthetic solutions injected locally in order to cause vasoconstriction. Adrenaline absorbed into the circulation may induce unwanted cardiovascular effects such as tachycardia and vasoconstriction and felypressin may cause coronary artery constriction. Their use in patients with cardiovascular disease is contraindicated.

NEW APPROACHES

Blocking specific sodium-channel subtypes is seen as a promising therapeutic strategy for a variety of clinical conditions, including epilepsy (see Ch. 45), neurodegenerative diseases and stroke (see Ch. 40), neuropathic pain (see Ch. 42) and myopathies. As our understanding of the role of specific sodium-channel subtypes in different pathophysiological situations increases, so too will be the likelihood that selective blocking agents can be developed for use in different clinical situations.

---

[1]Benzocaine is also used in 'endurance' condoms to delay ejaculation.

Table 43.2 Methods of administration, uses and adverse effects of local anaesthetics

Method	Uses	Drug(s)	Notes and adverse effects
Surface anaesthesia	Nose, mouth, bronchial tree (usually in spray form), cornea, urinary tract, uterus (for hysteroscopy) Not very effective for skin[a]	Lidocaine, tetracaine, (amethocaine), dibucaine, benzocaine	Risk of systemic toxicity when high concentrations and large areas are involved
Infiltration anaesthesia	Direct injection into tissues to reach nerve branches and terminals Used in minor surgery	Most	Adrenaline (epinephrine) or felypressin often added as vasoconstrictors (not with fingers or toes, for fear of causing ischaemic tissue damage) Suitable for only small areas, otherwise serious risk of systemic toxicity
Intravenous regional anaesthesia	LA injected intravenously distal to a pressure cuff to arrest blood flow; remains effective until the circulation is restored Used for limb surgery	Mainly lidocaine, prilocaine	Risk of systemic toxicity when cuff is released prematurely; risk is small if cuff remains inflated for at least 20 min
Nerve block anaesthesia	LA is injected close to nerve trunks (e.g. brachial plexus, intercostal or dental nerves) to produce a loss of sensation peripherally Used for surgery, dentistry, analgesia	Most	Less LA needed than for infiltration anaesthesia Accurate placement of the needle is important Onset of anaesthesia may be slow Duration of anaesthesia may be increased by addition of vasoconstrictor
Spinal anaesthesia[b]	LA injected into the subarachnoid space (containing cerebrospinal fluid) to act on spinal roots and spinal cord Sometimes formulated with glucose ('hyperbaricity') so that spread of LA can be controlled by tilting patient Used for surgery to abdomen, pelvis or leg LA can be used alone or in conjunction with a general anaesthetic to reduce stress Provides good postoperative pain relief	Mainly lidocaine	Main risks are bradycardia and hypotension (owing to sympathetic block), respiratory depression (owing to effects on phrenic nerve or respiratory centre); avoided by minimising cranial spread Postoperative urinary retention (block of pelvic autonomic outflow) is common
Epidural anaesthesia[c]	LA injected into epidural space, blocking spinal roots Uses as for spinal anaesthesia; also for painless childbirth	Mainly lidocaine, bupivacaine	Unwanted effects similar to those of spinal anaesthesia but less probable, because longitudinal spread of LA is reduced Postoperative urinary retention common

LA, local anaesthetic.

[a]Surface anaesthesia does not work well on the skin, although a non-crystalline mixture of lidocaine and prilocaine (eutectic mixture of local anaesthetics or EMLA) has been developed for application to the skin, producing complete anaesthesia in about 1 h. Lidocaine is available in a patch preparation that can be applied to the skin to reduce pain in conditions such as post-herpetic neuralgia (shingles).

[b]Use of spinal anaesthesia is declining in favour of epidural administration.

[c]Intrathecal or epidural administration of LA in combination with an opioid (see Ch. 42) produces more effective analgesia than can be achieved with the opioid alone. Only a small concentration of LA is needed, insufficient to produce appreciable loss of sensation or other side effects. The mechanism of this synergism is unknown, but the procedure has proved useful in pain treatment.

▼ Charged local anaesthetics do not cross the plasma membrane and thus when applied to the outside of nerves do not inhibit action potential firing. They can, however, enter cells via the pore of TRP channels such as TRPV1 (see Ch. 42). As TRPV1 channels are primarily localised on sensory neurons carrying pain information this raises the possibility of applying a charged local anaesthetic such as QX-314 along with a TRPV1 activator thus allowing the local anaesthetic to enter and block sodium channels only on nociceptive neurons resulting in the block of pain sensation without affecting motor, autonomic or other sensory nerves.

OTHER DRUGS THAT AFFECT SODIUM CHANNELS

TETRODOTOXIN AND SAXITOXIN

▼ Tetrodotoxin (TTX) is produced by a marine bacterium and accumulates in the tissues of a poisonous Pacific fish, the puffer fish. The puffer fish is regarded in Japan as a special delicacy partly because of the mild tingling sensation that follows eating its flesh. To serve it in public restaurants, however, the chef must be registered as

Unwanted effects and pharmacokinetics of local anaesthetics

- Local anaesthetics are either esters or amides. Esters are rapidly hydrolysed by plasma and tissue esterases, and amides are metabolised in the liver. Plasma half-lives are generally short, about 1–2 h.
- Unwanted effects are due mainly to escape of local anaesthetics into the systemic circulation.
- Main unwanted effects are:
  - central nervous system effects, namely agitation, confusion, tremors progressing to convulsions and respiratory depression
  - cardiovascular effects, namely myocardial depression and vasodilatation, leading to fall in blood pressure
  - occasional hypersensitivity reactions.
- Local anaesthetics vary in the rapidity with which they penetrate tissues, and in their duration of action. **Lidocaine** (lignocaine) penetrates tissues readily and is suitable for surface application; **bupivacaine** has a particularly long duration of action.

sufficiently skilled in removing the toxic organs (especially liver and ovaries) so as to make the flesh safe to eat. Accidental TTX poisoning is quite common, nonetheless. Historical records of long sea voyages often contained reference to attacks of severe weakness, progressing to complete paralysis and death, caused by eating puffer fish. It was suggested that the powders used by voodoo practitioners to induce zombification may contain TTX but this is disputed.

Saxitoxin (STX) is produced by a marine microorganism that sometimes proliferates in very large numbers and even colours the sea, giving the 'red tide' phenomenon. At such times, marine shellfish can accumulate the toxin and become poisonous to humans.

These toxins, unlike conventional local anaesthetics, act exclusively from the outside of the membrane. Both are complex molecules, bearing a positively charged guanidinium moiety. The guanidinium ion is able to permeate voltage-sensitive sodium channels, and this part of the TTX or STX molecule lodges in the channel, while the rest of the molecule blocks its outer mouth. In the manner of its blockade of sodium channels, TTX can be likened to a champagne cork. In contrast to the local anaesthetics, there is no interaction between the gating and blocking reactions with TTX or STX—their association and dissociation are independent of whether the channel is open or closed. Some voltage-sensitive sodium channels expressed in cardiac muscle or upregulated in sensory neurons in neuropathic

pain (i.e. $Na_V1.5$, $Na_V1.8$ and $Na_V1.9$) are relatively insensitive to TTX (see Ch. 42).

Both TTX and STX are unsuitable for clinical use as local anaesthetics, being expensive to obtain from their exotic sources and poor at penetrating tissues because of their very low lipid solubility. They have, however, been important as experimental tools for the isolation and cloning of sodium channels (see Ch. 4).

AGENTS THAT AFFECT SODIUM CHANNEL GATING

▼ Various substances modify sodium-channel gating in such a way as to *increase* the probability of opening of the channels (see Hille, 2001). They include various toxins, mainly from frog skin (e.g. batrachotoxin), scorpion or sea anemone venoms; plant alkaloids such as **veratridine**; and insecticides such as DDT and the pyrethrins. They facilitate sodium-channel activation so that sodium channels open at more negative potentials close to the normal resting potential; they also inhibit inactivation, so that the channels fail to close if the membrane remains depolarised. The membrane thus becomes hyperexcitable, and the action potential is prolonged. Spontaneous discharges occur at first, but the cells eventually become permanently depolarised and inexcitable. All these substances affect the heart, producing extrasystoles and other dysrhythmias, culminating in fibrillation; they also cause spontaneous discharges in nerve and muscle, leading to twitching and convulsions. The very high lipid solubility of substances like DDT makes them effective as insecticides, for they are readily absorbed through the integument. Drugs in this class are useful as experimental tools for studying sodium channels but have no clinical uses.

Clinical uses of local anaesthetics

- Local anaesthetics may be injected into soft tissue (e.g. of gums) or to block a nerve or nerve plexus.
- Co-administration of a vasoconstrictor (e.g. **adrenaline**) prolongs the local effect.
- Lipid-soluble drugs (e.g. **lidocaine**) are absorbed from mucous membranes and are used as surface anaesthetics.
- **Bupivacaine** has a slow onset but long duration. It is often used for epidural blockade (e.g. to provide continuous epidural blockade during labour) and spinal anaesthesia. Its isomer **levobupivacaine** is less cardiotoxic if it is inadvertently administered into a blood vessel.

REFERENCES AND FURTHER READING

Becker, D.E., Reed, K.L., 2012. Local anesthetics: review of pharmacological considerations. Anesth. Progr. 59, 90–102. (*Brief review of LA pharmacology from a dental perspective*)

Hille, B., 2001. Ionic channels of excitable membranes. Sinauer, Sunderland. (*Excellent, clearly written textbook for those wanting more than the basic minimum*)

Ragsdale, D.R., McPhee, J.C., Scheuer, T., Catterall, W.A., 1994. Molecular determinants of state-dependent block of Na⁺ channels by local anesthetics. Science 265, 1724–1728. (*Use of site-directed mutations*

of the sodium channel to show that local anaesthetics bind to residues in the S6 transmembrane domain*)

Strichartz, G.R., Ritchie, J.M., 1987. The action of local anaesthetics on ion channels of excitable tissues. Handb. Exp. Pharmacol. 81, 21–52. (*Excellent review of actions of local anaesthetics – other articles in the same volume cover more clinical aspects*)

Yanagidate, F., Stricharz, G.R., 2007. Local anesthetics. Handb. Exp. Pharmacol. 177, 95–127. (*Review of sodium-channel block by local anaesthetics and description of other actions of these drugs that might also be important*)

44

Anxiolytic and hypnotic drugs

OVERVIEW

In this chapter we discuss the nature of anxiety and the drugs used to treat it (anxiolytic drugs), as well as drugs used to treat insomnia (hypnotic drugs). Historically there was overlap between these two groups, reflecting the fact that older anxiolytic drugs commonly caused a degree of sedation and drowsiness. Newer anxiolytic drugs show much less sedative effect and other hypnotic drugs have been introduced that lack specific anxiolytic effects. Many of the drugs now used to treat anxiety were first developed, and are still used, to treat other disorders such as depression (Ch. 47), epilepsy (Ch. 45) and schizophrenia (Ch. 46). Here we will focus on their use as anxiolytics.

THE NATURE OF ANXIETY AND ITS TREATMENT

The normal fear response to threatening stimuli comprises several components, including defensive behaviours, autonomic reflexes, arousal and alertness, corticosteroid secretion and negative emotions. In anxiety states, these reactions occur in an anticipatory manner, independently of external events. The distinction between a 'pathological' and a 'normal' state of anxiety is not clear-cut but represents the point at which the symptoms interfere with normal productive activities. The term 'anxiety' is applied to several distinct disorders. A useful division of anxiety disorders that may help to explain why different types of anxiety respond differently to different drugs is into (i) disorders that involve *fear* (panic attacks and phobias) and (ii) those that involve a more general feeling of *anxiety* (often categorised as general anxiety disorder).

Anxiety disorders recognised clinically include the following:

- *generalised anxiety disorder* (an ongoing state of excessive anxiety lacking any clear reason or focus)
- *social anxiety disorder* (fear of being with and interacting with other people)
- *phobias* (strong fears of specific objects or situations, e.g. snakes, open spaces, flying)
- *panic disorder* (sudden attacks of overwhelming fear that occur in association with marked somatic symptoms, such as sweating, tachycardia, chest pains, trembling and choking). Such attacks can be induced even in normal individuals by infusion of sodium lactate, and the condition appears to have a genetic component
- *post-traumatic stress disorder* (anxiety triggered by recall of past stressful experiences)
- *obsessive–compulsive disorder* (compulsive ritualistic behaviour driven by irrational anxiety, e.g. fear of contamination).

Extensive descriptions of anxiety disorders can be found in DSM-5.[1]

It should be stressed that the treatment of such disorders generally involves psychological approaches as well as drug treatment. Over the last decade the drug treatment of anxiety has changed from using traditional anxiolytic/hypnotic agents (i.e. benzodiazepines and barbiturates) to using a range of drugs that are also used to treat other central nervous system (CNS) disorders (e.g. antidepressant, antiepileptic and antipsychotic drugs) or 5-hydroxytryptamine $(5\text{-HT})_{1A}$ receptor agonists (e.g. buspirone) that have no hypnotic effect. Furthermore, benzodiazepines, while being effective anxiolytic drugs, have the disadvantages of producing unwanted side effects such as amnesia, and of inducing tolerance and physical dependence, as well as being drugs of abuse. They are also ineffective in treating any depression that may occur along with anxiety. Antidepressants and **buspirone** do, however, require three or more weeks to show any therapeutic effect and must be taken continuously, whereas benzodiazepines can be useful for patients who need acute treatment, as they reduce anxiety within 30 min, and can be taken on an 'as needed' basis.

In recent years a number of over the counter 'relaxation' drinks containing CNS neurotransmitters, their precursors or other hormones and amino acids have been marketed, without any evidence of efficacy.[2]

MEASUREMENT OF ANXIOLYTIC ACTIVITY

ANIMAL MODELS OF ANXIETY

In addition to the subjective (emotional) component of human anxiety, there are measurable behavioural and physiological effects that also occur in experimental animals. In biological terms, anxiety induces a particular form of behavioural inhibition that occurs in response to novel environmental events that are threatening or painful. In animals, this behavioural inhibition may take the form of immobility or suppression of a behavioural response, such as bar pressing to obtain food (see p. 537). A rat placed in an unfamiliar environment normally responds by remaining immobile although alert (behavioural suppression) for a time, which may represent 'anxiety' produced by the strange environment. This immobility is reduced if anxiolytic drugs are administered. The 'elevated cross maze' is a widely used test model (see Fig 44.1). Two arms of the raised horizontal cross are closed in, and the others are open. Normally, rats spend most of their time in the closed arms and avoid the open arms (afraid, possibly, of falling off or being attacked). Administration of anxiolytic

---

[1]DSM-5: Diagnostic and Statistical Manual of Mental Disorders, Fifth Edition 2013. American Psychiatric Association, Washington, DC.
[2]Because 'relaxation' drinks are classified as dietary supplements they are not subject to the same efficacy and safety tests as drugs (see Editorial in Nature Neuroscience, 2012, vol. 15, p. 497).

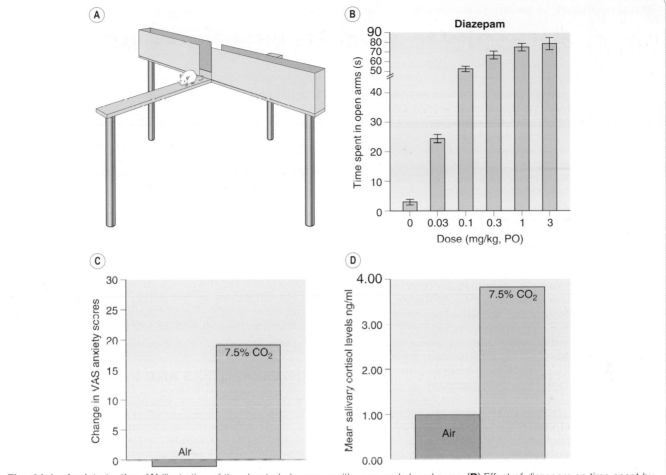

Fig. 44.1 Anxiety testing. [**A**] Illustration of the elevated plus maze with open and closed arms. [**B**] Effect of diazepam on time spent by rats in the open arms of the elevated plus maze. Each bar represents time spent with movement in the open arms during a 5 min test period. [**C**] and [**D**] Effect of a 7.5% CO$_2$ challenge for 20 min on anxiety, measured on a visual analogue scale (VAS), and salivary cortisol levels in human subjects. *(Panel [B], data taken from Kapus et al. 2008 Psychopharmacology 198, 2231–2241; panels [C] and [D], data taken from Seddon et al. 2011 J Psychopharmacol 25, 43–51.)*

drugs increases the time spent in the open arms and also increases the number of entries made into the open arm but without an increase in motor activity.

Conflict tests can also be used. For example, a rat trained to press a bar repeatedly to obtain a food pellet normally achieves a high and consistent response rate. A conflict element is then introduced: at intervals, indicated by an auditory signal, bar pressing results in an occasional 'punishment' in the form of an electric shock in addition to the reward of a food pellet. Normally, the rat ceases pressing the bar (behavioural inhibition), and thus avoids the shock, while the signal is sounding. The effect of an anxiolytic drug is to relieve this suppressive effect, so that the rats continue bar pressing for reward despite the 'punishment'. Other types of psychotropic drug are not effective, nor are analgesic drugs. Other evidence confirms that anxiolytic drugs affect the level of behavioural inhibition produced by the 'conflict situation', rather than simply raising the pain threshold.

Some of these 'anxiety' models may measure fear rather than general anxiety, which occurs in humans in the absence of specific stimuli. To develop new anxiolytic drugs, it is important to have animal tests that give a good guide to efficacy in humans, and much ingenuity has gone into developing and validating such tests (see Ramos, 2008).

TESTS ON HUMANS

Various subjective 'anxiety scale' tests have been devised based on standard patient questionnaires. Galvanic skin reactions – a measure of sweat secretion – are also used to monitor anxiety. Neuropsychological tests have been developed to investigate emotional and attentional biases associated with responses to emotive faces and words. An experience akin to a panic attack can be induced in many subjects by breathing an increased level of CO$_2$, usually prolonged breathing of 7.5% CO$_2$ or a single inhalation of 35% CO$_2$ (see Fig. 44.1). Such tests have confirmed the efficacy of many anxiolytic drugs, but placebo treatment often also produces highly significant responses.

A human version of the conflict test described above involves the substitution of money for food pellets, and the use of graded electric shocks as punishment. As with rats, administration of diazepam increases the rate of button pressing for money during the periods when the punishment was in operation, although the subjects reported no change in the painfulness of the electric shock.

Measurement of anxiolytic activity

- Behavioural tests in animals are based on measurements of the behavioural inhibition (considered to reflect 'anxiety') in response to conflict or novelty.
- Human tests for anxiolytic drugs employ psychiatric rating scales or measures of autonomic responses, such as the galvanic skin response.
- Tests such as these can distinguish between anxiolytic drugs (benzodiazepines, **buspirone**, etc.) and sedatives (e.g. barbiturates).

DRUGS USED TO TREAT ANXIETY

The main groups of drugs (see review by Hoffman & Mathew, 2008) are as follows:

- Antidepressants (see Ch. 47 for details). Selective serotonin (5-HT) reuptake inhibitors (SSRIs; e.g. **fluoxetine**, **paroxetine** and **sertraline**) and serotonin/noradrenaline reuptake inhibitors (SNRIs; e.g. **venlafaxine and duloxetine**) are effective in the treatment of generalised anxiety disorder, phobias, social anxiety disorder and post-traumatic stress disorder. Older antidepressants (tricyclic antidepressants [TCAs] and monoamine oxidase inhibitors [MAOIs]) are also effective but a lower side effect profile favours the use of SSRIs. These agents have the additional advantage of reducing depression, which is not uncommonly associated with anxiety.
- **Benzodiazepines.** Used to treat acute anxiety. Those used to treat anxiety have a long biological half-life (see Table 44.1). They may be co-administered during stabilisation of a patient on an SSRI. There is some evidence that in panic disorders the combination of a benzodiazepine with an SSRI may be better than an SSRI alone.
- **Buspirone.** This 5-HT$_{1A}$ receptor agonist is effective in generalised anxiety disorder but ineffective in the treatment of phobias or social anxiety disorder.
- **Gabapentin, pregabalin, tiagabine, valproate** and **levetiracetam**, antiepileptic drugs (see Ch. 45), are also effective in treating generalised anxiety disorder.
- Some atypical antipsychotic agents (see Ch. 46) such as **olanzapine**, **risperidone**, **quetiapine** and **ziprasidone** may be effective in some forms of anxiety, including generalised anxiety disorder and post-traumatic stress disorder.
- β-Adrenoceptor antagonists (e.g. **propranolol**; Ch. 14). These are used to treat some forms of anxiety, particularly where physical symptoms such as sweating, tremor and tachycardia are troublesome.[3] Their effectiveness depends on block of peripheral sympathetic responses rather than on any central effects.

Antidepressants (Ch. 47), antiepileptics (Ch. 45), antipsychotics Ch. 46), β-adrenoceptor antagonists (Ch. 14) and antihistamines (Ch. 26) are described in detail elsewhere in this book. Some discussion of how SSRIs exert their anxiolytic activity is included in the section on buspirone (see p. 543). Here we focus on drugs whose primary use is to treat anxiety.

Classes of anxiolytic drugs

- Antidepressant drugs (SSRIs, SNRIs, TCAs and MAOIs – see Ch. 47) are effective anxiolytic agents.
- Benzodiazepines are used for treating acute anxiety and insomnia.
- **Buspirone** is a 5-HT$_{1A}$ receptor agonist with anxiolytic activity but little sedative effect.
- Some antiepileptic drugs (e.g. **gabapentin, pregabalin, tiagabine, valproate** and **levetiracetam**) have anxiolytic properties.
- Some atypical antipsychotic agents can be useful to treat some forms of anxiety, but have significant unwanted effects.
- β-Adrenoceptor antagonists are used mainly to reduce physical symptoms of anxiety (tremor, palpitations, etc.); no effect on affective component.

BENZODIAZEPINES AND RELATED DRUGS

▼ The first benzodiazepine, **chlordiazepoxide**, was synthesised by accident in 1961, the unusual seven-membered ring having been produced as a result of a reaction that went wrong in the laboratories of Hoffman–La Roche. Its unexpected pharmacological activity was recognised in a routine screening procedure, and benzodiazepines quite soon became the most widely prescribed drugs in the pharmacopoeia.

The basic chemical structure of benzodiazepines consists of a seven-membered ring fused to an aromatic ring, with four main substituent groups that can be modified without loss of activity. Thousands of compounds have been made and tested, and about 20 are available for clinical use, the most important ones being listed in Table 44.1. They are basically similar in their pharmacological actions, although some degree of selectivity has been reported. For example, some, such as **clonazepam**, show anticonvulsant activity with less marked sedative effects. From a clinical point of view, differences in pharmacokinetic behaviour among different benzodiazepines (see Table 44.1) are more important than differences in profile of activity. Drugs with a similar structure have been discovered that specifically antagonise the effects of the benzodiazepines, for example **flumazenil** (see p. 540).

The term 'benzodiazepine' refers to a distinct chemical structure. Drugs such as **zolpidem** and **zopiclone** as well as **abecarnil** – a β-carboline (not licensed for clinical use) – have different chemical structures and are therefore not benzodiazepines. However, since they bind to the same sites, often referred to as the 'benzodiazepine receptor', they are discussed along with the benzodiazepines.

MECHANISM OF ACTION

Benzodiazepines act selectively on GABA$_A$ receptors (Ch. 38), which mediate inhibitory synaptic transmission throughout the central nervous system. Benzodiazepines enhance the response to GABA by facilitating the opening of GABA-activated chloride channels (Ch. 38, Fig. 38.5). They bind specifically to a regulatory site on the receptor, distinct from the GABA-binding sites (see Fig. 44.3), and act allosterically to increase the affinity of GABA for the receptor. Single-channel recordings show an increase

---

[3]β-Blockers are sometimes used by actors and musicians to reduce the symptoms of stage fright, but their use by snooker players to minimise tremor is banned as unsportsmanlike.

Table 44.1 **Characteristics of benzodiazepines in humans**

Drug(s)	Half-life of parent compound (h)	Active metabolite	Half-life of metabolite (h)	Overall duration of action	Main use(s)
Midazolam[a]	2–4	Hydroxylated derivative	2	Ultrashort (<6 h)	Hypnotic Midazolam used as intravenous anaesthetic
Zolpidem[b]	2	No	–	Ultrashort (~4 h)	Hypnotic
Lorazepam, oxazepam, temazepam, lormetazepam	8–12	No	–	Short (12–18 h)	Anxiolytic, hypnotic
Alprazolam	6–12	Hydroxylated derivative	6	Medium (24 h)	Anxiolytic, antidepressant
Nitrazepam	16–40	No	–	Medium	Anxiolytic
Diazepam, chlordiazepoxide	20–40	Nordazepam	60	Long (24–48 h)	Anxiolytic, muscle relaxant Diazepam used as anticonvulsant
Flurazepam	1	Desmethyl-flurazepam	60	Long	Anxiolytic
Clonazepam	50	No	–	Long	Anticonvulsant, anxiolytic (especially mania)

[a]Another short-acting benzodiazepine, triazolam has been withdrawn from use in the UK on account of side effects.
[b]Zolpidem is not a benzodiazepine but acts in a similar manner. Zopiclone and zaleplon are similar.

in the frequency of channel opening by a given concentration of GABA, but no change in the conductance or mean open time, consistent with an effect on GABA binding rather than the channel-gating mechanism. Benzodiazepines do not affect receptors for other amino acids, such as glycine or glutamate (Fig. 44.2).

▼ The GABA$_A$ receptor is a ligand-gated ion channel (see Ch. 3) consisting of a pentameric assembly of different subunits, the main ones being α, β and γ (see Ch. 38). The GABA$_A$ receptor should actually be thought of as a family of receptors as there are six different subtypes of α subunit, three subtypes of β and three subtypes of γ. Although the potential number of combinations is therefore large, certain combinations predominate in the adult brain (see Ch. 38). The various combinations occur in different parts of the brain, have different physiological functions and have subtle differences in their pharmacological properties.

Benzodiazepines bind across the interface between the α and γ subunits but only to receptors that contain γ2 and α1, α2, α3 or α5 subunits. Genetic approaches have been used to study the roles of different subunits in the different behavioural effects of benzodiazepines. Behavioural analysis of mice with various mutations of the GABA$_A$ receptor subunit indicates that α1-containing receptors mediate the anticonvulsant, sedative/hypnotic and addictive effects but not the anxiolytic effect of benzodiazepines whereas α2-containing receptors mediate the anxiolytic effect, α2-, α3- and α5-containing receptors mediate muscle relaxation and α1- and α5-containing receptors mediate the amnesic effects (Tan et al., 2011).

The obvious next step was to try to develop subunit-selective drugs. Unfortunately, this has proved difficult, due to the structural similarity between the benzodiazepine binding site on different α subunits. The α-subunit selectivity of some benzodiazepines is given in Table 44.2. It was hoped that selective efficacy at α2-containing receptors would produce anxiolytic drugs lacking the unwanted effects of sedation and amnesia. However, such compounds have not yet translated into human therapeutic agents (Skolnick, 2012). **Pagoclone**, reported to be a full agonist at α3 with less efficacy at α1, α2 and α5, has little or no sedative/hypnotic or amnesic actions.

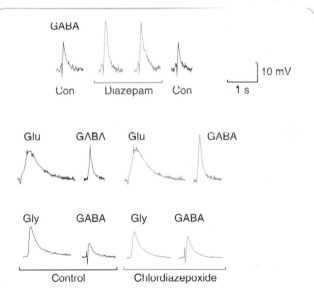

Fig. 44.2 **Potentiating effect of benzodiazepines and chlordiazepoxide on the action of GABA.** Drugs were applied by iontophoresis to mouse spinal cord neurons grown in tissue culture, from micropipettes placed close to the cells. The membrane was hyperpolarised to −90 mV, and the cells were loaded with Cl⁻ from the recording microelectrode, so inhibitory amino acids (GABA and glycine, Gly), as well as excitatory ones (glutamate, Glu), caused depolarising responses. The potentiating effect of diazepam is restricted to GABA responses, glutamate and glycine responses being unaffected. Con, control.

Table 44.2 GABA$_A$-receptor α-subunit selectivity of some therapeutically used benzodiazepines

Drug	Subunit selectivity
Diazepam	α1, α2, α3, α4, α5, α6
Flunitrazepam	α1, α2, α5
Midazolam	α1, α2, α3, α4, α5, α6
Zolpidem	α1
Flumazenil	Antagonist at α1, α2, α3, α4, α5, α6

(Adapted from Tan KR, Rudolph U, Lüscher C 2011 Hooked on benzodiazepines: GABA$_A$ receptor subtypes and addiction. Trends Neurosci 34, 188–197)

Peripheral benzodiazepine-binding sites, not associated with GABA receptors, are present in many tissues. The target is a protein known as *translocator protein* located primarily on mitochondrial membranes.

BENZODIAZEPINE ANTAGONISTS AND INVERSE AGONISTS

Competitive antagonists of benzodiazepines were first discovered in 1981. The best-known compound is flumazenil. This compound was originally reported to lack effects on behaviour or on drug-induced convulsions when given on its own, although it was later found to possess some 'anxiogenic' and proconvulsant activity. Flumazenil can be used to reverse the effect of benzodiazepine overdosage (normally used only if respiration is severely depressed), or to reverse the effect of benzodiazepines such as midazolam used for minor surgical procedures. Flumazenil acts quickly and effectively when given by injection, but its action lasts for only about 2 h, so drowsiness tends to return. Convulsions may occur in patients treated with flumazenil, and this is more common in patients receiving tricyclic antidepressants (Ch. 47). Reports that flumazenil improves the mental state of patients with severe liver disease (hepatic encephalopathy) and alcohol intoxication have not been confirmed in controlled trials, although partial inverse agonists do appear to be effective in animal models of hepatic encephalopathy (Ahboucha & Butterworth, 2005).

▼ The term *inverse agonist* (Ch. 2) is applied to drugs that bind to benzodiazepine receptors and exert the opposite effect to that of conventional benzodiazepines, producing signs of increased anxiety and convulsions. Ethyl-β-carboline-3-carboxylate (βCCE) and diazepam-binding inhibitor (see p. 541), as well as some benzodiazepine analogues, show inverse agonist activity. It is possible (see Fig. 44.3) to explain these complexities in terms of the two-state model discussed in Chapter 2, by postulating that the benzodiazepine receptor exists in two distinct conformations, only one of which [A] can bind GABA molecules and open the chloride channel. The other conformation [B] cannot bind GABA. Normally, with no benzodiazepine receptor ligand present, there is an equilibrium between these two conformations; sensitivity to GABA is present but submaximal. Benzodiazepine agonists (e.g. diazepam) are postulated to bind preferentially to conformation [A], thus shifting the equilibrium in favour of [A] and enhancing GABA sensitivity. Inverse agonists bind selectively to [B] and have the opposite effect. Competitive antagonists would bind equally to [A] and [B], and consequently would not disturb the conformational equilibrium but antagonise the effect of both agonists and inverse agonists

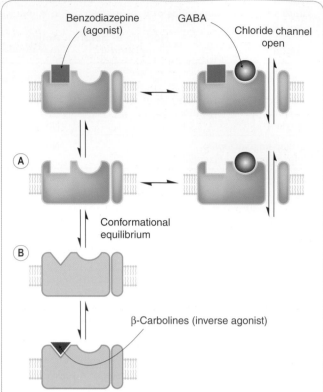

Fig. 44.3 Model of benzodiazepine/GABA receptor interaction. Benzodiazepine agonists, antagonists and inverse agonists are believed to bind to a site on the GABA receptor distinct from the GABA-binding site. A conformational equilibrium exists between states in which the benzodiazepine receptor exists in its agonist-binding conformation [**A**] and in its inverse agonist-binding conformation [**B**]. In the latter state, the GABA receptor has a much reduced affinity for GABA; consequently, the chloride channel remains closed.

PHARMACOLOGICAL EFFECTS AND USES

The main effects of benzodiazepines are:

- reduction of anxiety and aggression
- induction of sleep (see section on hypnotic drugs, p. 544)
- reduction of muscle tone
- anticonvulsant effect
- anterograde amnesia.

Reduction of anxiety and aggression

Benzodiazepines show anxiolytic effects in animal tests, as described above, and also exert a marked 'taming' effect, allowing animals to be handled more easily.[4] With the possible exception of alprazolam (Table 44.1), benzodiazepines do not have antidepressant effects. Benzodiazepines may paradoxically produce an increase in irritability and aggression in some individuals. This appears to be particularly pronounced with the ultrashort-acting drug triazolam (and led to its withdrawal in the UK and some other countries), and is generally more common with short-acting compounds. It is probably

[4]This depends on the species. Cats actually become more excitable, as a colleague of one of the authors discovered to his cost when attempting to sedate a tiger in the Baltimore zoo.

a manifestation of the benzodiazepine withdrawal syndrome, which occurs with all these drugs (see p. 542) but is more acute with drugs whose action wears off rapidly.

Benzodiazepines are now used mainly for treating acute anxiety states, behavioural emergencies and during procedures such as endoscopy. They are also used as premedication before surgery (both medical and dental). Under these circumstances their anxiolytic, sedative and amnesic properties may be beneficial. Intravenous midazolam can be used to induce anaesthesia (see Ch. 41).

Reduction of muscle tone

Benzodiazepines reduce muscle tone by a central action on $GABA_A$ receptors, primarily in the spinal cord.

Increased muscle tone is a common feature of anxiety states in humans and may contribute to the aches and pains, including headache, that often trouble anxious patients. The relaxant effect of benzodiazepines may therefore be clinically useful. A reduction of muscle tone appears to be possible without appreciable loss of coordination. However, with intravenous administration in anaesthesia and in overdose when these drugs are being abused, airway obstruction may occur. Other clinical uses of muscle relaxants are discussed in Chapter 13.

Anticonvulsant effects

All the benzodiazepines have anticonvulsant activity in experimental animal tests. They are highly effective against chemically induced convulsions caused by **pentylenetetrazol**, **bicuculline** and similar drugs that act by blocking $GABA_A$ receptors (see Chs 38 and 45) but less so against electrically induced convulsions.

Clonazepam (see Table 44.1), **diazepam** and **lorazepam** are used to treat epilepsy (Ch. 45). They can be given intravenously to control life-threatening seizures in status epilepticus. Diazepam can be administered rectally to children to control acute seizures. Tolerance develops to the anticonvulsant actions of benzodiazepines (see p. 542).

Anterograde amnesia

Benzodiazepines prevent memory of events experienced while under their influence, an effect not seen with other CNS depressants. Minor surgical or invasive procedures can thus be performed without leaving unpleasant memories. **Flunitrazepam** (better known to the general public by one of its trade names, Rohypnol) is infamous as a date rape drug and victims frequently have difficulty in recalling exactly what took place during the attack.

Amnesia is thought to be due to benzodiazepines binding to $GABA_A$ receptors containing the $\alpha5$ subunit. $\alpha5$-Knockout mice show an enhanced learning and memory phenotype. This raises the possibility that an $\alpha5$ subunit-selective inverse agonist could be memory enhancing.

IS THERE AN ENDOGENOUS BENZODIAZEPINE-LIKE MEDIATOR?

▼ Despite considerable scientific effort, the question of whether or not there are endogenous ligands for the benzodiazepine receptors, whose function is to regulate the action of GABA, remains unanswered.

That the antagonist **flumazenil** produces responses both *in vivo* and *in vitro* in the absence of any exogenous benzodiazepines is frequently cited to support the view that there must be ongoing benzodiazepine receptor activation by endogenous ligand(s). Although flumazenil was originally described as a neutral antagonist, it is possible that it has agonist or inverse agonist activity at subtypes of $GABA_A$ receptor (depending on the α subunit present) or in some

pathological conditions in which the $GABA_A$ receptors have become modified.

Several endogenous compounds that act on benzodiazepine receptors have been isolated, including *β-carbolines* (e.g. βCCE), structurally related to tryptophan, and *diazepam-binding inhibitor*, a 10-kDa peptide. Whether these molecules exist in the brain (i.e. are endogenous) or are generated during the processes involved in extracting them from the tissue is an open issue. Interestingly, both βCCE and diazepam-binding inhibitor have the opposite effect to benzodiazepines, i.e. they are inverse agonists and inhibit chloride channel opening by GABA and, in the whole animal, exert anxiogenic and proconvulsant effects. There was also a suggestion that benzodiazepines themselves may occur naturally in the brain but the origin of these compounds and how biosynthesis occurs is unclear. At present there is no general agreement on the identity and function of endogenous ligands for the benzodiazepine receptor. Other possible endogenous modulators of $GABA_A$ receptors include steroid metabolites but they bind to a different site from benzodiazepines (see Ch. 38).

PHARMACOKINETIC ASPECTS

Benzodiazepines are well absorbed when given orally, usually giving a peak plasma concentration in about 1 h. Some (e.g. oxazepam, lorazepam) are absorbed more slowly. They bind strongly to plasma protein, and their high lipid solubility causes many of them to accumulate gradually in body fat. They are normally given by mouth but can be given intravenously (e.g. diazepam in status epilepticus, midazolam in anaesthesia) or rectally. Intramuscular injection often results in slow absorption.

Benzodiazepines are all metabolised and eventually excreted as glucuronide conjugates in the urine. They vary greatly in duration of action and can be roughly divided into short-, medium- and long-acting compounds (Table 44.1). Duration of action influences their use, short-acting compounds being useful hypnotics with reduced hangover effect on wakening, long-acting compounds being more useful for use as anxiolytic and anticonvulsant drugs. Several are converted to active metabolites such as *N*-desmethyldiazepam (**nordiazepam**), which has a half-life of about 60 h, and which accounts for the tendency of many benzodiazepines to produce cumulative effects and long hangovers when they are given repeatedly. The short-acting compounds are those that are metabolised directly by conjugation with glucuronide. Figure 44.4 shows the gradual build up and slow disappearance of nordiazepam from the plasma of a human subject given diazepam daily for 15 days.

▼ Advancing age affects the rate of oxidative reactions more than that of conjugation reactions. Thus the effect of the long-acting benzodiazepines tends to increase with age, and it is common for drowsiness and confusion to develop insidiously for this reason.[5]

UNWANTED EFFECTS

These may be divided into:

- toxic effects resulting from acute overdosage
- unwanted effects occurring during normal therapeutic use
- tolerance and dependence.

---

[5]At the age of 91, the grandmother of one of the authors was growing increasingly forgetful and mildly dotty, having been taking nitrazepam for insomnia regularly for years. To the author's lasting shame, it took a canny general practitioner to diagnose the problem. Cancellation of the nitrazepam prescription produced a dramatic improvement.

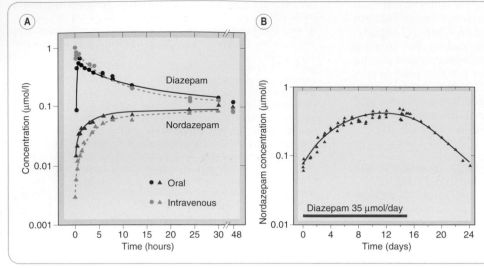

Fig. 44.4 Pharmacokinetics of diazepam in humans. **[A]** Concentrations of diazepam and nordazepam following a single oral or intravenous dose. Note the very slow disappearance of both substances after the first 20 h. **[B]** Accumulation of nordazepam during 2 weeks' daily administration of diazepam, and slow decline (half-life about 3 days) after cessation of diazepam administration. (*Data from Kaplan SA et al. 1973 J Pharmacol Sci 62, 1789.*)

Acute toxicity

Benzodiazepines in acute overdose are considerably less dangerous than other anxiolytic/hypnotic drugs. Because such agents are often used in attempted suicide, this is an important advantage. In overdose, benzodiazepines cause prolonged sleep, without serious depression of respiration or cardiovascular function. However, in the presence of other CNS depressants, particularly alcohol, benzodiazepines can cause severe, even life-threatening, respiratory depression. This is a frequent problem when benzodiazepines are abused (see Chs 49 and 58). The availability of an effective antagonist, flumazenil, means that the effects of an acute overdose can be counteracted,[6] which is not possible for most CNS depressants.

Side effects during therapeutic use

The main side effects of benzodiazepines are drowsiness, confusion, amnesia and impaired coordination, which considerably impairs manual skills such as driving performance. Benzodiazepines enhance the depressant effect of other drugs, including alcohol, in a more than additive way. The long and unpredictable duration of action of many benzodiazepines is important in relation to side effects. Long-acting drugs such as nitrazepam are no longer used as hypnotics, and even shorter-acting compounds such as lorazepam can produce a substantial day-after impairment of job performance and driving skill.

Tolerance and dependence

Tolerance (i.e. a gradual escalation of dose needed to produce the required effect) occurs with all benzodiazepines, as does dependence, which is their main drawback. They share these properties with other sedatives. Tolerance appears to represent a change at the receptor level, but the mechanism is not well understood. There may be selective loss of membrane GABA$_A$ receptors containing the α2 subunit (Jacob et al., 2012).

At the receptor level, the degree of tolerance will be governed both by the number of receptors occupied (i.e. the dose) and the duration of receptor occupancy (which may vary according to the therapeutic use). Therefore, marked tolerance develops when benzodiazepines are used continuously to treat epilepsy whereas less tolerance occurs to the sleep-inducing effect when the subject is relatively drug free during the day. It is not clear to what degree tolerance develops to the anxiolytic effect.

Benzodiazepines produce dependence, and this is a major problem. In human subjects and patients, abrupt cessation of benzodiazepine treatment after weeks or months causes a rebound heightened anxiety, together with tremor, dizziness, tinnitus, weight loss and disturbed sleep due to enhanced REM sleep (see p. 544). It is recommended that benzodiazepines be withdrawn gradually by stepwise lowering of the dose. Animals show only a weak tendency to self-administer benzodiazepines. Withdrawal after chronic administration causes physical symptoms, namely nervousness, tremor, loss of appetite and sometimes convulsions.[7] The withdrawal syndrome, in both animals and humans, is slower in onset than with opioids, probably because of the long plasma half-life of most benzodiazepines. With diazepam, the withdrawal symptoms may take up to 3 weeks to become apparent. Short-acting benzodiazepines cause more abrupt withdrawal effects.

The physical and psychological withdrawal symptoms make it difficult for patients to give up taking benzodiazepines, but craving (i.e. severe psychological dependence that outlasts the physical withdrawal syndrome), which occurs with many drugs of abuse (Ch. 49), is not a major problem.

Abuse potential

Benzodiazepines are widely abused drugs, often taken in combination with other drugs such as opioids or alcohol. Most illicit use comes from diversion of prescribed benzodiazepines. They induce a feeling of calm and reduced anxiety, with users describing a dream state where they are cushioned from reality. The risk of overdose is greatly increased when used in combination with alcohol. Tolerance and physical dependence occur as described above.

---

[6]In practice, patients are usually left to sleep it off, because there is a risk of seizures with flumazenil; however, flumazenil may be useful diagnostically to rule out coma of other causes.

[7]Withdrawal symptoms can be more severe. A relative of one of the authors, advised to stop taking benzodiazepines after 20 years, suffered hallucinations and one day tore down all the curtains, convinced that they were on fire.

> ## Benzodiazepines
>
> - Act by binding to a specific regulatory site on the $GABA_A$ receptor, thus enhancing the inhibitory effect of GABA. Subtypes of the $GABA_A$ receptor exist in different regions of the brain and differ in their functional effects.
> - Anxiolytic benzodiazepines are agonists at this regulatory site. Other benzodiazepines (e.g. **flumazenil**) are antagonists or weak inverse agonists and prevent the actions of the anxiolytic benzodiazepines. Inverse agonists (not used clinically) are anxiogenic.
> - Anxiolytic effects are mediated by $GABA_A$ receptors containing the $\alpha2$ subunit, while sedation occurs through those with the $\alpha1$ subunit.
> - Benzodiazepines cause:
>   - reduction of anxiety and aggression
>   - sedation, leading to improvement of insomnia
>   - muscle relaxation and loss of motor coordination
>   - suppression of convulsions (antiepileptic effect)
>   - anterograde amnesia.
> - Differences in the pharmacological profile of different benzodiazepines are minor; **clonazepam** appears to have more anticonvulsant action in relation to its other effects.
> - Benzodiazepines are active orally and differ mainly in respect of their duration of action. Short-acting agents (e.g. **lorazepam** and **temazepam**, half-lives 8–12 h) are metabolised to inactive compounds and are used mainly as sleeping pills. Some long-acting agents (e.g. **diazepam** and **chlordiazepoxide**) are converted to a long lasting active metabolite (**nordazepam**).
> - Some are used intravenously, for example **diazepam** in status epilepticus, **midazolam** in anaesthesia.
> - **Zolpidem** is a short-acting drug that is not a benzodiazepine but acts similarly and is used as a hypnotic.
> - Benzodiazepines are relatively safe in overdose. Their main disadvantages are interaction with alcohol, long-lasting 'hangover' effects and the development of tolerance and physical dependence – characteristic withdrawal syndrome on cessation of use.

BUSPIRONE

Buspirone is used to treat generalised anxiety disorders. It is less effective in controlling panic attacks or severe anxiety states.

Buspirone is a partial agonist at $5\text{-}HT_{1A}$ receptors (Ch. 15) and also binds to dopamine receptors, but it is likely that its 5-HT-related actions are important in relation to anxiety suppression, because related experimental compounds (e.g. ipsapirone and gepirone), which are highly specific for $5\text{-}HT_{1A}$ receptors, show similar anxiolytic activity in experimental animals. However, buspirone takes days or weeks to produce its effect in humans, suggesting a more complex mechanism of action than simply activation of $5\text{-}HT_{1A}$ receptors. SSRIs also have a delayed onset to their anxiolytic actions.

$5\text{-}HT_{1A}$ receptors are expressed on the soma and dendrites of 5-HT-containing neurons, where they function as inhibitory autoreceptors, as well as being expressed on other types of neuron (e.g. noradrenergic locus coeruleus neurons) where, along with other types of 5-HT receptor (see Ch. 39), they mediate the postsynaptic actions of 5-HT. Postsynaptic $5\text{-}HT_{1A}$ receptors are highly expressed within the cortico-limbic circuits implicated in emotional behaviour. One theory of how buspirone and SSRIs produce their delayed anxiolytic effect is that over time they induce desensitisation of somatodendritic $5\text{-}HT_{1A}$ autoreceptors, resulting in heightened excitation of serotonergic neurons and enhanced 5-HT release. This might also explain why early in treatment anxiety can be worsened by these drugs due to the initial activation of $5\text{-}HT_{1A}$ autoreceptors and inhibition of 5-HT release. This receptor desensitisation theory would predict that a $5\text{-}HT_{1A}$ antagonist that would rapidly block the action of 5-HT at $5\text{-}HT_{1A}$ autoreceptors and thus swiftly enhance 5-HT release, might be anxiolytic without delayed onset. Drugs with combined $5\text{-}HT_{1A}$ antagonism and SSRI properties have been developed but have not been found to be effective in man, perhaps because they block both $5HT_{1A}$ autoreceptors and postsynaptic receptors, the latter effect occluding the beneficial effect of the former. Elevated 5-HT levels may also induce other postsynaptic adaptations. $5\text{-}HT_2$ receptors have also been implicated, downregulation of which may be important for anxiolytic action. Drugs with $5\text{-}HT_2$ and $5\text{-}HT_3$ receptor antagonist activity are in clinical trials for treating anxiety.

Buspirone inhibits the activity of noradrenergic locus coeruleus neurons (Ch. 39) and thus interferes with arousal reactions. It has side effects quite different from those of benzodiazepines. It does not cause sedation or motor incoordination, nor have tolerance or withdrawal effects been reported. Its main side effects are nausea, dizziness, headache and restlessness, which generally seem to be less troublesome than the side effects of benzodiazepines. Buspirone does not suppress the benzodiazepine withdrawal syndrome, presumably because it acts by a different mechanism. Hence, when switching from benzodiazepine treatment to buspirone treatment, the benzodiazepine dose still needs to be reduced gradually.

> ## Antidepressants and $5\text{-}HT_{1A}$ agonists as anxiolytic drugs
>
> - Anxiolytic effects take days or weeks to develop.
> - Antidepressants (SSRIs, SNRIs, TCAs and MAOIs – see Ch. 47):
>   - effective treatments for generalised anxiety disorder, phobias, social anxiety disorder and post-traumatic stress disorder
>   - may also reduce depression associated with anxiety.
> - **Buspirone** is a potent agonist at $5\text{-}HT_{1A}$ receptors:
>   - it is an effective treatment for generalised anxiety disorder but not phobias
>   - side effects appear less troublesome than with benzodiazepines; they include dizziness, nausea, headache, but not sedation or loss of coordination.

OTHER POTENTIAL ANXIOLYTIC DRUGS

Besides the GABA and 5-HT mechanisms discussed above, many other transmitters and hormones have been implicated in anxiety and panic disorders, particularly noradrenaline, glutamate, corticotrophin-releasing factor, cholecystokinin (CCK), substance P, neuropeptide Y, galanin, orexins and neurosteroids. Anxiolytic drugs aimed at these targets are in development (see Mathew et al., 2009).

An exciting recent development is the realisation that the unpleasant, negative memories that underlie fear are not necessarily permanent. When such memories are reactivated (recalled) they return transiently to a labile state that can be disrupted. In humans, propranolol administered before memory reactivation may erase negative memories (see Lonergan et al., 2013). NMDA receptor antagonists may have a similar effect. Disrupting unpleasant memories in this way may provide a new treatment for post-traumatic stress disorder.

Clinical use of drugs as anxiolytics

- Antidepressants are now the main drugs used to treat anxiety, especially when this is associated with depression. Their effects are slow in onset (>2 weeks).
- Benzodiazepines are now usually limited to acute relief of severe and disabling anxiety.
- **Buspirone** (5-HT$_{1A}$ agonist) has a different pattern of adverse effects from benzodiazepines and much lower abuse potential. Its effect is slow in onset (>2 weeks). It is licensed for short-term use, but specialists may use it for several months.

DRUGS USED TO TREAT INSOMNIA (HYPNOTIC DRUGS)

Insomnia can be *transient*, in people who normally sleep well but have to do shift work or have jet lag, *short-term*, usually due to illness or emotional upset, or *chronic*, where there is an underlying cause such as anxiety, depression, drug abuse, pain, pruritus or dyspnoea. While in anxiety and depression the underlying psychiatric condition should be treated, improvement of sleep patterns can improve the underlying condition. The drugs used to treat these conditions are:

- Benzodiazepines. Short-acting benzodiazepines (e.g. lorazepam and temazepam) are used for treating insomnia as they have little hangover effect. Diazepam, which is longer-acting, can be used to treat insomnia associated with daytime anxiety.
- **Zaleplon**, **zolpidem** and **zopiclone**. Although chemically distinct, these short-acting hypnotics act similarly to benzodiazepines. They lack appreciable anxiolytic activity (see p. 540).
- **Chlormethiazole.** It acts as a positive allosteric modulator of GABA$_A$ receptors acting at a site distinct from the benzodiazepines.
- Melatonin receptor agonists. **Melatonin** and **ramelteon** are agonists at MT$_1$ and MT$_2$ receptors (see Ch. 39). They are effective in treating insomnia in the elderly and autistic children.
- Orexin receptor antagonist. **Suvorexant** is in development as a hypnotic. It is an antagonist of OX$_1$ and OX$_2$ receptors which mediate the actions of

the orexins, peptide transmitters in the CNS that are important in setting diurnal rhythm (see Ch. 39). Orexin levels are normally high in daylight and low at night, so the drug reduces wakefulness.

- Antihistamines[8] (see Ch. 26; e.g. **diphenhydramine** and **promethazine**) can be used to induce sleep. They are included in various over-the-counter preparations. **Doxepin** is an SNRI antidepressant (see Ch. 46) with histamine H$_1$- and H$_2$-receptor antagonist properties that can be used to treat insomnia.
- Miscellaneous other drugs (e.g. **chloral hydrate** and **meprobamate**). They are no longer recommended, but therapeutic habits die hard and they are occasionally used. **Methaqualone**, used as a hypnotic and once popular as a drug of abuse, has been discontinued.

Induction of sleep by benzodiazepines

Benzodiazepines decrease the time taken to get to sleep, and increase the total duration of sleep, although the latter effect occurs only in subjects who normally sleep for less than about 6 h each night. With agents that have a short duration of action (e.g. zolpidem or temazepam), a pronounced hangover effect on wakening can be avoided.

▼ On the basis of electroencephalography measurements, several levels of sleep can be recognised. Of particular psychological importance are rapid-eye-movement (REM) sleep, which is associated with dreaming, and slow-wave sleep, which corresponds to the deepest level of sleep when the metabolic rate and adrenal steroid secretion are at their lowest and the secretion of growth hormone is at its highest (see Ch. 33). Most hypnotic drugs reduce the proportion of REM sleep, although benzodiazepines affect it less than other hypnotics, and zolpidem least of all. Artificial interruption of REM

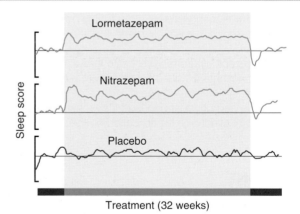

Fig. 44.5 **Effects of long-term benzodiazepine treatment on sleep quality.** A group of 100 poor sleepers were given, under double-blind conditions, lormetazepam 5 mg, nitrazepam 2 mg or placebo nightly for 24 weeks, the test period being preceded and followed by 4 weeks of placebo treatment. They were asked to assess, on a subjective rating scale, the quality of sleep during each night, and the results are expressed as a 5-day rolling average of these scores. The improvement in sleep quality was maintained during the 24-week test period, and was followed by a 'rebound' worsening of sleep when the test period ended. *(From Oswald I et al. 1982 Br Med J 284, 860–864.)*

---

[8]This is an interesting example of an initial unwanted side effect – sedation is undesired when treating hay fever – subsequently becoming a therapeutic use.

sleep causes irritability and anxiety, even if the total amount of sleep is not reduced, and the lost REM sleep is made up for at the end of such an experiment by a rebound increase. The same rebound in REM sleep is seen at the end of a period of administration of benzodiazepines or other hypnotics. The proportion of slow-wave sleep is significantly reduced by benzodiazepines, although growth hormone secretion is unaffected.

Figure 44.5 shows the improvement of subjective ratings of sleep quality produced by a benzodiazepine, and the rebound decrease at the end of a 32-week period of drug treatment. It is notable that, although tolerance to objective effects such as reduced sleep latency occurs within a few days, this is not obvious in the subjective ratings.

Benzodiazepines are now, however, only recommended for short courses of treatment of insomnia. Tolerance develops over 1–2 weeks with continuous use, and on cessation rebound insomnia and withdrawal occurs.

Hypnotic drugs

- Drugs that potentiate the action of GABA at GABA$_A$ receptors (e.g. benzodiazepines, **zolpidem**, **zopiclone**, **zaleplon** and **chlormethiazole**) are used to induce sleep.
- Drugs with shorter half-lives in the body reduce the incidence of hangover the next morning.
- H$_1$-receptor antagonists induce sedation and sleep.
- Drugs with novel mechanisms of action have been developed, e.g. melatonin receptor agonists and orexin receptor antagonists.

Clinical use of hypnotics ('sleeping tablets')

- The cause of insomnia should be established before administering hypnotic drugs. Common causes include alcohol or other drug misuse (see Ch. 49) and physical or psychiatric disorders (especially depression).
- Tricyclic antidepressants (Ch. 47) cause drowsiness, so can kill two birds with one stone if taken at night by depressed patients with sleep disturbance.
- Optimal treatment of chronic insomnia is often by changing behaviour (e.g. increasing exercise, staying awake during the day) rather than with drugs.
- Benzodiazepines should be used only for short periods (<4 weeks) and for severe insomnia. They can be useful for a few nights when transient factors such as

admission to hospital, jet lag or an impending procedure cause insomnia.
- Drugs used to treat insomnia include:
  - benzodiazepines (e.g. **temazepam**) and related drugs (e.g. **zolpidem**, **zopiclone**, which also work on the benzodiazepine receptor)
  - **chloral hydrate** and **triclofos**, which were used formerly in children, but this is seldom justified
  - sedating antihistamines (e.g. **promethazine**), which cause drowsiness (see Ch. 26) are less suitable for treating insomnia. They can impair performance the next day.

REFERENCES AND FURTHER READING

Ahboucha, S., Butterworth, R.F., 2005. Role of endogenous benzodiazepine ligands and their GABA$_A$-associated receptors in hepatic encephalopathy. Metab. Brain Dis. 20, 425–437.

Hoffman, E.J., Mathew, S.J., 2008. Anxiety disorders: a comprehensive review of pharmacotherapies. Mt Sinai J. Med. 75, 248–262. (*Describes the clinical usefulness of various drugs effective against different forms of anxiety*)

Jacob, T.C., Michels, G., Silayeva, L., Haydonm, J., Succol, F., Moss, S.J., 2012. Benzodiazepine treatment induces subtype-specific changes in GABA$_A$ receptor trafficking and decreases synaptic inhibition. Proc. Natl Acad. Sci. 109, 18595–18600. (*At last the mechanism of benzodiazepine tolerance is beginning to be explained*)

Lonergan, M.H., Olivera-Figueroa, L.A., Pitman, R.K., Brunet, A., 2013. Propranolol's effects on the consolidation and reconsolidation of long-term emotional memory in healthy participants: a meta-analysis. J. Psychiatry Neurosci. 38, 222–231. (*A meta analysis of a*

number of trials examining the ability of propranolol to disrupt negative memories)

Mathew, S.J., Price, R.B., Charney, D.S., 2009. Recent advances in the neurobiology of anxiety disorders: implications for novel therapeutics. Am. J. Med. Genet. C Semin. Med. Genet. 148C, 89–98. (*This review focuses on the potential for development of novel treatments for anxiety*)

Ramos, A., 2008. Animal models of anxiety: do I need multiple tests? Trends Pharmacol. Sci. 29, 493–498. (*Describes the need for animal models in the testing of anxiolytic drugs*)

Skolnick, P., 2012. Anxioselective anxiolytics: on a quest for the Holy Grail. Trends Pharmacol. Sci. 33, 611–620.

Tan, K.R., Rudolph, U., Lüscher, C., 2011. Hooked on benzodiazepines: GABA$_A$ receptor subtypes and addiction. Trends Neurosci. 34, 188–197. (*Don't be fooled by the title, this review also contains information on how different GABA$_A$-receptor subunits mediate the different effects of benzodiazepines*)

45

Antiepileptic drugs

OVERVIEW

In this chapter we describe the nature of epilepsy, the neurobiological mechanisms underlying it and the animal models that can be used to study it. We then proceed to describe the various classes of drugs that are used to treat it, the mechanisms by which they work and their pharmacological characteristics.

Centrally acting muscle relaxants are discussed briefly at the end of the chapter.

INTRODUCTION

Epilepsy is a very common disorder, characterised by *seizures*, which take various forms and result from episodic neuronal discharges, the form of the seizure depending on the part of the brain affected. Epilepsy affects 0.5–1% of the population i.e. ~50 million people worldwide. Often, there is no recognisable cause, although it may develop after brain damage, such as trauma, stroke, infection or tumour growth, or other kinds of neurological disease, including various inherited neurological syndromes. Epilepsy is treated mainly with drugs, although brain surgery may be used for suitable severe cases. Current antiepileptic drugs are effective in controlling seizures in about 70% of cases, but their use is often limited by side effects. In addition to their use in patients with epilepsy, antiepileptic drugs are used to treat or prevent convulsions caused by other brain disorders, for example trauma (including following neurosurgery), infection (as an adjunct to antibiotics), brain tumours and stroke. For this reason, they are sometimes termed anticonvulsants rather than antiepileptics. Increasingly, some antiepileptic drugs have been found to have beneficial effects in non-convulsive disorders such as neuropathic pain (Ch. 42), bipolar depression (Ch. 47) and anxiety (Ch. 44). Many new antiepileptic drugs have been developed over the past 20 or so years in attempts to improve their efficacy and side-effect profile, for example by modifying their pharmacokinetics. Improvements have been steady rather than spectacular, and epilepsy remains a difficult problem, despite the fact that controlling reverberative neuronal discharges would seem, on the face of it, to be a much simpler problem than controlling those aspects of brain function that determine emotions, mood and cognitive function.

THE NATURE OF EPILEPSY

The term 'epilepsy' is used to define a group of neurological disorders all of which exhibit periodic seizures. For information on the underlying causes of epilepsy and factors that precipitate periodic seizures see Browne & Holmes (2008). As explained later, not all seizures involve convulsions. Seizures are associated with episodic high-frequency discharge of impulses by a group of neurons (sometimes referred to as the *focus*) in the brain. What starts as a local abnormal discharge may then spread to other areas of the brain. The site of the primary discharge and the extent of its spread determine the symptoms that are produced, which range from a brief lapse of attention to a full convulsive fit lasting for several minutes, as well as odd sensations or behaviours. The particular symptoms produced depend on the function of the region of the brain that is affected. Thus, involvement of the motor cortex causes convulsions, involvement of the hypothalamus causes peripheral autonomic discharge, and involvement of the reticular formation in the upper brain stem leads to loss of consciousness.

Abnormal electrical activity during and following a seizure can be detected by electroencephalography (EEG) recording from electrodes distributed over the surface of the scalp. Various types of seizure can be recognised on the basis of the nature and distribution of the abnormal discharge (Fig. 45.1). Modern brain imaging techniques, such as magnetic resonance imaging and positron emission tomography, are now routinely used in the evaluation of patients with epilepsy (see Fig. 45.2) to identify structural abnormalities (e.g. ischaemic lesions, tumours; see Deblaere & Achten, 2008).

TYPES OF EPILEPSY

The clinical classification of epilepsy is done on the basis of the characteristics of the seizure rather than on the cause or underlying pathology. There are two major seizure categories, namely *partial* (localised to part of the brain) and *generalised* (involving the whole brain).

PARTIAL SEIZURES

Partial seizures are those in which the discharge begins locally and often remains localised. The symptoms depend on the brain region or regions involved, and include involuntary muscle contractions, abnormal sensory experiences or autonomic discharge, or effects on mood and behaviour, often termed *psychomotor epilepsy* – which may arise from a focus within a temporal lobe. The EEG discharge in this type of epilepsy is normally confined to one hemisphere (Fig. 45.1D). Partial seizures can often be attributed to local cerebral lesions, and their incidence increases with age. In complex partial seizures, loss of consciousness may occur at the outset of the attack, or somewhat later, when the discharge has spread from its site of origin to regions of the brain stem reticular formation. In some individuals, a partial seizure can, during the seizure, become generalised when the abnormal neuronal activity spreads across the whole brain.

---

[1]After Hughlings Jackson, a distinguished 19th-century Yorkshire neurologist who published his outstanding work in the *Annals of the West Riding Lunatic Asylum*.

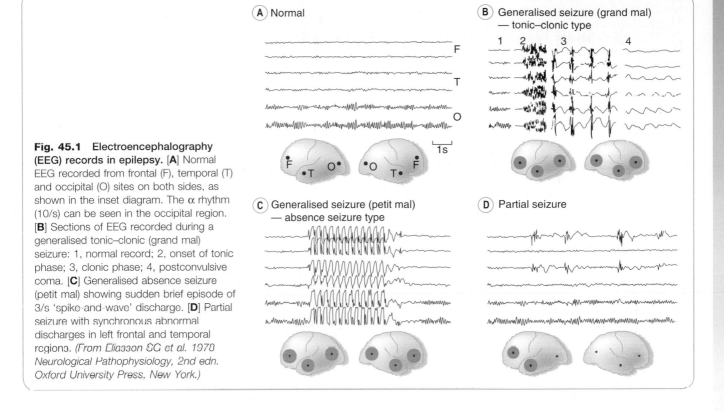

Fig. 45.1 Electroencephalography (EEG) records in epilepsy. **[A]** Normal EEG recorded from frontal (F), temporal (T) and occipital (O) sites on both sides, as shown in the inset diagram. The α rhythm (10/s) can be seen in the occipital region. **[B]** Sections of EEG recorded during a generalised tonic–clonic (grand mal) seizure: 1, normal record; 2, onset of tonic phase; 3, clonic phase; 4, postconvulsive coma. **[C]** Generalised absence seizure (petit mal) showing sudden brief episode of 3/s 'spike-and-wave' discharge. **[D]** Partial seizure with synchronous abnormal discharges in left frontal and temporal regions. *(From Eliasson SG et al. 1978 Neurological Pathophysiology, 2nd edn. Oxford University Press, New York.)*

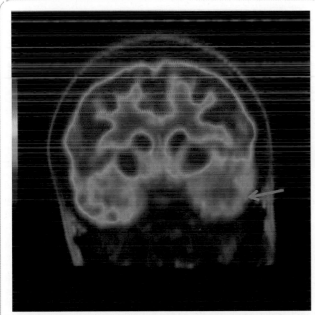

Fig. 45.2 Positron emission tomography (PET) image using [¹⁸F]-fluoro-2-deoxyglucose (FDG) of the brain of a female patient suffering from temporal lobe epilepsy. The interictal area of hypometabolism in the left temporal lobe (indicated by the arrow) is suggestive of the site of the epileptic focus. *(Image kindly provided by Prof. John Duncan and Prof. Peter Ell, UCL Institute of Neurology, London.)*

An epileptic focus in the motor cortex results in attacks, sometimes called *Jacksonian epilepsy*,[1] consisting of repetitive jerking of a particular muscle group, beginning on one side of the body, often in the thumb, big toe or angle of the mouth, which spreads and may involve much of the body within about 2 min before dying out. The patient loses voluntary control of the affected parts of the body but does not necessarily lose consciousness. In *psychomotor epilepsy* the attack may consist of stereotyped purposive movements such as rubbing or patting movements, or much more complex behaviour such as dressing, walking or hair combing. The seizure usually lasts for a few minutes, after which the patient recovers with no recollection of the event. The behaviour during the seizure can be bizarre and accompanied by a strong emotional response.

GENERALISED SEIZURES

Generalised seizures involve the whole brain, including the reticular system, thus producing abnormal electrical activity throughout both hemispheres. Immediate loss of consciousness is characteristic of generalised seizures. There are a number of types of generalised seizure – two important categories are *tonic–clonic* seizures (formerly referred to as grand mal, Fig. 45.1B) and *absence seizures* (petit mal, Fig. 45.1C); others include myoclonic, tonic, atonic and clonic seizures.

A *tonic–clonic seizure* consists of an initial strong contraction of the whole musculature, causing a rigid extensor spasm and an involuntary cry. Respiration stops, and defecation, micturition and salivation often occur. This tonic phase lasts for about 1 min, during which the face is suffused and becomes blue (an important clinical distinction from syncope, the main disorder from which fits must be distinguished, where the face is ashen pale), and is followed by a series of violent, synchronous jerks that gradually die out in 2–4 min. The patient stays unconscious for a few more minutes and then gradually recovers, feeling ill and confused. Injury may occur during the convulsive episode. The EEG shows generalised continuous high-frequency activity in the tonic phase and an intermittent discharge in the clonic phase (Fig. 45.1B).

Absence seizures occur in children; they are much less dramatic but may occur more frequently (many seizures each day) than tonic–clonic seizures. The patient abruptly ceases whatever he or she was doing, sometimes stopping speaking in mid-sentence, and stares vacantly for a few seconds, with little or no motor disturbance. Patients are unaware of their surroundings and recover abruptly with no after effects. The EEG pattern shows a characteristic rhythmic discharge during the period of the seizure (Fig. 45.1C). The rhythmicity appears to be due to oscillatory feedback between the cortex and the thalamus, the special properties of the thalamic neurons being dependent on the T-type calcium channels that they express (see Shin, 2006). The pattern differs from that of partial seizures, where a high-frequency asynchronous discharge spreads out from a local focus. Accordingly, the drugs used specifically to treat absence seizures act mainly by blocking T-type calcium channels, whereas drugs effective against other types of epilepsy act mainly by blocking sodium channels or enhancing GABA-mediated inhibition.

A particularly severe kind of epilepsy, *Lennox–Gastaut syndrome*, occurs in children and is associated with progressive mental retardation, possibly a reflection of excitotoxic neurodegeneration (see Ch. 40).

About one-third of cases of epilepsy are familial and involve genetic mutations. While some are due to a single mutation, most result from polygenetic mutations (see Pandolfo, 2011). Most genes associated with familial epilepsies encode neuronal ion channels closely involved in controlling action potential generation (see Ch. 4), such as voltage-gated sodium and potassium channels, GABA receptors and nicotinic acetylcholine receptors. Some other genes encode proteins that interact with ion channels.

Status epilepticus refers to continuous uninterrupted seizures, requiring emergency medical treatment.

NEURAL MECHANISMS AND ANIMAL MODELS OF EPILEPSY

▼ The underlying neuronal abnormality in epilepsy is poorly understood. In general, excitation will naturally tend to spread throughout a network of interconnected neurons but is normally prevented from doing so by inhibitory mechanisms. Thus, *epileptogenesis* can arise if excitatory transmission is facilitated or inhibitory transmission is reduced (exemplified by GABA$_A$ receptor antagonists causing convulsions; see Ch. 38). In certain respects, epileptogenesis resembles long-term potentiation (Ch. 38), and similar types of use-dependent synaptic plasticity may be involved. Neurons from which the epileptic discharge originates display an unusual type of electrical behaviour termed the paroxysmal depolarising shift (PDS), during which the membrane potential suddenly decreases by about 30 mV and remains depolarised for up to a few seconds before returning to normal. A burst of action potentials often accompanies this depolarisation (Fig. 45.3). This event

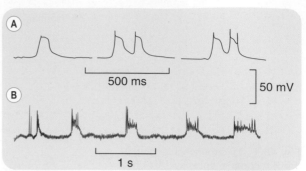

Fig. 45.3 'Paroxysmal depolarising shift' (PDS) compared with experimental activation of glutamate receptors of the NMDA type. [A] PDS recorded with an intracellular microelectrode from cortical neurons of anaesthetised cats. Seizure activity was induced by topical application of penicillin. [B] Intracellular recording from the caudate nucleus of an anaesthetised cat. The glutamate analogue NMDA was applied by ionophoresis from a nearby micropipette. *(Panel [A] from Matsumoto H, Marsan CA 1964 Exp Neurol 9, 286; panel [B] from Herrling PL et al. 1983 J Physiol 339, 207.)*

probably results from the abnormally exaggerated and prolonged action of an excitatory transmitter. Activation of NMDA receptors (see Ch. 38) produces 'plateau-shaped' depolarising responses very similar to the PDS. It is known that repeated seizure activity can lead to neuronal degeneration, possibly due to excitotoxicity (Ch. 40).

Because detailed studies are difficult to carry out on epileptic patients, many different animal models of epilepsy have been investigated (see Bialer & White, 2010). Several transgenic mouse strains have been reported that show spontaneous seizures. They include knockout mutations of various ion channels, receptors and other synaptic proteins. Local application of penicillin crystals results in focal seizures, probably by interfering with inhibitory synaptic transmission. Convulsant drugs (e.g. **pentylenetetrazol** [PTZ]) are often used as are seizures caused by electrical stimulation of the whole brain. Drugs that inhibit PTZ-induced convulsions and raise the threshold for production of electrically induced seizures are generally effective against absence seizures, whereas those that reduce the duration and spread of electrically induced convulsions are effective in focal types of epilepsy such as tonic–clonic seizures. In the *kainate model* a single injection of the glutamate receptor agonist kainic acid into the amygdaloid nucleus of a rat can produce spontaneous seizures 2–4 weeks later that continue indefinitely. This is believed to result from excitotoxic damage to inhibitory neurons.

In the *kindling model* brief low-intensity electrical stimulation of certain regions of the limbic system, such as the amygdala, normally produces no seizure response but if repeated daily for several days the response gradually increases until very low levels of stimulation will evoke a full seizure, and eventually seizures occur spontaneously. This kindled state can persist indefinitely but is prevented by NMDA receptor antagonists or deletion of the neurotrophin receptor, TrkB.

In human focal epilepsies, surgical removal of a damaged region of cortex may fail to cure the condition, as though the abnormal discharge from the region of primary damage had somehow produced a secondary hyperexcitability elsewhere in the brain. Furthermore, following severe head injury prophylactic treatment with antiepileptic drugs reduces the incidence of post-traumatic epilepsy, which suggests that a phenomenon similar to kindling may underlie this form of epilepsy.

Nature of epilepsy

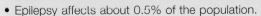

- Epilepsy affects about 0.5% of the population.
- The characteristic event is the seizure, which may be associated with convulsions but may take other forms.
- The seizure is caused by an asynchronous high-frequency discharge of a group of neurons, starting locally and spreading to a varying extent to affect other parts of the brain. In absence seizures, the discharge is regular and oscillatory.
- Partial seizures affect localised brain regions, and the attack may involve mainly motor, sensory or behavioural phenomena. Unconsciousness occurs when the reticular formation is involved.
- Generalised seizures affect the whole brain. Two common forms of generalised seizure are the tonic–clonic fit and the absence seizure. Status epilepticus is a life-threatening condition in which seizure activity is uninterrupted.

- Partial seizures can become secondarily generalised if the localised abnormal neuronal activity subsequently spreads across the whole brain.
- Many animal models have been devised, including electrically and chemically induced generalised seizures, production of local chemical damage and kindling. These provide good prediction of antiepileptic drug effects in humans.
- The neurochemical basis of the abnormal discharge is not well understood. It may be associated with enhanced excitatory amino acid transmission, impaired inhibitory transmission or abnormal electrical properties of the affected cells. Several susceptibility genes, mainly encoding neuronal ion channels, have been identified.
- Repeated epileptic discharge can cause neuronal death (excitotoxicity).
- Current drug therapy is effective in 70–80% of patients.

ANTIEPILEPTIC DRUGS

Antiepileptic (sometimes known as *anticonvulsant*) drugs are used to treat epilepsy as well as non-epileptic convulsive disorders.

With optimal drug therapy, epilepsy is controlled completely in about 75% of patients, but about 10% (50 000 in Britain) continue to have seizures at intervals of 1 month or less, which severely disrupts their life and work. There is therefore a need to improve the efficacy of therapy.

Patients with epilepsy usually need to take drugs continuously for many years, so avoidance of side effects is particularly important. Nevertheless, some drugs that have considerable adverse effects are still quite widely used even though they are not drugs of choice for newly diagnosed patients.[2] There is a need for more specific and effective drugs, and a number of new drugs have recently been introduced for clinical use or are in late stages of clinical trials. Long-established antiepileptic drugs are listed in Table 45.1. Newer drugs (see Table 45.2) with similar mechanisms of action to older drugs or novel mechanisms of action may offer advantages in terms of efficacy in drug-resistant epilepsies, better pharmacokinetic profile, improved tolerability, lower potential for interaction with other drugs (see Ch. 57) and fewer adverse effects. The appropriate use of drugs from this large available menu depends on many clinical factors (see Macleod & Appleton, 2007; Azar & Abou-Khalil, 2008).

MECHANISM OF ACTION

Antiepileptic drugs aim to inhibit the abnormal neuronal discharge rather than to correct the underlying cause. Three main mechanisms of action appear to be important:

1. Enhancement of GABA action.
2. Inhibition of sodium channel function.
3. Inhibition of calcium channel function.

More recently newer drugs with other, novel mechanisms of action have been developed.

Antiepileptic drugs may exert more than one beneficial action, prime examples being **valproate** and **topiramate** (see Table 45.1). The relative importance and contribution of each of these actions to the therapeutic effect is somewhat uncertain.

As with drugs used to treat cardiac dysrhythmias (Ch. 21), the aim is to prevent the paroxysmal discharge without affecting normal transmission. It is clear that properties such as use dependence and voltage-dependence of channel-blocking drugs (see Ch. 4) are important in achieving this selectivity, but our understanding remains fragmentary.

Enhancement of GABA action

Several antiepileptic drugs (e.g. **phenobarbital** and **benzodiazepines**) enhance the activation of GABA$_A$ receptors, thus facilitating the GABA-mediated opening of chloride channels (see Chs 3 and 44).[3] **Vigabatrin** acts by irreversibly inhibiting the enzyme GABA transaminase that is responsible for inactivating GABA (see Ch. 38) in astrocytes and GABAergic nerve terminals. Tiagabine is an equipotent inhibitor of both the neuronal and glial GABA transporter GAT1, thus inhibiting the removal of GABA from the synapse. It enhances the extracellular GABA concentration, as measured in microdialysis experiments, and also potentiates and prolongs GABA-mediated synaptic responses in the brain.

---

[2]Bromide was the first antiepileptic agent. Its propensity to induce sedation and other unwanted side effects has resulted in it being largely withdrawn from human medicine, although it is still approved for human use in some countries (e.g. Germany) and may have uses in childhood epilepsies. It is still widely used in veterinary practice to treat epilepsy in dogs and cats.

[3]Absence seizures, paradoxically, are often exacerbated by drugs that enhance GABA activity and better treated by drugs acting by different mechanisms such as T-type calcium channel inhibition.

Table 45.1 Properties of long-established antiepileptic drugs

Drug	Sodium channel	GABA$_A$ receptor	Calcium channel	Other	Main uses	Main unwanted effect(s)	Pharmacokinetics
Carbamazepine[a]	+				All types except absence seizures Especially temporal lobe epilepsy Also trigeminal neuralgia Most widely used antiepileptic drug	Sedation, ataxia, blurred vision, water retention, hypersensitivity reactions, leukopenia, liver failure (rare)	Half-life 12–18 h (longer initially) Strong induction of liver enzymes, so risk of drug interactions
Phenytoin	+				All types except absence seizures	Ataxia, vertigo, gum hypertrophy, hirsutism, megaloblastic anaemia, fetal malformation, hypersensitivity reactions	Half-life ~24 h Saturation kinetics, therefore unpredictable plasma levels Plasma monitoring often required
Valproate[b]	+	?+	+	GABA transaminase inhibition	Most types, including absence seizures	Generally less than with other drugs Nausea, hair loss, weight gain, fetal malformations	Half-life 12–15 h
Ethosuximide[c]			+		Absence seizures May exacerbate tonic–clonic seizures	Nausea, anorexia, mood changes, headache	Long plasma half-life (~60 h)
Phenobarbital[d]	?+	+			All types except absence seizures	Sedation, depression	Long plasma half-life (>60 h) Strong induction of liver enzymes, so risk of drug interactions (e.g. with phenytoin)
Benzodiazepines (e.g. clonazepam, clobazam, lorazepam, diazepam)		+			Lorazepam used intravenously to control status epilepticus	Sedation Withdrawal syndrome (see. Ch. 44)	See Ch. 44

[a]Oxcarbazepine, recently introduced, is similar; claimed to have fewer side effects.

[b]Valproate is effective against both partial and generalised seizures, including absence seizures.

[c]Trimethadione is similar to ethosuximide in that it acts selectively against absence seizures but has greater toxicity (especially the risk of severe hypersensitivity reactions and teratogenicity).

[d]Primidone is pharmacologically similar to phenobarbital and is converted to phenobarbital in the body. It has no clear advantages and is more liable to produce hypersensitivity reactions, so is now rarely used.

Inhibition of sodium channel function

Many antiepileptic drugs (e.g. **carbamazepine, phenytoin** and **lamotrigine**; see Tables 45.1 & 45.2) affect membrane excitability by an action on voltage-dependent sodium channels (see Chs 4 and 43), which carry the inward membrane current necessary for the generation of an action potential. Their blocking action shows the property of use-dependence; in other words, they block preferentially the excitation of cells that are firing repetitively, and the higher the frequency of firing, the greater the block produced. This characteristic, which is relevant to the ability of drugs to block the high-frequency discharge that occurs in an epileptic fit without unduly interfering with the low-frequency firing of neurons in the normal state, arises

Table 45.2 Properties of newer antiepileptic drugs

Drug	Site of action				Main uses	Main unwanted effect(s)	Pharmacokinetics
	Sodium channel	GABA$_A$ receptor	Calcium channel	Other			
Vigabatrin				GABA transaminase inhibition	All types Appears to be effective in patients resistant to other drugs	Sedation, behavioural and mood changes (occasionally psychosis) Visual field defects	Short plasma half-life, but enzyme inhibition is long-lasting
Lamotrigine	+		?+	Inhibits glutamate release	All types	Dizziness, sedation, rashes	Plasma half-life 24–36 h
Gabapentin Pregabalin			+		Partial seizures	Few side effects, mainly sedation	Plasma half-life 6–9 h
Felbamate	+	+	?+	?NMDA receptor block	Used mainly for severe epilepsy (Lennox–Gastaut syndrome) because of risk of adverse reaction	Few acute side effects but can cause aplastic anaemia and liver damage (rare but serious)	Plasma half-life ~20 h Excreted unchanged
Tiagabine				Inhibits GABA uptake	Partial seizures	Sedation Dizziness, lightheadedness	Plasma half-life ~7 h Liver metabolism
Topiramate	+	?+	?+	AMPA receptor block	Partial and generalised tonic–clonic seizures. Lennox–Gastaut syndrome	Sedation Fewer pharmacokinetic interactions than phenytoin Fetal malformation	Plasma half life ~20 h Excreted unchanged
Levetiracetam				Binds to SV2A protein	Partial and generalised tonic–clonic seizures	Sedation (slight)	Plasma half-life ~7 h Excreted unchanged
Zonisamide	+	?+	+		Partial seizures	Sedation (slight) Appetite suppression, weight loss	Plasma half-life ~70 h
Rufinamide	+			?+ Inhibits GABA reuptake	Partial seizures	Headache, dizziness, fatigue	Plasma half-life 6–10 h
Lacosamide	+				Partial seizures	Nausea, vomiting, dizziness, visual disturbances, impaired coordination, mood changes	Plasma half-life 13 h
Retigabine				Activates K$_v$7.2 (KCNQ2) potassium channels	Partial seizures	Prolongs QT interval, weight gain	Plasma half-life 6–11 h
Perampanel				Non-competitive AMPA antagonist	Partial seizures	Dizziness, weight gain, sedation, impaired coordination changes in mood and behaviour	Plasma half-life 70–100 h

SV2A, synaptic vesicle protein 2A.

from the ability of blocking drugs to discriminate between sodium channels in their resting, open and inactivated states (see Chs 4 and 43). Depolarisation of a neuron (such as occurs in the PDS described above) increases the proportion of the sodium channels in the inactivated state. Antiepileptic drugs bind preferentially to channels in this state, preventing them from returning to the resting state, and thus reducing the number of functional channels available to generate action potentials. **Lacosamide** enhances sodium channel inactivation, but unlike other antiepileptic drugs it appears to affect slow rather than rapid inactivation processes.

Inhibition of calcium channels

Drugs that are used to treat absence seizures (e.g. **ethosuximide** and **valproate**) all appear to share the ability to block T-type low-voltage-activated calcium channels. T-type channel activity is important in determining the rhythmic discharge of thalamic neurons associated with absence seizures (Khosravani et al., 2004).

Gabapentin, though designed as a simple analogue of GABA that would be sufficiently lipid soluble to penetrate the blood–brain barrier, owes its antiepileptic effect mainly to an action on P/Q-type calcium channels. By binding to a particular channel subunit ($\alpha 2\delta 1$), both gabapentin and **pregabalin** (a related analogue) reduce the trafficking to the plasma membrane of calcium channels containing this subunit, thereby reducing calcium entry into the nerve terminals and reducing the release of various neurotransmitters and modulators.

Other mechanisms

Many of the newer antiepileptic drugs were developed empirically on the basis of activity in animal models. Their mechanism of action at the cellular level is not fully understood.

Levetiracetam is believed to interfere with neurotransmitter release by binding to synaptic vesicle protein 2A (SV2A), which is involved in synaptic vesicle docking and fusion. **Brivaracetam**, a related potential antiepileptic agent, also binds to SV2A with ten-fold higher affinity: positive results have been noted in clinical trials.

While a drug may appear to work by one of the major mechanisms described above, close scrutiny often reveals other actions that may also be therapeutically relevant. For example, **phenytoin** not only causes use-dependent block of sodium channels (see p. 550) but also affects other aspects of membrane function, including calcium channels and post-tetanic potentiation, as well as intracellular protein phosphorylation by calmodulin-activated kinases, which could also interfere with membrane excitability and synaptic function.

Antagonism at ionotropic excitatory amino acid receptors has been a major focus in the search for new antiepileptic drugs. Despite showing efficacy in animal models, by and large they did not prove useful in the clinic, because the margin between the desired anticonvulsant effect and unacceptable side effects, such as loss of motor coordination, was too narrow. However, **perampanel**, a non-competitive AMPA-receptor antagonist, has recently been approved as adjunctive treatment for partial seizures.

Neuronal membrane excitability is controlled by potassium channel activity. Increasing potassium conductance hyperpolarises neurons making them less excitable. A new antiepileptic drug, **retigabine**, licensed for treatment of focal seizures, activates the 'M current' through channels containing $K_v 7.2$ subunits and is used in refractory cases.

> **Mechanism of action of antiepileptic drugs**
>
> - The major antiepileptic drugs are thought to act by three main mechanisms:
>   - reducing electrical excitability of cell membranes, mainly through use-dependent block of sodium channels
>   - enhancing GABA-mediated synaptic inhibition; this may be achieved by an enhanced postsynaptic action of GABA, by inhibiting GABA transaminase or by inhibiting GABA uptake into neurons and glial cells
>   - inhibiting T-type calcium channels (important in controlling absence seizures).
> - Newer drugs act by other mechanisms, some yet to be elucidated.

CARBAMAZEPINE

Carbamazepine, one of the most widely used antiepileptic drugs, is chemically related to the tricyclic antidepressant drugs (see Ch. 47) and was found in a routine screening test to inhibit electrically evoked seizures in mice. Pharmacologically and clinically, its actions resemble those of phenytoin, although it appears to be particularly effective in treating certain partial seizures (e.g. psychomotor epilepsy). It is also used to treat other conditions, such as neuropathic pain (Ch. 42) and manic-depressive illness (Ch. 47).

Pharmacokinetic aspects

Carbamazepine is slowly but well absorbed after oral administration. Its plasma half-life is about 30 h when it is given as a single dose, but it is a strong inducer of hepatic enzymes, and the plasma half-life shortens to about 15 h when it is given repeatedly. Some of its metabolites have antiepileptic properties. A slow-release preparation is used for patients who experience transient side effects coinciding with plasma concentration peaks following oral dosing.

Unwanted effects

Carbamazepine produces a variety of unwanted effects ranging from drowsiness, dizziness and ataxia to more severe mental and motor disturbances.[4] It can also cause water retention (and hence hyponatraemia; Ch. 29) and a variety of gastrointestinal and cardiovascular side effects. The incidence and severity of these effects is relatively low, however, compared with other drugs. Treatment is usually started with a low dose, which is built up gradually to avoid dose-related toxicity. Severe bone marrow

---

[4]One of the authors who was a keen hockey player played in a team with a goalkeeper who sometimes made silly errors early in the match. It turned out that he suffered from epilepsy and had taken his dose of carbamazepine too close to the start of the match.

depression, causing neutropenia, and other severe forms of hypersensitivity reaction can occur, especially in people of Asian origin (see Ch. 11).

Carbamazepine is a powerful inducer of hepatic microsomal enzymes, and thus accelerates the metabolism of many other drugs, such as phenytoin, oral contraceptives, warfarin and corticosteroids, as well as of itself. When starting treatment, the opposite of a 'loading dose' strategy is employed: small initial doses are gradually increased since when dosing is initiated metabolising enzymes are not induced and so even low doses may give rise to adverse effects (notably ataxia); as enzyme induction occurs, increasing doses are needed to maintain therapeutic plasma concentrations. In general, it is inadvisable to combine it with other antiepileptic drugs, and interactions with other drugs (e.g. warfarin) metabolised by cytochrome P450 (CYP) enzymes are common and clinically important. **Oxcarbazepine** is a prodrug that is metabolised to a compound closely resembling carbamazepine, with similar actions but less tendency to induce drug-metabolising enzymes. Another related drug, **eslicarbazepine**, is in development and may also have less effect on metabolising enzymes.

PHENYTOIN

Phenytoin is the most important member of the hydantoin group of compounds, which are structurally related to the barbiturates. It is highly effective in reducing the intensity and duration of electrically induced convulsions in mice, although ineffective against PTZ-induced convulsions. Despite its many side effects and unpredictable pharmacokinetic behaviour, phenytoin is widely used, being effective against various forms of partial and generalised seizures, although not against absence seizures, which it may even worsen.

Pharmacokinetic aspects

Phenytoin has certain pharmacokinetic peculiarities that need to be taken into account when it is used clinically. It is well absorbed when given orally, and about 80–90% of the plasma content is bound to albumin. Other drugs, such as salicylates, phenylbutazone and valproate, inhibit this binding competitively (see Ch. 57). This increases the free phenytoin concentration but also increases hepatic clearance of phenytoin, so may enhance or reduce the effect of the phenytoin in an unpredictable way. Phenytoin is metabolised by the hepatic mixed function oxidase system and excreted mainly as glucuronide. It causes enzyme induction, and thus increases the rate of metabolism of other drugs (e.g. oral anticoagulants). The metabolism of phenytoin itself can be either enhanced or competitively inhibited by various other drugs that share the same hepatic enzymes. **Phenobarbital** produces both effects, and because competitive inhibition is immediate whereas induction takes time, it initially enhances and later reduces the pharmacological activity of phenytoin. **Ethanol** has a similar dual effect.

The metabolism of phenytoin shows the characteristic of saturation (see Ch. 10), which means that over the therapeutic plasma concentration range the rate of inactivation does not increase in proportion to the plasma concentration. The consequences of this are that:

- the plasma half-life (approximately 20 h) increases as the dose is increased
- the steady-state mean plasma concentration, achieved when a patient is given a constant daily dose, varies disproportionately with the dose. Figure 45.4 shows that, in one patient, increasing the dose by 50% caused the steady-state plasma concentration to increase more than four-fold.

The range of plasma concentration over which phenytoin is effective without causing excessive unwanted effects is quite narrow (approximately 40–100 μmol/l). The very steep relationship between dose and plasma concentration, and the many interacting factors, mean that there is considerable individual variation in the plasma concentration achieved with a given dose. Regular monitoring of plasma concentration has helped considerably in achieving an optimal therapeutic effect. The past tendency was to add further drugs in cases where a single drug failed to give adequate control. It is now recognised that much of the unpredictability can be ascribed to pharmacokinetic variability, and regular monitoring of plasma concentration has reduced the use of polypharmacy.

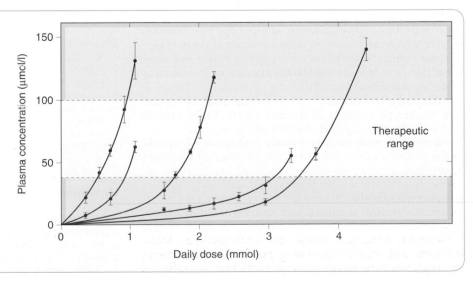

Fig. 45.4 Non-linear relationship between daily dose of phenytoin and steady-state plasma concentration in five individual human subjects. The daily dose required to achieve the therapeutic range of plasma concentrations (40–100 μmol/l) varies greatly between individuals, and for any one individual the dose has to be adjusted rather precisely to keep within the acceptable plasma concentration range. *(Redrawn from Richens A, Dunlop A 1975 Lancet 2, 247.)*

Unwanted effects

Side effects of phenytoin begin to appear at plasma concentrations exceeding 100 μmol/l and may be severe above about 150 μmol/l. The milder side effects include vertigo, ataxia, headache and nystagmus, but not sedation. At higher plasma concentrations, marked confusion with intellectual deterioration occurs; a paradoxical increase in seizure frequency is a particular trap for the unwary prescriber. These effects occur acutely and are quickly reversible. Hyperplasia of the gums often develops gradually, as does hirsutism and coarsening of the features, which probably result from increased androgen secretion. Megaloblastic anaemia, associated with a disorder of folate metabolism, sometimes occurs, and can be corrected by giving folic acid (Ch. 25). Hypersensitivity reactions, mainly rashes, are quite common. Phenytoin has also been implicated as a cause of the increased incidence of fetal malformations in children born to epileptic mothers, particularly the occurrence of cleft palate, associated with the formation of an epoxide metabolite. Severe idiosyncratic reactions, including hepatitis, skin reactions and neoplastic lymphocyte disorders, occur in a small proportion of patients.

VALPROATE

Valproate is a simple monocarboxylic acid, chemically unrelated to any other class of antiepileptic drug, and in 1963 it was discovered quite accidentally to have anticonvulsant properties in mice. It inhibits most kinds of experimentally induced convulsions and is effective in many kinds of epilepsy, being particularly useful in certain types of infantile epilepsy, where its low toxicity and lack of sedative action are important, and in adolescents who exhibit both tonic–clonic or myoclonic seizures as well as absence seizures, because valproate (unlike most antiepileptic drugs) is effective against each. Like carbamazepine, valproate is also used in psychiatric conditions such as bipolar depressive illness (Ch. 47).

Valproate works by several mechanisms (see Table 45.1), the relative importance of which remains to be clarified. It causes a significant increase in the GABA content of the brain and is a weak inhibitor of the enzyme system that inactivates GABA, namely GABA transaminase and succinic semialdehyde dehydrogenase (Ch. 38), but *in vitro* studies suggest that these effects would be very slight at clinical dosage. Other more potent inhibitors of these enzymes (e.g. **vigabatrin**; see p. 555) also increase GABA content and have an anticonvulsant effect in experimental animals. There is some evidence that it enhances the action of GABA by a postsynaptic action, but no clear evidence that it affects inhibitory synaptic responses. It inhibits sodium channels, but less so than phenytoin, and inhibits T-type calcium channels, which might explain why it is effective against absence seizures.

Valproate is well absorbed orally and excreted, mainly as the glucuronide, in the urine, the plasma half-life being about 15 h.

Unwanted effects

Valproate causes thinning and curling of the hair in about 10% of patients. The most serious side effect is hepatotoxicity. An increase in plasma glutamic oxaloacetic transaminase, which signals liver damage of some degree, commonly occurs, but proven cases of valproate-induced hepatitis are rare. The few cases of fatal hepatitis in valproate-treated patients may well have been caused by other factors. Valproate is a potent teratogen (even more so than other anticonvulsants that tend to share this secondary pharmacology) (see p. 557), causing spina bifida and other neural tube defects. Analogues of valproate with potentially reduced side effects are in development.

ETHOSUXIMIDE

Ethosuximide is another drug developed empirically by modifying the barbituric acid ring structure. Pharmacologically and clinically, however, it is different from the drugs so far discussed, in that it is active against PTZ-induced convulsions in animals and against absence seizures in humans, with little or no effect on other types of epilepsy. It supplanted **trimethadione**, the first drug found to be effective in absence seizures, which had major side effects. Ethosuximide is used clinically for its selective effect on absence seizures.

The mechanism of action of ethosuximide and trimethadione appears to differ from that of other antiepileptic drugs. The main effect is inhibition of T-type calcium channels, which may play a role in generating the firing rhythm in thalamic relay neurons that generates the 3/second spike-and-wave EEG pattern characteristic of absence seizures.

Ethosuximide is well absorbed, and metabolised and excreted much like phenobarbital, with a plasma half-life of about 60 h. Its main side effects are nausea and anorexia, sometimes lethargy and dizziness, and it is said to precipitate tonic–clonic seizures in susceptible patients. Very rarely, it can cause severe hypersensitivity reactions.

PHENOBARBITAL

▼ Phenobarbital was one of the first barbiturates to be developed. Its clinical effectiveness closely resembles that of phenytoin; it affects the duration and intensity of artificially induced seizures, rather than the seizure threshold, and is (like phenytoin) ineffective in treating absence seizures. **Primidone**, now rarely used, acts by being metabolised to phenobarbital. It often causes hypersensitivity reactions. The clinical uses of phenobarbital are virtually the same as those of phenytoin, but it is seldom used now because it causes sedation. Phenytoin does not produce this effect and is therefore the preferred option. For some years, phenobarbital was widely used in children, including as prophylaxis following febrile convulsions in infancy, but it can cause behavioural disturbances and hyperkinesias. It is, however, widely used in veterinary practice.

Pharmacokinetic aspects

▼ Phenobarbital is well absorbed, and about 50% of the drug in the blood is bound to plasma albumin. It is eliminated slowly from the plasma (half-life 50–140 h). About 25% is excreted unchanged in the urine. Because phenobarbital is a weak acid, its ionisation and hence renal elimination are increased if the urine is made alkaline (see Ch. 9). The remaining 75% is metabolised, mainly by oxidation and conjugation, by hepatic microsomal enzymes. Phenobarbital is a powerful inducer of liver CYP enzymes, and it lowers the plasma concentration of several other drugs (e.g. steroids, oral contraceptives, warfarin, tricyclic antidepressants) to an extent that is clinically important.

Unwanted effects

▼ The main unwanted effect of phenobarbital is sedation, which often occurs at plasma concentrations within the therapeutic range for seizure control. This is a serious drawback, because the drug may have to be used for years on end. Some degree of tolerance to the sedative effect seems to occur, but objective tests of cognition and motor performance show impairment even during long-term treatment. Other unwanted effects that may occur with clinical dosage include megaloblastic anaemia (similar to that caused by phenytoin), mild hypersensitivity reactions and osteomalacia. Like other barbiturates, it must not be given to patients with porphyria (see Ch. 11). In overdose, phenobarbital depresses brain stem function, producing coma and respiratory and circulatory failure, as do all barbiturates.

BENZODIAZEPINES

Benzodiazepines can be used to treat both acute seizures, especially in children – **diazepam** often being administered rectally – and status epilepticus (a life-threatening condition in which epileptic seizures occur almost without a break) for which agents such as **lorazepam**, diazepam, or **clonazepam** are administered intravenously. The advantage in status epilepticus is that they act very rapidly compared with other antiepileptic drugs. With most benzodiazepines (see Ch. 44), the sedative effect is too pronounced for them to be used for maintenance therapy and tolerance develops over 1–6 months. **Clonazepam** is unique among the benzodiazepines in that in addition to acting at the GABA$_A$ receptor, it also inhibits T-type calcium channels. Both it and the related compound **clobazam** are claimed to be relatively selective as antiepileptic drugs. Sedation is the main side effect of these compounds, and an added problem may be the withdrawal syndrome, which results in an exacerbation of seizures if the drug is stopped abruptly.

NEWER ANTIEPILEPTIC DRUGS

VIGABATRIN

Vigabatrin, the first 'designer drug' in the epilepsy field, is a vinyl-substituted analogue of GABA that was designed as an irreversible inhibitor of the GABA-metabolising enzyme GABA transaminase. In animal studies, vigabatrin increases the GABA content of the brain and also increases the stimulation-evoked release of GABA, implying that GABA transaminase inhibition can increase the releasable pool of GABA and effectively enhance inhibitory transmission. In humans, vigabatrin increases the content of GABA in the cerebrospinal fluid. Although its plasma half-life is short, it produces a long-lasting effect because the enzyme is blocked irreversibly, and the drug can be given by mouth once daily.

Vigabatrin has been reported to be effective in a substantial proportion of patients resistant to the established drugs. However, a drawback of vigabatrin is the development of peripheral visual field defects in a proportion of patients on long-term therapy. Therefore the benefit of using this drug in refractory epilepsy must be weighed against the potential risk of developing visual problems. Vigabatrin may cause depression, and occasionally psychotic disturbances and hallucinations, in a minority of patients.

LAMOTRIGINE

Lamotrigine, although chemically unrelated, resembles phenytoin and carbamazepine in its pharmacological effects but it appears that, despite its similar mechanism of action, lamotrigine has a broader therapeutic profile than the earlier drugs, with significant efficacy against absence seizures (it is also used to treat unrelated psychiatric disorders). Its main side effects are nausea, dizziness and ataxia, and hypersensitivity reactions (mainly mild rashes, but occasionally more severe). Its plasma half-life

is about 24 h, with no particular pharmacokinetic anomalies, and it is taken orally.

FELBAMATE

Felbamate is an analogue of an obsolete anxiolytic drug, **meprobamate**. It is active in many animal seizure models and has a broader clinical spectrum than earlier antiepileptic drugs, but its mechanism of action at the cellular level is uncertain. Its acute side effects are mild, mainly nausea, irritability and insomnia, but it occasionally causes severe reactions resulting in aplastic anaemia or hepatitis. For this reason, its recommended use is limited to intractable epilepsy (e.g. in children with Lennox–Gastaut syndrome) that is unresponsive to other drugs. Its plasma half-life is about 24 h, and it can enhance the plasma concentration of other antiepileptic drugs given concomitantly. **Carisbamate**, a sodium channel blocker, is a new drug currently in clinical trials that was originally designed with the intention of producing a drug similar to felbamate that does not cause aplastic anaemia.

GABAPENTIN AND PREGABALIN

Gabapentin is effective against partial seizures. Its side effects (sleepiness, headache, fatigue, dizziness and weight gain) are less severe than with many antiepileptic drugs. The absorption of gabapentin from the intestine depends on the L-amino acid carrier system and shows the property of saturability, which means that increasing the dose does not proportionately increase the amount absorbed. This makes gabapentin relatively safe and free of side effects associated with overdosing. Its plasma half-life is about 6 h, requiring dosing two to three times daily. It is free of interactions with other drugs. It is also used as an analgesic to treat neuropathic pain (Ch. 42). Pregabalin, an analogue of gabapentin, is more potent but otherwise very similar. As these drugs are excreted unchanged in the urine they must be used with care in patients whose renal function is impaired.

TIAGABINE

Tiagabine is an analogue of GABA that is able to penetrate the blood–brain barrier. It has a short plasma half-life and is mainly used as an add-on therapy for partial seizures. Its main side effects are drowsiness and confusion, dizziness, fatigue, agitation and tremor.

TOPIRAMATE

Topiramate is a drug that appears to do a little of everything, blocking sodium and calcium channels, enhancing the action of GABA, blocking AMPA receptors and, for good measure, weakly inhibiting carbonic anhydrase. Its clinical effectiveness resembles that of phenytoin, and it is claimed to produce less severe side effects, as well as being devoid of the pharmacokinetic properties that cause trouble with phenytoin. Currently, it is mainly used as add-on therapy in refractory cases of partial and generalised seizures.

LEVETIRACETAM

Levetiracetam was developed as an analogue of **piracetam**, a drug used to improve cognitive function, and discovered by accident to have antiepileptic activity in animal models. Unusually, it lacks activity in conventional models such as electroshock and PTZ tests, but is effective in the audiogenic and kindling models (see p. 548). Leveti-racetam is excreted unchanged in the urine. Common side effects include headaches, inflammation of the nose and throat, sleepiness, vomiting and irritability. Brivaracetam and **seletracetam** are similar to levetiracetam.

ZONISAMIDE

Zonisamide is a sulfonamide compound originally intended as an antibacterial drug and found accidentally to have antiepileptic properties. It is mainly free of major unwanted effects, although it causes drowsiness, and of serious interaction with other drugs. It tends to suppress appetite and cause weight loss, and is sometimes used for this purpose. Zonisamide has a long plasma half-life of 60–80 h, and is partly excreted unchanged and partly converted to a glucuronide metabolite. It is licensed for use as an adjunct treatment of partial and generalised seizures but may be effective as a monotherapy.

RUFINAMIDE

Rufinamide is a triazole derivative structurally unrelated to other antiepileptic drugs. It is licensed for treating Lennox–Gastaut syndrome and may also be effective in partial seizures. It has low plasma protein binding and is not metabolised by CYP enzymes.

RETIGABINE

Retigabine is used as an adjunct treatment for partial seizures. Side effects include weight gain, sedation and motor incoordination. It prolongs the QT interval so there is a theoretical possibility that it might provoke ventricular arrhythmia (see Ch. 21). As a precaution, the prescribing information recommends that an ECG is recorded before starting retigabine in patients who are taking other medication(s) that may prolong the QT interval.

PERAMPANEL

Perampanel is effective in refractory partial seizures. Side effects include dizziness, sedation, fatigue, irritability, weight gain, and loss of motor coordination. There is a risk of serious psychiatric problems (violent, even homicidal, thoughts and threatening behavior) in some individuals.

LACOSAMIDE

Lacosamide is used to treat partial seizures. Side effects include nausea, dizziness, sedation and fatigue. It produces relief of pain due to diabetic neuropathy.

STIRIPENTOL

Stiripentol has some efficacy as an adjunctive therapy in children. It enhances GABA release and prolongs GABA-mediated synaptic events in a manner similar to phenobarbital.

DEVELOPMENT OF NEW DRUGS

There are a number of new antiepileptic agents currently being evaluated in clinical trials (see Bialer & White, 2010). **Ganaxolone**, structurally resembling endogenous neurosteroids (see Ch. 38), is a positive allosteric modulator of GABA$_A$ receptors containing δ subunits. **Tonabersat** is a neuronal gap junction inhibitor.

The identification of epileptogenic mutations of genes encoding specific ion channels and other functional proteins (see Weber & Lerche, 2008) is expected to lead to new drugs aimed at these potential targets.

The major antiepileptic drugs

The main drugs in current use are carbamazepine, phenytoin, valproate, ethosuximide and benzodiazepines.

- **Carbamazepine**
  - acts mainly by use-dependent block of sodium channels
  - effective in most forms of epilepsy (except absence seizures); particularly effective in psychomotor epilepsy
  - also useful in neuropathic pain such as trigeminal neuralgia, and in bipolar disorder
  - strong liver-inducing agent, therefore many drug interactions
  - low incidence of unwanted effects, principally sedation, ataxia, mental disturbances, water retention
  - widely used in treatment of epilepsy.
- **Phenytoin**
  - acts mainly by use-dependent block of sodium channels
  - effective in many forms of epilepsy, but not absence seizures
  - metabolism shows saturation kinetics, so plasma concentration can vary widely; monitoring is therefore recommended
  - drug interactions are common
  - main unwanted effects are confusion, gum hyperplasia, skin rashes, anaemia, teratogenesis.
- **Valproate**
  - chemically unrelated to other antiepileptic drugs
  - effective in most forms of epilepsy including absence seizures
  - multiple possible mechanisms of action, including weak inhibition of GABA transaminase, some effect on sodium and T-type calcium channels
  - relatively few unwanted effects: baldness, teratogenicity, liver damage (rare, but serious).
- **Ethosuximide**
  - the main drug used to treat absence seizures; may exacerbate other forms
  - acts by blocking T-type calcium channels
  - relatively few unwanted effects, mainly nausea and anorexia.
- **Benzodiazepines** (mainly **clonazepam** and **diazepam**)
  - effective in the treatment of acute seizures
  - **lorazepam** used in treating status epilepticus.
- Other agents include **vigabatrin**, **lamotrigine**, **felbamate**, **gabapentin**, **pregabalin**, **tiagabine**, **topiramate**, **levetiracetam**, **zonisamide**, **rufinamide**, **retigabine**, **perampanel**, **lacosamide** and **stiripentol**.

OTHER USES OF ANTIEPILEPTIC DRUGS

Antiepileptic drugs have proved to have much wider clinical applications than was originally envisaged, and clinical trials have shown many of them to be effective in the following conditions:

- cardiac dysrhythmias (e.g. **phenytoin** – not used clinically, however; Ch. 21)
- bipolar disorder (**valproate, carbamazepine, oxcarbazepine, lamotrigine, topiramate**; Ch. 47)
- migraine prophylaxis (**valproate, gabapentin, topiramate**; Ch. 15)
- anxiety disorders (**gabapentin**; Ch. 44)
- neuropathic pain (**gabapentin, pregabalin, carbamazepine, lamotrigine**; Ch. 42).

This surprising multiplicity of clinical indications may reflect the fact that similar neurobiological mechanisms, involving synaptic plasticity and increased excitability of interconnected populations of neurons, underlie each of these disorders.

ANTIEPILEPTIC DRUGS AND PREGNANCY

There are several important implications for women taking antiepileptic drugs. By inducing hepatic CYP3A4 enzymes, some antiepileptic drugs may increase oral contraceptive metabolism, thus reducing their effectiveness. Taken during pregnancy, drugs such as phenytoin, carbamazepine, lamotrigine, topiramate and valproate are thought to produce teratogenic effects. It remains to be clarified if newer agents also have this problem. Induction of CYP enzymes may result in vitamin K deficiency in the newborn (Ch. 25).

> **Clinical uses of antiepileptic drugs**
>
> - Generalised tonic–clonic seizures:
>   - **carbamazepine** (preferred because of a relatively favourable effectiveness : risk ratio), **phenytoin, valproate**
>   - use of a single drug is preferred, when possible, to avoid pharmacokinetic interactions
>   - newer agents include **vigabatrin, lamotrigine, topiramate, levetiracetam**.
> - Partial (focal) seizures: **carbamazepine, valproate**; alternatives include **clonazepam, phenytoin, gabapentin, pregabalin, lamotrigine, topiramate, levetircetam, zonisamide**.
> - Absence seizures: **ethosuximide, valproate, lamotrigine**:
>   - **valproate** is useful when absence seizures coexist with tonic–clonic seizures, because most other drugs used for tonic–clonic seizures can worsen absence seizures.
> - Myoclonic seizures and status epilepticus: **diazepam** intravenously or (in absence of accessible veins) rectally.
> - Neuropathic pain: for example **carbamazepine, gabapentin** (see Ch. 42).
> - To stabilise mood in mono- or bipolar affective disorder (as an alternative to **lithium**): for example **carbamazepine, valproate** (see Ch. 47).

MUSCLE SPASM AND MUSCLE RELAXANTS

Many diseases of the brain and spinal cord produce an increase in muscle tone, which can be painful and disabling. Spasticity resulting from birth injury or cerebral vascular disease, and the paralysis produced by spinal cord lesions, are examples. Multiple sclerosis is a neurodegenerative disease that is triggered by inflammatory attack on the CNS. When the disease has progressed for some years it can cause muscle stiffness and spasms as well as other symptoms such as pain, fatigue, difficulty passing urine and tremors. Local injury or inflammation, as in arthritis, can also cause muscle spasm, and chronic back pain is also often associated with local muscle spasm.

Certain centrally acting drugs are available that have the effect of reducing the background tone of the muscle without seriously affecting its ability to contract transiently under voluntary control. The distinction between voluntary movements and 'background tone' is not clear-cut, and the selectivity of those drugs is not complete. Postural control, for example, is usually jeopardised by centrally acting muscle relaxants. Furthermore, drugs that affect motor control generally produce rather widespread effects on the central nervous system, and drowsiness and confusion turn out to be very common side effects of these agents.

Baclofen (see Ch. 38) is a chlorophenyl derivative of GABA originally prepared as a lipophilic GABA-like agent in order to assist penetration of the blood–brain barrier, which is impermeable to GABA itself. Baclofen is a selective agonist at $GABA_B$ receptors (see Ch. 38). The antispastic action of baclofen is exerted mainly on the spinal cord, where it inhibits both monosynaptic and polysynaptic activation of motor neurons. It is effective when given by mouth, and is used in the treatment of spasticity associated with multiple sclerosis or spinal injury. However, it is ineffective in cerebral spasticity caused by birth injury.

Baclofen produces various unwanted effects, particularly drowsiness, motor incoordination and nausea, and it may also have behavioural effects. It is not useful in epilepsy.

Benzodiazepines are discussed in detail in Chapter 44. They produce muscle relaxation by an effect in the spinal cord. They are also anxiolytic.

Tizanidine is an α_2-adrenoceptor agonist that relieves spasticity associated with multiple sclerosis and spinal cord injury.

Sativex. For many years anecdotal evidence suggested that smoking **cannabis** (Ch. 19) relieves the painful muscle spasms associated with multiple sclerosis. **Sativex**, a cannabis extract containing Δ^9-tetrahydrocannabinol (also known as THC or **dronabinol**; see Ch. 19) and cannabidiol, is licensed in some countries as a treatment for spasticity in multiple sclerosis. It also has pain-relieving properties (see Chs 19 and 42).

Dantrolene acts peripherally rather than centrally to produce muscle relaxation (see Ch. 4).

Botulinum toxin (see Ch. 13) injected into a muscle, this neurotoxin causes long-lasting paralysis confined to the site of injection; its use to treat local muscle spasm is increasing. Its non-medicinal use as a 'beauty' treatment has become widespread.

REFERENCES AND FURTHER READING

General

Browne, T.R., Holmes, G.L., 2008. Handbook of Epilepsy. Lippincott, Williams & Wilkins, Philadelphia. (*A compact textbook covering most areas of epilepsy and its treatment*)

Pathogenesis and types of epilepsy

Deblaere, K., Achten, E., 2008. Structural magnetic resonance imaging in epilepsy. Eur. Radiol. 18, 119–129. (*Describes the use of brain imaging in the diagnosis of epilepsy*)

Khosravani, H., Altier, C., Simms, B., et al., 2004. Gating effects of mutations in the Ca$_v$3.2 T-type calcium channel associated with childhood absence epilepsy. J. Biol. Chem. 279, 9681–9684. (*Study showing that calcium channel mutations seen in childhood absence seizures cause abnormal neuronal discharges in transgenic mice*)

Pandolfo, M., 2011. Genetics of epilepsy. Semin. Neurol. 31, 506–518.

Shin, H.-S., 2006. T-type Ca^{2+} channels and absence epilepsy. Cell Calcium 40, 191–196.

Weber, Y.G., Lerche, H., 2008. Genetic mechanisms in idiopathic epilepsies. Dev. Med. Child Neurol. 50, 648–654. (*Reviews how mutations in voltage- and ligand-gated ion channels are associated with idiopathic epilepsy syndromes*)

Antiepileptic drugs

Azar, N.J., Abou-Khalil, B.W., 2008. Considerations in the choice of an antiepileptic drug in the treatment of epilepsy. Semin. Neurol. 28, 305–316. (*Describes the current Food and Drug Administration approval for antiepileptic drug use in the USA*)

Bialer, M., White, H.S., 2010. Key factors in the discovery and development of new antiepileptic drugs. Nat. Rev. Drug Discov. 9, 68–82. (*Interesting account of new avenues for antiepileptic drug discovery*)

Macleod, S., Appleton, R.E., 2007. The new antiepileptic drugs. Arch. Dis. Child. Educ. Pract. Ed. 92, 182–188. (*Focuses on the clinical usefulness of newer antiepileptic drugs*)

Antipsychotic drugs **46**

OVERVIEW

In this chapter we focus on schizophrenia and the drugs used to treat it. We start by describing the illness and what is known of its pathogenesis, including the various neurochemical hypotheses and their relation to the actions of the main types of antipsychotic drugs that are in use or in development. Further information can be found in Gross & Geyer (2012).

INTRODUCTION

Psychotic illnesses include various disorders, but the term antipsychotic drugs – previously known as *neuroleptic drugs*, *antischizophrenic drugs* or *major tranquillisers* – conventionally refers to those used to treat schizophrenia, one of the most common and debilitating forms of mental illness. These same drugs are also used to treat mania (Ch. 47) and other acute behavioural disturbances (see clinical box, p. 568). Pharmacologically, most are dopamine receptor antagonists, although many of them also act on other targets, particularly 5-hydroxytryptamine (5-HT) receptors, which may contribute to their clinical efficacy. Existing drugs have many drawbacks in terms of their efficacy and side effects. Gradual improvements have been achieved with newer drugs, but radical new approaches will require a better understanding of the causes and underlying pathology of the disease, which are still poorly understood.[1]

THE NATURE OF SCHIZOPHRENIA

Schizophrenia[2] (see Stahl, 2008) affects about 1% of the population. It is one of the most important forms of psychiatric illness, because it affects young people, is often chronic and is usually highly disabling.[3] There is a strong hereditary factor in its aetiology, and evidence suggestive of a fundamental biological disorder. The main clinical features of the disease are as follows.

Positive symptoms
- Delusions (often paranoid in nature).
- Hallucinations (often in the form of voices, which may be exhortatory in their message).
- Thought disorder (comprising wild trains of thought, delusions of grandeur, garbled sentences and irrational conclusions).
- Abnormal, disorganised behaviour (such as stereotyped movements, disorientation and occasionally aggressive behaviours).
- Catatonia (can be apparent as immobility or purposeless motor activity).

Negative symptoms
- Withdrawal from social contacts.
- Flattening of emotional responses.
- Anhedonia (an inability to experience pleasure).
- Reluctance to perform everyday tasks.

Cognition
- Deficits in cognitive function (e.g. attention, memory).

In addition, anxiety, guilt, depression and self punishment are often present, leading to suicide attempts in up to 50% of cases, about 10% of which are successful. The clinical phenotype varies greatly, particularly with respect to the balance between positive and negative symptoms, and this may have a bearing on the efficacy of antipsychotic drugs in individual cases. Schizophrenia can present dramatically, usually in young people, with predominantly positive features such as hallucinations, delusions and uncontrollable behaviour, or more insidiously in older patients with negative features such as flat mood and social withdrawal. The latter may be more debilitated than those with a florid presentation, and the prognosis is generally worse. There is debate about whether cognitive impairment can develop even before the onset of other symptoms. Schizophrenia can follow a relapsing and remitting course, or be chronic and progressive, particularly in cases with a later onset. Chronic schizophrenia used to account for most of the patients in long-stay psychiatric hospitals; following the closure of many of these in the UK, it now accounts for many of society's outcasts.

A characteristic feature of schizophrenia is a defect in 'selective attention'. Whereas a normal individual quickly accommodates to stimuli of a familiar or inconsequential nature, and responds only to stimuli that are unexpected or significant, the ability of schizophrenic patients to discriminate between significant and insignificant stimuli seems to be impaired. Thus, the ticking of a clock may command as much attention as the words of a companion; a chance thought, which a normal person would dismiss as inconsequential, may become an irresistible imperative.

---

[1]In this respect, the study of schizophrenia lags some years behind that of Alzheimer's disease (Ch. 40), where understanding of the pathogenesis has progressed rapidly to the point where promising drug targets have been identified. On the other hand, pragmatists can argue that drugs against Alzheimer's disease are so far only marginally effective, whereas current antipsychotic drugs deliver great benefits even though we do not quite know how they work.

[2]Schizophrenia is a condition where the patient exhibits symptoms of psychosis (e.g. delusions, hallucinations and disorganized behaviour). Psychotic episodes may also occur as a result of taking certain recreational drugs (see Ch. 48); as an adverse effect of drug treatment, for example steroid-induced psychoses; or in disorders such as mania, depression (see Ch. 47) and Alzheimer's disease (see Ch. 40).

[3]A compelling account of what it is to suffer from schizophrenia is contained in Kean (2009) Schizophrenia Bulletin 35, 1034-1036. The author is now a pharmacology graduate.

AETIOLOGY AND PATHOGENESIS OF SCHIZOPHRENIA

GENETIC AND ENVIRONMENTAL FACTORS

The causes of schizophrenia remain unclear but involve a combination of genetic and environmental factors. Thus a person may have a genetic makeup that predisposes them to schizophrenia, but exposure to environmental factors may be required for schizophrenia to develop.

The disease shows a strong, but incomplete, hereditary tendency. In first-degree relatives, the risk is about 10%, but even in monozygotic (identical) twins, one of whom has schizophrenia, the probability of the other being affected is only about 50%, pointing towards the importance of environmental factors. Genetic linkage studies have identified more than 100 potential susceptibility genes (see Aberg et al., 2013; Ripke et al. 2014), but it is clear that no single gene is responsible. There are significant associations between polymorphisms in individual genes and the likelihood of an individual developing schizophrenia but there appears to be no single gene that has an overriding influence. Some of the genes implicated in schizophrenia are also associated with bipolar disorder (see Ch. 47).

▼ The most robust associations are with genes that control neuronal development, synaptic connectivity and glutamatergic neurotransmission. These include *neuregulin*, *dysbindin*, *DISC-1*, *TCF4* and *NOTCH4*. Transgenic mice that underexpress neuregulin 1, a protein involved in synaptic development and plasticity and which controls NMDA receptor expression, show a phenotype resembling human schizophrenia in certain respects. Malfunction of NMDA receptors is further implicated by genetic association with the genes for D-amino acid oxidase (DAAO), the enzyme responsible for metabolising D-serine, an allosteric modulator of NMDA receptors (see Ch. 38), and for DAAO activator (G72). Dysbindin is located in postsynaptic density domains and may be involved in tethering receptors including NMDA receptors. DISC-1 – which stands for **d**isrupted **in s**chizophrenia-1 – is a protein that associates with cytoskeletal proteins and is involved with cell migration, neurite outgrowth and receptor trafficking. Population genetic studies have suggested that *NOTCH4*, a developmentally expressed gene, and TCF-4, a gene also associated with mental retardation, are strongly associated with susceptibility for schizophrenia (Lennertz et al., 2011; Ikeda et al., 2013) but their precise roles in its aetiology remain to be elucidated. Among other suggested susceptibility genes, some (such as the genes for monoamine oxidase A [MAO-A], tyrosine hydroxylase and the D_2 dopamine receptor) are involved in monoamine transmission in the CNS. However, the weight of current evidence seems to suggest that schizophrenia may result from abnormal glutamatergic transmission, involving a decrease in NMDA receptor function (see p. 561).

Some environmental influences early in development have been identified as possible predisposing factors, particularly maternal virus infections. This and other evidence suggests that schizophrenia is associated with a neurodevelopmental disorder affecting mainly the cerebral cortex and occurring in the first few months of prenatal development. This view is supported by brain-imaging studies showing cortical atrophy apparent in the early course of the disease which may increase with time and correlate with the progression of the disorder (van Haren et al., 2007). Studies of postmortem schizophrenic brains show evidence of misplaced cortical neurons with abnormal morphology. Other environmental factors such as cannabis consumption in adolescence and early adulthood (see Chs 19 and 48) may also reveal schizophrenia.

THE NEUROANATOMICAL AND NEUROCHEMICAL BASIS OF SCHIZOPHRENIA

Different symptoms of schizophrenia appear to result from malfunctions in different neuronal circuits. Changes in the mesolimbic pathway (the neuronal projection from the ventral tegmental area (VTA) to the nucleus accumbens, amygdala and hippocampus) being associated with positive symptoms, whereas negative symptoms are associated with changes in the mesocortical pathway (the projection from the VTA to areas of the prefrontal cortex).

The main neurotransmitters thought to be involved in the pathogenesis of schizophrenia are dopamine and glutamate.

Dopamine

The original dopamine theory of schizophrenia was proposed by Carlson – awarded a Nobel Prize in 2000 – on the basis of indirect pharmacological evidence in humans and experimental animals. **Amphetamine** releases dopamine in the brain and can produce in humans a behavioural syndrome reminiscent of an acute schizophrenic episode. Also, hallucinations are a side effect of levodopa and dopamine agonists used for Parkinson's disease (see Ch. 40). In animals, dopamine release causes a specific pattern of stereotyped behaviour that resembles the repetitive behaviours sometimes seen in schizophrenic patients. Potent D_2-receptor agonists, such as **bromocriptine**, produce similar effects in animals, and these drugs, like amphetamine, exacerbate the symptoms of schizophrenic patients. Furthermore, dopamine antagonists and drugs that block neuronal dopamine storage (e.g. **reserpine**) are effective in controlling the positive symptoms of schizophrenia, and in preventing amphetamine-induced behavioural changes.

▼ It is now believed that positive symptoms result from *overactivity* in the mesolimbic dopaminergic pathway activating D_2 receptors (for a more detailed description of the dopamine pathways in the brain, see Ch. 39) whereas negative symptoms may result from a *decreased activity* in the mesocortical dopaminergic pathway where D_1 receptors predominate. Other dopaminergic pathways in the brain (i.e. nigrostriatal and tuberoinfundibular; see Ch. 39) appear to function normally in schizophrenia.

There is a strong correlation between antipsychotic potency in reducing positive symptoms and activity in blocking D_2 receptors (Fig. 46.1) and receptor-imaging studies have shown that clinical efficacy of antipsychotic drugs is consistently achieved when D_2-receptor occupancy reaches about 80%.[4] Furthermore, brain imaging studies have revealed an increased dopamine synthesis and release in the striatum of schizophrenic patients (Laruelle et al., 1999).[5] Similar changes have also been reported in non-schizophrenic close relatives indicating that such changes may indicate predisposition to schizophrenia rather than the exhibition of symptoms. Injection of amphetamine caused dopamine release that was greater by a factor of two or more in schizophrenic subjects compared with control subjects. The effect was greatest in schizophrenic individuals during acute attacks, and absent during spontaneous remissions – clear evidence linking dopamine release to the symptomatology.

Thus, therapeutically it might be desirable to *inhibit* dopaminergic transmission in the limbic system yet *enhance* dopaminergic transmission in the prefrontal cortex (how this might be achieved is discussed further below, p. 561).

---

[4]There are, however, exceptions to this simple rule. Up to one-third of schizophrenic patients fail to respond even when D_2-receptor blockade exceeds 90%, and clozapine (see Table 46.1) can be effective at much lower levels of block.

[5]An increase in dopamine receptor density in schizophrenia has been reported in some studies, but not consistently, and the interpretation is complicated by the fact that chronic antipsychotic drug treatment is known to increase dopamine receptor expression.

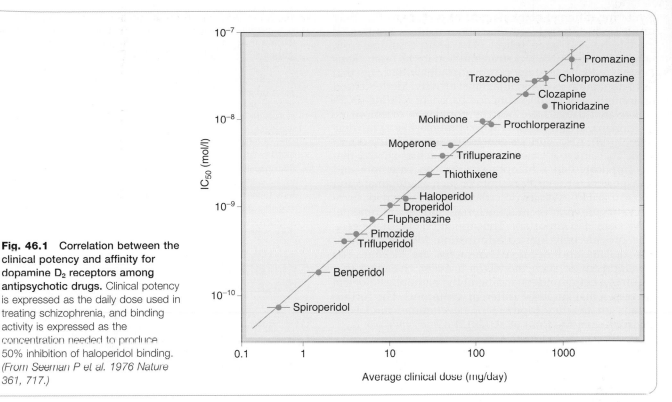

Fig. 46.1 Correlation between the clinical potency and affinity for dopamine D_2 receptors among antipsychotic drugs. Clinical potency is expressed as the daily dose used in treating schizophrenia, and binding activity is expressed as the concentration needed to produce 50% inhibition of haloperidol binding. *(From Seeman P et al. 1976 Nature 361, 717.)*

Glutamate

In humans, NMDA receptor antagonists such as **phencyclidine**, **ketamine** and **dizocilpine** (Ch. 38) can produce positive, negative and cognitive deficit symptoms – in contrast to amphetamine, which produces only positive symptoms. In the brains from schizophrenic patients expression of the glutamate uptake transporter VGLUT1 is reduced, which may indicate a disruption of glutamatergic nerve terminals. It has therefore been postulated that schizophrenia may result from disruption of glutamatergic neurotransmission, evident as a reduction in the function of NMDA receptors (the NMDA hypofunction hypothesis; see Coyle et al., 2012). Consistent with this hypothesis, transgenic mice in which NMDA receptor expression is reduced (not abolished, because this is fatal) show stereotypic behaviours and reduced social interaction that are features of human schizophrenia and that respond to antipsychotic drugs.

▼ Glutamatergic neurons and GABAergic neurons play complex roles in controlling the level of activity in neuronal pathways involved in schizophrenia. NMDA receptor hypofunction is thought to *reduce* the level of activity in mesocortical dopaminergic neurons. This would result in a decrease in dopamine release in the prefrontal cortex and could thus give rise to negative symptoms of schizophrenia. NMDA receptor hypofunction in the cortex may affect GABAergic interneurons and alter cortical processing, giving rise to cognitive impairment. In addition, NMDA-receptor hypofunction on GABAergic neurons would reduce inhibition of the excitatory cortical input to the VTA and thus *enhance* activity in the mesolimbic dopaminergic pathway. Thus NMDA-receptor hypofunction could give rise to enhanced dopamine release in limbic areas such as the nucleus accumbens, resulting in the production of positive symptoms.

Given the evidence that schizophrenic symptoms may be due to a reduction in NMDA-receptor function, efforts have been made to develop new drugs to enhance NMDA-receptor function but not to a level where it becomes neurotoxic (see Ch. 40), e.g. by activating the facilitatory glycine site on the NMDA receptor (see Ch. 38) with

an agonist or by raising extracellular glycine levels by inhibiting the GlyT1 transporter.[6]

Other glutamate pathways thought to be involved in schizophrenia are the corticostriatal, thalamocortical, corticothalamic and corticobrainstem pathways. The thalamus normally functions as a sensory filter to limit unnecessary sensory input to the cortex. Disruption of the normal inputs to the thalamus, for example from a reduction in glutamatergic or GABAergic transmission, disables this 'sensory gate' function, allowing uninhibited input to reach the cortex. The role of the thalamus in schizophrenia is reviewed by Sim et al. (2006).

Neurodegeneration

Factors such as structural abnormalities in the brains of schizophrenics and progression of the disease – absence of symptoms in early childhood, the likelihood of positive symptoms becoming apparent before negative symptoms, progressive worsening, reduced responsiveness to drugs with time and the development of dementia – are all suggestive of ongoing neurodegeneration in the disease. The causes of such neurodegeneration are unclear at present but may involve glutamate-induced excitotoxicity (see Ch. 40).

The hope is that a fuller understanding of the altered function of glutamate transmission in schizophrenia will lead to the development of new, improved antipsychotic drugs.

Animal models

There is a need for the development of animal models of schizophrenia that simulate the positive, negative and cognitive deficit components of this disorder. Schizophrenia presents as a heterogeneous disorder with sufferers

---

[6]Sadly the GlyT1 transporter inhibitor **bitopertin** failed in clinical trials as an antipsychotic, although it may still have potential as a treatment for obsessive–compulsive disorder.

exhibiting different combinations of symptoms that may result from different neuronal abnormalities. Traditional models by and large reflect behaviours resulting from heightened dopaminergic transmission in the brain. Thus they were likely to show positive results with drugs that have dopamine receptor antagonist activity. Models based on inhibition of NMDA function by phencyclidine (PCP) and related drugs have become popular in recent years. In humans, PCP causes a schizophrenia-like syndrome (see Ch. 48). Also, various genetic models are being examined. These have focused on proteins such as DISC-1 that are implicated in schizophrenia and on receptors and transporters for neurotransmitters such as glutamate and dopamine. However, as described above, the genetic basis of schizophrenia is multifactorial and environmental factors are also important. Thus mutation of a single gene may provide only limited information. Models of cognitive deficits and negative symptoms are lacking. The development of such models is a major challenge that requires a better understanding of the pathophysiological processes that underlie different symptoms. For further details on the development of new animal models of schizophrenia see Pratt et al. (2012).

The nature of schizophrenia

- Psychotic illness characterised by delusions, hallucinations and thought disorder (positive symptoms), together with social withdrawal and flattening of emotional responses (negative symptoms), and cognitive impairment.
- Acute episodes (mainly positive symptoms) frequently recur and may develop into chronic schizophrenia, with predominantly negative symptoms.
- Incidence is about 1% of the population, with a significant hereditary component. Genetic linkage studies suggest involvement of multiple genes, but no single 'schizophrenia gene'.
- Pharmacological evidence is generally consistent with dopamine dysregulation and glutamate underactivity hypotheses, supported by biochemical findings, clinical efficacy and imaging studies.

ANTIPSYCHOTIC DRUGS

CLASSIFICATION OF ANTIPSYCHOTIC DRUGS

More than 40 different antipsychotic drugs are available for clinical use. These have been divided into two groups – those drugs that were originally developed (e.g. **chlorpromazine**, **haloperidol** and many similar compounds), often referred to as *first-generation*, *typical* or *conventional antipsychotic drugs*, and more recently developed agents (e.g. **clozapine**, **risperidone**), which are termed *second-generation* or *atypical antipsychotic drugs*. Table 46.1 summarises the main drugs that are in clinical use.

▼ The term 'atypical' has been widely used but not clearly defined. In effect, it refers to the diminished tendency of later compounds to cause unwanted motor side effects, but it is also used to describe compounds with a different pharmacological profile from first-generation compounds. In practice, however, it often serves – not very usefully – to distinguish the large group of similar first-generation dopamine antagonists from the more diverse group of later compounds described below.

The therapeutic activity of the prototype drug, **chlorpromazine**, in schizophrenic patients was discovered through the acute observations of a French surgeon, Laborit, in 1947. He tested various substances, including **promethazine**, for their ability to alleviate signs of stress in patients undergoing surgery, and concluded that promethazine had a calming effect that was different from mere sedation. Elaboration of the phenothiazine structure led to chlorpromazine, the antipsychotic effect of which was demonstrated in man, at Laborit's instigation, by Delay and Deniker in 1953. This drug was unique in controlling the symptoms of psychotic patients. The clinical efficacy of phenothiazines was discovered long before their mechanism was guessed at (let alone understood).

Pharmacological investigation showed that phenothiazines, the first-generation antipsychotic agents, block many different mediators, including histamine, catecholamines, acetylcholine and 5-HT, and this multiplicity of actions led to the trade name Largactil for chlorpromazine. It is now clear (see Fig. 46.1) that antagonism of dopamine is the main determinant of antipsychotic action.

Classification of antipsychotic drugs

- Main categories are:
  - first-generation ('typical', 'classical' or 'conventional') antipsychotics (e.g. **chlorpromazine**, **haloperidol**, **fluphenazine**, **flupentixol**, **clopentixol**)
  - second-generation ('atypical') antipsychotics (e.g. **clozapine**, **risperidone**, **sertindole**, **quetiapine**, **amisulpride**, **aripiprazole**, **zotepine**, **ziprasidone**).
- Distinction between first- and second-generation drugs is not clearly defined but rests on:
  - receptor profile
  - incidence of extrapyramidal side effects (less in second-generation group)
  - efficacy (specifically of **clozapine**) in 'treatment-resistant' group of patients
  - efficacy against negative symptoms.

CLINICAL EFFICACY

The clinical efficacy of antipsychotic drugs in enabling schizophrenic patients to lead more normal lives has been demonstrated in many controlled trials. The inpatient population (mainly chronic schizophrenics) of mental hospitals declined sharply in the 1950s and 1960s. The introduction of antipsychotic drugs was a significant enabling factor, as well as the changing public and professional attitudes towards hospitalisation of the mentally ill.

Antipsychotic drugs have severe drawbacks that include:

- Not all schizophrenic patients respond to drug therapy. It is recommended to try **clozapine** in patients who are resistant to other antipsychotic drugs. The 30% of patients who do not respond are classed as 'treatment resistant' and present a major therapeutic problem. The reason for the difference between responsive and unresponsive patients is unknown at present, although there is some evidence (not conclusive) that polymorphisms within the family of dopamine and 5-HT receptors may be involved.
- While they control the positive symptoms (thought disorder, hallucinations, delusions, etc.) effectively, most are ineffective in relieving the negative

Table 46.1 Characteristics of some major antipsychotic drugs

Drug	Receptor affinity						Main side effects				Notes
	D_1	D_2	α_1	H_1	mACh	$5\text{-}HT_{2A}$	EPS	Sed	Hypo	Other	
Chlorpromazine	++	++	+++	+++	++	+++	++	+++	++	Increased prolactin (gynaecomastia)	Phenothiazine class
										Hypothermia Anticholinergic effects Hypersensitivity reactions	Fluphenazine, trifluperazine are similar but: • do not cause jaundice • cause less hypotension • cause more EPS
										Obstructive jaundice	Fluphenazine available as depot preparation
											Pericyazine, pipotiazine cause less EPS probably due to their greater muscarinic antagonist actions
Haloperidol	++	+++	++	+	−	++	+++	−	+	As chlorpromazine but does not cause jaundice	Butyrophenone class
										Fewer anticholinergic side effects	Widely used antipsychotic drug
											Strong EPS tendency
											Available as depot preparation
Flupentixol	+++	+++		+++	−	+	++	+	+	Increased prolactin (gynaecomastia)	Thioxanthine class
										Restlessness	Clopentixol is similar
											Available as depot preparation
Sulpiride	−	++	−	−	−	−	+			Increased prolactin (gynaecomastia)	Benzamide class
											Selective D_2/D_3 antagonist
											Less EPS than haloperidol (reason for this unclear, but could result from action at D_3 or very weak partial agonism at D_2)
											Increases alertness in apathetic patients
											Poorly absorbed
											Amisulpride and pimozide (long-acting) are similar
Clozapine	+	+	+++	++++	++	+++	−	++	++	Risk of agranulocytosis (~1%): regular blood counts required	Dibenzodiazepine class
										Seizures	No EPS (first second-generation antipsychotic)

Table 46.1 Continued

Drug	Receptor affinity						Main side effects					Notes
	D_1	D_2	α_1	H_1	mACh	5-HT$_{2A}$	EPS	Sed	Hypo	Other	
Clozapine, cont'd										Salivation	Shows efficacy in 'treatment-resistant' patients and reduces incidence of suicide
										Anticholinergic side effects	Effective against negative and positive symptoms
										Weight gain	Olanzapine is somewhat less sedative, without risk of agranulocytosis, but questionable efficacy in treatment-resistant patients
Risperidone	+	+++	+++	++	−	++++ (IA?)	+	++	++	Weight gain	Significant risk of EPS
										EPS at high doses	?Effective against negative symptoms
										Hypotension	Potent on D_4 receptors
											Available as depot preparation
											Paliperidone is a metabolite of risperidone
Quetiapine	+	+	+++	+++	+	+	−	++	++	Tachycardia	Low incidence of EPS
										Drowsiness	No increase in prolactin secretion
										Dry mouth	5-HT$_{1A}$ partial agonist
										Constipation	Short-acting (plasma half-life ~6 h)
										Weight gain	
Aripiprazole	+	++++ (PA)	++	++	−	+++	−	+	−	−	Long-acting (plasma half-life ~3 days)
											Unusual D_2 partial agonist profile may account for paucity of side effects
											Also a 5HT$_{1A}$ partial agonist
											No effect on prolactin secretion
											No weight gain
											Available as a depot preparation
Ziprasidone	++	+++	+++	++	−	++++	+	−	+	Tiredness	Low incidence of EPS
										Nausea	No weight gain
											?Effective against negative symptoms
											Short-acting (plasma half-life ~8 h) but a depot preparation is available

+, pKi 5–7; ++, pKi 7–8; +++, pKi 8–9; +++, pKi >9.

5-HT$_{1A}$, 5-HT$_{2A}$, 5-hydroxytryptamine types 1A and 2A receptors; α_1, α_1 adrenoceptor; D_1, D_2, D_3, D_4, dopamine types 1, 2, 3 and 4 receptor, respectively; ECG, electrocardiograph; EPS, extrapyramidal side effects; H$_1$, histamine type 1 receptor; Hypo, hypotension; mACh, muscarinic acetylcholine receptor; IA, inverse agonist; PA, partial agonist; Sed, sedation.

Table based on data contained in Guide to Pharmacology (www.guidetopharmacology.org/) and NIMH Psychoactive Drug Screening Program database (http://pdsp.med.unc.edu/). Where available, data obtained on human receptors are given.

symptoms (emotional flattening, social isolation) and cognitive impairment.

- They induce a range of side effects that include extrapyramidal motor, endocrine and sedative effects (see Table 46.1) that can be severe and limit patient compliance.
- They may shorten survival through cardiac (pro-arrhythmic) effects (see Ch. 21).

Second-generation antipsychotic drugs were believed to overcome these shortcomings to some degree. However, a meta-analysis (Leucht et al., 2009) concluded that only some of the second-generation antipsychotic drugs examined, showed better overall efficacy. There is a definite need for the development of new treatments.

Abrupt cessation of antipsychotic drug administration may lead to a rapid onset psychotic episode distinct from the underlying illness.

PHARMACOLOGICAL PROPERTIES

DOPAMINE RECEPTORS

The classification of dopamine receptors in the central nervous system is discussed in Chapter 39 (see Table 39.1). There are five subtypes, which fall into two functional classes: the D_1 type, comprising D_1 and D_5, and the D_2 type, comprising D_2, D_3 and D_4. Antipsychotic drugs owe their therapeutic effects mainly to blockade of D_2 receptors.[7] As stated above, antipsychotic effects require about 80% block of D_2 receptors. The first-generation compounds show some preference for D_2 over D_1 receptors, whereas some of the later agents (e.g. **sulpiride, amisulpride, remoxipride**) are highly selective for D_2 receptors. D_2 antagonists that dissociate rapidly from the receptor (e.g. **quetiapine**) and D_2 partial agonists (e.g. **aripiprazole**) have been introduced in an attempt to reduce extrapyramidal motor side effects (see p. 566).

It is the antagonism of D_2 receptors in the mesolimbic pathway that is believed to relieve the positive symptoms of schizophrenia. Unfortunately, systemically administered antipsychotic drugs do not discriminate between D_2 receptors in distinct brain regions and D_2 receptors in other brain pathways will also be blocked. Thus, antipsychotic drugs produce unwanted motor effects (block of D_2 receptors in the nigrostriatal pathway), enhance prolactin secretion (block of D_2 receptors in the tuberoinfundibular pathway), reduce pleasure (block of D_2 receptors in the reward component of the mesolimbic pathway) and perhaps even worsen the negative symptoms of schizophrenia (block of D_2 receptors in the prefrontal cortex, although these are only expressed at a low density – D_1 receptors being in greater abundance). While all antipsychotic drugs block D_2 receptors and should therefore in theory induce all of these unwanted effects, some have additional pharmacological activity (e.g. mACh receptor antagonism and 5-HT_{2A} receptor antagonism) that, to varying degrees, ameliorate unwanted effects. 5-HT_{2A} antagonism may also help to alleviate the negative and cognitive impairments of schizophrenia.

Antipsychotic drugs have classically been thought to have a delayed onset to their therapeutic actions, even though their dopamine receptor-blocking action is immediate. This view has, however, been called into question (Kapur et al., 2005; Leucht et al., 2005). In animal studies, chronic antipsychotic drug administration does produce compensatory changes in the brain, for example a reduction in the activity of dopaminergic neurons and proliferation of dopamine receptors, detectable as an increase in haloperidol binding, with a pharmacological supersensitivity to dopamine reminiscent of the phenomenon of denervation supersensitivity (Ch. 12). The mechanism(s) of these delayed effects are poorly understood. They are likely to contribute to the development of unwanted *tardive dyskinesias*. The sedating effect of antipsychotic drugs is immediate, allowing them to be used in acute behavioural emergencies.

Mechanism of action of antipsychotic drugs

- Most antipsychotic drugs are antagonists or partial agonists at D_2 dopamine receptors, but they also block a variety of other receptors.
- Antipsychotic potency generally runs parallel to activity on D_2 receptors, but activities at other receptors (e.g. 5-HT_{2A} and muscarinic) may reduce extrapyramidal side effects.
- Activity at muscarinic, H_1 and α receptors may determine unwanted side effect profile.
- Imaging studies suggest that therapeutic effect requires about 80% occupancy of D_2 receptors.

5 HYDROXYTRYPTAMINE RECEPTORS

The idea that 5-HT dysfunction could be involved in schizophrenia has drifted in and out of favour many times (see Busatto & Kerwin, 1997). It was originally based on the fact that LSD, a partial agonist at 5-HT_{2A} receptors (see Chs 15 and 48), produces hallucinations. Nowadays, conventional wisdom is that 5-HT is not directly involved in the pathogenesis of schizophrenia. Nevertheless, pharmacological manipulation of 5-HT receptor activity, combined with D_2 receptor antagonism, has resulted in new drugs with improved therapeutic profiles.[8] There is a plethora of 5-HT receptors (see Chs 15 and 39), with disparate functions in the body. It is the 5-HT_{2A} receptor and, to a lesser extent, the 5-HT_{1A} receptor that are important in the treatment of schizophrenia.

5-HT_{2A} receptors are G_i/G_o-coupled receptors and their activation produces neuronal inhibition (through decreased neuronal excitability at the soma and decreased transmitter release at the nerve terminals; see Ch. 39). In this way, in the nigrostriatal pathway, 5-HT_{2A} receptors control the release of dopamine. Drugs with 5-HT_{2A} antagonist properties (e.g. **olanzapine** and risperidone)

---

[7]The D_4 receptor attracted attention on account of the high degree of genetic polymorphism that it shows in human subjects, and because some of the newer antipsychotic drugs (e.g. clozapine) have a high affinity for this receptor subtype. However, a specific D_4-receptor antagonist proved ineffective in clinical trials.

[8]Early antipsychotic drugs (e.g. chlorpromazine) had actions at various receptors but also had unwanted side effects that resulted from activity at other receptors. Towards the end of the 20th century, drug development, not just of antipsychotic drugs, was focused largely on developing agents with a single action with the intention of reducing unwanted side effects. This philosophy drove the search for selective D_4-receptor antagonists, which proved ineffective. What is now apparent is that drugs with selected multiple actions (e.g. a combination of D_2 antagonism and 5-HT_{2A} antagonism) may have a better therapeutic profile.

enhance dopamine release in the striatum by reducing the inhibitory effect of 5-HT. This will reduce extrapyramidal side effects (see below). In contrast, in the mesolimbic pathway, the combined effects of D_2 and 5-HT$_{2A}$ antagonism are thought to counteract the increased dopamine function that gives rise to positive symptoms of schizophrenia. Further, enhancing both dopamine and glutamate release in the mesocortical circuit, 5-HT$_{2A}$ receptor antagonism may improve the negative symptoms of schizophrenia (Stahl, 2008).

5-HT$_{1A}$ receptors are somatodendritic autoreceptors that inhibit 5-HT release (see Ch. 39). Antipsychotic drugs that are agonists or partial agonists at 5-HT$_{1A}$ receptors (e.g. **quetiapine**; see Table 46.1) may work by decreasing 5-HT release thus enhancing dopamine release in the striatum and prefrontal cortex.

The concept of 5-HT receptors as targets for novel antipsychotic drug development is discussed at the end of this chapter.

MUSCARINIC ACETYLCHOLINE RECEPTORS

Some phenothiazine antipsychotic drugs (e.g. **pericyazine**) have been reported to produce fewer extrapyramidal side effects than others, and this was thought to correlate with their muscarinic antagonist actions. Also, some second-generation drugs possess muscarinic antagonist properties (e.g. olanzapine). In the striatum, dopaminergic nerve terminals are thought to innervate cholinergic interneurons that express inhibitory D_2 receptors (Pisani et al., 2007). It is suggested that there is normally a balance between D_2 receptor activation and muscarinic receptor activation. Blocking D_2 receptors in the striatum with an antipsychotic agent will result in enhanced acetylcholine release on to muscarinic receptors, thus producing extrapyramidal side effects, which are counteracted if the D_2 antagonist also has muscarinic antagonist activity. Maintaining the dopamine/acetylcholine balance was also the rationale for the use of the muscarinic antagonist **benztropine** to reduce extrapyramidal effects of antipsychotic drugs (see Ch. 40). Muscarinic antagonist activity does, however, induce side effects such as constipation, dry mouth and blurred vision.

UNWANTED EFFECTS

EXTRAPYRAMIDAL MOTOR DISTURBANCES

Antipsychotic drugs produce two main kinds of motor disturbance in humans: *acute dystonias* and *tardive dyskinesias*, collectively termed *extrapyramidal side effects*. These all result directly or indirectly from D_2 receptor blockade in the nigrostriatal pathway. Extrapyramidal side effects constitute one of the main disadvantages of first-generation antipsychotic drugs. Second-generation drugs were thought to have less tendency to produce extrapyramidal side effects. However, a long-term study of olanzapine, risperidone, quetiapine and **ziprasidone** concluded that they too can induce extrapyramidal side effects (see Lieberman & Stroup, 2011). Even aripiprazole, which is a D_2 partial agonist, has been reported to produce this unwanted effect.

Acute dystonias are involuntary movements (restlessness, muscle spasms, protruding tongue, fixed upward gaze, neck muscle spasm), often accompanied by symptoms of Parkinson's disease (Ch. 40). They occur commonly in the first few weeks, often declining with time, and are reversible on stopping drug treatment. The timing

is consistent with block of the dopaminergic nigrostriatal pathway. Concomitant block of muscarinic receptors and 5-HT$_{2A}$ receptors mitigates the motor effects of dopamine receptor antagonists (see above).

Tardive dyskinesia (see Klawans et al., 1988) develops after months or years (hence 'tardive') in 20–40% of patients treated with first-generation antipsychotic drugs, and is one of the main problems of antipsychotic therapy. Its seriousness lies in the fact that it is a disabling and often irreversible condition, which often gets worse when antipsychotic therapy is stopped and is resistant to treatment. The syndrome consists of involuntary movements, often of the face and tongue, but also of the trunk and limbs, which can be severely disabling. It resembles that seen after prolonged treatment of Parkinson's disease with **levodopa** (see Ch. 40). The incidence depends greatly on drug, dose and age (being commonest in patients over 50).

▼ There are several theories about the mechanism of tardive dyskinesia (see Casey, 1995). One is that it is associated with a gradual increase in the number of D_2 receptors in the striatum, which is less marked during treatment with second-generation than with first-generation antipsychotic drugs. Another possibility is that chronic block of inhibitory dopamine receptors enhances catecholamine and/or glutamate release in the striatum, leading to excitotoxic neurodegeneration (Ch. 40).

Drugs that rapidly dissociate from D_2 receptors (e.g. clozapine, olanzapine, **sertindole**) induce less severe extrapyramidal side effects. A possible explanation for this (see Kapur & Seeman, 2001) is that with a rapidly dissociating compound, a brief surge of dopamine can effectively overcome the block by competition (see Ch. 2), whereas with a slowly dissociating compound, the level of block takes a long time to respond to the presence of endogenous dopamine, and is in practice non-competitive. Adverse motor effects may be avoided if fractional receptor occupation falls during physiological surges of dopamine. An extension of this idea is that perhaps a little D_2 receptor activation may be beneficial. This could be produced, for example, by drugs that are D_2 partial agonists (e.g. aripiprazole) in contrast to simple antagonists. It is thought that partial agonists reduce D_2 hyperactivation in the mesolimbic pathway, thus alleviating positive symptoms of schizophrenia, but provide enough D_2 receptor stimulation in the mesocortical pathway to prevent negative symptoms, and in the nigrostriatal pathway to lower the incidence of extrapyramidal side effects. Newer D_2 partial agonists were being developed, although questions about their efficacy and safety have arisen.

ENDOCRINE EFFECTS

Dopamine, released in the median eminence by neurons of the tuberohypophyseal pathway (see Chs 33 and 39), acts physiologically via D_2 receptors to inhibit prolactin secretion. Blocking D_2 receptors by antipsychotic drugs can therefore increase the plasma prolactin concentration (Fig. 46.2), resulting in breast swelling, pain and lactation (known as 'galactorrhea'), which can occur in men as well as in women. As can be seen from Figure 46.2, the effect is maintained during chronic antipsychotic administration, without any habituation. Other less pronounced endocrine changes have also been reported, including a decrease of growth hormone secretion, but these, unlike the prolactin response, are believed to be relatively unimportant clinically. Because of its D_2 receptor partial agonist action aripiprazole, unlike other antipsychotic drugs, reduces prolactin secretion.

OTHER UNWANTED EFFECTS

Most antipsychotic drugs block a variety of receptors, particularly acetylcholine (muscarinic), histamine (H_1), noradrenaline (α) and 5-HT receptors (Table 46.1). This gives rise to a wide range of side effects.

Antipsychotic-induced motor disturbances

- Major problem of antipsychotic drug treatment.
- Two main types of disturbance occur:
  - acute, reversible dystonias and Parkinson-like symptoms (indeed, antipsychotic drugs generally worsen Parkinson's disease and block the actions of drugs used to treat the disorder)
  - slowly developing tardive dyskinesia, often irreversible.
- Acute symptoms comprise involuntary movements, tremor and rigidity, and are probably the direct consequence of block of nigrostriatal dopamine receptors.
- Tardive dyskinesia comprises mainly involuntary movements of the face and limbs, appearing after months or years of antipsychotic treatment. It may be associated with proliferation of dopamine receptors in the corpus striatum. Treatment is generally unsuccessful.
- Incidence of acute dystonias and tardive dyskinesia is less with newer, second-generation antipsychotics, and particularly low with **clozapine**, **aripiprazole** and **zotepine**.

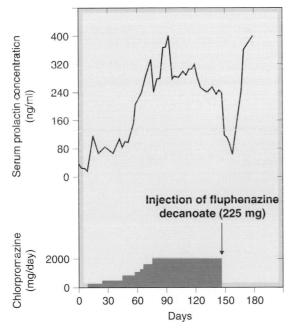

Fig. 46.2 **Effects of antipsychotic drugs on prolactin secretion in a schizophrenic patient.** When daily dosage with chlorpromazine was replaced with a depot injection of fluphenazine, the plasma prolactin initally dropped, because of the delay in absorption, and then returned to a high level. *(From Meltzer HY et al. 1978 In: Lipton et al. (eds) Psychopharmacology: A Generation in Progress. Raven Press, New York.)*

They can produce sexual dysfunction – decreased libido and decreased arousal as well as erection and ejaculation difficulties in men – through block of dopamine, muscarinic and α_1 receptors.

Drowsiness and sedation, which tend to decrease with continued use, occur with many antipsychotic drugs.

Antihistamine (H_1) activity is a property of some phenothiazine antipsychotics (e.g. chlorpromazine and **methotrimeprazine**) and contributes to their sedative and antiemetic properties (Chs 39 and 44), but not to their antipsychotic action.

While block of muscarinic receptors produces a variety of peripheral effects, including blurring of vision and increased intraocular pressure, dry mouth and eyes, constipation and urinary retention (see Ch. 13), it may, however, also be beneficial in relation to extrapyramidal side effects (see p. 566).

Blocking α adrenoceptors causes *orthostatic hypotension* (see Ch. 14) but does not seem to be important for their antipsychotic action.

Weight gain is a common and troublesome side effect. Increased risk of diabetes and cardiovascular disease occurs with several second-generation antipsychotic drugs. These effects are probably related to their antagonist actions at H_1, 5-HT and muscarinic receptors.

Antipsychotic drugs can prolong the QT interval in the heart (see Ch. 21) giving rise to arrhythmia and risk of sudden death (Jolly et al., 2009).

Various idiosyncratic and hypersensitivity reactions can occur, the most important being the following:

- *Jaundice*, which occurs with older phenothiazines such as chlorpromazine. The jaundice is usually mild, associated with elevated serum alkaline phosphatase activity (an 'obstructive' pattern), and disappears quickly when the drug is stopped or substituted by a chemically unrelated antipsychotic.
- *Leukopenia* and *agranulocytosis* are rare but potentially fatal, and occur in the first few weeks of treatment. The incidence of leukopenia (usually reversible) is less than 1 in 10000 for most antipsychotic drugs, but much higher (1–2%) with clozapine, whose use therefore requires regular monitoring of blood cell counts. Provided the drug is stopped at the first sign of leukopenia or anaemia, the effect is reversible. Olanzapine appears to be free of this disadvantage.
- *Urticarial skin reactions* are common but usually mild. Excessive sensitivity to ultraviolet light may also occur.
- *Antipsychotic malignant syndrome* is a rare but serious complication similar to the malignant hyperthermia syndrome seen with certain anaesthetics (see Ch. 41). Muscle rigidity is accompanied by a rapid rise in body temperature and mental confusion. It is usually reversible, but death from renal or cardiovascular failure occurs in 10–20% of cases.

PHARMACOKINETIC ASPECTS

Chlorpromazine, in common with other phenothiazines, is erratically absorbed after oral administration. Figure 46.3 shows the wide range of variation of the peak plasma concentration as a function of dosage in 14 patients. Among four patients treated at the high dosage level of 6–8 mg/kg, the variation in peak plasma concentration was nearly 90-fold; two showed marked side effects, one was well controlled and one showed no clinical response.

The relationship between the plasma concentration and the clinical effect of antipsychotic drugs is highly variable, and the dosage has to be adjusted on a trial-and-error basis. This is made even more difficult by the fact that at

Unwanted effects of antipsychotic drugs

- Important side effects common to many drugs are:
  – motor disturbances (see *Antipsychotic-induced motor disturbances* box)
  – endocrine disturbances (increased prolactin release)
  – these are secondary to dopamine receptor block.
- Sedation, hypotension and weight gain are common.
- Obstructive jaundice sometimes occurs with phenothiazines.
- Other side effects (dry mouth, blurred vision, hypotension, etc.) are due to block of other receptors, particularly muscarinic receptors and α adrenoceptors.
- Some antipsychotic drugs cause agranulocytosis as a rare and serious idiosyncratic reaction. With **clozapine**, leukopenia is common and requires routine monitoring.
- Antipsychotic malignant syndrome is a rare but potentially dangerous idiosyncratic reaction.

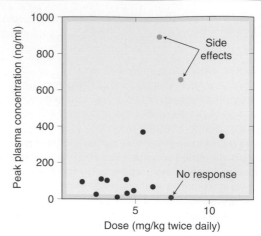

Fig. 46.3 Individual variation in the relation between dose and plasma concentration of chlorpromazine in a group of schizophrenic patients. *(Data from Curry SH et al. 1970 Arch Gen Psychiatry 22, 289.)*

least 40% of schizophrenic patients fail to take drugs as prescribed. It is remarkably fortunate that the acute toxicity of antipsychotic drugs is slight, given the unpredictability of the clinical response.

The plasma half-life of most antipsychotic drugs is 15–30h, clearance depending entirely on hepatic transformation by a combination of oxidative and conjugative reactions.

Most antipsychotic drugs can be given orally or in urgent situations by intramuscular injection. Slow-release (depot) preparations of many are available, in which the active drug is esterified with heptanoic or decanoic acid and dissolved in oil. Given as an intramuscular injection, the drug acts for 2–4 weeks, but initially may produce acute side effects. These preparations are widely used to minimise compliance problems.

FUTURE DEVELOPMENTS

The cognition enhancer **modafinil** (see Ch. 48) may be useful in treating the cognitive deficit in schizophrenia.

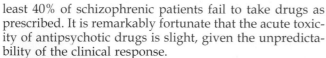

Clinical uses of antipsychotic drugs

- *Behavioural emergencies* (e.g. violent patients with a range of psychopathologies including *mania*, *toxic delirium*, *schizophrenia* and others):
  – antipsychotic drugs (e.g. **chlorpromazine**, **haloperidol**, **olanzapine**, **risperidone**) can rapidly control hyperactive psychotic states
  – note that the intramuscular dose is lower than the oral dose of the same drug because of presystemic metabolism.
- *Schizophrenia*:
  – many chronic schizophrenic patients are treated with first-generation antipsychotic drugs. Depot injections (e.g. **flupentixol decanoate**) may be useful for maintenance treatment when compliance with oral treatment is a problem
  – **flupentixol** has antidepressant properties distinct from its antipsychotic action
  – newer antipsychotic drugs (e.g. **amisulpride**, **olanzapine**, **risperidone**) are used if extrapyramidal symptoms are troublesome or if symptom control is inadequate
  – **clozapine** can cause *agranulocytosis* but is distinctively effective against 'negative' features of schizophrenia. It is reserved for patients whose condition remains inadequately controlled despite previous use of two or more antipsychotic drugs, of which at least one is a second-generation drug. Blood count is monitored weekly for the first 18 weeks, and less frequently thereafter.
- *Other clinical uses*: to some extent, the term 'antipsychotic drug' is misleading as some of these drugs are used to treat disorders other than schizophrenia. These include:
  – bipolar disorder, mania and depression (see Ch. 47)
  – short-term treatment of psychomotor agitation and severe anxiety (**chlorpromazine** and **haloperidol**)
  – agitation and restlessness in the elderly (**risperidone**), although this is highly questionable
  – restlessness and pain in palliative care (**levomepromazine**)
  – nausea and vomiting (e.g. **chlorpromazine** and **haloperidol**) reflecting antagonism at dopamine, muscarinic, histamine and possibly 5-HT receptors
  – motor tics and intractable hiccup (**chlorpromazine** and **haloperidol**)
  – antisocial sexual behavior (**benperidol**)
  – the treatment of involuntary movements caused by Huntington's disease (mainly haloperidol; see Ch. 40).

Preclinical and clinical studies have provided encouraging evidence that orthosteric and allosteric agonists of mGluR$_2$ and mGluR$_3$ metabotropic glutamate receptors (see Ch. 38) are effective in the treatment of the positive symptoms of schizophrenia. Paradoxically, activating presynaptic mGluR$_2$ and mGluR$_3$ autoreceptors reduces glutamate release but this may result in a compensatory upregulation of NMDA receptors which might be beneficial. mGluR$_2$ receptors form heteromers with 5-HT$_{2A}$ receptors (see Ch. 3) with altered intracellular signalling properties and targeting the dimer may offer hope for future drug development. Agonists at postsynaptic mGluR$_5$ receptors may improve positive and negative symptoms as well as cognitive function. mGluR$_5$ receptors are closely associated with NMDA receptors and activation of mGluR$_5$ may enhance NMDA receptor function by increasing NMDA receptor phosphorylation.

A number of current antipsychotic drugs have among their myriad of actions 5-HT$_6$ and 5-HT$_7$ receptor antagonist properties; more specific antagonists at these receptors are being investigated; their ability to produce cognitive improvement is controversial.

Also in various stages of development are inhibitors of phosphodiesterase (PDE10), α_7 nicotinic receptor agonists, histamine H$_3$ antagonists and 5-HT$_6$ antagonists. Selective agonist action at M$_1$ muscarinic receptors (either orthosteric or allosteric) has significant potential for cognition enhancement in both schizophrenia and Alzheimer's disease but to date drug development has been hampered by a lack of selectivity across muscarinic receptor subtypes (e.g. **xanomeline** is an M$_1$ and M$_4$ agonist and M$_5$ antagonist) that gives rise to significant unwanted effects.

Further information about novel targets can be found in Ellenbroek (2012) and Geyer & Gross (2012).

REFERENCES AND FURTHER READING

General reading

Geyer, M.A., Gross, G., 2012. Novel antischizophrenia treatments. Handb. Exp. Pharmacology 213. Springer Verlag (*Multi-authored volume containing individual chapters on the potential for development of new drugs*)

Gross, G., Geyer, M.A., 2012. Current antipsychotics. Handb. Exp. Pharmacology 212. Springer Verlag (*Multi-authored volume containing individual chapters on current drugs*)

Stahl, S.M., 2008. Antipsychotics and mood stabilizers, third ed. Cambridge University Press, New York. (*Highly readable, yet detailed, description of the biology of schizophrenia and of the mechanisms of action of the drugs used to treat the disorder*)

Pathogenesis of schizophrenia

Aberg, K.A., Liu, Y., Bukszár, J., et al., 2013. A comprehensive family-based replication study of schizophrenia genes. JAMA Psychiatry 70, 1–9. (*Study of genetic linkages to schizophrenia*)

Harrison, P.J., 1997. Schizophrenia: a disorder of development. Curr. Opin. Neurobiol. 7, 285–289. (*Reviews persuasively the evidence favouring abnormal early brain development as the basis of schizophrenia*)

Ikeda, M., Aleksic, B., Yamada, K., et al., 2013. Genetic evidence for association between NOTCH4 and schizophrenia supported by a GWAS follow-up study in a Japanese population. Mol. Psychiatry 18, 636–638. (*Recent population genetic study implicating mutation of this gene in aspects of schizophrenia*)

Lennertz, L., Quednow, B.B., Benninghoff, J., Wagner, M., Maier, W., Mössner, R., 2011. Impact of TCF4 on the genetics of schizophrenia. Eur. Arch. Psychiatry Clin. Neurosci. 261, S161–S165. (*A population genetic study implicating this gene, already thought to be involved in mental retardation, in aspects of schizophrenia*)

Ripke, S., Neale, B.M., Corvin, A., et al., 2014. Biological insights from 108 schizophrenia-associated genetic loci. Nature 511, 421–427. (*Extensive study on the human genetic basis of schizophrenia*)

Sim, K., Cullen, T., Ongur, D., Heckers, S., 2006. Testing models of thalamic dysfunction in schizophrenia using neuroimaging. J. Neural Transm. 113, 907–928.

van Haren, N.E., Hulshoff Pol, H.E., Schnack, H.G., et al., 2007. Focal gray matter changes in schizophrenia across the course of the illness: a 5-year follow-up study. Neuropsychopharmacology 32, 2057–2066.

Dopamine, glutamate and 5-hydroxytryptamine

Busatto, G.F., Kerwin, R.W., 1997. Perspectives on the role of serotonergic mechanisms in the pharmacology of schizophrenia. J. Psychopharmacol. 11, 3–12. (*Assesses the evidence implicating 5-HT as well as dopamine in the action of antipsychotic drugs*)

Coyle, J.T., Basu, A., Benneyworth, M., et al., 2012. Glutamatergic synaptic dysregulation in schizophrenia: therapeutic implications. Handb. Exp. Pharmacol. 213, 267–295. (*Describes the emerging view of the importance of glutamate in schizophrenia*)

Laruelle, M., Abi-Dargham, A., Gil, R., et al., 1999. Increased dopamine transmission in schizophrenia: relationship to illness phases. Biol. Psychiatry 46, 56–72. (*The first direct evidence for increased dopamine function as a cause of symptoms in schizophrenia*)

Animal models

Pratt, J., Winchester, C., Dawson, N., Morris, B., 2012. Advancing schizophrenia drug discovery: optimizing rodent models to bridge the translational gap. Nat. Rev. Drug Discov. 11, 560–579.

Antipsychotic drugs

Ellenbroek, B.A., 2012. Psychopharmacological treatment of schizophrenia: what do we have, and what could we get? Neuropharmacology 62, 1371–1380. (*Review of the current state of antipsychotic drug development*)

Jolly, K., Gammage, M.D., Cheng, K.K., Bradburn, P., Banting, M.V., Langman, M.J., 2009. Sudden death in patients receiving drugs tending to prolong the QT interval. Br. J. Clin. Pharmacol. 68, 743–751. (*Compares the risk of sudden death in patients receiving various antipsychotic and antidepressant therapies*)

Kapur, S., Seeman, P., 2001. Does fast dissociation from the dopamine D$_2$ receptor explain the action of atypical antipsychotics? A new hypothesis. Am. J. Psychiatry 158, 360–369. (*Suggests that differences in dissociation rates, rather than receptor selectivity profiles, may account for differing tendency of drugs to cause motor side effects*)

Kapur, S., Arenovich, T., Agid, O., et al., 2005. Evidence for onset of antipsychotic effects within the first 24 hours of treatment. Am. J. Psychiatry 162, 939–946.

Leucht, S., Busch, R., Hamann, J., Kissling, W., Kane, J.M., 2005. Early-onset hypothesis of antipsychotic drug action: a hypothesis tested, confirmed and extended. Biol. Psychiatry 57, 1543–1549.

Leucht, S., Corves, C., Arbter, D., et al., 2009. Second-generation versus first-generation antipsychotic drugs for schizophrenia: a meta-analysis. Lancet 373, 31–41. (*A comparison of the clinical effectiveness of new and old antipsychotic drugs*)

Extrapyramidal side effects

Casey, D.E., 1995. Tardive dyskinesia: pathophysiology. In: Bloom, F.E., Kupfer, D.J. (Eds.), Psychopharmacology: A Fourth Generation of Progress. Raven Press, New York.

Klawans, H.L., Tanner, C.M., Goetz, C.G., 1988. Epidemiology and pathophysiology of tardive dyskinesias. Adv. Neurol. 49, 185–197.

Lieberman, J.A., Stroup, T.S., 2011. The NIMH-CATIE Schizophrenia Study: what did we learn? Am. J. Psychiatry 68, 770–775. (*A comprehensive review of the effectiveness and side effect profiles of antipsychotic drugs*)

Pisani, A., Bernardi, G., Ding, J., Surmeier, D.J., 2007. Re-emergence of striatal cholinergic interneurons in movement disorders. Trends Neurosci. 30, 545–553.

47

Antidepressant drugs

OVERVIEW

Depression is an extremely common psychiatric condition, about which a variety of neurochemical theories exist, and for which a corresponding variety of different types of drug are used in treatment. It is a field in which therapeutic empiricism has led the way, with mechanistic understanding tending to lag behind, part of the problem being that it has been difficult to develop animal models that replicate the characteristics that define the human condition. In this chapter, we discuss the current understanding of the nature of the disorder, and describe the major drugs that are used to treat it.

THE NATURE OF DEPRESSION

Depression is the most common of the *affective disorders* (defined as disorders of mood); it may range from a very mild condition, bordering on normality, to severe (psychotic) depression accompanied by hallucinations and delusions. Worldwide, depression is a major cause of disability and premature death. In addition to the significant suicide risk, depressed individuals are more likely to die from other causes, such as heart disease or cancer. Depression is a heterogeneous disorder, with patients presenting with one or more core symptoms, and depression is often associated with other psychiatric conditions, including anxiety, eating disorders and drug addiction.

The symptoms of depression include emotional and biological components. Emotional symptoms include:

- low mood, excessive rumination of negative thought, misery, apathy and pessimism
- low self-esteem: feelings of guilt, inadequacy and ugliness
- indecisiveness, loss of motivation
- anhedonia, loss of reward.

Biological symptoms include:

- retardation of thought and action
- loss of libido
- sleep disturbance and loss of appetite.

There are two distinct types of depressive syndrome, namely *unipolar depression*, in which the mood changes are always in the same direction, and *bipolar disorder*, in which depression alternates with mania. Mania is in most respects exactly the opposite, with excessive exuberance, enthusiasm and self-confidence, accompanied by impulsive actions, these signs often being combined with irritability, impatience and aggression, and sometimes with grandiose delusions of the Napoleonic kind. As with depression, the mood and actions are inappropriate to the circumstances.

Unipolar depression is commonly (about 75% of cases) non-familial, clearly associated with stressful life events, and usually accompanied by symptoms of anxiety and agitation; this type is sometimes termed *reactive depression*. Other cases (about 25%, sometimes termed *endogenous depression*) show a familial pattern, unrelated to obvious external stresses, and with a somewhat different symptomatology. This distinction is made clinically, but there is little evidence that antidepressant drugs show significant selectivity between these conditions.

Bipolar disorder, which usually appears in early adult life, is less common and results in oscillating depression and mania over a period of a few weeks. It can be difficult to differentiate between mild bipolar disorder and unipolar depression. Also, bipolar manic episodes can be confused with episodes of schizophrenic psychosis (see Ch. 46). There is a strong hereditary tendency, but no specific susceptibility genes have been identified either by genetic linkage studies of affected families, or by comparison of affected and non-affected individuals.

Depression cannot be attributed to altered neuronal activity within a single brain region; rather, the circuitry linking different parts of the brain may be affected. Brain imaging studies have indicated that the prefrontal cortex, amygdala and hippocampus may all be involved in different components of these disorders.

THEORIES OF DEPRESSION

THE MONOAMINE THEORY

The monoamine theory of depression, first proposed by Schildkraut in 1965, states that depression is caused by a functional deficit of the monoamine transmitters, noradrenaline and 5-hydroxytryptamine (5-HT) at certain sites in the brain, while mania results from a functional excess.

The monoamine hypothesis grew originally out of associations between the clinical effects of various drugs that cause or alleviate symptoms of depression and their known neurochemical effects on monoaminergic transmission in the brain. This pharmacological evidence, which is summarised in Table 47.1, gives general support to the monoamine hypothesis, although there are several anomalies. Attempts to obtain more direct evidence, by studying monoamine metabolism in depressed patients or by measuring changes in the number of monoamine receptors in postmortem brain tissue, have tended to give inconsistent and equivocal results, and the interpretation of these studies is often problematic, because the changes described are not specific to depression. Similarly, investigation by functional tests of the activity of known monoaminergic pathways (e.g. those controlling pituitary hormone release) in depressed patients have also given equivocal results.

The pharmacological evidence does not enable a clear distinction to be drawn between the noradrenaline and 5-HT theories of depression. Clinically, it seems that inhibitors of noradrenaline reuptake and of 5-HT reuptake are

Table 47.1 Pharmacological evidence supporting the monoamine hypothesis of depression

Drug(s)	Principal action	Effect in depressed patients
Tricyclic antidepressants	Block noradrenaline and 5-HT reuptake	Mood ↑
Monoamine oxidase (MAO) inhibitors	Increase stores of noradrenaline and 5-HT	Mood ↑
Reserpine	Inhibits noradrenaline and 5-HT storage	Mood ↓
α-Methyltyrosine	Inhibits noradrenaline synthesis	Mood ↓ (calming of manic patients)
Methyldopa	Inhibits noradrenaline synthesis	Mood ↓
Electroconvulsive therapy	? Increases central nervous system responses to noradrenaline and 5-HT	Mood ↑
Tryptophan (5-hydroxytryptophan)	Increases 5-HT synthesis	Mood ? ↑ in some studies
Tryptophan depletion	Decreases brain 5-HT synthesis	Induces relapse in SSRI-treated patients

5-HT, 5-hydroxytryptamine; SSRI, selective serotonin reuptake inhibitor.

equally effective as antidepressants, although individual patients may respond better to one or the other.

Other evidence in support of the monoamine theory is that agents known to block noradrenaline or 5-HT synthesis consistently lower mood and reverse the therapeutic effects of antidepressant drugs that act selectively on these two transmitter systems (see Table 47.1).

Any theory of depression has to take account of the fact that the direct neurochemical effects of antidepressant drugs appear very rapidly (minutes to hours), whereas their antidepressant effects take weeks to develop. A similar situation exists in relation to antipsychotic drugs (Ch. 46) and some anxiolytic drugs (Ch. 44), suggesting that secondary, adaptive changes in the brain, rather than the primary drug effect, are responsible for the clinical improvement. Rather than thinking of the monoamine deficiency as causing direct changes in the activity of putative 'happy' or 'sad' neurons in the brain, we should think of the monoamines as regulators of longer-term trophic effects, whose time course is paralleled by mood changes.

Recent studies in healthy volunteers and depressed patients as well as in rodents suggest that antidepressant drugs may exert acute effects on the way information is processed (cognitive processing), leading to a positive effect on emotional behaviour. Whilst subjects may not be consciously aware of these acute effects, the drugs, by altering cognitive processes, will influence new learning and behaviour. Thus, over time and with chronic drug administration, these effects develop until the patient becomes subjectively aware of the improvement in their mood.

With improved neuroimaging methods for studying neurotransmitter function in the living human brain, as described in Chapter 36, our understanding of the causes of depression and how drugs can alleviate depression should improve.

NEUROENDOCRINE MECHANISMS

Various attempts have been made to test for a functional deficit of monoamine pathways in depression. Hypothalamic neurons controlling pituitary function receive noradrenergic and 5-HT inputs, which control the discharge of these cells. Hypothalamic cells release corticotrophin-releasing hormone (CRH), which stimulates pituitary cells to secrete adrenocorticotrophic hormone (ACTH), leading in turn to cortisol secretion (Ch. 33). The plasma cortisol concentration is usually high in depressed patients. Other hormones in plasma are also affected, for example growth hormone concentration is reduced and prolactin is increased. While these changes are consistent with deficiencies in monoamine transmission, they are not specific to depressive syndromes.

Corticotrophin-releasing hormone (CRH) is widely distributed in the brain and has behavioural effects that are distinct from its endocrine functions. Injected into the brain of experimental animals, CRH mimics some aspects of depression in humans, such as diminished activity, loss of appetite and increased signs of anxiety. Furthermore, CRH concentrations in the brain and cerebrospinal fluid of depressed patients are increased. Therefore CRH hyperfunction, as well as monoamine hypofunction, may be associated with depression. Raised CRH levels are associated with stress and, in many cases, depression is preceded by periods of chronic stress.

TROPHIC EFFECTS AND NEUROPLASTICITY

It has been suggested that lowered levels of brain-derived neurotrophic factor (BDNF) or malfunction of its receptor, TrkB, plays a significant role in the pathology of this condition (see Baudry et al., 2011). Depressive behaviour is often associated with a reduction in BDNF expression and treatment with antidepressants elevates BDNF levels. Glycogen synthase kinase 3 (GSK3β) has been implicated in the pathogenesis of depression following its identification as a target of the mood stabiliser **lithium** (see p. 587).

Changes in glutamatergic neurotransmission may also be involved in depression. Sufferers from depression have been shown to have elevated cortical levels of glutamate. Antidepressant treatment may reduce glutamate release and depress NMDA receptor function. The effects of antidepressants on activity-induced long-term potentiation (LTP; see Ch. 38) at hippocampal glutamatergic synapses is complex – both depression and facilitation have been observed and may occur quickly after antidepressant administration, thus calling into question the relevance to the therapeutic response.

Another view (see Racagni & Popoli, 2008) is that major depression is associated with neuronal loss in the hippocampus and prefrontal cortex, and that antidepressant therapies of different kinds act by inhibiting or actually reversing this loss by stimulating neurogenesis.[1] This surprising idea is supported by various lines of evidence:

- Brain imaging and postmortem studies show ventricular enlargement as well as shrinkage of the hippocampus and prefrontal cortex of depressed patients, with loss of neurons and glia. Functional imaging reveals reduced neuronal activity in these regions.
- In animals, the same effect is produced by chronic stress of various kinds, or by administration of glucocorticoids, mimicking the increased cortisol secretion in human depression. Excessive glucocorticoid secretion in humans (Cushing's syndrome; see Ch. 33) often causes depression.
- In experimental animals, antidepressant drugs, or other treatments such as electroconvulsions (see later section on Brain Stimulation Therapies), promote neurogenesis in these regions, and (as in humans) restore functional activity. Preventing hippocampal neurogenesis prevents the behavioural effects of antidepressants in rats.
- 5-HT and noradrenaline, whose actions are enhanced by many antidepressants, promote neurogenesis, probably through activation of 5-HT_{1A} receptors and α_2 adrenoceptors, respectively. This effect may be mediated by BDNF.

Monoamine theory of depression

- The monoamine theory, first proposed in 1965, suggests that depression results from functionally deficient monoaminergic (noradrenaline and/or 5-hydroxytryptamine) transmission in the central nervous system.
- The theory is based on the ability of known antidepressant drugs (tricyclic antidepressants and monoamine oxidase inhibitors) to facilitate monoaminergic transmission, and of drugs such as **reserpine** to cause depression.
- Biochemical studies on depressed patients do not clearly support the monoamine hypothesis in its simple form.
- Although the monoamine hypothesis in its simple form is insufficient as an explanation of depression, pharmacological manipulation of monoamine transmission remains the most successful therapeutic approach.
- Recent evidence suggests that depression may be associated with neurodegeneration and reduced neurogenesis in the hippocampus.
- Current approaches focus on other mediators (e.g. corticotrophin-releasing hormone), signal transduction pathways, growth factors, etc., but theories remain imprecise.

- Exercise has been shown to promote neurogenesis in animals and to be effective in some patients with mild to moderate depression.

Figure 47.1 summarises the possible mechanisms involved. It should be stressed that these hypotheses are far from proven, but the diagram emphasises the way in which the field has moved on since the formulation of the monoamine hypothesis, suggesting a range of possible targets for the next generation of antidepressant drugs.[2]

ANTIDEPRESSANT DRUGS

TYPES OF ANTIDEPRESSANT DRUG

Antidepressant drugs fall into the following categories.

Inhibitors of monoamine uptake
- Selective serotonin (5-HT) reuptake inhibitors (SSRIs) (e.g. **fluoxetine, fluvoxamine, paroxetine, sertraline, citalopram, escitalopram, vilazodone**).
- Classic tricyclic antidepressants (TCAs) (e.g. **imipramine, desipramine, amitriptyline, nortriptyline, clomipramine**). These vary in their activity and selectivity with respect to inhibition of noradrenaline and 5-HT reuptake.
- Newer, mixed 5-HT and noradrenaline reuptake inhibitors (e.g. **venlafaxine** [somewhat selective for 5-HT, although less so than SSRIs], **desvenlafaxine, duloxetine**).
- Noradrenaline reuptake inhibitors (e.g. **bupropion, reboxetine, atomoxetine**).
- The herbal preparation St John's wort, whose main active ingredient is hyperforin: it has similar clinical efficacy to most of the prescribed antidepressants. It is a weak monoamine uptake inhibitor but also has other actions.[3]

Monoamine receptor antagonists
- Drugs such as **mirtazapine, trazodone, mianserin** are non-selective and inhibit a range of amine receptors including α_2 adrenoceptors and 5-HT_2 receptors. They may also have weak effects on monoamine uptake.

Monoamine oxidase inhibitors (MAOIs)
- Irreversible, non-competitive inhibitors (e.g. **phenelzine, tranylcypromine**), which are non-selective with respect to the MAO-A and -B subtypes.
- Reversible, MAO-A-selective inhibitors (e.g. **moclobemide**).

---

[2]Cynics may feel that these mechanisms, in which glutamate, neurotrophic factors, monoamines and steroids all interact to control neuronal death, survival and plasticity, are being invoked just as enthusiastically to account for almost every neurological and psychiatric disorder that you can think of, from stroke and Parkinson's disease to schizophrenia. 'Are we missing something,' they may feel, 'or are all these diseases basically the same? If so, why are their effects so different? Is this just a scientific bandwagon, or does this mechanistic convergence point to some fundamental principles of neural organisation?' We do not have the answers, of course, but it is a field worth watching.
[3]Although relatively free of acute side effects, hyperforin activates cytochrome P450, resulting in loss of efficacy (Ch. 9), with serious consequences, of several important drugs, including ciclosporin, oral contraceptives, some anti-HIV and anticancer drugs, and oral anticoagulants – underlining the principle that herbal remedies are not inherently safe, and must be used with the same degree of informed caution as any other drug.

[1]Neurogenesis (see Ch. 40) – the formation of new neurons from stem cell precursors – occurs to a significant degree in the adult hippocampus, and possibly elsewhere in the brain, contradicting the old dogma that it occurs only during brain development.

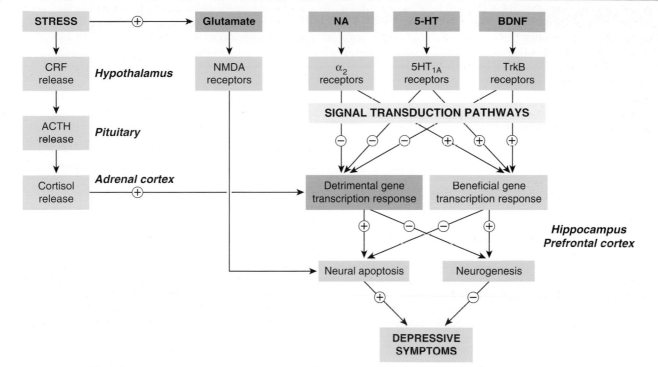

Fig. 47.1 Simplified diagram showing mechanisms believed to be involved in the pathophysiology of depression. The main prodepressive pathways involve the hypothalamic–pituitary–adrenal axis, which is activated by stress and in turn enhances the excitotoxic action of glutamate, mediated by NMDA receptors (see Ch. 38), and switches on the expression of genes that promote neural apoptosis in the hippocampus and prefrontal cortex. The antidepressive pathways involve the monoamines noradrenaline (NA) and 5-hydroxytryptamine (5-HT), which act on G protein-coupled receptors, and the brain-derived neurotrophic factor (BDNF), which acts on a kinase-linked receptor (TrkB), switching on genes that protect neurons against apoptosis and also promote neurogenesis. For further detail, see Charney & Manji (2004). ACTH, adrenocorticotrophic hormone; CRF, corticotrophin-releasing factor.

Types of antidepressant drugs

- Main types are:
  - monoamine uptake inhibitors (tricyclic antidepressants, selective serotonin reuptake inhibitors, newer inhibitors of noradrenaline and 5-HT reuptake)
  - monoamine receptor antagonists
  - monoamine oxidase (MAO) inhibitors.
- Monoamine uptake inhibitors act by inhibiting uptake of noradrenaline and/or 5-HT by monoaminergic nerve terminals.
- α_2-Adrenoceptor antagonists can indirectly elevate 5-HT release.
- MAO inhibitors inhibit one or both forms of brain MAO, thus increasing the cytosolic stores of noradrenaline and

5-HT in nerve terminals. Inhibition of type A MAO correlates with antidepressant activity. Most are non-selective; **moclobemide** is specific for MAO-A.
- All types of antidepressant drug appear to take at least 2 weeks to produce any perceived beneficial effects, even though their pharmacological effects are produced immediately, indicating that secondary adaptive changes are important.
- Recent evidence suggests that antidepressants may act by increasing neurogenesis in the hippocampus and other brain areas.

Melatonin receptor agonist
- **Agomelatine** is an agonist at MT_1 and MT_2 melatonin receptors, and a weak $5\text{-}HT_{2C}$ antagonist.

Table 47.2 summarises the main features of these types of drug. Mention should also be made of electroconvulsive therapy (ECT), electromagnetic therapy, deep brain stimulation and vagus stimulation, which are effective and usually act more rapidly than antidepressant drugs (see p. 585).

TESTING OF ANTIDEPRESSANT DRUGS

ANIMAL MODELS

Progress in unravelling the neurochemical mechanisms is, as in so many areas of psychopharmacology, limited by the lack of good animal models of the clinical condition. There is no known animal condition corresponding to the inherited form of depression in humans, but various procedures have been described that produce in animals

Table 47.2 Types of antidepressant drugs and their characteristics

Type and examples	Action(s)	Unwanted effects	Risk of overdose	Pharmacokinetics	Notes
Monoamine uptake inhibitors					
(1) SSRIs	All highly selective for 5-HT	Nausea, diarrhoea, agitation, insomnia, anorgasmia Inhibit metabolism of other drugs, so risk of interactions	Low risk in overdose but must not be used in combination with MAO inhibitors	–	–
Fluoxetine	As above	As above	As above	Long $t_{1/2}$ (24–96 h)	–
Fluvoxamine	As above	As above	As above	$t_{1/2}$ 18–24 h	Less nausea than with other SSRIs
Paroxetine	As above	As above	As above	$t_{1/2}$ 18–24 h	Withdrawal reaction
Citalopram	As above	As above	As above	$t_{1/2}$ 24–36 h	–
Escitalopram	As above	As above	As above	$t_{1/2}$ 24–36 h	Active S isomer of citalopram Fewer side effects
Vilazodone	As above. Also has 5-HT$_{1A}$ receptor partial agonist activity	As above	As above	$t_{1/2}$ 25 h	–
Sertraline	As above	As above	As above	$t_{1/2}$ 24–36 h	–
(2) **Classical TCA group**[a]	Inhibition of NA and 5-HT reuptake	Sedation Anticholinergic effects (dry mouth, constipation, blurred vision, urinary retention, etc.) Postural hypotension Seizures Impotence Interaction with CNS depressants (especially alcohol, MAO inhibitors)	Ventricular dysrhythmias High risk in combination with CNS depressants	–	'First-generation' antidepressants, still very widely used, although newer compounds generally have fewer side effects and lower risk with overdose
Imipramine	Non-selective Converted to desipramine	As above	As above	$t_{1/2}$ 4–18 h	–
Desipramine	NA selective	As above	As above	$t_{1/2}$ 12–24 h	–
Amitriptyline	Non-selective	As above	As above	$t_{1/2}$ 12–24 h; converted to nortriptyline	Widely used, also for neuropathic pain (Ch. 42)
Nortriptyline	NA selective (slight)	As above	As above	Long $t_{1/2}$ (24–96 h)	Long duration, less sedative
Clomipramine	Non-selective	As above	As above	$t_{1/2}$ 18–24 h	Also used for anxiety disorders

[a]Other TCAs include dosulepin, doxepin, lofepramine, trimipramine.

Table 47.2 Continued

Type and examples	Action(s)	Unwanted effects	Risk of overdose	Pharmacokinetics	Notes
(3) Other 5-HT/NA uptake inhibitors					
Venlafaxine	Weak non-selective NA/5-HT uptake inhibitor Also non-selective receptor-blocking effects	As SSRIs Withdrawal effects common and troublesome if doses are missed	Safe in overdose	Short $t_{1/2}$ (~5 h) Converted to desvenlafaxine which inhibits NA uptake	Claimed to act more rapidly than other antidepressants, and to work better in 'treatment-resistant' patients Usually classed as non-selective NA/5-HT uptake blocker, although *in vitro* data show selectivity for 5-HT
Duloxetine	Potent non-selective NA/5-HT uptake inhibitor No action on monoamine receptors	Fewer side effects than venlafaxine Sedation, dizziness, nausea Sexual dysfunction	See SSRIs above	$t_{1/2}$ ~14 h	Also used to treat urinary incontinence (see Ch. 29) and for anxiety disorders
St John's wort (active principle: hyperforin)	Weak non-selective NA/5-HT uptake inhibitor Also non-selective receptor-blocking effects	Few side effects reported Risk of drug interactions due to enhanced drug metabolism (e.g. loss of efficacy of ciclosporin, antidiabetic drugs, etc.)		$t_{1/2}$ ~12 h	Freely available as crude herbal preparation Similar efficacy to other antidepressants, with fewer acute side effects but risk of serious drug interactions
NA-selective inhibitors					
Bupropion	Selective inhibitor of NA over 5-HT uptake but also inhibits dopamine uptake Converted to active metabolites (e.g. radafaxine)	Headache, dry mouth, agitation, insomnia	Seizures at high doses	$t_{1/2}$ ~12 h Plasma half-life ~20 h	Used in depression associated with anxiety Slow-release formulation used to treat nicotine dependence (Ch. 49)
Maprotiline	Selective NA uptake inhibitor	As TCAs; no significant advantages	As TCAs	Long $t_{1/2}$ ~40 h	No significant advantages over TCAs
Reboxetine	Selective NA uptake inhibitor	Dizziness Insomnia Anticholinergic effects	Safe in overdose (low risk of cardiac dysrhythmia)	$t_{1/2}$ ~12 h	Less effective than TCAs The related drug atomoxetine now used mainly to treat ADHD (Ch. 48)

Table 47.2 Continued

Type and examples	Action(s)	Unwanted effects	Risk of overdose	Pharmacokinetics	Notes
(4) Monoamine receptor antagonists					
Mirtazapine	Blocks α_2, 5-HT_{2C} and 5-HT_3 receptors	Dry mouth Sedation Weight gain	No serious drug interactions	$t_{1/2}$ 20–40 h	Claimed to have faster onset of action than other antidepressants
Trazodone	Blocks 5-HT_{2A} and 5-HT_{2C} receptors as well as H_1 receptors Weak 5-HT uptake inhibitor (enhances NA/5-HT release)	Sedation Hypotension Cardiac dysrhythmias	Safe in overdose	$t_{1/2}$ 6–12 h	Nefazodone is similar
Mianserin	Blocks α_1, α_2, 5-HT_{2A} and H_1 receptors	Milder antimuscarinic and cardiovascular effects than TCAs Agranulocytosis, aplastic anaemia	–	$t_{1/2}$ 10–35 h	Blood count advised in early stages of use
MAO inhibitors	Inhibit MAO-A and/or MAO-B Earlier compounds have long duration of action due to covalent binding to enzyme				
Phenelzine	Non-selective	'Cheese reaction' to tyramine-containing foods (see text) Anticholinergic side effects Hypotension Insomnia Weight gain Liver damage (rare)	Many interactions (TCAs, opioids, sympathomimetic drugs) – risk of severe hypertension due to 'cheese reaction'	$t_{1/2}$ 1–2 h Long duration of action due to irreversible binding	–
Tranylcypromine	Non-selective	As phenelzine	As phenelzine	$t_{1/2}$ 1–2 h Long duration of action due to irreversible binding	–
Isocarboxazid	Non-selective	As phenelzine	As phenelzine	Long $t_{1/2}$ ~36 h	–
Moclobemide	MAO-A selective Short acting	Nausea, insomnia, agitation	Interactions less severe than with other MAO inhibitors; no 'cheese reactions' reported	$t_{1/2}$ 1–2 h	Safer alternative to earlier MAO inhibitors
Melatonin agonist					
Agomelatine	MT_1 and MT_2 receptor agonist. Weak 5-HT_{2C} antagonist	Headache, dizziness, drowsiness, fatigue, sleep disturbance, anxiety, nausea, GI disturbances, sweating	Limited data available at present	$t_{1/2}$ 1–2 h	Should not be combined with ethanol Usually taken once daily before bed

5-HT, 5-hydroxytryptamine; ADHD, attention deficit/hyperactivity disorder; CNS, central nervous system; MAO, monoamine oxidase; NA, noradrenaline; SSRI, selective serotonin reuptake inhibitor; TCA, tricyclic antidepressant.

behavioural states (withdrawal from social interaction, loss of appetite, reduced motor activity, etc.) typical of human depression (see Neumann et al., 2011; O'Leary & Cryan, 2013). The use of genetically modified mice (e.g. 5-HT transporter knockdown) to mimic various aspects of the disorder may provide useful models. However, the similarity of these animal models to human depression is questionable.

TESTS ON HUMANS

Clinically, the effect of antidepressant drugs is usually measured by a subjective rating scale such as the 17-item Hamilton Rating Scale. Clinical depression takes many forms, and the symptoms vary between patients and over time. Quantitation is therefore difficult, and the many clinical trials of antidepressants have generally shown rather weak effects, after allowance for quite large placebo responses. There is also a high degree of individual variation, with 30–40% of patients failing to show any improvement, possibly due to genetic factors (see later section on Clinical Effectiveness).

MECHANISM OF ACTION OF ANTIDEPRESSANT DRUGS

CHRONIC ADAPTIVE CHANGES

Given the discrepancy between the fast onset of the neurochemical effects of antidepressant drugs and the slow onset of their antidepressant effects, efforts have been made to determine whether the therapeutic benefits arise from slow adaptive changes induced by chronic exposure to these drugs (Racagni & Popoli, 2008).

This approach led to the discovery that certain monoamine receptors, in particular β_1 and α_2 adrenoceptors, are consistently downregulated following chronic antidepressant treatment and, in some cases, by electroconvulsive therapy too. This can be demonstrated in experimental animals as a reduction in the number of binding sites, as well as by a reduction in the functional response to agonists (e.g. stimulation of cAMP formation by β-adrenoceptor agonists). Receptor downregulation probably also occurs in humans, because endocrine responses to **clonidine**, an α_2-adrenoceptor agonist, are reduced by long-term antidepressant treatment. However, the relevance of these findings to the antidepressant response is unclear. Loss of β adrenoceptors as a factor in alleviating depression does not fit comfortably with theory, because β-adrenoceptor antagonists are not antidepressant.

On acute administration, one would expect inhibition of 5-HT uptake (e.g. by SSRIs) to increase the level of 5-HT at the synapse by inhibiting reuptake into the nerve terminals. However, the increase in synaptic 5-HT levels has been observed to be less than expected. This is because increased activation of 5-HT_{1A} receptors on the soma and dendrites of 5-HT-containing raphe neurons (Fig. 47.2A) inhibits these neurons and thus reduces 5-HT release, thus cancelling out to some extent the effect of inhibiting reuptake into the terminals. On prolonged drug treatment, the elevated level of 5-HT in the somatodendritic region desensitises the 5-HT_{1A} receptors, reducing their inhibitory effect on 5-HT release from the nerve terminals. The need to desensitise somatodendritic 5-HT_{1A} receptors could thus explain in part the slow onset of antidepressant action of 5-HT uptake inhibitors.

NORADRENERGIC CONTROL OF 5-HT RELEASE

Block of presynaptic α_2 autoreceptors on noradrenergic nerve terminals throughout the central nervous system (CNS) will reduce the negative feedback from released noradrenaline and thus enhance further noradrenaline release (see Chs 14 and 37). In addition, α_2-adrenoceptor antagonists can indirectly enhance 5-HT release.

The effect of α_2-adrenoceptor antagonists on synaptic noradrenaline and 5-HT levels would be rapid in onset and so these changes must somehow induce other, slower adaptive responses that give rise to the slowly developing antidepressant effects.

GENE EXPRESSION AND NEUROGENESIS

More recently, interest has centred on intracellular signalling pathways, changes in gene expression and neurogenesis. Much attention has been focused on how antidepressants may activate the transcription factor, CREB, a cAMP response element-binding protein. The role of other transcription factors, such as those of the Fos family and NF-κB, have been less extensively studied. As described above, several antidepressant drugs appear to promote neurogenesis in the hippocampus, a mechanism that could account for the slow development of the therapeutic effect. The role of raised synaptic noradrenaline and 5-HT levels in inducing changes in gene expression and neurogenesis, and the mechanisms involved, await further elucidation.

MONOAMINE UPTAKE INHIBITORS

SELECTIVE 5-HYDROXYTRYPTAMINE UPTAKE INHIBITORS (SSRIs)

These are the most commonly prescribed group of antidepressants. Examples include **fluoxetine**, **fluvoxamine**, **paroxetine**, **citalopram**, **escitalopram** and **sertraline** (see Table 47.2). As well as showing selectivity with respect to 5-HT over noradrenaline uptake (Fig. 47.3), they are less likely than TCAs to cause anticholinergic side effects and are less dangerous in overdose. In contrast to MAOIs, they do not cause 'cheese reactions'. They are also used to treat anxiety disorders (see Ch. 44) and premature ejaculation. **Vortioxetine**, recently approved in the US, is a novel SSRI that also has partial agonist activity at 5-HT_{1A} and 5-HT_{1B} receptors and is an antagonist at 5-HT_{3A} and 5-HT_7 receptors.

Individual patients may respond more favourably to one SSRI than another. This may reflect other pharmacological properties of each individual drug as none is devoid of other actions. Fluoxetine has 5-HT_{2C} antagonist activity, a property it shares with other non-SSRI antidepressants such as **mirtazapine**. Sertraline is a weak inhibitor of dopamine uptake. Escitalopram is the *S* isomer of racemic citalopram. It lacks the antihistamine and CYP2D6 inhibitory properties of the *R* isomer.

Pharmacokinetic aspects

The SSRIs are well absorbed when given orally, and most have plasma half-lives of 18–24 h (fluoxetine is longer acting: 24–96 h). Paroxetine and fluoxetine are not used in combination with TCAs, whose hepatic metabolism they inhibit through an interaction with CYP2D6, for fear of increasing TCA toxicity.

Unwanted effects

Common side effects include nausea, anorexia, insomnia, loss of libido and failure of orgasm.[4] Some of these unwanted effects result from the enhanced stimulation of postsynaptic 5-HT receptors as a result of the drugs increasing the levels of extracellular 5-HT. This can be either stimulation of the wrong type of 5-HT receptor (e.g. $5\text{-}HT_2$, $5\text{-}HT_3$ and $5\text{-}HT_4$ receptors) or stimulation of the same receptor that gives therapeutic benefit (e.g.

postsynaptic $5\text{-}HT_{1A}$ receptors) but in the wrong brain region (i.e. enhanced stimulation of 5-HT receptors can result in both therapeutic and adverse responses).

In combination with MAOIs, SSRIs can cause a 'serotonin syndrome' characterised by tremor, hyperthermia and cardiovascular collapse, from which deaths have occurred.

There have been reports of increased aggression, and occasionally violence, in patients treated with fluoxetine, but these have not been confirmed by controlled studies. The use of SSRIs is not recommended for treating depression in children under 18, in whom efficacy is doubtful

---

[4]Thus, conversely, SSRIs can be used to treat premature ejaculation. Dapoxetine has a short half-life and is taken 1–3 hours before sex.

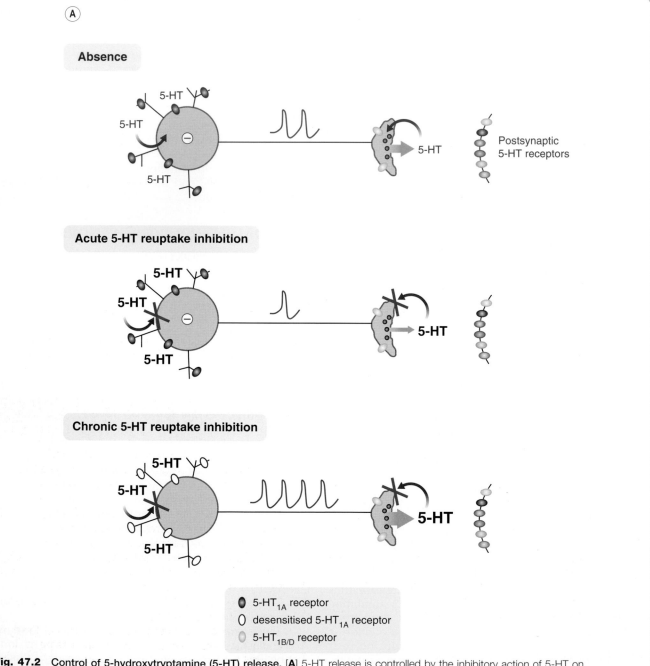

Fig. 47.2 Control of 5-hydroxytryptamine (5-HT) release. **[A]** 5-HT release is controlled by the inhibitory action of 5-HT on somatodendritic $5\text{-}HT_{1A}$ receptors. Acute inhibition of 5-HT reuptake results in increased extracellular levels of 5-HT but this increases somatodendritic $5\text{-}HT_{1A}$ receptor-mediated inhibition, hence synaptic 5-HT levels do not rise as much as expected. $5\text{-}HT_{1A}$ receptors eventually desensitise, resulting in reduced inhibition and thus greater 5-HT release.

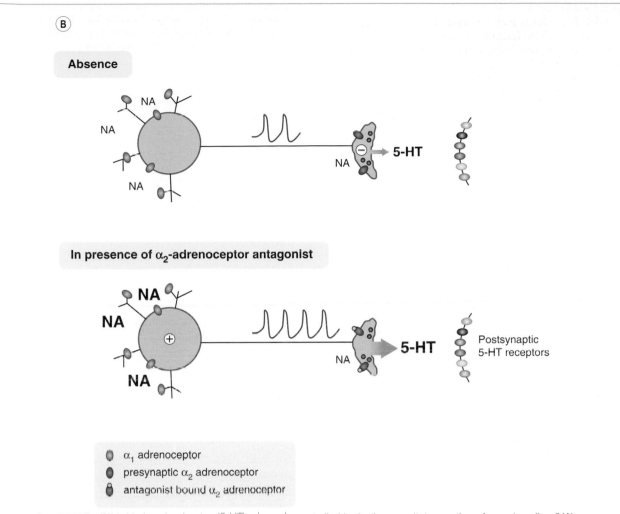

Absence

In presence of α₂-adrenoceptor antagonist

Postsynaptic
5-HT receptors

- α₁ adrenoceptor
- presynaptic α₂ adrenoceptor
- antagonist bound α₂ adrenoceptor

Fig. 47.2, Continued [B] 5-Hydroxytryptamine (5-HT) release is controlled by both an excitatory action of noradrenaline (NA) on somatodendritic α₁ adrenoceptors and an inhibitory action on α₂ adrenoceptors on serotonergic nerve terminals. Block of α₂ adrenoceptors located on noradrenergic neurons (not shown) enhances noradrenaline release resulting in further excitation of serotonergic neurons, while block of α₂ adrenoceptors on serotonergic neurons removes presynaptic inhibition and thus 5-HT release is enhanced.

and adverse effects, including excitement, insomnia and aggression in the first few weeks of treatment, may occur. The possibility of increased suicidal ideation is a concern in this age group (see p. 586).

Despite the apparent advantages of 5-HT uptake inhibitors over TCAs in terms of side effects, the combined results of many trials show little overall difference in terms of patient acceptability (Song et al., 1993; Cipriani et al., 2009).

They are relatively safe in overdose, compared with TCAs (see p. 580-581) but can prolong the cardiac QT interval, giving rise to ventricular arrhythmias (see Ch. 21) and risk of sudden death (Jolly et al., 2009).

5-HT uptake inhibitors are used in a variety of other psychiatric disorders, as well as in depression, including anxiety disorders and obsessive–compulsive disorder (see Ch. 44).

TRICYCLIC ANTIDEPRESSANT DRUGS

Tricyclic antidepressants (TCAs; **imipramine, desipramine, amitriptyline, nortriptyline, clomipramine**) are still widely used. They are, however, far from ideal in practice, and it was the need for drugs that act more quickly and reliably,

Selective serotonin reuptake inhibitors (SSRIs)

- Examples include **fluoxetine, fluvoxamine, paroxetine, sertraline, citalopram, escitalopram**.
- Antidepressant actions are similar in efficacy and time course to TCAs.
- Acute toxicity (especially cardiotoxicity) is less than that of MAOIs or TCAs, so overdose risk is reduced.
- Side effects include nausea, insomnia and sexual dysfunction. SSRIs are less sedating and have fewer antimuscarinic side effects than the older TCAs.
- No food reactions, but dangerous 'serotonin reaction' (hyperthermia, muscle rigidity, cardiovascular collapse) can occur if given with MAOIs.
- There is concern about the use of SSRIs in children and adolescents, due to reports of an increase in suicidal thoughts on starting treatment.
- Also used for some other psychiatric indications, e.g. anxiety.

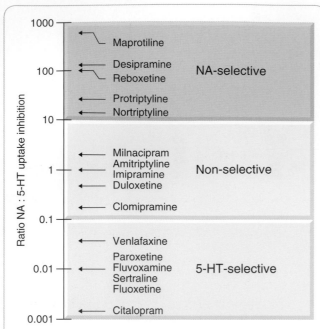

Fig. 47.3 Selectivity of inhibition of noradrenaline (NA) and 5-hydroxytryptamine (5-HT) uptake by various antidepressants.

Table 47.3 Inhibition of neuronal noradrenaline and 5-hydroxytryptamine (5-HT) uptake by tricyclic antidepressants and their metabolites

Drug/metabolite	NA uptake	5-HT uptake
Imipramine	+++	++
Desmethylimipramine (DMI) (also known as desipramine)	++++	+
Hydroxy-DMI	+++	–
Clomipramine (CMI)	++	+++
Desmethyl-CMI	+++	+
Amitriptyline (AMI)	++	++
Nortriptyline (desmethyl-AMI)	+++	++
Hydroxynortriptyline	++	++

produce fewer side effects and are less hazardous in overdose that led to the introduction of newer 5-HT reuptake inhibitors and other antidepressants.

TCAs are closely related in structure to the phenothiazines (Ch. 46) and were initially synthesised (in 1949) as potential antipsychotic drugs. Several are tertiary amines and are quite rapidly demethylated *in vivo* (Fig. 47.4) to the corresponding secondary amines (e.g. imipramine to desipramine, amitriptyline to nortriptyline), which are themselves active and may be administered as drugs in their own right. Other tricyclic derivatives with slightly modified bridge structures include **doxepin**. The pharmacological differences between these drugs are not very great and relate mainly to their side effects, which are discussed below.

Some TCAs are also used to treat neuropathic pain (see Ch. 42).

Mechanism of action

As discussed above, the main immediate effect of TCAs is to block the uptake of amines by nerve terminals, by competition for the binding site of the amine transporter (Ch. 14). Most TCAs inhibit noradrenaline and 5-HT uptake (Fig. 47.3) but have much less effect on dopamine uptake. It has been suggested that improvement of emotional symptoms reflects mainly an enhancement of 5-HT-mediated transmission, whereas relief of biological symptoms results from facilitation of noradrenergic transmission. Interpretation is made difficult by the fact that the major metabolites of TCAs have considerable pharmacological activity (in some cases greater than that of the parent drug) and often differ from the parent drug in respect of their noradrenaline/5-HT selectivity (Table 47.3).

In addition to their effects on amine uptake, most TCAs affect other receptors, including muscarinic acetylcholine receptors, histamine receptors and 5-HT receptors. The antimuscarinic effects of TCAs do not contribute to their antidepressant effects but are responsible for various side effects (see below).

Unwanted effects

In non-depressed human subjects, TCAs cause sedation, confusion and motor incoordination. These effects occur also in depressed patients in the first few days of treatment, but tend to wear off in 1–2 weeks as the antidepressant effect develops.

Tricyclic antidepressants produce a number of troublesome side effects, mainly due to interference with autonomic control.

Anti-muscarinic effects include dry mouth, blurred vision, constipation and urinary retention. These effects are strong with amitriptyline and much weaker with desipramine. Postural hypotension occurs with TCAs. This may seem anomalous for drugs that enhance noradrenergic transmission, and possibly results from an effect on adrenergic transmission in the medullary vasomotor centre. The other common side effect is sedation, and the long duration of action means that daytime performance is often affected by drowsiness and difficulty in concentrating.

TCAs, particularly in overdose, may cause ventricular dysrhythmias associated with prolongation of the QT interval (see Ch. 21). Usual therapeutic doses of TCAs increase, slightly but significantly, the risk of sudden cardiac death.

Interactions with other drugs

TCAs are particularly likely to cause adverse effects when given in conjunction with other drugs (see Ch. 57). They rely on hepatic metabolism by microsomal cytochrome P450 (CYP) enzymes for elimination, and this may be inhibited by competing drugs (e.g. antipsychotic drugs and some steroids).

TCAs potentiate the effects of alcohol and anaesthetic agents, for reasons that are not well understood, and deaths have occurred as a result of this, when severe respiratory depression has followed a bout of drinking. TCAs also interfere with the action of various antihypertensive drugs (see Ch. 22), with potentially dangerous consequences, so their use in hypertensive patients requires close monitoring.

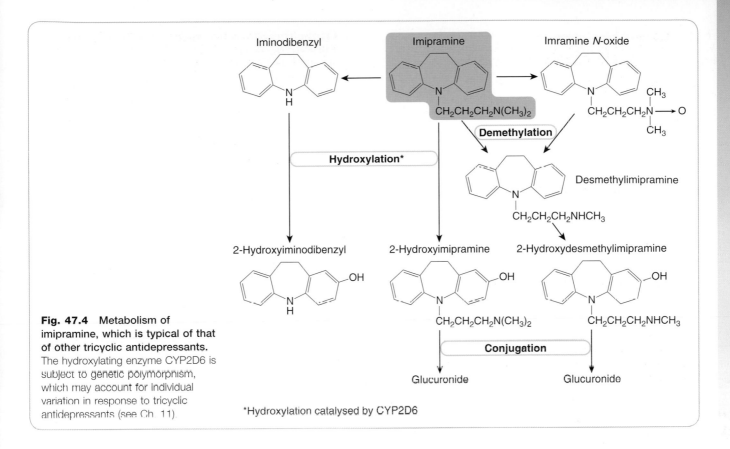

Fig. 47.4 Metabolism of imipramine, which is typical of that of other tricyclic antidepressants. The hydroxylating enzyme CYP2D6 is subject to genetic polymorphism, which may account for individual variation in response to tricyclic antidepressants (see Ch. 11).

*Hydroxylation catalysed by CYP2D6

Acute toxicity

TCAs are dangerous in overdose, and were at one time commonly used for suicide attempts, which was an important factor prompting the introduction of safer antidepressants. The main effects are on the central nervous system and the heart. The initial effect of TCA overdosage is to cause excitement and delirium, which may be accompanied by convulsions. This is followed by coma and respiratory depression lasting for some days. Atropine-like effects are pronounced, including dry mouth and skin, mydriasis and inhibition of gut and bladder. Anticholinesterase drugs have been used to counter atropine-like effects but are no longer recommended. Cardiac dysrhythmias are common, and sudden death (rare) may occur from ventricular fibrillation.

Pharmacokinetic aspects

TCAs are all rapidly absorbed when given orally and bind strongly to plasma albumin, most being 90–95% bound at therapeutic plasma concentrations. They also bind to extravascular tissues, which accounts for their generally very large distribution volumes (usually 10–50 l/kg; see Ch. 8) and low rates of elimination. Extravascular sequestration, together with strong binding to plasma albumin, means that haemodialysis is ineffective as a means of increasing drug elimination.

TCAs are metabolised in the liver by two main routes, *N*-demethylation and ring hydroxylation (Fig. 47.4). Both the desmethyl and the hydroxylated metabolites commonly retain biological activity (see Table 47.3). During prolonged treatment with TCAs, the plasma concentration of these metabolites is usually comparable to that of the parent drug, although there is wide variation between

individuals. Inactivation of the drugs occurs by glucuronide conjugation of the hydroxylated metabolites, the glucuronides being excreted in the urine.

The overall half-times for elimination of TCAs are generally long, ranging from 10 to 20 h for imipramine and desipramine to about 80 h for **protriptyline**. They are even longer in elderly patients. Therefore, gradual accumulation is possible, leading to slowly developing side effects. The relationship between plasma concentrations and the therapeutic effect is not simple. Indeed, a study on nortriptyline (Fig. 47.5) showed that too high a plasma concentration actually reduces the antidepressant effect, and there is a narrow 'therapeutic window'.

SEROTONIN AND NORADRENALINE UPTAKE INHIBITORS (SNRIs)

These drugs are relatively non-selective for 5-HT and NA uptake. They include **venlafaxine**, **desvenlafaxine** and **duloxetine** (see Table 47.2). These have become extensively used antidepressant drugs due to manufacturers' claims of greater therapeutic efficacy and low side effect profiles, the evidence for which is rather weak.

As the dose of venlafaxine is increased, its efficacy also increases, which has been interpreted as demonstrating that its weak action to inhibit noradrenaline reuptake may add to its 5-HT uptake inhibition that occurs at lower doses, the combination providing additional therapeutic benefit. They are all active orally; venlafaxine is available in a slow-release formulation that reduces the incidence of nausea. Venlafaxine, desvenlafaxine and duloxetine are effective in some anxiety disorders (see Ch. 44). Desvenlafaxine may be useful in treating some perimenopausal

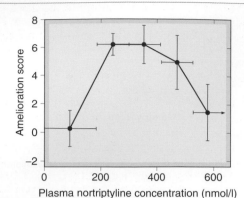

Fig. 47.5 'Therapeutic window' for nortriptyline. The antidepressant effect, determined from subjective rating scales, is optimal at plasma concentrations between 200 nmol/l and 400 nmol/l, and declines at higher levels.

Tricyclic antidepressants

- Tricyclic antidepressants are chemically related to phenothiazines, and some have similar non-selective receptor-blocking actions.
- Important examples are **imipramine**, **amitriptyline** and **clomipramine**.
- Most are long acting, and they are often converted to active metabolites.
- Important side effects: sedation (H_1 block); postural hypotension (α-adrenoceptor block); dry mouth, blurred vision, constipation (muscarinic block); occasionally mania and convulsions. Risk of ventricular dysrhythmias.
- Dangerous in acute overdose: confusion and mania, cardiac dysrhythmias.
- Liable to interact with other drugs (e.g. alcohol, anaesthetics, hypotensive drugs and non-steroidal anti-inflammatory drugs; should not be given with monoamine oxidase inhibitors).
- Also used to treat neuropathic pain.

---

symptoms such as hot flushes and insomnia. Duloxetine is also used in the treatment of neuropathic pain and fibromyalgia (see Ch. 42) and urinary incontinence.

Venlafaxine and duloxetine are metabolised by CYP2D6. Venlafaxine is converted to desvenlafaxine, which shows greater inhibition of noradrenaline reuptake. Unwanted effects of these drugs – largely due to enhanced activation of adrenoceptors – include headache, insomnia, sexual dysfunction, dry mouth, dizziness, sweating and decreased appetite. The most common symptoms in overdose are CNS depression, serotonin toxicity, seizure and cardiac conduction abnormalities. Duloxetine has been reported to cause hepatotoxicity and is contraindicated for patients with hepatic impairment.

OTHER NORADRENALINE UPTAKE INHIBITORS

Bupropion inhibits both noradrenaline and dopamine (but not 5-HT) uptake but, unlike cocaine and amphetamine (see Ch. 48), does not induce euphoria and has so far not been observed to have abuse potential. It is

---

Other monoamine uptake inhibitors

- **Venlafaxine** is a 5-HT uptake inhibitor, but less selective for 5-HT versus noradrenaline than SSRIs. It is metabolised to **desvenlafaxine**, which is also antidepressant.
- **Duloxetine** inhibits NA and 5-HT uptake.
- **Bupropion** is a noradrenaline and dopamine uptake inhibitor.
- Generally similar to tricyclic antidepressants but lack major receptor-blocking actions, so fewer side effects.
- Less risk of cardiac effects, so safer in overdose than tricyclic antidepressants.
- Can be used to treat other disorders:
  - **venlafaxine**, **desvenlafaxine** and **duloxetine** – anxiety disorders
  - **duloxetine** and **milnacipran** – neuropathic pain and fibromyalgia
  - **duloxetine** – urinary incontinence
  - **bupropion** – nicotine dependence.

---

metabolised to active metabolites. It is also used to treat nicotine dependence (see Ch. 49). At high doses it may induce seizures. **Reboxetine** and **atomoxetine** are highly selective inhibitors of noradrenaline uptake but their efficacy in depression is less than that of TCAs. Atomoxetine is approved for the treatment of attention deficit/hyperactivity disorder (see Ch. 48).

MONOAMINE RECEPTOR ANTAGONISTS

Mirtazapine blocks not only α_2 adrenoreceptors but also other receptors, including 5-HT_{2C} receptors, which may contribute to its antidepressant actions. Block of α_2 adrenoceptors will not only increase noradrenaline release but will also enhance 5-HT release (see Fig 47.2B); however, by simultaneously blocking 5-HT_{2A} and 5-HT_3 receptors it will reduce unwanted effects mediated through these receptors (e.g. sexual dysfunction and nausea) but leave intact stimulation of postsynaptic 5-HT_{1A} receptors. It also blocks histamine H_1 receptors, which may cause sedation. **Trazodone** combines 5-HT_{2A} and 5-HT_{2C} receptor antagonism with 5-HT reuptake inhibition.

Mianserin, another α_2-adrenoceptor antagonist that also blocks H_1, 5-HT_{2A} and α_1 adrenoreceptors, can cause bone marrow depression, requiring regular blood counts, so its use has declined in recent years.

MONOAMINE OXIDASE INHIBITORS

Monoamine oxidase inhibitors (MAOIs) were among the first drugs to be introduced clinically as antidepressants but were largely superseded by other types of antidepressants, whose clinical efficacies were considered better and whose side effects are generally less than those of MAOIs. The main examples are **phenelzine**, **tranylcypromine** and **iproniazid**. These drugs cause irreversible inhibition of the enzyme and do not distinguish between the two main isozymes (see below). The discovery of reversible inhibitors that show isozyme selectivity has rekindled interest in this class of drug. Although several studies have shown a reduction in platelet MAO activity in certain groups of depressed

Table 47.4 Substrates and inhibitors for type A and type B monoamine oxidase

	Type A	Type B
Preferred substrates	Noradrenaline 5-Hydroxytryptamine	Phenylethylamine Benzylamine
Non-specific substrates	Dopamine Tyramine	Dopamine Tyramine
Specific inhibitors	Clorgyline Moclobemide	Selegiline
Non-specific inhibitors	Pargyline Tranylcypromine Isocarboxazid	Pargyline Tranylcypromine Isocarboxazid

Other antidepressant drugs

- **Mirtazapine** blocks α_2 adrenoceptors and 5-HT$_{2C}$ receptors, enhancing noradrenaline and 5-HT release.
- **Mirtazapine** may act more rapidly than other antidepressants, and causes less nausea and sexual dysfunction than SSRIs.
- **Trazodone** blocks 5-HT$_{2A}$ and 5-HT$_{2C}$ receptors and blocks 5-HT reuptake.
- **Mianserin** is an antagonist at multiple 5-HT receptors (including 5-HT$_{2A}$) as well as at α_1 and α_2 receptors. It is also an inverse agonist at H$_1$ receptors. Use is declining because of risk of bone marrow depression. Regular blood counts are advisable.
- Cardiovascular side effects of these drugs are fewer than those of tricyclic antidepressants.
- **Agomelatine** is an agonist at MT$_1$ and MT$_2$ melatonin receptors.

patients, there is no clear evidence that abnormal MAO activity is involved in the pathogenesis of depression.

Monoamine oxidase (see Ch. 14) is found in nearly all tissues, and exists in two similar molecular forms coded by separate genes (see Table 47.4). MAO-A has a substrate preference for 5-HT and is the main target for the antidepressant MAOIs. MAO-B has a substrate preference for phenylethylamine and dopamine. Type B is selectively inhibited by **selegiline**, which is used in the treatment of Parkinson's disease (see Ch. 40). Disruption of the MAO-A gene in mice causes increased brain accumulation of 5-HT and, to a lesser extent, noradrenaline, along with aggressive behaviour. A family has been reported with an inherited mutation leading to loss of MAO-A activity, whose members showed mental retardation and violent behaviour patterns. Most antidepressant MAOIs act on both forms of MAO, but clinical studies with subtype-specific inhibitors have shown clearly that antidepressant activity, as well as the main side effects of MAOIs, is associated with MAO-A inhibition. MAO is located intracellularly, mostly associated with mitochondria, and has two main functions:

1. Within nerve terminals, MAO regulates the free intraneuronal concentration of noradrenaline or 5-HT. It is not involved in the inactivation of released transmitter.

2. MAO in the gut wall is important in the inactivation of endogenous and ingested amines such as tyramine that would otherwise produce unwanted effects.

Chemical aspects

Monoamine oxidase inhibitors are substrate analogues with a phenylethylamine-like structure, and most contain a reactive group (e.g. hydrazine, propargylamine, cyclopropylamine) that enables the inhibitor to bind covalently to the enzyme, resulting in a non-competitive and long-lasting inhibition. Recovery of MAO activity after inhibition takes several weeks with most drugs, but is quicker after **tranylcypromine**, which forms a less stable bond with the enzyme. **Moclobemide** acts as a reversible competitive inhibitor.

Monoamine oxidase inhibitors are not specific in their actions, and inhibit a variety of other enzymes as well as MAO, including many enzymes involved in the metabolism of other drugs. This is responsible for some of the many clinically important drug interactions associated with MAOIs.

Pharmacological effects

Monoamine oxidase inhibitors cause a rapid and sustained increase in the 5-HT, noradrenaline and dopamine content of the brain, 5-HT being affected most and dopamine least. Similar changes occur in peripheral tissues such as heart, liver and intestine, and increases in the plasma concentrations of these amines are also detectable. Although these increases in tissue amine content are largely due to accumulation within neurons, transmitter release in response to nerve activity is not increased. In contrast to the effect of TCAs, MAOIs do not increase the response of peripheral organs, such as the heart and blood vessels, to sympathetic nerve stimulation. The main effect of MAOIs is to increase the cytoplasmic concentration of monoamines in nerve terminals, without greatly affecting the vesicular stores that are releasable by nerve stimulation. The increased cytoplasmic pool results in an increased rate of spontaneous leakage of monoamines, and also an increased release by indirectly acting sympathomimetic amines such as amphetamine and tyramine (see Ch. 14 and Fig. 14.8). Tyramine thus causes a much greater rise in blood pressure in MAOI-treated animals than in controls. This mechanism is important in relation to the 'cheese reaction' produced by MAOIs in humans (see below).

In normal human subjects, MAOIs cause an immediate increase in motor activity, and euphoria and excitement develop over the course of a few days. This is in contrast to TCAs, which cause only sedation and confusion when given to non-depressed subjects. The effects of MAOIs on amine metabolism develop rapidly, and the effect of a single dose lasts for several days. There is a clear discrepancy, as with SSRIs and TCAs, between the rapid biochemical response and the delayed antidepressant effect.

Unwanted effects and toxicity

Many of the unwanted effects of MAOIs result directly from MAO inhibition, but some are produced by other mechanisms.

Hypotension is a common side effect; indeed, **pargyline** was at one time used as an antihypertensive drug. One possible explanation for this effect – the opposite of what might have been expected – is that amines such as dopamine or octopamine accumulate within peripheral sympathetic nerve terminals and displace noradrenaline from the storage vesicles, thus reducing noradrenaline release associated with sympathetic activity.

Excessive central stimulation may cause tremors, excitement, insomnia and, in overdose, convulsions.

Increased appetite, leading to weight gain, can be so extreme as to require the drug to be discontinued.

Atropine-like side effects (dry mouth, blurred vision, urinary retention, etc.) are common with MAOIs, although they are less of a problem than with TCAs.

MAOIs of the hydrazine type (e.g. phenelzine and iproniazid) produce, very rarely (less than 1 in 10 000), severe hepatotoxicity, which seems to be due to the hydrazine moiety of the molecule. Their use in patients with liver disease is therefore unwise.

Interaction with other drugs and foods

Interaction with other drugs and foods is the most serious problem with MAOIs and is the main factor that caused their clinical use to decline. The special advantage claimed for the new reversible MAOIs, such as moclobemide, is that these interactions are reduced.

The 'cheese reaction' is a direct consequence of MAO inhibition and occurs when normally innocuous amines (mainly tyramine) produced during fermentation are ingested. Tyramine is normally metabolised by MAO in the gut wall and liver, and little dietary tyramine reaches the systemic circulation. MAO inhibition allows tyramine to be absorbed, and also enhances its sympathomimetic effect, as discussed above. The result is acute hypertension, giving rise to a severe throbbing headache and occasionally even to intracranial haemorrhage. Although many foods contain some tyramine, it appears that at least 10 mg of tyramine needs to be ingested to produce such a response, and the main danger is from ripe cheeses and from concentrated yeast products such as Marmite. Administration of indirectly acting sympathomimetic amines (e.g. **ephedrine** – a nasal decongestant – or amphetamine – a drug of abuse) also causes severe hypertension in patients receiving MAOIs; directly acting agents such as noradrenaline (used, for example, in conjunction with local anaesthetics; see Ch. 43) are not hazardous. Moclobemide, a specific MAO-A inhibitor, does not cause the 'cheese reaction', probably because tyramine can still be metabolised by MAO-B.

Hypertensive episodes have been reported in patients given TCAs and MAOIs simultaneously. The probable explanation is that inhibition of noradrenaline reuptake further enhances the cardiovascular response to dietary tyramine, thus accentuating the 'cheese reaction'. This combination of drugs can also produce excitement and hyperactivity.

Monoamine oxidase inhibitors can interact with **pethidine** (see Ch. 42) to cause severe hyperpyrexia, with restlessness, coma and hypotension. The mechanism is uncertain, but it is likely that an abnormal pethidine metabolite is produced because of inhibition of demethylation.

MELATONIN AGONIST

Agomelatine is an agonist at MT_1 and MT_2 receptors (see Ch. 39), and has a short biological half-life. It is used to treat severe depression, usually taken once daily before bed. It may work by correcting disturbances in circadian rhythms often associated with depression. There are

reports of hepatotoxicity in a few patients, and it should not be used in patients with liver disease.

> ## Monoamine oxidase inhibitors (MAOIs)
>
> - Main examples are **phenelzine**, **tranylcypromine**, **isocarboxazid** (irreversible, long-acting, non-selective between MAO-A and B) and **moclobemide** (reversible, short-acting, MAO-A selective).
> - Long-acting MAOIs:
>   - main side effects: postural hypotension (sympathetic block); atropine-like effects (as with TCAs); weight gain; CNS stimulation, causing restlessness, insomnia; hepatotoxicity and neurotoxicity (rare)
>   - acute overdose causes CNS stimulation, sometimes convulsions
>   - 'cheese reaction', i.e. severe hypertensive response to tyramine-containing foods (e.g. cheese, beer, wine, well-hung game, yeast or soy extracts); such reactions can occur up to 2 weeks after treatment is discontinued.
> - Interaction with other amines (e.g. **ephedrine** in over-the-counter decongestants, **clomipramine** and other TCAs) and some other drugs (e.g. **pethidine**) are also potentially lethal.
> - **Moclobemide** is used for major depression and social phobia. 'Cheese reaction' and other drug interactions are less severe and shorter lasting than with irreversible MAOIs.
> - MAOIs are used much less than other antidepressants because of their adverse effects and serious interactions. They are indicated for major depression in patients who have not responded to other drugs.

MISCELLANEOUS AGENTS

Methylfolate, given as a dietary supplement, may be effective in depressed individuals who have lowered folate levels.

Oestrogen, which is known to elevate mood in perimenopausal women, may also be of value for the treatment of postnatal depression. Its effectiveness in treating other forms of depression is unclear. In addition to its well-documented hormonal actions in the body (see Ch. 35), it also has actions on monoaminergic, GABAergic and glutamatergic systems in the brain (see Chs 38 and 39).

FUTURE ANTIDEPRESSANT DRUGS

After a fallow period, there are now several promising new drugs in development (see Lodge & Li, 2008; Mathew et al., 2008).[5] These can be classified broadly into the following:

- Broad spectrum monoamine uptake inhibitors, i.e. affecting 5-HT, NA and DA uptake. One such drug, **tedatioxetine**, is in clinical trials.

---

[5]Hopes for an antidepressant drug targeting nicotinic receptors have been dashed by the failure of an α4β2 subtype antagonist in Phase III clinical trials.

- Drugs inhibiting 5-HT, NA and DA uptake as well as having one or more of the following properties: β_3-adrenoreceptor agonism, D_2 dopamine-receptor agonism or antagonism, $5-HT_{1A}$-receptor agonism or partial agonism and $5-HT_{2A}$-receptor antagonism.
- Interest in drugs acting at the NMDA receptor has been stimulated by the observation that a single, intravenous, subanaesthetic dose of **ketamine** (see Ch. 41) rapidly alleviates depression, an effect that lasts for days.
- Antagonists at the κ opioid receptor are in clinical trials as antidepressants (see Ch. 42). κ opioid receptor agonists have long been known to induce dysphoria, anhedonia and hallucinations.
- Drugs acting at novel receptor targets – such as GRII cortisol receptor antagonists, melanocyte inhibiting factor (MIF-1) analogues, $GABA_B$ receptor antagonists.

Other avenues of research are into the development of compounds that act on the signal transduction pathways responsible for neurogenesis, neural plasticity and apoptosis (see Baudry et al., 2011).

Clinical uses of drugs in depression

- Mild depression is often best treated initially with non-drug measures, with antidepressant drugs being used in addition if the response is poor.
- The use of antidepressant drugs is advisable in the treatment of moderate to severe depression.
- The clinical efficacy of antidepressant drugs is limited, and varies between individuals. Clinical trials have produced inconsistent results, because of placebo responses and spontaneous fluctuations in the level of depression.
- Different classes of antidepressant drugs have similar efficacy but different side effects.
- Choice of drug is based on individual aspects including concomitant disease (TCAs in particular have several indications) and treatment (MAOIs and TCAs cause important interactions), suicide risk and previous response to treatment. Other things being equal, an SSRI is preferred as these are usually better tolerated and are less dangerous in overdose.
- Antidepressant drugs take several weeks before taking effect, so decisions on dose increment or switching to another class should not be made precipitately. Use of MAOIs is by specialists.
- An effective regimen should be continued for at least 2 years.
- In urgent situations, specialist consideration should be given to possible use of electroconvulsive therapy.
- Anxiolytic (e.g. benzodiazepine, Ch. 44), or antipsychotic drugs (Ch. 46) are useful adjuncts in some patients.

BRAIN STIMULATION THERAPIES

A number of brain stimulation techniques are now being used or developed to treat depression. Bright light stimulation has been proposed as a treatment for seasonal affective disorder. The most established brain stimulation techniques are electroconvulsive therapy (ECT) and repetitive transcranial magnetic stimulation (TMS). Brain stimulation treatments are often used as the therapeutic approach of last resort for patients who have not responded to antidepressant drugs.

ECT involves stimulation through electrodes placed on either side of the head, with the patient lightly anaesthetised, paralysed with a short-acting neuromuscular-blocking drug (e.g. **suxamethonium**; Ch. 13) so as to avoid physical injury, and artificially ventilated. Controlled trials have shown ECT to be at least as effective as antidepressant drugs, with response rates ranging between 60% and 80%; it appears to be an effective treatment for severe suicidal depression and has the advantage of producing a fast-onset response. The main disadvantage of ECT is that it often causes confusion and memory loss lasting for days or weeks. TMS gives electrical stimulation without anaesthesia or convulsion and does not produce cognitive impairment, but comparative studies suggest that its antidepressant efficacy is less than that of conventional ECT.

The effect of ECT on experimental animals has been carefully analysed to see if it provides clues as to the mode of action of antidepressant drugs, but the clues it gives are enigmatic. 5-HT synthesis and uptake are unaltered, and noradrenaline uptake is somewhat increased (in contrast to the effect of TCAs). Decreased β adrenoceptor responsiveness, both biochemical and behavioural, occurs with both ECT and long-term administration of antidepressant drugs, but changes in 5-HT-mediated responses tend to go in opposite directions.

There have been reports that deep brain stimulation, which has also been used in the treatment of Parkinson's disease (see Ch. 40), in which stimulation is delivered in a specific brain region through surgically implanted electrodes, is effective in patients not responding to other treatments (see Mayberg et al., 2005). The effectiveness of another technique, vagal stimulation, in producing long-term benefit in depression is still unclear (see Grimm & Bajbouj, 2010).

CLINICAL EFFECTIVENESS OF ANTIDEPRESSANT TREATMENTS

The overall clinical efficacy of antidepressants is generally accepted for severe depression, though there is concern that the published clinical trials evidence may be misleading, because many negative trials have gone unreported. Trials data suggest that 30–40% of depressed patients fail to show improvement, and those that do show only limited improvement. Clear evidence of benefit in mild to moderate depression is lacking. Interpretation of trials data is complicated by a high placebo response, and spontaneous recovery independent of any treatment. Current trials data do not suggest that drugs currently in use differ in terms of efficacy. Nevertheless, clinical experience suggests that individual patients may, for unknown reasons, respond better to one drug than another. Overall, it is now believed that antidepressant drugs are less effective than was originally thought, though they remain among the most commonly prescribed. Current treatment guidelines recommend evidence-based psychological procedures as first-line treatments in most cases, before antidepressant drugs.

Pharmacogenetic factors

▼ The individual variation in response to antidepressants may be partly due to genetic factors, as well as to heterogeneity of the clinical condition. Two genetic factors have received particular attention, namely:

- polymorphism of the cytochrome P450 gene, especially *CYP2D6* (see Kirchheiner et al., 2004), which is responsible for hydroxylation of TCAs
- polymorphism of monoamine transporter genes (see Glatt & Reus, 2003).

Up to 10% of Caucasians possess a dysfunctional *CYP2D6* gene, and consequently may be susceptible to side effects of TCAs and various other drugs (see Ch. 11) that are metabolised by this route. The opposite effect, caused by duplication of the gene, is common in Eastern European and East African populations, and may account for a lack of clinical efficacy in some individuals. There is some evidence to suggest that responsiveness to SSRIs is related to polymorphism of one of the serotonin transporter genes (see Gerretsen & Pollock, 2008).

Although genotyping may prove to be a useful approach in the future to individualising antidepressant therapy, its practical realisation is still some way off.

Suicide and antidepressants

▼ There have been reports that antidepressants increased the risk of 'suicidality' in depressed patients, especially in children and adolescents (see Licinio & Wong, 2005). The term *suicidality* encompasses suicidal thoughts and planning as well as unsuccessful attempts; actual suicide, although one of the major causes of death in young people, is much rarer than suicidality. Clinical trials to determine the relationship between antidepressants and suicidality are difficult, because of the clear association between depression and suicide, and have given variable results, with some studies suggesting that suicidality may be increased during the first few weeks of antidepressant treatment, although not thereafter, and some showing a small increase in the risk of actual suicide (see Cipriani et al., 2005). Although antidepressants, including SSRIs, may carry a small risk of inducing suicidal thoughts and suicide attempts in young people, the risk is less in older age groups. There is no evidence to suggest that SSRIs carry any greater risk than other antidepressants. Furthermore, the risk has to be balanced against the beneficial effects of these drugs, not only on depression but also on anxiety, panic and obsessive–compulsive disorders (see Ch. 44).

OTHER CLINICAL USES OF ANTIDEPRESSANT DRUGS

To some extent, the term 'antidepressant drug' is misleading, as many of these drugs are now used to treat disorders other than depression. These include:

- neuropathic pain (e.g. **amytriptyline**, **nortryptyline**, duloxetine; Ch. 42)
- anxiety disorders (e.g. SSRIs, venlafaxine, duloxetine; Ch. 44)
- fibromyalgia (e.g. duloxetine, venlafaxine, SSRIs, TCAs; Ch. 42)
- bipolar disorder (e.g. fluoxetine in conjunction with **olanzapine**; see below)
- smoking cessation (e.g. buproprion; Ch. 49)
- attention deficit/hyperactivity disorder (e.g. atomoxetine; Ch. 48).

DRUG TREATMENT OF BIPOLAR DISORDER

A range of drugs are now used to control the mood swings characteristic of manic-depressive (bipolar) illness. The major drugs are:

- **lithium**
- several antiepileptic drugs, e.g. **carbamazepine**, **valproate**, **lamotrogine**
- some antipsychotic drugs, e.g. **olanzapine**, **risperidone**, **quetiapine**, **aripiprazole**.

When used to treat bipolar disorder, lithium and antiepileptic agents are often referred to as *mood-stabilising* drugs.

Other agents that may have some beneficial effects in the treatment of bipolar disorder are benzodiazepines (to calm, induce sleep and reduce anxiety), **memantine**, **amantadine** and **ketamine**. The use of antidepressant drugs in bipolar disorder is somewhat controversial. It is recommended that they are given in combination with an antimanic agent because, in some patients, they may induce or enhance mania.

Used prophylactically in bipolar disorder, drugs prevent the swings of mood and thus can reduce both the depressive and the manic phases of the illness. They are given over long periods, and their beneficial effects take 3–4 weeks to develop. Given in an acute attack, they are effective only in reducing mania, but not the depressive phase (although lithium is sometimes used as an adjunct to antidepressants in severe cases of unipolar depression).

LITHIUM

The psychotropic effect of lithium was discovered in 1949 by Cade, who had predicted that urate salts should prevent the induction by uraemia of a hyperexcitability state in guinea pigs. He found lithium urate to produce an effect, quickly discovered that it was due to lithium rather than urate, and went on to show that lithium produced a rapid improvement in a group of manic patients.

Antiepileptic and atypical antipsychotic drugs (see below) are equally effective in treating acute mania; they act more quickly and are considerably safer, so the clinical use of lithium is mainly confined to prophylactic control of manic-depressive illness. The use of lithium is declining.[6] It is relatively difficult to use, as plasma concentration monitoring is required, and there is the potential for problems in patients with renal impairment and for drug interactions, for example with diuretics (see Ch. 57). Lithium may have beneficial effects in neurodegenerative diseases such as Alzheimer's disease (see Ch. 40).

Pharmacological effects and mechanism of action

Lithium is clinically effective at a plasma concentration of 0.5–1 mmol/l, and above 1.5 mmol/l it produces a variety of toxic effects, so the therapeutic window is narrow. In normal subjects, 1 mmol/l lithium in plasma has no appreciable psychotropic effects. It does, however, produce many detectable biochemical changes, and it is still unclear how these may be related to its therapeutic effect.

Lithium is a monovalent cation that can mimic the role of Na^+ in excitable tissues, being able to permeate the voltage-gated Na^+ channels that are responsible for action potential generation (see Ch. 4). It is, however, not pumped out by the Na^+-K^+-ATPase, and therefore tends to accumulate inside excitable cells, leading to a partial loss of intracellular K^+, and depolarisation of the cell.

---

[6]The decline in lithium use may have been influenced by the imbalance in the marketing of this simple inorganic ion versus more profitable pharmacological agents.

The biochemical effects of lithium are complex, and it inhibits many enzymes that participate in signal transduction pathways. Those that are thought to be relevant to its therapeutic actions are as follows:

- Inhibition of inositol monophosphatase, which blocks the phosphatidyl inositol (PI) pathway (see Ch. 3) at the point where inositol phosphate is hydrolysed to free inositol, resulting in depletion of PI. This prevents agonist-stimulated inositol trisphosphate formation through various PI-linked receptors, and therefore blocks many receptor-mediated effects.
- Inhibition of glycogen synthase kinase 3 (GSK3) isoforms, possibly by competing with magnesium for its association with these kinases. GSK3 isoforms phosphorylate a number of key enzymes involved in pathways leading to apoptosis and amyloid formation (see Phiel & Klein, 2001). Lithium can also affect GSK3 isoforms indirectly by interfering with their regulation by Akt, a closely related serine/threonine kinase regulated through PI-mediated signalling and by arrestins (see Ch. 3; Beaulieu et al., 2009).

Lithium also inhibits hormone-induced cAMP production and blocks other cellular responses (e.g. the response of renal tubular cells to antidiuretic hormone, and of the thyroid to thyroid-stimulating hormone; see Chs 29 and 34, respectively). This is not, however, a pronounced effect in the brain.

The cellular selectivity of lithium appears to depend on its selective uptake, reflecting the activity of sodium channels in different cells. This could explain its relatively selective action in the brain and kidney, even though many other tissues use the same second messengers. Notwithstanding such insights, our ignorance of the nature of the disturbance underlying the mood swings in bipolar disorder leaves us groping for links between the biochemical and prophylactic effects of lithium.

Pharmacokinetic aspects and toxicity

Lithium is given by mouth as the carbonate salt and is excreted by the kidney. About half of an oral dose is excreted within about 12 h – the remainder, which presumably represents lithium taken up by cells, is excreted over the next 1–2 weeks. This very slow phase means that, with regular dosage, lithium accumulates slowly over 2 weeks or more before a steady state is reached. The narrow therapeutic window means that monitoring of the plasma concentration is essential. Na^+ depletion reduces the rate of excretion by increasing the reabsorption of lithium by the proximal tubule, and thus increases the likelihood of toxicity. Diuretics that act distal to the proximal tubule (Ch. 29) also have this effect, and renal disease also predisposes to lithium toxicity.

The main toxic effects that may occur during treatment are as follows:

- nausea, vomiting and diarrhoea
- tremor
- renal effects: polyuria (with resulting thirst) resulting from inhibition of the action of antidiuretic hormone. At the same time, there is some Na^+ retention associated with increased aldosterone secretion. With prolonged treatment, serious renal tubular damage may occur, making it essential to monitor renal function regularly in lithium-treated patients
- thyroid enlargement, sometimes associated with hypothyroidism
- weight gain
- hair loss.

Acute lithium toxicity results in various neurological effects, progressing from confusion and motor impairment to coma, convulsions and death if the plasma concentration reaches 3–5 mmol/l.

ANTIEPILEPTIC DRUGS

Carbamazepine, **valproate** and **lamotrogine** (see Ch. 45) have fewer side effects than lithium and have proved efficacious in the treatment of bipolar disorder.

It is assumed that the mechanisms of action of anticonvulsant drugs in reducing bipolar disorder are related to their anticonvulsant activity. While each drug has multiple actions (see Table 45.1), the antiepileptic drugs effective in bipolar disorder share the property of sodium channel blockade, although there are subtle differences in their effectiveness against the different phases of bipolar disorder. Valproate and carbamazepine are effective in treating acute attacks of mania and in the long-term treatment of the disorder, although carbamazepine may not be as effective in treating the depression phase. Valproate is sometimes given along with other drugs such as lithium. Lamotrogine is effective in preventing the recurrence of both mania and depression.

ATYPICAL ANTIPSYCHOTIC DRUGS

Atypical antipsychotic drugs (e.g. **olanzapine**, **risperidone**, **quetiapine**, **aripiprazole**) are second-generation drugs developed for the treatment of schizophrenia (see Ch. 46). These agents have D_2-dopamine and 5-HT_{2A}-receptor antagonist properties as well as actions on other receptors and amine transporters that may contribute to their effectiveness in bipolar depression. All appear to be effective against mania while some may also be effective against bipolar depression. In bipolar depression, atypical antipsychotics are often used in combination with lithium or valproate. Olanzapine is given in combination with the antidepressant fluoxetine.

Treatment of bipolar disorder

- **Lithium**, an inorganic ion, taken orally as lithium carbonate.
- Mechanism of action is not understood. The main biochemical possibilities are:
  - interference with inositol trisphosphate formation
  - inhibition of kinases.
- Antiepileptic drugs (e.g. **carbamazepine**, **valproate**, **lamotrogine**):
  - better side effect and safety profile.
- Atypical antipsychotic drugs (e.g. **olanzapine**, **risperidone**, **quetiapine**, **aripiprazole**).

Clinical uses of mood-stabilising drugs

- **Lithium** (as the carbonate) is the classical drug. It is used:
  - in prophylaxis and treatment of *mania*, and in the prophylaxis of *bipolar* or *unipolar disorder* (manic depression or recurrent depression).
- Points to note include the following:
  - there is a narrow therapeutic window and long duration of action
  - acute toxic effects include cerebellar effects, nephrogenic *diabetes insipidus* (see Ch. 29) and *renal failure*
  - dose must be adjusted according to the plasma concentration
  - elimination is via the kidney and is reduced by proximal tubular reabsorption. Diuretics increase the activity of

the reabsorptive mechanism and hence can precipitate lithium toxicity
  - *thyroid disorders* and mild *cognitive impairment* occur during chronic use.
- **Carbamazepine valproate** and **lamotrogine** (sodium-channel blockers with antiepileptic actions; Ch. 45) are used for:
  - the prophylaxis and treatment of manic episodes in patients with *bipolar disorder*
  - the treatment of *bipolar disorder* (**valproate, lamotrogine**).
- **Olanzapine**, **risperidone**, **quetiapine**, **aripiprazole** (atypical antipsychotic drugs) are used to treat *mania*.

REFERENCES AND FURTHER READING

Pathogenesis of depressive illness

Baudry, A., Mouillet-Richard, S., Launay, J.M., Kellermann, O., 2011. New views on antidepressant action. Curr. Opin. Neurobiol. 21, 858–865. (*Reviews new theories of depression and how antidepressant drugs might work*)

Charney, D.S., Manji, M.K., 2004. Life stress, genes and depression: multiple pathways lead to increased risk and new opportunities for intervention. Sci. STKE 2004, re5. <www.stke.org> (*Detailed review of current understanding of the pathophysiology of depression, emphasising the role of neural plasticity, neurogenesis and apoptosis*)

Neumann, I.D., Wegener, G., Homberg, J.R., et al., 2011. Animal models of depression and anxiety: what do they tell us about human condition? Prog. Neuropsychopharmacol Biol. Psychiatry 35, 1357–1375. (*Detailed discussion of animal models of depression*)

O'Leary, O.F., Cryan, J.F., 2013. Towards translational rodent models of depression. Cell Tissue Res. 354, 141–153.

Antidepressant treatments

Cipriani, A., Barbui, C., Geddes, J.R., 2005. Suicide, depression, and antidepressants. Br. Med. J. 330, 373–374. (*Comment on detailed trials data in the same issue of the journal*)

Cipriani, A., Santilli, C., Furukawa, T.A., et al., 2009. Escitalopram versus other antidepressive agents for depression. Cochrane Database Syst. Rev. (2), Art. No.: CD006532, doi:10.1002/14651858.CD006532.pub2.

Gerretsen, P., Pollock, B.G., 2008. Pharmacogenetics and the serotonin transporter in late-life depression. Exp. Opin. Drug Metab. Toxicol. 4, 1465–1478.

Glatt, C.E., Reus, V.I., 2003. Pharmacogenetics of monoamine transporters. Pharmacogenomics 4, 583–596. (*Discusses prospects for correlating transporter gene polymorphism to variation in response to psychoactive drugs*)

Grimm, S., Bajbouj, M., 2010. Efficacy of vagus nerve stimulation in the treatment of depression. Expert Rev. Neurother. 10, 87–92.

Jolly, K., Gammage, M.D., Cheng, K.K., Bradburn, P., Banting, M.V., Langman, M.J., 2009. Sudden death in patients receiving drugs tending to prolong the QT interval. Br. J. Clin. Pharmacol. 68, 743–751. (*Compares the risk of sudden death in patients receiving various antipsychotic and antidepressant therapies*)

Kirchheiner, J., Nickchen, K., Bauer, M., et al., 2004. Pharmacogenetics of antidepressants and antipsychotics: the contribution of allelic variations to the phenotype of drug response. Mol. Psychiatry 9, 442–473. (*Discusses effect of gene polymorphisms on antidepressant actions; principles are not yet incorporated into clinical practice*)

Licinio, J., Wong, M.-L., 2005. Depression, antidepressants and suicidality: a critical appraisal. Nat. Rev. Drug Discov. 4, 165–171. (*Review of the equivocal evidence linking antidepressant use to suicide*)

Lodge, N.J., Li, Y.-W., 2008. Ion channels as potential targets for the treatment of depression. Curr. Opin. Drug Discov. Devel. 11, 633–641.

Mathew, S.J., Manji, H.K., Charney, D.S., 2008. Novel drugs and therapeutic targets for severe mood disorders. Neuropsychopharmacology 33, 2080–2092.

Mayberg, H.S., Lozano, A.M., Voon, V., et al., 2005. Deep brain stimulation for treatment-resistant depression. Neuron 45, 651–660.

Racagni, G., Popoli, M., 2008. Cellular and molecular mechanisms in the long-term action of antidepressants. Dialogues Clin. Neurosci. 10, 385–400. (*An extensive review of long-term changes induced in the brain by antidepressant drugs that may be responsible for producing the therapeutic benefit*)

Song, F., Freemantle, N., Sheldon, T.A., et al., 1993. Selective serotonin reuptake inhibitors: meta-analysis of efficacy and acceptability. Br. Med. J. 306, 683–687. (*Summary of clinical trials data, showing limitations as well as advantages of SSRIs*)

Lithium

Beaulieu, J.M., Gainetdinov, R.R., Caron, M.G., 2009. Akt/GSK3 signaling in the action of psychotropic drugs. Annu. Rev. Pharmacol. Toxicol. 49, 327–347.

Phiel, C.J., Klein, P.S., 2001. Molecular targets of lithium action. Annu. Rev. Pharmacol. Toxicol. 41, 789–813. (*Review of a topic that is still little understood*)

CNS stimulants and psychotomimetic drugs

48

OVERVIEW

In this chapter we describe drugs that have a pre-dominantly stimulant effect on the central nervous system (CNS); these fall into two broad categories:

1. psychomotor stimulants
2. psychotomimetic (hallucinogenic) drugs.

Drugs in the first category (see Table 48.1) have a marked effect on mental function and behaviour, producing excitement and euphoria, reduced sensation of fatigue, and an increase in motor activity. Some enhance cognitive function.

Drugs in the second category (see Table 48.2) mainly affect thought patterns and perception, distorting cognition in a complex way.

Several of these drugs have no clinical uses but are used for recreational purposes and are recognised as drugs of abuse. This aspect is also discussed in Chapters 49 and 58.

For more detailed information see Iversen et al. (2009).

PSYCHOMOTOR STIMULANTS

AMPHETAMINES

DL-amphetamine (speed or billy whizz), its active dextro-isomer dextroamphetamine (dexies), and methamphetamine (crystal meth or ice) have very similar chemical and pharmacological properties (see Fig. 48.1). Methylphenidate (Ritalin) and MDMA (3,4-methylenedioxymethamphetamine, ecstasy) are chemically related but considered separately below as they differ in the neurochemical and behavioural effects they produce.

Pharmacological effects

The amphetamines act by releasing monoamines, primarily dopamine and noradrenaline, from nerve terminals in the brain (see Green et al., 2003). They do this in a number of ways. They are substrates for the neuronal plasma membrane monoamine uptake transporters DAT and NET but not SERT (see Chs 14, 15 and 39), and thus act as competitive inhibitors, reducing the reuptake of dopamine and noradrenaline. In addition, they enter nerve terminals via the uptake processes or by diffusion and interact with the vesicular monoamine pump VMAT-2 to inhibit the uptake into synaptic vesicles of cytoplasmic dopamine and noradrenaline. The amphetamines are taken up into the storage vesicles by VMAT-2 and displace the endogenous monoamines from the vesicles into the cytoplasm. At high concentrations amphetamines can inhibit monoamine oxidase, which otherwise would break down cytoplasmic monoamines, and monoamine oxidase inhibitors (see Ch. 47) potentiate the effects of amphetamine. The cytoplasmic monoamines can then be transported out of the nerve endings via the plasma membrane DAT and

NET transporters working in reverse, a process that is thought to be facilitated by amphetamine binding to these transporters. All of the above will combine to increase the concentration of extracellular dopamine and noradrenaline in the vicinity of the synapse (see Chs 14 and 39).

In animals, prolonged administration results in degeneration of monoamine-containing nerve terminals and eventually cell death. This effect is observed with toxic doses and is probably due to the accumulation of reactive metabolites of the parent compounds within the nerve terminals. In human brain imaging studies a reduction in the levels of DAT and D_2 receptors has been observed in the brains of amphetamine users. It is unclear, however, whether this is due to long-term exposure to the drug inducing nerve damage or is an underlying pathology that was responsible for drug-seeking in the first instance.

The main central effects of amphetamine-like drugs are:

- locomotor stimulation
- euphoria and excitement
- insomnia
- increased stamina
- anorexia
- long-term psychological effects: psychotic symptoms, anxiety, depression and cognitive impairment.

In addition, amphetamines have peripheral sympathomimetic actions (Ch. 14), producing a rise in blood pressure and inhibition of gastrointestinal motility.

In humans, amphetamines cause euphoria; with intravenous injection, this can be so intense as to be described as 'orgasmic'. Rats quickly learn to press a lever in order to obtain a dose of amphetamine – an indication that the drug is rewarding. Humans become confident, hyperactive and talkative, and sex drive is said to be enhanced. Fatigue, both physical and mental, is reduced. Amphetamines cause marked anorexia, but with continued administration this effect wears off and food intake returns to normal.

Adverse effects of amphetamines include feelings of anxiety, irritability and restlessness. High doses may induce panic and paranoia.

The locomotor and rewarding effects of amphetamine are due mainly to release of dopamine rather than noradrenaline since destruction of the dopamine-containing nucleus accumbens (see Ch. 39) or administration of D_2-receptor antagonists (see Ch. 46) inhibit these responses, which are absent in mice genetically engineered to lack DAT.

Chronic use, tolerance and dependence

If amphetamines are taken repeatedly over a few days a state of 'amphetamine psychosis' can develop, resembling an acute schizophrenic attack (see Ch. 46), with hallucinations, paranoia and aggressive behaviour. At the same time, repetitive stereotyped behaviour may develop. The close similarity of this condition to schizophrenia, and the effectiveness of antipsychotic drugs in controlling it, is

Table 48.1   Central nervous system stimulants

Drugs	Mode(s) of action	Clinical significance
Amphetamine and related compounds (e.g. dexamphetamine, methamphetamine)	Release of catecholamines Inhibition of catecholamine uptake	Dexamphetamine used to treat attention deficit/hyperactivity disorder in children; otherwise very limited clinical use Some use to treat narcolepsy and as appetite suppressants Risk of dependence, sympathomimetic side effects and pulmonary hypertension Mainly important as drugs of abuse para-Methoxymethamphetamine acts similarly
Methylphenidate	Inhibition of catecholamine uptake	Used to treat attention deficit/hyperactivity disorder in children
Modafinil	Still unclear, possibly acts by inhibiting dopamine reuptake	May have use to reduce fatigue and enhance cognition
Cocaine	Inhibition of catecholamine uptake Local anaesthetic	Important as drug of abuse Risk of fetal damage Occasionally used for nasopharyngeal and ophthalmic anaesthesia (see Ch. 43)
Mephedrone	Inhibition of dopamine and 5-HT uptake	It is considered a drug of abuse in many countries
Methylxanthines (e.g. caffeine, theophylline)	Inhibition of phosphodiesterase Antagonism of adenosine A_2 receptors	Clinical uses unrelated to stimulant activity Theophylline used for action on cardiac and bronchial muscle (see Chs 21, 28) Caffeine is a constituents of beverages and tonics. It is also available in tablet form

5-HT, 5-hydroxytryptamine.

Table 48.2   Psychotomimetic drugs

Drugs	Mode(s) of action	Clinical significance
LSD	Agonist at 5-HT_{2A} receptors (see Chs 15 and 39)	No clinical use Important as drug of abuse
MDMA (ecstasy)	Releases 5-HT and blocks reuptake	No current clinical use. May have potential in the treatment of post traumatic stress disorder Important as drug of abuse
Mescaline	Not known Chemically similar to amphetamine	–
Psilocybin	Chemically related to 5-HT; acts on 5-HT_{2A} receptors	–
Ketamine	Phencyclidine (PCP) and methoxetamine are chemically similar Blocks NMDA receptor-operated ion channels (see Ch. 38)	Dissociative anaesthetic, antidepressant action Important as drug of abuse PCP used as a model for schizophrenia
Δ^9-tetrahydrocannabinol	Activates CB_1 and CB_2 receptors (see Ch. 19)	Has analgesic and antiemetic properties (see Ch. 19) Active ingredient in cannabis
Salvinorin A	κ Opioid receptor agonist	No clinical use Drug of abuse

5-HT, 5-hydroxytryptamine; LSD, lysergic acid diethylamide; MDMA, methylenedioxymethamphetamine.

consistent with the dopamine theory of schizophrenia (see Ch. 46). When the drug is stopped after a few days, there is usually a period of deep sleep and on awakening the subject feels lethargic, depressed, anxious (sometimes even suicidal) and hungry. These after-effects may be the result of depletion of the normal stores of dopamine and noradrenaline, but the evidence is not clear-cut.

Tolerance develops rapidly to euphoric and anorexic effects of amphetamines, but more slowly to the other effects.

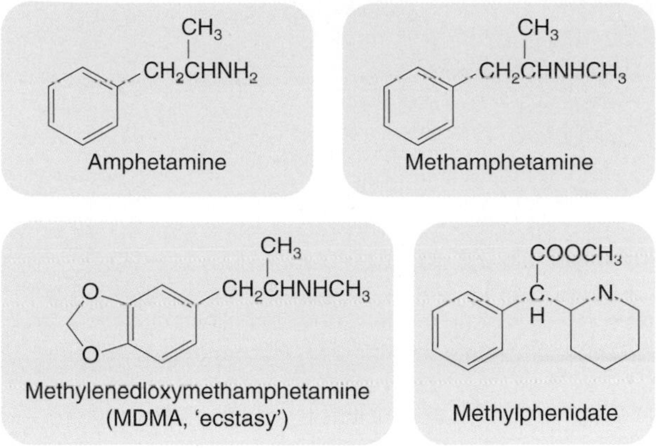

Amphetamine

Methamphetamine

Methylenedioxymethamphetamine
(MDMA, 'ecstasy')

Methylphenidate

Fig. 48.1 Structures of amphetamine-like drugs.

Dependence on amphetamines appears to be a consequence of the insistent memory of euphoria. There is no clear-cut physical withdrawal syndrome such as occurs with opioids. It is estimated that about 10–15% of users progress to full dependence, the usual pattern being that the dose is increased as tolerance develops, and then uncontrolled 'binges' occur in which the user takes the drug repeatedly over a period of a day or more, remaining continuously intoxicated. Large doses may be consumed in such binges, with a high risk of acute toxicity, and the demand for the drug displaces all other considerations.

Experimental animals, given unlimited access to amphetamine, take it in such large amounts that they die from the cardiovascular effects within a few days. Given limited amounts, they too develop a binge pattern of dependence.

Pharmacokinetic aspects

Amphetamines are readily absorbed from the gastrointestinal tract, but to increase the intensity of the hit the drugs can be snorted or injected. In crystal form, the free base of methamphetamine can be ignited and smoked in a manner similar to crack cocaine (see p. 593). Amphetamines freely penetrate the blood–brain barrier. They do this more readily than other indirectly acting sympathomimetic amines such as **ephedrine** or **tyramine** (Ch. 14), which probably explains why they produce more marked central effects than those drugs. Amphetamines are mainly excreted unchanged in the urine, and the rate of excretion is increased when the urine is made more acidic (see Ch. 9). The plasma half-life of amphetamines varies from 5 to 30 hours, depending on urine flow and urinary pH (see Fig. 9.6).

METHYLPHENIDATE

Like the amphetamines, **methylphenidate** inhibits the NET and DAT transporters on the neuronal plasma membrane (and, with much lower potency, inhibits the 5-HT transporter, SERT). Unlike the amphetamines, methylphenidate is not a substrate for these transporters and thus does not enter the nerve terminals to facilitate noradrenaline (NA) and dopamine (DA) release (Heal et al., 2009). It produces a profound and sustained elevation of extracellular NA and DA.

Methylphenidate is orally active, being absorbed from the intestine and colon, but it undergoes presystemic

metabolism such that only ~20% enters the systemic circulation. Absorption is slow following oral administration – peak level after ~2 hours – which may limit the intensity of any euphoric response to the drug. It is metabolised by carboxylesterase and has a half life of ~2–4 h. It is used therapeutically (see clinical box below).

> #### Clinical uses of CNS stimulants
>
> - CNS stimulants have few legitimate therapeutic indications. Where appropriate they are usually initiated by experts.
> - Attention deficit/hyperactivity disorder (ADHD): **methylphenidate**, **atomoxetine** (see Ch. 47). **Dexamphetamine** is an alternative in children who do not respond.
> - Narcolepsy: **modafinil** for the excessive sleepiness; **oxybate** to reduce cataplexy (which can be associated with narcolepsy).
> - Apnoea of prematurity: *xanthine alkaloids* (under expert supervision in hospital) are effective; **caffeine** is preferred to **theophylline**.

MODAFINIL

Modafinil is the primary metabolite of **adrafinil**, a drug that was introduced as a treatment for narcolepsy in the 1980s. Since 1994 modafinil has been available as a drug in its own right. It inhibits dopamine reuptake by binding to DAT but with low potency. In a human brain imaging study modafinil was shown to block DAT and increase extracellular dopamine levels in the caudate, putamen and nucleus accumbens (Volkow et al., 2009). It also produces a number of other effects including α_1-drenoceptor activation, enhanced release of 5-HT, glutamate and histamine and inhibition of GABA release, as well as enhanced electrotonic coupling between neurons. The contribution of each action to the behavioural effects of modafinil remains to be clarified. Modafinil is claimed to enhance cognitive performance (see p. 594), and is gaining popularity as a 'lifestyle drug' (see Ch. 58) for this reason.

Modafinil is well absorbed from the gut, metabolised in the liver and has a half-life of 10–14 h. While reported to 'brighten mood' there is little evidence that modafinil produces significant levels of euphoria when administered by mouth, but tablets can be crushed and snorted to obtain a quicker onset of effect. Modafinil is too insoluble for intravenous injection to be practical.

CLINICAL USE OF STIMULANTS

Attention deficit/hyperactivity disorder (ADHD)

The main use of amphetamines and methylphenidate is in the treatment of ADHD, a common and increasingly diagnosed condition, estimated as occurring in up to 9% of children whose overactivity and limited attention span disrupt their education and social development. The efficacy of drug treatment (e.g. with methylphenidate) has been confirmed in controlled trials, but there is concern as to possible long-term adverse effects since treatment may need to be continued into adolescence and beyond. Drug treatment should be part of a programme that includes psychological intervention if available, and is started after the diagnosis has been confirmed by an expert. Disorders of noradrenaline and dopamine pathways in the frontal cortex and basal ganglia are thought to underlie ADHD symptomatology, but there is still controversy over the relative importance of each monoamine and the specific brain regions involved in the actions of drugs to alleviate the symptoms of ADHD.

Slow-release formulations of amphetamine and methylphenidate have been developed to deliver more stable levels of drug, lower than that required to produce euphoria. D-amphetamine conjugated to lysine (**lisdexamphetamine**) is an inactive prodrug that, following oral administration, is cleaved enzymatically to release D-amphetamine, resulting in a slower onset of action and potentially a reduced abuse potential.

▼ Other drug treatments for ADHD include the noradrenaline reuptake inhibitor **atomoxetine** (Ch. 47), and α₂-adrenoceptor agonists such as **clonidine** and **guanfacine**. The monoamine uptake inhibitor modafinil is not approved for paediatric use but may be effective in adult ADHD. **Melatonin** (Ch. 39) improves sleep patterns in ADHD sufferers. The pharmacology of drugs used to treat ADHD is reviewed by Heal et al. (2009).

Narcolepsy

This is a rare, disabling sleep disturbance in which the patient suddenly and unpredictably falls asleep at frequent intervals during the day, while suffering nocturnal insomnia. It is often accompanied by *cataplexy* (abrupt onset of paralysis of variable extent often triggered by emotion, sometimes with 'frozen' posture). Amphetamine is helpful but not completely effective. Modafinil is also effective in reducing the need for sleep. **Sodium oxybate**, the sodium salt of γ-hydroxybutyrate (also known as GHB and frequently abused, see Ch. 38), is a CNS depressant that paradoxically is licensed for the prevention of cataplexy.

Appetite suppression

Amphetamines and similar drugs such as dexphenfluramine reduce appetite, but are no longer used for this purpose. They are ineffective in producing maintained weight loss, and have harmful CNS and cardiovascular side effects, in particular pulmonary hypertension, which can be so severe as to necessitate heart–lung transplantation.

COCAINE

Cocaine (see Streatfeild, 2002) is found in the leaves of the South American shrub coca. These leaves are used for their stimulant properties by natives of South America, particularly those in mountainous areas, who use it to reduce fatigue during work at high altitude.

Considerable mystical significance was attached to the powers of cocaine to boost the flagging human spirit, and Freud tested it extensively on his patients and his family, publishing an influential monograph in 1884 advocating its use as a psychostimulant.[1] Freud's ophthalmologist colleague Köller obtained supplies of the drug and discovered its local anaesthetic action (Ch. 43), but the psychostimulant effects of cocaine have not proved to be

---

[1] In the 1860s, a Corsican pharmacist, Mariani, devised cocaine-containing beverages, Vin Mariani and Thé Mariani, which were sold very successfully as tonics. Imitators soon moved in, and Thé Mariani became the forerunner of Coca-Cola. In 1903, cocaine was removed from Coca-Cola because of its growing association with addiction and criminality (see Courtwright, 2001, for a lively account).

> **Amphetamines**
>
> - The main effects are:
>   - increased motor activity
>   - euphoria and excitement
>   - insomnia
>   - anorexia
>   - with prolonged administration, stereotyped and psychotic behaviour.
> - Effects are due mainly to release of catecholamines, especially dopamine and noradrenaline.
> - Stimulant effect lasts for a few hours and is followed by depression and anxiety.
> - Tolerance to the stimulant effects develops rapidly, although peripheral sympathomimetic effects may persist.
> - Amphetamines induce strong psychological dependence.
> - Amphetamine psychosis, which closely resembles schizophrenia, can develop after prolonged use.
> - Amphetamines may be useful in treating narcolepsy, and also (paradoxically) to control hyperkinetic children. They are no longer prescribed as appetite suppressants.
> - Their main importance is in drug abuse.

clinically useful. On the other hand, they led to it becoming a widespread drug of abuse in Western countries. The mechanisms and treatment of cocaine abuse are discussed in Chapter 49.

Pharmacological effects

Cocaine binds to and inhibits the transporters NET, DAT and SERT (see Chs 14, 15 and 39), thereby producing a marked psychomotor stimulant effect, and enhancing the peripheral effects of sympathetic nerve activity.

In humans, cocaine produces euphoria, garrulousness, increased motor activity and a magnification of pleasure. Users feel alert, energetic and physically strong and believe they have enhanced mental capabilities. Its effects resemble those of amphetamines, although it has less tendency to produce stereotyped behaviour, delusions, hallucinations and paranoia. Evidence from transgenic knockout mice indicate that the euphoric effects of cocaine involve inhibition of both dopamine and 5-HT reuptake. With excessive dosage, tremors and convulsions, followed by respiratory and vasomotor depression, may occur. The peripheral sympathomimetic actions lead to tachycardia, vasoconstriction and an increase in blood pressure. Body temperature may increase, owing to the increased motor activity coupled with reduced heat loss.

Experimental animals rapidly learn to press a lever to self-administer cocaine and will consume toxic amounts of the drug if access is not limited. In transgenic mice lacking the D₂ receptor, the enhanced locomotor effects of cocaine are reduced, but surprisingly self-administration of cocaine is increased, in contrast to what is found with other self-administered drugs such as ethanol and morphine (see De Mei et al., 2009).

Chronic use, dependence and tolerance

Cocaine undoubtedly causes strong psychological dependence (see Ch. 49), but there is some debate about whether or not its continued use induces tolerance and physical dependence. Users may increase their intake of the drug but this may reflect a desire for an increased effect rather than the development of tolerance. In experimental animals, sensitisation (the opposite of tolerance) can be observed but the relevance of this to the situation in humans is unclear. Like amphetamine, cocaine produces no clear-cut withdrawal syndrome but depression, dysphoria and fatigue may be experienced following the initial stimulant effect. Cocaine induces psychological dependence where users crave the drug's euphoric and stimulatory effects. The cellular mechanisms underlying craving, and pharmacological approaches to reduce craving, are discussed in Chapter 49. The pattern of dependence, evolving from occasional use through escalating dosage to compulsive binges, is similar to that seen with amphetamines.

Pharmacokinetic aspects

Cocaine is readily absorbed by many routes. For many years illicit supplies have consisted of the hydrochloride salt, which could be given by nasal inhalation or intravenously. The latter route produces an intense and immediate euphoria, whereas nasal inhalation produces a less dramatic sensation and also tends to cause atrophy and necrosis of the nasal mucosa and septum.

Cocaine use increased dramatically when the free-base form ('crack') became available as a street drug. When an aqueous solution of cocaine hydrochloride is heated with sodium bicarbonate, then free-base cocaine, water, CO_2 and NaCl are produced. The free-base cocaine is insoluble in water, precipitates out and can then be rolled into 'rocks' of crack. Free-base cocaine vaporises at around 90°C, much lower than the melting point of cocaine hydrochloride (190°C) which burns rather than vaporises. Thus crack can be smoked, with the uncharged free-base being rapidly absorbed across the large surface area of the alveolae, giving rise to a greater CNS effect than that obtained by snorting cocaine. Indeed, the effect is nearly as rapid as that of intravenous administration. The social, economic and even political consequences of this small change in formulation have been far-reaching.

The duration of its stimulant effect, about 30 min, is much shorter than that of amphetamine. It is rapidly metabolised in the liver.

A cocaine metabolite is deposited in hair, and analysis of its content along the hair shaft allows the pattern of cocaine consumption to be monitored, a technique that has revealed a much higher incidence of cocaine use than was voluntarily reported. Cocaine exposure *in utero* can be estimated from analysis of the hair of neonates.

Cocaine is still occasionally used topically as a local anaesthetic, mainly in ophthalmology and minor nose and throat surgery, where its local vasoconstrictor action is an advantage, but has no other clinical uses.

Adverse effects

Toxic effects occur commonly in cocaine abusers. The main acute dangers are serious cardiovascular events (cardiac dysrhythmias, aortic dissection, and myocardial or cerebral infarction or haemorrhage). Progressive myocardial damage can lead to heart failure, even in the absence of a history of acute cardiac effects.

Cocaine can severely impair brain development *in utero* (see Volpe, 1992). The brain size is significantly

reduced in babies exposed to cocaine in pregnancy, and neurological and limb malformations are increased. The incidence of ischaemic and haemorrhagic brain lesions, and of sudden infant death, is also higher in cocaine-exposed babies. Interpretation of the data is difficult because many cocaine abusers also take other illicit drugs that may affect fetal development, but the probability is that cocaine is highly detrimental.

Dependence, the main psychological adverse effect of amphetamines and cocaine, has potentially severe effects on quality of life (Ch. 49).

> **Cocaine**
>
> - **Cocaine** acts by inhibiting catecholamine uptake (especially dopamine) by nerve terminals.
> - Behavioural effects of cocaine are very similar to those of amphetamines, although psychotomimetic effects are rarer. Duration of action is shorter.
> - **Cocaine** used in pregnancy impairs fetal development and may produce fetal malformations.
> - **Cocaine** produces strong psychological dependence.

METHYLXANTHINES

Various beverages, particularly tea, coffee and cocoa, contain methylxanthines, to which they owe their mild central stimulant effects. The main compounds responsible are **caffeine** and **theophylline**. The nuts of the cola plant also contain caffeine, which is present in cola-flavoured soft drinks. However, the most important sources, by far, are coffee and tea, which account for more than 90% of caffeine consumption. A cup of instant coffee or strong tea contains 50–70 mg of caffeine, while filter coffee contains about twice as much. Among adults in tea- and coffee-drinking countries, the average daily caffeine consumption is about 200 mg. Further information on the pharmacology and toxicology of caffeine is presented by Fredholm et al. (1999).

Pharmacological effects

Methylxanthines have the following major pharmacological actions:

- CNS stimulation
- diuresis (see Ch. 29)
- stimulation of cardiac muscle (see Ch. 21)
- relaxation of smooth muscle, especially bronchial muscle (see Ch. 28).

The latter two effects resemble those of β-adrenoceptor stimulation (see Chs 14, 21 and 28). This is thought to be because methylxanthines (especially **theophylline**) inhibit phosphodiesterase, which is responsible for the intracellular metabolism of cAMP (Ch. 3). They thus increase intracellular cAMP and produce effects that mimic those of mediators that stimulate adenylyl cyclase. Methylxanthines also antagonise many of the effects of adenosine, acting on both A_1 and A_2 receptors (see Ch. 16). Transgenic mice lacking functional A_2 receptors are abnormally active and aggressive, and fail to show increased motor activity in response to caffeine, suggesting that antagonism at A_2 receptors accounts for part, at least, of its CNS stimulant action. Caffeine also sensitises ryanodine receptors (see Ch. 4) but this effect occurs at higher concentrations (>10 mmol/l) than those achieved by recreational intake of caffeine. The concentration of caffeine reached in plasma and brain after two or three cups of strong coffee – about 100 µmol/l – is sufficient to produce appreciable adenosine receptor block and a small degree of phosphodiesterase inhibition. The diuretic effect probably results from vasodilatation of the afferent glomerular arteriole, causing an increased glomerular filtration rate.

Caffeine and theophylline have very similar stimulant effects on the CNS. Human subjects experience a reduction of fatigue, with improved concentration and a clearer flow of thought. This is confirmed by objective studies, which have shown that caffeine reduces reaction time and produces an increase in the speed at which simple calculations can be performed (although without much improvement in accuracy). Performance at motor tasks, such as typing and simulated driving, is also improved, particularly in fatigued subjects. Mental tasks, such as syllable learning, association tests and so on, are also facilitated by moderate doses (up to about 200 mg of caffeine, or about two cups of coffee) but impaired by larger doses. Insomnia is common. By comparison with amphetamines, methylxanthines produce less locomotor stimulation and do not induce euphoria, stereotyped behaviour patterns or a psychotic state, but their effects on fatigue and mental function are similar.

Tolerance and habituation develop to a small extent, but much less than with amphetamines, and withdrawal effects are modest. Caffeine is not self-administered by animals, and it cannot be classified as a dependence-producing drug.

Clinical use and unwanted effects

There are few clinical uses for caffeine. It is included with aspirin in some preparations for treating headaches and other aches and pains, and with ergotamine in some antimigraine preparations, the objective being to produce a mildly agreeable sense of alertness. Methylxanthines are effective respiratory stimulants in the treatment of apnea of prematurity (a developmental disorder caused by immaturity of central respiratory control), for which indication caffeine is preferred to theophylline because of its long half-life and safety. Theophylline (formulated as **aminophylline**) is used mainly as a bronchodilator in treating severe asthmatic attacks (see Ch. 28). *In vitro* tests show that it has mutagenic activity, and large doses are teratogenic in animals. However, epidemiological studies have shown no evidence of carcinogenic or teratogenic effects of tea or coffee drinking in humans.

CATHINONES

Cathinone and **cathine** are the active ingredients in the khat shrub. Chewing the leaves is popular in parts of Africa, such as Ethiopia and Somalia, and its use is spreading through immigrant populations in Western countries.

Some cathinone derivatives have recently appeared as recreational drugs that produce feelings of elevated mood and improved mental function. **Mephedrone** elevates extracellular levels of both dopamine and 5-HT, possibly by inhibiting reuptake and enhancing release. Drugs with similar action include **methedrone** and **methylone**. The latter is reported anecdotally to be more MDMA-like in the effects it produces.

> ### Methylxanthines
>
> - **Caffeine** and **theophylline** produce psychomotor stimulant effects.
> - Average **caffeine** consumption from beverages is about 200 mg/day.
> - Main psychological effects are reduced fatigue and improved mental performance, without euphoria. Even large doses do not cause stereotyped behaviour or psychotomimetic effects.
> - Methylxanthines act mainly by antagonism at A_2 purine receptors, and partly by inhibiting phosphodiesterase, thus producing effects similar to those of β-adrenoceptor agonists.
> - Peripheral actions are exerted mainly on heart, smooth muscle and kidney.
> - **Theophylline** is used clinically as a bronchodilator; **caffeine** is used as a respiratory stimulant for apnea of prematurity and as an additive in many beverages and over-the-counter analgesics.

OTHER STIMULANTS

Benzylpiperazine (BZP), another banned recreational drug, produces stimulation and euphoria similar to amphetamine. It has a 'rich' pharmacology, inhibiting 5-HT reuptake as well as dopamine and noradrenaline reuptake but with lower potency. It is also an antagonist at α_2 adrenoceptors and a 5-HT_{2A} agonist.

Arecoline, a cholinergic agonist, is a mild stimulant contained in the betel nut, which improves learning and memory. Its use is widespread in India, Thailand, Indonesia and other Asian cultures.

COGNITION-ENHANCING DRUGS

'Cognition enhancers' are drugs that:

- reduce fatigue (stimulants), thus permitting the user to function for longer (i.e. perform complex tasks, study for examinations, overcome jet lag)
- increase motivation and concentration
- alter memory processing (i.e. enhance memory).

In this regard it is important to distinguish between drugs that only improve a subject's abilities when they are fatigued and those that might improve cognitive ability even in non-fatigued individuals.

Cognition enhancers have therapeutic potential in the treatment of psychiatric conditions associated with cognitive impairment, such as Alzheimer's disease (Ch 40), schizophrenia (Ch. 46), depression (Ch. 47) and drug addiction (Ch. 49), or (controversially) to make normal people more 'intelligent'.

The main drugs used to enhance cognitive performance, often in the absence of medical advice, are caffeine, amphetamines, methylphenidate, modafinil, arecoline and **piracetam**. While their effectiveness is often trumpeted by individuals who use them, and in the media, their actual effectiveness as assessed in scientific studies is inconclusive and ambiguous (Repantis et al., 2010; Smith and Farah, 2011).

Many studies have shown that amphetamines improve mental performance in fatigued subjects. Mental performance is improved for simple tedious tasks much more than for difficult tasks. Amphetamines are thought to increase ability to focus and maintain self control. In addition to reducing fatigue, methylphenidate has a positive effect on long-term memory consolidation. Modafinil improves attention in rested individuals, while improving wakefulness, memory and executive functions in sleep-deprived individuals.

Amphetamines and modafinil have been used to improve the performance of soldiers, military pilots and others who need to remain alert under extremely fatiguing conditions. They have also been in vogue as a means of helping students to concentrate before and during examinations, but the improvement caused by reduction of fatigue are said sometimes to be offset by the mistakes of overconfidence and a decreased ability to deal with large amounts of information.[2]

Piracetam, which is a positive allosteric modulator at AMPA receptors, enhances memory in non-fatigued adults, and there is limited clinical evidence of reading improvement in dyslexic children.

A number of other drugs have been proposed to possess cognition-enhancing activity but firm evidence of their efficacy is still awaited. A wide range of novel targets are being investigated. As with many CNS disorders, the importance of glutamate and its receptors is widely speculated but new, effective drugs acting on the glutamatergic system are still awaited (see, for example, Collingridge et al., 2013; Harms et al., 2013).

PSYCHOTOMIMETIC DRUGS

Psychotomimetic drugs (also referred to as *psychedelic* or *hallucinogenic* drugs) affect thought, perception and mood, without causing marked psychomotor stimulation or depression (see Nichols, 2004). Thoughts and perceptions tend to become distorted and dream-like, rather than being merely sharpened or dulled, and the change in mood is likewise more complex than a simple shift in the direction of euphoria or depression. Importantly, psychotomimetic drugs do not cause dependence, even though their psychological effects overlap those of highly addictive major psychostimulants such as cocaine and amphetamines.

Psychotomimetic drugs include the following:

- Drugs that act on 5-hydroxytryptamine (5-HT) receptors and transporters. These include **lysergic acid diethylamide** (**LSD**), **psilocybin** and **mescaline**, which are agonists at 5-HT$_2$ receptors (see Chs 15 and 39), and **MDMA** (ecstasy), which acts by inhibiting 5-HT uptake. MDMA also acts on several other receptors and transporters, and has powerful psychostimulant effects typical of amphetamines, as well as psychotomimetic effects.
- **Ketamine** and **phencyclidine**, antagonists at NMDA-type glutamate receptors.
- **Δ^9-Tetrahydrocannabinol** (THC, Ch.19), the active ingredient in cannabis, produces a mixture of psychotomimetic and depressant effects similar to, but less pronounced than, those of LSD.
- **Salvinorin A,** a κ-opioid-receptor agonist (Ch. 42).

LSD, PSILOCYBIN AND MESCALINE

LSD is an exceptionally potent psychotomimetic drug capable of producing strong effects in humans in doses less than 1 µg/kg. It is a chemical derivative of lysergic acid, which occurs in the cereal fungus ergot (see Ch. 15).

▼ LSD was first synthesised by Hoffman in 1943. Hoffman deliberately swallowed about 250 µg of LSD (the threshold dose is now known to be around 20 µg) and wrote 30 years later of the experience: 'the faces of those around me appeared as grotesque coloured masks … marked motoric unrest, alternating with paralysis … heavy feeling in the head, limbs and entire body, as if they were filled with lead … clear recognition of my condition, in which state I sometimes observed, in the manner of an independent observer, that I shouted half insanely.' These effects lasted for a few hours, after which Hoffman fell asleep, 'and awoke next morning feeling perfectly well'. Apart from these dramatic psychological effects, LSD has few physiological effects.

Mescaline, which is derived from a Mexican cactus and has been known as a hallucinogenic agent for many centuries, was made famous by Aldous Huxley in *The Doors of Perception*. It is chemically related to amphetamine.

Psilocybin is obtained from fungi ('magic mushrooms'). Its effects are similar to those experienced with LSD.

Pharmacological effects

The main effects of these drugs are on mental function, most notably an alteration of perception in such a way that sights and sounds appear distorted and fantastic. Hallucinations – visual, auditory, tactile or olfactory – also occur, and sensory modalities may become confused, so that sounds are perceived as visions. Thought processes tend to become illogical and disconnected, but subjects retain insight into the fact that their disturbance is drug-induced, and generally find the experience exhilarating. Occasionally, especially if the user is already anxious, LSD produces a syndrome that is extremely disturbing (the 'bad trip'), in which the hallucinatory experience takes on a menacing quality and may be accompanied by paranoid delusions. 'Flashbacks' of the hallucinatory experience have been reported weeks or months later.

LSD acts on various 5-HT-receptor subtypes (see Chs 15 and 39); its psychotomimetic effects are thought to be mediated mainly by its 5-HT$_{2A}$-receptor agonist actions (see Nichols, 2004). It inhibits the firing of 5-HT-containing neurons in the raphe nuclei (see Ch. 39), apparently by acting as an agonist on the inhibitory autoreceptors of these cells. The significance of this response to its psychotomimetic effects is unclear. Psilocybin is dephosphorylated to psilocin, which is an agonist at several 5-HT receptors including the 5-HT$_{2A}$ receptor. The mechanism of action of mescaline is less well defined. There are contradictory reports about its activity at 5-HT$_{2A}$ receptors. It has also been reported to act as an inhibitor of monoamine transport.

The main effects of psychotomimetic drugs are subjective, so it is not surprising that animal tests that reliably predict psychotomimetic activity in humans have not been devised.[3]

---

[2]Pay heed to the awful warning of the medical student who, it is said, having taken copious amounts of dextroamphetamine, left the examination hall in confident mood, having spent 3 hours writing his name over and over again – a good example of amphetamine-induced stereotyped behaviour.

[3]One of the more bizarre attempts involves spiders, whose normal elegantly symmetrical webs become jumbled and erratic if the animals are treated with LSD. Search the Web (World Wide rather than arachnid) for 'spiders LSD' to see images.

Dependence and adverse effects

Psychotomimetic agents are seldom self-administered by experimental animals. Indeed, in contrast to most of the drugs that are widely abused by humans, they have aversive rather than reinforcing properties in behavioural tests. Tolerance to their effects develops quite quickly, but there is no physical withdrawal syndrome in animals or humans.

MDMA (ECSTASY)

MDMA (3,4-methylenedioxymethamphetamine) is widely used as a 'party drug' because of the euphoria, loss of inhibitions and energy surge that it induces. It is a stimulant drug that also has mild hallucinogenic effects. Users describe feelings of empathy and emotional closeness to others and the terms 'empathogen' and 'enactogen' have been coined to describe MDMA and related drugs. There is ongoing debate about whether MDMA, in conjunction with psychotherapy, may be useful in treating post-traumatic stress disorder.

Pharmacological effects

Although an amphetamine derivative (Fig. 48.1), MDMA affects monoamine function in a different manner from the amphetamines. It inhibits monoamine transporters, principally the 5-HT transporter, and also releases 5-HT, the net effect being a large increase in free 5-HT in certain brain regions, followed by depletion. Similar changes occur in relation to dopamine and noradrenaline. Simplistically, the effects on 5-HT function determine the psychotomimetic effects, while dopamine and noradrenaline changes account for the initial euphoria and later rebound dysphoria. Although not addictive, MDMA carries serious risks, both acute and long term.

Sudden illness and death can occur even after small doses of MDMA. This can be due to several factors:

- Acute hyperthermia (see Fig. 48.2), resulting in damage to skeletal muscle and consequent renal failure. It is still unclear how hyperthermia is produced in humans. It may be mediated centrally through release of 5-HT, dopamine and noradrenaline acting on various receptors for these monoamines (Docherty & Green, 2010). It could also reflect an action of MDMA on mitochondrial function. It is exacerbated by energetic dancing and high ambient temperature and certain individuals may be particularly susceptible to this danger.
- Excess water intake and water retention. Users may consume large amounts of water as a result of increased physical activity and feeling hot. In addition MDMA causes inappropriate secretion of antidiuretic hormone (see Ch. 33). This can lead to overhydration and hyponatraemia ('water intoxication'). Symptoms include dizziness and disorientation, leading to collapse into coma.
- Heart failure in individuals with an undiagnosed heart condition.

The after-effects of MDMA persist for a few days and comprise depression, anxiety, irritability and increased aggression – the 'mid-week blues'. There is also evidence of long-term deleterious effects on memory and cognitive function in heavy MDMA users. In animal studies, MDMA can cause degeneration of 5-HT and dopamine neurons, but whether this occurs in humans is uncertain (see Green et al., 2012).

Illicit 'ecstasy' tablets and powder are sometimes contaminated or entirely substituted with **para-methoxyamphetamine**, which produces similar behavioural effects but which may be more dangerous to the user. Other related drugs are **4-bromo-2,5-dimethoxyphenethylamine** (2CB) and **4-methylthioamphetamine** (4-MTA).

KETAMINE AND PHENCYCLIDINE

Ketamine ('*Special K*') is a dissociative anaesthetic (Ch. 41) now also used as a recreational drug (see Morgan & Curran, 2012). An analogue, **phencyclidine** (PCP, '*angel dust*'), was a popular hallucinogen in the 1970s but its use has declined. These drugs produce a feeling of euphoria. At higher doses they cause hallucinations and a feeling of detachment, disorientation and numbness. PCP was reported to cause psychotic episodes and is used in experimental animals to produce a model of schizophrenia (see Ch. 46 and Morris et al., 2005).

Pharmacological effects

Their main pharmacological effect is block of the NMDA-receptor channel (see Ch. 38). This was at one time mistakenly described as 'acting at σ opioid receptors'. **Methoxetamine**, a chemical derivative of ketamine, is an NMDA antagonist as well as an inhibitor of 5-HT reuptake, which may contribute to its CNS effects.

Adverse effects

Tolerance develops with repeated use of ketamine, resulting in higher doses being taken to achieve the same effect. Repeated use is associated with serious and persistent toxic effects, including abdominal pain, ulcerative cystitis (with associated severe bladder pain), liver damage and cognitive impairment (Morgan & Curran, 2012). Combination of ketamine with depressant drugs such as **alcohol, barbiturates** and **heroin** can result in dangerous overdose.

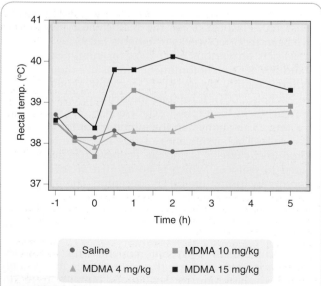

Fig. 48.2 A single injection of MDMA causes a dose-related increase in body temperature in rats. Drug administered at time zero. *(Reproduced with permission from Green et al., 2004.)*

- Saline
- MDMA 10 mg/kg
- MDMA 4 mg/kg
- MDMA 15 mg/kg

OTHER PSYCHOTOMIMETIC DRUGS

Salvinorin A is a hallucinogenic agent contained in the American sage plant *Salvia divinorum*, a member of the mint family. It was originally used by the Mazatecs in Mexico; in recent years its use has spread and it has become known as *herbal ecstasy*. It is a κ-opioid-receptor agonist (see Ch. 42).[4] At high doses, delirium may be produced.

DMT (dimethyltryptamine), **DPT** (dipropyltryptamine) and **DOM** (2,5-dimethoxy-4-methylamphetamine) are synthetic hallucinogenic drugs that produce effects similar to LSD.

Muscarinic receptor antagonists (see Chs 13 and 39), **hyoscine**, **hyoscyamine** and **atropine** are contained in various plants, including henbane and mandrake. Consumption can cause hallucinations, drowsiness and disorientation.

Ibogaine is contained in the root bark of iboga shrubs in Africa, South America and Australia. At high doses, it is hallucinogenic. Users have reported experiencing a reduced desire to take other drugs such as cocaine and heroin, leading to ibogaine being investigated as a potential treatment for drug craving (see Ch. 49).

---

[4]In Phase I clinical trials of synthetic κ-opioid-receptor agonists as potential analgesic agents, the drugs were reported to induce a feeling of dysphoria. Perhaps the 'normal' volunteers in those trials were disturbed by the hallucinations they probably experienced. Interesting then that a naturally occurring κ agonist has now become a recreational drug.

> ## Psychotomimetic drugs
>
> - The main types are:
>   - **lysergic acid diethylamide** (**LSD**), **psilocybin** and **mescaline**
>   - **methylenedioxymethamphetamine** (**MDMA**, 'ecstasy')
>   - **ketamine** and **phencyclidine**.
> - Their main effect is to cause sensory distortion and hallucinatory experiences.
> - **LSD** is exceptionally potent, producing a long-lasting sense of dissociation and disordered thought, sometimes with frightening hallucinations and delusions, which can lead to violence. Hallucinatory episodes can recur after a long interval.
> - **LSD** and **phencyclidine** precipitate schizophrenic attacks in susceptible patients, and **LSD** may cause long-lasting psychopathological changes.
> - **LSD** appears to act as an agonist at 5-HT$_{2A}$ receptors.
> - **MDMA** is an amphetamine analogue that has powerful psychostimulant as well as mild psychotomimetic effects.
> - **MDMA** can cause an acute hyperthermic reaction as well as over-hydration and hyponatraemia, sometimes fatal.
> - Psychotomimetic drugs do not cause physical dependence and tend to be aversive, rather than reinforcing, in animal models.
> - **Ketamine** and **phencyclidine** act by blocking the glutamate-activated NMDA receptor channel.

REFERENCES AND FURTHER READING

General reference

Courtwright, D.T., 2001. Forces of Habit: Drugs and the Making of the Modern World. Harvard University Press, Cambridge. (*A lively historical account of habit-forming drugs*)

Iversen, L.L., Iversen, S.D., Bloom, F.E., Roth, R.H., 2009. Introduction to Neuropsychopharmacology. Oxford University Press, New York. (*Clear and well-written textbook giving more detailed information on many topics covered in this chapter*)

Psychostimulants

Collingridge, G.L., Volianskis, A., Bannister, N., France, G., Hanna, L., et al., 2013. The NMDA receptor as a target for cognitive enhancement. Neuropharmacology 64, 13–26.

De Mei, C., Ramos, M., Iitaka, C., Borrelli, E., 2009. Getting specialized: presynaptic and postsynaptic dopamine D$_2$ receptors. Curr. Opin. Pharmacol. 9, 53–58.

Fredholm, B.B., Battig, K., Holmes, J., et al., 1999. Actions of caffeine in the brain with special reference to factors that contribute to its widespread use. Pharmacol. Rev. 51, 83–133. (*Comprehensive review article covering pharmacological, behavioural and social aspects*)

Harms, J.E., Benveniste, M., Maclean, J.K., Partin, K.M., Jamieson, C., 2013. Functional analysis of a novel positive allosteric modulator of AMPA receptors derived from a structure-based drug design strategy. Neuropharmacology 64, 45–52.

Heal, D.J., Cheetham, S.C., Smith, S.L., 2009. The neuropharmacology of ADHD drugs in vivo: insights on efficacy and safety. Neuropharmacology 57, 608–618. (*Reviews various aspects of the pharmacology of drugs used to treat ADHD*)

Iversen, L.L., 2006. Speed, Ecstasy, Ritalin. The Science of Amfetamines. Oxford University Press, Oxford and New York. (*Authoritative book on all aspects of the properties, use and abuse of amphetamines*)

Repantis, D., Schlattmann, P., Laisney, O., Heuser, I., 2010. Modafinil and methylphenidate for neuroenhancement in healthy individuals: a systematic review. Pharmacol. Res. 62, 187–206. (*A critical appraisal of previous studies on cognition enhancement by drugs*)

Smith, M.E., Farah, M.J., 2011. Are prescription stimulants 'smart pills'? The epidemiology and cognitive neuroscience of prescription stimulant use by normal healthy individuals. Psychol. Bull. 137, 717–741.

Streatfeild, D., 2002. Cocaine: A Definitive History. Diane Publishing Co., Derby, PA.

Volpe, J.J., 1992. Effect of cocaine on the fetus. N. Engl. J. Med. 327, 399–407.

Volkow, N.D., Fowler, J.S., Logan, J., et al., 2009. Effects of modafinil on dopamine and dopamine transporters in the male human brain: clinical implications. JAMA 301, 1148–1154.

Psychotomimetics

Docherty, J.R., Green, A.R., 2010. The role of monoamines in the changes in body temperature induced by 3,4-methylenedioxymethamphetamine (MDMA, ecstasy) and its derivatives. Br. J. Pharmacol. 160, 1029–1044.

Green, A.R., Mechan, A.O., Elliott, J.M., et al., 2003. The pharmacology and clinical pharmacology of 3,4-methylenedioxymethamphetamine (MDMA, 'ecstasy'). Pharm. Rev. 55, 463–508.

Green, A.R., O'Shea, E., Colado, I., 2004. A review of the mechanisms involved in the acute MDMA (ecstasy)-induced hyperthermic response. Eur. J. Pharmacol. 500, 3–13.

Green, A.R., King, M.V., Shortall, S.E., Fone, K.C., 2012. Lost in translation: preclinical studies on 3,4-methylenedioxymethamphetamine provide information on mechanisms of action, but do not allow accurate prediction of adverse events in humans. Br. J. Pharmacol. 166, 1523–1536.

Morgan, C.J., Curran, H.V., 2012. Ketamine use: a review. Addiction 107, 27–38. (*Extensive review of current use of ketamine and the harms associated with its use*)

Morris, B.J., Cochran, S.M., Pratt, J.A., 2005. PCP: from pharmacology to modelling schizophrenia. Curr. Opin. Pharmacol. 5, 101–106. (*Review arguing that NMDA channel block by phencyclidine closely models human schizophrenia*)

Nichols, D.E., 2004. Hallucinogens. Pharmacol. Ther. 101, 131–181. (*Comprehensive review article focusing on 5-HT$_{2A}$ receptors as the target of psychotomimetic drugs*)

49 Drug addiction, dependence and abuse

OVERVIEW

In this chapter we consider drugs that are consumed because people choose to, and not because they are advised to by their doctor. Drugs in sport are discussed in Ch. 58. Largely, the drugs described in this chapter are taken because they are pleasurable (hedonic). A list of the more frequently used drugs is given in Table 49.1. It includes drugs that are also used for medicinal purposes (e.g. general anaesthetics, benzodiazepines, opioids and some psychostimulants), non-therapeutic drugs that are legal in many countries (e.g. nicotine and ethanol) and many other drugs that are widely used although their manufacture, sale and consumption have been declared illegal in most Western countries.

The reasons why the use of a particular drug is viewed as a problem to society – and hence may be considered 'drug abuse' – are complex and largely outside the scope of this book. The drug and its pharmacological activity are only the starting point. For many, but not all, drugs of abuse, continued use leads to dependence. Here, we briefly review the relevant classes of drug and the biological processes underlying drug dependence. We also describe in detail the pharmacology of two important drugs that are consumed in large amounts, namely **nicotine** and **ethanol**. Other drugs that are abused are described elsewhere in this book (see Table 49.1). 'Lifestyle' and 'sport' drugs are discussed in Chapter 58.

For further information on various aspects of drug abuse, see Koob & Le Moal (2006).

DRUG USE AND ABUSE

A number of terms are used, sometimes interchangeably and sometimes incorrectly, to describe drug use and the consequences of administration of drugs. Terms that are best avoided are listed in Table 49.2. Other, more useful, terms are defined in the text below.

A vast and ever-increasing array of drugs is used to alter mood and perception. These range from drugs that are also used as medicines, through non-medicinal synthetic drugs to herbal preparations (Table 49.1). The popularity of each varies between different societies across the world, and within societies popularity differs among different groups of individuals.[1] Frequently, users will take more than one drug concomitantly or sequentially. Polydrug use is a very under-researched area in regard to why it is done, how different drugs may interact and the potential harm that may arise from such practices. For example, ethanol alters cocaine metabolism, resulting in the production of *cocaethylene*, which is more potent than

cocaine and has greater cardiovascular toxicity. Sequential use is often intended to reduce adverse effects when coming down off the first drug (e.g. use of benzodiazepines when coming down from stimulants).

At first sight, the drugs listed in Table 49.1 form an extremely heterogeneous pharmacological group; we can find little in common at the molecular and cellular level between say, **morphine**, **cocaine** and **LSD** (lysergic acid diethylamide). What links them is that people find their effects pleasurable (hedonic) and tend to want to repeat the experience. The drug experience may take the form of intense euphoria, mood elevation, hallucinations, stimulation, sedation or calming depending upon the specific drug taken. In this regard drug use can be described as *thrill seeking*. Many drug users, however, have existing mental health problems and for them drug taking is a means of escaping reality and this can be described as *self-medicating*.

Abuse of prescription drugs, largely opioid analgesics such as **oxycodone** and **fentanyl** (see Ch. 42) as well as benzodiazepines (Ch. 44), has dramatically increased in recent years, especially in the USA. Thus a person may initially be prescribed an opioid drug to treat mild to moderate pain but continue to take the drug when the pain has receded, thus experiencing the pleasurable effects of the drug leading to addiction. In the USA, deaths from overdose of prescription drugs have tripled since 1990 – of over 38 000 deaths due to drug overdoses in 2010, 60% were due to prescription drugs. These overdose deaths include both prescription drug users and illicit **heroin** users who have obtained diverted supplies of these medicines. Illicit drugs such as heroin and cocaine are no longer the number one cause of drug overdose deaths.

Drug use involves effects on the brain that can be both acute and chronic (Fig. 49.1). The immediate, acute effect on mood is the reason the drug is taken. For some drugs (e.g. **amphetamines**, Ch. 48), this may be followed by a rebound negative or depressed phase. Persistent use of a drug may lead to compulsive drug use (addiction/dependence – a complex state that involves both psychological and physiological dependence) and to the development of tolerance. Psychological dependence can give rise to intense craving even when the user has been drug-free for months or years.

DRUG ADMINISTRATION

For drugs that induce strong feelings of euphoria, there are two components to the experience: an initial rapid effect (the *rush* or *buzz*) and a more prolonged pleasurable effect (the *high*). The intensity of the initial effect is determined by how fast the drug enters the brain and activates its effector mechanism. For many casual drug users, ease of administration defines how the drug is taken (e.g. smoking, swallowing or snorting a drug is relatively easy). However, for other drug users chasing a more intense experience, the route of administration and the

---

[1] A survey in one UK city showed that among Friday-night clubbers the choice of drug was associated with the type of music the clubs played (Measham & Moore, 2009).

Table 49.1 The main drugs of abuse

Type	Examples	Dependence liability	See Chapter
Opioids	Morphine	Very strong	42
	Diamorphine (heroin)	Very strong	42
	Methadone	Very strong	42
	Oxycodone	Very strong	42
	Hydrocodone	Very strong	42
General central nervous system depressants	Ethanol	Strong	This chapter
	Barbiturates	Strong	44
	General anaesthetics (e.g. N₂O, propofol)	Moderate	41
	Ketamine	Moderate	41, 48
	Organic solvents (e.g. glue sniffing)	Strong	–
Anxiolytic and hypnotic drugs	Benzodiazepines	Moderate	44
	GHB	Probably moderate	38
Psychomotor stimulants	Amphetamines	Strong	48
	Cocaine	Very strong	48
	MDMA (ecstasy)	Weak or absent	48
	Cathinones	Weak or absent	48
	Nicotine	Very strong	This chapter
Psychotomimetic agents	Lysergic acid diethylamide (LSD)	Weak or absent	48
	Mescaline	Weak or absent	48
	Cannabis and synthetic derivatives	Weak	19, 47

Table 49.2 Glossary of frequently used and 'abused' terms

Addict	Person for whom the desire to experience a drug's effects overrides any consideration for the serious physical, social or psychological problems that the drug may cause to the individual or others. Often used in non-scientific circles to convey criminal intent and so has fallen out of favour with those involved in treating people with drug problems
Drug misuse	Non-medicinal drug use (although some would not consider taking drugs to alter mood/induce hallucinations as 'misuse' or 'abuse')
Junkie	Pejorative term for someone who is dependent upon a drug
Narcotics	Originally used as a term to describe opioids as they induce sleep (narcosis). Subsequently this term has been used by non-scientists to describe a wide range of drugs of abuse (including cocaine which is a stimulant!)
Recreational drug use	Originally used to describe all drug abuse, it is now sometimes used to describe drug use in the bar/club/dance scene
Substance use	Some governments do not consider ethanol to be a drug, hence 'substance use' (or 'substance abuse') is used to include ethanol

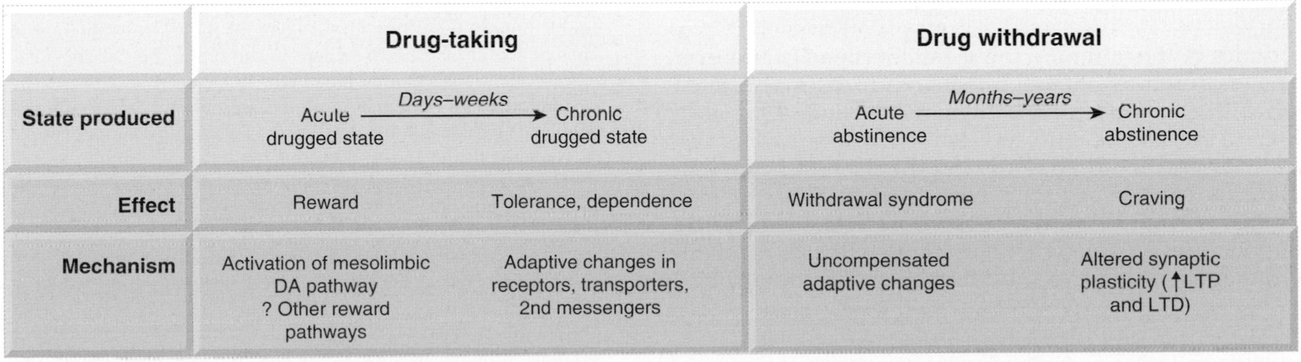

	Drug-taking		Drug withdrawal	
State produced	Acute drugged state → *Days–weeks* → Chronic drugged state		Acute abstinence → *Months–years* → Chronic abstinence	
Effect	Reward	Tolerance, dependence	Withdrawal syndrome	Craving
Mechanism	Activation of mesolimbic DA pathway ? Other reward pathways	Adaptive changes in receptors, transporters, 2nd messengers	Uncompensated adaptive changes	Altered synaptic plasticity (↑LTP and LTD)

Fig. 49.1 Cellular and physiological mechanisms involved in drug dependence showing the relationship between the immediate and delayed effects of drug taking and drug withdrawal. DA, dopamine; LTD, long-term depression; LTD, long-term potentiation.

choice of individual drug become important. Intravenous injection or smoking results in faster absorption of a drug than when it is taken orally. Heroin (official name diamorphine), cocaine, amphetamines, tobacco and **cannabis** are all taken by one or other of these routes. Heroin is more popular as a drug of abuse than morphine. This is because it enters the brain more rapidly than morphine. However, heroin itself does not interact with opioid receptors but is rapidly deacetylated to 6-acetylmorphine and morphine, μ-opioid-receptor agonists (see Ch. 42).

DRUG HARM

All drugs of abuse are harmful to a varying extent. Adverse effects can be the result of drug overdose (e.g. respiratory depression produced by opioids), of effects on tissues other than the brain (e.g. necrosis of the nasal septum resulting from chronic cocaine use), of the route of administration (e.g. HIV and other infections in drug users who share needles), of effects unrelated to the specific actions of the drug (e.g. carcinogenicity of tobacco smoke, severe bladder pain in regular ketamine users) or of use for illegal purposes (e.g. **flunitrazepam** or **γ-hydroxybutyrate** (**GHB**) as date-rape drugs). Many major harms relate to the ability of some drugs to induce dependence (e.g. psychostimulants, opioids, ethanol and tobacco) or to reveal a susceptibility to psychotic illness in some individuals (e.g. amphetamines and cannabis).

An attempt to produce a rational scale of harm, based on assessment by an expert panel of physical risk, dependence liability and social cost, was reported by Nutt et al. (2010), who have argued that such ratings should influence how governments police and punish people for supplying and using particular drugs. As expected, ethanol, heroin and cocaine were judged to be the most harmful, with cannabis, LSD and ecstasy (**MDMA**, see Ch. 48) much less so – an order that is not reflected in the classification of these drugs under UK law.[2]

DRUG DEPENDENCE

Drug dependence describes the human condition in which drug taking becomes compulsive, taking precedence over other needs, often with serious adverse consequences. Dependence becomes a problem when:

- the want becomes so insistent that it dominates the lifestyle of the individual and damages his or her quality of life
- the habit itself causes actual harm to the individual or the community.

Examples of the latter are the mental incapacity and liver damage caused by ethanol, the many diseases associated with smoking tobacco, the high risk of infection when injecting intravenously (especially HIV), the serious risk of overdose with most opioids and the criminal behaviour resorted to when drug users need to finance their habit.

Dependence involves both psychological and physical components. Family studies show clearly that susceptibility to dependence is an inherited characteristic. Around

50% of the risk of becoming dependent is genetic, with the remainder being developmental (adolescents are more at risk than adults) and environmental, e.g. stress, social pressures and drug availability. Variants of many different genes may each make a small contribution to the overall susceptibility of an individual to addiction – a familiar scenario that provides few pointers for therapeutic intervention. Polymorphisms in ethanol-metabolising genes (see later section on ethanol) are the best example of genes that directly affect the tendency to abuse a drug.

DRUG-INDUCED REWARD

The common feature of the various types of psychoactive drugs that are addictive is that all produce a *rewarding* experience (e.g. an elevation of mood or a feeling of euphoria or calmness).

In animal studies, where the state of mood cannot be inferred directly, reward is manifest as *positive reinforcement*, i.e. an increase in the probability of occurrence of any behaviour that is associated with the drug experience. In *conditioned place preference* studies, animals receive a drug or placebo and are then placed in different environments. Subsequently, when tested in a drug-free state, they will spend more time in the environment associated with a previous rewarding drug experience. Another way of determining if a drug is rewarding is to test whether or not animals will self-administer the drug by pressing a lever to obtain it. All dependence-producing drugs are self-administered by experimental animals. Hallucinogenic drugs are not, however, normally self-administered by experimental animals, which may indicate that, unlike humans, they find the experience non-rewarding.

Humans have a choice as to whether or not they wish to experiment with and continue taking drugs – there may therefore be an element of risk-taking when experimenting with drugs. In behavioural tests, some rats are observed to be much more impulsive than others (Dalley et al., 2007). These impulsive rats show a higher rate of cocaine self-administration and have a lower level of expression of D_2 and D_3 dopamine receptors in the nucleus accumbens (see below for the importance of this brain region in drug use). Impulsive rats are not, however, more prone to self-administering opioids.

Reward pathways

▼ Virtually all dependence-producing drugs so far tested, including opioids, nicotine, amphetamines, ethanol and cocaine, activate the *reward pathway* – the mesolimbic dopaminergic pathway (see Ch. 39), that runs, via the medial forebrain bundle, from the ventral tegmental area (VTA) of the midbrain to the nucleus accumbens and limbic region. Even though for some of these drugs their primary sites of action may be elsewhere in the brain, they all increase the extracellular level of dopamine in the nucleus accumbens, as shown by microdialysis in animals and *in vivo* brain imaging techniques in humans. Opioids enhance the firing of VTA dopaminergic neurons by reducing the level of GABAergic inhibition (disinhibition) within the VTA, whereas amphetamine and cocaine act on dopaminergic nerve terminals in the nucleus accumbens to release dopamine or prevent its reuptake (see Ch. 14). Given that dopamine release in the nucleus accumbens is also enhanced by naturally rewarding stimuli, such as food, water, sex and nurturing, it would appear that drugs are simply activating, or overactivating, the body's own pleasure system. In experienced drug users the anticipation of the effect may become sufficient to elicit the release of dopamine. Paradoxically, brain imaging studies have revealed that in chronic users the increase in dopamine may be less than expected when compared to what is seen in naïve subjects even although the subjective high is

---

[2]In determining society's attitude towards drugs, the media play an influential role. In the UK, deaths following consumption of ecstasy (around 60 per year) are often widely reported in the press and on television, but deaths due to heroin overdose (much more prevalent, at around 700 per year) are largely ignored unless the victim is famous.

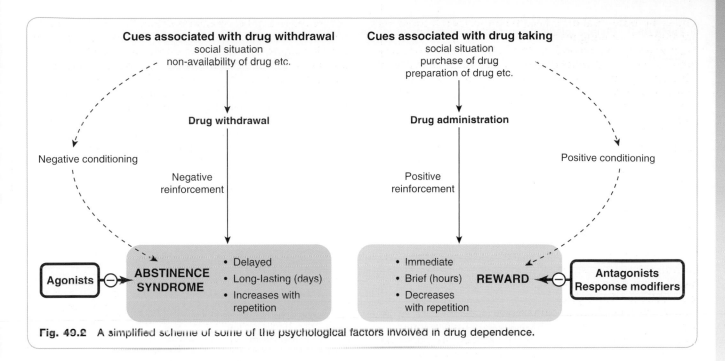

Fig. 49.2 A simplified scheme of some of the psychological factors involved in drug dependence.

still intense. This may reflect some degree of sensitisation but the mechanism is not well understood.

Chemical or surgical interruption of the VTA–accumbens dopaminergic pathway impairs drug-seeking behaviours in many experimental situations. Deletion of D_2 receptors in a transgenic mouse strain eliminated the rewarding properties of morphine administration without eliminating other opioid effects, and it did not prevent the occurrence of physical withdrawal symptoms in morphine-dependent animals (Maldonado et al., 1997), suggesting that the dopaminergic pathway is responsible for the positive reward but not for the negative withdrawal effects. However, D_2-receptor antagonists (antipsychotic drugs; see Ch. 46) have not been successful in treating addiction, and more recent evidence suggests that D_1 and possibly D_3 receptors play important roles. The development of D_3-receptor antagonists or partial agonists as treatments for drug abuse is awaited (see Newman et al., 2012).

PSYCHOLOGICAL DEPENDENCE

Having experienced the rewarding effects of a drug, an individual may desire to repeat the experience. The memory of previous drug-induced experiences can be very intense and long-lasting, giving rise to *craving*; it may drive an individual to take the drug again – referred to as *relapse* – even after a prolonged period of abstinence (see Weiss, 2005).

Craving may be triggered by stress or by cues such as experiencing the environment that a person associates with previously taking the drug or the sight of drug administration paraphernalia (e.g. a crack pipe or syringe). Coupled with the direct rewarding effect of the drug, cessation of drug use may be associated with an aversive psychological effect from which the subject will attempt to escape by self-administering the drug.

The psychological factors in drug dependence are discussed in detail by Koob & Le Moal (2006) and summarised in Figure 49.2.

PHYSICAL DEPENDENCE

This condition is characterised by a *withdrawal* or *abstinence syndrome* whereby on cessation of drug administration or on administering an antagonist, adverse physiological effects are experienced. On cessation of drug administration the withdrawal effects can persist for a period of days or weeks, the precise withdrawal responses being characteristic of the type of drug taken. Withdrawal responses can be observed in animals after chronic drug administration. The intensity of the withdrawal syndrome also varies between drugs of the same type but different pharmacokinetic characteristics. Pharmacological intervention can be used to reduce the intensity of the withdrawal (see Table 49.3). Several types of therapeutic drug, including antidepressant and antipsychotic agents, also produce withdrawal symptoms on cessation of administration but it is important to distinguish this type of commonly observed 'rebound' phenomenon from the physical dependence associated with drugs of abuse.

Physical dependence is less important in sustaining drug-seeking behaviour than psychological dependence. A degree of physical dependence is common when patients receive opioid analgesics in hospital for several days, but this rarely leads to addiction. On the other hand, heroin users who are nursed through and recover fully from the physical abstinence syndrome are still extremely likely to revert to drug taking later. Therefore although physical dependence may influence the drive to retake a drug, it is not the major factor in long-term drug dependence and relapse following a prolonged period of abstinence.

TOLERANCE

Tolerance (see Ch. 2) describes the decrease in pharmacological effect on repeated administration of a drug – it develops over time, as does the state of dependence. It does not occur with all drugs of abuse.

MECHANISMS OF DEPENDENCE AND TOLERANCE

▼ Drug users report that visual cues – such as the sight of a crack pipe or of a syringe – can evoke intense memories of the drug experience and induce strong craving for the drug, which may

Table 49.3 Pharmacological approaches to treating drug dependence

Mechanism	Example(s)
To alleviate withdrawal symptoms	Methadone (orally active) used short term to blunt opioid withdrawal Ibogaine (a naturally occurring psychoactive agent) used by some to reduce opioid withdrawal α_2-Adrenoceptor agonists (e.g. clonidine, lofexidine) to diminish opioid, alcohol and nicotine withdrawal symptoms β-Adrenoceptor antagonists (e.g. propranolol) to diminish excessive peripheral sympathetic activity Benzodiazepines, clomethiazole, topiramate and γ-hydroxybutyric acid (GHB) to blunt alcohol withdrawal
Long-term substitution	Methadone, buprenorphine or legal heroin to maintain opioid-dependent patients Nicotine patches or chewing gum Varenicline ($\alpha4\beta2$ nicotinic receptor partial agonist)
Blocking response	Naltrexone to block opioid effects in drug-withdrawn patients Naltrexone and nalmefene to reduce ethanol use Mecamylamine to block nicotine effects Immunisation against cocaine and nicotine to produce circulating antibody (still being developed)
Aversive therapies	Disulfiram to induce unpleasant response to ethanol
Reducing continued drug use (may act by reducing craving)	Bupropion (antidepressant with some nicotinic receptor antagonist activity) to reduce tobacco use Clonidine (α_2-adrenoceptor agonist) to reduce craving for nicotine[a] Acamprosate (NMDA-receptor antagonist) to treat alcoholism[a] Topiramate and lamotrogine (antiepileptic agents) to treat alcoholism and cocaine use[a] γ-Hydroxybutyric acid (GHB) reported to reduce craving for alcohol and cocaine[a] Baclofen reported to reduce opioid, alcohol and stimulant use[a] Modafinil to reduce cocaine use[a] Ibogaine reported to reduce craving for stimulants and opioids[a]

[a]How effective these agents are at reducing the continued use of other drugs of abuse over and above the ones listed remains to be determined.

Notes: Antidepressant, mood stabilising, anxiolytic and antipsychotic medications are useful when treating patients who, in addition to their drug use, also suffer from other mental disorders. The cannabinoid CB_1-receptor antagonist rimonabant, in addition to its antiobesity effects, also reduces nicotine, ethanol, stimulant and opioid consumption. However, it also induces depression and its use has been discontinued.

See Web links in the reference list for further information on treatments of drug dependence.

Drug dependence

- Dependence occurs when, as a result of repeated administration of the drug, the desire to experience the effects of a drug again becomes compulsive.
- Dependence occurs with a wide range of psychotropic drugs, acting by many different mechanisms.
- Dependence can be subdivided into psychological dependence and physical dependence.
- Psychological dependence (craving) is the major factor leading to relapse among treated addicts.
- The common feature of psychological dependence-inducing drugs is that they have a positive reinforcing action ('reward') associated with activation of the mesolimbic dopaminergic pathway.
- Physical dependence is characterised by an abstinence syndrome, which varies in type and intensity for different classes of drug.
- On repeated administration, tolerance may occur to the effects of the drug.
- Although genetic factors contribute to drug-seeking behaviour, no specific genes have yet been identified.

precipitate relapse. This suggests that associative learning may be a major factor in psychological dependence (Robbins et al., 2008). It has been suggested that drugs alter memory formation to enhance the recollection of previous drug experience. In this regard, it is of interest that several drugs produce changes in synaptic plasticity, a cellular correlate of memory formation (see Ch. 38). While cocaine, morphine, nicotine and ethanol enhance long-term potentiation (LTP) in the VTA by increasing the expression of AMPA receptors on the plasma membrane, cocaine also increases long-term depression (LTD) in the nucleus accumbens (Hyman et al., 2006).

Contrary to earlier thinking, physical dependence and tolerance are now though to involve different mechanisms (see Bailey & Connor, 2005).

The mechanisms responsible for the withdrawal syndrome have been most fully characterised for opioid dependence but similar mechanisms may apply to cocaine and ethanol withdrawal. At the cellular level, opioids inhibit cAMP formation, and withdrawal results in a rebound increase as a result of 'superactivation' of adenylyl cyclase, as well as upregulation of the amount of this enzyme. This results in activation of protein kinase A (PKA), in an increase in adenosine as a consequence of the conversion of cAMP to adenosine, and in activation of a transcription factor – cAMP response element binding protein (CREB). The rise in PKA activity increases the excitability of nerve terminals by phosphorylating neurotransmitter transporters to increase their ionic conductance (see Bagley et al., 2005) as well as increasing neurotransmitter release by a direct action on the secretory process (Williams et al., 2001). Withdrawal results in enhanced GABA release in various parts of the brain, probably through the mechanisms described above (see Bagley et al., 2011).

The release of other neurotransmitters is also likely to be enhanced. On the other hand, the enhanced extracellular levels of adenosine, acting on presynaptic A_1 receptors (see Ch. 16), inhibits glutamate release at excitatory synapses, and thus counteracts the neuronal hyperexcitability that occurs during drug withdrawal, suggesting the possibility – not yet clinically proven – that adenosine agonists might prove useful in treating drug dependence. CREB, which is upregulated in the nucleus accumbens by prolonged administration of opioids or cocaine, plays a key role in regulating various components of cAMP signalling pathways, and transgenic animals lacking CREB show reduced withdrawal symptoms (see Chao & Nestler, 2004).

For drugs such as opioids that are agonists at specific receptors (see Ch. 42), cellular tolerance results in part from desensitisation of the receptors. On prolonged activation by an agonist, the μ opioid receptor (MOPr) is phosphorylated by various intracellular kinases (Williams et al., 2013) – which either directly desensitises the receptor or causes the binding to the receptor of other proteins, such as arrestins, that uncouple the receptor from its G protein (see Ch. 3). In the intact animal, inhibition or knockout of these kinases reduces the level of tolerance.

Clinical use of drugs in substance dependence

Tobacco dependence
- Short-term **nicotine** is an adjunct to behavioural therapy in smokers committed to giving up; **varenicline** is also used as an adjunct but has been linked to suicidal ideation.
- **Bupropion** is also effective but lowers seizure threshold, so is contraindicated in people with risk factors for seizures (and also if there is a history of eating disorder).

Alcohol dependence
- Long-acting benzodiazepines (e.g. **chlordiazepoxide**) can be used to reduce withdrawal symptoms and the risk of seizures; they should be tapered over 1–2 weeks and then discontinued because of their abuse potential.
- **Disulfiram** is used as an adjunct to behavioural therapy in suitably motivated alcoholics after detoxification; it is contraindicated for patients in whom hypotension would be dangerous (e.g. those with coronary or cerebral vascular disease).
- **Acamprosate** can help to maintain abstinence; it is started as soon as abstinence has been achieved and maintained if relapse occurs, and it is continued for 1 year.

Opioid dependence
- Opioid agonists or partial agonists (e.g., respectively, **methadone** or **buprenorphine**) administered orally or sublingually may be substituted for injectable narcotics, many of whose harmful effects are attributable to the route of administration.
- **Naltrexone**, a long-acting opioid antagonist, is used as an adjunct to help prevent relapse in detoxified addicts (opioid free for at least 1 week).
- **Lofexidine**, an α_2 agonist (cf. **clonidine**; Ch. 14), is used short term (usually up to 10 days) to ameliorate symptoms of opioid withdrawal, and is then tapered over a further 2–4 days.

PHARMACOLOGICAL APPROACHES TO TREATING DRUG ADDICTION

From the discussion above, it will be clear that drug abuse involves many psychosocial and some genetic factors, as well as neuropharmacological mechanisms, so drug treatment is only one component of the therapeutic approaches that are used. The main pharmacological approaches (see Heidbreder & Hagan, 2005) are summarised in Table 49.3. For information on other approaches to the treatment of drug addiction, readers are advised to consult the National Institute on Drug Abuse (NIDA) website at www.nida.nih.gov/.

NICOTINE AND TOBACCO

Tobacco growing, chewing and smoking was indigenous throughout the American subcontinent and Australia at the time that European explorers first visited these places. Smoking spread through Europe during the 16th century, coming to England mainly as a result of its enthusiastic espousal by Walter Raleigh at the court of Elizabeth I. James I strongly disapproved of both Raleigh and tobacco, and in the early 17th century initiated the first antismoking campaign, with the support of the Royal College of Physicians. Parliament responded by imposing a substantial duty on tobacco, thereby giving the state an economic interest in the continuation of smoking at the same time that its official expert advisers were issuing emphatic warnings about its dangers.

Until the latter half of the 19th century, tobacco was smoked in pipes, and primarily by men. Cigarette manufacture began at the end of the 19th century, and now cigarettes account for 98% of tobacco consumption. Filter cigarettes (which give a somewhat lower delivery of tar and nicotine than standard cigarettes) and 'low tar' cigarettes (which are also low in nicotine) constitute an increasing proportion of the total.[3] Cigarette consumption across the globe continues to rise (Fig. 49.3), although it is decreasing in some countries such as the UK[4] and Australia. There are about 1.1 billion smokers in the world (18% of the population), and the number in developing countries is increasing rapidly. Six trillion (6×10^{12}) cigarettes are sold each year, more than 900 cigarettes for every man, woman and child on the planet. In 2010, 12 million cigarettes per minute were smoked around the world.

PHARMACOLOGICAL EFFECTS OF SMOKING

Nicotine[5] is the main pharmacologically active substance in tobacco smoke. The acute effects of smoking can be mimicked by injection of nicotine and are blocked by

---

[3]Smokers, however, adapt by smoking more low-tar cigarettes and inhaling more deeply so as to maintain their nicotine consumption.
[4]In the UK consumption has dropped by over 50% from its peak in the 1970s, the main factors being increased price, adverse publicity, restrictions on advertising, the compulsory publication of health warnings and a ban on smoking in public places. Still, however, around 9.4 million adults (just over 20% of the adult population) in the UK smoke, with little difference between men and women. About 10% of children aged 10–15 are regular smokers.
[5]From the plant *Nicotiana*, named after Jean Nicot, French ambassador to Portugal, who presented seeds to the French king in 1560, having been persuaded by natives of South America of the medical value of smoking tobacco leaves. Smoking was believed to protect against illness, particularly the plague.

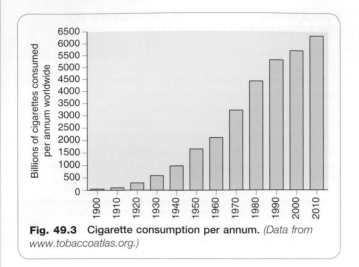

Fig. 49.3 Cigarette consumption per annum. *(Data from www.tobaccoatlas.org.)*

Tobacco smoking

- Cigarette consumption across the world continues to rise, although in the UK it is now declining after reaching a peak in the mid-1970s.
- The worldwide prevalence of smoking is now about 18% of the adult population, each smoker using on average 5000 cigarettes per year.
- **Nicotine** is the main pharmacologically active agent in tobacco, apart from carcinogenic tars and carbon monoxide.
- The amount of **nicotine** absorbed from an average cigarette is about 1–1.5 mg, which causes the plasma **nicotine** concentration to reach 130–200 nmol/l. These values depend greatly on the type of cigarette and on the extent of inhalation of the smoke.

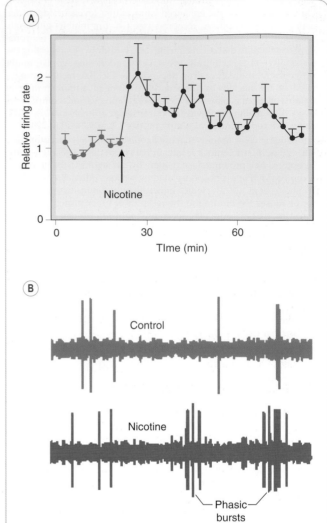

Fig. 49.4 Nicotine alters action potential firing characteristics of VTA dopaminergic neurons in freely moving rats. [**A**] Neuronal firing rate increases after nicotine injection i.p. [**B**] Action potential firing is phasic after nicotine injection. *(Adapted from De Biasi et al. 2011.)*

mecamylamine, an antagonist at neuronal nicotinic acetylcholine receptors (nAChRs; see Ch. 13). For reviews on nicotine and addiction see (De Biasi et al., 2011; Leslie et al., 2013).

Effects on the central nervous system

At the neuronal level, nicotine acts on nAChRs (see Ch. 39), which are widely expressed in the brain, particularly in the cortex and hippocampus, and are believed to play a role in cognitive function, as well as in the VTA, from which dopaminergic neurons project to the nucleus accumbens (the reward pathway, see Fig 39.3). nAChRs are ligand-gated cation channels located both pre- and postsynaptically, causing, respectively, enhanced transmitter release and neuronal excitation (see Wonnacott et al., 2005). Nicotine increases the firing rate and phasic activity of VTA dopaminergic neurons (Fig. 49.4). Of the various subtypes of nAChR (see Table 39.2), the α4β2, α6β2 and α7 subtypes have received most attention, but other subtypes may also be involved in the rewarding effects of nicotine. As well as activating the receptors, nicotine also causes desensitisation, so the effects of a dose of nicotine are diminished in animals after sustained exposure to the drug. Chronic nicotine administration leads to a substantial increase in the number of nAChRs

(an effect opposite to that produced by sustained administration of most receptor agonists), which may represent an adaptive response to prolonged receptor desensitisation. It is likely that the overall effect of nicotine reflects a balance between activation of nAChRs, causing neuronal excitation, and desensitisation, causing synaptic block.

At the spinal level, nicotine inhibits spinal reflexes, causing skeletal muscle relaxation that can be measured by electromyography. This may be due to stimulation of the inhibitory Renshaw cells in the ventral horn of the spinal cord. The higher level functioning of the brain, as reflected in the subjective sense of alertness or by the electroencephalography (EEG) pattern, can be affected in either direction by nicotine, according to dose and circumstances. Smokers report that smoking wakes them up when they are drowsy and calms them down when they are tense, and EEG recordings broadly bear this out. It also seems that small doses of nicotine tend to cause arousal, whereas large doses do the reverse. Tests of motor and sensory performance (e.g. reaction time measurements or vigilance tests) in humans generally show improvement after smoking, and nicotine enhances learning in rats. Nicotine and other nicotinic agonists such as **epibatidine** (Ch. 42) have significant analgesic activity.

Peripheral effects

The peripheral effects of small doses of nicotine result from stimulation of autonomic ganglia (see Ch. 13) and of peripheral sensory receptors, mainly in the heart and lungs. Stimulation of these receptors produces tachycardia, increased cardiac output and increased arterial pressure, reduction of gastrointestinal motility and sweating. When people smoke for the first time, they usually experience nausea and sometimes vomit, probably because of stimulation of sensory receptors in the stomach. All these effects decline with repeated dosage, although the central effects remain. Secretion of adrenaline and noradrenaline from the adrenal medulla contributes to the cardiovascular effects, and release of antidiuretic hormone from the posterior pituitary causes a decrease in urine flow.[6] The plasma concentration of free fatty acids is increased, probably owing to sympathetic stimulation and adrenaline secretion.

Smokers weigh, on average, about 4 kg less than non-smokers, mainly because of reduced food intake; giving up smoking usually causes weight gain associated with increased food intake.

PHARMACOKINETIC ASPECTS

An average cigarette contains about 0.8 g of tobacco and 9–17 mg of nicotine, of which about 10% is normally absorbed by the smoker. This fraction varies greatly with the habits of the smoker and the type of cigarette.

Nicotine in cigarette smoke is rapidly absorbed from the lungs but poorly from the mouth and nasopharynx. Therefore, inhalation is required to give appreciable absorption of nicotine, each puff delivering a distinct bolus of drug to the CNS. Pipe or cigar smoke is less acidic than cigarette smoke, and the nicotine tends to be absorbed from the mouth and nasopharynx rather than the lungs. Absorption is considerably slower than from inhaled cigarette smoke, resulting in a later and longer-lasting peak in the plasma nicotine concentration (Fig. 49.5). An average cigarette, smoked over 10 min, causes the plasma nicotine concentration to rise to 15–30 ng/ml (100–200 nmol/l), falling to about half within 10 min and then more slowly over the next 1–2 h. The rapid decline results mainly from redistribution between the blood and other tissues; the slower decline is due to hepatic metabolism, mainly by oxidation to an inactive ketone metabolite, *cotinine*. This has a long plasma half-life, and measurement of cotinine concentration provides a useful measure of smoking behaviour. A nicotine patch applied for 24 h causes the plasma concentration of nicotine to rise to 75–150 nmol/l over 6 h and to remain fairly constant for about 20 h. Administration by nasal spray or chewing gum results in a time course intermediate between that of smoking and the nicotine patch.

TOLERANCE AND DEPENDENCE

As with other dependence-producing drugs, three separate processes – psychological dependence, physical

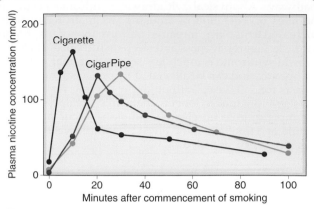

Fig 49.5 Nicotine concentration in plasma during smoking. The subjects were habitual smokers who smoked a cigarette, cigar or pipe according to their usual habit. *(From Bowman WC, Rand M 1980 Chapter 4. In: Textbook of Pharmacology. Blackwell, Oxford.)*

dependence and tolerance – contribute to the overall state of dependence, in which taking the drug becomes compulsive.

The effects of nicotine associated with peripheral ganglionic stimulation show rapid tolerance, perhaps as a result of desensitisation of nAChRs. With large doses of nicotine, this desensitisation produces a block of ganglionic transmission (see Ch. 13). Tolerance to the central effects of nicotine (e.g. in the arousal response) is much less than in the periphery. The increase in the number of nAChRs in the brain produced by chronic nicotine administration in animals (see p. 604) also occurs in heavy smokers. Because the cellular effects of nicotine are diminished, it is possible that the additional binding sites represent desensitised rather than functional receptors.

The addictiveness of smoking is due to the effects of nicotine combined with the ritual of smoking (see Le Foll & Goldberg, 2005). Rats choose to drink dilute nicotine solution in preference to water if given a choice, and in a situation in which lever pressing causes an injection of nicotine to be delivered – admittedly at high doses – they quickly learn to self-administer it. Similarly, monkeys who have been trained to smoke, by providing a reward in response to smoking behaviour, will continue to do so spontaneously (i.e. unrewarded) if the smoking medium contains nicotine, but not if nicotine-free tobacco is offered instead. Humans, however, are unlikely to become addicted to nicotine delivered from patches suggesting that other factors are also involved, such as the controlled pulsatile delivery associated with smoking.

Like other addictive drugs, nicotine causes excitation of the mesolimbic reward pathway and increased dopamine release in the nucleus accumbens. Transgenic mice lacking the β2 subunit of the nAChR lose the rewarding effect of nicotine and its dopamine-releasing effect, confirming the importance of the β2-containing nAChR subtypes and mesolimbic dopamine release in the response to nicotine. In contrast to normal mice, the mutant mice could not be induced to self-administer nicotine, even though they did so with cocaine.

In contrast to euphoria, induction of physical dependence involves nicotinic receptors containing α5 and β4 subunits in the medial habenula–interpeduncular nucleus

---

[6]This may explain why, in years gone by, men smoked cigars while chatting over drinks after dinner.

605

pathway. A physical withdrawal syndrome occurs in humans on cessation of smoking. Its main features are increased irritability, impaired performance of psychomotor tasks, aggressiveness and sleep disturbance. The withdrawal syndrome is much less severe than that produced by opioids, and can be alleviated by replacement nicotine. It lasts for 2–3 weeks, although the craving for cigarettes persists for much longer than this; relapses during attempts to give up cigarette smoking occur most commonly at a time when the physical withdrawal syndrome has long since subsided.

Pharmacology of nicotine

- At the cellular level, **nicotine** acts on nicotinic acetylcholine receptors (nAChRs) to enhance neurotransmitter release and increase neuronal excitation. Its central effects are blocked by receptor antagonists such as **mecamylamine**.
- At the behavioural level, nicotine produces a mixture of inhibitory and excitatory effects.
- **Nicotine** shows reinforcing properties, associated with increased activity in the mesolimbic dopaminergic pathway, and self-administration can be elicited in animal studies.
- Electroencephalography changes show an arousal response, and subjects report increased alertness accompanied by a reduction of anxiety and tension.
- Learning, particularly under stress, is facilitated by **nicotine**.
- Peripheral effects of **nicotine** are due mainly to ganglionic stimulation: tachycardia, increased blood pressure and reduced gastrointestinal motility. Tolerance develops rapidly to these effects.
- **Nicotine** is metabolised, mainly in the liver, within 1–2 h.
- The inactive metabolite, cotinine, has a long elimination half-life. Urinary cotinine excretion can be used as a measure of smoking habits.
- **Nicotine** gives rise to tolerance, physical dependence and psychological dependence (craving). Attempts at long-term cessation succeed in only about 20% of cases.
- **Nicotine** replacement therapy (chewing gum or skin patch preparations) improves the chances of giving up smoking when combined with active counselling.

HARMFUL EFFECTS OF SMOKING

The life expectancy of smokers is shorter than that of non-smokers. Smoking causes almost 90% of deaths from lung cancer, about 80% of deaths from bronchitis and emphysema, and 17% of deaths from heart disease. About one-third of all cancer deaths can be attributed to smoking. Smoking is, by a large margin, the biggest preventable cause of death, responsible for about 1 in 10 adult deaths worldwide. Deaths from smoking are continuing to rise. In 2011, smoking was responsible for about 6 million deaths worldwide (and approximately 600 000 non-smokers died in 2011 from involuntary secondary inhalation); by 2030, deaths are expected to increase to 10 million, mainly due to the growth of smoking in Asia, Africa and Latin America.

The main health risks are as follows:

- *Cancer, particularly of the lung and upper respiratory tract but also of the oesophagus, pancreas and bladder.* Smoking 20 cigarettes per day is estimated to increase the risk of lung cancer about 10-fold. Pipe and cigar smoking carry much less risk than cigarette smoking, although the risk is still appreciable. Tar, rather than nicotine, is responsible for the cancer risk. Genetic variants of nicotinic-receptor subunits have been associated with lung cancer although the mechanisms behind this association are unclear (see Hung et al., 2008).
- *Coronary heart disease and other forms of peripheral vascular disease.* The mortality among men aged 55–64 from coronary thrombosis is about 60% greater in men who smoke 20 cigarettes per day than in non-smokers. Although the increase in risk is less than it is for lung cancer, the actual number of excess deaths associated with smoking is larger, because coronary heart disease is so common. Other kinds of vascular disease (e.g. stroke, intermittent claudication and diabetic gangrene) are also strongly smoking-related. A causal link between nicotine and cardiovascular risk has not been demonstrated. Indeed nicotine preparations, used to help smokers give up cigarettes, are not thought to carry a serious risk. Carbon monoxide (see p. 607) could be a factor. However, there is no clear increase in ischaemic heart disease in pipe and cigar smokers, even though similar blood nicotine and carboxyhaemoglobin concentrations are reached, suggesting that other factors may be responsible for the risk associated with cigarettes.
- *Chronic obstructive pulmonary disease* (COPD; see Ch. 28) is a major global health problem. Cigarette smoking is the main cause. Stopping smoking slows the progression of the disease. Bronchitis, inflammation of the mucous membranes of the bronchi, is much more common in smokers than in non-smokers. These effects are probably due to tar and other irritants rather than nicotine.
- *Harmful effects in pregnancy.* Smoking, particularly during the latter half of pregnancy, significantly reduces birth weight (by about 8% in women who smoke 25 or more cigarettes per day during pregnancy) and increases perinatal mortality (by an estimated 28% in babies born to mothers who smoke in the last half of pregnancy). There is evidence that children born to smoking mothers remain behind, in both physical and mental development, for at least 7 years. By 11 years of age, the difference is no longer significant. These effects of smoking, although measurable, are much smaller than the effects of other factors, such as social class and birth order. Various other complications of pregnancy are also more common in women who smoke, including spontaneous abortion (increased 30–70% by smoking), premature delivery (increased about 40%) and placenta praevia (increased 25–90%). Nicotine is excreted in breast milk in sufficient amounts to cause tachycardia in the infant.

The agents probably responsible for the harmful effects are as follows:

- Tar and irritants, such as nitrogen dioxide and formaldehyde. Cigarette smoke tar contains many known carcinogenic hydrocarbons, as well as tumour promoters, which account for the high cancer risk. It is likely that the various irritant substances are also responsible for the increase in bronchitis and emphysema.
- Nicotine probably accounts for retarded fetal development because of its vasoconstrictor properties.
- Carbon monoxide. Cigarette smoke contains about 3% carbon monoxide. Carbon monoxide has a high affinity for haemoglobin, and the average carboxyhaemoglobin content in the blood of cigarette smokers is about 2.5% (compared with 0.4% for non-smoking urban dwellers). In very heavy smokers, up to 15% of haemoglobin may be carboxylated, a level that affects fetal development in rats. Fetal haemoglobin has a higher affinity for carbon monoxide than adult haemoglobin, and the proportion of carboxyhaemoglobin is higher in fetal than in maternal blood.
- Increased oxidative stress may be responsible for atherogenesis (Ch. 23) and chronic obstructive pulmonary disease (Ch. 28).

OTHER EFFECTS OF SMOKING

Parkinson's disease is approximately twice as common in non-smokers as in smokers. It is possible that this reflects a protective effect of nicotine. Ulcerative colitis appears to be a disease of non-smokers. Former smokers are at high risk for developing ulcerative colitis, while current smokers have the least risk. This tendency indicates that smoking cigarettes may prevent the onset of ulcerative colitis. In contrast, smoking tends to worsen the effects of Crohn's disease. Earlier reports that Alzheimer's disease is less common in smokers have not been confirmed; indeed there is evidence that smoking may increase the occurrence of Alzheimer's disease in some genetic groups.

Effects of smoking

- Smoking accounts for more than 10% of deaths worldwide, mainly due to:
  - cancer, especially lung cancer, of which about 90% of cases are smoking related; carcinogenic tars are responsible
  - chronic bronchitis; tars are mainly responsible.
- Smoking in pregnancy reduces birth weight and retards childhood development. It also increases abortion rate and perinatal mortality. **Nicotine** and possibly carbon monoxide are responsible.
- The incidence of Parkinson's disease is lower in smokers than in non-smokers.

PHARMACOLOGICAL APPROACHES TO TREATING NICOTINE DEPENDENCE

Most smokers would like to quit, but few succeed.[7] The most successful smoking cure clinics, using a combination of psychological and pharmacological treatments, achieve a success rate of about 25%, measured as the percentage of patients still abstinent after 1 year. The main pharmacological treatments are **nicotine replacement therapy**, **varenicline** and **bupropion** (originally used to treat depression; see Ch. 47, Table 47.2).

Nicotine replacement therapy is used mainly to assist smokers to quit by reducing craving and physical withdrawal symptoms. Because nicotine is relatively short-acting and not well absorbed from the gastrointestinal tract, it is given in the form of chewing gum, lozenges and oral or nasal sprays that can be used several times a day or as a transdermal patch that is replaced daily.[8]

These preparations cause various side effects, particularly nausea and gastrointestinal cramps, cough, insomnia and muscle pains. There is a risk that nicotine may cause coronary spasm in patients with heart disease. Transdermal patches may cause local irritation and itching. Combined with professional counselling and supportive therapy, nicotine replacement therapy roughly doubles the chances of successfully breaking the smoking habit. Nicotine on its own, without counselling and support, is no more effective than placebo. In Sweden, the use of 'smokeless tobacco' is encouraged and the smoking-related death rate is much lower than elsewhere in Europe or North America.

nAChR subtypes containing the α4β2 subunits are thought to mediate the rewarding properties of tobacco smoking, which may allow selective agonists to be developed as nicotine substitutes with fewer side effects. Varenicline is a partial agonist at the α4β2 nAChR subtype and has differing levels of efficacy at other subtypes. Being a partial agonist it may provide a level of substitution while at the same time blocking the rewarding effect of smoking. It is effective in preventing relapse but there was concern that it may induce suicidal thoughts, suicide attempts, aggression and homicide. However, a large retrospective study (Gunnell et al., 2009) found no evidence of increased suicide or suicidal thoughts with varenicline, compared with other antismoking treatments.

Bupropion (see Ch. 47) is a nicotinic antagonist. It may also act by increasing dopamine activity in the nucleus accumbens as it is a weak blocker of dopamine and noradrenaline uptake, but it is not clear that this accounts for its efficacy in treating nicotine dependence. It is usually given as a slow-release formulation. It appears to be as effective as nicotine replacement therapy, even in non-depressed patients, and has fewer side effects. However, bupropion lowers the seizure threshold so should not be prescribed if there are other risk factors for seizures (including other drugs that lower seizure threshold). It is also contraindicated if there is a history of eating disorders or of bipolar mood disorder, and is used only with caution in patients with liver or renal disease. Because of these problems, nicotine remains the pharmacological treatment of choice in most cases.

Although an early method of making the body produce antibodies that bind and inactivate nicotine was shown to be no better than placebo in clinical trials, it is still hoped that the use of genetically modified viruses to induce higher levels of circulating antibodies will prove to be more effective.

---

[7]Sigmund Freud tried unsuccessfully to give up cigars for 45 years before dying of cancer of the mouth at the age of 83.

[8]Electronic cigarettes – basically inhalers that deliver nicotine – are designed to mimic cigarettes in their use and appearance. The dose of nicotine delivered/inhaled is variable and their effectiveness remains to be determined.

ETHANOL

Judged on a molar basis, the consumption of ethanol far exceeds that of any other drug. The ethanol content of various drinks ranges from about 2.5% (weak beer) to about 55% (strong spirits), and the size of the normal measure is such that a single drink usually contains about 8–12 g (0.17–0.26 mol) of ethanol. Its low pharmacological potency is reflected in the range of plasma concentrations needed to produce pharmacological effects: minimal effects occur at about 10 mmol/l (46 mg/100 ml), and 10 times this concentration may be lethal. The average per capita consumption of ethanol in the UK doubled between 1970 and 2007, falling slightly since then. The main changes have been a growing consumption of wine in preference to beer among adults, greater consumption in the home and an increasing tendency for binge drinking, especially among young people.

For practical purposes, ethanol intake is often expressed in terms of units. One unit is equal to 8 g (10 ml) of ethanol, and is the amount contained in half a pint of normal strength beer, one measure of spirits or one small glass of wine. Based on the health risks described below, the recommendation is a maximum of 21–28 units/week for men and 14–21 units/week for women. It is estimated that in the UK, about 33% of men and 13% of women exceed these levels. The annual spend on drinks is £15 billion, providing a tax revenue of about £9 billion. The health cost is estimated at £3 billion, and the social cost as £8 billion for crime and disruptive behaviour plus £2 billion in absenteeism from work. Governments in most developed countries are attempting to curb alcohol consumption.

An excellent detailed review of all aspects of alcohol and alcoholism is provided by Spanagel (2009).

PHARMACOLOGICAL EFFECTS OF ETHANOL

Effects on central nervous system neurons

The main effects of ethanol are on the CNS (see review Spanagel, 2009), where its depressant actions resemble those of volatile anaesthetics (Ch. 41). At a cellular level, the effect of ethanol is depressant, although it increases neuronal activity – presumably by disinhibition – in some parts of the CNS, notably in the mesolimbic dopaminergic pathway that is involved in reward. The main acute cellular effects of ethanol that occur at concentrations (5–100 mmol/l) relevant to alcohol consumption by humans are:

- enhancement of both GABA- and glycine-mediated inhibition
- inhibition of Ca^{2+} entry through voltage-gated calcium channels
- activation of certain types of K^+ channel
- inhibition of ionotropic glutamate receptor function
- inhibition of adenosine transport.

For review see Harris et al. (2008).

Ethanol enhances the action of GABA on $GABA_A$ receptors in a similar way to benzodiazepines (see Ch. 44). Its effect is, however, smaller and less consistent than that of benzodiazepines, and no clear effect on inhibitory synaptic transmission in the CNS has been demonstrated for ethanol. This may be because the effect of ethanol is seen only on some subtypes of $GABA_A$ receptor (see Ch. 38).

Exactly which $GABA_A$ receptor subtypes are sensitive to ethanol is still unclear but those containing δ subunits appear to be important. Ethanol may also act presynaptically to enhance GABA release. The benzodiazepine inverse agonist **flumazenil** (see Ch. 44) reverses the central depressant actions of ethanol by a non-competitive interaction on the $GABA_A$ receptor. The use of flumazenil to reverse ethanol intoxication and treat dependence has not found favour for several reasons. Because flumazenil is an inverse agonist (see Ch. 2) at benzodiazepine receptors, it carries a risk of causing seizures, and it could cause an increase in ethanol consumption and thus increase long-term toxic manifestations.

Ethanol produces a consistent enhancement of glycine receptor function. This effect is likely to be due both to a direct interaction of ethanol with the α1 subunit of the glycine receptor and to indirect effects of ethanol mediated through PKC activation. Ethanol can also enhance glycine release from nerve terminals.

Ethanol reduces transmitter release in response to nerve terminal depolarisation by inhibiting the opening of voltage-gated calcium channels in neurons. It also reduces neuronal excitability by activating G protein-activated inwardly rectifying K^+ (GIRK) channels as well as potentiating calcium-activated potassium (BK) channel activity.

The excitatory effects of glutamate are inhibited by ethanol at concentrations that produce CNS depressant effects *in vivo*. NMDA receptor activation is inhibited at lower ethanol concentrations than are required to affect AMPA receptors (see Ch. 38). Other effects produced by ethanol include an enhancement of the excitatory effects produced by activation of nAChRs and 5-HT$_3$ receptors. The relative importance of these various effects in the overall effects of ethanol on CNS function is not clear.

The depressant effects of ethanol on neuronal function resemble those of adenosine acting on A_1 receptors (see Ch. 16). Ethanol in cell culture systems increases extracellular adenosine by inhibiting adenosine uptake, and there is some evidence that inhibition of the adenosine transporter may account for some of its CNS effects (Melendez & Kalivas, 2004).

Endogenous opioids also play a role in the CNS effects of ethanol, because both human and animal studies show that the opioid receptor antagonist **naltrexone** reduces the reward associated with ethanol.

Behavioural effects

The effects of acute ethanol intoxication in humans are well known and include slurred speech, motor incoordination, increased self-confidence and euphoria. The effect on mood varies among individuals, most becoming louder and more outgoing, but some becoming morose and withdrawn. At higher levels of intoxication, the mood tends to become highly labile, with euphoria and melancholy, aggression and submission, often occurring successively. The association between alcohol and violence is well documented.

Intellectual and motor performance and sensory discrimination are impaired by ethanol, but subjects are generally unable to judge this for themselves. For example, bus drivers were asked to drive through a gap that they selected as the minimum for their bus to pass through; ethanol caused them not only to hit the barriers more often at any given gap setting, but also to set the gap to a narrower dimension, often narrower than the bus.

Much effort has gone into measuring the effect of ethanol on driving performance in real life, as opposed to artificial tests under experimental conditions. In an American study of city drivers, it was found that the probability of being involved in an accident was unaffected at blood ethanol concentrations up to 50 mg/100 ml (10.9 mmol/l); by 80 mg/100 ml (17.4 mmol/l) the probability was increased about four-fold, and by 150 mg/100 ml (32.6 mmol/l) about 25-fold. In the UK, driving with a blood ethanol concentration greater than 80 mg/100 ml is illegal.

The relationship between plasma ethanol concentration and effect is highly variable. A given concentration produces a larger effect when the concentration is rising than when it is steady or falling. A substantial degree of cellular tolerance develops in habitual drinkers, with the result that a higher plasma ethanol concentration is needed to produce a given effect. In one study, 'gross intoxication' (assessed by a battery of tests that measured speech, gait and so on) occurred in 30% of subjects between 50 and 100 mg/100 ml and in 90% of subjects with more than 150 mg/100 ml. Coma generally occurs at about 400 mg/100 ml, and death from respiratory failure is likely at levels exceeding 500 mg/100 ml.

Ethanol significantly enhances – sometimes to a dangerous extent – the CNS depressant effects of many other drugs, including benzodiazepines, antidepressants, antipsychotic drugs and opioids.

Neurotoxicity

In addition to the acute effects of ethanol on the nervous system, chronic administration also causes irreversible neurological damage (see Harper & Matsumoto, 2005). This may be due to ethanol itself, or to metabolites such as acetaldehyde or fatty acid esters, or to dietary deficiencies (e.g. of thiamine) that are common in alcoholics. Binge drinking is thought to produce greater damage, probably due to the high brain concentrations of ethanol achieved and to repeated phases of withdrawal between binges. Heavy drinkers often exhibit convulsions and may develop irreversible dementia and motor impairment associated with thinning of the cerebral cortex (apparent as ventricular enlargement) detectable by brain-imaging techniques. Degeneration of the cerebellar vermis, the mammillary bodies and other specific brain regions can also occur, as well as peripheral neuropathy.

Effects on other systems

The main acute cardiovascular effect of ethanol is to produce cutaneous vasodilatation, central in origin, which causes a warm feeling but actually increases heat loss.[9] Paradoxically, there is a positive correlation between ethanol consumption and hypertension, possibly because ethanol withdrawal causes increased sympathetic activity. The beneficial effect of moderate drinking on cardiovascular function is discussed below.

Diuresis is a familiar effect of ethanol. It is caused by inhibition of antidiuretic hormone secretion, and tolerance develops rapidly, so that the diuresis is not sustained. There is a similar inhibition of oxytocin secretion, which can delay parturition.

Ethanol increases salivary and gastric secretion, perhaps a reason in some cultures for the popularity of a glass of sherry before dinner. However, heavy consumption of spirits causes damage directly to the gastric mucosa, causing chronic gastritis. Both this and the increased acid secretion are factors in the high incidence of gastric bleeding in alcoholics. CNS depression predisposes to aspiration pneumonia and lung abscess formation. Acute pancreatitis may become chronic with pseudocyst formation (collections of fluid in the peritoneal sac), fat malabsorption and ultimately loss of B-cell function and insulin-dependent diabetes mellitus.

Ethanol produces a variety of endocrine effects. In particular, it increases the output of adrenal steroid hormones by stimulating the anterior pituitary gland to secrete adrenocorticotrophic hormone. However, the increase in plasma hydrocortisone usually seen in alcoholics (producing a 'pseudo-Cushing's syndrome'[Ch. 33]) is due partly to inhibition by ethanol of hydrocortisone metabolism in the liver.

Acute toxic effects on muscle are exacerbated by seizures and prolonged immobility; severe myositis ('rhabdomyolysis') with myoglobinuria can cause acute renal failure. Chronic toxicity affects particularly cardiac muscle, giving rise to alcoholic cardiomyopathy and chronic heart failure.

Chronic ethanol consumption may also result in immunosuppression, leading to increased incidence of infections such as pneumonia (immunisation with pneumococcal vaccine is important in chronic alcoholics); and increased cancer risk, particularly of the mouth, larynx and oesophagus.

Male alcoholics are often impotent and show signs of feminisation. This is associated with impaired testicular steroid synthesis, but induction of hepatic microsomal enzymes by ethanol, and hence an increased rate of testosterone inactivation, also contributes.

Effects of ethanol on the liver

Together with brain damage, liver damage is the most common serious long-term consequence of excessive ethanol consumption (see Lieber, 1995). Increased fat accumulation (fatty liver) progresses to hepatitis (i.e. inflammation of the liver) and eventually to irreversible hepatic necrosis and fibrosis. Cirrhosis is an end stage, with extensive fibrosis and foci of regenerating hepatocytes that are not correctly 'plumbed in' to the blood and biliary systems. Diversion of portal blood flow around the cirrhotic liver often causes oesophageal varices to develop, which can bleed suddenly and catastrophically. Increased fat accumulation in the liver occurs, in rats or in humans, after a single large dose of ethanol. The mechanism is complex, the main factors being:

- increased release of fatty acids from adipose tissue, which is the result of increased stress, causing sympathetic discharge
- impaired fatty acid oxidation, because of the metabolic load imposed by the ethanol itself.

With chronic ethanol consumption, many other factors contribute to the liver damage. One is malnutrition, for alcoholic individuals may satisfy much of their calorie requirement from ethanol itself. Three hundred grams of

---

[9]The image of a large St Bernard dog carrying a small keg of brandy around its neck to revive avalanche victims is an apocryphal one created by the English painter Edwin Landseer, who in 1820 produced a painting called 'Alpine Mastiffs Reanimating a Distressed Traveller'. With their keen sense of smell, such dogs were useful in searching for people buried in the snow, but taking a tot of brandy would only have enhanced the victim's heat loss.

ethanol (equivalent to one bottle of whisky) provides about 2000 kcal but, unlike a normal diet, it provides no vitamins, amino acids or fatty acids. Thiamine deficiency is an important factor in causing chronic neurological damage.

The overall incidence of chronic liver disease is a function of cumulative ethanol consumption over many years. An increase in the plasma concentration of the liver enzyme γ-glutamyl transpeptidase (a marker of cytochrome P450 [CYP] induction, Ch. 9) often raises the suspicion of alcohol-related liver damage, although not specific to ethanol.

Effects on lipid metabolism, platelet function and atherosclerosis

Moderate drinking reduces mortality associated with coronary heart disease, the maximum effect – about 30% reduction of mortality overall – being achieved at a level of 2–3 units/day (see Groenbaek et al., 1994). The effect is much more pronounced (>50% reduction) in men with high plasma concentrations of low-density-lipoprotein cholesterol (see Ch. 23).[10] Most evidence suggests that ethanol, rather than any specific beverage, such as red wine, is the essential factor.

Two mechanisms have been proposed. The first involves the effect of ethanol on the plasma lipoproteins that are the carrier molecules for cholesterol and other lipids in the bloodstream (see Ch. 23). Epidemiological studies, as well as studies on volunteers, have shown that ethanol, in daily doses too small to produce obvious CNS effects, can over the course of a few weeks increase plasma high-density-lipoprotein concentration, thus exerting a protective effect against atheroma formation.

Ethanol may also protect against ischaemic heart disease by inhibiting platelet aggregation. This effect occurs at ethanol concentrations in the range achieved by normal drinking in humans (10–20 mmol/l) and probably results from inhibition of arachidonic acid formation from phospholipid. In humans, the magnitude of the effect depends critically on dietary fat intake, and it is not yet clear how important it is clinically.

The effect of ethanol on fetal development

The adverse effect of ethanol consumption during pregnancy on fetal development was demonstrated in the early 1970s, when the term *fetal alcohol syndrome* (FAS) was coined.

The features of full FAS include:

- abnormal facial development, with wide-set eyes, short palpebral fissures and small cheekbones
- reduced cranial circumference
- retarded growth
- mental retardation and behavioural abnormalities, often taking the form of hyperactivity and difficulty with social integration
- other anatomical abnormalities, which may be major or minor (e.g. congenital cardiac abnormalities, malformation of the eyes and ears).

A lesser degree of impairment, termed *alcohol-related neurodevelopmental disorder* (ARND), results in behavioural

problems, and cognitive and motor deficits, often associated with reduced brain size. Full FAS occurs in about 3 per 1000 live births and affects about 30% of children born to alcoholic mothers. It is rare with mothers who drink less than about 5 units/day, and most common in binge drinkers who sporadically consume much larger amounts, resulting in high peak levels of ethanol. ARND is about three times as common. Although there is no clearly defined safe threshold, there is no evidence that amounts less than about 2 units/day are harmful. There is no critical period during pregnancy when ethanol consumption is likely to lead to FAS, although one study suggests that FAS incidence correlates most strongly with ethanol consumption very early in pregnancy, even before pregnancy is recognised, implying that not only pregnant women, but also women who are likely to become pregnant, must be advised not to drink heavily. Experiments on rats and mice suggest that the effect on facial development may be produced very early in pregnancy (up to 4 weeks in humans), while the effect on brain development is produced rather later (up to 10 weeks).

Effects of ethanol

- **Ethanol** consumption is generally expressed in units of 10 ml (8 g) of pure **ethanol**. Per capita consumption in the UK is more than 10 l/year.
- **Ethanol** acts as a general central nervous system depressant, similar to volatile anaesthetic agents, producing the familiar effects of acute intoxication.
- Several cellular mechanisms are postulated: enhancement of GABA and glycine action, inhibition of calcium channel opening, activation of potassium channels and inhibition at NMDA-type glutamate receptors.
- Effective plasma concentrations:
  - threshold effects: about 20 mg/100 ml (5 mmol/l)
  - severe intoxication: about 150 mg/100 ml
  - death from respiratory failure: about 500 mg/100 ml.
- Main peripheral effects are self-limiting diuresis (reduced antidiuretic hormone secretion), cutaneous vasodilatation and delayed labour (reduced oxytocin secretion).
- Neurological degeneration occurs with heavy and binge drinking, causing dementia and peripheral neuropathies.
- Long-term ethanol consumption causes liver disease, progressing to cirrhosis and liver failure.
- Moderate **ethanol** consumption has a protective effect against ischaemic heart disease.
- Excessive consumption in pregnancy causes impaired fetal development, associated with small size, abnormal facial development and other physical abnormalities, and mental retardation.
- Psychological dependence, physical dependence and tolerance all occur with **ethanol**.
- Drugs used to treat alcohol dependence include **disulfiram** (aldehyde dehydrogenase inhibitor), **naltrexone** (opiate antagonist) and **acamprosate** (NMDA receptor antagonist). **Topiramate** and **bupropion** are also used.

---

[10]This beneficial effect of moderate drinking outweighs the risk of adverse effects (e.g. accidents, cancers, liver damage) only in men over 45 and women over 55.

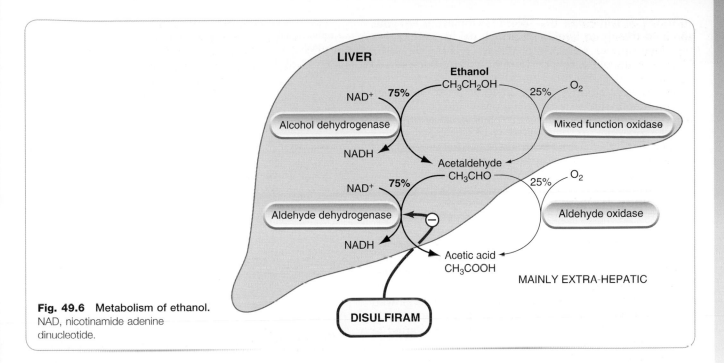

Fig. 49.6 Metabolism of ethanol. NAD, nicotinamide adenine dinucleotide.

PHARMACOKINETIC ASPECTS

Metabolism of ethanol

Ethanol is rapidly absorbed, an appreciable amount being absorbed from the stomach. A substantial fraction is cleared by first-pass hepatic metabolism. Hepatic metabolism of ethanol shows saturation kinetics (see Chs 9 and 10) at quite low ethanol concentrations, so the fraction of ethanol removed decreases as the concentration reaching the liver increases. Thus, if ethanol absorption is rapid and portal vein concentration is high, most of the ethanol escapes into the systemic circulation, whereas with slow absorption more is removed by first-pass metabolism. This is one reason why drinking ethanol on an empty stomach produces a much greater pharmacological effect. Ethanol is quickly distributed throughout the body water, the rate of its redistribution depending mainly on the blood flow to individual tissues, as with volatile anaesthetics (see Ch. 41).

Ethanol is about 90% metabolised, 5–10% being excreted unchanged in expired air and in urine. This fraction is not pharmacokinetically significant but provides the basis for estimating blood ethanol concentration from measurements on breath or urine. The ratio of ethanol concentrations in blood and alveolar air, measured at the end of deep expiration, is relatively constant, 80 mg/100 ml of ethanol in blood producing 35 µg/100 ml in expired air, this being the basis of the breathalyser test. The concentration in urine is more variable and provides a less accurate measure of blood concentration.

Ethanol metabolism occurs almost entirely in the liver, and mainly by a pathway involving successive oxidations, first to acetaldehyde and then to acetic acid (Fig. 49.6). Since ethanol is often consumed in large quantities (compared with most drugs), 1–2 mol daily being by no means unusual, it constitutes a substantial load on the hepatic oxidative systems. The oxidation of 2 mol of ethanol consumes about 1.5 kg of the co-factor nicotinamide adenine dinucleotide (NAD+). Availability of NAD+ limits the rate of ethanol oxidation to about 8 g/h

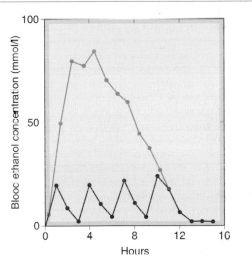

Fig. 49.7 Zero-order kinetics of ethanol elimination in rats. Rats were given ethanol orally (104 mmol/kg) either as a single dose or as four divided doses. The single dose results in a much higher and more sustained blood ethanol concentration than the same quantity given as divided doses. Note that, after the single dose, ethanol concentration declines linearly, the rate of decline being similar after a small or large dose, because of the saturation phenomenon. *(From Kalant H et al. 1975 Biochem Pharmacol 24, 431.)*

in a normal adult, independently of ethanol concentration (Fig. 49.7), causing the process to show saturating kinetics (Ch. 10). It also leads to competition between the ethanol and other metabolic substrates for the available NAD+ supplies, which may be a factor in ethanol-induced liver damage (see Ch. 57). The intermediate metabolite, acetaldehyde, is a reactive and toxic compound, and this may also contribute to the hepatotoxicity. A small degree of esterification of ethanol with various fatty acids also occurs in the tissues, and these esters may also contribute to long-term toxicity.

Alcohol dehydrogenase is a soluble cytoplasmic enzyme, confined mainly to liver cells, which oxidises ethanol at the same time as reducing NAD^+ to NADH (Fig. 49.6). Ethanol metabolism causes the ratio of NAD^+ to NADH to fall, and this has other metabolic consequences (e.g. increased lactate and slowing down of the Krebs cycle). The limitation on ethanol metabolism imposed by the limited rate of NAD^+ regeneration has led to attempts to find a 'sobering up' agent that works by regenerating NAD^+ from NADH. One such agent is fructose, which is reduced by an NADH-requiring enzyme. In large doses, it causes a measurable increase in the rate of ethanol metabolism, but not enough to have a useful effect on the rate of return to sobriety.

Normally, only a small amount of ethanol is metabolised by the microsomal mixed function oxidase system (see Ch. 9), but induction of this system occurs in alcoholics. Ethanol can affect the metabolism of other drugs that are metabolised by the mixed function oxidase system (e.g. **phenobarbitone**, **warfarin** and **steroids**), with an initial inhibitory effect produced by competition, followed by enhancement due to enzyme induction.

Nearly all the acetaldehyde produced is converted to acetate in the liver by *aldehyde dehydrogenase* (Fig. 49.6). Normally, only a little acetaldehyde escapes from the liver, giving a blood acetaldehyde concentration of 20–50 μmol/l after an intoxicating dose of ethanol in humans. The circulating acetaldehyde usually has little or no effect, but the concentration may become much larger under certain circumstances and produce toxic effects. This occurs if aldehyde dehydrogenase is inhibited by drugs such as **disulfiram**. In the presence of disulfiram, which produces no marked effect when given alone, ethanol consumption is followed by a severe reaction comprising flushing, tachycardia, hyperventilation, and considerable panic and distress, which is due to excessive acetaldehyde accumulation in the bloodstream. This reaction is extremely unpleasant but not harmful, and disulfiram can be used as aversion therapy to discourage people from taking ethanol. Some other drugs (e.g. **metronidazole**; see Ch. 51) produce similar reactions to ethanol. Interestingly, a Chinese herbal medicine used traditionally to cure alcoholics contains **daidzin**, a specific inhibitor of aldehyde dehydrogenase.[11]

Genetic factors
In 50% of Asian people, an inactive genetic variant of one of the aldehyde dehydrogenase isoforms (ALDH-2) is expressed; these individuals experience a disulfiram-like reaction after alcohol, and the incidence of alcoholism in this group is extremely low (see Tyndale, 2003).

Metabolism and toxicity of methanol and ethylene glycol
▼ Methanol is metabolised in the same way as ethanol but produces formaldehyde instead of acetaldehyde from the first oxidation step. Formaldehyde is more reactive than acetaldehyde and reacts rapidly with proteins, causing the inactivation of enzymes involved in the tricarboxylic acid cycle. It is converted to another toxic metabolite, formic acid. This, unlike acetic acid, cannot be utilised in the tricarboxylic acid cycle and is liable to cause tissue damage. Conversion of alcohols to aldehydes occurs not only in the liver but also in the retina, catalysed by the dehydrogenase responsible for retinol–retinal conversion. Formation of formaldehyde in the retina accounts for one of the main toxic effects of methanol, namely blindness, which can occur after ingestion of as little as 10 g. Formic acid production and derangement of the tricarboxylic acid cycle also produce severe acidosis.

Methanol is used as an industrial solvent and also to adulterate industrial ethanol in order to make it unfit to drink. Methanol poisoning is quite common, and used to be treated by administration of large doses of ethanol, which acts to retard methanol metabolism by competition for alcohol dehydrogenase. **Fomepizole** inhibits alcohol dehydrogenase and is now preferred if available. Such treatment may be in conjunction with haemodialysis to remove unchanged methanol, which has a small volume of distribution.

Poisoning with ethylene glycol, used in automobile antifreeze and brake fluid, is a medical emergency. It is rapidly absorbed from the gut and metabolised to glycolate and then more slowly to oxalate. Glycolate interferes with metabolic processes and produces metabolic acidosis. It affects the brain, heart and kidneys. Treatment is with fomepizole or, with caution, ethanol,[12] and haemodialysis.

Metabolism of ethanol

- **Ethanol** is metabolised mainly by the liver, first by alcohol dehydrogenase to acetaldehyde, then by aldehyde dehydrogenase to acetate. About 25% of the acetaldehyde is metabolised extrahepatically.
- Small amounts of **ethanol** are excreted in urine and expired air.
- Hepatic metabolism shows saturation kinetics, mainly because of limited availability of nicotinamide adenine dinucleotide (NAD^+). Maximal rate of **ethanol** metabolism is about 10 ml/h. Thus plasma concentration falls linearly rather than exponentially.
- Acetaldehyde may produce toxic effects. Inhibition of aldehyde dehydrogenase by **disulfiram** accentuates nausea, etc., caused by acetaldehyde, and can be used in aversion therapy.
- **Methanol** is similarly metabolised to formic acid, which is toxic, especially to the retina.
- Asian people show a high rate of genetic polymorphism of alcohol and aldehyde dehydrogenase, associated with alcoholism and alcohol intolerance, respectively.

TOLERANCE AND DEPENDENCE

Tolerance to the effects of ethanol can be demonstrated in both humans and experimental animals, to the extent of a two- to three-fold reduction in potency occurring over 1–3 weeks of continuing ethanol administration. A small component of this is due to the more rapid elimination of ethanol. The major component is cellular tolerance, which accounts for a roughly two-fold decrease in potency and which can be observed *in vitro* (e.g. by measuring the inhibitory effect of ethanol on transmitter release from synaptosomes) as well as *in vivo*. The mechanism of this tolerance is not known for certain. Ethanol tolerance is

---

[11]In hamsters (which spontaneously consume alcohol in amounts that would defeat even the hardest two-legged drinker, while remaining, as far as one can tell in a hamster, completely sober), daidzin markedly inhibits alcohol consumption.

[12]When presented with a late evening emergency poisoning of a dog with ethylene glycol a veterinarian colleague of one of the authors ran to the local supermarket and purchased a bottle of vodka – the dog survived!

associated with tolerance to many anaesthetic agents, and alcoholics are often difficult to anaesthetise.

Chronic ethanol administration produces various changes in CNS neurons, which tend to oppose the acute cellular effects that it produces. There is a small reduction in the density of $GABA_A$ receptors, and a proliferation of voltage-gated calcium channels and NMDA receptors.

A well-defined physical abstinence syndrome develops in response to ethanol withdrawal. As with most other dependence-producing drugs, this is probably important as a short-term factor in sustaining the drug habit, but other (mainly psychological) factors are more important in the longer term (see p. 601). The physical abstinence syndrome usually subsides in a few days, but the craving for ethanol and the tendency to relapse last for very much longer.

The physical abstinence syndrome in humans, in severe form, develops after about 8h. In the first stage, the main symptoms are tremor, nausea, sweating, fever and sometimes hallucinations. These last for about 24h. This phase may be followed by seizures ('rum fits'). Over the next few days, the condition of 'delirium tremens' develops, in which the patient becomes confused, agitated and often aggressive, and may suffer much more severe hallucinations. Treatment of this medical emergency is by sedation with large doses of a benzodiazepine such as **chlordiazepoxide** (Ch. 44) together with large doses of thiamine.

PHARMACOLOGICAL APPROACHES TO TREATING ALCOHOL DEPENDENCE

Alcohol dependence ('alcoholism') is common (4–5% of the population) and, as with smoking, difficult to treat effectively. The main pharmacological approaches (see Garbutt, 2009; Table 49.3) are the following:

- To alleviate the acute abstinence syndrome during 'drying out', **benzodiazepines** (see Ch. 44) and **clomethiazole** are effective; **clonidine** and **propranolol** are also useful. Clonidine (α_2-adrenoceptor agonist) is believed to act by inhibiting the exaggerated transmitter release that occurs during withdrawal, while propranolol (β-adrenoceptor antagonist) blocks some of the effects of excessive sympathetic activity.
- To render alcohol consumption unpleasant, **disulfiram**.
- The non-selective opioid antagonists **naltrexone** and **nalmefene** are effective in reducing alcohol consumption, indicating the possible involvement of endorphins (see Ch. 42) in the rewarding properties of alcohol.
- To reduce craving, **acamprosate** is used. This taurine analogue is a weak antagonist at NMDA receptors, and may work by interfering in some way with synaptic plasticity. Several clinical trials have shown it to improve the success rate in achieving alcohol abstinence, with few unwanted effects.
- To alleviate both withdrawal and craving, the antiepileptic agent **topiramate**, which has multiple effects on the brain (see Ch. 45), shows promise as does γ-hydroxybutyric acid (GHB), a short-chain fatty acid structurally similar to the inhibitory neurotransmitter γ-aminobutyric acid (see Ch. 38).

REFERENCES AND FURTHER READING

General

Bagley, E.E., Gerke, M.B., Vaughan, C.W., et al., 2005. GABA transporter currents activated by protein kinase A excite midbrain neurons during opioid withdrawal. Neuron 45, 433–445.

Bagley, E.E., Hacker, J., Chefer, V.I., et al., 2011. Drug-induced GABA transporter currents enhance GABA release to induce opioid withdrawal behaviors. Nat. Neurosci. 14, 1548–1554. (*Describes the cellular mechanism underlying the opioid withdrawal response*)

Bailey, C.P., Connor, M., 2005. Opioids: cellular mechanisms of tolerance and physical dependence. Curr. Opin. Pharmacol. 5, 60–68.

Chao, J., Nestler, E.J., 2004. Molecular neurobiology of addiction. Annu. Rev. Med. 55, 113–132. (*Useful review article by leading scientists in addiction research*)

Dalley, J.W., Fryer, T.D., Brichard, L., et al., 2007. Nucleus accumbens $D_{2/3}$ receptors predict trait impulsivity and cocaine reinforcement. Science 315, 1267–1270. (*An exciting first description of the role of dopamine receptors and impulsivity in drug self-administration*)

Heidbreder, C.A., Hagan, J.J., 2005. Novel pharmacological approaches for the treatment of drug addiction and craving. Curr. Opin. Pharmacol. 5, 107–118. (*Describes the numerous theoretical strategies, based mainly on monoamine pharmacology, for treating addiction*)

Hyman, S.E., Malenka, R.C., Nestler, E.J., 2006. Neural mechanisms of addiction: the role of reward-related learning and memory. Annu. Rev. Neurosci. 29, 565–598. (*Extensive review on how drugs of abuse can alter memory and learning processes*)

Koob, G.F., Le Moal, M., 2006. Neurobiology of Addiction. Academic Press, London. (*A very extensive book covering many aspects of addiction from the neuroscientist's perspective*)

Maldonado, R., Saiardi, A., Valverde, O., et al., 1997. Absence of opiate rewarding effects in mice lacking dopamine D_2 receptors. Nature 388, 586–589. (*Use of transgenic animals to demonstrate role of dopamine receptors in reward properties of opiates*)

Measham, F., Moore, K., 2009. Repertoires of distinction. Exploring patterns of weekend polydrug use within local leisure scenes across the English night time economy. Criminol. Crim. Justice. 9, 437–464.

Newman, A.H., Blaylock, B.L., Nader, M.A., Bergman, J., Sibley, D.R., Skolnick, P., 2012. Medication discovery for addiction: translating the dopamine D_3 receptor hypothesis. Biochem. Pharmacol. 84, 882–890. (*Discusses the potential use of established drugs that have D_3 antagonism as well as other activities and selective D_3 antagonists*)

Nutt, D., King, L.A., Phillips, L.D., 2010. Drug harms in the UK: a multicriteria decision analysis. Lancet 376, 558–565.

Robbins, T.W., Ersche, K.D., Everitt, B.J., 2008. Drug addiction and the memory systems of the brain. Ann. N. Y. Acad. Sci. 1141, 1–21. (*Review of how different forms of memory play important roles in drug dependence*)

Weiss, F., 2005. Neurobiology of craving, conditioned reward and relapse. Curr. Opin. Pharmacol. 5, 9–19. (*Review of recent studies on the neurobiology of addiction, focusing mainly on animal models*)

Williams, J.T., Christie, M.J., Manzoni, O., 2001. Cellular and synaptic adaptations mediating opioid dependence. Physiol. Rev. 81, 299–343.

Williams, J.T., Ingram, S.L., Henderson, G., et al., 2013. Regulation of µ-opioid receptors: desensitization, phosphorylation, internalization, and tolerance. Pharmacol. Rev. 65, 223–254.

Nicotine

De Biasi, M., Dani, J.A., 2011. Reward, addiction, withdrawal to nicotine. Annu. Rev. Neurosci. 34, 105–130.

Gunnell, D., Irvine, D., Wise, L., Davies, C., Martin, R.M., 2009. Varenicline and suicidal behaviour: a cohort study based on data from the General Practice Research Database. BMJ 339, b3805.

Hung, R.J., McKay, J.D., Gaborieau, V., et al., 2008. A susceptibility locus for lung cancer maps to nicotinic acetylcholine receptor subunit genes on 15q25. Nature 452, 633–637. (*Original paper showing a genetic link between cancer and single nucleotide polymorphisms in the nicotinic receptor*)

Le Foll, B., Goldberg, S.R., 2005. Control of the reinforcing effects of nicotine by associated environmental stimuli in animals and humans. Trends Pharmacol. Sci. 26, 287–293.

Leslie, F.M., Mojica, C.Y., Reynaga, D.D., 2013. Nicotinic receptors in addiction pathways. Mol. Pharmacol. 83, 753–758.

Wonnacott, S., Sidhpura, N., Balfour, D.J.K., 2005. Nicotine: from molecular mechanisms to behaviour. Curr. Opin. Pharmacol. 5, 53–59. (*Useful review on the acute and long-term CNS effects of nicotine*)

Ethanol

Garbutt, J.C., 2009. The state of pharmacotherapy for the treatment of alcohol dependence. J. Subst. Abuse Treat. 36 (Suppl.), S15–S21. (*Reviews current drugs and potential new approaches*)

Groenbaek, M., Deis, A., Sørensen, T.I., et al., 1994. Influence of sex, age, body mass index and smoking on alcohol intake and mortality. BMJ 308, 302–306. (*Large-scale Danish study showing reduced coronary mortality at moderate levels of drinking, with increase at high levels*)

Harper, C., Matsumoto, I., 2005. Ethanol and brain damage. Curr. Opin. Pharmacol. 5, 73–78. (*Describes deleterious effects of long-term alcohol abuse on brain function*)

Harris, R.A., Trudell, J.R., Mihic, S.J., 2008. Ethanol's molecular targets. Sci. Signal. 1, re7. (*Short review of potential molecular actions of alcohol relevant to its effects on the brain*)

Lieber, C.S., 1995. Medical disorders of alcoholism. N. Engl. J. Med. 333, 1058–1065. (*Review focusing on ethanol-induced liver damage in relation to ethanol metabolism*)

Melendez, R.I., Kalivas, P.W., 2004. Last call for adenosine transporters. Nat. Neurosci. 7, 795–796. (*Commentary on a study supporting a role for adenosine in the CNS effects of ethanol*)

Spanagel, R., 2009. Alcoholism: a systems approach from molecular physiology to addictive behaviour. Physiol. Rev. 89, 649–705. (*Comprehensive review article, very useful for reference*)

Tyndale, R.F., 2003. Genetics of alcohol and tobacco use in humans. Ann. Med. 35, 94–121. (*Detailed review of the many genetic factors implicated in alcohol and nicotine consumption habits*)

Useful Web resources

(*ASH, an antismoking organisation*)

(*DrugScope, an independent organisation providing advice on various aspects of drug abuse*)

(*National Institute on Drug Abuse [NIDA], US government organisation providing information to scientists and the general public on various aspects of drug abuse*)

<www.drugabuse.gov/PODAT/PODATIndex.html> (*Provides access to the NIDA publication Principles of Drug Addiction Treatment: A Research Based Guide, second edn*)

<www.ias.org.uk> (*The Institute of Alcohol Studies [UK] provides a Knowledge Centre offering an excellent range of factsheets relating to all aspects of alcohol consumption and its consequences*)

Basic principles of antimicrobial chemotherapy

50

OVERVIEW

Chemotherapy is the term originally used to describe the use of drugs that are 'selectively toxic' to invading microorganisms while having minimal effects on the host. It also refers to the use of drugs to treat tumours, and in the public mind at least, 'chemotherapy' is usually associated with cytotoxic anticancer drugs that cause unwanted effects such as loss of hair, nausea and vomiting. In this chapter, we focus on antimicrobial chemotherapy. Anticancer drugs are covered in Ch. 56.

All living organisms are vulnerable to infection. Humans, being no exception, are susceptible to diseases caused by viruses, bacteria, protozoa, fungi and helminths (collectively referred to as pathogens). The use of chemotherapeutic agents dates back to the work of Ehrlich and others and to the development of selectively toxic arsenical drugs such as salvarsan for the treatment of syphilis.[1] The successful development of such agents during the past 80 years, particularly the 'antibiotic revolution', which began in the 1940s with the advent of penicillin, constitutes one of the most important therapeutic advances in the history of medicine.

The feasibility of the selective toxicity strategy depends on the ability to exploit such biochemical differences as may exist between the infecting organism and the host. While the bulk of the chapters in this section of the book describe the drugs used to combat such infections, in this introductory chapter we consider the nature of these biochemical differences and outline the molecular targets of drug action.

BACKGROUND

The term *chemotherapy* was coined by Ehrlich himself at the beginning of the 20th century to describe the use of synthetic chemicals to destroy infective pathogens. In recent years the definition of the term has been broadened to include *antibiotics* – substances produced by some microorganisms (or by pharmaceutical chemists) that kill or inhibit the growth of other microorganisms.

Unhappily, our success in developing drugs to attack these invaders has been paralleled by their own success in counteracting the effects of the drugs, resulting in the emergence of drug resistance. And at present, the invaders – particularly some bacteria – seem close to getting the upper hand. This is a very important problem, and we will devote some space to the mechanisms of resistance and the means by which it is spread.

THE MOLECULAR BASIS OF CHEMOTHERAPY

Chemotherapeutic agents, then, are chemicals intended to be toxic to the pathogenic organism but innocuous to the host. It is important to remember that many microorganisms share our body spaces (e.g. the gut[2]) without causing disease (these are called *commensals*), although they may become pathogenic under adverse circumstances (i.e. if the host is immunocompromised or if barrier breakdown results in them setting up shop elsewhere in our bodies).

All living organisms can be classified as either *prokaryotes*, cells without nuclei (e.g. bacteria), or *eukaryotes*, cells with nuclei (e.g. protozoa, fungi, helminths). In a separate category are the viruses, which need to utilise the metabolic machinery of the host cell to replicate, and they thus present a particular kind of problem for chemotherapeutic attack. There remain those mysterious proteinaceous agents, *prions* (see Ch. 40), which cause disease but resist all attempts at classification and treatment.

Virtually all creatures, host and parasite alike, have the same basic DNA blueprint (an exception being the RNA viruses), so some biochemical processes are common to most, if not all, organisms. Finding agents that affect pathogens but not other human cells necessitates finding either qualitative or quantitative biochemical differences between them.

Bacteria cause most infectious diseases, and Figure 50.1 shows, in simplified diagrammatic form, the main components of a 'generalised' bacterial cell and their functions. Surrounding the cell is the *cell wall*, which characteristically contains *peptidoglycan* in all forms of bacteria except *Mycoplasma*. Peptidoglycan is unique to prokaryotic cells and has no counterpart in eukaryotes. Within the cell wall is the *plasma membrane*, which, like that of eukaryotic cells, consists of a phospholipid bilayer and proteins. It functions as a selectively permeable membrane with specific transport mechanisms for various nutrients. However, in bacteria the plasma membrane does not contain any *sterols* (e.g. cholesterol), and this may alter the penetration of some chemicals.

The cell wall supports the underlying plasma membrane, which is subject to an internal osmotic pressure of about 5 atmospheres in *Gram-negative* organisms, and about 20 atmospheres in *Gram-positive* organisms. The plasma membrane and cell wall together comprise the *bacterial envelope*.

As in eukaryotic cells, the plasma membrane contains the *cytoplasm* but bacterial cells have no nucleus; instead, the genetic material, in the form of a single *chromosome* containing all the genetic information, lies in the cytoplasm with no surrounding nuclear membrane. In further contrast to eukaryotic cells, there are no *mitochondria*

---

[1] Mercury-containing compounds were also once used for treating syphilis. 'One night with Venus, a lifetime with Mercury' was a saying prior to the advent of the antibiotic era.

[2] Humans harbour about 2 kg of bacteria in the gut, comprising a large 'forgotten organ' in the body with important metabolic functions.

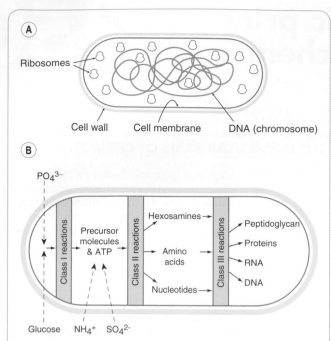

Fig. 50.1 Diagram of the structure and metabolism of a 'typical' bacterial cell. [**A**] Schematic representation of a bacterial cell. [**B**] Flow diagram showing the synthesis of the main types of macromolecule of a bacterial cell. Class I reactions result in the synthesis of the precursor molecules necessary for class II reactions, which result in the synthesis of the constituent molecules; these are then assembled into macromolecules by class III reactions. *(Modified from Mandelstam J, McQuillen K, Dawes I (eds) 1982 Biochemistry of Bacterial growth. Blackwell Scientific, Oxford.)*

– cellular energy is generated by enzyme systems located in the plasma membrane.

Some bacteria have additional components relevant to chemotherapy, including an *outer membrane* on the outside of the cell wall. This determines whether they take up *Gram's stain* ('Gram-positive') or not ('Gram-negative'; for more details, see Ch. 51). In Gram-negative bacteria, this membrane prevents penetration of some antibacterial agents.

Biochemical reactions that are potential targets for antibacterial drugs are shown in Figure 50.1. There are three groups:

- *Class I*: the utilisation of glucose, or some alternative carbon source, for the generation of energy (ATP) and synthesis of simple carbon compounds used as precursors in the next class of reactions.
- *Class II*: the utilisation of these precursors in an energy-dependent synthesis of all the amino acids, nucleotides, phospholipids, amino sugars, carbohydrates and growth factors required by the cell for survival and growth.
- *Class III*: assembly of small molecules into macromolecules – proteins, RNA, DNA, polysaccharides and peptidoglycan.

Other potential drug targets are *formed structures*, for example the cell membrane, the *microtubules* in fungi or muscle tissue in helminths. In considering these targets, emphasis will be placed on bacteria, but reference will also be made to protozoa, helminths, fungi and viruses.

The classification that follows is not rigid; a drug may affect more than one class of reactions or more than one subgroup of reactions within a class.

The molecular basis of antibacterial chemotherapy

- Chemotherapeutic drugs should be toxic to invading organisms and innocuous to the host. Such selective toxicity depends on the discovery of biochemical differences between the pathogen and the host that can be appropriately exploited.
- Three general classes of biochemical reaction are potential targets for chemotherapy of bacteria:
  - *class I*: reactions that utilise glucose and other carbon sources to produce ATP and simple carbon compounds
  - *class II*: pathways utilising energy and class I compounds to make small molecules (e.g. amino acids and nucleotides)
  - *class III*: pathways that convert small molecules into macromolecules such as proteins, nucleic acids and peptidoglycan.

BIOCHEMICAL REACTIONS AS POTENTIAL TARGETS

CLASS I REACTIONS

Class I reactions are not promising targets for two reasons. First, bacterial and human cells use similar mechanisms to obtain energy from glucose (the *Embden–Meyerhof pathway* and the *tricarboxylic acid cycle*). Second, even if glucose oxidation is blocked, many other compounds (amino acids, lactate, etc.) can be utilised by bacteria as an alternative energy source.

CLASS II REACTIONS

Class II reactions are better targets because some pathways exist in pathogens, but not human, cells. There are several examples.

Folate

The folate biosynthesitic pathway is found in bacteria but not in humans. Folate is required for DNA synthesis in both bacteria and in humans (see Chs 25 and 51). As it cannot be synthesised by humans it must be obtained from the diet and concentrated in cells by specific uptake mechanisms. By contrast, most species of bacteria, as well as the asexual forms of malarial protozoa, lack these essential transport mechanisms. Therefore they cannot make use of preformed folate but must synthesise this *de novo*. **Sulfonamides** contain the sulfanilamide moiety – a structural analogue of *p*-aminobenzoic acid (PABA), which is essential in bacterial synthesis of folate (see Ch. 51, Fig. 51.1). Sulfonamides compete with PABA, and thus inhibit bacterial growth without impairing mammalian cell function.

The utilisation of folate, in the form of *tetrahydrofolate*, as a co-factor in thymidylate synthesis is a good example of a pathway where human and bacterial enzymes exhibit a differential sensitivity to chemicals (Table 50.1; see Volpato & Pelletier, 2009). Although the pathway is

Table 50.1 Specificity of inhibitors of dihydrofolate reductase

Inhibitor	IC$_{50}$ (µmol/l) for dihydrofolate reductase		
	Human	Protozoal	Bacterial
Trimethoprim	260	0.07	0.005
Pyrimethamine	0.7	0.0005	2.5
Methotrexate	0.001	~0.1[a]	Inactive

[a]Tested on *Plasmodium berghei*, a rodent malaria.

virtually identical in microorganisms and humans, one of the key enzymes, *dihydrofolate reductase*, which reduces dihydrofolate to tetrahydrofolate (Ch. 51, Fig. 51.2), is many times more sensitive to the inhibitor **trimethoprim** in bacteria than in humans. In some malarial protozoa, this enzyme is somewhat less sensitive than the bacterial enzyme to trimethoprim but more sensitive to **pyrimethamine** and **proguanil**, which are used as antimalarial agents (Ch. 54). The relative IC$_{50}$ values (the concentration causing 50% inhibition) for bacterial, malarial, protozoal and mammalian enzymes are given in Table 50.1. The human enzyme, by comparison, is very sensitive to the effect of the folate analogue **methotrexate**, which is used to treat inflammatory arthritis (Ch. 26), severe psoriasis (Ch. 27) and cancer (Ch. 56).

▼ The use of sequential blockade with a combination of two drugs that affect the same pathway at different points, for example sulfonamides and the folate antagonists, may be more successful than the use of either alone. Thus, pyrimethamine and a sulfonamide (**sulfadoxine**) are used to treat *falciparum* malaria. **Co-trimoxazole** is an antibacterial formulation that contains both a sulfonamide and trimethoprim. Once widely used, this combination has become less popular for treating bacterial infections because trimethoprim alone is similarly effective and does not cause sulfonamide-specific adverse effects; its use is now mainly restricted to treatment of *Pneumocystis jirovecii*, for which high doses are required (Ch. 54).

CLASS III REACTIONS

As pathogen cells cannot take up their own unique macromolecules, class III reactions are particularly good targets for selective toxicity, and there are distinct differences between mammalian cells and parasitic cells in this respect.

The synthesis of peptidoglycan

The cell wall of bacteria contains peptidoglycan, a substance that does not occur in eukaryotes. It is the equivalent of a non-stretchable string bag enclosing the whole bacterium. In Gram-negative bacteria, this bag consists of a single thickness, but in Gram-positive bacteria there may be as many as 40 layers of peptidoglycan. Each layer consists of multiple backbones of amino sugars – alternating *N*-acetylglucosamine and *N*-acetylmuramic acid residues (Fig. 50.2) – the latter having short peptide side-chains that are cross-linked to form a polymeric lattice, which may constitute up to 10–15% of the dry weight of the cell and is strong enough to resist the high internal osmotic pressure. The cross-links differ in different species. In staphylococci, they consist of five glycine residues.

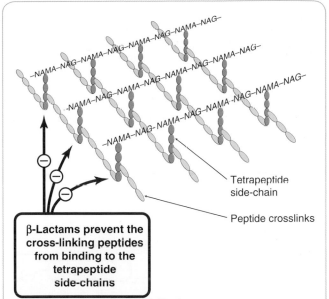

β-Lactams prevent the cross-linking peptides from binding to the tetrapeptide side-chains

Fig. 50.2 Schematic diagram of a single layer of peptidoglycan from a bacterial cell (e.g. *Staphylococcus aureus*), showing the site of action of the β-lactam antibiotics. In *S. aureus* the peptide crosslinks consist of five glycine residues. Gram-positive bacteria have several layers of peptidoglycan. NAG, *N*-acetylglucosamine; NAMA, *N*-acetylmuramic acid (more detail in Fig. 50.3).

▼ To build up this very large insoluble peptidoglycan layer on the outside of the cell membrane, the bacterial cell has the problem of how to transport the hydrophilic cytoplasmic 'building blocks' through the hydrophobic cell membrane structure. This is accomplished by linking them to a very large lipid carrier, containing 55 carbon atoms, which 'tows' them across the membrane. The process of peptidoglycan synthesis is outlined in Figure 50.3. First, *N*-acetylmuramic acid, attached to uridine diphosphate (UDP) and a pentapeptide, is transferred to the C$_{55}$ lipid carrier in the membrane, with the release of uridine monophosphate. This is followed by a reaction with UDP–*N*-acetylglucosamine, resulting in the formation of a disaccharide pentapeptide complex attached to the carrier. This complex is the basic building block of the peptidoglycan. In *Staphylococcus aureus*, the five glycine residues are attached to the peptide chain at this stage. The building block is now transported out of the cell and added to the growing end of the peptidoglycan, the 'acceptor', with the release of the C$_{55}$ lipid, which still has two phosphates attached. The lipid carrier then loses one phosphate group and thus becomes available for another cycle. Crosslinking between the peptide side-chains of the sugar residues in the peptidoglycan layer then occurs, the hydrolytic removal of the terminal alanine supplying the requisite energy.

This synthesis of peptidoglycan is a vulnerable step and can be blocked at several points by antibiotics (Fig. 50.3 and see Ch. 51). **Cycloserine**, which is a structural analogue of D-alanine, prevents the addition of the two terminal alanine residues to the initial tripeptide side-chain on *N*-acetylmuramic acid by competitive inhibition. **Vancomycin** inhibits the release of the building block unit from the carrier, thus preventing its addition to the growing end of the peptidoglycan. **Bacitracin** interferes with the regeneration of the lipid carrier by blocking its dephosphorylation. **Penicillins**, **cephalosporins** and other β-lactams inhibit the final transpeptidation by forming covalent bonds with *penicillin binding proteins* that have transpeptidase and carboxypeptidase activities, thus preventing formation of the crosslinks.

617

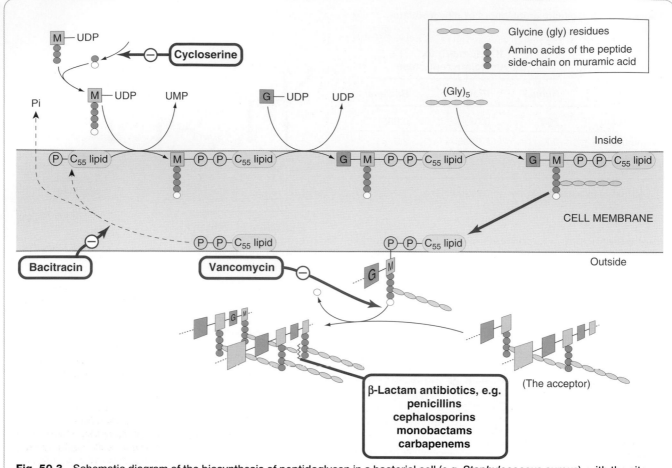

Fig. 50.3 Schematic diagram of the biosynthesis of peptidoglycan in a bacterial cell (e.g. *Staphylococcus aureus*), with the sites of action of various antibiotics. The hydrophilic disaccharide–pentapeptide is transferred across the lipid cell membrane attached to a large lipid (C_{55} lipid) by a pyrophosphate bridge (–P–P–). On the outside, it is enzymically attached to the 'acceptor' (the growing peptidoglycan layer). The final reaction is a transpeptidation, in which the loose end of the (Gly) 5 chain is attached to a peptide side-chain of an M in the acceptor and during which the terminal amino acid (alanine) is lost. The lipid is regenerated by loss of a phosphate group (Pi) before functioning again as a carrier. G, *N*-acetylglucosamine; M, *N*-acetylmuramic acid; UDP, uridine diphosphate; UMP, uridine monophosphate.

Protein synthesis

Protein synthesis takes place on the ribosomes. Eukaryotic and prokaryotic ribosomes are different, and this provides the basis for the selective antimicrobial action of some antibiotics. The bacterial ribosome consists of a 50S subunit and a 30S subunit (Fig. 50.4), whereas in the mammalian ribosome the subunits are 60S and 40S. The other elements involved in peptide synthesis are messenger RNA (mRNA), which forms the template for protein synthesis, and transfer RNA (tRNA), which specifically transfers the individual amino acids to the ribosome. The ribosome has three binding sites for tRNA, termed the A, P and E sites.

A simplified version of protein synthesis in bacteria is shown in Figure 50.4. To initiate translation, mRNA, transcribed from the DNA template, is attached to the 30S subunit of the ribosome. The 50S subunit then binds to the 30S subunit to form a 70S subunit,[3] which moves along the mRNA such that successive codons of the messenger

pass along the ribosome from the A position to the P position. Antibiotics may affect protein synthesis at any one of these stages (Fig. 50.4 and see Ch. 51).

Nucleic acid synthesis

Gene expression and cell division also require nucleic acid synthesis, interference with which is an important mechanism of action of many chemotherapeutic drugs. It is possible to interfere with nucleic acid synthesis in five different ways:

- by inhibiting the synthesis of the nucleotides
- by altering the base-pairing properties of the DNA template
- by inhibiting either DNA or RNA polymerase
- by inhibiting DNA gyrase, which uncoils supercoiled DNA to allow transcription
- by a direct effect on DNA itself. Some anticancer drugs, but no antimicrobial drugs work in this way.

Inhibition of the synthesis of the nucleotides

This can be accomplished by an effect on the metabolic pathways that generate nucleotide precursors. Examples of agents that have such an effect have been described under class II reactions.

---

[3]You query whether 30S + 50S = 70S? Yes it does, because we are talking about *Svedberg units*, which measure sedimentation *rate*, not *mass*.

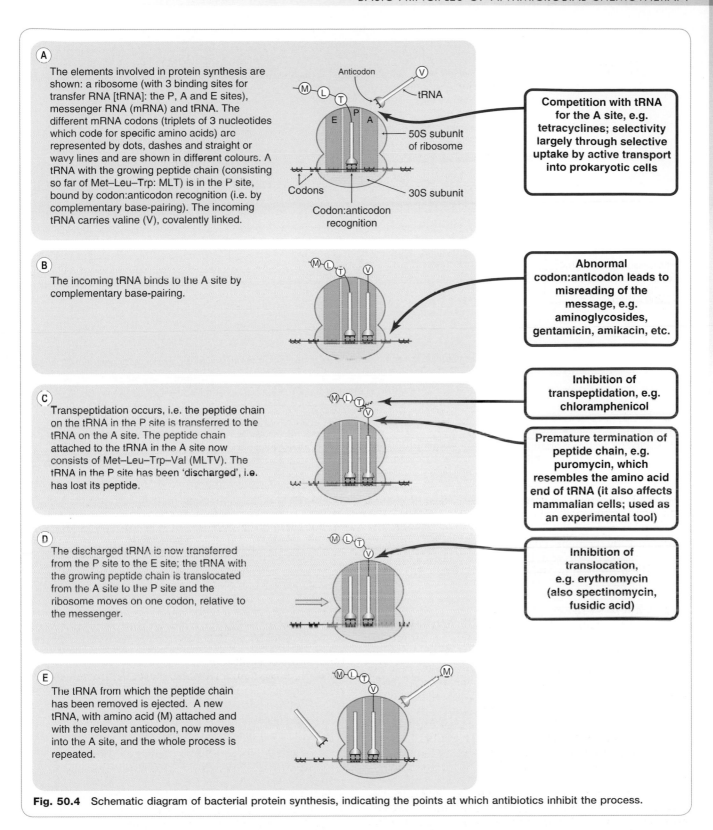

A

The elements involved in protein synthesis are shown: a ribosome (with 3 binding sites for transfer RNA [tRNA]: the P, A and E sites), messenger RNA (mRNA) and tRNA. The different mRNA codons (triplets of 3 nucleotides which code for specific amino acids) are represented by dots, dashes and straight or wavy lines and are shown in different colours. A tRNA with the growing peptide chain (consisting so far of Met–Leu–Trp: MLT) is in the P site, bound by codon:anticodon recognition (i.e. by complementary base-pairing). The incoming tRNA carries valine (V), covalently linked.

Anticodon · V · tRNA · M · L · T · E · P · A · 50S subunit of ribosome · Codons · 30S subunit · Codon:anticodon recognition

Competition with tRNA for the A site, e.g. tetracyclines; selectivity largely through selective uptake by active transport into prokaryotic cells

B

The incoming tRNA binds to the A site by complementary base-pairing.

Abnormal codon:anticodon leads to misreading of the message, e.g. aminoglycosides, gentamicin, amikacin, etc.

C

Transpeptidation occurs, i.e. the peptide chain on the tRNA in the P site is transferred to the tRNA on the A site. The peptide chain attached to the tRNA in the A site now consists of Met–Leu–Trp–Val (MLTV). The tRNA in the P site has been 'discharged', i.e. has lost its peptide.

Inhibition of transpeptidation, e.g. chloramphenicol

Premature termination of peptide chain, e.g. puromycin, which resembles the amino acid end of tRNA (it also affects mammalian cells; used as an experimental tool)

D

The discharged tRNA is now transferred from the P site to the E site; the tRNA with the growing peptide chain is translocated from the A site to the P site and the ribosome moves on one codon, relative to the messenger.

Inhibition of translocation, e.g. erythromycin (also spectinomycin, fusidic acid)

E

The tRNA from which the peptide chain has been removed is ejected. A new tRNA, with amino acid (M) attached and with the relevant anticodon, now moves into the A site, and the whole process is repeated.

Fig. 50.4 Schematic diagram of bacterial protein synthesis, indicating the points at which antibiotics inhibit the process.

Alteration of the base-pairing properties of the template
Agents that intercalate in the DNA have this effect. Examples include acridines (**proflavine** and **acriflavine**), which are used topically as antiseptics. The acridines double the distance between adjacent base pairs and cause a *frameshift mutation*, whereas some purine and pyrimidine analogues cause base *mispairing*.

Inhibition of either DNA or RNA polymerase
Specific inhibitors of bacterial RNA polymerase that act by binding to this enzyme in prokaryotic but not in eukaryotic cells include **rifamycin** and **rifampicin**, which are particularly useful for treating tuberculosis (see Ch. 51). **Aciclovir** (an analogue of guanine) is phosphorylated in cells infected with herpes virus, the initial

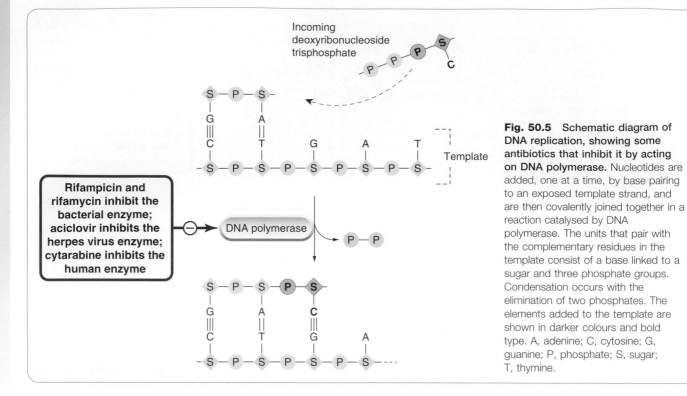

Fig. 50.5 Schematic diagram of DNA replication, showing some antibiotics that inhibit it by acting on DNA polymerase. Nucleotides are added, one at a time, by base pairing to an exposed template strand, and are then covalently joined together in a reaction catalysed by DNA polymerase. The units that pair with the complementary residues in the template consist of a base linked to a sugar and three phosphate groups. Condensation occurs with the elimination of two phosphates. The elements added to the template are shown in darker colours and bold type. A, adenine; C, cytosine; G, guanine; P, phosphate; S, sugar; T, thymine.

phosphorylation being by a virus-specific kinase to give the aciclovir trisphosphate, which has an inhibitory action on the DNA polymerase of the herpes virus (Ch. 52; Fig. 50.5).

RNA retroviruses have a *reverse transcriptase* (*viral RNA-dependent DNA polymerase*) that copies the viral RNA into DNA that integrates into the host cell genome as a provirus. Various agents (**zidovudine, didanosine**) are phosphorylated by cellular enzymes to the trisphosphate forms, which compete with the host cell precursors essential for the formation by the viral reverse transcriptase of proviral DNA.

Inhibition of DNA gyrase

Figure 50.6 is a simplified scheme showing the action of DNA gyrase. The *fluoroquinolones* (**cinoxacin, ciprofloxacin, nalidixic acid** and **norfloxacin**) act by inhibiting DNA gyrase, and these chemotherapeutic agents are particularly useful for treating infections with Gram-negative organisms (Ch. 51). They are selective for the bacterial enzyme.

THE FORMED STRUCTURES OF THE CELL AS POTENTIAL TARGETS

THE MEMBRANE

The plasma membrane of bacterial cells is similar to that in mammalian cells in that it consists of a phospholipid bilayer in which proteins are embedded, but it can be more easily disrupted in certain bacteria and fungi.

Polymixins are cationic peptide antibiotics, containing both hydrophilic and lipophilic groups, which have a selective effect on bacterial cell membranes. They act as detergents, disrupting the phospholipid components of the membrane structure, thus killing the cell.

Unlike mammalian and bacterial cells, fungal cell membranes comprise large amounts of *ergosterol*. This

Biochemical reactions as potential targets for chemotherapy

- Class I reactions are poor targets.
- Class II reactions are better targets:
  - *folate synthesis* in bacteria is inhibited by sulfonamides
  - *folate utilisation* is inhibited by folate antagonists, for example **trimethoprim** (bacteria), **pyrimethamine** (malarial parasite).
- Class III reactions are important targets:
  - *peptidoglycan synthesis* in bacteria can be selectively inhibited by β-lactam antibiotics (e.g. **penicillin**)
  - *bacterial protein synthesis* can be selectively inhibited by antibiotics that prevent binding of tRNA (e.g. tetracyclines), promote misreading of mRNA (e.g. aminoglycosides), inhibit transpeptidation (e.g. **chloramphenicol**) or inhibit translocation of tRNA (e.g. **erythromycin**)
  - *nucleic acid synthesis* can be inhibited by altering base pairing of DNA template (e.g. the antiviral **vidarabine**), by inhibiting DNA polymerase (e.g. the antivirals **aciclovir** and **foscarnet**) or by inhibiting DNA gyrase (e.g. the antibacterial **ciprofloxacin**).

facilitates the attachment of *polyene antibiotics* (e.g. **nystatin** and **amphotericin**; Ch. 53), which act as ionophores and cause leakage of cations from the cytoplasm.

Azoles such as **itraconazole** kill fungal cells by inhibiting ergosterol synthesis, thereby disrupting the function of membrane-associated enzymes. The azoles also affect Gram-positive bacteria, their selectivity being associated with the presence of high levels of free fatty acids in the membrane of susceptible organisms (Ch. 53).

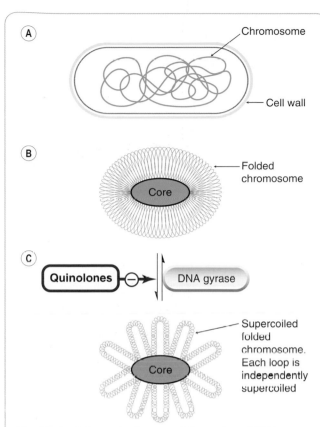

Fig. 50.6 Schematic diagram of the action of DNA gyrase: the site of action for quinolone antibacterials. [A] Conventional diagram used to depict a bacterial cell and chromosome (e.g. *Escherichia coli*). Note that the *E. coli* chromosome is 1300 mm long and is contained in a cell envelope of 2 μm × 1 μm; this is approximately equivalent to a 50 m length of cotton folded into a matchbox, [B] Chromosome folded around RNA core, and then [C], supercoiled by DNA gyrase (topoisomerase II). Quinolone antibacterials interfere with the action of this enzyme. *(Modified from Smith JT 1985 In: Greenwood D, O'Grady F (eds) Scientific Basis of Antimicrobial Therapy. Cambridge University Press, Cambridge, p. 69.)*

INTRACELLULAR ORGANELLES

Microtubules and/or microfilaments

The benzimidazoles (e.g. **albendazole**) exert their anthelmintic action by binding selectively to parasite tubulin and preventing microtubule formation (Ch. 55).

Food vacuoles

The erythrocytic form of the malaria plasmodium feeds on host haemoglobin, which is digested by proteases in the parasite food vacuole, the final product, haem, being detoxified by polymerisation. **Chloroquine** exerts its antimalarial action by inhibiting plasmodial haem polymerase (Ch. 54).

MUSCLE FIBRES

Some anthelmintic drugs have a selective action on helminth muscle cells (Ch. 55). **Piperazine** acts as an agonist on parasite-specific chloride channels gated by GABA in nematode muscle, hyperpolarising the muscle fibre membrane and paralysing the worm; **avermectins** increase Cl⁻ permeability in helminth muscle – possibly by a similar mechanism. **Pyrantel** (now seldom used) and

levamisole are agonists at nematode acetylcholine nicotinic receptors on muscle, causing contraction followed by paralysis (Ch. 55).

> ## Formed structures of the cell that are targets for chemotherapy
>
> - The plasma membrane is affected by:
>   - **amphotericin**, which acts as an ionophore in fungal cells
>   - azoles, which inhibit fungal membrane ergosterol synthesis.
> - Microtubule function is disrupted by:
>   - benzimidazoles (anthelmintics).
> - Muscle fibres are affected by:
>   - avermectins (anthelmintics), which increase Cl⁻ permeability
>   - **pyrantel** (anthelmintic), which stimulates nematode nicotinic receptors, eventually causing muscle paralysis.

RESISTANCE TO ANTIBACTERIAL DRUGS

Since the 1940s, the development of effective and safe drugs to deal with bacterial and other infections has revolutionised medical treatment, and the morbidity and mortality associated with these diseases has been dramatically reduced. Unfortunately, the development of effective antibacterial drugs has been accompanied by the emergence of drug-resistant organisms.

However, the bacterial 'resistome' (as the pool of genes that determines resistance is called) actually predates the advent of pharmaceutical antibiotics. It originally evolved to counteract naturally occurring bactericidal compounds encountered in their natural habitats and has changed to meet the challenges posed by modern antibiotic drugs used in the clinic (Cox & Wright, 2013). The short generation time of many bacterial species affords ample opportunity for such evolutionary adaptations. The phenomenon of resistance imposes serious constraints on the options available for the medical treatment of many bacterial infections. Resistance to chemotherapeutic agents can also develop in protozoa, in multicellular parasites (and also in populations of malignant cells, discussed in Ch. 56). Here, however, we will confine our discussion mainly to the mechanisms of resistance in bacteria.

Antibiotic resistance may be *innate* or *acquired*. There are three basic mechanisms by which resistance is spread:

1. by transfer of resistant bacteria between people
2. by transfer of resistance genes between bacteria (usually on plasmids)
3. by transfer of resistance genes between genetic elements within bacteria, on transposons.

Understanding the mechanisms involved in antibiotic resistance is crucial for the sensible clinical use of existing medicines ('antibiotic stewardship') and in the design of new antibacterial drugs. One byproduct of the studies of resistance in bacteria was the development of plasmid-based techniques for DNA cloning, leading to the use of bacteria to produce recombinant proteins for therapeutic use (see Ch. 59).

GENETIC DETERMINANTS OF ANTIBIOTIC RESISTANCE

CHROMOSOMAL DETERMINANTS: MUTATIONS

▼ The spontaneous mutation rate in bacterial populations for any particular gene is very low, and the probability is that approximately only 1 cell in 10 million will, on division, give rise to a daughter cell containing a mutation in that gene. However, as there are likely to be very many more cells than this over the course of an infection, the probability of a mutation causing a change from drug sensitivity to drug resistance can be quite high. Fortunately, the presence of a few mutants is not generally sufficient to produce resistance: despite the selective advantage that the resistant mutants possess, the drastic reduction of the population by the antibiotic usually enables the host's natural defences (see Ch. 6) to prevail at least in acute, if not chronic, infections. However, the outcome may not be quite so happy if the primary infection is caused by a drug-resistant strain.

GENE AMPLIFICATION

▼ *Gene duplication* and *amplification* are important mechanisms for resistance in some organisms (Sandegren & Andersson, 2009). According to this idea, treatment with antibiotics can induce an increased number of copies for pre-existing resistance genes such as antibiotic-destroying enzymes and efflux pumps.

EXTRACHROMOSOMAL DETERMINANTS: PLASMIDS

▼ In addition to the chromosome itself, many species of bacteria contain extrachromosomal genetic elements called *plasmids* that exist free in the cytoplasm. These are also genetic elements that can replicate independently. Structurally, they are closed loops of DNA that may comprise a single gene or as many as 500 or even more. Only a few plasmid copies may exist in the cell but often multiple copies are present, and there may also be more than one type of plasmid in each bacterial cell. Plasmids that carry genes for resistance to antibiotics (*r genes*) are referred to as *R plasmids*. Much of the drug resistance encountered in clinical medicine is plasmid-determined. It is not known how these genes arose.

The whole process can occur with frightening speed. *Staphylococcus aureus*, for example, is a past master of the art of antibiotic resistance. Having become completely resistant to penicillin through plasmid-mediated mechanisms, this organism, within only 1–2 years, was able to acquire resistance to its replacement, **meticillin** (de Lencastre et al., 2007).

THE TRANSFER OF RESISTANCE GENES BETWEEN GENETIC ELEMENTS WITHIN THE BACTERIUM

Transposons

▼ Some stretches of DNA are readily transferred (transposed) from one plasmid to another and also from plasmid to chromosome or vice versa. This is because integration of these segments of DNA, which are called *transposons*, into the acceptor DNA can occur independently of the normal mechanism of homologous genetic recombination. Unlike plasmids, transposons are not able to replicate independently, although some may replicate during the process of integration (Fig. 50.7), resulting in a copy in both the donor and the acceptor DNA molecules. Transposons may carry one or more resistance genes and can 'hitch-hike' on a plasmid to a new species of bacterium. Even if the plasmid is unable to replicate in the new host, the transposon may integrate into the new host's chromosome or into its indigenous plasmids. This probably accounts for the widespread distribution of certain of the resistance genes on different R plasmids and among unrelated bacteria.

Gene cassettes and integrons

▼ Plasmids and transposons do not complete the tally of mechanisms that natural selection has provided to confound the hopes of the microbiologist/chemotherapist. Resistance – in fact, *multidrug resistance* – can also be spread by another mobile element, the *gene cassette*, which consists of a resistance gene attached to a small recognition site. Several cassettes may be packaged together in a

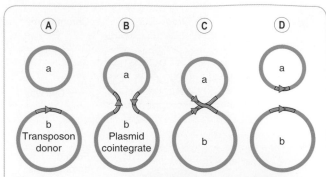

Fig. 50.7 An example of the transfer and replication of a transposon (which may carry genes coding for resistance to antibiotics). [**A**] Two plasmids, a and b, with plasmid b containing a transposon (shown in brown). [**B**] An enzyme encoded by the transposon cuts DNA of both donor plasmid and target plasmid a to form a cointegrate. During this process, the transposon replicates. [**C**] An enzyme encoded by the transposon resolves the cointegrate. [**D**] Both plasmids now contain the transposon DNA.

multicassette array, which can, in turn, be integrated into a larger mobile DNA unit termed an *integron*. The integron (which may be located on a transposon) contains a gene for an enzyme, *integrase* (*recombinase*), which inserts the cassette(s) at unique sites on the integron. This system – transposon/integron/multiresistance cassette array – allows particularly rapid and efficient transfer of multidrug resistance between genetic elements both within and between bacteria.

THE TRANSFER OF RESISTANCE GENES BETWEEN BACTERIA

▼ The transfer of resistance genes between bacteria of the same and indeed of different species is of fundamental importance in the spread of antibiotic resistance. The most important mechanism in this context is *conjugation*. Another gene transfer mechanism, *transduction* is less important in spreading resistance genes.

Conjugation

▼ Conjugation involves cell-to-cell contact during which chromosomal or extrachromosomal DNA is transferred from one bacterium to another, and is the main mechanism for the spread of resistance. The ability to conjugate is encoded in *conjugative plasmids*; these are plasmids that contain transfer genes that, in coliform bacteria, code for the production by the host bacterium of proteinaceous surface tubules, termed *sex pili*, which connect the two cells. The conjugative plasmid then passes across from one bacterial cell to another (generally of the same species). Many Gram-negative and some Gram-positive bacteria can conjugate. Some *promiscuous plasmids* can cross the species barrier, accepting one host as readily as another. Many R plasmids are conjugative. Non-conjugative plasmids, if they co-exist in a 'donor' cell with conjugative plasmids, can hitch-hike from one bacterium to the other with the conjugative plasmids. The transfer of resistance by conjugation is significant in populations of bacteria that are normally found at high densities, as in the gut.

Transduction

▼ *Transduction* is a process by which plasmid DNA is enclosed in a bacterial virus (or *phage*) and transferred to another bacterium of the same species. It is a relatively ineffective means of transfer of genetic material but is clinically important in the transmission of resistance genes between strains of staphylococci and of streptococci.

Transformation

▼ A few species of bacteria can, under natural conditions, undergo *transformation* by taking up DNA from the environment and incorporating it into the genome by normal homologous recombination. However, this mechanism is probably not of importance clinically.

Resistance to antibiotics

- Drug resistance in bacterial populations can be spread from person to person by bacteria, from bacterium to bacterium by plasmids and from plasmid to plasmid (or chromosome) by transposons.
- Multicassette arrays of drug resistance genes can be transferred between bacteria, leading to spread of multidrug resistant strains.
- Plasmids are extrachromosomal genetic elements that can replicate independently and can carry genes coding for resistance to antibiotics (r genes).
- The main method of transfer of r genes from one bacterium to another is by conjugative plasmids. The bacterium forms a connecting tube with other bacteria through which the plasmids pass.
- A less common method of transfer is by transduction, i.e. the transmission by a bacterial virus (phage) of a plasmid bearing an r gene into another bacterium.
- Transposons are stretches of DNA that can be transposed from one plasmid to another, from a plasmid to a chromosome or vice versa. A plasmid containing an r gene-bearing transposon may code for enzymes that cause the plasmid to be integrated with another. Following their separation, this transposon replicates so that both plasmids then contain the r gene.

BIOCHEMICAL MECHANISMS OF RESISTANCE TO ANTIBIOTICS

THE PRODUCTION OF AN ENZYME THAT INACTIVATES THE DRUG

Inactivation of β-lactam antibiotics

The most important example of resistance caused by inactivation is that of the *β-lactam antibiotics*. The enzymes concerned are *β-lactamases*, which cleave the β-lactam ring of penicillins and **cephalosporins** (see Ch. 51). Cross-resistance between the two classes of antibiotic is not complete, because some β-lactamases have a preference for penicillins and some for cephalosporins.

▼ Staphylococci are the principal bacterial species producing β-lactamase, and the genes coding for the enzymes are on plasmids that can be transferred by transduction. In staphylococci, the enzyme is inducible (i.e. it is not expressed in the absence of the drug) and minute, sub-inhibitory, concentrations of antibiotics de-repress the gene and result in a 50- to 80-fold increase in expression. The enzyme passes through the bacterial envelope and inactivates antibiotic molecules in the surrounding medium. The grave clinical problem posed by resistant staphylococci secreting β-lactamase was tackled by developing semisynthetic penicillins (such as meticillin) and new β-lactam antibiotics (the **monobactams** and **carbapenems**), and cephalosporins (such as **cephamandole**), that are less susceptible to inactivation. The growing problem of meticillin-resistant *Staphylococcus aureus* (MRSA) infection is discussed below.

Gram-negative organisms can also produce β-lactamases, and this is a significant factor in their resistance to the semisynthetic broad-spectrum β-lactam antibiotics. In these organisms, the enzymes may be coded by either chromosomal or plasmid genes. In the former case, the enzymes may be inducible, but in the latter they are produced constitutively. When this occurs, the enzyme does not inactivate the drug in the surrounding medium but instead remains attached to the cell wall, preventing access of the drug to membrane-associated target sites. Many of these β-lactamases are encoded by transposons, some of which may also carry resistance determinants to several other antibiotics.

Inactivation of chloramphenicol

Chloramphenicol is inactivated by *chloramphenicol acetyltransferase*, an enzyme produced by resistant strains of both Gram-positive and Gram-negative organisms, the resistance gene being plasmid borne. In Gram-negative bacteria, the enzyme is produced constitutively, resulting in levels of resistance five-fold higher than in Gram-positive bacteria, in which the enzyme is inducible.

Inactivation of aminoglycosides

Aminoglycosides are inactivated by phosphorylation, adenylation or acetylation, and the requisite enzymes are found in both Gram-negative and Gram-positive organisms. The resistance genes are carried on plasmids, and several are found on transposons.

Many other examples of this kind are given by Wright (2005) and Giedraitiene et al (2011).

ALTERATION OF DRUG-SENSITIVE OR DRUG-BINDING SITE

The aminoglycoside-binding site on the 30S subunit of the ribosome may be altered by chromosomal mutation. A plasmid-mediated alteration of the binding site protein on the 50S subunit also underlies resistance to **erythromycin**, and decreased binding of fluoroquinolones because of a point mutation in DNA gyrase A has also been described. An altered DNA dependent RNA polymerase determined by a chromosomal mutation is reported to be the basis for **rifampicin** resistance.

In addition to acquiring resistance to β-lactams susceptible to β-lactamase, some strains of *S. aureus* have even become resistant to some antibiotics that are not significantly inactivated by β-lactamase (e.g. meticillin), because they express an additional β-lactam-binding protein coded for by a mutated chromosomal gene. See Lambert (2005) for other examples of this type of action.

DECREASED DRUG ACCUMULATION IN THE BACTERIUM

An important example of decreased drug accumulation is the plasmid-mediated resistance to **tetracyclines** encountered in both Gram-positive and Gram-negative bacteria. In this case, resistance genes in the plasmid code for inducible proteins in the bacterial membrane, which promote energy-dependent efflux of the tetracyclines, and hence resistance. This type of resistance is common and has greatly reduced the therapeutic value of the tetracyclines in human and veterinary medicine. Resistance of *S. aureus* to erythromycin and the other macrolides, and to fluoroquinolones, is also brought about by energy-dependent efflux. Inhibitors of such pumps may be useful adjuncts to antibiotics (Van Bambeke et al., 2006).

There is also recent evidence of plasmid-determined inhibition of *porin* synthesis, which could affect those hydrophilic antibiotics that enter the bacterium through these water-filled channels in the outer membrane. Altered permeability as a result of chromosomal mutations involving the polysaccharide components of the outer membrane of Gram-negative organisms may confer enhanced resistance to **ampicillin**. Mutations affecting envelope components have been reported to affect the accumulation of aminoglycosides, β-lactams, chloramphenicol, peptide antibiotics and tetracycline.

ALTERATION OF ENZYME PATHWAYS

Resistance to trimethoprim is the result of plasmid-directed synthesis of a *dihydrofolate reductase* with low or zero affinity for trimethoprim. It is transferred by transduction and may be spread by transposons.

Sulfonamide resistance in many bacteria is plasmid-mediated and results from the production of a form of *dihydropteroate synthetase* with a low affinity for sulfonamides but no change in affinity for PABA. Bacteria causing serious infections have been found to carry plasmids with resistance genes to both sulfonamides and trimethoprim.

Biochemical mechanisms of resistance to antibiotics

The principal mechanisms are as follow:

- *Production of enzymes that inactivate the drug*: for example, β-lactamases, which inactivate **penicillin**; acetyltransferases, which inactivate **chloramphenicol**; kinases and other enzymes, which inactivate aminoglycosides.
- *Alteration of the drug-binding sites*: this occurs with aminoglycosides, **erythromycin**, **penicillin**.
- *Reduction of drug uptake by the bacterium*: for example, tetracyclines.
- *Alteration of enzyme pathways*: for example, dihydrofolate reductase becomes insensitive to **trimethoprim**.

CURRENT STATUS OF ANTIBIOTIC RESISTANCE IN BACTERIA

The most disturbing development of resistance has been in staphylococci, one of the commonest causes of hospital bloodstream infections, many strains of which are now resistant to almost all currently available antibiotics (de Lencastre et al., 2007). In addition to resistance to some β-lactams through production of β-lactamase and the production of an additional β-lactam-binding protein that also renders them resistant to meticillin, *S. aureus* may also manifest resistance to other antibiotics as follows:

- to **streptomycin** (because of chromosomally determined alterations of target site)
- to aminoglycosides in general (because of altered target site and plasmid-determined inactivating enzymes)
- to chloramphenicol and the macrolides (because of plasmid-determined enzymes)
- to trimethoprim (because of transposon-encoded drug-resistant dihydrofolate reductase)
- to sulfonamides (because of chromosomally determined increased production of PABA)
- to rifampicin (because of chromosomally and plasmid determined increases in efflux of the drug)
- to **fusidic acid** (because of chromosomally determined decreased affinity of the target site or a

plasmid-encoded decreased permeability to the drug)
- to quinolones, for example **ciprofloxacin** and norfloxacin (because of chromosomally determined reduced uptake).

Infections with MRSA are a major problem, particularly in hospitals, where they can spread rapidly among elderly and/or seriously ill patients, and patients with burns or wounds. Until recently, the glycopeptide **vancomycin** was the antibiotic of last resort against MRSA but, ominously, strains of MRSA showing decreased susceptibility to this drug were isolated from hospitalised patients in the USA and Japan in 1997 and, more recently, in the community. MRSA infections are rising globally.

The fact that vancomycin resistance seems to have developed spontaneously could have major clinical implications – and not only for hospital-acquired MRSA infections. It had been thought that antibiotic-resistant bacteria were dangerous only to seriously ill, hospitalised patients, in that the genetic burden of multiple resistance genes would lead to reduced virulence. Distressingly, however, there is now evidence that the spectrum and frequency of disease produced by meticillin-susceptible and meticillin-resistant staphylococci are similar.

▼ In the past few years, *enterococci* have been rapidly developing resistance to many chemotherapeutic agents and have emerged as the second most common hospital-acquired pathogen. Nonpathogenic enterococci are ubiquitous in the intestine, have intrinsic resistance to many antibacterial drugs and can readily become resistant to other agents by taking up plasmids and transposons carrying the relevant resistance genes. Such resistance is easily transferred to invading pathogenic enterococci.

Enterococci, already multiresistant, have recently developed resistance to vancomycin (see Arias & Murray, 2012). This is apparently achieved by substitution of D-Ala-D-Ala with D-Ala-D-lactate in the peptide chain attached to *N*-acetylglucosamine-*N*-acetylmuramic acid (G-M) during the first steps of peptidoglycan synthesis (see Fig. 50.3; Ch. 51). A particular concern is the possibility of transfer of vancomycin resistance from enterococci to staphylococci, because they can co-exist in the same patient.

Many other pathogens are developing or have developed resistance to commonly used drugs. This list includes *Pseudomonas aeruginosa*, *Streptococcus pyogenes*, *S. pneumoniae*, *Neisseria meningitidis*, *N. gonorrhoeae*, *Haemophilius influenzae* and *H. ducreyi*, as well as *Mycobacterium*, *Campylobacter* and *Bacteroides* species. Some strains of *Mycobacterium tuberculosis* are now able to evade every antibiotic in the clinician's armamentarium, and tuberculosis, once easily treatable, is now once again a major killer. Fortunately, some glycopeptide and other antibiotics (e.g. **teicoplanin**, **daptomycin** and **linezolide**, see Ch. 51) that are used to treat resistant Gram-positive strains have largely maintained their potency. Even so, there is a danger of resistance arising if they are wrongly utilised.

Prescribers and consumers must also bear a responsibility for the burgeoning problem of resistance. Indiscriminate use of antibiotics in human and veterinary medicine, and their use in animal foodstuffs, has undoubtedly encouraged the growth of resistant strains. Some governmental and regulatory bodies (e.g. the European Union) have devised political and social measures to curb such excesses, and these have been at least partly successful.

The issue around declining antibiotic efficacy is, however, not solely to do with bacterial countermeasures. Historically, antibiotics were one of the mainstays of the pharmaceutical industry, and by 1970 it was thought that infectious diseases had been effectively vanquished.[4]

Most of the drugs developed since are the result of incremental changes in the structures of a relatively small number of well-known molecular structures, such as the β-lactams, to which resistance has developed rapidly. Many pharmaceutical companies scaled down their efforts in the area, despite the continuing need for compounds acting by novel mechanisms to keep pace with the adaptive potential of pathogens. Drug-resistant infections are now seen as a serious global threat by the World Health Organization, needful of major incentives for research in what has become a somewhat neglected area.

---

[4]In 1967 the US Surgeon General announced (in effect) that infectious diseases had been vanquished, and that the researchers should turn their attention to chronic diseases instead.

> ### Multidrug resistance
>
> Many pathogenic bacteria have developed resistance to the commonly used antibiotics. Examples include the following:
> - Some strains of staphylococci and enterococci that are resistant to virtually all current antibiotics, the resistance being transferred by transposons and/or plasmids; such organisms can cause serious and virtually untreatable nosocomial infections.
> - Some strains of *Mycobacterium tuberculosis* that have become resistant to most antituberculosis agents.

REFERENCES AND FURTHER READING

Amyes, S.G.B., 2001. Magic Bullets, Lost Horizons: The Rise and Fall of Antibiotics. Taylor & Francis, London. (*Thought-provoking book by a bacteriologist with wide experience in bacterial resistance and genetics; he opines that unless the problem of antibiotic resistance is solved within 5 years, 'we are going to slip further into the abyss of uncontrollable infection'*)

Arias, C.A., Murray, B.E., 2012. The rise of the *Enterococcus*: beyond vancomycin resistance. Nat. Rev. Microbiol. 10, 266–278. (*A comprehensive review dealing with many aspects of vancomycin resistance in enterococci and other species. Highly recommended*)

Barrett, C.T., Barrett, J.F., 2003. Antibacterials: are the new entries enough to deal with the emerging resistance problem? Curr. Opin. Biotechnol. 14, 621–626. (*Good general review with some compelling examples and a round-up of new drug candidates*)

Bax, R., Mullan, N., Verhoef, J., 2000. The millennium bugs – the need for and development of new antibacterials. Int. J. Antimicrob. Agents 16, 51–59. (*Excellent review of the problem of resistance and some potential new antibiotics*)

Cox, G., Wright, G.D., 2013. Intrinsic antibiotic resistance: mechanisms, origins, challenges and solutions. Int. J. Med. Microbiol. 303, 287–292. (*This paper reviews general mechanisms of bacterial resistance based upon the notion that resistance is a naturally occurring defence in bacteria. Recommended*)

de Lencastre, H., Oliveira, D., Tomasz, A., 2007. Antibiotic resistant *Staphylococcus aureus*: a paradigm of adaptive power. Curr. Opin. Microbiol. 10, 428–435. (*A little specialised, but worth reading. It details the extraordinary ability of this organism to survive attack by virtually all the drugs in our antibiotic arsenal*)

Giedraitiene, A., Vitkauskiene, A., Naginiene, R., Pavilonis, A., 2011. Antibiotic resistance mechanisms of clinically important bacteria. Medicina 47, 137–146. (*Good review of resistance mechanisms*)

Hawkey, P.M., 1998. The origins and molecular basis of antibiotic resistance. Br. Med. J. 7159, 657–659. (*Succinct overview of resistance; useful, simple diagrams; this is one of 12 papers on resistance in this issue of the journal*)

Knodler, L.A., Celli, J., Finlay, B.B., 2001. Pathogenic trickery: deception of host cell processes. Mol. Cell. Biol. 2, 578–588. (*Discusses bacterial ploys to subvert or block normal host cellular processes: mimicking the ligands for host cell receptors or signalling pathways. Useful list of examples*)

Lambert, P.A., 2005. Bacterial resistance to antibiotics: modified target sites. Adv. Drug Deliv. Rev. 57, 1471–1485. (*Excellent review dealing with this important topic. Numerous examples drawn from studies with many different bacterial species*)

Levy, S.B., 1998. The challenge of antibiotic resistance. Sci. Am. March, 32–39. (*Simple, clear review by an expert in the field; excellent diagrams*)

Michel, M., Gutman, L., 1997. Methicillin-resistant *Staphylococcus aureus* and vancomycin-resistant enterococci: therapeutic realities and possibilities. Lancet 349, 1901–1906. (*Good review article; useful diagram; suggests schemes for medical management of infections caused by resistant organisms*)

Noble, W.C., Virani, Z., Cree, R.G., 1992. Co-transfer of vancomycin and other resistance genes from *Enterococcus faecalis* NCTC 12201 to *Staphylococcus aureus*. FEMS Microbiol. Lett. 72, 195–198.

Recchia, G.D., Hall, R.M., 1995. Gene cassettes: a new class of mobile element. Microbiology 141, 3015–3027. (*Detailed coverage of this unusual mechanism*)

Sandegren, L., Andersson, D.I., 2009. Bacterial gene amplification: implications for the evolution of antibiotic resistance. Nat. Rev. Microbiol. 7, 578–588.

Shlaes, D.M., 2003. The abandonment of antibacterials: why and wherefore? Curr. Opin. Pharmacol. 3, 470–473. (*A good review that explains the reasons underlying the resistance problem and the regulatory and other hurdles that must be overcome before new antibacterials appear on to the market; almost apocalyptic in tone*)

St Georgiev, V., 2000. Membrane transporters and antifungal drug resistance. Curr. Drug Targets 1, 184–261. (*Discusses various aspects of multidrug resistance in disease-causing fungi in the context of targeted drug development*)

Van Bambeke, F., Pages, J.M., Lee, V.J., 2006. Inhibitors of bacterial efflux pumps as adjuvants in antibiotic treatments and diagnostic tools for detection of resistance by efflux. Recent. Pat. Antiinfect. Drug Discov. 1, 157–175.

van Belkum, A., 2000. Molecular epidemiology of methicillin-resistant *Staphylococcus aureus* strains: state of affairs and tomorrow's possibilities. Microb. Drug Resist. 6, 173–187.

Volpato, J.P., Pelletier, J.N., 2009. Mutational 'hot-spots' in mammalian, bacterial and protozoal dihydrofolate reductases associated with antifolate resistance: sequence and structural comparison. Drug Resist. Updat. 12, 28–41.

Walsh, C., 2000. Molecular mechanisms that confer antibacterial drug resistance. Nature 406, 775–781. (*Excellent review outlining the mechanisms of action of antibiotics and the resistance ploys of bacteria; very good diagrams*)

Woodford, N., 2005. Biological counterstrike: antibiotic resistance mechanisms of Gram-positive cocci. Clin. Microbiol. Infect. 3, 2–21. (*A useful reference that classifies antibiotic resistance as one of the major public health concerns of the 21st century and discusses drug treatment for resistant strains*)

Wright, G.D., 2005. Bacterial resistance to antibiotics: enzymatic degradation and modification. Adv. Drug Deliv. Rev. 57, 1451–1470. (*This comprehensive review gives details of the many pathways that have evolved in bacteria to destroy antibiotics. A little complex, but fascinating reading*)

Zasloff, M., 2002. Antimicrobial peptides of multicellular organisms. Nature 415, 389–395. (*Thought-provoking article about the potent broad-spectrum antimicrobial peptides possessed by both animals and plants, which are used to fend off a wide range of microbes; it is suggested that exploiting these might be one answer to the problem of antibiotic resistance*)

51 Antibacterial drugs

OVERVIEW

In this chapter we continue to develop the ideas we introduced in the previous chapter. A detailed discussion of bacteriology is beyond the scope of this book but information about some clinically significant pathogens (see Table 51.1) is provided to give some context. The major classes of antibacterial[1] drugs are described (see Table 51.2), along with their mechanism of action, relevant pharmacokinetic properties and side effects. We conclude with an overview of new directions in research in this vital area.

INTRODUCTION

In 1928 Alexander Fleming, working at St Mary's Hospital in London, discovered that a culture plate on which staphylococci were being grown had become contaminated with a mould of the genus *Penicillium*. He made the crucial observation that bacterial growth in the vicinity of the mould had been inhibited. He subsequently isolated the mould in pure culture and demonstrated that it produced an antibacterial substance, which he called **penicillin**. This substance was subsequently prepared in bulk, extracted and its antibacterial effects analysed by Florey, Chain and their colleagues at Oxford in 1940. They showed that it was non-toxic to the host but killed the pathogens in infected mice, thus ushering in the 'antibiotic era'. Seventy years later, the number of different types of antibiotics had grown 10-fold and the practice of medicine would be unthinkable without them.

Gram staining and bacterial cell wall structure

Most bacteria can be classified as being either *Gram-positive* or *Gram-negative* depending on whether or not they stain with *Gram's stain*. This reflects fundamental differences in the structure of their cell walls, which has important implications for the action of antibiotics.

The cell wall of Gram-positive organisms is a relatively simple structure. It is some 15–50 nm thick and comprises about 50% peptidoglycan (see Ch. 50), 40–45% acidic polymer (which results in the cell surface being highly polar and negatively charged) together with 5–10% proteins and polysaccharides. The strongly polar polymer layer influences the penetration of ionised molecules and favours the penetration into the cell of positively charged compounds such as **streptomycin**.

The cell wall of Gram-negative organisms is much more complex. From the plasma membrane outwards, it consists of the following:

- A *periplasmic space* containing enzymes and other components.
- A *peptidoglycan layer* 2 nm in thickness, forming 5% of the cell wall mass, which is often linked to outwardly projecting lipoprotein molecules.
- An *outer membrane* consisting of a lipid bilayer, similar in some respects to the plasma membrane, that contains protein molecules and (on its inner aspect) lipoproteins linked to the peptidoglycan. Other proteins form transmembrane water-filled channels, termed *porins*, through which hydrophilic antibiotics can move freely.
- *Complex polysaccharides* forming important components of the outer surface. These differ between strains of bacteria and are the main determinants of their antigenicity. They are also the source of *endotoxin* which, when shed *in vivo*, triggers various aspects of the inflammatory reaction by activating complement and cytokines, causing fever, etc. (see Ch. 6).

Difficulty in penetrating this complex outer layer explains why some antibiotics are less active against Gram-negative than Gram-positive bacteria. It is also one reason for the extraordinary antibiotic resistance exhibited by *Pseudomonas aeruginosa*, a pathogen that can cause life-threatening infections in neutropenic patients and those with burns and wounds. The cell wall lipopolysaccharide is also a major barrier to penetration of some antibiotics, including **benzylpenicillin**, **meticillin**, the macrolides, **rifampicin**, **fusidic acid** and **vancomycin**.

In discussing the pharmacology of antibacterial drugs, it is convenient to divide them into different groups based upon their mechanism of action.

ANTIBACTERIAL AGENTS THAT INTERFERE WITH FOLATE SYNTHESIS OR ACTION

SULFONAMIDES

In a landmark discovery in the 1930s, before the advent of penicillin, Domagk demonstrated that it was possible for a drug to suppress a bacterial infection. The agent was prontosil,[2] a dye that proved to be an inactive prodrug that was metabolised *in vivo* to an active product, **sulfanilamide** (Fig. 51.1). Many sulfonamides have been developed since, but their importance has declined in the face of increasing resistance. The only sulfonamide drugs still commonly used as systemic antibacterials are **sulfamethoxazole** (usually in combination with **trimethoprim** as **co-trimoxazole**), **sulfasalazine** (poorly absorbed in the

---

[1]Strictly speaking, the term 'antibiotic' only applies to antibacterials that are produced by one organism to kill others (e.g. penicillin) in contrast to synthetic compounds such as the sulfonamides. In practice, however, this distinction is often ignored as many antibacterial drugs are 'semi-synthetic' (e.g. flucloxacillin).

[2]Domagk believed, wrongly, that the staining property of azo dyes, such as prontosil, was responsible for their antibacterial action. He used prontosil – a red dye – to treat his young daughter for a life-threatening streptococcal infection. She survived, but was left with permanently red-stained skin.

Table 51.1 Some clinically significant pathogenic bacteria

Genus	Morphology	Species	Disease
Gram-negative			
Bordetella	Cocci	*B. pertussis*	Whooping cough
Brucella	Curved rods	*B. abortus*	Brucellosis (cattle and humans)
Campylobacter	Spiral rods	*C. jejuni*	Food poisoning
Escherichia	Rods	*E. coli*	Septicaemia, wound infections, UTIs
Haemophilus	Rods	*H. influenzae*	Acute respiratory tract infection, meningitis
Helicobacter	Motile rods	*H. pylori*	Peptic ulcers, gastric cancer
Klebsiella	Capsulated rods	*K. pneumoniae*	Pneumonia, septicaemia
Legionella	Flagellated rods	*L. pneumophila*	Legionnaires' disease
Neisseria	Cocci, paired	*N. gonorrhea*	Gonorrhoea
Pseudomonas	Flagellated rods	*P. aeruginosa*	Septicaemia, respiratory infections, UTIs
Rickettsiae	Cocci or threads	Several spp.	Tick- and insect-borne infections
Salmonella	Motile rods	*S. typhimurium*	Food poisoning
Shigella	Rods	*S. dysenteriae*	Bacillary dysentry
Yersinia	Rods	*Y. pestis*	Bubonic plague
Vibrio	Flagellated rods	*V. cholerae*	Cholera
Gram-positive			
Bacillus	Rods, chains	*B. anthrax*	Anthrax
Clostridium	Rods	*C. tetani*	Tetanus
Corynebacterium	Rod	*C. diphtheriae*	Diphtheria
Mycobacterium	Rods	*M. tuberculosis*	Tuberculosis
		M. leprae	Leprosy
Staphylococcus	Cocci, clusters	*S. aureus*	Wound infections, boils, septicaemia
Streptococcus	Cocci, pairs	*S. pneumoniae*	Pneumonia, meningitis
	Cocci, chains	*S. pyogenes*	Scarlet fever, rheumatic fever, cellulitis
Other			
Chlamydia	Gram 'uncertain'	*C. trachomatis*	Eye disease, infertility
Treponema	Flagellated spiral rods	*T. pallidum*	Syphillis

UTI, urinary tract infection.

gastrointestinal tract, used to treat ulcerative colitis and Crohn's disease; see Chs 26 and 30). Silver **sulfadiazine** is used topically, for example to treat infected burns. Some drugs with quite different clinical uses (e.g. the antiplatelet drug **prasugrel**, Ch. 24, and the carbonic anhydrase inhibitor **acetazolamide**, Ch. 29), are sulfonamides and share some of the off-target adverse effects of this class.

Mechanism of action

Sulfanilamide is a structural analogue of *p*-aminobenzoic acid (PABA; see Fig. 51.1), which is an essential precursor in the synthesis of folic acid, required for the synthesis of DNA and RNA in bacteria (see Ch. 50). Sulfonamides

Clinical uses of sulfonamides

- Combined with **trimethoprim (co-trimoxazole)** for *Pneumocystis carinii* (now known as *P. jirovecii*), for toxoplamsosis and nocardiasis.
- Combined with **pyrimethamine** for drug-resistant malaria (Table 54.1) and for toxoplasmosis.
- In inflammatory bowel disease: **sulfasalazine** (sulfapyridine–aminosalicylate combination) is used (see Ch. 30).
- For infected burns (silver **sulfadiazine** given topically).

Table 51.2 A general overview of antibacterials and their mechanism of action

Family	Examples	Typical target organisms	Mechanism of action
Sulfonamides	Sulfadiazine, sulfamethoxazole, (trimethoprim)	*T. gondii, P. jirovecii*	Bacterial folate synthesis or action
β-lactams	PENICILLINS Benzylpenicillin, phenoxymethylpenicillin	Overall, mainly Gram-positive spp.; some Gram-negative spp.	Bacterial cell wall peptidoglycan synthesis
	Penicillinase-resistant penicillins Flucloxacillin, temocillin	Used for staphylococcal infections	
	Broad-spectrum penicillins Amoxicillin, ampicillin	A wide range of Gram-positive and Gram-negative spp.	
	Antipseudomonal penicillins Piperacillin, ticarcillin	Selected Gram-negative spp., especially *P. aeruginosa*	
	MECILLINAMS Pivmecillinam	Mainly Gram-negative spp.	
	CEPHALOSPORINS Cefalcor, cefadroxil, cefalexin, cefixime, cefotaxime, cefpodoxime, cefradine, ceftaroline, ceftazidime, ceftriaxone, cefuroxime	Broad spectrum of activity against Gram-negative and positive spp.	
	CARBAPENEMS Ertapenem, impenem, meropenem, doripenem.	Many Gram-negative and positive spp.	
	MONOBACTAMS Aztreonam	Gram-negative rods	
Glycopeptides	Vancomycin, teicoplanin, daptomycin	Gram-positive spp.	
Polymixins	Colistimethate, polymixin B	Gram-negative spp.	Bacterial outer cell membrane structure
Tetracyclines	Demeclocycline, doxycycline, lymecycline, minocycline, oxytetracycline, tetracycline tigecycline	Many Gram-negative and Gram-positive spp.	Bacterial protein synthesis (multiple mechanisms inhibited including initiation, transpeptidation and translocation; see text)
Aminogycosides	Amikacin, gentamicin, neomycin, tobramycin	Many Gram-negative, some Gram-positive spp.	
Macrolides	Azithromycin, clarithromycin, erythromycin, spiramycin, telithromycin	Similar to penicillin	
Oxazolidinones	Linezolid	Gram-positive spp.	
Lincosamides	Clindamycin	Gram-positive spp.	
Amphenicols	Chloramphenicol	Gram-negative and Gram-positive spp.	
Streptogramins	Quinupristin, dalfopristin	Gram-positive spp.	
Antimycobacterials	Capreomycin, clofazimine, cycloserine, dapsone, ethambutol, isoniazid, pyrazinamide, rifabutin, rifampicin	Most used for mycobacterial infections only	Various unrelated mechanisms (see text)
Quinolones	Ciprofloxacin, levofloxacin, moxifloxacin, nalidixic acid, norfloxacin, ofloxacin	Gram-negative and Gram-positive spp.	Bacterial DNA synthesis
Miscellaneous	Fusidic acid	Gram-positive spp.	Bacterial protein synthesis
	Nitrofurantoin	Gram-negative UTIs	Damages bacterial DNA
	Methenamine	Gram-negative UTIs	Formaldehyde pro-drug

Drug mixtures (e.g. co-fluampicil – flucloxacillin with ampicillin) are not shown.

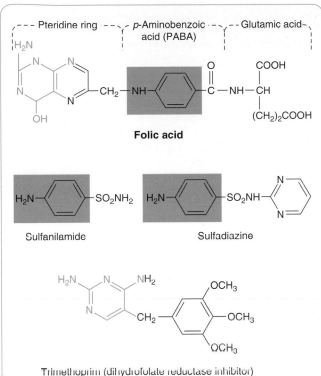

Fig. 51.1 Structures of two representative sulfonamides and trimethoprim. The structures illustrate the relationship between the sulfonamides and the *p*-aminobenzoic acid moiety in folic acid (orange box), as well as the possible relationship between the antifolate drugs and the pteridine moiety (orange). Co-trimoxazole is a mixture of sulfamethoxazole and trimethoprim.

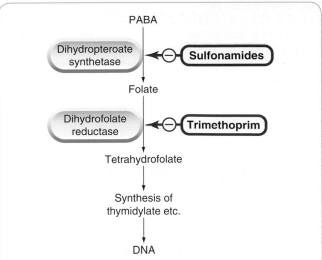

Fig. 51.2 The action of sulfonamides and trimethoprim on bacterial folate synthesis. See Chapter 25 for more detail of tetrahydrofolate synthesis, and Table 50.1 for comparisons of antifolate drugs. PABA, *p*-aminobenzoic acid.

compete with PABA for the enzyme *dihydropteroate synthetase*, and the effect of the sulfonamide may be overcome by adding excess PABA. This is why some local anaesthetics, which are PABA esters (such as **procaine**; see Ch. 43), can antagonise the antibacterial effect of these agents.

▼ While not necessarily clinically relevant, a general rule is that antibiotics that interfere with bacterial cell wall synthesis (e.g. penicillins: see Table 51.2) or inhibit crucial enzymes (such as the quinolones) generally kill bacteria (i.e. they are *bactericidal*). Those that inhibit protein synthesis such as the tetracyclines, tend to be *bacteriostatic*, that is they prevent growth and replication. Sulfonamides belong to the second group.

Sulfonamide action is vitiated in the presence of pus or products of tissue breakdown, because these contain thymidine and purines, which bacteria utilise directly, bypassing the requirement for folic acid. Resistance, which is common, is plasmid-mediated (see Ch. 50) and results from the synthesis of a bacterial enzyme insensitive to the drugs.

Pharmacokinetic aspects

Most sulfonamides are given orally and, apart from sulfasalazine, are well absorbed and widely distributed in the body. There is a risk of sensitisation or allergic reactions when these drugs are given topically.

The drugs pass into inflammatory exudates and cross both placental and blood–brain barriers. They are metabolised mainly in the liver, the major product being an acetylated derivative that lacks antibacterial action.

Unwanted effects

Serious adverse effects necessitating cessation of therapy include hepatitis, hypersensitivity reactions (rashes including Stevens–Johnson syndrome and toxic epidermal necrolysis, fever, anaphylactoid reactions – see Ch. 57), bone marrow depression and acute renal failure due to interstitial nephritis or crystalluria. This last effect results from the precipitation of acetylated metabolites in the urine (Ch. 29). Cyanosis caused by methaemoglobinaemia may occur but is a lot less alarming than it looks. Mild to moderate side effects include nausea and vomiting, headache and mental depression.

TRIMETHOPRIM

Mechanism of action

Trimethoprim is chemically related to the antimalarial drug **pyrimethamine** (Ch. 54), both being folate antagonists. Structurally (Fig. 51.1), it resembles the pteridine moiety of folate and the similarity is close enough to fool the bacterial dihydrofolate reductase, which is many times more sensitive to trimethoprim than is the equivalent enzyme in humans.

Trimethoprim, also bacteriostatic, is active against most common bacterial pathogens as well as protozoa, and is used to treat various urinary, pulmonary and other infections. It is sometimes given as a mixture with sulfamethoxazole as co-trimoxazole (Fig. 51.1). Because sulfonamides inhibit a different stage on the same bacterial metabolic pathway, they can potentiate the action of trimethoprim (see Fig. 51.2). In the UK, the use of co-trimoxazole is generally restricted to the treatment of *Pneumocystis carinii* (now known as *P. jirovecii*) pneumonia (a fungal infection), toxoplasmosis (a protozoan infection) or nocardiasis (a bacterial infection).

Pharmacokinetic aspects

Trimethoprim is well absorbed orally, and widely distributed throughout the tissues and body fluids. It reaches high concentrations in the lungs and kidneys, and fairly high concentrations in the cerebrospinal fluid (CSF). When given with sulfamethoxazole, about half the dose of each is excreted within 24 h. Because trimethoprim is a weak base, its elimination by the kidney increases with decreasing urinary pH.

Unwanted effects

Folate deficiency, with resultant *megaloblastic anaemia* (see Ch. 25) is a danger of long-term administration of trimethoprim. Other unwanted effects include nausea, vomiting, blood disorders and rashes.

Antimicrobial agents that interfere with the synthesis or action of folate

- Sulfonamides are bacteriostatic; they act by interfering with folate synthesis and thus with nucleotide synthesis. Unwanted effects include crystalluria and hypersensitivities.
- **Trimethoprim** is bacteriostatic. It acts by antagonising folate.
- **Co-trimoxazole** is a mixture of **trimethoprim** with **sulfamethoxazole**, which affects bacterial nucleotide synthesis at two points in the pathway.
- **Pyrimethamine** and **proguanil** are also antimalarial agents (see Ch. 54).

β-LACTAM ANTIBIOTICS

PENICILLINS

The remarkable antibacterial effects of systemic penicillin in humans were clearly demonstrated in 1941.[3] A small amount of penicillin, extracted laboriously from crude cultures in the laboratories of the Dunn School of Pathology in Oxford, was given to a desperately ill policeman who had septicaemia with multiple abscesses. Although sulfonamides were available, they would have had no effect in the presence of pus. Intravenous injections of penicillin were given every 3 h. All the patient's urine was collected, and each day the bulk of the excreted penicillin was extracted and reused. After 5 days, the patient's condition was vastly improved, and there was obvious resolution of the abscesses. Furthermore, there seemed to be no toxic effects of the drug. Unfortunately, when the supply of penicillin was finally exhausted his condition gradually deteriorated and he died a month later.

Penicillins, often combined with other antibiotics, remain crucially important in antibacterial chemotherapy, but they can be destroyed by bacterial *amidases* and *β-lactamases* (*penicillinases*; see Fig. 51.3). This forms the basis of one of the principal types of antibiotic resistance.

Mechanisms of action

All β-lactam antibiotics interfere with the synthesis of the bacterial cell wall peptidoglycan (see Ch. 50, Fig. 50.3). After attachment to *penicillin-binding proteins* on bacteria (there may be seven or more types in different organisms), they inhibit the transpeptidation enzyme that crosslinks the peptide chains attached to the backbone of the peptidoglycan.

---

[3]Although *topical* penicillin had actually been used with success in five patients with eye infections 10 years previously by Paine, a graduate of St Mary's who had obtained some penicillin mould from Fleming.

Clinical uses of the penicillins

- Penicillins are given by mouth or, in more severe infections, intravenously, and often in combination with other antibiotics.
- Uses are for sensitive organisms and may (but may not: individual sensitivity testing is often appropriate depending on local conditions) include:
  - *bacterial meningitis* (e.g. caused by *Neisseria meningitidis*, *Streptococcus pneumoniae*): **benzylpenicillin**, high doses intravenously
  - *bone* and *joint infections* (e.g. with *Staphylococcus aureus*): **flucloxacillin**
  - *skin* and *soft tissue infections* (e.g. with *Streptococcus pyogenes* or *S. aureus*): **benzylpenicillin**, **flucloxacillin**; animal bites: **co-amoxiclav**
  - *pharyngitis* (from *S. pyogenes*): **phenoxylmethylpenicillin**
  - *otitis media* (organisms commonly include *S. pyogenes*, *Haemophilus influenzae*): **amoxicillin**
  - *bronchitis* (mixed infections common): **amoxicillin**
  - *pneumonia*: **amoxicillin**
  - *urinary tract infections* (e.g. with *Escherichia coli*): **amoxicillin**
  - *gonorrhea*: **amoxicillin** (plus **probenecid**)
  - *syphilis*: **procaine benzylpenicillin**
  - *endocarditis* (e.g. with *Streptococcus viridans* or *Enterococcus faecalis*): high-dose intravenous **benzylpenicillin** sometimes with an aminoglycoside
  - *serious infections with Psuedomonas aeruginosa*: **ticarcillin**, **piperacillin**.

  This list is not exhaustive. Treatment with penicillins is sometimes started empirically, if the likely causative organism is one thought to be susceptible to penicillin, while awaiting the results of laboratory tests to identify the organism and determine its antibiotic susceptibility.

The final bactericidal event is the inactivation of an inhibitor of autolytic enzymes in the cell wall, leading to lysis of the bacterium. Some organisms, referred to as 'tolerant', have defective autolytic enzymes in which case lysis does not occur in response to the drug. Resistance to penicillin may result from a number of different causes and is discussed in detail in Chapter 50.

Types of penicillin and their antimicrobial activity

The first penicillins were the naturally occurring **benzylpenicillin** (**penicillin G**) and its congeners, including **phenoxymethylpenicillin** (**penicillin V**). Benzylpenicillin is active against a wide range of organisms and is the drug of first choice for many infections (see clinical box, above). Its main drawbacks are poor absorption in the gastrointestinal tract (which means it must be given by injection) and its susceptibility to bacterial β-lactamases.

Semisynthetic penicillins, incorporating different side-chains attached to the penicillin nucleus (at R_1 in Fig. 51.3),

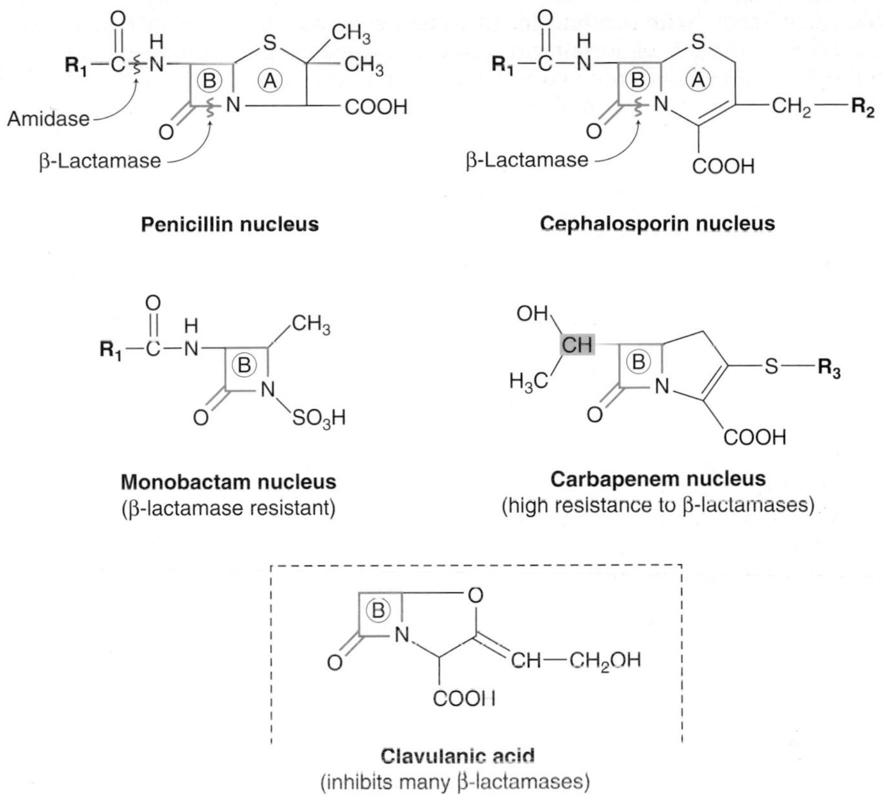

Fig. 51.3 Basic structures of four groups of β-lactam antibiotics and clavulanic acid. The structures illustrate the β-lactam ring (marked B) and the sites of action of bacterial enzymes that inactivate these antibiotics (A, thiazolidine ring). Various substituents are added at R_1, R_2 and R_3 to produce agents with different properties. In carbapenems, the stereochemical configuration of the part of the β-lactam ring shown shaded in orange here is different from the corresponding part of the penicillin and cephalosporin molecules; this is probably the basis of the β-lactamase resistance of the carbapenems. The β-lactam ring of clavulanic acid is thought to bind strongly to β-lactamase, meanwhile protecting other β-lactams from the enzyme.

include *β-lactamase-resistant* penicillins (e.g. **meticillin,**[4] **flucloxacillin, temocillin**) and *broad-spectrum* penicillins (e.g. **ampicillin, amoxicillin**). *Extended-spectrum* penicillins (e.g. **ticarcillin, piperacillin**) with antipseudomonal activity have gone some way to overcoming the problem of serious infections caused by *P. aeruginosa*. Amoxicillin and ticarcillin are sometimes given in combination with the β-lactamase inhibitor **clavulanic acid** (e.g. **co-amoxiclav**). **Pivmecillinam** is a prodrug of mecillinam, which also has a wide spectrum of action.

Pharmacokinetic aspects

Oral absorption of penicillins varies, depending on their stability in acid and their adsorption to foodstuffs in the gut. Penicillins can also be given by intravenous injection. Preparations for intramuscular injection are also available, including slow-release preparations such as **benzathine benzylpenicillin** is useful for treating syphilis since *Treponema pallidum* is a very slowly dividing organism. Intrathecal administration of benzylpenicillin (used historically to treat meningitis) is no longer used, as it can cause convulsions.[5]

The penicillins are widely distributed in body fluids, passing into joints; into pleural and pericardial cavities; into bile, saliva and milk; and across the placenta. Being lipid-insoluble, they do not enter mammalian cells, and

cross the blood–brain barrier only if the meninges are inflamed, in which case they may reach therapeutically effective concentrations in the cerebrospinal fluid.

Elimination of most penicillins occurs rapidly and is mainly renal, 90% being through tubular secretion. The relatively short plasma half-life is a potential problem in the clinical use of benzylpenicillin, although because penicillin works by preventing cell wall synthesis in dividing organisms, intermittent rather than continuous exposure to the drug can be an advantage.

Unwanted effects

Penicillins are relatively free from direct toxic effects (other than their proconvulsant effect when given intrathecally). The main unwanted effects are hypersensitivity reactions caused by the degradation products of penicillin, which combine with host protein and become antigenic. Skin rashes and fever are common; a delayed type of serum sickness occurs infrequently. Much more serious is acute anaphylactic shock which, although rare, may be fatal. When given orally, penicillins, particularly the broad-spectrum type, alter the bacterial flora in the gut. This can be associated with gastrointestinal disturbances and in some cases with suprainfection by other, penicillin-insensitive, microorganisms leading to problems such as pseudomembranous colitis (caused by *Clostridium difficile*, see below).

CEPHALOSPORINS AND CEPHAMYCINS

Cephalosporins and cephamycins are β-lactam antibiotics, first isolated from fungi. They all have the same mechanism of action as penicillins.

---

[4]Meticillin (previous name: methicillin) was the first β-lactamase-resistant penicillin. It is not now used clinically because it was associated with interstitial nephritis, but is remembered in the acronym 'MRSA' – meticillin-resistant *Staphylococcus aureus*.

[5]Indeed, penicillins applied topically to the cortex are used to induce convulsions in an animal model of epilepsy (see Ch. 45).

Semisynthetic broad-spectrum cephalosporins have been produced by addition, to the cephalosporin C nucleus, of different side-chains at R_1 and/or R_2 (see Fig. 51.3). These agents are water-soluble and relatively acid stable. They vary in susceptibility to β-lactamases. Many cephalosporins and cephamycins are now available for clinical use (see list in Table 51.2). Resistance to this group of drugs has increased because of plasmid-encoded or chromosomal β-lactamase. The latter is present in nearly all Gram-negative bacteria and it is more active in hydrolysing cephalosporins than penicillins. In several organisms a single mutation can result in high-level constitutive production of this enzyme. Resistance also occurs when there is decreased penetration of the drug as a result of alterations to outer membrane proteins, or mutations of the binding-site proteins.

Clinical uses of the cephalosporins

Cephalosporins are used to treat infections caused by sensitive organisms. As with other antibiotics, patterns of sensitivity vary geographically, and treatment is often started empirically. Many different kinds of infection may be treated, including:

- *septicaemia* (e.g. **cefuroxime**, **cefotaxime**)
- *pneumonia* caused by susceptible organisms
- *meningitis* (e.g. **ceftriaxone**, **cefotaxime**)
- *biliary tract infection*
- *urinary tract infection* (especially in pregnancy or in patients unresponsive to other drugs)
- *sinusitis* (e.g. **cefadroxil**).

Pharmacokinetic aspects

Some cephalosporins may be given orally, but most are given parenterally, intramuscularly (which may be painful) or intravenously. After absorption, they are widely distributed in the body and some, such as **cefotaxime**, **cefuroxime** and **ceftriaxone**, cross the blood–brain barrier. Excretion is mostly via the kidney, largely by tubular secretion, but 40% of ceftriaxone is eliminated in the bile.

Unwanted effects

Hypersensitivity reactions, very similar to those seen with penicillin, may occur, and there may be some cross-sensitivity; about 10% of penicillin-sensitive individuals will have allergic reactions to cephalosporins. Nephrotoxicity has been reported (especially with **cefradine**), as has drug-induced alcohol intolerance. Diarrhoea is common and can be due to *C. difficile*.

OTHER β-LACTAM ANTIBIOTICS

Carbapenems and monobactams (see Fig. 51.3) were developed to deal with β-lactamase-producing Gram-negative organisms resistant to penicillins.

CARBAPENEMS

Imipenem, an example of a carbapenem, acts in the same way as the other β-lactams (see Fig. 51.3). It has a very broad spectrum of antimicrobial activity, being active against many aerobic and anaerobic Gram-positive and Gram-negative organisms. However, many of the 'meticillin-resistant' staphylococci are less susceptible, and resistant strains of *P. aeruginosa* have emerged during therapy. Resistance to imipenem was low, but is increasing as some organisms now have chromosomal genes that code for imipenem-hydrolysing β-lactamases. It is sometimes given together with **cilastatin**, which inhibits its inactivation by renal enzymes. **Meropenem** is similar but is not metabolised by the kidney. **Ertapenem** has a broad spectrum of antibacterial actions but is licensed only for a limited range of indications. Most carbapenems are not orally active, and are used only in special situations.

Unwanted effects are generally similar to those seen with other β-lactams, nausea and vomiting being the most frequently seen. Neurotoxicity can occur with high plasma concentrations.

MONOBACTAMS

The main monobactam is **aztreonam** (see Fig. 51.3), which is resistant to most β-lactamases. It is given by injection and has a plasma half-life of 2 h. Aztreonam has an unusual spectrum of activity and is effective only against Gram-negative aerobic bacilli such as pseudomonas species, *Neisseria meningitidis* and *Haemophilus influenzae*. It has no action against Gram-positive organisms or anaerobes.

Unwanted effects are, in general, similar to those of other β-lactam antibiotics, but this agent does not necessarily cross-react immunologically with penicillin and its products, and so does not usually cause allergic reactions in penicillin-sensitive individuals.

GLYCOPEPTIDES

Vancomycin is a glycopeptide antibiotic, and **teicoplanin** is similar but longer lasting. Vancomycin inhibits cell wall synthesis (Ch. 50, Fig. 50.3). It is effective mainly against Gram-positive bacteria. Vancomycin is not absorbed from the gut and is only given by the oral route for treatment of gastrointestinal infection with *C. difficile*. For systemic use, it is given intravenously and has a plasma half-life of about 8 h.

The main clinical use of vancomycin is the treatment of MRSA (it is often the drug of last resort for this condition) and some other serious infections. It is also valuable in severe staphylococcal infections in patients allergic to both penicillins and cephalosporins.

Unwanted effects include fever, rashes and local phlebitis at the site of injection. Ototoxicity and nephrotoxicity can occur, and hypersensitivity reactions are occasionally seen.

Daptomycin is a new lipopeptide antibacterial with a similar spectrum of actions to vancomycin. It is usually used, in combination with other drugs, for the treatment of MRSA.

ANTIMICROBIAL AGENTS AFFECTING BACTERIAL PROTEIN SYNTHESIS

TETRACYCLINES

The tetracyclines are broad-spectrum antibiotics. The group includes **tetracycline**, **oxytetracycline**, **demeclocycline**, **lymecycline**, **doxycycline**, **minocycline** and **tigecycline**.

β-Lactam antibiotics

Bactericidal because they inhibit peptidoglycan synthesis.

Penicillins

- The first choice for many infections.
- **Benzylpenicillin**:
  - given by injection, short half-life and is destroyed by β-lactamases
  - spectrum: Gram-positive and Gram-negative cocci and some Gram-negative bacteria
  - many staphylococci are now resistant.
- β-Lactamase-resistant penicillins (e.g. **flucloxacillin**):
  - given orally
  - spectrum: as for benzylpenicillin
  - many staphylococci are now resistant.
- Broad-spectrum penicillins (e.g. **amoxicillin**):
  - given orally; they are destroyed by β-lactamases
  - spectrum: as for **benzylpenicillin** (although less potent); they are also active against Gram-negative bacteria.
- Extended-spectrum penicillins (e.g. **ticarcillin**):
  - given orally; they are susceptible to β-lactamases
  - spectrum: as for broad-spectrum penicillins; they are also active against pseudomonads.

- Unwanted effects of penicillins: mainly hypersensitivities.
- A combination of **clavulanic acid** plus **amoxicillin** or **ticarcillin** is effective against many β-lactamase-producing organisms.

Cephalosporins and cephamycins

- Second choice for many infections.
- Oral drugs (e.g. **cefaclor**) are used in urinary infections.
- Parenteral drugs (e.g. **cefuroxime**, which is active against *S. aureus*, *H. influenzae*, Enterobacteriaceae).
- Unwanted effects: mainly hypersensitivities.

Carbapenems

- **Imipenem** is a broad-spectrum antibiotic.
- Imipenem is used with **cilastin**, which prevents its breakdown in the kidney.

Monobactams

- **Aztreonam**: Active only against Gram-negative aerobic bacteria and resistant to most β-lactamases.

Miscellaneous antibacterial agents that prevent cell wall or membrane synthesis

- *Glycopeptide antibiotics* (e.g. **vancomycin**). **Vancomycin** is bactericidal, acting by inhibiting cell wall synthesis. It is used intravenously for multiresistant staphylococcal infections and orally for pseudomembranous colitis. Unwanted effects include ototoxicity and nephrotoxicity.
- *Polymixins* (e.g. **colistimethate**). They are bactericidal, acting by disrupting bacterial cell membranes. They are highly neurotoxic and nephrotoxic, and are only used topically.

Mechanism of action

Following uptake into susceptible organisms by active transport, tetracyclines act by inhibiting protein synthesis (see Ch. 50, Fig. 50.4). They are regarded as bacteriostatic, not bactericidal.

Antibacterial spectrum

The spectrum of antimicrobial activity of the tetracyclines is very wide and includes Gram-positive and Gram-negative bacteria, *Mycoplasma*, *Rickettsia*, *Chlamydia* spp., spirochaetes and some protozoa (e.g. amoebae). Minocycline is also effective against *N. meningitidis* and has been used to eradicate this organism from the nasopharynx of carriers. However, widespread resistance to these agents has decreased their usefulness. Resistance is transmitted mainly by plasmids and, because the genes controlling resistance to tetracyclines are closely associated with genes for resistance to other antibiotics, organisms may develop resistance to many drugs simultaneously.

Clinical uses of tetracyclines

- The use of tetracyclines declined because of widespread drug resistance, but has staged a comeback, e.g. for respiratory infections, as resistance has receded with reduced use. Most members of the group are microbiologically similar; **doxycycline** is given once daily and may be used in patients with renal impairment. Uses (sometimes in combination with other antibiotics) include:
  - rickettsial and chlamydial infections, brucellosis, anthrax and Lyme disease
  - as useful second choice, for example in patients with allergies, for several infections (see Table 51.1), including mycoplasma and leptospira
  - respiratory tract infections (e.g. exacerbations of chronic bronchitis, community-acquired pneumonia)
  - acne
  - inappropriate secretion of antidiuretic hormone (e.g. by some malignant lung tumours), causing hyponatraemia: **demeclocycline** inhibits the action of this hormone by an entirely distinct action from its antibacterial effect (Ch. 33).

Pharmacokinetic aspects

The tetracyclines are generally given orally but can also be administered parenterally. Minocycline and doxycycline are well absorbed orally. The absorption of most other tetracyclines is irregular and incomplete but is improved in the absence of food. Because tetracyclines chelate metal ions (calcium, magnesium, iron, aluminium), forming non-absorbable complexes, absorption is decreased in the presence of milk, certain antacids and iron preparations.

Unwanted effects

The commonest unwanted effects are gastrointestinal disturbances caused initially by direct irritation and later by modification of the gut flora. Vitamin B complex deficiency can occur, as can suprainfection. Because they chelate Ca^{2+}, tetracyclines are deposited in growing bones and teeth, causing staining and sometimes dental hypoplasia and bone deformities. They should therefore not be given to children, pregnant women or nursing mothers. Another hazard to pregnant women is hepatotoxicity. Phototoxicity (sensitisation to sunlight) has also been seen, particularly with demeclocycline. Minocycline can produce vestibular disturbances (dizziness and nausea). High doses of tetracyclines can decrease protein synthesis in host cells, an antianabolic effect that may result in renal damage. Long-term therapy can cause disturbances of the bone marrow.

CHLORAMPHENICOL

Chloramphenicol was originally isolated from cultures of *Streptomyces*. It inhibits bacterial protein synthesis by binding to the 50S ribosomal subunit (see Ch. 50, Fig. 50.4).

Antibacterial spectrum

Chloramphenicol has a wide spectrum of antimicrobial activity, including Gram-negative and Gram-positive organisms and rickettsiae. It is bacteriostatic for most organisms but kills *H. influenzae*. Resistance, caused by the production of *chloramphenicol acetyltransferase*, is plasmid-mediated.

Clinical uses of chloramphenicol

- Systemic use should be reserved for serious infections in which the benefit of the drug outweighs its uncommon but serious haematological toxicity. Such uses may include:
  - infections caused by *Haemophilus influenzae* resistant to other drugs
  - *meningitis* in patients in whom penicillin cannot be used
  - *typhoid fever*, but **ciprofloxacin** or **amoxicillin** and **co-trimoxazole** are similarly effective and less toxic.
- Topical use safe and effective in bacterial conjunctivitis.

Pharmacokinetic aspects

Given orally, chloramphenicol is rapidly and completely absorbed and reaches its maximum concentration in the plasma within 2 h. It can also be given parenterally. The drug is widely distributed throughout the tissues and body fluids including the CSF. Its half-life is approximately 2 h. About 10% is excreted unchanged in the urine, and the remainder is inactivated in the liver.

Unwanted effects

The most important unwanted effect of chloramphenicol is severe, idiosyncratic depression of the bone marrow, resulting in *pancytopenia* (a decrease in all blood cell elements) – an effect that, although rare, can occur even with low doses in some individuals. Chloramphenicol must be used with great care in newborns, with monitoring of plasma concentrations, because inadequate inactivation and excretion of the drug can result in the 'grey baby syndrome' – vomiting, diarrhoea, flaccidity, low temperature and an ashen-grey colour – which carries 40% mortality. Hypersensitivity reactions can occur, as can gastrointestinal disturbances secondary to alteration of the intestinal microbial flora.

AMINOGLYCOSIDES

The aminoglycosides are a group of antibiotics of complex chemical structure, resembling each other in antimicrobial activity, pharmacokinetic characteristics and toxicity. The main agents are **gentamicin**, **streptomycin**, **amikacin**, **tobramycin** and **neomycin**.

Mechanism of action

Aminoglycosides inhibit bacterial protein synthesis (see Ch. 50). There are several possible sites of action. Their penetration through the cell membrane of the bacterium depends partly on oxygen-dependent active transport by a polyamine carrier system (which, incidentally, is blocked by chloramphenicol) and they have minimal action against anaerobic organisms. The effect of the aminoglycosides is bactericidal and is enhanced by agents that interfere with cell wall synthesis (e.g. penicillins).

Resistance

Resistance to aminoglycosides is becoming a problem. It occurs through several different mechanisms, the most important being inactivation by microbial enzymes, of which nine or more are known. Amikacin was designed as a poor substrate for these enzymes, but some organisms can inactivate this agent as well. Resistance as a result of failure of penetration can be largely overcome by the concomitant use of penicillin and/or vancomycin, at the cost of an increased risk of severe adverse effects.

Antibacterial spectrum

The aminoglycosides are effective against many aerobic Gram-negative and some Gram-positive organisms. They are most widely used against Gram-negative enteric organisms and in sepsis. They may be given together with a penicillin in streptococcal infections and those caused by *Listeria* spp. and *P. aeruginosa* (see Table 51.1). Gentamicin is the aminoglycoside most commonly used, although tobramycin is the preferred member of this group for *P. aeruginosa* infections. Amikacin has the widest antimicrobial spectrum and can be effective in infections with organisms resistant to gentamicin and tobramycin.

Pharmacokinetic aspects

The aminoglycosides are polycations and therefore highly polar. They are not absorbed from the gastrointestinal tract and are usually given intramuscularly or intravenously. They cross the placenta but do not cross the blood–brain barrier, although high concentrations can be attained in joint and pleural fluids. The plasma half-life is 2–3 h. Elimination is virtually entirely by glomerular filtration in the kidney, 50–60% of a dose being excreted unchanged within 24 h. If renal function is impaired, accumulation occurs rapidly, with a resultant increase in those toxic effects (such as ototoxicity and nephrotoxicity) that are dose related.

Unwanted effects

Serious, dose-related toxic effects, which may increase as treatment proceeds, can occur with the aminoglycosides, the main hazards being ototoxicity and nephrotoxicity.

The ototoxicity involves progressive damage to, and eventually destruction of, the sensory cells in the cochlea and vestibular organ of the ear. The result, usually irreversible, may manifest as vertigo, ataxia and loss of balance in the case of vestibular damage, and auditory disturbances or deafness in the case of cochlear damage. Any aminoglycoside may produce both types of effect, but streptomycin and gentamicin are more likely to interfere with vestibular function, whereas neomycin and amikacin mostly affect hearing. Ototoxicity is potentiated by the concomitant use of other ototoxic drugs (e.g. loop diuretics; Ch. 29) and susceptibility is genetically determined via mitochondrial DNA (see Ch. 11).

The nephrotoxicity consists of damage to the kidney tubules and may necessitate dialysis, although function usually recovers when administration ceases. Nephrotoxicity is more likely to occur in patients with pre-existing renal disease or in conditions in which urine volume is reduced, and concomitant use of other nephrotoxic agents (e.g. first-generation cephalosporins, vancomycin) increases the risk. As the elimination of these drugs is almost entirely renal, this nephrotoxic action can impair their own excretion and a vicious cycle may develop. Plasma concentrations should be monitored regularly and the dose adjusted accordingly.

A rare but serious toxic reaction is paralysis caused by neuromuscular blockade. This is usually seen only if the agents are given concurrently with neuromuscular-blocking agents. It results from inhibition of the Ca^{2+} uptake necessary for the exocytotic release of acetylcholine (see Ch. 13).

MACROLIDES

The term *macrolide* relates to the structure – a many-membered lactone ring to which one or more deoxy sugars are attached. The main macrolide and related antibiotics are **erythromycin**, **clarithromycin** and **azithromycin**. **Spiramycin** and **telithromycin** are of minor utility.

Mechanism of action
The macrolides inhibit bacterial protein synthesis by an effect on ribosomal translocation (Ch. 50, Fig. 50.4). The drugs bind to the same 50S subunit of the bacterial ribosome as chloramphenicol and **clindamycin**, and any of these drugs may compete if given concurrently.

Antimicrobial spectrum
The antimicrobial spectrum of erythromycin is very similar to that of penicillin, and it is a safe and effective alternative for penicillin-sensitive patients. Erythromycin is effective against Gram-positive bacteria and spirochaetes but not against most Gram-negative organisms, exceptions being *N. gonorrhoeae* and, to a lesser extent, *H. influenzae*. *Mycoplasma pneumoniae*, *Legionella* spp. and some chlamydial organisms are also susceptible (see Table 51.1). Resistance can occur and results from a plasmid-controlled alteration of the binding site for erythromycin on the bacterial ribosome (Ch. 50, Fig. 50.4).

Azithromycin is less active than erythromycin against Gram-positive bacteria but is considerably more effective against *H. influenzae* and may be more active against *Legionella*. It can be used to treat *Toxoplasma gondii*, as it kills the cysts. Clarithromycin is as active, and its metabolite is twice as active, against *H. influenzae* as

erythromycin. It is also effective against *Mycobacterium avium-intracellulare* (which can infect immunologically compromised individuals and elderly patients with chronic lung disease), and it may also be useful in leprosy and against *Helicobacter pylori* (see Ch. 30). Both these macrolides are also effective in *Lyme disease*.

Pharmacokinetic aspects
The macrolides are administered orally or parenterally, although intravenous injections can be followed by local thrombophlebitis. They diffuse readily into most tissues but do not cross the blood–brain barrier, and there is poor penetration into synovial fluid. The plasma half-life of erythromycin is about 90 min; that of clarithromycin is three times longer, and that of azithromycin 8–16 times longer. Macrolides enter and indeed are concentrated within phagocytes – azithromycin concentrations in phagocyte lysosomes can be 40 times higher than in the blood – and they can enhance intracellular killing of bacteria by phagocytes.

Erythromycin is partly inactivated in the liver; azithromycin is more resistant to inactivation, and clarithromycin is converted to an active metabolite. Inhibition of the P450 cytochrome system by these agents can affect the bioavailability of other drugs leading to clinically important interactions, for example with theophylline. The major route of elimination is in the bile.

Unwanted effects
Gastrointestinal disturbances are common and unpleasant but not serious. With erythromycin, the following have also been reported: hypersensitivity reactions such as rashes and fever, transient hearing disturbances and rarely, following treatment for longer than 2 weeks, cholestatic jaundice. Opportunistic infections of the gastrointestinal tract or vagina can occur.

ANTIMICROBIAL AGENTS AFFECTING TOPOISOMERASE

QUINOLONES

The quinolones include the broad-spectrum agents **ciprofloxacin**, **levofloxacin**, **ofloxacin**, **norfloxacin** and **moxifloxacin** as well as **nalidixic acid**, a narrow-spectrum drug used in urinary tract infections. Most are fluorinated (fluoroquinolones). These agents inhibit topoisomerase II (a bacterial DNA gyrase), the enzyme that produces a negative supercoil in DNA and thus permits transcription or replication (see Fig. 51.4).

Antibacterial spectrum and clinical use
Ciprofloxacin is the most commonly used and typical of the group. It is a broad-spectrum antibiotic effective against both Gram-positive and Gram-negative organisms, including the *Enterobacteriaceae* (enteric Gram-negative bacilli), many organisms resistant to penicillins, cephalosporins and aminoglycosides, and against *H. influenzae*, penicillinase-producing *N. gonorrhoeae*, *Campylobacter* spp. and pseudomonads. Of the Gram-positive organisms, streptococci and pneumococci are only weakly inhibited, and there is a high incidence of staphylococcal resistance. Ciprofloxacin should be avoided in MRSA infections. Clinically, the fluoroquinolones are best reserved for infections with facultative and aerobic

Antimicrobial agents affecting bacterial protein synthesis

- *Tetracyclines* (e.g. **minocycline**). These are orally active, bacteriostatic, broad-spectrum antibiotics. Resistance is increasing. Gastrointestinal disorders are common. They also chelate calcium and are deposited in growing bone. They are contraindicated in children and pregnant women.
- *Chloramphenicol*. This is an orally active, bacteriostatic, broad-spectrum antibiotic. Serious toxic effects are possible, including bone marrow depression and 'grey baby syndrome'. It should be reserved for life-threatening infections.
- *Aminoglycosides* (e.g. **gentamicin**). These are given by injection. They are bactericidal, broad-spectrum antibiotics (but with low activity against anaerobes, streptococci and pneumococci). Resistance is increasing. The main unwanted effects are dose-related nephrotoxicity and ototoxicity. Serum levels should be monitored. (**Streptomycin** is an anti-tuberculosis aminoglycoside.)

- *Macrolides* (e.g. **erythromycin**). Can be given orally and parenterally. They are bactericidal/bacteriostatic. The antibacterial spectrum is the same as for penicillin. **Erythromycin** can cause jaundice. Newer agents are **clarithromycin** and **azithromycin**.
- *Lincosamides* (e.g. **clindamycin**). Can be given orally and parenterally. It can cause pseudomembranous colitis.
- *Streptogramins* (e.g. **quinupristin/dalfopristin**). Given by intravenous infusion as a combination. Considerably less active when administered separately. Active against several strains of drug-resistant bacteria.
- *Fusidic acid*. This is a narrow-spectrum antibiotic that acts by inhibiting protein synthesis. It penetrates bone. Unwanted effects include gastrointestinal disorders.
- *Linezolid*. Given orally or by intravenous injection. Active against several strains of drug-resistant bacteria.

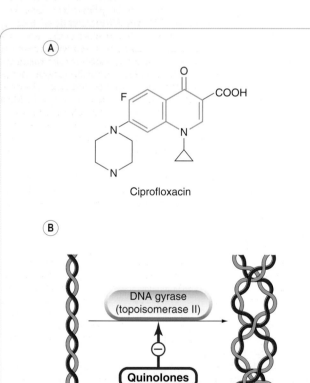

Fig. 51.4 A simplified diagram of the mechanism of action of the fluoroquinolones. [**A**] An example of a quinolone (the quinolone moiety is shown in orange). [**B**] Schematic diagram of (left) the double helix and (right) the double helix in supercoiled form (see also Fig. 50.6). In essence, the DNA gyrase unwinds the RNA-induced positive supercoil (not shown) and introduces a negative supercoil.

Gram-negative bacilli and cocci.[6] Resistant strains of *Staphylococcus aureus* and *P. aeruginosa* have emerged.

Clinical uses of the fluoroquinolones

- Complicated *urinary tract infections* (**norfloxacin, ofloxacin**).
- *Pseudomonas aeruginosa* respiratory infections in patients with cystic fibrosis.
- Invasive external otitis ('malignant otitis') caused by *P. aeruginosa*.
- Chronic Gram-negative bacillary osteomyelitis.
- Eradication of *Salmonella typhi* in carriers.
- *Gonorrhoea* (**norfloxacin, ofloxacin**).
- Bacterial *prostatitis* (**norfloxacin**).
- *Cervicitis* (**ofloxacin**).
- *Anthrax*.

Pharmacokinetic aspects

Fluoroquinolones are well absorbed orally. The drugs accumulate in several tissues, particularly in the kidney, prostate and lung. All quinolones are concentrated in phagocytes. Most fail to cross the blood–brain barrier, but ofloxacin does so. Aluminium and magnesium antacids interfere with the absorption of the quinolones. Elimination of ciprofloxacin and norfloxacin is partly by hepatic metabolism by P450 enzymes (which they can

---

[6]When ciprofloxacin was introduced, clinical pharmacologists and microbiologists sensibly suggested that it should be reserved for organisms already resistant to other drugs so as to prevent emergence of resistance. However, by 1989 it was already estimated that it was prescribed for 1 in 44 of Americans, so it would seem that the horse had not only left the stable but had bolted into the blue!

inhibit, giving rise to interactions with other drugs) and partly by renal excretion. Ofloxacin is excreted in the urine.

Unwanted effects

In hospitals, infection with *C. difficile* may prove hazardous but otherwise unwanted effects are infrequent, usually mild and reversible. The most frequent manifestations are gastrointestinal disorders and skin rashes. Arthropathy has been reported in young individuals. Central nervous system symptoms – headache and dizziness – have occurred, as have, less frequently, convulsions associated with central nervous system pathology or concurrent use of **theophylline** or an non-steroidal anti-inflammatory drug (NSAID) (Ch. 26).

There is a clinically important interaction between ciprofloxacin and theophylline (through inhibition of P450 enzymes), which can lead to theophylline toxicity in asthmatics treated with the fluoroquinolones. The topic is discussed further in Chapter 28. Moxifloxacin prolongs the electrocardiographic QT interval and is used extensively, following Food and Drug Administration guidance, as a positive control in studies in healthy volunteers examining possible effects of new drugs on cardiac repolarisation.

Antimicrobial agents affecting DNA topoisomerase II

- The quinolones interfere with the supercoiling of DNA.
- **Ciprofloxacin** has a wide antibacterial spectrum, being especially active against Gram-negative enteric coliform organisms, including many organisms resistant to penicillins, cephalosporins and aminoglycosides; it is also effective against *H. influenzae*, penicillinase-producing *N. gonorrhoeae*, *Campylobacter* spp. and pseudomonads. There is a high incidence of staphylococcal resistance.
- Unwanted effects include gastrointestinal tract upsets, hypersensitivity reactions and, rarely, central nervous system disturbances.

MISCELLANEOUS AND LESS COMMON ANTIBACTERIAL AGENTS

METRONIDAZOLE

▼ **Metronidazole** was introduced as an antiprotozoal agent (see Ch. 54), but it is also active against anaerobic bacteria such as *Bacteroides*, *Clostridia* spp. and some streptococci. It is effective in the therapy of *pseudomembranous colitis*, and is important in the treatment of serious anaerobic infections (e.g. sepsis secondary to bowel disease). It has a disulfiram-like action (see Ch. 49), so patients must avoid alcohol while taking metronidazole.

STREPTOGRAMINS

▼ **Quinupristin** and **dalfopristin** are cyclic peptides, which inhibit bacterial protein synthesis by binding to the 50S subunit of the bacterial ribosome. Dalfopristin changes the structure of the ribosome so as to promote the binding of quinupristin. Individually, they exhibit only very modest bacteriostatic activity, but combined together as an intravenous injection they are active against many Gram-positive bacteria. The combination is used to treat serious infections, usually where no other antibacterial is suitable. For example, the combination is effective against MRSA and vancomycin-resistant *Enterococcus faecium*. They are not currently used in the UK. Both drugs undergo extensive first-pass hepatic metabolism and must therefore be given as an intravenous infusion. The half-life of each compound is 1–2 h.

Unwanted effects include inflammation and pain at the infusion site, arthralgia, myalgia and nausea, vomiting and diarrhoea. To date, resistance to quinupristin and dalfopristin does not seem to be a major problem.

CLINDAMYCIN

▼ The lincosamide clindamycin is active against Gram-positive cocci, including many penicillin-resistant staphylococci and many anaerobic bacteria such as *Bacteroides* spp. It acts in the same way as macrolides and chloramphenicol (Ch. 50, Fig. 50.4). In addition to its use in infections caused by *Bacteroides* organisms, it is used to treat staphylococcal infections of bones and joints. It is also given topically, as eye drops, for staphylococcal conjunctivitis and as an anti-protozoal drug (see Ch. 54).

Unwanted effects consist mainly of gastrointestinal disturbances, ranging from uncomfortable diarrhoea to potentially lethal pseudomembranous colitis, caused by a toxin-forming *C. difficile*.[7]

OXAZOLIDINONES

▼ Originally hailed as the 'first truly new class of antibacterial agents to reach the marketplace in several decades' (Zurenko et al., 2001), the oxazolidinones inhibit bacterial protein synthesis by a novel mechanism: inhibition of *N*-formylmethionyl-tRNA binding to the 70S ribosome. **Linezolid** is the first member of this new antibiotic family to be introduced. It is active against a wide variety of Gram-positive bacteria and is particularly useful for the treatment of drug-resistant bacteria such as MRSA, penicillin-resistant *Streptococcus pneumoniae* and vancomycin-resistant enterococci. The drug is also effective against some anaerobes, such as *C. difficile*. Most common Gram-negative organisms are not susceptible to the drug. Linezolid can be used to treat pneumonia, septicaemia, and skin and soft tissue infections. Its use is restricted to serious bacterial infections where other antibiotics have failed, and there have so far been few reports of resistance.

Unwanted effects include thrombocytopenia, diarrhoea, nausea and, rarely, rash and dizziness. Linezolid is a non-selective inhibitor of monoamine oxidase, and appropriate precautions need to be observed (see Ch. 47).

FUSIDIC ACID

▼ Fusidic acid is a narrow-spectrum steroid antibiotic active mainly against Gram-positive bacteria. It acts by inhibiting bacterial protein synthesis (Ch. 50, Fig. 50.4). As the sodium salt, the drug is well absorbed from the gut and is distributed widely in the tissues. Some is excreted in the bile and some metabolised. It is used in combination with other antistaphylococcal agents in staphylococcal sepsis, and is very widely used topically for staphylococcal infections (e.g. as eye drops or cream).

Unwanted effects such as gastrointestinal disturbances are fairly common. Skin eruptions and jaundice can occur. Resistance occurs if it is used systemically as a single agent so it is always combined with other antibacterial drugs when used systemically.

NITROFURANTOIN

▼ **Nitrofurantoin** is a synthetic compound active against a range of Gram-positive and Gram-negative organisms. The development of resistance in susceptible organisms is rare, and there is no cross-resistance. Its mechanism of action is probably related to its ability to damage bacterial DNA. It is given orally and is rapidly and totally

---

[7]This may also occur with broad-spectrum penicillins and cephalosporins.

absorbed from the gastrointestinal tract and just as rapidly excreted by the kidney. Its use is confined to the treatment of urinary tract infections.

Unwanted effects such as gastrointestinal disturbances are relatively common, and hypersensitivity reactions involving the skin and the bone marrow (e.g. leukopenia) can occur. Hepatotoxicity and peripheral neuropathy have also been reported.

Methanamine has a similar clinical utility to nitrofurantoin and shares several of its unwanted effects. It exerts its effects following slow conversion (in acidic urine) to formaldehyde.

POLYMIXINS

▼ The polymixin antibiotics in use are **polymixin B** and **colistimeth-ate**. They have cationic detergent properties and disrupt the bacterial outer cell membrane (Ch. 50). They have a selective, rapidly bactericidal action on Gram-negative bacilli, especially pseudomonads and coliform organisms. They are not absorbed from the gastrointestinal tract. Clinical use of these drugs is limited by their toxicity and is confined largely to gut sterilisation and topical treatment of ear, eye or skin infections caused by susceptible organisms.

Unwanted effects may be serious and include neurotoxicity and nephrotoxicity.

ANTIMYCOBACTERIAL AGENTS

The main mycobacterial infections in humans are tuberculosis and leprosy, chronic infections caused by *Mycobacterium tuberculosis* and *M. leprae*, respectively. Another mycobacterial infection of less significance here is *M. avium-intracellulare* (actually two organisms), which can infect some AIDS patients. A particular problem with mycobacteria is that they can survive inside macrophages after phagocytosis, unless these cells are 'activated' by cytokines produced by T-helper (Th)1 lymphocytes (see Chs 6 and 18).

DRUGS USED TO TREAT TUBERCULOSIS

For centuries, tuberculosis was a major killer disease, but the introduction of **streptomycin** in the late 1940s followed by **isoniazid** and, in the 1960s, of **rifampicin** and **ethambutol** revolutionised therapy. Tuberculosis came to be regarded as an easily treatable condition but, regrettably, this is so no longer true and strains with increased virulence or exhibiting multidrug resistance are now common (Bloom & Small, 1998). It now causes more deaths than any other single agent even though infection rates are slowly falling. In 2012, the World Health Organization (WHO) estimated that 8.6 million people contracted the disease and some 1.3 million died as a result of the infection. One-third of the world's population (2 billion people) harbour the bacillus, 10% of whom will develop the disease at some point in their lifetime. Poverty-stricken countries in Africa and Asia bear the brunt of the disease, partly because of an ominous synergy between mycobacteria (e.g. *M. tuberculosis, M. avium-intercellulare*) and HIV. About a quarter of HIV-associated deaths are caused by tuberculosis.

Treatment is led by the first-line drugs isoniazid, rifampicin, **rifabutin**, ethambutol and **pyrazinamide**. Second-line drugs include **capreomycin**, **cycloserine**, streptomycin (rarely used now in the UK), **clarithromycin** and ciprofloxacin. These are used to treat infections likely to be resistant to first-line drugs, or when the first-line agents have to be abandoned because of unwanted reactions.

To decrease the probability of the emergence of resistant organisms, combination drug therapy is a frequent strategy. This commonly involves:

- an initial phase of treatment (about 2 months) with a combination of isoniazid, rifampicin and pyrazinamide (plus ethambutol if the organism is suspected to be resistant)
- a second, continuation phase (about 4 months) of therapy, with isoniazid and rifampicin; longer-term treatment is needed for patients with meningitis, bone/joint involvement or drug-resistant infection.

ISONIAZID

The antibacterial activity of isoniazid is limited to mycobacteria. It halts the growth of resting organisms (i.e. is bacteriostatic) but can kill dividing bacteria. It passes freely into mammalian cells and is thus effective against intracellular organisms. Isoniazid is a prodrug that must be activated by bacterial enzymes before it can exert its inhibitory activity on the synthesis of *mycolic acids*, important constituents of the cell wall peculiar to mycobacteria. Resistance to the drug, secondary to reduced penetration into the bacterium, may be present, but cross-resistance with other tuberculostatic drugs does not occur.

Isoniazid is readily absorbed from the gastrointestinal tract and is widely distributed throughout the tissues and body fluids, including the CSF. An important point is that it penetrates well into 'caseous' tuberculous lesions (i.e. necrotic lesions with a cheese-like consistency). Metabolism, which involves acetylation, depends on genetic factors that determine whether a person is a slow or rapid acetylator of the drug (see Ch. 11), with slow inactivators enjoying a better therapeutic response. The half-life in slow inactivators is 3 h and in rapid inactivators, 1 h. Isoniazid is excreted in the urine partly as unchanged drug and partly in the acetylated or otherwise inactivated form.

Unwanted effects depend on the dosage and occur in about 5% of individuals, the commonest being allergic skin eruptions. A variety of other adverse reactions have been reported, including fever, hepatotoxicity, haematological changes, arthritic symptoms and vasculitis. Adverse effects involving the central or peripheral nervous systems are largely consequences of pyridoxine deficiency and are common in malnourished patients unless prevented by administration of this substance. Isoniazid may cause haemolytic anaemia in individuals with glucose 6-phosphate dehydrogenase deficiency, and it decreases the metabolism of the antiepileptic agents **phenytoin**, **ethosuximide** and **carbamazepine**, resulting in an increase in the plasma concentration and toxicity of these drugs.

RIFAMPICIN

Rifampicin (also called **rifampin**) acts by binding to, and inhibiting, DNA-dependent RNA polymerase in prokaryotic but not in eukaryotic cells (Ch. 50). It is one of the most active antituberculosis agents known, and is also effective against leprosy and most Gram-positive bacteria as well as many Gram-negative species. It enters phagocytic cells and can therefore kill intracellular microorganisms including the tubercle bacillus. Resistance can develop rapidly in a one-step process in which a chromosomal mutation changes its target site on microbial DNA-dependent RNA polymerase (see Ch. 50).

Rifampicin is given orally and is widely distributed in the tissues and body fluids (including CSF), giving an orange tinge to saliva, sputum, tears and sweat. It is excreted partly in the urine and partly in the bile, some of it undergoing enterohepatic cycling. The metabolite retains antibacterial activity but is less well absorbed from the gastrointestinal tract. The half-life is 1–5 h, becoming shorter during treatment because of induction of hepatic microsomal enzymes.

Unwanted effects are relatively infrequent. The commonest are skin eruptions, fever and gastrointestinal disturbances. Liver damage with jaundice has been reported and has proved fatal in a very small proportion of patients, and liver function should be assessed before treatment is started. Rifampicin causes induction of hepatic metabolising enzymes (Ch. 10), resulting in an increase in the degradation of warfarin, glucocorticoids, narcotic analgesics, oral antidiabetic drugs, **dapsone** and oestrogens, the last effect leading to failure of oral contraception.

ETHAMBUTOL

Ethambutol has no effect on organisms other than mycobacteria. It is taken up by the bacteria and exerts a bacteriostatic effect after a period of 24 h, probably by inhibiting mycobacterial cell wall synthesis. Resistance emerges rapidly if the drug is used alone. Ethambutol is given orally and is well absorbed. It can reach therapeutic concentrations in the CSF in tuberculous meningitis. In the blood, it is taken up by erythrocytes and slowly released. Ethambutol is partly metabolised and is excreted in the urine.

Unwanted effects are uncommon, the most significant being optic neuritis, which is dose-related and is more likely to occur if renal function is decreased. This results in visual disturbances manifesting initially as red–green colour blindness progressing to a decreased visual acuity. Colour vision should be monitored before and during prolonged treatment.

PYRAZINAMIDE

Pyrazinamide is inactive at neutral pH but tuberculostatic at acid pH. It is effective against the intracellular organisms in macrophages because, after phagocytosis, the organisms are contained in phagolysosomes where the pH is low. The drug probably inhibits bacterial fatty acid synthesis. Resistance develops rather readily, but cross-resistance with isoniazid does not occur. The drug is well absorbed after oral administration and is widely distributed, penetrating the meninges. It is excreted through the kidney, mainly by glomerular filtration.

Unwanted effects include gout, which is associated with high concentrations of plasma urates. Gastrointestinal upsets, malaise and fever have also been reported. Serious hepatic damage due to high doses was once a problem but is less likely with lower dose/shorter course regimens now used; nevertheless, liver function should be assessed before treatment.

CAPREOMYCIN

▼ Capreomycin is a peptide antibiotic given by intramuscular injection. Unwanted effects include kidney damage and injury to the auditory nerve, with consequent deafness and ataxia. The drug should not be given at the same time as streptomycin or other drugs that may cause deafness.

CYCLOSERINE

▼ Cycloserine is a broad-spectrum antibiotic that inhibits the growth of many bacteria, including coliforms and mycobacteria. It is water-soluble and destroyed at acid pH. It acts by competitively inhibiting bacterial cell wall synthesis. It does this by preventing the formation of D-alanine and the D-Ala-D-Ala dipeptide that is added to the initial tripeptide side-chain on *N*-acetylmuramic acid, i.e. it prevents completion of the major building block of peptidoglycan (Ch. 50, Fig. 50.3). It is absorbed orally and distributed throughout the tissues and body fluids, including CSF. Most of the drug is eliminated in active form in the urine, but approximately 35% is metabolised.

Cycloserine has unwanted effects, mainly on the central nervous system. A wide variety of disturbances may occur, ranging from headache and irritability to depression, convulsions and psychotic states. Its use is limited to tuberculosis that is resistant to other drugs.

> ## Antituberculosis drugs
>
> To avoid the emergence of resistant organisms, compound therapy is used (e.g. three drugs initially, followed by a two-drug regimen later).
>
> ### First-line drugs
> - **Isoniazid** kills actively growing mycobacteria within host cells. Given orally, it penetrates necrotic lesions, also the cerebrospinal fluid (CSF). 'Slow acetylators' (genetically determined) respond well. It has low toxicity. Pyridoxine deficiency increases risk of neurotoxicity. No cross resistance with other agents.
> - **Rifampicin** is a potent, orally active drug that inhibits mycobacterial RNA polymerase. It penetrates CSF. Unwanted effects are infrequent (but serious liver damage has occurred). It induces hepatic drug-metabolising enzymes. Resistance can develop rapidly.
> - **Ethambutol** inhibits growth of mycobacteria. It is given orally and can penetrate CSF. Unwanted effects are uncommon, but optic neuritis can occur. Resistance can emerge rapidly.
> - **Pyrazinamide** is tuberculostatic against intracellular mycobacteria. Given orally, it penetrates CSF. Resistance can develop rapidly. Unwanted effects include increased plasma urate and liver toxicity with high doses.
>
> ### Second-line drugs
> - **Capreomycin** is given intramuscularly. Unwanted effects include damage to the kidney and to the auditory nerve.
> - **Cycloserine** is a broad-spectrum agent. It inhibits an early stage of peptidoglycan synthesis. Given orally, it penetrates the CSF. Unwanted effects affect mostly the central nervous system.
> - **Streptomycin**, an aminoglycoside antibiotic, acts by inhibiting bacterial protein synthesis. It is given intramuscularly. Unwanted effects are ototoxicity (mainly vestibular) and nephrotoxicity.

DRUGS USED TO TREAT LEPROSY

Leprosy is one of the most ancient diseases known to mankind and has been mentioned in texts dating back to 600 BC. The causative organism is *M. leprae*. It is a chronic disfiguring illness with a long latency, and historically sufferers have been ostracised and forced to live apart from their communities even though the disease is not actually particularly contagious. Once viewed as incurable, the introduction in the 1940s of dapsone, and subsequently rifampicin and **clofazimine** in the 1960s, completely changed our perspective on leprosy. It is now generally curable, and the global figures show that the prevalence rates for the disease have dropped by 90% over the last 20 years as a result of public health measures and **M**ulti**d**rug **T**reatment (MDT) regimens (to avoid drug resistance) implemented by WHO and supported by some pharmaceutical companies. The disease has been eliminated from 119 out of 122 countries where it was considered to be a major health problem. In 2012, some 180 000 new cases were reported mainly in Asia and Africa.

Paucibacillary leprosy, leprosy characterised by one to five numb patches, is mainly *tuberculoid*[8] in type and is treated for 6 months with dapsone and rifampicin. *Multibacillary leprosy*, characterised by more than five numb skin patches, is mainly *lepromatous* in type and is treated for at least 2 years with rifampicin, dapsone and clofazimine.

DAPSONE

Dapsone is chemically related to the sulfonamides and, because its action is antagonised by PABA, probably acts through inhibition of bacterial folate synthesis. Resistance to the drug has steadily increased since its introduction and treatment in combination with other drugs is now recommended.

Dapsone is given orally; it is well absorbed and widely distributed through the body water and in all tissues. The plasma half-life is 24–48 h, but some drug persists in liver, kidney (and, to some extent, skin and muscle) for much longer periods. There is enterohepatic recycling of the drug, but some is acetylated and excreted in the urine. Dapsone is also used to treat *dermatitis herpetiformis*, a chronic blistering skin condition associated with coeliac disease.

Unwanted effects occur fairly frequently and include haemolysis of red cells (usually not severe enough to lead to frank anaemia), methaemoglobinaemia, anorexia, nausea and vomiting, fever, allergic dermatitis and neuropathy. *Lepra reactions* (an exacerbation of lepromatous lesions) can occur, and a potentially fatal syndrome resembling infectious mononucleosis has occasionally been seen.

CLOFAZIMINE

Clofazimine is a dye of complex structure. Its mechanism of action against leprosy bacilli may involve an action on DNA. It also has anti-inflammatory activity and is useful in patients in whom dapsone causes inflammatory side effects.

Clofazimine is given orally and accumulates in the body, being sequestered in the mononuclear phagocyte system. The plasma half-life may be as long as 8 weeks.

The anti-leprotic effect is delayed and is usually not evident for 6–7 weeks.

Unwanted effects may be related to the fact that clofazimine is a dye. The skin and urine can develop a reddish colour and the lesions a blue–black discoloration. Dose-related nausea, giddiness, headache and gastrointestinal disturbances can also occur.

> ### Antileprosy drugs
>
> - For *tuberculoid leprosy*: **dapsone** and **rifampicin (rifampin)**.
>   - **Dapsone** is sulfonamide-like and may inhibit folate synthesis. It is given orally. Unwanted effects are fairly frequent; a few are serious. Resistance is increasing.
>   - **Rifampicin** (see *Antituberculosis drugs* box).
> - For *lepromatous leprosy*: dapsone, **rifampicin** and **clofazimine**.
>   - **Clofazimine** is a dye that is given orally and can accumulate by sequestering in macrophages. Action is delayed for 6–7 weeks, and its half-life is 8 weeks. Unwanted effects include red skin and urine, sometimes gastrointesinal disturbances.

POSSIBLE NEW ANTIBACTERIAL DRUGS

In contrast to the rapid discoveries and developments that characterised the 'heroic' years of antibiotic research spanning approximately 1950–1980, and which produced virtually all our existing drugs, the flow has since dried up, with only two totally novel antibiotics introduced during this period (Jagusztyn-Krynicka & Wysznska, 2008). At the same time, resistance has been increasing, with about half the infection-related deaths in Europe now attributable to drug resistance (Watson, 2008).[9]

Resistance normally appears within 2 years or so of the introduction of a new agent (Bax et al., 2000). In a disquieting review and meta-analysis, Costelloe et al. (2010) concluded that most patients prescribed antibiotics for a respiratory or urinary tract infection develop individual resistance to the drug within a few weeks and that this may persist for up to a year after treatment. Since about half the antibiotic use is for veterinary purposes, it is not just human medicine that is implicated in this phenomenon.

The reason for the failure to develop new drugs is complex and has been analysed in detail by Coates et al. (2011), who also evaluate many new leads arising from academic and industrial research. Their overall message is rather depressing, however: they point out that another 20 new classes of antibiotics would need to be discovered in the next 50 years to keep up with the challenges posed by the increasing prevalence of drug resistance.

On a more optimistic note, novel antibiotic candidates continue to be discovered in plants (Limsuwan et al., 2009) and bacteria (Sit & Vederas, 2008) as well as through

---

[8]The difference between *tuberculoid* and *lepromatous* disease appears to be that the T cells from patients with the former vigorously produce interferon-γ, which enables macrophages to kill intracellular microbes, whereas in the latter case the immune response is dominated by interleukin-4, which blocks the action of interferon-γ (see Ch. 18).

[9]The worst offenders are sometimes collectively referred to, rather fittingly, as 'ESKAPE pathogens'. The acronym is formed of the initial letters of *E. faecium, S. aureus, K. pneumonia, A. baumanii, P. aeruginosa* and *Enterobacter* spp.

traditional medicinal chemistry approaches. In addition, researchers in the front line of this important field are recruiting all the latest conceptual technologies into the fray: bioinformatics, utilising information derived from pathogen genome sequencing, is one such approach (Bansal, 2008). The hunt for, and targeting of, bacterial *virulence factors* is showing some promise (Escaich, 2008). New types of screening procedures have been devised (Falconer & Brown, 2009) which would reveal novel targets, and sophisticated pharmacodynamic profiling is being brought to bear on the problem (Lister, 2006).

The world awaits developments with bated breath.

REFERENCES AND FURTHER READING

Antibacterial drugs

Allington, D.R., Rivey, M.P., 2001. Quinupristine/dalfopristin: a therapeutic review. Clin. Ther. 23, 24–44.

Ball, P., 2001. Future of the quinolones. Semin. Resp. Infect. 16, 215–224. (*Good overview of this class of drugs*)

Blondeau, J.M., 1999. Expanded activity and utility of the new fluoroquinolones: a review. Clin. Ther. 21, 3–15. (*Good overview*)

Bryskier, A., 2000. Ketolides – telithromycin, an example of a new class of antibacterial agents. Clin. Microbiol. Infect. 6, 661–669.

Duran, J.M., Amsden, G.W., 2000. Azithromycin: indications for the future? Expert Opin. Pharmacother. 1, 489–505.

Greenwood, D. (Ed.), 1995. Antimicrobial Chemotherapy, third ed. Oxford University Press, Oxford. (*Good all-round textbook*)

Lowy, F.D., 1998. *Staphylococcus aureus* infections. N. Engl. J. Med. 339, 520–541. (*Basis of S. aureus pathogenesis of infection, resistance; extensive references; impressive diagrams*)

Perry, C.M., Jarvis, B., 2001. Linezolid: a review of its use in the management of serious gram positive infections. Drugs 61, 525–551.

Sato, K., Hoshino, K., Mitsuhashi, S., 1992. Mode of action of the new quinolones: the inhibitory action on DNA gyrase. Prog. Drug Res. 38, 121–132.

Shimada, J., Hori, S., 1992. Adverse effects of fluoroquinolones. Prog. Drug Res. 38, 133–143.

Tillotson, G.S., 1996. Quinolones: structure–activity relationships and future predictions. J. Med. Microbiol. 44, 320–324.

Zurenko, G.E., Gibson, J.K., Shinabarger, D.L., et al., 2001. Oxazolidinones: a new class of antibacterials. Curr. Opin. Pharmacol. 1, 470–476. (*Easy-to-assimilate review that discusses this relatively new group of antibacterials*)

Resistance (see also reading list in Ch. 50)

Bax, R., Mullan, N., Verhoef, J., 2000. The millennium bugs – the need for and development of new antibacterials. Int. J. Antimicrob. Agents 16, 51–59. (*Good review that includes an account of the development of 'resistance' and a round-up of potential new drugs*)

Bloom, B.R., Small, P.M., 1998. The evolving relation between humans and *Mycobacterium tuberculosis*. Lancet 338, 677–678. (*Editorial comment*)

Coates, A.R., Halls, G., Hu, Y., 2011. Novel classes of antibiotics or more of the same? Br. J. Pharmacol. 163, 184–194. (*A comprehensive review that sets out the challenges we face because of antibiotic resistance. Also includes a survey of potential new leads. Easy to read and highly recommended*)

Costelloe, C., Metcalfe, C., Lovering, A., Mant, D., Hay, A.D., 2010. Effect of antibiotic prescribing in primary care on antimicrobial resistance in individual patients: systematic review and meta-analysis. BMJ 340, c2096. (*Details the incidence of resistance following simple antibiotic regimes. Truly depressing*)

Courvalin, P., 1996. Evasion of antibiotic action by bacteria. J. Antimicrob. Chemother. 37, 855–869. (*Covers developments in the understanding of the genetics and biochemical mechanisms of resistance*)

Gold, H.S., Moellering, R.C., 1996. Antimicrobial drug resistance. N. Engl. J. Med. 335, 1445–1453. (*Excellent well-referenced review; covers mechanisms of resistance of important organisms to the main drugs; has useful table of therapeutic and preventive strategies, culled from the literature*)

Heym, B., Honoré, N., Truffot-Pernot, C., et al., 1994. Implications of multidrug resistance for the future of short-course chemotherapy of tuberculosis: a molecular study. Lancet 344, 293–298.

Iseman, M.D., 1993. Treatment of multidrug-resistant tuberculosis. N. Engl. J. Med. 329, 784–791.

Livermore, D.M., 2000. Antibiotic resistance in staphylococci. J. Antimicrob. Agents 16, S3–S10. (*Overview of problems of bacterial resistance*)

Michel, M., Gutman, L., 1997. Methicillin-resistant *Staphylococcus aureus* and vancomycin-resistant enterococci: therapeutic realities and possibilities. Lancet 349, 1901–1906. (*Excellent review article; good diagrams*)

Nicas, T.I., Zeckel, M.L., Braun, D.K., 1997. Beyond vancomycin: new therapies to meet the challenge of glycopeptide resistance. Trends Microbiol. 5, 240–249.

Watson, R., 2008. Multidrug resistance responsible for half of deaths from healthcare associated infections in Europe. BMJ 336, 1266–1267.

New approaches to antibacterial drug discovery

(*These papers have been provided for those who want to learn more about the work under way to develop novel antibacterial drugs. Some are quite technical in nature*)

Bansal, A.K., 2008. Role of bioinformatics in the development of new antibacterial therapy. Expert Rev. Anti Infect. Ther. 6, 51–65.

Escaich, S., 2008. Antivirulence as a new antibacterial approach for chemotherapy. Curr. Opin. Chem. Biol. 12, 400–408.

Falconer, S.B., Brown, E.D., 2009. New screens and targets in antibacterial drug discovery. Curr. Opin. Microbiol. 12, 497–504.

Jagusztyn-Krynicka, E.K., Wyszynska, A., 2008. The decline of antibiotic era – new approaches for antibacterial drug discovery. Pol. J. Microbiol. 57, 91–98.

Limsuwan, S., Trip, E.N., Kouwen, T.R., et al., 2009. Rhodomyrtone: a new candidate as natural antibacterial drug from *Rhodomyrtus tomentosa*. Phytomedicine 16, 645–651.

Lister, P.D., 2006. The role of pharmacodynamic research in the assessment and development of new antibacterial drugs. Biochem. Pharmacol. 71, 1057–1065.

Loferer, H., 2000. Mining bacterial genomes for antimicrobial targets. Mol. Med. Today 6, 470–474. (*An interesting article focusing on the way in which a better understanding of the bacterial genome may lead to new drugs*)

O'Neill, A.J., 2008. New antibacterial agents for treating infections caused by multi-drug resistant Gram-negative bacteria. Expert. Opin. Invest. Drugs 17, 297–302.

Sit, C.S., Vederas, J.C., 2008. Approaches to the discovery of new antibacterial agents based on bacteriocins. Biochem. Cell Biol. 86, 116–123.

Useful website

<www.who.int>. (*Once again, the World Health Organization website is a mine of information about the demographics and treatment of infectious diseases. The sections on leprosy and tuberculosis are especially worthwhile studying. The site includes photographs, maps and much statistical information, as well as information on drug resistance. Highly recommended*)

52 Antiviral drugs

OVERVIEW

This chapter deals with drugs used to treat infections caused by viruses. We provide some basic information about viruses: a simple outline of their structure, a list of the main pathogenic species and a brief summary of the life history of an infectious virus. We then continue with a consideration of the host–virus interaction: the defences deployed by the human host against viruses and the strategies employed by viruses to evade these measures. We then discuss the various types of antiviral drugs and their mechanisms of action, with particular reference to the treatment of acquired immunodeficiency syndrome (AIDS), an infection caused by the human immunodeficiency virus (HIV).

BACKGROUND INFORMATION ABOUT VIRUSES

AN OUTLINE OF VIRUS STRUCTURE

Viruses are small (usually in the range 20–30 nm) infective agents that are incapable of reproduction outside their host cells. The free-living (e.g. outside its host) virus particle is termed a *virion*, and consists of segments of nucleic acid (either RNA or DNA) enclosed in a protein coat comprised of symmetrical repeating structural units and called a *capsid* (Fig. 52.1). The viral coat, together with the nucleic acid core, is termed the *nucleocapsid*. Some viruses have a further external lipoprotein envelope, which may be decorated with antigenic viral glycoproteins or phospholipids acquired from its host when the nucleocapsid buds through the membranes of the infected cell. Certain viruses also contain enzymes that initiate their replication in the host cell.

Viruses are generally characterised either as *DNA* or *RNA viruses* depending on the nature of their nucleic acid content. These two broad categories are conventionally subdivided into some six subgroups, which classify viruses according to whether they contain single- or double-stranded nucleic acids and how this functions during replication.

EXAMPLES OF PATHOGENIC VIRUSES

Viruses can infect virtually all living organisms, and they are common causes of disease in humans. Some important examples are as follows:

- ▼ *DNA viruses*: poxviruses (smallpox), herpesviruses (chickenpox, shingles, cold sores, glandular fever), adenoviruses (sore throat, conjunctivitis) and papillomaviruses (warts).
- *RNA viruses*: orthomyxoviruses (influenza), paramyxoviruses (measles, mumps, respiratory tract infections), rubella virus (German measles), rhabdoviruses (rabies), picornaviruses (colds, meningitis, poliomyelitis), retroviruses (AIDS, T-cell

leukaemia), arenaviruses (meningitis, Lassa fever), hepadnaviruses (serum hepatitis) and arboviruses (various <u>ar</u>thropod-<u>bo</u>rne illnesses, e.g. encephalitis, yellow fever).

VIRUS FUNCTION AND LIFE HISTORY

As viruses have no metabolic machinery of their own, they have to attach to and penetrate a living host cell – animal, plant or bacterial – and hijack the victim's own metabolic processes to replicate. The first step in this process is facilitated by polypeptide binding sites on the envelope or *capsid* which interact with receptors on the host cell. These 'receptors' are normal membrane constituents, for example receptors for cytokines, neurotransmitters or hormones, ion channels, integral membrane glycoproteins, etc. Some examples are listed in Table 52.1.

Following attachment, the receptor–virus complex enters the cell (often by receptor-mediated endocytosis), during which time the virus coat may be removed by host cell enzymes (often lysosomal in nature). Some viruses bypass this route. Once inside the host cell, the viral nucleic acid then uses the host cell's machinery to synthesise nucleic acids and proteins that are assembled into new virus particles. The actual way in which this occurs differs between DNA and RNA viruses.

Replication of DNA viruses

Viral DNA enters the host cell nucleus, where transcription into mRNA occurs catalysed by the host cell *RNA polymerase*. Translation of the mRNA into virus-specific proteins then takes place. Some of these proteins are enzymes that then synthesise more viral DNA, as well as structural proteins comprising the viral coat and envelope. After assembly of coat proteins around the viral DNA, complete *virions* are released by budding or after host cell lysis.

Replication of RNA viruses

Enzymes within the virion synthesise its mRNA from the viral RNA template, or sometimes the viral RNA serves as its own mRNA. This is translated by the host cell into various enzymes, including *RNA polymerase* (which directs the synthesis of more viral RNA), and also into structural proteins of the virion. Assembly and release of virions occurs as explained above. The host cell nucleus is usually not involved in replication of RNA viruses, although some (e.g. *orthomyxoviruses*) replicate exclusively within the host nuclear compartment.

Replication in retroviruses

The virion in *retroviruses*[1] contains a *reverse transcriptase enzyme* (virus RNA-dependent DNA polymerase), which makes a DNA copy of the viral RNA. This DNA copy is

---

[1]Viruses that can synthesise DNA from an RNA template – the reverse of the normal situation.

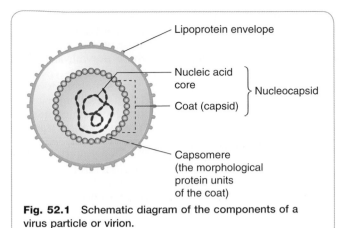

Fig. 52.1 Schematic diagram of the components of a virus particle or virion.

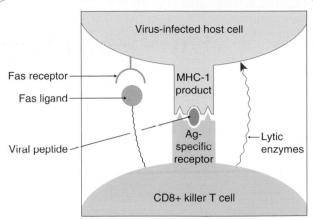

Fig. 52.2 How a CD8[+] T cell kills a virus-infected host cell. The virus-infected host cell expresses a complex of virus peptides plus major histocompatibility complex class I product (MHC-I) on its surface. This is recognised by the CD8[+] T cell, which then releases lytic enzymes into the virus-infected cell and also expresses a Fas ligand. This triggers apoptosis in the infected cell by stimulating its Fas 'death receptor'.

Table 52.1 Some host cell structures that can function as receptors for viruses

Host cell structure[a]	Virus(es)
Helper T lymphocytes CD4 glycoprotein	HIV (causing AIDS)
CCR5 receptor for chemokines MCP-1 and RANTES	HIV (causing AIDS)
CXCR4 chemokine receptor for cytokine SDF-1	HIV (causing AIDS)
Acetylcholine receptor on skeletal muscle	Rabies virus
B lymphocyte complement C3d receptor	Glandular fever virus
T lymphocyte interleukin-2 receptor	T-cell leukaemia viruses
β Adrenoceptors	Infantile diarrhoea virus
MHC molecules	Adenovirus (causing sore throat and conjunctivitis) T-cell leukaemia viruses

MCP-1, monocyte chemoattractant protein-1; MHC, major histocompatibility complex; RANTES, regulated on activation normal T-cell expressed and secreted; SDF-1, stromal cell-derived factor-1.

[a]For more detail on complement, interleukin-2, the CD4 glycoprotein on helper T lymphocytes, MHC molecules, etc., see Chapter 6.

chickenpox and shingles), which can recur when viral replication is reactivated by some factor (or when the immune system is compromised in some way). Some RNA retroviruses (e.g. the *Rous sarcoma* virus) can transform normal cells into malignant cells (a serious concern with use of retroviral vectors for gene therapy, see Ch. 59).

THE HOST–VIRUS INTERACTION

HOST DEFENCES AGAINST VIRUSES

The first defence is the simple barrier function of intact skin, which most viruses are unable to penetrate. However, broken skin (e.g. at sites of wounds or insect bites) and mucous membranes are more vulnerable to viral attack. Should the virus gain entry to the body, then the host will deploy both the innate and subsequently the adaptive immune response (Ch. 6) to limit the incursion. The infected cell presents viral peptides, complexed with major histocompatibility complex (MHC) class I molecules on its surface. This is recognised by T lymphocytes, which then kill the infected cell (Fig. 52.2). Killing may be accomplished by the release of lytic proteins (such as *perforins*, *granzymes*) or by triggering the apoptotic pathway in the infected cell by activation of its Fas receptor ('death receptor', see Ch. 5). The latter may also be triggered indirectly through the release of a cytokine such as tumour necrosis factor (TNF)-α. The virus may escape immune detection by cytotoxic lymphocytes by modifying the expression of the peptide–MHC complex (see Ch. 6), but still fall victim to natural killer (NK) cells. This reaction to the absence of normal MHC molecules is called the 'mother turkey' strategy (kill everything that does not sound exactly like a baby turkey; see Ch. 6). Some viruses also have a device for evading NK cells as well.

Within the cell itself, *gene silencing* provides a further level of protection (see Schutze, 2004). Short double-stranded fragments of RNA, such as those that could arise as a result of the virus's attempts to recruit the host's

integrated into the genome of the host cell, and it is then termed a *provirus*. The provirus DNA is transcribed into both new viral genome RNA as well as mRNA for translation in the host into viral proteins, and the completed viruses are released by budding. Many retroviruses can replicate without killing the host cell.

The ability of several viruses to remain dormant within, and be replicated together with, the host genome is responsible for the periodic nature of some viral diseases, such as those caused by *herpes labialis* (cold sores) or *varicella zoster* – another type of herpes virus (which causes transcription/translational machinery, actually cause the gene coding for the RNA to be 'silenced' – to be switched off – probably by DNA phosphorylation. This means that the gene is no longer able to direct further viral protein synthesis and replication is halted. This mechanism can be exploited for experimental purposes in many areas of biology, and tailored siRNA (*small- or short-interfering RNA*) is a cheap and useful technique to suppress temporarily the expression of a particular gene of interest. Attempts to harness the technique for viricidal purposes have met with some success (see Barik, 2004), and are beginning to find their way into therapeutics (see Ch. 59).

VIRAL PLOYS TO CIRCUMVENT HOST DEFENCES

Viruses have evolved a variety of strategies to ensure successful infection, some entailing redirection of the host's response for the advantage of the virus (discussed by Tortorella et al., 2000). Some examples are discussed below.

Subversion of the immune response
Viruses can inhibit the synthesis or action of the cytokines, such as interleukin-1, TNF-α and the antiviral interferons (IFNs) that normally coordinate the innate and adaptive immune responses. For example, following infection, some poxviruses express proteins that mimic the extracellular ligand-binding domains of cytokine receptors. These *pseudoreceptors* bind cytokines, preventing them from reaching their natural receptors on cells of the immune system and thus moderating the normal immune response to virus-infected cells. Other viruses that can interfere with cytokine signalling include human cytomegalovirus, Epstein–Barr virus, herpesvirus and adenovirus.

Evasion of immune detection and attack by killer cells
Once within host cells, viruses may also escape immune detection and evade lethal attack by cytotoxic lymphocytes and NK cells in various ways, such as:

- *Interference with the surface protein markers on the infected cells necessary for killer cell recognition and attack.* Some viruses inhibit generation of the antigenic peptide and/or the presentation of MHC–peptide molecules that signals that the cells are infected. In this way, the viruses remain undetected. Examples of viruses that can do this are adenovirus, herpes simplex virus, human cytomegalovirus, Epstein–Barr virus and influenza virus.
- *Interference with the apoptotic pathway.* Some viruses (e.g. adenovirus, human cytomegalovirus, Epstein–Barr virus) can subvert this pathway to ensure their own survival.
- *Adopting the 'baby turkey' ploy.* Some viruses (e.g. cytomegalovirus) get round the mother turkey approach of NK cells by expressing a homologue of MHC class I (the equivalent of a turkey chick's chirping) that is close enough to the real thing to hoodwink NK cells.

It is evident that natural selection has equipped pathogenic viruses with many efficacious tactics for circumventing host defences, and understanding these in more detail is likely to suggest new types of antiviral therapy. Fortunately, the biological arms race is not one-sided, and evolution has also equipped the host with sophisticated countermeasures. In most cases these prevail, and most viral infections eventually resolve spontaneously, except in an immunocompromised host. The situation does not always end happily though; some viral infections, such as Lassa fever and Ebola virus infection, have a high mortality, and we now discuss a further, grave example: the HIV virus. This is appropriate because, whilst the infection develops more slowly than (e.g.) Ebola virus, HIV exhibits many of the features common to other viral infections, and the sheer scale of the global AIDS problem has pushed HIV to the top of the list of antiviral targets.

> ### Viruses
>
> - Viruses are small infective agents consisting of nucleic acid (RNA or DNA) enclosed in a protein coat.
> - They are not cells and, having no metabolic machinery of their own, are obligate intracellular parasites, utilising the metabolic processes of the host cell they infect to replicate.
> - *DNA viruses* usually enter the host cell nucleus and dirct the generation of new viruses.
> - *RNA viruses* direct the generation of new viruses usually without involving the host cell nucleus (the influenza virus is an exception).
> - *RNA retroviruses* (e.g. HIV, T-cell leukaemia virus) contain an enzyme, reverse transcriptase, which makes a DNA copy of the viral RNA. This DNA copy is integrated into the host cell genome and directs the generation of new virus particles.

HIV AND AIDS

HIV is an RNA retrovirus. Two forms are known. *HIV-1* is the organism responsible for human AIDS. The *HIV-2* organism is similar to the HIV-1 virus in that it also causes immune suppression, but it is less virulent. HIV-1 is distributed around the world, whereas the HIV-2 virus is confined to parts of Africa.

▼ Thanks to increased availability of effective drug therapy the global situation is improving and the number of AIDS-related deaths is falling. Even so, the World Health Organization (2013 report) estimated that almost 34 million people were living with AIDS and that some 1.7 million people die of the disease each year. The epidemic is overwhelmingly centred on sub-Saharan Africa, which accounts for two-thirds of the total global number of infected persons, and where the adult prevalence is over 10 times greater than in Europe. For a review of the pathogenesis (and many other aspects) of AIDS, see Moss (2013).

The interaction of HIV with the host's immune system is complex, and although it involves mainly cytotoxic T lymphocytes (CTLs, CD8⁺ T cells) and CD4⁺ helper T lymphocytes (CD4⁺ cells), other immune cells, such as macrophages, dendritic cells and NK cells, also play a part. Antibodies are produced by the host to various HIV components, but it is the action of the CTLs and CD4⁺ cells that initially prevents the spread of HIV.

Cytotoxic T lymphocytes directly kill virally infected cells and produce and release antiviral cytokines (Fig. 52.2). The lethal event is lysis of the target cell, but induction of apoptosis by interaction of Fas ligand (see Ch. 5, Fig. 5.5) on the CTL with Fas receptors on the virally infected cell can also play a part. **CD4$^+$ cells** have an important role as helper cells, and may have a direct role (e.g. lysis of target cells), in the control of HIV replication (Norris et al., 2004). It is the progressive loss of these cells that is the defining characteristic of HIV infection (see Fig. 52.4 below).

The priming of naive T cells to become CTLs during the induction phase involves interaction of the T-cell receptor complex with antigenic HIV peptide in association with MHC class I molecules on the surface of antigen-presenting cells (APCs; see Ch. 6, Figs 6.3 and 6.4). Priming also requires the presence and participation of CD4$^+$ cells. It is thought that both types of cell need to recognise antigen on the surface of the same APC (Fig. 6.3).

The CTLs thus generated are effective during the initial stages of the infection but are not able to stop the progression of the disease. It is believed that this is because they become 'exhausted' and unable to maintain their protective function. Different mechanisms may be involved (see Jansen et al., 2004, and Barber et al., 2006, for further details).

▼ The HIV virion cannily attaches to proteins on the host cell surface to gain entry to the cells. The main targets are CD4 (the glycoprotein marker of a particular group of helper T lymphocytes) and CCR5 (a co-receptor for certain chemokines, including monocyte chemoattractant protein-1 and RANTES; see Ch. 6). CD4$^+$ cells normally orchestrate the immune response to viruses, but by entering these cells and using them as virion factories, HIV virtually cripples this aspect of the immune response. Figure 52.3 shows an HIV virion infecting a CD4$^+$ T cell. Such infected activated cells in lymphoid tissue form the major source of HIV production in HIV-infected individuals; infected macrophages are another source.

As for CCR5, evidence from exposed individuals who somehow evade infection indicates that this surface protein has a central role in HIV pathogenesis. Compounds that inhibit the entry of HIV into cells by blocking CCR5 are now available.

When immune surveillance breaks down, other strains of HIV arise that recognise other host cell surface molecules such as CD4 and CXCR4. A surface glycoprotein, gp120, on the HIV envelope binds to CD4 and also to the T-cell chemokine co-receptor CXCR4. Another viral glycoprotein, gp41, then causes fusion of the viral envelope with the plasma membrane of the cell (Fig. 52.3).

Once within the cell, HIV is integrated with the host DNA (the provirus form), undergoing transcription and generating new virions when the cell is activated (Fig. 52.3). In an untreated subject, a staggering 10^{10} new virus particles may be produced each day. Intracellular HIV can remain silent (latent) for a long time.

Viral replication is highly error-prone. Many mutations occur daily at each site in the HIV genome, so HIV soon escapes recognition by the original cytotoxic lymphocytes. Although other cytotoxic lymphocytes arise that recognise the altered virus protein(s), further mutations, in turn, allow escape from surveillance by these cells too. It is suggested that wave after wave of cytotoxic lymphocytes act against new mutants as they arise, gradually depleting a T-cell repertoire already seriously compromised by the loss of CD4$^+$ helper T cells, until eventually the immune response fails.

There is considerable variability in the progress of the disease, but the usual clinical course of an untreated HIV infection is shown in Figure 52.4. An initial acute influenza-like illness is associated with an increase in the number of virus particles in the blood, their widespread dissemination through the tissues and the seeding of lymphoid tissue with the virion particles. Within a few weeks, this *viraemia* is reduced by the action of cytotoxic lymphocytes as specified above.

The acute initial illness is followed by a symptom-free period during which there is reduction in the viraemia accompanied by silent virus replication in the lymph nodes, associated with damage to lymph node architecture and the loss of CD4$^+$ lymphocytes and dendritic cells. Clinical latency (median duration 10 years) comes to an end when the immune response finally fails and the signs and symptoms of AIDS appear – opportunistic infections (e.g. *Pneumocystis* pneumonia or tuberculosis), neurological disease (e.g. confusion, paralysis, dementia), bone marrow depression and cancers. Chronic gastrointestinal infections contribute to the severe weight loss. Cardiovascular and kidney damage can also occur. In an untreated patient, death usually follows within 2 years. The advent of effective drug regimens has greatly improved the prognosis in countries that are able to deploy them and the treated disease is now compatible with a normal life expectancy.

There is evidence that genetic factors play an important role in determining the susceptibility – or resistance – to HIV (see Flores-Villanueva et al., 2003).

ANTIVIRAL DRUGS

Because viruses hijack many of the metabolic processes of the host cell itself, it is difficult to find drugs that are selective for the pathogen. However, there are some enzymes that are virus-specific and these have proved to be useful drug targets. Most currently available antiviral agents are effective only while the virus is replicating. Because the initial phases of viral infection are often asymptomatic, treatment is often not initiated until the infection is well established. As is often the case with infectious diseases, an ounce of prevention is worth a pound of cure.

Antiviral drugs, of which many are now available, may be conveniently grouped according to their mechanisms of action and side effects. Table 52.2 shows the commonest antiviral drugs, classified in this manner together with some of the diseases they are used to treat and common side effects.

REVERSE TRANSCRIPTASE INHIBITORS

The majority are *nucleoside analogues*, typified by **zidovudine**, all of which are phosphorylated by host cell enzymes to give the 5′-triphosphate derivative. In retroviral replication this moiety competes with the equivalent host cellular triphosphate substrates for proviral DNA synthesis by viral reverse transcriptase (viral RNA-dependent DNA polymerase). Eventually, the incorporation of the 5′-triphosphate moiety into the growing viral DNA chain results in chain termination. Mammalian α-DNA polymerase is relatively resistant to the effect. However, γ-DNA polymerase in the host cell mitochondria is more susceptible, and this may be the basis of some unwanted effects. The main utility of these drugs is the treatment of HIV, but a number of them have useful activity against other viruses also (e.g. hepatitis B, which, though not a retrovirus, uses reverse transcriptase for replication).

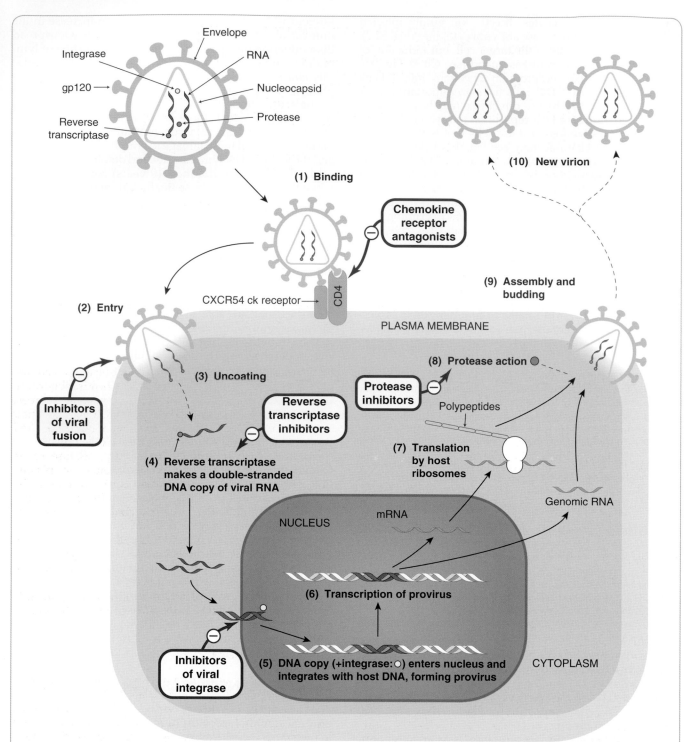

Fig. 52.3 Schematic diagram of infection of a CD4$^+$ T cell by an HIV virion, with the sites of action of the two main classes of anti-HIV drugs. The 10 steps of HIV infection, from attachment to the cell to release of new virions, are shown. The virus uses the CD4 co-receptor and the chemokine (ck) receptors CCR5/CXCR4 as binding sites to facilitate entry into the cell, where it becomes incorporated into host DNA (steps 1–5). When transcription occurs (step 6), the T cell itself is activated and the transcription factor nuclear factor κB initiates transcription of both host cell and provirus DNA. A viral protease cleaves the nascent viral polypeptides (steps 7 and 8) into structural proteins and enzymes (integrase, reverse transcriptase, protease) for the new virion. The new virions are assembled and released from the cells, initiating a fresh round of infection (steps 9 and 10). The sites of action of the currently used anti-HIV drugs are shown.

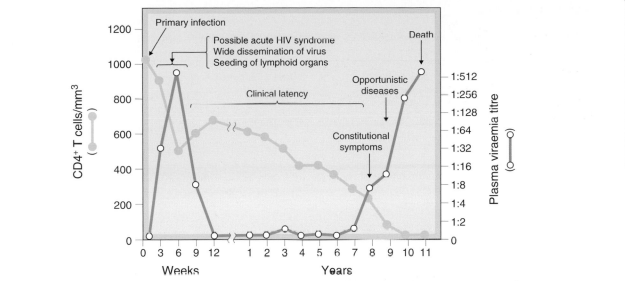

Fig. 52.4 Schematic outline of the course of HIV infection. The CD4⁺ T-cell titre is often expressed as cells/mm³. *(Adapted from Pantaleo et al. 1993.)*

Zidovudine

Zidovudine (or **azidothymidine**, AZT) was the first drug to be introduced for the treatment of HIV and retains an important place. It can prolong life in HIV-infected individuals and diminish HIV-associated dementia. Given during pregnancy and labour and then to the newborn infant, it can reduce mother- to-baby transmission by more than 20%. It is generally administered orally 2–3 times each day but can also be given by intravenous infusion. Its plasma half-life is 1 h, but the intracellular half-life of the active trisphosphate is 3 h. The concentration in cerebrospinal fluid (CSF) is 65% of the plasma level. Most of the drug is metabolised to the inactive glucuronide in the liver, only 20% of the active form being excreted in the urine.

Because of rapid mutation, the virus is a constantly moving target, and resistance develops with long-term use of zidovudine, particularly in late stage disease. Furthermore, resistant strains can be transferred between individuals. Other factors that underlie the loss of efficacy of the drug are decreased activation of zidovudine to the trisphosphate and increased virus load as the host immune response fails.

Unwanted effects include gastrointestinal disturbances (e.g. nausea, vomiting, abdominal pain), blood disorders (sometimes anaemia or neutropenia) and central nervous system (CNS) effects (e.g. insomnia, dizziness, headache) as well as the risk of lactic acidosis in some patients, which are shared by this entire group of drugs to a greater or lesser extent.

Other, currently approved, antiviral drugs in this group include **abacavir, adefovir, dipivoxil, didanosine, emtricitabine, entecavir, lamivudine, stavudine, telbivudine** and **tenofovir**.

NON-NUCLEOSIDE REVERSE TRANSCRIPTASE INHIBITORS

Non-nucleoside reverse transcriptase inhibitors are chemically diverse compounds that bind to the reverse transcriptase enzyme near the catalytic site and inactivate it. Most non-nucleoside reverse transcriptase inhibitors are also inducers, substrates or inhibitors, to varying degrees, of the liver cytochrome P450 enzymes (Ch. 9). Currently available drugs include **efavirenz** and **nevirapine**, and the related compounds **etravirine** and **rilpivarine**.

Efavirenz is given orally, once daily, because of its plasma half-life (~50 h). It is 99% bound to plasma albumin, and its CSF concentration is ~1% of that in the plasma. Nevertheless, its major adverse effects are insomnia, bad dreams and sometimes psychotic symptoms. It is teratogenic.

Nevirapine has good oral bioavailability, and penetrates into the CSF. It is metabolised in the liver, and the metabolite is excreted in the urine. Nevirapine can prevent mother-to-baby transmission of HIV.

Unwanted effects common to both of these drugs include rash (common) as well as a cluster of other effects (see Table 52.2).

PROTEASE INHIBITORS

In HIV and many other viral infections, the mRNA transcribed from the provirus is translated into two biochemically inert *polyproteins*. A virus-specific protease then converts the polyproteins into various structural and functional proteins by cleavage at the appropriate positions (see Fig. 52.3). Because this protease does not occur in the host, it is a useful target for chemotherapeutic intervention. HIV-specific protease inhibitors bind to the site where cleavage occurs, and their use, in combination with reverse transcriptase inhibitors, has transformed the therapy of AIDS. Examples of current protease inhibitors are shown in Table 52.2.

Ritonavir, a typical example, binds to and thus inactivates proteases from HIV-1 or HIV-2. It is often given in combination with other protease inhibitors (e.g. **lopinavir**) as it potentiates their action. Ritonavir is given orally, usually twice a day. It is usual to start at a low dose and increase gradually to a maximum over a period of a few days.

Table 52.2 Antiviral drugs

Type	Drug	Common therapeutic indication	Principal unwanted effects
Nucleoside reverse transcriptase inhibitors	Abacavir, didanosine, emtricitabine, lamivudine, stavudine, tenofovir, zidovudine	Mainly HIV, generally in combination with other retrovirals	Multiple effects including: GI disturbances; CNS and related effects; musculoskeletal and dermatological effects; blood disorders; metabolic effects including pancreatitis, liver damage, lactic acidosis and lipodystrophy
	Adefovir, entecavir, lamivudine, telbivudine, tenvofir	Hepatitis B	
Non-nucleoside reverse transcriptase inhibitors	Efavirenz, etravirine, nevirapine, rilpivirine	HIV, generally in combination with other retrovirals	Multiple effects including: dermatological effects; GI disturbances; CNS and related effects; musculoskeletal and blood disorders; metabolic effects including pancreatitis, liver damage and lipodystrophy. Efavirenz is teratogenic
Protease inhibitors	Atazanavir, darunavir, fosamprenavir, indinavir, lopinavir, ritonavir, saquinavir, timpranavir	HIV, generally in combination with other retrovirals	Multiple effects including: GI disturbances; CNS and related effects; musculoskeletal and dermatological effects; blood disorders; metabolic effects including pancreatitis, liver damage and lipodystrophy
	Boceprevir, telaprevir	Hepatitis C	
Viral DNA polymerase inhibitors	Cidofovir, foscarnet, ganciclovir, valganciclovir	Cytomegalovirus	Nephrotoxicity, blood disorders, ocular problems
	Aciclovir, famciclovir, idoxuridine, penciclovir, valaciclovir	Herpes	Mainly GI and dermatological disorders
Inhibitor of HIV fusion with host cells	Enfurvitide	HIV, generally in combination with other retrovirals	CNS, metabolic and GI effects
Inhibitors of viral coat disassembly and neuraminidase inhibitors	Amantadine	Influenza A	GI disturbances, CNS effects
	Oseltamivir	Influenza A and B	GI disturbances, headache
	Zanamivir		Brochospasm (unusual)
Integrase inhibitor	Ratelgravir	HIV (refractory to other treatments)	Mainly GI and metabolic disturbances
Chemokine receptor antagonist (CCR5)	Maraviroc	HIV (CCR5 dependent)	Mainly GI and CNS disturbances
Biopharmaceuticals and immunomodulators	Interferon-α, pegylated interferon-α	Hepatitis B and C	Flu-like symptoms, anorexia and fatigue
	Ribavirin, palivizumab	Respiratory syncytial virus	Fever, some GI effects
	Inosine prabonex	Herpes	Hyperuricaemia, GI effects

CNS, central nervous system; GI, gastrointestinal.

The plasma half-life of ritonavir is 3–5 h but oral absorption may be delayed in the presence of food. The drug is mainly (>80%) excreted in the faeces with some 10% excreted in the urine. A major metabolite accounts for approximately one-third of all excreted drug.

Unwanted effects that are shared among this group include gastrointestinal disturbances (e.g. nausea, vomiting, abdominal pain), blood disorders (sometimes anaemia or neutropenia) and CNS effects (e.g. insomnia, dizziness, headache) as well as the risk of hyperglycaemia.

Drug interactions are numerous, clinically important and unpredictable. As with other antiretroviral drugs it is essential to look up possible interactions before prescribing any other drugs in patients receiving anti-retroviral treatment.

DNA POLYMERASE INHIBITORS

Aciclovir

The development of the landmark drug **aciclovir** launched the era of effective selective antiviral therapy. Typical of drugs of this type, it is a guanosine derivative that is converted to the monophosphate by viral thymidine kinase, which is very much more effective in carrying out the phosphorylation than the enzyme of the host cell; it is therefore only activated in infected cells. The host cell kinases then convert the monophosphate to the trisphosphate, the active form that inhibits viral DNA polymerase, terminating the nucleotide chain. It is 30 times more potent against the herpes virus enzyme than the host enzyme. Aciclovir trisphosphate is inactivated within the host cells, presumably by cellular phosphatases. Resistance caused by changes in the viral genes coding for thymidine kinase or DNA polymerase has been reported, and aciclovir-resistant herpes simplex virus has been the cause of pneumonia, encephalitis and mucocutaneous infections in immunocompromised patients.

Aciclovir can be given orally, intravenously or topically. When it is given orally, only 20% of the dose is absorbed. The drug is widely distributed, and reaches effective concentrations in the CSF. It is excreted by the kidneys, partly by glomerular filtration and partly by tubular secretion.

Unwanted effects are minimal. Local inflammation can occur during intravenous injection if there is extravasation of the solution. Renal dysfunction has been reported when aciclovir is given intravenously; slow infusion reduces the risk. Nausea and headache can occur and, rarely, encephalopathy.

There are now many other drugs with a similar action to aciclovir (see list in Table 52.2). **Foscarnet** achieves the same effect through a slightly different mechanism.

Clinical uses of drugs for herpes viruses (e.g. aciclovir, famciclovir, valaciclovir)

- *Varicella zoster* infections (chickenpox, shingles):
  - orally in immunocompetent patients.
  - intravenously in immunocompromised patients.
- *Herpes simplex* infections (*genital* herpes, *mucocutaneous* herpes and herpes *encephalitis*).
- Prophylactically:
  - patients who are to be treated with immunosuppressant drugs or radiotherapy and who are at risk of herpesvirus infection owing to reactivation of a latent virus
  - in individuals who suffer from frequent recurrences of genital infection with herpes simplex virus.

NEURAMINIDASE INHIBITORS AND INHIBITORS OF VIRAL COAT DISASSEMBLY

Viral neuraminidase is one of three transmembrane proteins coded by the influenza genome. Infection with these RNA viruses begins with the attachment of the viral haemaglutinin to neuraminic (sialic) acid residues on host cells. The viral particle then enters the cell by endocytosis. The endosome is acidified following influx of H^+ through another viral protein, the *M2 ion channel*. This facilitates the disassembly of the viral structure, allowing the RNA

to enter the host nucleus, thus initiating a round of viral replication. Newly replicated virions escape from the host cell by budding from the cell membrane. Viral neuraminidase promotes this by severing the bonds linking the particle coat and host sialic acid.

The neuraminidase inhibitors **zanamivir** and **oseltamivir** are active against both influenza A and B viruses, and are licensed for use at early stages in the infection or when use of the vaccine is impossible. Zanamivir is available as a powder for inhalation, and oseltamivir as an oral preparation. Though oseltamivir has been 'stockpiled' by governments when flu pandemics (e.g. 'swine' flu – H1N1) are forecast, clinical trials suggest that its efficacy in reducing disease severity is very limited.

Unwanted effects of both include gastrointestinal symptoms (nausea, vomiting, dyspepsia and diarrhoea), but these are less frequent and severe in the inhaled preparation.

Amantadine,[2] quite an old drug (1966) and seldom recommended today, effectively blocks viral M2 ion channels, thus inhibiting disassembly. It is active against influenza A virus (an RNA virus) but has no action against influenza B virus. Given orally, amantadine is well absorbed, reaches high levels in secretions (e.g. saliva) and most is excreted unchanged via the kidney. Aerosol administration is feasible.

Unwanted effects are relatively infrequent, occurring in 5–10% of patients, and are not serious. Dizziness, insomnia and slurred speech are the most common adverse effects.

DRUGS ACTING THROUGH OTHER MECHANISMS

Enfurvitide inhibits the fusion of HIV with host cells. It is generally given by subcutaneous injection in combination with other drugs to treat HIV when resistance becomes a problem or when the patient is intolerant of other anti-retroviral drugs.

Unwanted effects include flu-like symptoms, central effects such as headache, dizziness, alterations in mood, gastrointestinal effects and sometimes hypersensitivity reactions.

Ratelgravir acts by inhibiting HIV DNA integrase, the enzyme that splices viral DNA into the host genome when forming the provirus. It is used for the treatment of HIV as part of combination therapy, and is generally reserved for cases that are resistant to other antiretroviral agents.

MARAVIROC

CCR5, together with CXCR4, are cell surface chemokine receptors that have been exploited by some strains of HIV to gain entry to the cell. In patients who harbour 'R5' strains, the chemokine receptor antagonist **maraviroc** may be used, in combination with more conventional antiretroviral drugs. Maraviroc – a novel concept in HIV therapy (see Dhami et al., 2009) – is the only drug of its type currently available. Its use, in combination with other antiretroviral drugs, is currently restricted to CCR5-tropic HIV infection in patients previously treated with other antiretrovirals.

---

[2]Also used for its mildly beneficial effects in Parkinson's disease (see Ch. 40).

BIOPHARMACEUTICAL ANTIVIRAL DRUGS

Biopharmaceuticals that have been recruited in the fight against virus infections include immunoglobulin preparations, interferons (IFNs) and monoclonal antibodies.

Immunoglobulin

Pooled immunoglobulin contains antibodies against various viruses present in the population. The antibodies are directed against the virus envelope and can 'neutralise' some viruses and prevent their attachment to host cells. If used before the onset of signs and symptoms, it may attenuate or prevent measles, German measles, infectious hepatitis, rabies or poliomyelitis. *Hyperimmune* globulin, specific against particular viruses, is used against hepatitis B, varicella zoster and rabies.

Palivisumab

Related in terms of its mechanism of action to immunoglobulins is **palivisumab**, a monoclonal antibody (see Chs 18 and 59) directed against a glycoprotein on the surface of respiratory syncytial virus. It is used as an intramuscular injection, under specialist supervision, in children at high risk to prevent infection by this organism.

Interferons

IFNs are a family of inducible proteins synthesised by mammalian cells and now generally produced commercially by recombinant DNA technology. There are at least three types, α, β and γ, constituting a family of hormones involved in cell growth and regulation and the modulation of immune reactions. IFN-γ, termed *immune interferon*, is produced mainly by T lymphocytes as part of an immunological response to both viral and non-viral antigens, the latter including bacteria and their products, rickettsiae, protozoa, fungal polysaccharides and a range of polymeric chemicals and other cytokines. IFN-α and IFN-β are produced by B and T lymphocytes, macrophages and fibroblasts in response to the presence of viruses and cytokines. The general actions of the IFNs are described briefly in Chapter 18.

The IFNs bind to specific ganglioside receptors on host cell membranes. They induce, in host cell ribosomes, the production of enzymes that inhibit the translation of viral mRNA into viral proteins, thus halting viral replication. They have a broad spectrum of action and inhibit the replication of most viruses *in vitro*. Given intravenously, IFNs have a half-life of 2–4 h. They do not cross the blood–brain barrier.

IFN-α-2a is used for treatment of hepatitis B infections and AIDS-related Kaposi sarcomas; **IFN-α-2b** is used for hepatitis C (a chronic viral infection which can progress insidiously in apparently healthy people, leading to end-stage liver disease or liver cancer). There are reports that IFNs can prevent reactivation of herpes simplex after trigeminal root section in animals and can prevent spread of herpes zoster in cancer patients. Preparations of IFNs conjugated with polyethylene glycol (pegylated IFNs) have a longer lifetime in the circulation.

Unwanted effects are common and resemble the symptoms of influenza (which are mediated by cytokine release) including fever, lassitude, headache and myalgia. Repeated injections cause chronic malaise. Bone marrow depression, rashes, alopecia and disturbances in cardiovascular, thyroid and hepatic function can also occur.

OTHER AGENTS

Immunomodulators are drugs that act by moderating the immune response to viruses or use an immune mechanism to target a virus or other organism. **Inosine pranobex** may interfere with viral nucleic acid synthesis but also has immunopotentiating actions on the host. It is sometimes used to treat herpes infections of mucosal tissues or skin.

Tribavirin (ribavirin) is a synthetic nucleoside, similar in structure to guanosine. It is thought to act either by altering virus nucleotide pools or by interfering with the synthesis of viral mRNA. While it inhibits a wide range of DNA and RNA viruses, including many that affect the lower airways, it is mainly used in aerosol or tablet form to treat infections with *respiratory syncytial virus* (an RNA paramyxovirus). It has also been shown to be effective in hepatitis C as well as Lassa fever, an extremely serious *arenavirus* infection. When given promptly to victims of the latter disease, it has been shown to reduce to fatality rates (usually about 76%) by approximately 8-fold.

> ### Antiviral drugs
>
> Most antiviral drugs generally fall into the following groups:
> - *Nucleoside analogues* that inhibit the viral reverse transcriptase enzyme, preventing replication (e.g. **lamivudine**, **zidovudine**).
> - *Non-nucleoside analogues* that have the same effect (e.g. **efavirenz**).
> - *Inhibitors of proteases* that prevent viral protein processing (e.g. **saquinavir**, **indinavir**).
> - *Inhibitors of viral DNA polymerase* that prevent replication (e.g. **aciclovir**, **famciclovir**).
> - *Inhibitors of viral capsule disassembly* (e.g. **amantidine**).
> - *Inhibitors of neuraminidase* that prevent viral escape from infected cells (e.g. **oseltamivir**).
> - *Inhibitors of HIV integrase* that prevent the incorporation of viral DNA into the host genome (**ratelgravir**).
> - *Inhibitors of viral entry* that block the use of host cell surface receptors, which are used as entry points by viruses (**maraviroc**).
> - *Immunomodulators* that enhance host defences (e.g. interferons and **inosine pranobex**).
> - *Immunoglobulin and related preparations* that contain neutralising antibodies to various viruses.

COMBINATION THERAPY FOR HIV

Two main classes of antiviral drugs are used to treat HIV: reverse transcriptase inhibitors and protease inhibitors. As they have different mechanisms of action (Fig. 52.3), they can usefully be deployed in combinations and this has dramatically improved the prognosis of the disease. The combination treatment is known as **h**ighly **a**ctive **a**ntiretroviral **t**herapy (HAART). A typical HAART three- or four-drug combination would involve two nucleoside reverse transcriptase inhibitors with either a non-nucleoside reverse transcriptase inhibitor or one or two protease inhibitors.

Using a HAART protocol, HIV replication is inhibited, the presence in the plasma of HIV RNA is reduced to undetectable levels and patient survival is greatly prolonged. But the regimen is complex and has many unwanted effects. Compliance is difficult and lifelong treatment is necessary. The virus is not eradicated but lies latent in the host genome of memory T cells, ready to reactivate if therapy is stopped.

Unwelcome interactions can occur between the component drugs of HAART combinations, and there may be inter-individual variations in absorption. Metabolic and cardiovascular complications attend the usage of these drugs and pose a problem to patients who may require lifelong therapy (see Hester, 2012). Some drugs penetrate poorly into the brain, and this could lead to local proliferation of the virus. So far there is no cross-resistance between the three groups of drugs, but it needs to be borne in mind that the virus has a high mutation rate – so resistance could be a problem in the future. The AIDS virus has certainly not yet been outsmarted. Even with full compliance – which is often not achieved for long periods, given the complexity of the regimen and side effects – the virus can only be kept in check, not eliminated.

The choice of drugs to treat pregnant or breastfeeding women is difficult. The main aims are to avoid damage to the fetus and to prevent transmission of the disease to the neonate. Therapy with zidovudine alone is often used in these cases. Another area that requires special consideration is prophylaxis for individuals who may have been exposed to the virus accidentally. Specific guidelines have been developed for such cases, but they are beyond the scope of this chapter.

Other drugs such as enfurvitide, maraviroc and ratelgravir are used in combination therapy regimens and are seldom deployed alone.

PROSPECTS FOR NEW ANTIVIRAL DRUGS

At the beginning of the 1990s there were only five drugs available to treat viral infections; 20 years later, this number has increased some 10-fold. Our understanding of the biology of pathogenic viruses and their action on, and in, host cells has grown enormously (see for example, Stevenson, 2012). New strategies could, if vigorously implemented, have the potential to target the viruses causing most viral diseases (see de Clercq, 2002). One such example has been the recent introduction of drugs that prevent CCR5 from serving as an entry portal for HIV. Work is under way to develop CXCR4 inhibitors for similar purposes, as are other approaches to disrupting this function of CCR5 (reviewed by Dhami et al., 2009).

However, the ultimate weapon in the fight against HIV would be vaccination. This has proved to be highly effective in the past against diseases such as polio and smallpox, and more recently against influenza (both types) and hepatitis B. Unfortunately, despite some encouraging results in animal models (and even some very modest success with one human trial) the prospect of a vaccine

against HIV (and sadly many other viruses) still seems rather remote (Girard et al., 2011). Part of the problem is *antigenic drift*, a process whereby the virus mutates, thus presenting different antigenic structures and minimising the chance of an effective and long-lasting immune response or the production of a vaccine.. The problem of HIV vaccines is the subject of numerous reviews (see Kaufman & Barouch, 2009; Rhee & Barouch, 2009; Girard et al., 2011).

Drugs for HIV infections

- Reverse transcriptase inhibitors (RTIs):
  - *nucleoside RTIs* are phosphorylated by host cell enzymes to give the 5'-trisphosphate, which competes with the equivalent host cellular trisphosphates that are essential substrates for the formation of proviral DNA by viral reverse transcriptase (examples are **zidovudine** and **abacavir**); they are used in combination with protease inhibitors
  - *non-nucleoside RTIs* are chemically diverse compounds that bind to the reverse transcriptase near the catalytic site and denature it; an example is **nevirapine**.
- Protease inhibitors inhibit cleavage of the nascent viral protein into functional and structural proteins. They are often used in combination with reverse transcriptase inhibitors. An example is **saquinavir**.
- Combination therapy is essential in treating HIV; this characteristically comprises two nucleoside RTIs with either a non-nucleoside RTI or one or two protease inhibitors. Other drugs, such as the HIV integrase inhibitor **ratelgravir**, the chemokine receptor antagonist **maraviroc** and the HIV fusion inhibitor **enfurvitide**, may also be used in such combination therapy regimens.

Treatment of HIV/AIDS

A consensus on the use of retroviral therapy in AIDS has emerged based on the following principles:

- Monitor plasma viral load and CD4$^+$ cell count.
- Start treatment before immunodeficiency becomes evident.
- Aim to reduce plasma viral concentration as much as possible for as long as possible.
- Use combinations of at least three drugs (e.g. two reverse transcriptase inhibitors and one protease inhibitor).
- Change to a new regimen if plasma viral concentration increases.

REFERENCES AND FURTHER READING

Viral infections in general

Hanazaki, K., 2004. Antiviral therapy for chronic hepatitis B: a review. Curr. Drug Targets Inflamm. Allergy 3, 63–70. (*Reviews the use of IFN and lamivudine, alone or in combination, in the treatment of this viral infection*)

Lauer, G.M., Walker, B.D., 2001. Hepatitis C virus infection. N. Engl. J. Med. 345, 41–52. (*Comprehensive review of pathogenesis, clinical characteristics, natural history and treatment of hepatitis C infection*)

Schmidt, A.C., 2004. Antiviral therapy for influenza: a clinical and economic comparative review. Drugs 64, 2031–2046. (*A useful review of influenza biology, together with a comprehensive evaluation of drug treatments, their mechanisms of action and relative economic costs*)

Whitley, R.J., Roizman, B., 2001. Herpes simplex virus infections. Lancet 357, 1513–1518. (*A concise review of the viral replication cycle and the pathogenesis and treatment of herpes simplex virus infections*)

HIV infections

Barber, D.L., Wherry, E.J., Masopust, D., et al., 2006. Restoring function in exhausted CD8 T cells during chronic viral infection. Nature 439, 682–687. (*Deals with a potential mechanism whereby the exhaustion of T cells may be reversed*)

Jansen, C.A., Piriou, E., Bronke, C., et al., 2004. Characterisation of virus-specific CD8(+) effector T cells in the course of HIV-1 infection: longitudinal analyses in slow and rapid progressors. Clin. Immunol. 11, 299–309.

Levy, J.A., 2001. The importance of the innate immune system in controlling HIV infection and disease. Trends Immunol. 22, 312–316. (*Stresses the role of innate immunity in the response to HIV; clear exposition of the various components of the innate and adaptive immune systems, as well as the role of non-cytotoxic CD8$^+$ cell response to HIV*)

Moss, J.A., 2013. HIV/AIDS review. Radiol. Technol. 84, 247–267. (*This paper was written to update radiologists and radiographers and is therefore an excellent introduction to all matters related to HIV/AIDS. Highly recommended*)

Murphy, P.M., 2001. Viral exploitation and subversion of the immune system through chemokine mimicry. Nat. Immunol. 2, 116–122. (*Excellent description of virus–immune system interaction*)

Norris, P.J., Moffett, H.F., Brander, C., et al., 2004. Fine specificity and cross-clade reactivity of HIV type 1 Gag-specific CD4$^+$ T cells. AIDS Res. Hum. Retroviruses 20, 315–325.

Pantaleo, G., Graziosi, C., Fauci, A.S., 1993. New concepts in the immunopathogenesis of human immunodeficiency virus infection. N. Engl. J. Med. 328, 327–335.

Schutze, N., 2004. siRNA technology. Mol. Cell. Endocrinol. 213, 115–119. (*An article explaining the siRNA concept*)

Tortorella, D., Gewurz, B.E., Furman, M.H., et al., 2000. Viral subversion of the immune system. Annu. Rev. Immunol. 18, 861–926. (*A comprehensive and clearly written review of the various mechanisms by which viruses elude detection and destruction by the host immune system*)

Mechanisms of antiviral drug action

Balfour, H.H., 1999. Antiviral drugs. N. Engl. J. Med. 340, 1255–1268. (*An excellent and comprehensive review of antiviral agents other than those used for HIV therapy; describes their mechanisms of action, adverse effects and clinical use*)

de Clercq, E., 2002. Strategies in the design of antiviral drugs. Nat. Rev. Drug Discov. 1, 13–24. (*Outstanding article describing the rationale behind current and future strategies for antiviral drug development*)

Hester, E.K., 2012. HIV medications: an update and review of metabolic complications. Nutr. Clin. Pract. 27, 51–64. (*Deals with the problems encountered by many patients who may have to take HAART medication for years*)

Flexner, C., 1998. HIV-protease inhibitors. N. Engl. J. Med. 338, 1281–1292. (*Excellent and comprehensive review covering mechanisms of action, clinical and pharmacokinetic properties, potential drug resistance and possible treatment failure*)

Gubareva, L., Kaiser, L., Hayden, F.G., 2000. Influenza virus neuraminidase inhibitors. Lancet 355, 827–835. (*Admirable coverage of this topic; lucid summary and clear diagrams of the influenza virus and its replication cycle; description of the structure and the action of, and resistance to, zanamivir and oseltamivir, and the relevant pharmacokinetic aspects and clinical efficacy*)

Combination treatment for HIV

Flexner, C., 2000. Dual protease inhibitor therapy in HIV-infected patients: pharmacologic rationale and clinical benefits. Annu. Rev. Pharmacol. Toxicol. 40, 649–674. (*Review emphasising interactions between individual protease inhibitors and the potential benefits and disadvantages of dual therapy*)

Richman, D.D., 2001. HIV chemotherapy. Nature 410, 995–1001. (*Outstanding article; covers pathogenesis and natural history of HIV infection and the impact on viral dynamics and immune function of antiretroviral therapy; discusses the main antiretroviral drugs, drug resistance of HIV and targets for new drugs; excellent figures and comprehensive references*)

New leads in antiviral drug therapy

Barik, S., 2004. Control of nonsegmented negative-strand RNA virus replication by siRNA. Virus Res. 102, 27–35. (*Interesting article explaining how siRNA technology might be used to inhibit viral replication*)

Dhami, H., Fritz, C.E., Gankin, B., et al., 2009. The chemokine system and CCR5 antagonists: potential in HIV treatment and other novel therapies. J. Clin. Pharm. Ther. 34, 147–160. (*Excellent and easy-to-read review of this area. Helpful diagrams*)

Flores-Villanueva, P.O., Hendel, H., Caillat-Zucman, S., et al., 2003. Associations of MHC ancestral haplotypes with resistance/susceptibility to AIDS disease development. J. Immunol. 170, 1925–1929. (*A paper that deals with the hereditary component of HIV susceptibility/resistance; interesting, but complex for the non-geneticist*)

Girard, M.P., Osmanov, S., Assossou, O.M., Kieny, M.P., 2011. Human immunodeficiency virus (HIV) immunopathogenesis and vaccine development: a review. Vaccine 29, 6191–6218. (*This paper reviews the progress made towards an effective HIV vaccine and, in the light of the widespread failures encountered, the major challenges facing the field in the future*)

Kaufman, D.R., Barouch, D.H., 2009. Translational mini-review series on vaccines for HIV: T lymphocyte trafficking and vaccine-elicited mucosal immunity. Clin. Exp. Immunol. 157, 165–173. (*This paper, together with the paper by Rhee et al. below, review new research that seeks to design better HIV vaccines through an increased understanding of the innate and adaptive immune systems. They are fairly advanced but worthwhile if you are interested in the topic*)

Kilby, J.M., Eron, J.J., 2003. Novel therapies based on mechanisms of HIV-1 cell entry. N. Engl. J. Med. 348, 2228–2238. (*Excellent review on this innovative strategy*)

Kitabwalla, M., Ruprecht, R.M., 2002. RNA interference: a new weapon against HIV and beyond. N. Engl. J. Med. 347, 1364–1368. (*An article in the series 'Clinical implications of basic research'*)

Moore, J.P., Stevenson, M., 2000. New targets for inhibitors of HIV-1 replication. Nat. Rev. Mol. Cell Biol. 1, 40–49. (*Excellent coverage of stages of the viral life cycle that might be susceptible to new drugs. Introduces various potentially promising chemical compounds*)

Rhee, E.G., Barouch, D.H., 2009. Translational mini-review series on vaccines for HIV: harnessing innate immunity for HIV vaccine development. Clin. Exp. Immunol. 157, 174–180. (*See review of Kaufman & Barouch above*)

Stevenson, M., 2012. Review of basic science advances in HIV. Top. Antivir. Med. 20, 26–29. (*An account of a conference on retroviruses that dealt with new therapeutic opportunities arising from basic research into HIV mechanisms. Advanced*)

Books

Pisani, E., 2008. The Wisdom of Whores. Granta Books, London. (*An entertaining and informative account of efforts made to pioneer HIV programmes in developing countries and the many bureaucratic and other obstacles that had to be overcome. See also www.wisdomofwhores.com/. Highly recommended*)

Useful Web resources

. (*The official HIV/AIDS site of the US National Institutes of Health. Authoritative and up-to-date information on every aspect of this disease and its treatment, including data on drugs and drug action as well as the results of recent clinical trials and the latest progress in developing a vaccine. Superb*)

<www.unaids.org/en/default.asp>. (*The official site of the United Nations Programme on HIV/AIDS. It focuses on the demographics of the epidemic with various resources that bring home the enormous problems in dealing with this disease. Prepare to be appalled*)

Antifungal drugs

53

OVERVIEW

Fungal infections (*mycoses*) are widespread in the population. In temperate climates, such as the UK, they are generally associated with the skin (e.g. 'athlete's foot') or mucous membranes (e.g. 'thrush').[1] In otherwise healthy people, these infections are mainly minor, being more of a nuisance than a threat. However, they become a more serious problem when the immune system is compromised or when the organism gains access to the systemic circulation. When this occurs, fungal infections can be fatal. In this chapter, we will briefly review the main types of fungal infections and discuss the drugs that can be used to treat them.

FUNGI AND FUNGAL INFECTIONS

Fungi are non-motile eukaryotic cells. Unlike plants, they cannot photosynthesise and many are parasitic or saprophytic in nature. Thousands of species have been characterised. Many are of economic importance, either because they are edible (e.g. mushrooms), useful in manufacturing other products (e.g. yeast in brewing and in the production of antibiotics) or because of the damage they cause to other animals, crops or to foodstuffs.

Approximately 50 species are pathogenic in humans. These organisms are present in the environment or may co-exist with humans as *commensals* without causing any overt risks to health. However, since the 1970s there has been a steady increase in the incidence of serious secondary systemic fungal infections. One of the contributory factors has been the widespread use of broad-spectrum antibiotics, which eradicate the non-pathogenic bacterial populations that normally compete with fungi for nutritional resources. Other causes include the spread of AIDS and the use of immunosuppressant or cancer chemotherapy agents. The result has been an increased prevalence of *opportunistic infections*, i.e. infections that rarely cause disease in healthy individuals. Older people, diabetics, pregnant women and burn wound victims are particularly at risk of fungal infections such as *candidiasis*. Primary fungal infections, once rare in the temperate world, are also now encountered more often because of increased international travel.

Clinically important fungi may be classified into four main types on the basis of morphological and other characteristics. Of particular taxonomic significance is the presence of *hyphae* – filamentous projections that can knit together to form a complex *mycelium*, a mat-like structure

that is responsible for the characteristic appearance of moulds. Fungi are remarkably specific in their choice of preferred location. The main groups are:

- yeasts (e.g. *Cryptococcus neoformans*)
- yeast-like fungi that produce a structure resembling a mycelium (e.g. *Candida albicans*)
- filamentous fungi with a true mycelium (e.g. *Aspergillus fumigatus*)
- 'dimorphic' fungi that, depending on nutritional constraints, may grow as either yeasts or filamentous fungi (e.g. *Histoplasma capsulatum*).

Another organism, *Pneumocystis carinii* (also known as *P. jirovecii*), described in Ch. 54, shares characteristics of both protozoa and fungi; it is an important opportunistic pathogen in patients with compromised immune systems (e.g. those suffering from AIDS), but is not susceptible to antifungal drugs.

Drugs vary in their efficacy between the different fungal groups. Table 53.1 gives examples of each type of organism and lists some of the diseases they cause and the most common choice of drug.

Superficial fungal infections can be classified into the *dermatomycoses* and *candidiasis*. Dermatomycoses include infections of the skin, hair and nails (*onychomycosis*). They are most commonly caused by *Trichophyton*, *Microsporum* or *Epidermophyton*, giving rise to various types of 'ringworm' (not to be confused with genuine helminth infections; see Ch. 54) or tinea. *Tinea capitis* affects the scalp; *Tinea cruris*, the groin ('dhobie itch'); *Tinea pedis*, the feet ('athlete's foot'); and *Tinea corporis*, the body. In superficial candidiasis, the yeast-like organism may infect the mucous membranes of the mouth or vagina (thrush), or the skin. Secondary bacterial infections may complicate the course and treatment of these conditions.

Systemic (or 'disseminated') fungal diseases are much more serious than superficial infections. The commonest in the UK is candidiasis. Other serious conditions are cryptococcal meningitis, endocarditis, pulmonary aspergillosis, and rhinocerebral mucormycosis. Invasive pulmonary aspergillosis is now a leading cause of death in recipients of bone marrow transplants or those with neutropenia. Colonisation by *Aspergillus* of the lungs of patients with asthma or cystic fibrosis can lead to a condition termed allergic *bronchopulmonary aspergillosis*.

In other parts of the world, systemic fungal infections include blastomycosis, histoplasmosis (which is quite common as an asymptomatic finding usually of characteristic calcifications on chest X-ray in the American midwest), coccidiomycosis and paracoccidiomycosis; these are often primary infections, i.e. they are not secondary to reduced immunological function or altered commensal microorganisms.

---

[1]However, they may also 'infect' buildings too and contribute to the 'sick building syndrome'.

Table 53.1 Some clinically significant fungal infections and a typical first choice of antifungal drug therapy

Organism(s) responsible		Principal disease(s)	Common drug treatments
Yeasts	*Cryptococcus neoformans*	Meningitis	Amphotericin, flucytosine, fluoconazole
Yeast-like fungus	*Candida albicans*	Thrush (and other superficial infection)	Fluconazole, itraconazole
		Systemic candidiasis	Echinocandins, fluconazole, amphotericin, other azoles
Filamentous fungi	*Trichophyton* spp. *Epidermophyton floccosum* *Microsporum* spp.	All these organisms cause skin and nail infections and are referred to as tinea or 'ringworm'	Itraconazole, terbinafine, griseofulvin
	Aspergillus fumigatus	Pulmonary aspergillosis	Voriconazole, amphotericin, capsofungin, other azoles
Dimorphic fungi	*Histoplasma capsulatum*	Histoplasmosis	Itraconazole, amphotericin
	Coccidioides immitis	Coccidiomycosis	
	Blastomyces dermatides	Blastomycosis	

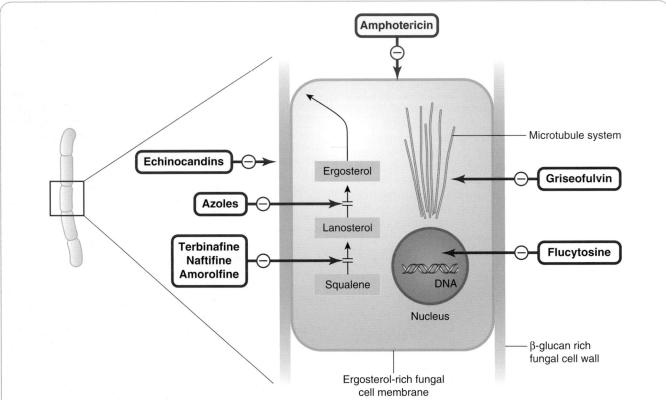

Fig. 53.1 Sites of action of common antifungal drugs. Fungi are morphologically very diverse organisms, and this diagram of a 'typical' fungus is not intended to be technically accurate. The principal sites of action of the main antifungal agents mentioned in this chapter (in red-bordered boxes) are indicated as shown.

DRUGS USED TO TREAT FUNGAL INFECTIONS

The current therapeutic agents can be broadly classified into two groups: first, the naturally occurring antifungal antibiotics such as the *polyenes* and *echinocandins*, and second, synthetic drugs including *azoles* and *fluorinated pyrimidines*. Because many infections are superficial, there are many topical preparations. Many antifungal agents are quite toxic, and when systemic therapy is required this is generally undertaken under strict medical supervision.

Figure 53.1 shows sites of action of common antifungal drugs.

ANTIFUNGAL ANTIBIOTICS

Amphotericin

Amphotericin (also called **amphotericin B**) is a mixture of antifungal substances derived from cultures of *Streptomyces*. Structurally, these are very large ('macrolide') molecules belonging to the polyene group of antifungal agents.

Like other polyene antibiotics (see Ch. 50), the site of amphotericin action is the fungal cell membrane, where it interferes with permeability and with transport functions by forming large pores in the membrane. The hydrophilic core of the doughnut-shaped molecule creates a transmembrane ion channel, causing gross disturbances in ion balance including the loss of intracellular K^+. Amphotericin has a selective action, binding avidly to the membranes of fungi and some protozoa, less avidly to mammalian cells and not at all to bacteria. The basis of this relative specificity is the drug's greater avidity for *ergosterol*, a fungal membrane sterol that is not found in animal cells (where cholesterol is the principal sterol). Amphotericin is active against most fungi and yeasts, and is the gold standard for treating disseminated infections caused by organisms including *Aspergillus* and *Candida*. Amphotericin also enhances the antifungal effect of **flucytosine**, providing a useful synergistic combination.

Pharmacokinetic aspects

Amphotericin is very poorly absorbed when given orally, and this route is used only for treating fungal infections of the upper gastrointestinal tract. It can be used topically, but for systemic infections it is generally administered, formulated in liposomes or other lipid-containing preparations, by slow intravenous infusion. This improves the pharmacokinetics and reduces the considerable burden of side effects.

Amphotericin is very highly protein-bound. It penetrates tissues and membranes (such as the blood–brain barrier) poorly, although it is found in fairly high concentrations in inflammatory exudates and may cross the blood–brain barrier more readily when the meninges are inflamed. Intravenous amphotericin is essential in the treatment of cryptococcal meningitis, often with flucytosine. It is excreted very slowly via the kidney, traces being found in the urine for 2 months or more after administration has ceased.

Unwanted effects

The commonest (indeed almost invariable) adverse effect of amphotericin is a reaction with rigors, fever, chills and headache during drug infusion; hypotension and anaphylactoid reactions occur in more severely affected individuals. The (considerably more expensive) liposome-encapsulated and lipid-complexed preparations have no greater efficacy than the native drug but cause much less frequent and less severe infusion reactions.

The most serious and common unwanted effect of amphotericin is renal toxicity. Some reduction of renal function occurs in more than 80% of patients receiving the drug; although this generally improves after treatment is stopped, some impairment of glomerular filtration may remain. Hypokalaemia occurs in 25% of patients, due to the primary action of the drug on fungi spilling over into renal tubular cells, causing potassium loss, which often requires potassium chloride supplementation. Hypomagnesaemia also occurs for the same reason. Acid-base disturbance and anaemia can be further problems. Other unwanted effects include impaired hepatic function and thrombocytopenia,. The drug is irritant to the endothelium of the veins, and can cause local thrombophlebitis. Intrathecal injections can cause neurotoxicity, and topical applications cause a skin rash.

Nystatin

Nystatin (also called **fungicidin**) is a polyene macrolide antibiotic similar in structure to amphotericin and with the same mechanism of action. It is given orally, but is not absorbed through mucous membranes or skin, and its use is mainly limited to *Candida* infections of the skin, mucous membranes and the gastrointestinal tract. *Unwanted effects* may include nausea, vomiting and diarrhoea.

Griseofulvin

Griseofulvin is a narrow-spectrum antifungal agent isolated from cultures of *Penicillium griseofulvum*. It interferes with mitosis by binding to fungal microtubules. It can be used to treat dermatophyte infections of skin or nails when local administration is ineffective, but treatment needs to be prolonged. It has largely been superseded by other drugs.

Pharmacokinetic aspects

Griseofulvin is given orally. It is poorly soluble in water, and absorption varies with the type of preparation, in particular with particle size. It is taken up selectively by newly formed skin and concentrated in the keratin. The plasma half-life is 24 h, but it is retained in the skin for much longer. It potently induces cytochrome P450 enzymes and causes several clinically important drug interactions.

Unwanted effects

Unwanted effects with griseofulvin use are infrequent, but the drug can cause gastrointestinal upsets, headache and photosensitivity. Allergic reactions (rashes, fever) may also occur. The drug should not be given to pregnant women.

Echinocandins

Echinocandins comprise a ring of six amino acids linked to a lipophilic side-chain. All drugs in this group are synthetic modifications of **echinocandin B**, which is found naturally in *Aspergillus nidulans*. As a group, the echinocandins are fungicidal for *Candida* and fungistatic for *Aspergillus*. The drugs inhibit the synthesis of 1,3-β-glucan, a glucose polymer that is necessary for maintaining the structure of fungal cell walls. In the absence of this polymer, fungal cells lose integrity and lyse. Resistance genes have been identified in *Candida* (Chen et al., 2011).

Caspofungin is active *in vitro* against a wide variety of fungi, and it has proved effective in the treatment of candidiasis and forms of invasive aspergillosis that are refractory to amphotericin. Oral absorption is poor, and it is given intravenously, once daily. **Anidulafungin** is used mainly for invasive candidiasis; again it is given intravenously. The principal side effects of both drugs include nausea, vomiting and diarrhoea, and skin rash. The relatively new **micafungin** is also mainly used for treating invasive candidiasis. It shares many of the side effects of the group but may also cause serious hepatotoxicity.

SYNTHETIC ANTIFUNGAL DRUGS

AZOLES

The azoles are a group of synthetic fungistatic agents with a broad spectrum of antifungal activity. **Clotrimazole, econazole, fenticonazole, ketoconazole, miconazole, tioconazole** and **sulconazole** (not UK) are based on the imidazole nucleus and **itraconazole, posaconazole, voriconazole** and **fluconazole** are triazole derivatives.

The azoles inhibit the fungal cytochrome P450 3A enzyme, lanosine 14α-demethylase, which is responsible for converting lanosterol to ergosterol, the main sterol in the fungal cell membrane. The resulting depletion of ergosterol alters the fluidity of the membrane, and this interferes with the action of membrane-associated enzymes. The net effect is an inhibition of replication. Azoles also inhibit the transformation of candidal yeast cells into hyphae – the invasive and pathogenic form of the parasite. Depletion of membrane ergosterol reduces the binding of amphotericin.

Ketoconazole

Ketoconazole was the first azole that could be given orally to treat systemic fungal infections. It is effective against several different types of organism (see Table 53.1). It is, however, toxic, and relapse is common after apparently successful treatment. It is well absorbed from the gastrointestinal tract. It is distributed widely throughout the tissues and tissue fluids but does not reach therapeutic concentrations in the central nervous system unless high doses are given. It is inactivated in the liver and excreted in bile and in urine. Its half-life in the plasma is 8 h.

Unwanted effects

The main hazard of ketoconazole is liver toxicity, which is rare but can prove fatal. Liver function is monitored before and during treatment. Other side effects that occur are gastrointestinal disturbances and pruritus. Inhibition of adrenocortical steroid and testosterone synthesis has been recorded with high doses, the latter resulting in gynaecomastia in some male patients. There may be adverse interactions with other drugs. **Ciclosporin** and **astemizole** all interfere with cytochrome P450 drug-metabolising enzymes, causing increased plasma concentrations of ketoconazole or the interacting drug, or both. **Rifampicin**, histamine H_2-receptor antagonists and antacids decrease the absorption of ketoconazole.

Fluconazole

Fluconazole is well absorbed and can be given orally or intravenously. It reaches high concentrations in the cerebrospinal fluid and ocular fluids, and is used to treat most types of fungal meningitis. Fungicidal concentrations are also achieved in vaginal tissue, saliva, skin and nails. It has a half-life of ~25 h, and is mainly excreted unchanged in the urine.

Unwanted effects

Unwanted effects, which are generally mild, include nausea, headache and abdominal pain. However, exfoliative skin lesions (including, on occasion, Stevens–Johnson syndrome[2]) have been seen in some individuals – primarily in AIDS patients who are being treated with multiple drugs. Hepatitis has been reported, although this is rare, and fluconazole, in the doses usually used, does not inhibit steroidogenesis and hepatic drug metabolism to the same extent as occurs with ketoconazole.

Itraconazole

Itraconazole is active against a range of dermatophytes. It may be given orally but, after absorption (which is variable) undergoes extensive hepatic metabolism. It is highly lipid-soluble (and water-insoluble), and a formulation in which the drug is retained within pockets of β-cyclodextrin is available. In this form, itraconazole can be administered intravenously, thereby overcoming the problem of variable absorption from the gastrointestinal tract. Administered orally, its half-life is about 36 h, and it is excreted in the urine. It does not penetrate the cerebrospinal fluid.

Unwanted effects

The most serious are hepatoxicity and Stevens–Johnson syndrome. Gastrointestinal disturbances, headache and allergic skin reactions can occur. Inhibition of steroidogenesis has not been reported. Drug interactions as a result of inhibition of cytochrome P450 enzymes occur (similar to ketoconazole).

Miconazole

Miconazole is generally used topically (often as a gel) for oral and other infections of the gastrointestinal tract or for skin or mucosal fungal infection. If significant systemic absorption occurs, drug interactions can present a problem.

Other azoles

Clotrimazole, econazole, tioconazole and sulconazole are used only for topical application. Clotrimazole interferes with amino acid transport into the fungus by an action on the cell membrane. It is active against a wide range of fungi, including candidal organisms. These drugs are sometimes combined with anti-inflammatory glucocorticoids (see Ch. 26). Posacanazole and voriconazole are used mainly for the treatment of invasive life-threatening infections such as aspergillosis.

OTHER ANTIFUNGAL DRUGS

Flucytosine is a synthetic, orally active antifungal agent that is effective against a limited range (mainly yeasts) of systemic fungal infections. If given alone, drug resistance commonly arises during treatment, so it is usually combined with amphotericin for severe systemic infections such as candidiasis and cryptococcal meningitis.

Flucytosine is converted to the antimetabolite 5-fluorouracil in fungal but not human cells. 5-Fluorouracil inhibits thymidylate synthetase and thus DNA synthesis (see Chs 5 and 56). Resistant mutants may emerge rapidly, so this drug should not be used alone.

Flucytosine is usually given by intravenous infusion (because such patients are often too ill to take medicine by mouth) but can also be given orally. It is widely distributed throughout the body fluids, including the cerebrospinal fluid. About 90% is excreted unchanged via the kidneys, and the plasma half-life is 3–5 h. The dosage should be reduced if renal function is impaired.

Unwanted effects include gastrointestinal disturbances, anaemia, neutropenia, thrombocytopenia and alopecia (possibly due to formation of fluorouracil [Ch. 56] from flucytosine by gut bacteria), but these are usually manageable. Uracil is reported to decrease the toxic effects on the bone marrow without impairing the antimycotic action. Hepatitis has been reported but is rare.

Terbinafine is a highly lipophilic, keratinophilic fungicidal compound active against a wide range of skin pathogens. It is particularly useful against nail infections.

---

[2]This is a severe and sometimes fatal condition involving blistering of the skin, mouth, gastrointestinal tract, eyes and genitalia, often accompanied by fever, polyarthritis and kidney failure.

It acts by selectively inhibiting the enzyme *squalene epoxidase*, which is involved in the synthesis of ergosterol from squalene in the fungal cell wall. The accumulation of squalene within the cell is toxic to the organism.

When used to treat ringworm or fungal infections of the nails, it is given orally. The drug is rapidly absorbed and is taken up by skin, nails and adipose tissue. Given topically, it penetrates skin and mucous membranes. It is metabolised in the liver by the cytochrome P450 system, and the metabolites are excreted in the urine.

Unwanted effects occur in about 10% of individuals and are usually mild and self-limiting. They include gastrointestinal disturbances, rashes, pruritus, headache and dizziness. Joint and muscle pains have been reported and, more rarely, hepatitis.

Naftifine is similar in action to terbinafine. Among other developments, a morpholine derivative, **amorolfine**, which interferes with fungal sterol synthesis, is available as a nail lacquer, being effective against onchomycoses.

FUTURE DEVELOPMENTS

Increasing numbers of fungal strains are becoming resistant to the current antifungal drugs (fortunately, drug resistance is not transferable in fungi), and toxicity and low efficacy also contribute to the need for better antifungal drugs. An additional problem is that new strains of commensal-turned-pathogenic fungi have emerged. Fungal infections are also on the rise because of the prevalence of cancer chemotherapy and transplant-associated immunosuppression.

Encouragingly, new compounds are in development, some with novel mechanisms of action. The development of new inhibitors of β-glucan has been reviewed by Hector and Bierer (2011), new targets such as V-ATPase are being assessed (Zhang & Rao, 2012) while the prospect of discovering new naturally occurring antifungals (like the antibiotic drugs already mentioned) continues to attract attention (Dhankhar et al., 2012). The prospect of using combination therapies has been explored in more depth (see Lupetti et al., 2003) and several groups have identified resistance genes that may improve the design and use of new drugs in the future (Chen et al., 2011; Hadrich et al., 2012; Noel, 2012).

Because fungal infections are often secondary to compromised host defence, attempts have been made to boost this by administration of the cytokine *granulocyte macrophage colony stimulating factor* (GM–CSF, see Ch. 18) and other factors that increase host leukocyte numbers or function (see also Lupetti et al., 2003). Finally, the possibility of developing an antifungal vaccine, first mooted in the 1960s, has recently met with limited success in animals (see Torosantucci et al., 2005 for an account of a *Candida* vaccine). It is hoped that such advances will soon find their way into clinical practice.

REFERENCES AND FURTHER READING

Chen, S.C., Slavin, M.A., Sorrell, T.C., 2011. Echinocandin antifungal drugs in fungal infections: a comparison. Drugs 71, 11–41. (*A very comprehensive review of the echinocandin drugs, including comments upon the phenomenon of drug resistance*)

Como, J.A., Dismukes, W.E., 1994. Oral azole drugs as systemic antifungal therapy. N. Engl. J. Med. 330, 263–272. (*A bit dated now but still worth reading for the review of ketoconazole, fluconazole and itraconazole*)

Deepe, G.S. Jr., 2004. Preventative and therapeutic vaccines for fungal infections: from concept to implementation. Expert Rev. Vaccines 3, 701–709. (*An interesting, and optimistic, overview of the quest for antifungal vaccines*)

Denning, D.W., 2003. Echinocandin antifungal drugs. Lancet 362, 1142–1151. (*General review on the echinocandins, focusing on their clinical use*)

Dhankhar, S., Dhankhar, S., Kumar, M., Ruhil, S., Balhara, M., Chhillar, A.K., 2012. Analysis toward innovative herbal antibacterial and antifungal drugs. Recent Pat. Antiinfect. Drug Discov. 7, 242–248. (*The quest for more naturally occurring antifungals continues with the identification of potential new active compounds*)

Dodds, E.S., Drew, R.H., Perfect, J.R., 2000. Antifungal pharmacodynamics: review of the literature and clinical applications. Pharmacotherapy 20, 1335–1355. (*Good review of antifungals used to treat systemic infections; somewhat clinical in tone*)

Gupta, A.K., Tomas, E., 2003. New antifungal agents. Dermatol. Clin. 21, 565–576. (*Quite a comprehensive review that deals mainly with the newer antifungals, their mechanisms of action and resistance*)

Hadrich, I., Makni, F., Neji, S., et al., 2012. Invasive aspergillosis: resistance to antifungal drugs. Mycopathologia 174, 131–141. (*Mainly deals with the mechanisms of resistance of aspergillus to conventional antifungal drugs*)

Hector, R.F., Bierer, D.E., 2011. New beta-glucan inhibitors as antifungal drugs. Expert Opin. Ther. Pat. 21, 1597–1610. (*A review of new patents in the area. Strictly for those who want to go into the subject in depth*)

Lupetti, A., Nibbering, P.H., Campa, M., et al., 2003. Molecular targeted treatments for fungal infections: the role of drug combinations. Trends Mol. Med. 9, 269–276. (*Interesting and accessible article that deals with the use of combination antifungal therapy. Some good diagrams*)

Noel, T., 2012. The cellular and molecular defense mechanisms of the Candida yeasts against azole antifungal drugs. J. Mycologie Med. 22, 173–178. (*Another paper that discusses resistance mechanisms, in this case to the azoles*)

Thursky, K.A., Playford, E.G., Seymour, J.F., et al., 2008. Recommendations for the treatment of established fungal infections. Intern. Med. J. 38, 496–520. (*A very comprehensive review of the treatment of fungal infections. Clinical in tone*)

Torosantucci, A., Bromuro, C., Chiani, P., et al., 2005. A novel glyco-conjugate vaccine against fungal pathogens. J. Exp. Med. 202, 597–606. (*An experimental paper demonstrating the development of a novel type of vaccine effective against Candida infections in mice*)

Zhang, Y., Rao, R., 2012. The V-ATPase as a target for antifungal drugs. Curr. Protein Peptide Sci. 13, 134–140. (*The title is self explanatory*)

Useful Web resources

<www.doctorfungus.org> (*This is an excellent site sponsored by a consortium of pharmaceutical companies. It covers all aspects of fungal infections and drug therapy, and has many compelling images and some video clips. Highly recommended – and fun!*)

54 Antiprotozoal drugs

OVERVIEW

Protozoa are motile, unicellular eukaryotic organisms that have colonised virtually every habitat and ecological niche. They may be conveniently classified into four main groups on the basis of their mode of locomotion: *amoebas*, *flagellates* and *sporozoa* are easily characterised but the final group comprises *ciliates* and other organisms of uncertain affiliation, such as the *Pneumocystis jirovecii* mentioned in the last chapter. Protozoa have diverse feeding behaviour, with some being parasitic. Many have extremely complex life cycles, sometimes involving several hosts, reminiscent of the helminths discussed in Chapter 55.

As a group, the protozoa are responsible for an enormous burden of illness in humans as well as domestic and wild animal populations. Table 54.1 lists some of these clinically important organisms, together with the diseases that they cause and an overview of anti-infective drugs. In this chapter we will first discuss some general features of protozoa–host interactions and then discuss the therapy of each group of diseases in turn. In view of its global importance, malaria is the main topic.

HOST–PARASITE INTERACTIONS

Mammals have developed very efficient mechanisms for defending themselves against invading parasites, but many parasites have, in turn, evolved sophisticated evasion tactics. One common parasite ploy is to take refuge within the cells of the host, where antibodies cannot reach them. Most protozoa do this, for example *Plasmodium* species take up residence in red cells, *Leishmania* species infect macrophages exclusively, while *Trypanosoma* species invade many other cell types. The host deals with these intracellular fugitives by deploying cytotoxic CD8[+] T cells and T helper (Th)1 pathway cytokines, such as interleukin (IL)-2, tumour necrosis factor (TNF)-α and interferon-γ. These cytokines (see Ch. 18) activate macrophages, which can then kill intracellular parasites.

As we explained in Chapter 6, the Th1 pathway responses can be downregulated by Th2 pathway cytokines (e.g. transforming growth factor-β, IL-4 and IL-10). Some intracellular parasites have exploited this fact by stimulating the production of Th2 cytokines thus reducing their vulnerability to Th1-driven activated macrophages. For example, the invasion of macrophages by *Leishmania* species induces transforming growth factor-β, IL-10, inactivates complement pathways, and downregulates many other intracellular defence mechanisms (Singh et al., 2012). Similar mechanisms operate during worm infestations (see Ch. 55).

Toxoplasma gondii has evolved a different gambit – *upregulation* of host defence responses. The definitive (i.e. where sexual recombination occurs) host of this protozoon is the cat, but humans can inadvertently become intermediate hosts, harbouring the asexual form of the parasite. In humans, *T. gondii* infects numerous cell types and has a highly virulent replicative stage. To ensure that its host survives, it stimulates production of interferon-γ, modulating the host's cell-mediated responses to promote encystment of the parasite in the tissues. The use of cytokine analogues and/or antagonists to treat disease caused by protozoa is a promising area for the development of new anti-parasite drugs (see Odeh, 2001).

MALARIA AND ANTIMALARIAL DRUGS

Malaria[1] is caused by parasites belonging to the genus *Plasmodium*. Four main species infect humans: *P. vivax*, *P. falciparum*, *P. ovale* and *P. malariae*. A related parasite that infects monkeys, *P. knowlesi*, can also infect humans and is causing increasing concern in some regions, such as South-East Asia. The insect vector in all cases is the female *Anopheles* mosquito. This breeds in stagnant water and the disease it spreads is one of the major killers on our planet.

Largely because of a massive increase in spending on public health campaigns such as the *Roll Back Malaria* programme (which is sponsored by a partnership of transnational organisations including the World Health Organization, WHO), the global malaria mortality rate has fallen by approximately a quarter over the last decade, but even so, the overall statistics make gloomy reading. According to the 2012 WHO report, malaria is a significant public health problem in more than 100 countries. In 2010, there were an estimated 219 million cases and some 660 000 deaths from the disease. More than 90% of these occur in sub-Saharan Africa, and most of the victims are children. Even those who survive may suffer from lasting mental impairment. Other high-risk groups include pregnant women, refugees and labourers entering endemic regions. Malaria also imposes a huge economic burden on countries where the disease is rife.

Also of concern is the fact that malaria has gained a foothold in other countries where it is not normally endemic.[2] The WHO recorded over 100 000 such cases in over 90 countries between 2001 and 2010. This phenomenon is partly due to international travel, partly due to immigration from countries where the disease is endemic and (possibly) partly caused by global warming.

The symptoms of malaria include fever, shivering, pain in the joints, headache, repeated vomiting, generalised

---

[1]The disease was once considered to arise from marshy land, hence the Latin name '*mal aria*', meaning bad or poisonous air.
[2]This is usually referred to as 'imported malaria'. 'Airport malaria' is caused by infected mosquitoes in aircraft arriving from areas where the disease is endemic; 'baggage malaria' is caused by their presence in luggage arriving from such areas; and 'runway malaria' has been contracted by passengers who have stopped in endemic areas, but have not even left the aircraft.

Table 54.1 Principal protozoal infections and common drug treatments

Organism	Disease	Common drug treatments
Amoeba		
Entamoeba histolytica	Amoebic dysentery	Metronidazole, tinidazole, diloxanide
Flagellates		
Trypanosoma brucei rhodesiense *Trypanosoma brucei gambiense*	Sleeping sickness	Suramin, pentamidine, melarpasol, eflornithine, nifurtimox
Trypanosoma cruzi	Chagas' disease	Nifurtimox, benzindazole
Leishmania tropica *Leishmania donovani* *Leishmania Mexicana* *Leishmania braziliensis*	'Kala-azar' 'Chiclero's ulcer' 'Espundia' 'Oriental sore'	Sodium stibogluconate, amphotericin, pentamidine isetionate
Trichomonas vaginalis	Vaginitis	Metronidazole, tinidazole
Giardia lamblia	Diarrhoea, steatorrhoea	Metronidazole, tinidazole, mepacrine
Sporozoa		
Plasmodium falciparum[a] *Plasmodium vivax* *Plasmodium ovale* *Plasmodium malarariae*	Malignant tertian malaria Benign tertian malaria Benign tertian malaria Quartan malaria	Artemether, atovaquone, chloroquine, clindamycin, dapsone, doxycycline, lumefantrine, mefloquine, primaquine, proguanil, pyrimethamine, quinine, sulfadoxine
Toxoplasma gondii	Encephalitis, congenital malformations, eye disease	Pyrimethamine-sulfadiazine
Ciliates and others		
Pneumocystis carinii[b]	Pneumonia	Co-trimoxazole, atovaquone, pentamidine isetionate

[a]See also Table 54.2.
[b]This organism is of uncertain classification. See text for details and Chapter 53 for further comments.

Malaria

- Malaria is caused by various species of plasmodia, which are carried by the female *Anopheles* mosquito. Sporozoites (the asexual form of the parasite) are introduced into the host following insect bite and these develop in the liver into:
  - schizonts (the pre-erythrocytic stage), which liberate merozoites – these infect red blood cells, forming motile trophozoites, which, after development, release another batch of erythrocyte-infecting merozoites, causing fever; this constitutes the erythrocytic cycle
  - dormant hypnozoites, which may liberate merozoites later (the exoerythrocytic stage).

- The main malarial parasites causing tertian ('every third day') malaria are:
  - *P. vivax*, which causes benign tertian malaria
  - *P. falciparum*, which causes malignant tertian malaria; unlike *P. vivax*, this plasmodium has no exoerythrocytic stage.
- Some merozoites develop into gametocytes, the sexual forms of the parasite. When ingested by the mosquito, these give rise to further stages of the parasite's life cycle within the insect.

---

convulsions and coma. Symptoms become apparent only 7–9 days after being bitten by an infected mosquito. By far the most dangerous parasite is *P. falciparum*.

Malaria was eradicated from most temperate countries in the 20th century, and the WHO attempted to eradicate malaria elsewhere using the powerful 'residual' insecticides and the highly effective antimalarial drugs, such as **chloroquine**, which had, by then, become available. By the end of the 1950s, the incidence of malaria had dropped dramatically. However, it was clear by the 1970s that the attempt at eradication had failed, largely because of the increasing resistance of the mosquito to the insecticides, and of the parasite to the drugs. Sadly, malaria has now re-emerged in several countries where it was previously under control or eradicated.

THE LIFE CYCLE OF THE MALARIA PARASITE

The life cycle of the parasite consists of a sexual cycle, which takes place in the female *Anopheles* mosquito, and

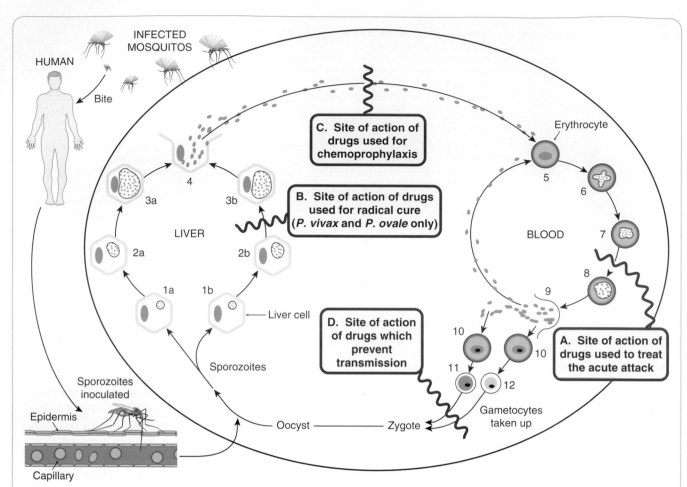

Fig. 54.1 **The life cycle of the malarial parasite and the site of action of antimalarial drugs.** The infection is initiated by the bite of an infected female *Anopheles* mosquito, which introduces the parasite into the blood. This then enters a pre- or exoerythrocytic cycle in the liver and an erythrocytic cycle in the blood: (**1a**) from the blood stream the sporozoite enters into liver cells (the parasite is shown as a small circle containing dots, and the liver cell nucleus as a blue oval); (**2a** and **3a**) the schizont develops in the liver cells; (**4**) these eventually rupture releasing merozoites (some may enter further liver cells and become resting forms of the parasite, hypnozoites). (**5**) Merozoites enter into red cells and form motile trophozoites (**6**); following division and multiplication (**7** and **8**) schizonts develop in red cells that eventually (**9**) rupture releasing further merozoites, most of which parasitise other red cells. Sometimes (**10–12**) merozoites develop into male and female gametocytes in red cells. These can constitute a fresh source of infective material if the blood is then consumed by another mosquito. (**1b**) Resting form of parasite in liver (hypnozoite). (**2b** and **3b**) Growth and multiplication of hypnozoites.

Sites of drug action are as follows. (**A**) Drugs used to treat the acute attack (also called 'blood schizonticidal agents' or 'drugs for suppressive or clinical cure'). (**B**) Drugs that affect the exoerythrocytic hypnozoites and result in a 'radical' cure of *P. vivax* and *P. ovale*. (**C**) Drugs that block the link between the exoerythrocytic stage and the erythrocytic stage; they are used for chemoprophylaxis (also termed causal prophylactics) and prevent the development of malarial attacks. (**D**) Drugs that prevent transmission and thus prevent increase of the human reservoir of the disease.

an asexual cycle, which occurs in humans (Fig. 54.1 and the 'Malaria' box). Therefore, the mosquito, not the human, is the definitive host for plasmodia. Indeed, it has been said that the only function of humans is to enable the parasite to infect more mosquitoes so that further sexual recombination can occur.

▼ The cycle in the mosquito involves fertilisation of the female *gametocyte* by the male gametocyte, with the formation of a *zygote*, which develops into an *oocyst* (*sporocyst*). A further stage of division and multiplication takes place, leading to rupture of the sporocyst with release of *sporozoites*, which then migrate to the mosquito's salivary glands and a few enter the human host with the mosquito's bite.

When sporozoites enter the human host they disappear from the bloodstream within 30 min and enter the parenchymal cells of the liver where, during the next 10–14 days, they undergo a *pre-erythrocytic* stage of

development and multiplication. The parasitised liver cells then rupture, and a host of fresh *merozoites* are released. These bind to and enter erythrocytes and form motile intracellular parasites termed *trophozoites*. During the erythrocytic stage the parasite remodels the host cell, inserting parasite proteins and phospholipids into the red cell membrane. The host's haemoglobin is transported to the parasite's food vacuole, where it is digested, providing a source of amino acids. Free haem, which would be toxic to the plasmodium, is rendered harmless by polymerisation to *haemozoin*. Some antimalarial drugs act by inhibiting the haem polymerase enzyme responsible for this step.

▼ Following mitotic replication, the parasite in the red cell is termed a schizont, and its rapid growth and division, *schizogony*. Another phase of multiplication results in the production of further merozoites, which are released when the red cell ruptures. These merozoites then bind to and enter fresh red cells, and the erythrocytic cycle begins again. In certain forms of malaria, some sporozoites entering the liver cells form *hypnozoites*, or 'sleeping' forms of the parasite, which can be reactivated months or years later to continue an *exoerythrocytic* cycle of multiplication.

Malaria parasites can multiply in the body at a phenomenal rate – a single parasite of *P. vivax* can give rise to 250 million merozoites in 14 days. To appreciate the action required of an antimalarial drug, note that destruction of 94% of the parasites every 48 h will serve only to maintain equilibrium and will not further reduce their number or their propensity for proliferation. Some merozoites, on entering red cells, differentiate into male and female *gametocytes*. These can complete their cycle only when taken up by the mosquito, when it sucks the blood from the infected host.

The periodic episodes of fever that characterise malaria result from the synchronised rupture of red cells with release of merozoites and cell debris. The rise in temperature is associated with a rise in the concentration of TNF-α in the plasma. Relapses of malaria are likely to occur with those forms of malaria that have an exoerythrocytic cycle, because the dormant hypnozoite form in the liver may emerge after an interval of weeks or months to start the infection again.

▼ The characteristic presentations of the different forms of human malaria are as follows (see Fig. 54.1 for details):

- *P. falciparum*, which has an erythrocytic cycle of 48 h in humans, produces *malignant tertian malaria* – 'tertian' because the fever was believed to recur every third day (actually it varies), 'malignant' because it is the most severe form of malaria and can be fatal. The plasmodium induces adhesion molecules on the infected cells, which then stick to uninfected red cells, forming clusters (rosettes), and also adhere to and pack the vessels of the microcirculation, interfering with tissue blood flow and causing organ dysfunction including renal failure and encephalopathy (cerebral malaria). *P. falciparum* does not have an exoerythrocytic stage, so if the erythrocytic stage is eradicated, relapses do not occur.
- *P. vivax* produces *benign tertian malaria*, less severe than falciparum malaria and rarely fatal. Exoerythrocytic forms may persist for years and cause relapses.
- *P. ovale*, which has a 48 h cycle and an exoerythrocytic stage, is the cause of a rare form of malaria.
- *P. malariae* has a 72 h cycle, causes *quartan malaria* and has no exoerythrocytic cycle.

Individuals living in areas where malaria is endemic may acquire a natural immunity, but this may be lost if the individual is absent from the area for more than 6 months. The best way to deal with malaria is to prevent mosquito bites by suitable clothing, insect repellents and bed nets. Bed nets sprayed with insecticides such as permethrin can be very effective.

ANTIMALARIAL DRUGS

Some drugs can be used prophylactically to prevent malaria (see Table 54.2), while others are directed towards treating acute attacks. In general, antimalarial drugs are classified in terms of the action against the different stages of the life cycle of the parasite (Fig. 54.1).

The use of drugs for the treatment of malaria has changed considerably during the last half-century mainly because resistance developed to chloroquine and other successful early drug combinations (see Butler et al., 2010). Monotherapy has largely been abandoned in favour of **artemisinin**-based combination therapy (ACT; see Table 54.3). Only antimalarial drugs in common use

---

Antimalarial therapy and the parasite life cycle

Drugs used in the treatment of malaria may have several sites of action:

- Drugs used to treat the acute attack of malaria act on the parasites in the blood; they can cure infections with parasites (e.g. *P. falciparum*) that have no exoerythrocytic stage.
- Drugs used for prophylaxis act on merozoites emerging from liver cells.
- Drugs used for radical cure are active against parasites in the liver.
- Some drugs act on gametocytes and prevent transmission by the mosquito.

Table 54.2 Examples of drug treatment and chemoprophylaxis of malaria[a]

To treat ...	Typical drug choices
Infection with *P. falciparum* or with unknown or mixed organisms	Quinine + doxycycline or clindamycin; or Proguanil + atovaquone;[b] or Artemether + lumefantrine[c]
Infection with *P. malariae*, *P. vivax* or *P. ovale*	Chloroquine, possibly followed by primaquine in the case of *P. vivax* or *P. ovale*
Chemoprophylaxis (short-term)	Proguanil + atovaquone[b] or doxycycline
Chemoprophylaxis (long-term)	Chloroquine + proguanil; mefloquine or doxycycline

[a]It must be appreciated that this is only a summary, not a definitive guide to prescription, as the recommended drug combinations vary depending on the patient, the area visited, the overall risk of infection, the presence of resistant forms of the disease and so on. This information is based on current UK recommendations (source: British National Formulary 2013).

[b]Malarone is a proprietary combination of atovaquone and proguanil hydrochloride.

[c]Riamet is a proprietary combination of artemether and lumefantrine.

---

are described in this chapter. For a brief summary of currently recommended treatment regimens, see the 'Antimalarial drugs' box and Table 54.1. Na-Bangchang and Karbwang (2009) give a more detailed coverage of current therapeutic options and their use in the treatment of malaria around the world.

Drugs used to treat the acute attack

Blood schizonticidal agents (Fig. 54.1, site A) are used to treat the acute attack but also produce a 'suppressive' or 'clinical' cure. They act on the erythrocytic forms of the plasmodium. In the case of *P. falciparum* or *P. malariae*, which have no exoerythrocytic stage, these drugs effect a cure; however, with *P. vivax* or *P. ovale*, the drugs suppress the actual attack but exoerythrocytic forms can re-emerge later to cause relapses.

This group of drugs includes:

- artemisinin and related compounds derived from the Chinese herb *qinghao*, which are usually used in combination with other drugs
- the quinoline–methanols (e.g. **quinine** and **mefloquine**) and various 4-aminoquinolines (e.g. chloroquine)
- agents that interfere either with the synthesis of folate (e.g. **dapsone**) or with its action (e.g. **pyrimethamine** and **proguanil**)
- **atovaquone**, which affects mitochondrial function.

Combinations of these agents are frequently used. Some antibiotics, such as the tetracycline **doxycycline** (see Ch. 51), have proved useful when combined with the above agents. They have an antiparasite effect in their own right but also control other concomitant infections.

Drugs that effect a radical cure

Tissue schizonticidal agents effect a 'radical' cure by eradicating *P. vivax* and *P. ovale* parasites in the liver (Fig. 54.1, site B). Only the 8-aminoquinolines (e.g. **primaquine** and **tafenoquine**) have this action. These drugs also destroy gametocytes and thus reduce the spread of infection.

Drugs used for chemoprophylaxis

Drugs used for chemoprophylaxis (also known as *causal prophylactic drugs*: see Table 54.2) block the link between the exoerythrocytic stage and the erythrocytic stage, and thus prevent the development of malarial attacks. True causal prophylaxis – the prevention of infection by the killing of the sporozoites on entry into the host – is not feasible with present drugs, although it may be feasible in the future with vaccines. Clinical attacks can be prevented by chemoprophylactic drugs that kill the parasites when they emerge from the liver after the pre-erythrocytic stage (Fig. 54.1, site C). The drugs used for this purpose are mainly artemisinin derivatives, chloroquine, **lumefantrine**, mefloquine, proguanil, pyrimethamine, dapsone and doxycycline. They are often used in combinations.

▼ Chemoprophylactic agents are given to individuals who intend travelling to an area where malaria is endemic. Administration should start at least 1 week before entering the area and should be continued throughout the stay and for at least a month afterwards. No chemoprophylactic regimen is 100% effective, and unwanted effects may occur. A further problem is the complexity of the regimens, which require different drugs to be taken at different times, and the fact that different agents may be required for different travel destinations. For a brief summary of currently recommended regimens of chemoprophylaxis, see Table 54.2.

Drugs used to prevent transmission

Some drugs (e.g. primaquine, proguanil and pyrimethamine) can also destroy gametocytes (Fig. 54.1, site D), preventing transmission by the mosquito and thus diminishing the human reservoir of the disease, although they are rarely used for this action alone.

Table 54.3 summarises what is known about the molecular targets of these drugs and Figure 54.2 shows chemical structures of some significant drugs.

CHLOROQUINE

The 4-aminoquinoline chloroquine dates from the 1940s but is still widely used as a blood schizonticidal agent (Fig. 54.1, site A), effective against the erythrocytic forms of all four plasmodial species (where resistance is not an issue), but it does not have any effect on sporozoites, hypnozoites or gametocytes. It is uncharged at neutral pH and can therefore diffuse freely into the parasite lysosome. At the acid pH of the lysosome, it is converted to a protonated, membrane-impermeable form and is 'trapped' inside the parasite. Its chief antimalarial action derives from an inhibition of *haem polymerase*, the enzyme that polymerises toxic free haem to haemozoin. This poisons the parasite and prevents it from utilising the amino acids from haemoglobin proteolysis. Chloroquine is also used as a disease-modifying antirheumatoid drug (Ch. 26) and also has some quinidine-like actions on the heart (Ch. 21).

Resistance

P. falciparum is now resistant to chloroquine in most parts of the world. Resistance appears to result from enhanced efflux of the drug from parasitic vesicles as a result of mutations in plasmodia transporter genes (Baird, 2005). Resistance of *P. vivax* to chloroquine is also a growing problem in many parts of the world.

Table 54.3 Drug targets of antimalarial drugs

Parasite organelle	Target	Chemical class	Drugs
Cytosolic compartment	Inhibit or antagonise folic acid metabolism	Diaminopyridines	Pyrimethamine
		Biguanides	Proguanil
		Sulfones	Dapsone
		Sulfonamides	Sulfadoxine
Mitochondrion	Block electron transport energy production	Hydroxynapthoquinones	Atovaquone, tafenoquine, pyridones
Apicoplast	Block protein synthetic machinery	Tetracyclines and others	Azithromycin, doxycycline, clindamycin other antibiotics
Digestive vacuole	Inhibit the detoxification of haem	Quinolones	Chloroquine, amodiaquine, mefloquine, quinine
		Aryl amino alcohols	Lumefantrine
Membranes?	Inhibition of Ca^{2+}-dependent ATPase	Sesquiterpene lactones	Artemisinin derivatives

After Fidock et al. 2004.

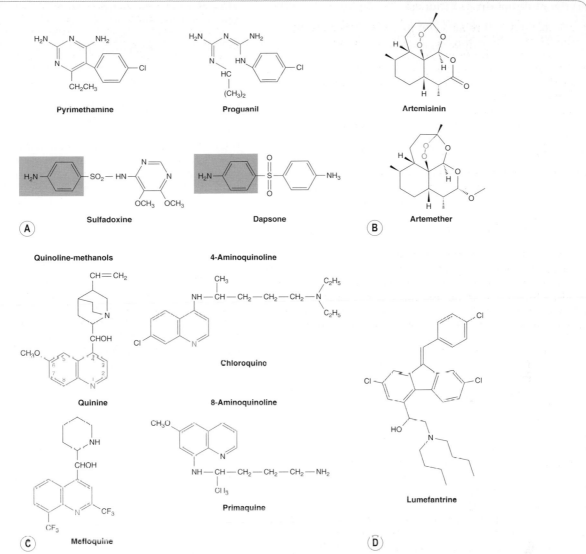

Fig. 54.2 Structures of some significant antimalarial drugs. [A] Drugs that act on the folic acid pathway of the plasmodia. Folate antagonists (pyrimethamine, proguanil) inhibit dihydrofolate reductase; the relationship between these drugs and the pteridine moiety is shown in orange. Sulfones (e.g. dapsone) and sulfonamides (e.g. sulfadoxine) compete with p-aminobenzoic acid for dihydropteroate synthetase (relationship shown in orange box, see also Ch. 50) [B] Artemisinin and a derivative artemether. Note the endoperoxide bridge structure (in orange) that is crucial to their action. [C] Some quinolone antimalarials. The quinoline moiety is shown in orange. [D] The aryl amino alcohol lumefantrine.

Administration and pharmacokinetic aspects

Chloroquine is generally administered orally, but severe falciparum malaria may be treated by frequent intramuscular or subcutaneous injection of small doses, or by slow continuous intravenous infusion. Following oral dosing, it is completely absorbed, extensively distributed throughout the tissues and concentrated in parasitised red cells. Release from tissues and infected erythrocytes is slow. The drug is metabolised in the liver and excreted in the urine, 70% as unchanged drug and 30% as metabolites. Elimination is slow, the major phase having a half-life of 50 h, and a residue persists for weeks or months.

Unwanted effects

Chloroquine has few adverse effects when given for chemoprophylaxis. However, unwanted effects, including nausea and vomiting, dizziness and blurring of vision, headache and urticarial symptoms, can occur when larger doses are administered to treat acute attacks of malaria. Large doses have also sometimes resulted in retinopathies and hearing loss. Bolus intravenous injections of chloroquine may cause hypotension and, if high doses are used, fatal dysrhythmias. Chloroquine is considered to be safe for use by pregnant women.

Amodiaquine has very similar action to chloroquine. It was withdrawn several years ago because of the risk of agranulocytosis, but has now been reintroduced in several areas of the world where chloroquine resistance is endemic.

QUININE

Quinine, derived from cinchona bark, has been used for the treatment of 'fevers' since the 16th century, when Jesuit missionaries brought the bark to Europe from Peru. It is a blood schizonticidal drug effective against the erythrocytic forms of all four species of plasmodium (Fig. 54.1, site A), but it has no effect on exoerythrocytic forms or on the gametocytes of *P. falciparum*. Its mechanism of action is the same as that of chloroquine, but quinine is not so extensively concentrated in the plasmodium as chloroquine, so other mechanisms could also be involved. With the emergence and spread of chloroquine resistance, quinine is now the main chemotherapeutic agent for *P. falciparum* in certain parts of the world. Pharmacological actions on host tissue include a depressant action on the heart, a mild oxytocic effect on the uterus in pregnancy, a slight blocking action on the neuromuscular junction and a weak antipyretic effect.

Some degree of resistance to quinine has developed because of increased expression of plasmodial drug efflux transporters.

Pharmacokinetic aspects

Quinine is well absorbed and is usually administered orally as a 7-day course, but it can also be given by slow intravenous infusion for severe *P. falciparum* infections and in patients who are vomiting. A loading dose may be required, but bolus intravenous administration is contraindicated because of the risk of cardiac dysrhythmias. The half-life of the drug is 10 h; it is metabolised in the liver and the metabolites are excreted in the urine within about 24 h.

Unwanted effects

Quinine has a bitter taste, and oral compliance is often poor.[3] It is irritant to the gastric mucosa and can cause nausea and vomiting. 'Cinchonism' – characterised by nausea, dizziness, tinnitus, headache and blurring of vision – is likely to occur if the plasma concentration exceeds 30–60 µmol/l. Excessive plasma levels may also cause hypotension, cardiac dysrhythmias and severe CNS disturbances such as delirium and coma.

Other, infrequent, unwanted reactions that have been reported are bone marrow depression (mainly thrombocytopenia) and hypersensitivity reactions. Quinine can stimulate insulin release. Patients with marked falciparum parasitaemia can have low blood sugar for this reason and also because of glucose consumption by the parasite. This can make a differential diagnosis between a coma caused by cerebral malaria and hypoglycaemia difficult. A rare result of treating malaria with quinine, or of erratic and inappropriate use of quinine, is Blackwater fever, a severe and often fatal condition in which acute haemolytic anaemia is associated with renal failure.

MEFLOQUINE

Mefloquine (Fig. 54.2) is a blood schizonticidal compound active against *P. falciparum* and *P. vivax* (Fig. 54.1, site A); however, it has no effect on hepatic forms of the parasites, so treatment of *P. vivax* infections should be followed by a course of primaquine to eradicate the hypnozoites. Mefloquine acts in the same way as quinine, and is frequently combined with pyrimethamine.

Resistance to mefloquine has occurred in *P. falciparum* in some areas – particularly in South-East Asia – and is thought to be caused, as with quinine, by increased expression in the parasite of drug efflux transporters.

Pharmacokinetic aspects and unwanted effects

Mefloquine is given orally and is rapidly absorbed. It has a slow onset of action and a very long plasma half-life (up to 30 days), which may be the result of enterohepatic cycling or tissue storage.

When mefloquine is used for treatment of the acute attack, about 50% of subjects complain of gastrointestinal disturbances. Transient CNS side effects – giddiness, confusion, dysphoria and insomnia – can occur, and there have been a few reports of aberrant atrioventricular conduction and serious, but rare, skin diseases. Rarely, mefloquine may provoke severe neuropsychiatric reactions. Mefloquine is contraindicated in pregnant women or in those liable to become pregnant within 3 months of stopping the drug, because of its long half-life and uncertainty about its teratogenic potential. When used for chemoprophylaxis, the unwanted actions are usually milder, but the drug should not be used in this way unless there is a high risk of acquiring chloroquine-resistant malaria.

LUMEFANTRINE

This aryl amino alcohol drug is related to an older compound, halofantrine, which is now seldom used. Lumefantrine is never used alone but in combination with **artemether**. Its mode of action is probably to prevent parasite detoxification of haem. The pharmacokinetics of the combination is complex and the reader is referred to Ezzet et al. (1998) for more details. Unwanted effects of the combination may include gastrointestinal and central nervous system (CNS) symptoms.

DRUGS AFFECTING FOLATE METABOLISM

Sulfonamides and sulfones, used as antibacterial drugs (see Ch. 51), inhibit the synthesis of folate in plasmodia by competing with p-aminobenzoic acid. Pyrimethamine and proguanil inhibit dihydrofolate reductase, which prevents the utilisation of folate in DNA synthesis. Used together, they block the folate pathway at different points, and thus act synergistically.

The main sulfonamide used in malaria treatment is **sulfadoxine**, and the only sulfone used is dapsone. Details of these drugs are given in Chapter 51. The sulfonamides and sulfones are active against the erythrocytic forms of *P. falciparum* but are less active against those of *P. vivax*; they have no activity against the sporozoite or hypnozoite forms of the plasmodia. Pyrimethamine–sulfadoxine has been extensively used for chloroquine-resistant malaria, but resistance to this combination has developed in many areas.

Pyrimethamine is similar in structure to the antibacterial drug **trimethoprim** (see Ch. 51). Proguanil has a slightly different structure but its (active) metabolite can assume a similar configuration. Both drugs have a greater affinity for the plasmodium enzyme than for the human enzyme. They have a slow action against the erythrocytic forms of the parasite (Fig. 54.1, site A), and proguanil is believed to have an additional effect on the initial hepatic stage (1a to 3a in Fig. 54.1) but not on the hypnozoites of *P. vivax* (Fig. 54.1, site B). Pyrimethamine is used only in combination with either a sulfone or a sulfonamide.

Pharmacokinetic aspects

Both pyrimethamine and proguanil are given orally and are well, although slowly, absorbed. Pyrimethamine has

---

[3]Hence the invention of palatable drinks containing the drug, including, of course, the famous 'tonic' drunk together with gin and other beverages.

a plasma half-life of 4 days, and effective 'suppressive' plasma concentrations may last for 14 days; it is taken once a week. The half-life of proguanil is 16 h. It is a prodrug and is metabolised in the liver to its active form, cycloguanil, which is excreted mainly in the urine. It must be taken daily.

Unwanted effects

These drugs have few untoward effects in therapeutic doses. Larger doses of the pyrimethamine–dapsone combination can cause serious reactions such as haemolytic anaemia, agranulocytosis and lung inflammation. The pyrimethamine–sulfadoxine combination can cause serious skin reactions, blood dyscrasias and allergic alveolitis; it is no longer recommended for chemoprophylaxis. In high doses, pyrimethamine may inhibit mammalian dihydrofolate reductase and cause a *megaloblastic anaemia* (see Ch. 25) and folic acid supplements should be given if this drug is used during pregnancy. Resistance to antifolate drugs arises from single-point mutations in the genes encoding parasite dihydrofolate reductase.

PRIMAQUINE

Primaquine is an 8-aminoquinoline drug, which is (almost uniquely among clinically available antimalarial drugs) active against liver hypnozoites (see Fig. 54.2). **Etaquine** and tafenoquine are more active and slowly metabolised analogues of primaquine. These drugs can effect a radical cure of *P. vivax* and *P. ovale* malaria in which the parasites have a dormant stage in the liver. Primaquine does not affect sporozoites and has little if any action against the erythrocytic stage of the parasite. However, it has a gametocidal action and is the most effective antimalarial drug for preventing transmission of all four species of plasmodia. It is almost invariably used in combination with another drug, usually chloroquine. Resistance to primaquine is rare, although evidence of a decreased sensitivity of some *P. vivax* strains has been reported. The pharmacology of primaquine and similar drugs has been reviewed by Shanks et al. (2001).

Pharmacokinetic aspects

Primaquine is given orally and is well absorbed. Its metabolism is rapid, and very little drug is present in the body after 10–12 h. The half-life is 3–6 h. Tafenoquine is metabolised much more slowly and therefore has the advantage that it can be given on a weekly basis.

Unwanted effects

Primaquine has few unwanted effects in most patients when used in normal therapeutic dosage. Dose-related gastrointestinal symptoms can occur, and large doses may cause methaemoglobinaemia with cyanosis.

Primaquine can cause haemolysis in individuals with the X chromosome-linked genetic metabolic condition, *glucose 6-phosphate dehydrogenase deficiency*, in red cells (Ch. 11). When this deficiency is present, the red cells are not able to regenerate NADPH, which is depleted by the oxidant metabolic derivatives of primaquine. As a consequence, the metabolic functions of the red cells are impaired and haemolysis occurs. The deficiency of the enzyme occurs in up to 15% of black males and is also fairly common in some other ethnic groups. Glucose 6-phosphate dehydrogenase activity should be estimated before giving primaquine.

ARTEMISININ AND RELATED COMPOUNDS

The importance of this group is that they are often the only drugs that can effectively treat resistant *P. falciparum*. These sesquiterpene lactones are derived from the herb *qinghao*, a traditional Chinese remedy for fevers. The scientific name, conferred on the herb by Linnaeus, is *Artemisia*.[4] Artemisinin, a poorly soluble chemical extract from *Artemisia*, is a fast-acting blood schizonticide effective in treating the acute attack of malaria (including chloroquine-resistant and cerebral malaria). Derivatives of artemisinin, which include **artesunate** (a water-soluble derivative available in some countries) and **artemether**, have higher activity and are better absorbed. The compounds are concentrated in parasitised red cells. The mechanism of action is probably through inhibition of a parasite Ca^{2+}-dependent ATPase (Eckstein-Ludwig et al., 2003) and it is likely that the unusual 'endoperoxide bridge' of this drug (see Fig. 54.2) has to be 'activated' in the presence of intracellular iron before it can exert its effects. These drugs are without effect on liver hypnozoites. Artemisinin can be given orally, intramuscularly or by suppository, artemether orally or intramuscularly, and artesunate intramuscularly or intravenously. They are rapidly absorbed and widely distributed, and are converted in the liver to the active metabolite dihydroartemisinin. The half-life of artemisinin is about 4 h, of artesunate, 45 min and of artemether, 4–11 h.

There are few unwanted effects. Transient heart block, decrease in blood neutrophil count and brief episodes of fever have been reported. In animal studies, artemisinin causes an unusual injury to some brain stem nuclei, particularly those involved in auditory function; however, there have been no reported incidences of neurotoxicity in humans. So far, resistance has not been a problem, but recent reports suggest that the parasite in some areas of the world is becoming less sensitive to these drugs. In rodent studies, artemisinin potentiated the effects of mefloquine, primaquine and tetracycline, was additive with chloroquine and antagonised the sulfonamides and the folate antagonists. For this reason, artemisinin derivatives are frequently used in combination with other antimalarial drugs; for example, artemether is often given in combination with lumefantrine.

In randomised trials, artemisinins have cured attacks of malaria, including cerebral malaria, more rapidly and with fewer unwanted effects than other antimalarial agents. Artemisinin and derivatives are effective against multidrug-resistant *P. falciparum* in sub-Saharan Africa and, combined with mefloquine, against multidrug-resistant *P. falciparum* in South-East Asia.

ATAVOQUONE

Atavoquone is a hydroxynaphthoquinone drug used prophylactically to prevent malaria, and to treat cases resistant to other drugs. It acts primarily to inhibit the parasite's mitochondrial electron transport chain,

---

[4]Having been used for thousands of years in China as a herbal extract for treating 'fevers', the active compound artemisinin was isolated by Chinese chemists in 1972. This was ignored in the West for more than 10 years, until the WHO recognised its importance and, in 2002, placed it on the WHO 'essential drugs' list for malaria treatment. The herbs are noted for their extreme bitterness, and their name derives from *Artemisia*, wife and sister of the 4th-century king of Halicarnassus; her sorrow on his death led her to mix his ashes with whatever she drank to make it bitter.

possibly by mimicking the natural substrate ubiquinone. Atavoquone is usually used in combination with the anti-folate drug proguanil, because they act synergistically. The mechanism underlying this synergism is not known, but it is specific for this particular pair of drugs, because other antifolate drugs or electron transport inhibitors have no such synergistic effect. When combined with pro-guanil, atavoquone is highly effective and well tolerated. Few unwanted effects of such combination treatment have been reported, but abdominal pain, nausea and vomiting can occur. Pregnant or breastfeeding women should not take atavoquone. Resistance to atavoquone alone is rapid and results from a single point mutation in the gene for cytochrome b. Resistance to combined treatment with atavoquone and proguanil is less common.

POTENTIAL NEW ANTIMALARIAL DRUGS

Malaria has been dubbed a 're-emerging disease' largely because of the ongoing development of resistant strains of the parasite. The quest for new drugs is urgent and there has been some progress in this area both in the search for new entities (see Muregi et al., 2012, and Tschan et al., 2012) as well as a better understanding of the phar-macokinetic aspects of current drugs (Na-Bangchang & Karbwang, 2009), enabling better treatment regimes. But perhaps the most significant advance has come through the application of synthetic biology to solve the problem of artemisinin production. Artemisinin is notoriously dif-ficult to synthesise by conventional chemical techniques and awkward to harvest in large amounts. Using geneti-cally modified yeast transfected with genes from *Artemisia* it has been possible to produce large amounts of the pre-cursor *artemisinic acid*, which can be easily converted into artemisinin (Paddon et al., 2013). This breakthrough tech-nique should relieve the desperate shortage of the drug.

The prospects for an effective malaria vaccine have increased dramatically over the last decade and some can-didate vaccines are undergoing field trials. Discussion is beyond the scope of this chapter but the reader is referred to Schwarz et al. (2012) and Epstein and Richie (2013) for more information.

AMOEBIASIS AND AMOEBICIDAL DRUGS

The main organism in this group to concern us here is *Entamoeba histolytica*, the causative agent of amoebiasis, which may manifest as a severe colitis (dysentery) and, sometimes, liver abscesses.

▼ The infection is encountered around the world, but more often in warmer climates. Approximately 500 million people are thought to harbour the disease, with 40000–100000 deaths occurring each year as a result (Stanley, 2003). It is considered to be the second leading cause of death from parasitic diseases worldwide.

The organism has a simple life cycle, and humans are the chief hosts. Infection, generally spread by poor hygiene, follows the ingestion of the mature cysts in water or food that is contaminated with human faeces. The infectious cysts pass into the colon, where they develop into trophozoites. These motile organisms adhere to colonic epithe-lial cells, utilising a galactose-containing lectin on the host cell mem-brane. Here, the trophozoites feed, multiply, encyst and eventually pass out in the faeces, thus completing their life cycle. Some indi-viduals are symptomless 'carriers' and harbour the parasite without developing overt disease, but cysts are present in their faeces and they can infect other individuals. The cysts can survive outside the body for at least a week in a moist and cool environment.

Antimalarial drugs

- **Chloroquine** is a blood schizonticide that is concentrated in the parasite and inhibits the haem polymerase. Orally active; half-life 50 h. *Unwanted effects*: gastrointestinal disturbances, dizziness and urticaria. Bolus intravenous injections can cause dysrhythmias. Resistance is now common.
- **Quinine** is a blood schizonticide. It may be given orally or intravenously; half-life 10 h. *Unwanted effects*: gastrointestinal tract disturbances, tinnitus, blurred vision and, in large doses, dysrhythmias and central nervous system disturbances. It is usually given in combination therapy with:
  - **pyrimethamine**, a folate antagonist that acts as a slow blood schizonticide (orally active; half-life 4 days), and either
  - **dapsone**, a sulfone (orally active; half-life 24–48 h), or
  - **sulfadoxine**, a long-acting sulfonamide (orally active; half-life 7–9 days).
- **Proguanil**, a folate antagonist, is a slow blood schizonticide with some action on the primary liver forms of *P. vivax*. Orally active; half-life 16 h.
- **Mefloquine** is a blood schizonticidal agent active against *P. falciparum* and *P. vivax*, and acts by inhibiting the parasite haem polymerase. Orally active; half-life 30 days. The onset of action is slow. *Unwanted effects*: gastrointestinal disturbances, neurotoxicity and psychiatric problems.
- **Primaquine** is effective against the liver hypnozoites and is also active against gametocytes. Orally active; half-life 36 h. *Unwanted effects*: gastrointestinal tract disturbances and, with large doses, methaemoglobinaemia. Erythrocyte haemolysis in individuals with genetic deficiency of glucose 6-phosphate dehydrogenase.
- **Artemisinin** derivatives are now widely used particularly in combination with other drugs such as **lumefantrine**. They are fast-acting blood schizonticidal agents that are effective against both *P. falciparum* and *P. vivax*.
- **Artesunate** is water-soluble and can be given orally or by intravenous, intramuscular or rectal administration. Side effects are rare. Resistance is so far uncommon.
- **Atavoquone** (in combination with **proguanil**) is used for prevention, and for the treatment of, acute uncomplicated *P. falciparum* malaria. The drug combination is effective orally. It is given at regular intervals over 3 to 4 days. *Unwanted effects*: diarrhoea, nausea and vomiting. Resistance to **atavoquone** develops rapidly if it is given alone.

The trophozoite lyses the colonic mucosal cells (hence 'histolytica') using proteases, *amoebapores* (peptides that form pores in cell mem-branes) or by inducing host cell apoptosis. The organism then invades the submucosa, where it secretes factors to modify the host response, which would otherwise prove lethal to the parasite. It is this process that produces the characteristic bloody diarrhoea and abdominal pain, although a chronic intestinal infection may be present in the absence of dysentery. In some patients, an *amoebic granuloma* (amoeboma) may be present in the intestinal wall. The trophozoites may also migrate through the damaged intestinal tissue into the portal blood and hence the liver, giving rise to the most common extra-intestinal symptom of the disease – amoebic liver abscesses.

The use of drugs to treat this condition depends largely on the site and type of infection. The drugs of choice for the various forms of amoebiasis are:

- **metronidazole** (or **tinidazole**) followed by **diloxanide** for acute invasive intestinal amoebiasis resulting in acute severe amoebic dysentery
- diloxanide for chronic intestinal amoebiasis
- metronidazole followed by diloxanide for hepatic amoebiasis
- diloxanide for the carrier state.

These agents are often used in combination.

METRONIDAZOLE

Metronidazole kills the trophozoites of *E. histolytica* but has no effect on the cysts. It is the drug of choice for invasive amoebiasis of the intestine or the liver, but it is less effective against organisms in the lumen of the gut. Metronidazole is activated by anaerobic organisms to a compound that damages DNA, leading to parasite apoptosis.

Metronidazole is usually given orally and is rapidly and completely absorbed. Rectal and intravenous preparations are also available. It is distributed rapidly throughout the tissues, reaching high concentrations in the body fluids, including the cerebrospinal fluid. Some is metabolised, but most is excreted in urine.

Unwanted effects are mild. The drug has a metallic, bitter taste in the mouth but causes few unwanted effects in therapeutic doses. Minor gastrointestinal disturbances have been reported, as have CNS symptoms (dizziness, headache, sensory neuropathies). Metronidazole causes a disulfiram-like reaction to alcohol (see Ch. 49), which should be strictly avoided. Metronidazole should not be used in pregnancy.

Tinidazole is similar to metronidazole in its mechanism of action and unwanted effects, but is eliminated more slowly, having a half-life of 12–14 h.

DILOXANIDE

Diloxanide or, more commonly, an insoluble ester, diloxanide furoate, are the drugs of choice for the asymptomatic infected patient, and are often given as a follow-up after the disease has been reversed with metronidazole. Both drugs have a direct amoebicidal action, affecting the parasites before encystment. Diloxanide furoate is given orally, and acts without being absorbed. Unwanted gastrointestinal or other effects may be seen but it has an excellent safety profile.

Other drugs that are sometimes used include the antibiotic **paromomycin**.

TRYPANOSOMIASIS AND TRYPANOCIDAL DRUGS

Trypanosomes belong to the group of pathogenic flagellate protozoa. Two subtypes of *Trypanosoma brucei* (*rhodesiense* and *gambiense*) cause sleeping sickness in Africa (also called *HAT* – human African trypanosomiasis). In South America,

Drugs used in amoebiasis

Amoebiasis is caused by infection with *E. histolytica*, which causes dysentery and liver abscesses. The organism may be present in motile invasive form or as a cyst. The main drugs are:

- **metronidazole** given orally (half-life 7 h). Active against the invasive form in gut and liver but not the cysts. Unwanted effects (rare); gastrointestinal disturbances and central nervous system symptoms. **Tinidazole** is similar.
- **diloxanide** is given orally with no serious unwanted effects. It is active, while unabsorbed, against the non-invasive form in the gastrointestinal tract.

another species *Trypanosoma cruzi*, causes *Chagas' disease* (also known as American trypanosomiasis). Almost eliminated by 1960, HAT has re-emerged. In 2009 WHO estimated about 30 000 cases, with about 70 million people at risk of contracting sleeping sickness. The disease caused by *T. b. rhodesiense* is the more aggressive form. Civil unrest, famine and AIDS encourage the spread of the disease by reducing the chances of distributing medication or because patients are immunocompromised, but despite this the incidence appears to be dropping. Related trypanosome infections also pose a major risk to livestock and thus have a secondary impact on human health and well-being.

▼ The vector of HAT is the tsetse fly. In both types of disease, there is an initial local lesion at the site of entry, which may (in the case of *T. b. rhodesiense*) develop into a painful *chancre* (ulcer or sore). This is followed by bouts of parasitaemia and fever as the parasite enters the haemolymphatic system. The parasites and the toxins they release during the second phase of the disease cause organ damage. This manifests as 'sleeping sickness' when parasites reach the CNS causing somnolence and progressive neurological breakdown. Left untreated, such infections are fatal.

T. cruzi is spread through other blood-sucking insects, including the 'kissing bugs'. The initial phases of the infection are similar but parasites damage the heart, muscles and sometimes liver, spleen, bone and intestine. Many people harbour chronic infections but the cure rate is good if treatment begins immediately after infection.

The main drugs used for HAT are **suramin**, with **pentamidine** as an alternative, in the haemolymphatic stage of the disease, and the arsenical **melarsoprol** for the late stage with CNS involvement and **eflornithine** (see Burchmore et al., 2002; Burri & Brun, 2003). All have toxic side effects. **Nifurtimox**, eflornithine and **benznidazole** are used in Chagas' disease: however, there is no totally effective treatment for this form of trypanosomiasis.

SURAMIN

Suramin was introduced into the therapy of trypanosomiasis in 1920. The drug binds firmly to host plasma proteins, and the complex enters the trypanosome by endocytosis, then liberated by lysosomal proteases. It inhibits key parasite enzymes inducing gradual destruction of organelles, such that the organisms are cleared from the circulation after a short interval.

The drug is given by slow intravenous injection. The blood concentration drops rapidly during the first few hours and then more slowly over the succeeding days. A residual concentration remains for 3–4 months. Suramin tends to accumulate in mononuclear phagocytes, and in the cells of the proximal tubule in the kidney.

Unwanted effects are common. Suramin is relatively toxic, particularly in a malnourished patient, the main organ affected being the kidney. Many other slowly developing adverse effects have been reported, including optic atrophy, adrenal insufficiency, skin rashes, haemolytic anaemia and agranulocytosis. A small proportion of individuals have an immediate idiosyncratic reaction to suramin injection that may include nausea, vomiting, shock, seizures and loss of consciousness.

PENTAMIDINE

Pentamidine has a direct trypanocidal action *in vitro*. It is rapidly taken up in the parasites by a high-affinity energy-dependent carrier and is thought to interact with their DNA. The drug is administered intravenously or by deep intramuscular injection, usually daily for 10–15 days. After absorption from the injection site, it binds strongly to tissues (especially the kidney) and is eliminated slowly, only 50% of a dose being excreted over 5 days. Fairly high concentrations of the drug persist in the kidney, the liver and the spleen for several months, but it does not penetrate the blood–brain barrier. It is also active in *Pneumocystis* pneumonia (Ch. 51). Its usefulness is limited by its unwanted effects – an immediate decrease in blood pressure, with tachycardia, breathlessness and vomiting, and later serious toxicity, such as kidney damage, hepatic impairment, blood dyscrasias and hypoglycaemia.

MELARPROSOL

▼ This is an organic arsenical compound that is used mainly when the CNS is involved. It is given intravenously and enters the CNS in high concentrations, where it is able to kill the parasite. It is a highly toxic drug that produces many unwanted effects including encephalopathy and, sometimes, immediate fatality. As such, it is only administered under strict supervision.

EFLORNITHINE

▼ Eflornithine inhibits the parasite ornithine decarboxylase enzyme. It shows good activity against *T. b. gambiense* and is used as a back-up for melarsoprol, although unfortunately it has limited activity against *T. b. rhodesiense*. Side effects are common and may be severe, but are readily reversed when treatment is discontinued.

There is an urgent need for new agents to treat trypanasome infections, partly because of the toxicity of existing drugs and partly because of developing drug resistance. There is some cause for optimism and new agents, and new treatment modalities, may be forthcoming in the medium term (Barrett, 2010; Brun et al., 2011).

OTHER PROTOZOAL INFECTIONS AND DRUGS USED TO TREAT THEM

LEISHMANIASIS

Leishmania organisms are flagellate protozoa and *leishmaniasis*, the infection that they cause, is spread by the sandfly. According to the WHO (2013 figures) the incidence of the disease is increasing with some 1.3 million new cases and 20000–30000 deaths recorded each year. With increasing international travel, leishmaniasis is being imported into new areas and opportunistic infections are now being reported (particularly in AIDS patients).

▼ The vector is the female sandfly. The parasite exists as a flagellated form (promastigote) in the gut of the infected insect, and a non-flagellated intracellular form (amastigote) in the mononuclear phagocytes of the infected mammalian host. Within these cells, the parasites thrive in modified phagolysosomes. By deploying an array of countermeasures (Singh et al., 2012), they promote the generation of Th2 cytokines and subvert the macrophage's microbiocidal systems to ensure their survival. The amastigotes multiply, and eventually the infected cell releases a new crop of parasites into the haemolymphatic system, where they can infect further macrophages and possibly other cells.

Different species of *Leishmania* exist in different geographical areas and cause distinctive clinical manifestations (see Table 54.1). Typical presentations include:

- a *cutaneous form*, which presents as an unpleasant chancre ('oriental sore', 'Chiclero's ulcer' and other names) that may heal spontaneously but can leave scarring. This is the most common form and is found in the Americas, some Mediterranean countries and parts of central Asia;
- a *mucocutaneous form* ('espundia' and other names), which presents as large ulcers of the mucous membranes of the mouth, nose and throat; most cases are seen in South America;
- a serious *visceral form* ('kala-azar' and other names), where the parasite spreads through the bloodstream and causes hepatomegaly, splenomegaly, anaemia and intermittent fever. This manifestation is encountered mainly in the Indian subcontinent and West Africa.

The main drugs used in visceral leishmaniasis are pentavalent antimony compounds such as **sodium stibogluconate** and pentamidine as well as **amphotericin** (see Ch. 53), which is sometimes used as a follow-up treatment. **Miltefosine**, an antitumour drug, is also used in some countries (not UK), as is **meglumine antimoniate**.

Sodium stibogluconate is given intramuscularly or by slow intravenous injection in a 10-day course. It is rapidly eliminated in the urine, 70% being excreted within 6 h. More than one course of treatment may be required.

Unwanted effects include anorexia, vomiting, bradycardia and hypotension. Coughing and substernal pain may occur during intravenous infusion. Reversible hepatitis and pancreatitis are common. The mechanism of action of sodium stibogluconate is not clear, but the drug may increase production of toxic oxygen free radicals in the parasite.

Miltefosine (hexadecylphosphocholine) is also effective in the treatment of both cutaneous and visceral leishmaniasis. The drug may be given orally and is well tolerated. Side effects are mild and include nausea and vomiting. *In vitro*, the drug induces DNA fragmentation and apoptosis in the parasites

Other drugs, such as antibiotics and antifungals, may be given concomitantly with the above agents. They may have some action on the parasite in their own right, but their main utility is to control the spread of secondary infections.

Resistance to current drugs, particularly the pentavalent antimonials (possibly caused by increased expression of an antimonial efflux pump), is a serious problem and there is no immediate prospect of a vaccine. The pharmacology of current drugs and prospects for new agents is reviewed by Singh et al. (2012).

TRICHOMONIASIS

The principal *Trichomonas* organism that produces disease in humans is *T. vaginalis*. Virulent strains cause inflammation of the vagina and sometimes of the urethra in males. The main drug used in therapy is metronidazole (Ch. 51), although resistance to this drug is on the increase.

High doses of tinidazole are also effective, with few side effects.

GIARDIASIS

Giardia lamblia colonises the upper gastrointestinal tract in its trophozoite form, and the cysts pass out in the faeces. Infection is then spread by ingestion of food or water contaminated with faecal matter containing the cysts. It is encountered worldwide, and epidemics caused by bad sanitation are not uncommon. Metronidazole is the drug of choice, and treatment is usually very effective. Tinidazole or **mepacrine** may be used as an alternative.

TOXOPLASMOSIS

The cat is the definitive host of *Toxoplasma gondii*, a pathogenic member of this group of organisms (i.e. it is the only host in which the sexual cycle can occur). It expels the infectious cysts in its faeces; humans can inadvertently become intermediate hosts, harbouring the asexual form of the parasite. Ingested oocysts develop into sporozoites, then to trophozoites, and finally encyst in the tissues. In most individuals, the disease is asymptomatic or self-limiting, although intrauterine infections can severely damage the developing fetus and it may cause fatal generalised infection in immunosuppressed patients or those with AIDS, in whom toxoplasmic encephalitis may occur. In humans, *T. gondii* infects numerous cell types and has a highly virulent replicative stage.

The treatment of choice is pyrimethamine–sulfadiazine (to be avoided in **pregnant** patients); trimethoprim–**sulfamethoxazole** (co-trimoxazole, see Ch. 51) or combinations of pyrimethamine with **clindamycin**, **clarithromycin** or **azithromycin** (see Ch. 51) have shown promise.

PNEUMOCYSTIS

First recognised in 1909, *Pneumocystis carinii* (now known as *P. jirovecii*; see also Ch. 53) shares structural features with both protozoa and fungi, leaving its precise classification uncertain. Previously considered to be a widely distributed but largely innocuous microorganism, it is now recognised as an important cause of opportunistic infections in immunocompromised patients. It is common in AIDS, where *P. carinii* pneumonia is often the presenting symptom as well as a leading cause of death.

High-dose **co-trimoxazole** (Ch. 50) is the drug of choice in serious cases, with parenteral pentamidine as an alternative. Treatment of milder forms of the disease (or prophylaxis) can be effected with atovaquone, trimethoprim–dapsone, or clindamycin–primaquine combinations.

FUTURE DEVELOPMENTS

This field is a huge global challenge, with each species posing its own distinct problems to the would-be designer of new antiprotozoal drugs.

Transnational initiatives (e.g. Medicines for Malaria Venture and Institute for OneWorld Health) are now major players in the development of new medicines for protozoal diseases. But it is not simply a lack of new drugs that is the problem: for economic reasons, the countries and populations most affected often lack an efficient infrastructure for the distribution and safe administration of the drugs that we already possess. Cultural attitudes, civil wars, famine, the circulation of counterfeit or defective drugs, drought and natural disasters also exacerbate this problem.

REFERENCES AND FURTHER READING

Host–parasite interactions

Brenier-Pinchart, M.-P., Pelloux, H., Derouich-Guergour, D., et al., 2001. Chemokines in host–parasite interactions. Trends Parasitol. 17, 292–296. (*Good review of role of immune system*)

Malaria

Baird, J.K., 2005. Effectiveness of antimalarial drugs. N. Engl. J. Med. 352, 1565–1577. (*An excellent overview covering many aspects of drug therapy, drug resistance and the socioeconomic factors affecting the treatment of this disease – thoroughly recommended*)

Butler, A.R., Khan, S., Ferguson, E., 2010. A brief history of malaria chemotherapy. J. R. Coll. Phys. Edinb. 40, 172–177. (*Deals with the subject from a historical perspective beginning with the discovery of quinine and including recent developments in artemisinin synthesis. Good overview*)

Eckstein-Ludwig, U., Webb, R.J., Van Goethem, I.D., et al., 2003. Artemisinins target the SERCA of Plasmodium falciparum. Nature 424, 957–961. (*Research paper that elucidates the site of action of artemisinin drugs*)

Epstein, J.E., Richie, T.L., 2013. The whole parasite, pre-erythrocytic stage approach to malaria vaccine development: a review. Curr. Opin. Infect. Dis. 26, 420–428. (*A largely optimistic assessment of the successes of a novel malaria candidate vaccine. Fascinating reading*)

Ezzet, F., Mull, R., Karbwang, J., 1998. Population pharmacokinetics and therapeutic response of CGP 56697 (artemether + benflumetol) in malaria patients. Br. J. Clin. Pharmacol. 46, 553–561. (*Deals with the pharmacokinetics of this increasingly important combination therapy*)

Fidock, D.A., Rosenthal, P.J., Croft, S.L., et al., 2004. Antimalarial drug discovery: efficacy models for compound screening. Nat. Rev. Drug Discov. 3, 509–520. (*Useful review dealing with mechanisms of antimalarial drug action and new concepts for screening future candidates*)

Foley, M., Tilley, L., 1997. Quinoline antimalarials: mechanisms of action and resistance. Int. J. Parasitol. 27, 231–240. (*Good, short review; useful diagrams*)

Greenwood, B.M., Fidock, D.A., Kyle, D.E., et al., 2008. Malaria: progress, perils, and prospects for eradication. J. Clin. Invest. 118, 1266–1276. (*Good overview of the disease, its current and future treatment*)

Lanteri, C.A., Johnson, J.D., Waters, N.C., 2007. Recent advances in malaria drug discovery. Recent. Pat. Antiinfect. Drug Discov. 2, 95–114. (*This comprehensive review focuses mainly upon chemical leads but also has a good section on drug targets and ways of optimising existing therapies*)

Muregi, F.W., Wamakima, H.N., Kimani, F.T., 2012. Novel drug targets in malaria parasite with potential to yield antimalarial drugs with long useful therapeutic lives. Cur. Pharm. Des. 18, 3505–3521. (*Good account of anti-malarial pharmacology and how their usage might be improved*)

Na-Bangchang, K., Karbwang, J., 2009. Current status of malaria chemotherapy and the role of pharmacology in antimalarial drug research and development. Fund. Clin. Pharmacol. 23, 387–409. (*Excellent overview of the whole area stressing the contribution that pharmacology makes to the development of new drugs. Highly recommended*)

O'Brien, C., 1997. Beating the malaria parasite at its own game. Lancet 350, 192. (*Clear, succinct coverage of mechanisms of action and resistance of current antimalarials and potential new drugs; useful diagram*)

Odeh, M., 2001. The role of tumour necrosis factor-alpha in the pathogenesis of complicated falciparum malaria. Cytokine 14, 11–18.

Paddon, C.J., Westfall, P.J., Pitera, D.J., et al., 2013. High-level semi-synthetic production of the potent antimalarial artemisinin. Nature 25, 528–532. (*The use of synthetic biology techniques to produce artemesinic acid in yeast so that the global supply of artemisinin can be increased. A real tour de force*)

Shanks, G.D., Kain, K.C., Keystone, J.S., 2001. Malaria chemoprophylaxis in the age of drug resistance. II. Drugs that may be available in the future. Clin. Infect. Dis. 33, 381–385. (*A useful look ahead to new drugs*)

Schwartz, L., Brown, G.V., Genton, B., Moorthy, V.S., 2012. A review of malaria vaccine clinical projects based on the WHO rainbow table. Mal. J. 11, 11.

Tschan, S., Kremsner, P.G., Mordmuller, B., 2012. Emerging drugs for malaria. Exp. Opin. Emerg. Drugs 17, 319–333. (*A critical account of the development of novel anti-malarials*)

Amoebiasis

Haque, R., Huston, C.D., Hughes, M., et al., 2003. Amebiasis. N. Engl. J. Med. 348, 1565–1573. (*Good review; concentrates on the pathogenesis of the disease but has a useful table of drugs and their side effects*)

Stanley, S.L., 2001. Pathophysiology of amoebiasis. Trends Parasitol. 17, 280–285. (*A good account of the human disease that incorporates some results from animal models also*)

Stanley, S.L., 2003. Amoebiasis. Lancet 361, 1025–1034. (*Comprehensive and easy-to-read account of this disease, covering all aspects from diagnosis to treatment. Excellent*)

Trypanosomiasis

Aksoy, S., Gibson, W.C., Lehane, M.J., 2003. Interactions between tsetse and trypanosomes with implications for the control of trypanosomiasis. Adv. Parasitol. 53, 1–83. (*A very substantial and comprehensive article covering the biology of the tsetse fly, which also discusses alternative methods from controlling the insect population. Less good on drug therapy, but if you are interested in the biology of the insect vector of trypanosomiasis, then this is for you*)

Barrett, M.P., 2010. Potential new drugs for human African trypanosomiasis: some progress at last. Curr. Opin. Infect. Dis. 23, 603–608. (*An account of the pharmacology of current trypanicides and ways in which their usage might be improved. Discusses how new agents might be developed using (for example) a systems biology approach*)

Brun, R., Don, R., Jacobs, R.T., Wang, M.Z., Barrett, M.P., 2011. Development of novel drugs for human African trypanosomiasis. Fut. Microbiol. 6, 677–691.

Burchmore, R.J., Ogbunude, P.O., Enanga, B., Barrett, M.P., 2002. Chemotherapy of human African trypanosomiasis. Curr. Pharm. Des. 8, 256–267. (*Very good concise article; nice discussion of future therapeutic possibilities*)

Burri, C., Brun, R., 2003. Eflornithine for the treatment of human African trypanosomiasis. Parasitol. Res. 90 (Suppl. 1), S49–S52. (*The title is self-explanatory*)

Denise, H., Barrett, M.P., 2001. Uptake and mode of action of drugs used against sleeping sickness. Biochem. Pharmacol. 61, 1–5. (*Good coverage of drug therapy*)

Gehrig, S., Efferth, T., 2008. Development of drug resistance in *Trypanosoma brucei rhodesiense* and *Trypanosoma brucei gambiense*. Treatment of human African trypanosomiasis with natural products (Review). Int. J. Mol. Med. 22, 411–419. (*Good overview of drug therapy including sections on mechanisms of drug resistance*)

Keiser, J., Stich, A., Burri, C., 2001. New drugs for the treatment of human African trypanosomiasis: research and development. Trends Parasitol. 17, 42–49. (*Excellent review on an increasingly threatening disease*)

Legros, D., Ollivier, G., Gastellu-Etchegorry, M., et al., 2002. Treatment of human African trypanosomiasis – present situation and needs for research and development. Lancet Infect. Dis. 2, 437–440.

Leishmaniasis

Handman, E., Bullen, D.V.R., 2002. Interaction of *Leishmania* with the host macrophage. Trends Parasitol. 18, 332–334. (*Very good article describing how this parasite colonises macrophages and evades intracellular killing; easy to read*)

Kumari, S., Kumar, A., Samant, M., et al., 2008. Discovery of novel vaccine candidates and drug targets against visceral leishmaniasis using proteomics and transcriptomics. Curr. Drug Targets 9, 938–947. (*Reviews the use of sophisticated bioinformatic tools to facilitate the development of new vaccines*)

Mishra, J., Saxena, A., Singh, S., 2007. Chemotherapy of leishmaniasis: past, present and future. Curr. Med. Chem. 14, 1153–1169. (*Self-explanatory title!*)

Singh, N., Kumar, M., Singh, R.K., 2012. Leishmaniasis: current status of available drugs and new potential drug targets. As. Pac. J. Trop. Med. 5, 485–497. (*Excellent article dealing with the use of drugs to combat leishmaniasis. Also deals with resistance mechanisms in some detail. Highly recommended*)

Pneumocystis pneumonia

Warren, E., George, S., You, J., Kazanjian, P., 1997. Advances in the treatment and prophylaxis of *Pneumocystis carinii* pneumonia. Pharmacotherapy 17, 900–916.

Useful Web resources

<http://malaria.who.int/> (*The WHO home page containing the major information on malaria – a terrific starting point for further investigation. Other who.int sites cover trypanosomiasis, leishmaniasis and other important protozozoal diseases*)

(*The Web page of the Medicines for Malaria Venture, a private–public partnership established to bring together funding and expertise from a number of sources to tackle malaria*)

<www.oneworldhealth.org> (*The Web page of the visionary 'non-profit pharmaceutical company', with details of their current programmes dealing with global health issues*)

Anthelmintic drugs

55

OVERVIEW

Some 2 billion people around the world suffer from *helminthiasis* **– infection with various species of parasitic** *helminths* **(worms). Inhabitants of tropical or subtropical low-income countries are most at risk; children often become infected at birth and may remain so throughout their lives and polyparasitaemia is common. Helminthiasis is often co-endemic with malaria, TB and HIV/AIDS, adding to the disease burden as well as interfering with vaccination campaigns. The clinical consequences of helminthiasis vary: for example, threadworm infections mainly cause discomfort but infection with** *schistosomiasis* **(***bilharzia***) or hookworm is associated with serious morbidity. Worm infections are an even greater cause for concern in veterinary medicine, affecting both domestic pets and farm animals. In some parts of the world,** *fascioliasis* **is associated with significant loss of livestock. Because of its prevalence and economic significance, the pharmacological treatment of helminthiasis is therefore of great practical therapeutic importance.**

HELMINTH INFECTIONS

The helminths comprise two major groups: the *nemathelminths* (nematodes, roundworms) and the *platyhelminths* (flatworms). The latter group is subdivided into the *trematodes* (flukes) and the *cestodes* (tapeworms). Almost 350 species of helminths have been found in humans, and most colonise the gastrointestinal tract. The global range and occurrence of helminthiasis has been reviewed by Lustigman et al. (2012).

Helminths have a complex life cycle, often involving several host species. Infection may occur in many ways, with poor hygiene a major contributory factor. Many enter by the mouth in unpurified drinking water or in undercooked flesh from infected animals or fish. However, species can enter through the skin following a cut, an insect bite or even after swimming or walking on infected soil. Humans are generally the *primary* (or *definitive*) host for helminth infections, in the sense that they harbour the sexually mature reproductive form. Eggs or larvae then pass out of the body and infect the *secondary* (*intermediate*) host. In some cases, the eggs or larvae may persist in the human host and become *encysted*, covered with granulation tissue, giving rise to *cysticercosis*. Encysted larvae may lodge in the muscles and viscera or, more seriously, in the eye or the brain.

Approximately 20 helminth species are considered to be clinically significant and these fall into two main categories – those in which the worm lives in the host's alimentary canal, and those in which the worm lives in other tissues of the host's body.

The main examples of intestinal worms are:

- *Tapeworms*: *Taenia saginata*, *Taenia solium*, *Hymenolepis nana* and *Diphyllobothrium latum*. Some 85 million people in Asia, Africa and parts of America harbour one or other of these tapeworm species. Only the first two are likely to be seen in the UK. Cattle and pigs are the usual intermediate hosts of the most common tapeworms (*T. saginata* and *T. solium*). Humans become infected by eating raw or undercooked meat containing the larvae, which have encysted in the animals' muscle tissue. *H. nana* may exist as both the adult (the intestinal worm) and the larval stage in the same host, which may be human or rodent, although some insects (fleas, grain beetles) can also serve as intermediate hosts. The infection is usually asymptomatic. *D. latum* has two sequential intermediate hosts: a freshwater crustacean and a freshwater fish. Humans become infected by eating raw or incompletely cooked fish containing the larvae.
- *Intestinal roundworms*: *Ascaris lumbricoides* (common roundworm), *Enterobius vermicularis* (threadworm, called pinworm in the USA), *Trichuris trichiura* (whipworm), *Strongyloides stercoralis* (threadworm in the USA), *Necator americanus* and *Ancylostoma duodenale* (hookworms). Again, undercooked meat or contaminated food is an important cause of infection by roundworm, threadworm and whipworm, whereas hookworm is generally acquired when their larvae penetrate the skin. Intestinal blood loss is a common cause of anaemia in regions where hookworm is endemic.

The main examples of worms that live elsewhere in host tissues are:

- *Flukes*: *Schistosoma haematobium*, *Schistosoma mansoni* and *Schistosoma japonicum*. These cause schistosomiasis (bilharzia). The adult worms of both sexes live and mate in the veins or venules of the bladder or the gut wall. The female lays eggs that pass into the bladder or gut triggering inflammation in these organs. This results in haematuria in the former case and, occasionally, loss of blood in the faeces in the latter. The eggs hatch in water after discharge from the body and thus enter the secondary host – a particular species of snail. After a period of development in this host, free-swimming *cercariae* emerge. These are capable of infecting humans by penetration of the skin. About 200 million people are infected with one or other of the schistosomes.
- *Tissue roundworms*: *Trichinella spiralis*, *Dracunculus medinensis* (*guinea worm*) and the *filariae*, which include *Wuchereria bancrofti*, *Loa loa*, *Onchocerca volvulus* and *Brugia malayi*. The adult filariae live in

671

the lymphatics, connective tissues or mesentery of the host and produce live embryos or *microfilariae*, which find their way into the bloodstream and may be ingested by mosquitoes or other biting insects. After a period of development within this secondary host, the larvae pass to the mouth parts of the insect and thus infect the next victim. Major filarial diseases are caused by *Wuchereria* or *Brugia*, which cause obstruction of lymphatic vessels, producing *elephantiasis* – hugely swollen legs. Other related diseases are *onchocerciasis* (in which the presence of microfilariae in the eye causes 'river blindness' – a leading preventable cause of blindness in Africa and Latin America) and *loiasis* (in which the microfilariae cause inflammation in the skin and other tissues). *Trichinella spiralis* causes trichinosis; the larvae from the viviparous female worms in the intestine migrate to skeletal muscle, where they become encysted. In *guinea worm disease*,[1] larvae of *D. medinensis* released from crustaceans in wells and waterholes are ingested and migrate from the intestinal tract to mature and mate in the tissues; the gravid female then migrates to the subcutaneous tissues of the leg or the foot, and may protrude through an ulcer in the skin. The worm may be up to a metre in length and has to be removed surgically or by slow mechanical winding of the worm on to a stick over a period of days.

- *Hydatid tapeworm.* These are cestodes of the *Echinococcus* species for which dogs are the primary hosts, and sheep the intermediate hosts. The primary, intestinal stage does not occur in humans, but under certain circumstances humans can function as the intermediate host, in which case the larvae develop into *hydatid cysts* within the tissues, sometimes with fatal consequences.

Some nematodes that generally live in the gastrointestinal tract of animals may infect humans and penetrate tissues. A skin infestation, termed *creeping eruption* or *cutaneous larva migrans*, is caused by the larvae of dog and cat hookworms which often enter through the foot. Visceral larva migrans is caused by larvae of cat and dog roundworms of the *Toxocara* genus.

ANTHELMINTIC DRUGS

The first effective anthelmintic drugs were discovered in the 20th century and incorporated toxic metals such as arsenic (*atoxyl*) or antimony (*tartar emetic*). They were used to treat trypanosome and schistosome infestations.

Current anthelmintic drugs act by paralysing the parasite (e.g. by preventing muscular contraction), by damaging the worm such that the host immune system can eliminate it, or by altering parasite metabolism (e.g. by affecting microtubule function). Because the metabolic requirements of these parasites vary greatly from one species to another, drugs that are highly effective against one type of worm may be ineffective against others. To bring about its action, the drug must penetrate the tough exterior cuticle of the worm or gain access to its alimentary tract. This may present difficulties, because some worms are exclusively *haemophagous* ('blood-eating'), while others are best described as 'tissue grazers'. A

further complication is that many helminths possess active drug efflux pumps that reduce the concentration of the drug in the parasite. The route of administration and dose of anthelmintic drugs are therefore important. In a reversal of the normal order of things, several anthelmintic drugs used in human medicine were originally developed for veterinary use.

Some individual anthelmintic drugs are described briefly below and indications for their use are given in Table 55.1. Several of these drugs (e.g. **albendazole, ivermectin, levamisole**) are unlicensed in the UK and used on a 'named patient' basis.[2]

BENZIMIDAZOLES

This group includes **mebendazole, tiabendazole** and **albendazole,** which are widely used broad-spectrum anthelmintics. They are thought to act by inhibiting the polymerisation of helminth β-tubulin, thus interfering with microtubule-dependent functions such as glucose uptake. They have a selective inhibitory action, being 250–400 times more effective in producing this effect in helminth, than in mammalian, tissue. However, the effect takes time to develop and the worms may not be expelled for several days. Cure rates are generally between 60% and 100% with most parasites.

Only 10% of mebendazole is absorbed after oral administration, but a fatty meal increases absorption. It is rapidly metabolised, the products being excreted in the urine and the bile within 24–48 h. It is generally given as a single dose for threadworm, and twice daily for 3 days for hookworm and roundworm infestations. Tiabendazole is rapidly absorbed from the gastrointestinal tract, very rapidly metabolised and excreted in the urine in conjugated form. It may be given twice daily for 3 days for guinea worm and *Strongyloides* infestations, and for up to 5 days for hookworm and roundworm infestations. Albendazole is also poorly absorbed but, as with mebendazole, absorption is increased by food, especially fats. It is metabolised extensively by presystemic metabolism to sulfoxide and sulfone metabolites. The former is likely to be the pharmacologically active species.

Unwanted effects are few with albendazole or mebendazole, although gastrointestinal disturbances can occasionally occur. Unwanted effects with tiabendazole are more frequent but usually transient, the commonest being gastrointestinal disturbances, although headache, dizziness and drowsiness have been reported and allergic reactions (fever, rashes) may also occur. Mebendazole is considered unsuitable for pregnant women or children less than 2 years old.

PRAZIQUANTEL

Praziquantel is a highly effective broad-spectrum anthelmintic drug that was introduced over 20 years ago. It is the drug of choice for all forms of schistosomiasis and is the agent generally used in large-scale schistosome eradication programmes. It is also effective in cysticercosis. The drug affects not only the adult schistosomes

---

[1]Now, happily, eliminated from many parts of the world.

[2]A situation in which the physician seeks access to an unlicensed drug from a pharmaceutical company to use in a named individual. The drug is either a 'newcomer' that has shown particular promise in clinical trials but has not yet been licensed or, as in these instances, an established drug that has not been licensed because the company has not applied for a product license for this indication (possibly for commercial reasons).

Table 55.1 Principal drugs used in helminth infections and some common indications

	Helminth	Principal drug(s) used
Threadworm (pinworm)	*Enterobius vermicularis*	Mebendazole, piperazine
	Strongyloides stercoralis (threadworm in the USA)	Albendazole
Common roundworm	*Ascaris lumbricoides*	Levamisole, mebendazole, piperazine
Other roundworm (filariae)	Lymphatic filariasis 'elephantiasis'. (*Wuchereria bancrofti*, *Brugia malayi*)	Diethylcarbamazine, ivermectin
	Subcutaneous filariasis 'eyeworm' (*Loa loa*)	Diethylcarbamazine
	Onchocerciasis 'river blindness' (*Onchocerca volvulus*)	Ivermectin
	Guinea worm (*Dracunculus medinensis*)	Praziquantel, mebendazole
	Trichiniasis (*Trichinella spiralis*)	Tiabendazole, mebendazole
	Cysticercosis (infection with larval *Taenia solium*)	Praziquantel, albendazole
	Tapeworm (*Taenia saginata*, *Taenia solium*)	Praziquantel, niclosamide
	Hydatid disease (*Echinococcus granulosus*)	Albendazole
	Hookworm (*Ancylostoma duodenale*, *Necator americanus*)	Mebendazole, albendazole
	Whipworm (*Trichuris trichiura*)	Mebendazole, albendazole, diethylcarbamazine
Blood flukes (*Schistosoma* spp.)	Bilharziasis: *S. haematobium*, *S. mansoni*, *S. japonicum*	Praziquantel
Cutaneous larva migrans	*Ancylostoma caninum*	Albendazole, tiabendazole, ivermectin
Visceral larva migrans	*Toxocara canis*	Albendazole, tiabendazole, diethylcarbamazine

but also the immature forms and the cercariae – the form of the parasite that infects humans by penetrating the skin.

It disrupts Ca^{2+} homeostasis in the parasite by binding to consensus protein kinase C-binding sites in a β subunit of schistosome voltage-gated calcium channels (Greenberg, 2005). This induces an influx of Ca^{2+}, a rapid and prolonged contraction of the musculature, and eventual paralysis and death of the worm. Praziquantel also disrupts the tegument of the parasite, unmasking novel antigens, and as a result it may become more susceptible to the host's normal immune responses.

Given orally, praziquantel is well absorbed; much of the drug is rapidly metabolised to inactive metabolites on first passage through the liver, and the metabolites are excreted in the urine. The plasma half-life of the parent compound is 60–90 min.

Praziquantel has minimal side effects in therapeutic dosage. Such unwanted effects as do occur are usually transitory and rarely of clinical importance. Effects may be more marked in patients with a heavy worm load because of products released from the dead worms. Praziquantel is considered safe for pregnant and lactating women, an important property for a drug that is commonly used in national disease control programmes. Some resistance has developed to the drug.

PIPERAZINE

Piperazine can be used to treat infections with the common roundworm (*A. lumbricoides*) and the threadworm (*E. vermicularis*). It reversibly inhibits neuromuscular transmission in the worm, probably by mimicking GABA (Ch. 38), at GABA-gated chloride channels in nematode muscle.

The paralysed worms are expelled alive by normal intestinal peristaltic movements. It is administered with a stimulant laxative such as **senna** (Ch. 30) to facilitate expulsion of the worms.

Piperazine is given orally and some, but not all, is absorbed. It is partly metabolised, and the remainder is eliminated, unchanged, via the kidney. The drug has little pharmacological action in the host. When used to treat roundworm, piperazine is effective in a single dose. For threadworm, a longer course (7 days) at lower dosage is necessary.

Unwanted effects may include gastrointestinal disturbances, urticaria and bronchospasm. Some patients experience dizziness, paraesthesias, vertigo and incoordination. The drug should not be given to pregnant patients or to those with compromised renal or hepatic function.

NICLOSAMIDE

Niclosamide is widely used for the treatment of tapeworm infections together with praziquantel. The *scolex* (the head of the worm that attaches to the host intestine) and a proximal segment are irreversibly damaged by the drug, such that the worm separates from the intestinal wall and is expelled. For *T. solium*, the drug is given in a single dose after a light meal, usually followed by a purgative 2 h later in case the damaged tapeworm segments release ova, which are not affected by the drug. For other tapeworm infections, this precaution is not necessary. There is negligible absorption of the drug from the gastrointestinal tract.

Unwanted effects: nausea, vomiting, pruritus and lightheadedness may occur but generally such effects are few, infrequent and transient.

DIETHYLCARBAMAZINE

Diethylcarbamazine is a piperazine derivative that is active in filarial infections caused by *B. malayi*, *W. bancrofti* and *L. loa*. Diethylcarbamazine rapidly removes the microfilariae from the blood circulation and has a limited effect on the adult worms in the lymphatics, but it has little action on microfilariae *in vitro*. It may act by changing the parasite such that it becomes susceptible to the host's normal immune responses. It may also interfere with helminth arachidonate metabolism.

The drug is absorbed following oral administration and is distributed throughout the cells and tissues of the body, excepting adipose tissue. It is partly metabolised, and both the parent drug and its metabolites are excreted in the urine, being cleared from the body within about 48 h.

Unwanted effects are common but transient, subsiding within a day or so even if the drug is continued. Side effects from the drug itself include gastrointestinal disturbances, joint pain, headache and a general feeling of weakness. Allergic side effects referable to the products of the dying filariae are common and vary with the species of worm. In general, these start during the first day's treatment and last 3–7 days; they include skin reactions, enlargement of lymph glands, dizziness, tachycardia, and gastrointestinal and respiratory disturbances. When these symptoms disappear, larger doses of the drug can be given without further problem. The drug is not used in patients with onchocerciasis, in whom it can have serious unwanted effects.

LEVAMISOLE

Levamisole is effective in infections with the common roundworm (*A. lumbricoides*). It has a nicotine-like action (Ch. 13), stimulating and subsequently blocking the neuromuscular junctions. The paralysed worms are then expelled in the faeces. Ova are not killed. The drug is given orally, is rapidly absorbed and is widely distributed. It crosses the blood–brain barrier. It is metabolised in the liver to inactive metabolites, which are excreted via the kidney. Its plasma half-life is 4 h. It has immunomodulatory effects and has in the past been used to treat various solid tumours.

It can cause gastrointestinal disturbance but also more serious effects, notably agranulocytosis, and it has been withdrawn from North American markets..

IVERMECTIN

First introduced in 1981 as a veterinary drug, **ivermectin** is a safe and highly effective broad-spectrum antiparasitic in humans. It is frequently used in global public health campaigns,[3] and is the first choice of drug for the treatment of many filarial infections. It has also given good results against *W. bancrofti*, which causes elephantiasis. A single dose kills the immature microfilariae of *O. volvulus* but not the adult worms. Ivermectin is also the drug of choice for onchocerciasis, which causes river blindness and reduces the incidence of this disease by up to 80%. It is also active against some roundworms: common roundworms, whipworms, and threadworms of both the UK (*E. vermicularis*) and the US variety (*S. stercoralis*), but not hookworms.

Chemically, ivermectin is a semisynthetic agent derived from a group of natural substances, the *avermectins*,

obtained from an actinomycete organism. The drug is given orally and has a half-life of 11 h. It is thought to kill the worm either by opening glutamate-gated chloride channels (found only in invertebrates) and increasing Cl^- conductance; by binding to a novel allosteric site on the acetylcholine nicotinic receptor to cause an increase in transmission, leading to motor paralysis; or by binding to GABA receptors.

Unwanted effects include skin rashes and itching but in general the drug is very well tolerated. One interesting exception in veterinary medicine is the central nervous system (CNS) toxicity seen in Collie dogs.[4]

RESISTANCE TO ANTHELMINTIC DRUGS

Resistance to anthelmintic drugs is a widespread and growing problem affecting not only humans but also the animal health market. During the 1990s, helminth infections in sheep (and, to a lesser extent, cattle) developed varying degrees of resistance to a number of different drugs. Parasites that develop such resistance pass this ability on to their offspring, leading to treatment failure. The widespread use of anthelmintic agents in farming has been blamed for the spread of resistant species.

There are probably several molecular mechanisms that contribute to drug resistance. The presence of the P-glycoprotein transporter (Ch. 9) in some species of nematode has already been mentioned, and agents such as **verapamil** that block the transporter in trypanosomes can partially reverse resistance to the benzimidazoles. However, some aspects of benzimidazole resistance may be attributed to alterations in their high-affinity binding to parasite β-tubulin. Likewise, resistance to levamisole is associated with changes in the structure of the target acetylcholine nicotinic receptor.

Of great significance is the way in which helminths evade the host's immune system. Even though they may reside in immunologically exposed sites such as the lymphatics or the bloodstream, many are long-lived and may co-exist with their hosts for many years without seriously affecting their health, or in some cases without even being noticed. It is striking that the two major families of helminths, while evolving separately, deploy similar strategies to evade destruction by the immune system. Clearly, this must be of major survival value for the species.

▼ It appears that many helminths can actually exploit this mechanism by steering the immune system away from a local Th1 response (see Ch. 6), which would be potentially more damaging to the parasite, and promoting instead a modified systemic Th2 type of response. This is associated with the production of 'anti-inflammatory' cytokines such as interleukin-10 favourable to, or at least better tolerated by, the parasites. The immunology underlying this is complex (see Pearce & MacDonald, 2002; Maizels et al., 2004; Harris, 2011).

Ironically, the ability of helminths to modify the host immune response in this way may confer some survival value on the hosts themselves. For example, in addition to the local anti-inflammatory effect exerted by helminth infections, rapid wound healing is also seen. Clearly, this is of advantage to parasites that must penetrate tissues without killing the host, but may also be beneficial to the host as well. It has been proposed that helminth infections may

---

[3]Ivermectin is supplied by the manufacturers free of charge in countries where river blindness is endemic. Because the worms develop slowly, a single annual dose of ivermectin is sufficient to prevent the disease.

[4]A multi-drug-resistance (MDR) gene (see Chs 3 and 51) coding for a transporter that expels ivermectins from the CNS, is mutated to an inactive form in Collie dogs.

mitigate some forms of malaria and other diseases, possibly conferring survival advantages in populations where these diseases are endemic. Indeed, ingestion of helminths by patients has been evaluated as an (admittedly unappealing) strategy to induce remission of Crohn's disease (see Ch. 30; Hunter & McKay, 2004; Reddy & Fried, 2007). On the negative side, helminth infections may undermine the efficacy of tuberculosis vaccination programmes that depend upon a vigorous Th1 response (Elias et al., 2006).

On the basis that Th2 responses reciprocally inhibit the development of Th1 diseases, it has also been hypothesised that the comparative absence of Crohn's disease, as well as some other autoimmune diseases, in the developing world may be associated with the high incidence of parasite infection, and that the rise of these disorders in the West is associated with superior sanitation and reduced helminth infection! This type of argument is generally known as the 'hygiene hypothesis'.

VACCINES AND OTHER NOVEL APPROACHES

Despite the enormity of the clinical problem, there are few novel anthelmintic drugs in development. New candidates such as **tribendimidine** are being assessed in a range of human infections and some new veterinary drugs (e.g. **derquantel**) also tested in humans (see Prichard et al., 2012).

The sequencing of the genomes of several helminths may facilitate the creation of a transgenic species that expresses mutations found in resistant parasitic worms, thus providing insights into the mechanisms underlying resistance. Such databases may also reveal new drug targets, as well as opening the way for other types of anthelmintic agent, such as those based on antisense DNA or small interfering RNA.

Ambitious research agendas have been published enumerating the steps that would be required to eliminate helminth infections (see Boatin et al., 2012, for example) and vaccines are often prominent on the list of essential objectives. Efficacious helminth vaccines would have major benefits. Protein antigens on the surface of the (highly infectious) larval stage have been cloned and used as immunogens, and considerable success has also been achieved in the veterinary field with vaccines to organisms such as *T. ovis* and *E. granulosus* (in sheep) as well as *T. saginata* (in cattle) and *T. solium* (in pigs), with cure rates of 90–100% often reported (see Dalton & Mulcahy, 2001; Garcia, 2007). Qualified success has also been obtained with vaccines to other helminth species (see Capron et al., 2005; McManus & Loukas, 2008). Looking further ahead, it may be possible to develop DNA vaccines rather than protein immunogens to control these organisms.

REFERENCES AND FURTHER READING

General papers on helminths and their diseases

Boatin, B.A., Basanez, M.G., Prichard, R.K., et al., 2012. A research agenda for helminth diseases of humans: towards control and elimination. PLoS Negl. Trop. Dis. 6, e1547. PubMed PMID: 22545161. Pubmed Central PMCID: 3335858. (*Discussion of the overall strategies that would be required to eliminate helminth infections*)

Horton, J., 2003. Human gastrointestinal helminth infections: are they now neglected diseases? Trends Parasitol. 19, 527–531. (*Accessible review on helminth infections and their treatments*)

Lustigman, S., Prichard, R.K., Gazzinelli, A., et al., 2012. A research agenda for helminth diseases of humans: the problem of helminthiases. PLoS Negl. Trop. Dis. 6, e1582. PubMed PMID: 22545164. Pubmed Central PMCID: 3335854. (*Another paper in this series, dealing mainly with the distribution of helminth diseases around the world*)

Anthelmintic drugs

Burkhart, C.N., 2000. Ivermectin: an assessment of its pharmacology, microbiology and safety. Vet. Hum. Toxicol. 42, 30–35. (*Useful paper that focuses on ivermectin pharmacology*)

Croft, S.L., 1997. The current status of antiparasite chemotherapy. Parasitology 114, S3–S15. (*Comprehensive coverage of current drugs and outline of approaches to possible future agents*)

Geary, T.G., Sangster, N.C., Thompson, D.P., 1999. Frontiers in anthelmintic pharmacology. Vet. Parasitol. 84, 275–295. (*Thoughtful account of the difficulties associated with drug treatment*)

Greenberg, R.M., 2005. Are Ca²⁺ channels targets of praziquantel action? Int. J. Parasitol. 35, 1–9. (*Interesting review on praziquantel action*)

Prichard, R., Tait, A., 2001. The role of molecular biology in veterinary parasitology. Vet. Parasitol. 98, 169–194. (*Excellent review of the application of molecular biology to understanding the problem of drug resistance and to the development of new anthelmintic agents*)

Prichard, R.K., Basanez, M.G., Boatin, B.A., et al., 2012. A research agenda for helminth diseases of humans: intervention for control and elimination. PLoS Negl. Trop. Dis. 6, e1549. PubMed PMID: 22545163. Pubmed Central PMCID: 3335868. (*Another paper in this series, providing a useful review of new anthelmintic drugs*)

Robertson, A.P., Bjorn, H.E., Martin, R.J., 2000. Pyrantel resistance alters nematode nicotinic acetylcholine receptor single channel properties. Eur. J. Pharmacol. 394, 1–8. (*A research paper that describing the interactions of praziquantel and levamisole with the nematode nicotinic receptor and a proposed mechanism of drug resistance*)

Anthelmintic vaccines

Capron, A., Riveau, G., Capron, M., Trottein, F., 2005. Schistosomes: the road from host–parasite interactions to vaccines in clinical trials.

Trends Parasitol. 21, 143–149. (*Good general review dealing with the immune response to parasite infection and vaccine development*)

Dalton, J.P., Brindley, P.J., Knox, D.P., et al., 2003. Helminth vaccines: from mining genomic information for vaccine targets to systems used for protein expression. Int. J. Parasitol. 33, 621–640. (*Very comprehensive but may be overcomplicated in parts for the non-specialist*)

Dalton, J.P., Mulcahy, G., 2001. Parasite vaccines – a reality? Vet Parasitol. 98, 149–167. (*Interesting discussion of the promise and pitfalls of vaccines*)

Garcia, H.H., Gonzalez, A.E., Del Brutto, O.H., et al., 2007. Strategies for the elimination of taeniasis/cysticercosis. J. Neurol. Sci. 262, 153–157. (*Discusses the successful attempts to vaccinate pigs against helminth infections and explains how these are applied in the field*)

Harris, N.L., 2011. Advances in helminth immunology: optimism for future vaccine design? Trends Parasitol. 27, 288–293. (*An easy-to-read paper reviewing the latest advances in helminth vaccine immunology. Some good diagrams*)

McManus, D.P., Loukas, A., 2008. Current status of vaccines for schistosomiasis. Clin. Microbiol. Rev. 21, 225–242. (*Very comprehensive survey of the theory and development of vaccines for schistosomiasis*)

Immune evasion by helminths

Cruz-Chan, J.V., Rosado-Vallado, M., Dumonteil, E., 2010. Malaria vaccine efficacy: overcoming the helminth hurdle. Expert Rev. Vaccines 9, 707–711.

Elias, D., Akuffo, H., Britton, S., 2006. Helminths could influence the outcome of vaccines against TB in the tropics. Parasite Immunol. 28, 507–513. (*Easy-to-read introduction to this phenomenon for those who want to follow up this topic*)

Hunter, M.M., McKay, D.M., 2004. Review article: helminths as therapeutic agents for inflammatory bowel disease. Aliment. Pharmacol. Ther. 19, 167–177. (*Fascinating review on potential therapeutic uses of helminths and why they work*)

Maizels, R.M., Balic, A., Gomez-Escobar, N., et al., 2004. Helminth parasites – masters of regulation. Immunol. Rev. 201, 89–116. (*Excellent and very comprehensive review dealing with mechanisms of immune evasion; complicated in parts for the non-specialist*)

Pearce, E.J., MacDonald, A.S., 2002. The immunobiology of schistosomiasis. Nat. Rev. Immunol. 2, 499–512. (*Deals mainly with the immunology of schistosome infections in mice*)

Reddy, A., Fried, B., 2007. The use of *Trichuris suis* and other helminth therapies to treat Crohn's disease. Parasitol. Res. 100, 921–927. (*Excellent review of this interesting therapeutic area*)

56 Anticancer drugs

OVERVIEW

In this chapter we deal with cancer[1] and anticancer drug therapy. We discuss first the pathogenesis of cancer and then describe the drugs that can be used to treat malignant disease. Finally, we consider the extent to which our new knowledge of cancer biology is leading to new therapies. The use of radioactive isotopes in cancer treatment is beyond the scope of this book.

INTRODUCTION

'Cancer' is characterised by uncontrolled multiplication and spread of abnormal forms of the body's own cells. It is the second most common cause of death in the developed nations (cardiovascular disease has the dubious distinction of heading that table) and one in three people will be diagnosed with cancer during their lifetime. According to Cancer Research UK (2013), over 325 000 new cases were reported in the UK in 2010 and mortality was in excess of 157 000 (global figure, 7.4 million). Cancer is responsible for approximately one-quarter of all deaths in the UK. Lung and bowel cancer are the commonest malignancies, closely followed by breast and prostate cancer. Statistics from most other countries in the developed world tell much the same story.

A comparison of the incidence of cancer over the past 100 years or so gives the impression that the disease is increasing in developed countries, but this is not so. Cancer occurs mainly in later life and, with advances in public health and medical science, many more people now live to an age where malignancy is common.

The terms *cancer*, *malignancy* and *malignant tumour* are often used synonymously.[2] Both benign and malignant tumours manifest uncontrolled proliferation, but the latter are distinguished by their capacity for *de-differentiation*, their *invasiveness* and their ability to *metastasise* (spread to other parts of the body). In this chapter, we shall be concerned only with the therapy of malignant disease. The appearance of these abnormal characteristics reflects altered patterns of gene expression in the cancer cells, resulting from inherited or acquired mutations.

There are three main approaches to treating established cancer – *surgical excision*, *irradiation* and *drug therapy* (previously often called *chemotherapy*, but now often including hormonal and biological agents as described below and

in Chs 35 and 59) – and the relative value of each of these approaches depends on the disease and the stage of its development. Drug therapy may be used on its own or as an adjunct to other forms of therapy.

Compared with that of bacterial diseases, cancer chemotherapy presents a difficult conceptual problem. In biochemical terms, microorganisms are both quantitatively and qualitatively different from human cells (see Ch. 50), but cancer cells and normal cells are so similar in most respects that it is more difficult to find general, exploitable, biochemical differences between them. Conventional *cytotoxic drugs* act on all cells and rely on a small margin of selectivity to be useful as anticancer agents, but the scope of cancer therapy has now broadened to include drugs that affect either the hormonal regulation of tumour growth, or the defective cell cycle controls that underlie malignancy (see Ch. 5 and Weinberg et al., 1996). Overall, this has been one of the most fruitful fields of drug development in recent years, and both genomics and biopharmaceuticals have played a major role. The flow of innovation seems set to continue.

THE PATHOGENESIS OF CANCER

To understand the action and drawbacks of current anticancer agents and to appreciate the therapeutic hurdles that must be surmounted by putative new drugs, it is important to consider the pathobiology in more detail.

Cancer cells manifest, to varying degrees, four characteristics that distinguish them from normal cells. These are:

- *uncontrolled proliferation*
- *de-differentiation and loss of function*
- *invasiveness*
- *metastasis*.

THE GENESIS OF A CANCER CELL

A normal cell turns into a cancer cell because of one or more mutations in its DNA. These can be inherited or acquired, usually through exposure to viruses or *carcinogens* (e.g. tobacco products, asbestos). A good example is breast cancer; women who inherit a single defective copy of either of the tumour suppressor genes *BRCA1* and *BRCA2* have a significantly increased *risk* of developing breast cancer. However, carcinogenesis is a complex multistage process, usually involving more than one genetic change as well as other, *epigenetic* factors (hormonal, co-carcinogen and tumour promoter effects, etc.) that do not themselves produce cancer but which increase the *likelihood* that the genetic mutation(s) will eventually result in cancer.

There are two main categories of relevant genetic change:

1. The activation of *proto-oncogenes* to *oncogenes*. Proto-oncogenes are genes that normally control cell

---

[1]The term 'cancer' actually embraces a range of different diseases, each with its own characteristic aetiology and clinical outcome, but all giving rise to uncontrolled cell growth. Whilst acknowledging this, we have retained this historical category here for convenience.
[2]Blood cell malignancies – lymphomas and leukaemias – are non-tumour-forming, and not usually referred to as cancers. In this account, 'cancer' is used to cover all malignancies.

division, apoptosis and differentiation (see Ch. 5), but which can be converted to oncogenes that induce malignant change by viral or carcinogen action.

2. The inactivation of *tumour suppressor genes*. Normal cells contain genes that suppress malignant change – termed tumour suppressor genes (*anti-oncogenes*) – and mutations of these genes are involved in many different cancers. The loss of function of tumour suppressor genes can be the critical event in carcinogenesis.

About 30 tumour suppressor genes and 100 dominant oncogenes have been identified. The changes that lead to malignancy are a result of point mutations, gene amplification or chromosomal translocation, often caused by viruses or chemical carcinogens.

THE SPECIAL CHARACTERISTICS OF CANCER CELLS

UNCONTROLLED PROLIFERATION

It is not generally true that cancer cells proliferate faster than normal cells. Many healthy cells, in the bone marrow and the epithelium of the gastrointestinal tract (for example), undergo continuous rapid division. Some cancer cells multiply slowly (e.g. those in plasma cell tumours) and some much more rapidly (e.g. the cells of

Burkitt's lymphoma). The significant issue is that cancer cells *have escaped from the mechanisms that normally regulate cell division and tissue growth*. It is this, rather than their rate of proliferation, that distinguishes them from normal cells.

What are the changes that lead to the uncontrolled proliferation of tumour cells? Inactivation of tumour suppressor genes or transformation of proto-oncogenes into oncogenes can confer autonomy of growth on a cell and thus result in uncontrolled proliferation by producing changes in cellular systems (see Fig. 56.1), including:

- *growth factors*, their receptors and signalling pathways
- the *cell cycle transducers*, for example cyclins, cyclin-dependent kinases (cdks) or the cdk inhibitors
- the *apoptotic machinery* that normally disposes of abnormal cells
- *telomerase expression*
- *local blood vessels*, resulting from tumour-directed angiogenesis.

Potentially all the genes coding for the above components could be regarded as oncogenes or tumour suppressor genes (see Fig. 56.2), although not all are equally prone to malignant transformation. It should be understood that

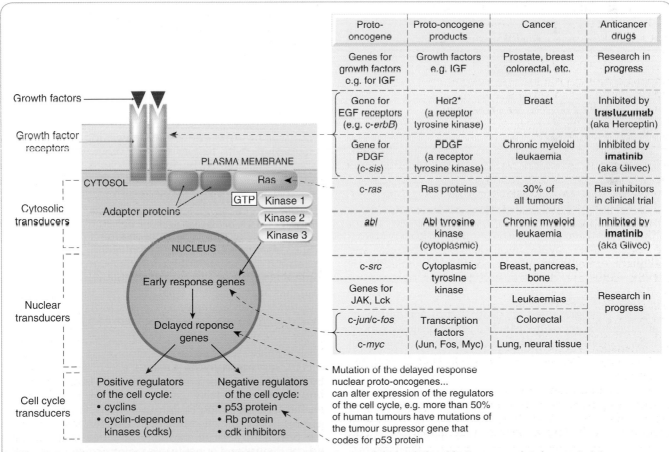

Proto-oncogene	Proto-oncogene products	Cancer	Anticancer drugs
Genes for growth factors e.g. for IGF	Growth factors e.g. IGF	Prostate, breast colorectal, etc.	Research in progress
Gene for EGF receptors (e.g. c-*erbB*)	Her2* (a receptor tyrosine kinase)	Breast	Inhibited by **trastuzumab** (aka Herceptin)
Gene for PDGF (c-*sis*)	PDGF (a receptor tyrosine kinase)	Chronic myeloid leukaemia	Inhibited by **imatinib** (aka Glivec)
c-*ras*	Ras proteins	30% of all tumours	Ras inhibitors in clinical trial
abl	Abl tyrosine kinase (cytoplasmic)	Chronic myeloid leukaemia	Inhibited by **imatinib** (aka Glivec)
c-*src*	Cytoplasmic tyrosine kinase	Breast, pancreas, bone	
Genes for JAK, Lck		Leukaemias	Research in progress
c-*jun*/c-*fos*	Transcription factors (Jun, Fos, Myc)	Colorectal	
c-*myc*		Lung, neural tissue	

Mutation of the delayed response nuclear proto-oncogenes... can alter expression of the regulators of the cell cycle, e.g. more than 50% of human tumours have mutations of the tumour suppressor gene that codes for p53 protein

Fig. 56.1 **Signal transduction pathways initiated by growth factors and their relationship to cancer development.** A few examples of proto-oncogenes and the products they code for are given in the table, with examples of the cancers that are associated with their conversion to oncogenes. Many growth factor receptors are receptor tyrosine kinases, the cytosolic transducers including adapter proteins that bind to phosphorylated tyrosine residues in the receptors. Ras proteins are guanine nucleotide-binding proteins and have GTPase action; decreased GTPase action means that Ras remains activated. EGF, epidermal growth factor; IGF, insulin-like growth factor; PDGF, platelet-derived growth factor; *Her2 is also termed *her2/neu*.

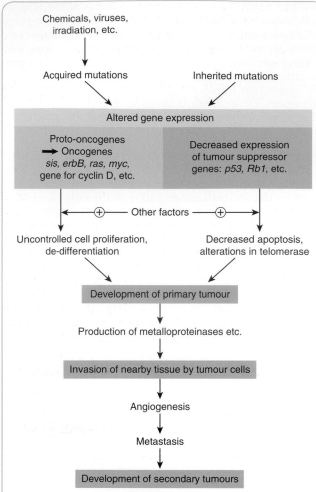

Fig. 56.2 Simplified outline of the genesis of cancer. The diagram summarises the information given in the text. The genesis of cancer is usually multifactorial, involving more than one genetic change. 'Other factors', as specified above, may involve the actions of promoters, co-carcinogens, hormones etc. which, while not themselves carcinogenic, increase the likelihood that genetic mutation(s) will result in cancer.

malignant transformation of several components is needed for the development of cancer.

Resistance to apoptosis
Apoptosis is programmed cell death (Ch. 5), and mutations in antiapoptotic genes are usually a prerequisite for cancer; indeed, resistance to apoptosis is a hallmark of malignant disease. It can be brought about by inactivation of proapoptotic factors or by activation of antiapoptotic factors.

Telomerase expression
Telomeres are specialised structures that cap the ends of chromosomes – like the small metal tubes on the end of shoelaces – protecting them from degradation, rearrangement and fusion with other chromosomes. Furthermore, DNA polymerase cannot easily duplicate the last few nucleotides at the ends of DNA, and telomeres prevent loss of the 'end' genes. With each round of cell division, a portion of the telomere is eroded, so that eventually it becomes non-functional. At this point, DNA replication ceases and the cell becomes senescent.

Rapidly dividing cells, such as stem and bone marrow cells, the germline and the epithelium of the gastrointestinal tract, express *telomerase*, an enzyme that maintains and stabilises telomeres. While it is absent from most fully differentiated somatic cells, about 95% of late-stage malignant tumours do express this enzyme, and it is this that may confer 'immortality' on cancer cells (see Buys, 2000; Keith et al., 2004).

The control of tumour-related blood vessels
The factors described above lead to the uncontrolled proliferation of individual cancer cells, but other factors, particularly blood supply, determine the actual growth of a solid tumour. Tumours 1–2 mm in diameter can obtain nutrients by diffusion, but their further expansion requires *angiogenesis*, the development of new blood vessels in response to growth factors produced by the growing tumour (see Griffioen & Molema, 2000).

DE-DIFFERENTIATION AND LOSS OF FUNCTION
The multiplication of normal cells in a tissue begins with division of the undifferentiated stem cells giving rise to *daughter cells* that differentiate to become the mature non-dividing cells, ready to perform functions appropriate to that tissue. For example, mature fibroblasts secrete and organise extracellular matrix; mature muscle cells are capable of contraction etc. One of the main characteristics of cancer cells is that they de-differentiate to varying degrees. In general, poorly differentiated cancers multiply faster and carry a worse prognosis than well-differentiated cancers.

INVASIVENESS
Normal cells, other than those of the blood and lymphoid tissues, are not generally found outside their 'designated' tissue of origin. This is because, during differentiation and tissue or organ growth, they develop certain spatial relationships with respect to each other. These relationships are maintained by various tissue-specific survival factors that prevent apoptosis (see Ch. 5). In this way, any cells that escape accidentally lose these survival signals and die.

For example, whilst the cells of the normal mucosal epithelium of the rectum proliferate continuously as the lining is shed, they remain as a lining epithelium. A cancer of the rectal mucosa, in contrast, invades other surrounding tissues. Cancer cells have not only lost, through mutation, the restraints that act on normal cells, but they also secrete enzymes (e.g. metalloproteinases; see Ch. 5) that break down the extracellular matrix, enabling them to move around.

METASTASIS
Metastases are *secondary tumours* ('secondaries') formed by cells that have been released from the initial or *primary tumour* and which have reached other sites through blood vessels or lymphatics, by transportation on other cells or as a result of being shed into body cavities. Metastases are the principal cause of mortality and morbidity in most solid tumours and constitute a major problem for cancer therapy (see Chambers et al., 2002).

As discussed above, displacement or aberrant migration of normal cells would lead to programmed cell death as a result of withdrawal of the necessary antiapoptotic factors. Cancer cells that metastasise have undergone a series of genetic changes that alter their responses to the regulatory factors that control the cellular architecture of normal tissues, enabling them to establish themselves 'extraterritorially'. Tumour-induced growth of new blood vessels locally favours metastasis.

Secondary tumours occur more frequently in some tissues than in others. For example, metastases of mammary cancers are often found in lung, bone and brain. The reason for this is that breast cancer cells express chemokine receptors such as CXCR4 (see Ch. 18) on their surfaces, and chemokines that recognise these receptors are expressed at high level in these tissues but not in others (e.g. kidney), facilitating the selective accumulation of cells at these sites.

GENERAL PRINCIPLES OF CYTOTOXIC ANTICANCER DRUGS

In experiments with rapidly growing transplantable leukaemias in mice, it has been found that a given therapeutic dose of a cytotoxic drug[3] destroys a constant fraction of the malignant cells. If used to treat a tumour with 10^{11} cells, a dose of drug that kills 99.99% of cells will still leave 10 million (10^7) viable malignant cells. As the same principle holds for fast-growing tumours in humans, schedules for chemotherapy are aimed at producing as near a total cell kill as possible because, in contrast to the situation that occurs in microorganisms, little reliance can be placed on the host's immunological defence mechanisms against the remaining cancer cells. If a tumour is removed (or at least *de-bulked*) surgically, any remaining *micro-metastases* are highly sensitive to chemotherapy, hence its use as adjuvant therapy in these circumstances.

One of the major difficulties in treating cancer is that tumour growth is usually far advanced before cancer is diagnosed. Let us suppose that a tumour arises from a single cell and that the growth is exponential, as it may well be during the initial stages. 'Doubling' times vary, being, for example, approximately 24 h with Burkitt's lymphoma, 2 weeks in the case of some leukaemias, and 3 months with mammary cancers. Approximately 30 doublings would be required to produce a cell mass with a diameter of 2 cm, containing 10^9 cells. Such a tumour is within the limits of diagnostic procedures, although it could easily go unnoticed. A further 10 doublings would produce 10^{12} cells, a tumour mass that is likely to be lethal, and which would measure about 20 cm in diameter if it were one solid mass.

However, continuous exponential growth of this sort does not usually occur. In the case of most solid tumours, as opposed to *leukaemias* (tumours of white blood cells), the growth rate falls as the neoplasm grows. This is partly because the tumour outgrows its blood supply, and partly because not all the cells proliferate continuously. The cells of a solid tumour can be considered as belonging to three compartments:

1. *Compartment A* consists of dividing cells, possibly being continuously in the cell cycle.

2. *Compartment B* consists of resting cells (G_0 phase) which, although not dividing, are potentially able to do so.

3. *Compartment C* consists of cells that are no longer able to divide but which contribute to the tumour volume.

Essentially, only cells in *compartment A*, which may form as little as 5% of some solid tumours, are susceptible to the main current cytotoxic drugs. The cells in *compartment C* do not constitute a problem, but the existence of *compartment B* makes cancer chemotherapy difficult, because these cells are not very sensitive to cytotoxic drugs and are liable to re-enter *compartment A* following chemotherapy.

Most current anticancer drugs, particularly cytotoxic agents, affect only one characteristic aspect of cancer cell biology – cell division – but have no specific inhibitory effect on invasiveness, the loss of differentiation or the tendency to metastasise. In many cases, the antiproliferative action results from an action during S phase of the cell cycle, and the resultant damage to DNA initiates apoptosis. Furthermore, because their main target is cell division, they will affect all rapidly dividing normal tissues, and therefore are likely to produce, to a greater or lesser extent, the following general toxic effects:

- *bone marrow toxicity* (myelosuppression) with decreased leukocyte production and thus decreased resistance to infection
- *impaired wound healing*
- *loss of hair* (alopecia)
- damage to *gastrointestinal epithelium* (including oral mucous membranes)
- *depression of growth* in children
- *sterility*
- *teratogenicity*
- *carcinogenicity* – because many cytotoxic drugs are mutagens.

Rapid cell destruction also entails extensive purine catabolism, and urates may precipitate in the renal tubules and cause kidney damage. Finally, in addition to specific toxic effects associated with individual drugs, virtually all cytotoxic drugs produce severe nausea and vomiting, an 'inbuilt deterrent' now thankfully largely overcome by modern antiemetic drug prophylaxis (Ch. 30).

ANTICANCER DRUGS

The main anticancer drugs can be divided into the following general categories:

- *Cytotoxic drugs*. These include:
  - *alkylating agents* and related compounds, which act by forming covalent bonds with DNA and thus impeding replication
  - *antimetabolites*, which block or subvert one or more of the metabolic pathways involved in DNA synthesis
  - *cytotoxic antibiotics*, i.e. substances of microbial origin that prevent mammalian cell division
  - *plant derivatives* (e.g. vinca alkaloids, taxanes, camptothecins): most of these specifically affect microtubule function and hence the formation of the mitotic spindle.

---

[3]The term *cytotoxic drug* applies to any drug that can damage or kill cells. In practice, it is used more restrictively to refer to drugs that inhibit cell division and are therefore potentially useful in cancer chemotherapy.

Cancer pathogenesis and cancer chemotherapy: general principles

- Cancer arises as a result of a series of genetic and epigenetic changes, the main genetic lesions being:
  - inactivation of tumour suppressor genes
  - the activation of oncogenes (mutation of the normal genes controlling cell division and other processes).
- Cancer cells have four characteristics that distinguish them from normal cells:
  - uncontrolled proliferation
  - loss of function because of lack of capacity to differentiate
  - invasiveness
  - the ability to metastasise.
- Cancer cells have uncontrolled proliferation often because of changes in:
  - growth factors and/or their receptors
  - intracellular signalling pathways, particularly those controlling the cell cycle and apoptosis
  - telomerase expression.
- Proliferation may be supported by tumour-related angiogenesis.
- Most anticancer drugs are antiproliferative – most damage DNA and thereby initiate apoptosis. They also affect rapidly dividing normal cells and are thus likely to depress bone marrow, impair healing and depress growth. Most cause nausea, vomiting, sterility, hair loss and teratogenicity.

- *Hormones*, of which the most important are steroids (e.g. glucocorticoids, Ch. 33) as well as drugs that suppress oestrogen synthesis (e.g. aromatase inhibitors) or the secretion of male sex hormones (e.g. gonadorelin analogues, Ch. 35) or antagonise hormone action (e.g. oestrogen and androgen antagonists, Ch. 35).
- *Protein kinase inhibitors:* these drugs inhibit the protein kinases (usually tyrosine kinases but sometimes others) involved in growth factor receptor signal transduction. They are increasingly used in a range of specific malignancies (see Krause & van Etten, 2005).
- *Monoclonal antibodies*: of growing importance in particular types of cancer.
- *Miscellaneous agents* that do not easily fit into the above categories.

The clinical use of anticancer drugs is the province of the specialist, who selects treatment regimens appropriate to the patient with the objective of curing, prolonging life or providing palliative therapy.[4] There are over 80 drugs available in the UK for this purpose and they are often used in combination. The principal treatments are listed in Table 56.1. For reasons of space, we restrict our discussion of mechanisms of action to common examples from each group. A textbook (Airley, 2009) provides detailed information.

---

[4]You will have gathered that many anticancer drugs are toxic. 'To be an oncologist,' one practitioner commented, 'one has to hate cancer more than one loves life.'

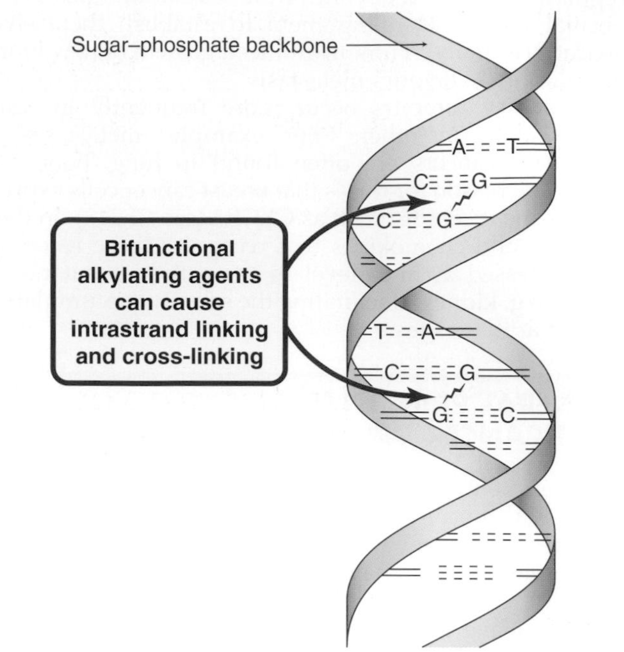

Sugar–phosphate backbone

Bifunctional alkylating agents can cause intrastrand linking and cross-linking

Fig. 56.3 The effects of bifunctional alkylating agents on DNA. Note the cross-linking of two guanines. A, adenine; C, cytosine; G, guanine; T, thymine.

ALKYLATING AGENTS AND RELATED COMPOUNDS

Alkylating agents and related compounds contain chemical groups that can form covalent bonds with particular nucleophilic substances in the cell (such as DNA). With alkylating agents themselves, the main step is the formation of a *carbonium ion* – a carbon atom with only six electrons in its outer shell. Such ions are highly reactive and react instantaneously with an electron donor such as an amine, hydroxyl or sulfhydryl group. Most of the cytotoxic anticancer alkylating agents are *bifunctional*, i.e. they have two alkylating groups (Fig. 56.3).

▼ The nitrogen at position 7 (N7) of guanine, being strongly nucleophilic, is probably the main molecular target for alkylation in DNA (Fig. 56.3), although N1 and N3 of adenine and N3 of cytosine may also be affected. A bifunctional agent, by reacting with two groups, can cause intra- or inter-chain cross-linking. This interferes not only with transcription, but also with DNA replication, which is probably the critical effect of anticancer alkylating agents. Other effects of alkylation at guanine N7 are excision of the guanine base with main chain scission, or pairing of the alkylated guanine with thymine instead of cytosine, and eventual substitution of the GC pair by an AT pair. Their main impact is seen during replication (S phase), when some zones of the DNA are unpaired and more susceptible to alkylation. This results in a block at G_2 and subsequent apoptotic cell death.

All alkylating agents depress bone marrow function and cause hair loss and gastrointestinal disturbances. With prolonged use, two further unwanted effects occur: depression of gametogenesis (particularly in men), leading to sterility, and an increased risk of acute non-lymphocytic leukaemia and other malignancies.

Alkylating agents are among the most commonly employed of all anticancer drugs (about 20 are approved in the UK at the time of writing). Only a few commonly used examples will be dealt with here.

Table 56.1 An overview of anticancer drugs

Type	Group	Examples	Main mechanism
Alkylating, and related, agents	Nitrogen mustards	Bendramustine, chlorambucil, cyclophosphamide, estramustine,[a] ifosfamide, melphalan	Intrastrand cross-linking of DNA
	Nitrosoureas	Carmustine, lomustine	
	Platinum compounds	Carboplatin, cisplatin, oxaliplatin	
	Other	Busulfan, dacarbazine, hydroxycarbamide, mitobronitol, procarbazine treosulfan, thiotepa, temozolimide	
Antimetabolites	Folate antagonists	Methotrexate, pemetrexed, raltitrexed	Blocking the synthesis of DNA and/or RNA
	Pyrimdine pathway	Azacitidine, capecitabine, cytarabine, decitabine, fluorouracil gemcitabine, tegafur	
	Purine pathway	Cladibrine, clofarabrine, fludarabine, mercaptopurine, nelarabine, pentostatin, tioguanine	
Cytotoxic antibiotics	Anthracyclines	(Amascrine), daunorubicin, doxorubicin, epirubicin, idarubicin, (mitoxantrine)	Multiple effects on DNA/RNA synthesis and topisomerase action
	Other	Bleomycin, dactinomycin, mitomycin, trabectedin	
Plant derivatives and similar compounds	Taxanes	Cabazitaxel, docetaxel, paclitaxel	Microtubule assembly; prevents spindle formation
	Vinca alkaloids	Vinblastine, vincristine, vindesine, vinflunine, vinorelbine. (eribulin)	
	Campothecins	Irinotecan, topotecan	Inhibition of topoisomerase
	Other	Etoposide	
Hormones/ antagonists	Hormones/analogues	Buserelin, diethylstilbestrol, ethinyloestradiol, goserelin, histrelin, lanreotide, leuporelin, medroxyprogesterone, megesterol, norhisterone, triptorelin, octreotide, pasreotide	Act as physiological agonists, antagonists or hormone synthesis inhibitors to disrupt hormone-dependent tumour growth
	Antagonists	Bicalutamide, cyproterone, degarelix, flutamide, fulvestrant, mitotane, tamoxifen, toremifine	
	Aromatase inhibitors	Anastrozole, exemastine, letrozole	
Protein kinase inhibitors	Tyrosine, or other kinase, inhibitors	Axitinib, crizotinib, dasatinib, erlotinib, gefitinib, imatinib, lapatinib, nilotinib, pazopanib, ruxolitinib, sunitinib, vandetanib, vemurafenib	Inhibition of kinases involved in growth factor receptor transduction
	Pan kinase inhibitors	Everolimus, sorafenib, temsirolimus	
Monoclonal antibodies	Anti-EGF, EGF-2	Panitumumab, trastuzumab	Blocks cell proliferation
	Anti-CD20/CD30/ CD52	Brentixumab, ofatumab, rituximab	Inhibition of lymphocyte proliferation
	Anti-CD3/EpCAM or CTLA-4	Catumexomab	Binds adhesion molecules promoting cell killing
	Anti-VEGF	Bevacizumab	Prevents angiogenesis
Miscellaneous	Retinoid X receptor antagonist	Bexarotene	Inhibits cell proliferation and differentiation
	Proteasome inhibitor	Bortezomib	Activation of programmed cell death
	Enzyme	Cristantaspase	Depletes asparagine
	Photoactivated cytotoxics	Porfimer, temoporfin	Accumulate in cells and kills them when activated by light

[a]A combination of oestrogen and chlormethine. Drugs in parentheses have similar pharmacological actions but are not necessarily chemically related.

Nitrogen mustards

Nitrogen mustards are related to the 'mustard gas' used during the First World War,[5] their basic formula (R-N-*bis*-(2-chloroethyl)) is shown in Figure 56.4. In the body, each 2-chloroethyl side-chain undergoes an intramolecular cyclisation with the release of a Cl⁻. The highly reactive *ethylene immonium* derivative so formed can interact with DNA (see Figs 56.3 and 56.4) and other molecules.

Cyclophosphamide is probably the most commonly used alkylating agent. It is inactive until metabolised in the liver by the P450 mixed function oxidases (see Ch. 9). It has a pronounced effect on lymphocytes and can also be used as an immunosuppressant (see Ch. 26). It is usually given orally or by intravenous injection. Important toxic effects are nausea and vomiting, bone marrow depression and haemorrhagic cystitis. This last effect (which also occurs with the related drug **ifosfamide**) is caused by the metabolite acrolein and can be ameliorated

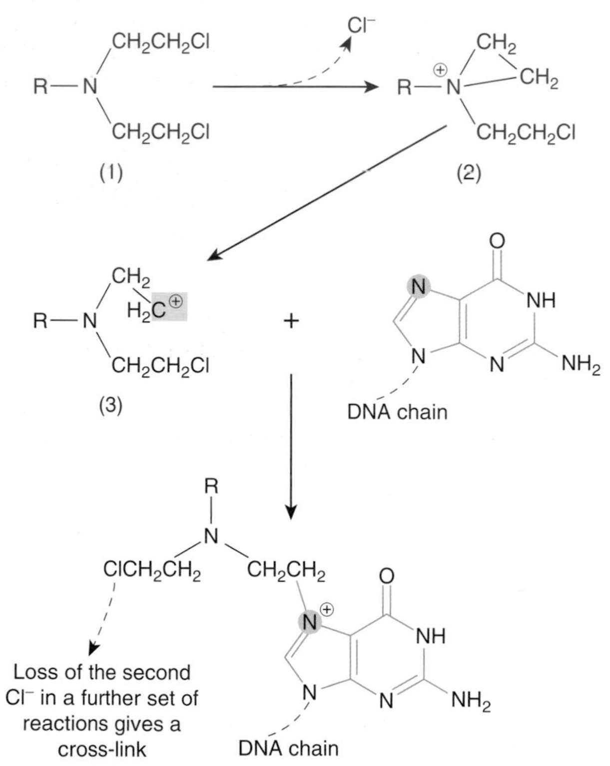

Fig. 56.4 An example of alkylation and cross-linking of DNA by a nitrogen mustard. A bis(chloroethyl)amine (1) undergoes intramolecular cyclisation, forming an unstable ethylene immonium cation (2) and releasing Cl⁻, the tertiary amine being transformed to a quaternary ammonium compound. The strained ring of the ethylene immonium intermediate opens to form a reactive carbonium ion (in yellow box) (3), which reacts immediately with N7 of guanine (in green circle) to give 7-alkylguanine (bond shown in blue), the N7 being converted to a quaternary ammonium nitrogen. These reactions can then be repeated with the other –CH₂CH₂Cl to give a cross-link.

by increasing fluid intake and administering compounds that are sulfhydryl donors, such as **N-acetylcysteine** or **mesna** (sodium-2-mercaptoethane sulfonate). These agents react with acrolein, forming a non-toxic compound. (See also Chs 9 and 57.)

▼ Other nitrogen mustards used include **bendramustine**, ifosfamide, **chlorambucil** and **melphalan**. **Estramustine** is a combination of **chlormethine** (mustine) with an oestrogen. It has both cytotoxic and hormonal action, and is used for the treatment of prostate cancer.

Nitrosoureas

Examples include **lomustine** and **carmustine**. As they are lipid soluble and cross the blood–brain barrier, they are used to treat tumours of the brain and meninges. However, most nitrosoureas have a severe cumulative depressive effect on the bone marrow that starts 3–6 weeks after initiation of treatment.

Other alkylating agents

Busulfan has a selective effect on the bone marrow, depressing the formation of granulocytes and platelets in low dosage and of red cells in higher dosage. It has little or no effect on lymphoid tissue or the gastrointestinal tract. It is used in chronic granulocytic leukaemia.

Dacarbazine, a prodrug, is activated in the liver, and the resulting compound is subsequently cleaved in the target cell to release an alkylating derivative. Unwanted effects include myelotoxicity and severe nausea and vomiting. **Temozolomide** is a related compound with a restricted usage (malignant glioma).

Procarbazine inhibits DNA and RNA synthesis and interferes with mitosis at interphase. Its effects may be mediated by the production of active metabolites. It is given orally, and its main use is in Hodgkin's disease. It causes **disulfiram**-like actions with alcohol (see Ch. 49), exacerbates the effects of central nervous system depressants and, because it is a weak monoamine oxidase inhibitor, can produce hypertension if given with certain sympathomimetic agents (see Ch. 47). Other alkylating agents in clinical use include **hydroxycarbamide**, **mitobronitol**, **thiotepa** and **treosulfan**.

Platinum compounds

Cisplatin is a water-soluble planar coordination complex containing a central platinum atom surrounded by two chlorine atoms and two ammonia groups. Its action is analogous to that of the alkylating agents. When it enters the cell, Cl⁻ dissociates, leaving a reactive complex that reacts with water and then interacts with DNA. It causes intra-strand cross-linking, probably between N7 and O6 of adjacent guanine molecules, which results in local denaturation of DNA.

Cisplatin has revolutionised the treatment of solid tumours of the testes and ovary. Therapeutically, it is given by slow intravenous injection or infusion. It is seriously nephrotoxic, and strict regimens of hydration and diuresis must be instituted. It has low myelotoxicity but causes very severe nausea and vomiting. The 5-HT₃ receptor antagonists (e.g. **ondansetron**; see Chs 15, 30 and 39) are very effective in preventing this and have transformed cisplatin-based chemotherapy. Tinnitus and hearing loss in the high-frequency range may occur, as may peripheral neuropathies, hyperuricaemia and anaphylactic reactions.

▼ **Carboplatin** is a derivative of cisplatin. Because it causes less nephrotoxicity, neurotoxicity, ototoxicity, nausea and vomiting than

---

[5]It was the clinical insight of Alfred Goodman and Louis Gilman that led to the testing of (what became the first effective anticancer drug) mustine, a modified and stable version of 'mustard gas', to treat lymphomas. They also wrote what was to become a famous textbook of pharmacology.

cisplatin (although it is more myelotoxic), it is sometimes given on an outpatient basis. **Oxaliplatin** is another platinum-containing compound with a restricted application.

ANTIMETABOLITES

Folate antagonists

The main folate antagonist is **methotrexate**, one of the most widely used antimetabolites in cancer chemotherapy. Folates are essential for the synthesis of purine nucleotides and thymidylate, which in turn are essential for DNA synthesis and cell division. (This topic is also dealt with in Chs 25, 50 and 54.) The main action of the folate antagonists is to interfere with thymidylate synthesis.

▼ Structurally, folates consist of three elements: a pteridine ring, *p*-aminobenzoic acid and glutamic acid (Fig. 56.5). Folates are actively taken up into cells, where they are converted to polyglutamates. In order to act as coenzymes, folates must be reduced to tetrahydrofolate (FH_4). This two-step reaction is catalysed by dihydrofolate reductase, which converts the substrate first to dihydrofolate (FH_2), then to FH_4 (Fig. 56.6). FH_4 functions as an essential co-factor carrying the methyl groups necessary for the transformation of 2'-deoxyuridylate (DUMP) to the 2'-deoxythymidylate (DTMP) required for the synthesis of DNA and purines. During the formation of DTMP from DUMP, FH_4 is converted back to FH_2, enabling the cycle to repeat. Methotrexate has a higher affinity than FH_2 for dihydrofolate reductase and thus inhibits the enzyme (Fig. 56.6), depleting intracellular FH_4. The binding of methotrexate to dihydrofolate reductase involves an additional bond not present when FH_2 binds. The reaction most sensitive to FH_4 depletion is DTMP formation.

Methotrexate is usually given orally but can also be given intramuscularly, intravenously or intrathecally. It has low lipid solubility and thus does not readily cross the blood–brain barrier. It is, however, actively taken up into cells by the folate transport system and is metabolised to polyglutamate derivatives, which are retained in the cell for weeks or months even in the absence of extracellular drug. Resistance to methotrexate may develop in tumour cells by a variety of mechanisms. Methotrexate is also used as an immunosuppressant drug to treat rheumatoid arthritis, psoriasis and other autoimmune conditions (see Ch. 26).

Unwanted effects include depression of the bone marrow and damage to the epithelium of the gastrointestinal tract. Pneumonitis can occur. In addition, high-dose regimens – doses 10 times greater than the standard doses, sometimes used in patients with methotrexate

---

Anticancer drugs: alkylating agents and related compounds

- Alkylating agents have groups that form covalent bonds with cell substituents; a carbonium ion is the reactive intermediate. Most have two alkylating groups and can cross-link DNA. This causes defective replication and chain breakage.
- Their principal effect occurs during DNA synthesis and the resulting damage triggers apoptosis
- Unwanted effects include myelosuppression, sterility and risk of non-lymphocytic leukaemia.
- The main alkylating agents are:
  – nitrogen mustards, for example **cyclophosphamide**, which is converted to phosphoramide mustard (the cytotoxic molecule); **cyclophosphamide** myelosuppression affects particularly the lymphocytes
  – nitrosoureas, for example **lomustine**, may act on non-dividing cells, can cross the blood–brain barrier and cause delayed, cumulative myelotoxicity.
- Platinum compounds (e.g. **cisplatin**) cause intrastrand linking in DNA. **Cisplatin** has low myelotoxicity but causes severe nausea and vomiting, and can be nephrotoxic. It has revolutionised the treatment of germ cell tumours.

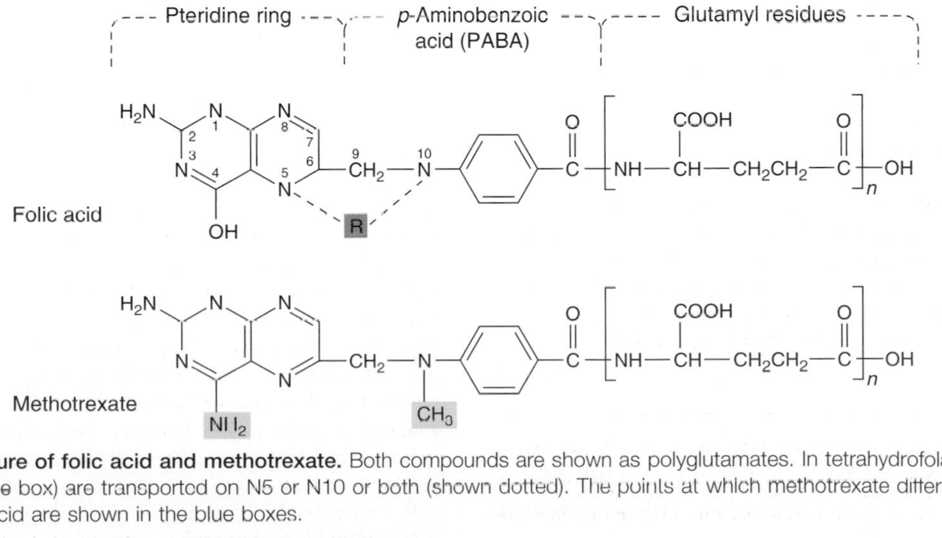

Fig. 56.5 **Structure of folic acid and methotrexate.** Both compounds are shown as polyglutamates. In tetrahydrofolate, one-carbon groups (R, in orange box) are transported on N5 or N10 or both (shown dotted). The points at which methotrexate differs from endogenous folic acid are shown in the blue boxes.

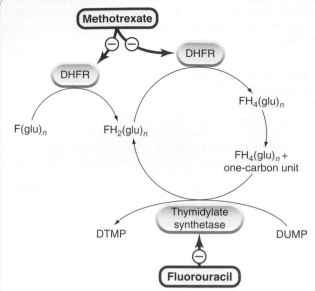

Fig. 56.6 Simplified diagram of action of methotrexate and fluorouracil on thymidylate synthesis. Tetrahydrofolate polyglutamate $FH_4(glu)_n$ functions as a carrier of a one-carbon unit, providing the methyl group necessary for the conversion of 2'-deoxyuridylate (DUMP) to 2'-deoxythymidylate (DTMP) by thymidylate synthetase. This one-carbon transfer results in the oxidation of $FH_4(glu)_n$ to $FH_2(glu)_n$. Fluorouracil is converted to FDUMP, which inhibits thymidylate synthetase. DHFR, dihydrofolate reductase.

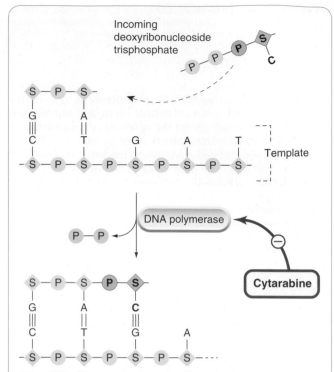

Fig. 56.7 The mechanism of action of cytarabine (cytosine arabinoside). For details of DNA polymerase action, see Figure 50.5. Cytarabine is an analogue of cytosine.

resistance – can lead to nephrotoxicity. This is caused by precipitation of the drug or a metabolite in the renal tubules. High-dose regimens must be followed by 'rescue' with folinic acid (a form of FH_4).

Also chemically related to folate are **raltitrexed**, which inhibits thymidylate synthetase, and **pemetrexed**, which inhibits thymidylate transferase.

Pyrimidine analogues

Fluorouracil, an analogue of uracil, also interferes with DTMP synthesis (Fig. 56.6). It is converted into a 'fraudulent' nucleotide, *fluorodeoxyuridine monophosphate* (FDUMP). This interacts with thymidylate synthetase but cannot be converted into DTMP. The result is inhibition of DNA but not RNA or protein synthesis.

Fluorouracil is usually given parenterally. The main unwanted effects are gastrointestinal epithelial damage and myelotoxicity. Cerebellar disturbances can also occur. Two other drugs, **capecitabine** and **tegafur**, are metabolised to fluorouracil.

Cytarabine (cytosine arabinoside) is an analogue of the naturally occurring nucleoside 2'-deoxycytidine. The drug enters the target cell and undergoes the same phosphorylation reactions as the endogenous nucleoside to give cytosine arabinoside trisphosphate, which inhibits DNA polymerase (see Fig. 56.7). The main unwanted effects are on the bone marrow and the gastrointestinal tract. It also causes nausea and vomiting.

Gemcitabine, an analogue of cytarabine, has fewer unwanted actions, mainly an influenza-like syndrome and mild myelotoxicity. It is often given in combination with other drugs such as cisplatin. **Azacitidine** and **decitabine** inhibit DNA methylase.

Purine analogues

The main anticancer purine analogues include **cladribine**, **clofarabine**, **fludarabine**, **pentostatin**, **nelarabine**, **mercaptopurine** and **tioguanine**.

Fludarabine is metabolised to the trisphosphate and inhibits DNA synthesis by actions similar to those of cytarabine. It is myelosuppressive. Pentostatin has a different mechanism of action. It inhibits adenosine deaminase, the enzyme that transforms adenosine to inosine. This action interferes with critical pathways in purine metabolism and can have significant effects on cell proliferation. Cladribine, mercaptopurine and tioguanine are used mainly in the treatment of leukaemia.

Anticancer drugs: antimetabolites

Antimetabolites block or subvert pathways of DNA synthesis.
- *Folate antagonists*. **Methotrexate** inhibits dihydrofolate reductase, preventing generation of tetrahydrofolate interfering with thymidylate synthesis.
- *Pyrimidine analogues*. **Fluorouracil** is converted to a 'fraudulent' nucleotide and inhibits thymidylate synthesis. **Cytarabine** in its trisphosphate form inhibits DNA polymerase. They are potent myelosuppressives.
- *Purine analogues*. **Mercaptopurine** is converted into fraudulent nucleotide. **Fludarabine** in its trisphosphate form inhibits DNA polymerase and is myelosuppressive. **Pentostatin** inhibits adenosine deaminase – a critical pathway in purine metabolism.

CYTOTOXIC ANTIBIOTICS

This is a widely used group of drugs that mainly produce their effects through direct action on DNA. As a rule, they should not be given together with radiotherapy, as the cumulative burden of toxicity is very high.

Doxorubicin and the anthracyclines

Doxorubicin, **idarubicin**, **daunorubicin** and **epirubicin** are widely used anthracycline antibiotics; **mitoxantrone** (**mitozantrone**) is a derivative.

Doxorubicin has several cytotoxic actions. It binds to DNA and inhibits both DNA and RNA synthesis, but its main cytotoxic action appears to be mediated through an effect on topoisomerase II (a DNA gyrase; see Ch. 50), the activity of which is markedly increased in proliferating cells. During replication of the DNA helix, reversible swivelling needs to take place around the replication fork in order to prevent the daughter DNA molecule becoming inextricably entangled during mitotic segregation. The 'swivel' is produced by topoisomerase II, which 'nicks' both DNA strands and subsequently reseals the breaks. Doxorubicin intercalates in the DNA, and its effect is, in essence, to stabilise the DNA–topoisomerase II complex after the strands have been nicked, thus halting the process at this point.

Doxorubicin is given by intravenous infusion. Extravasation at the injection site can cause local necrosis. In addition to the general unwanted effects, the drug can cause cumulative, dose-related cardiac damage, leading to dysrhythmias and heart failure. This action may be the result of generation of free radicals. Marked hair loss frequently occurs.

Dactinomycin

Dactinomycin intercalates in the minor groove of DNA between adjacent guanosine cytosine pairs, interfering with the movement of RNA polymerase along the gene and thus preventing transcription. There is also evidence that it has a similar action to that of the anthracyclines on topoisomerase II. It produces most of the toxic effects outlined above, except cardiotoxicity. It is mainly used for treating paediatric cancers.

Bleomycins

The bleomycins are a group of metal-chelating glycopeptide antibiotics that degrade preformed DNA, causing chain fragmentation and release of free bases. This action is thought to involve chelation of ferrous iron and interaction with oxygen, resulting in the oxidation of the iron and generation of superoxide and/or hydroxyl radicals. **Bleomycin** is most effective in the G_2 phase of the cell cycle and mitosis, but it is also active against non-dividing cells (i.e. cells in the G_0 phase; Ch. 5, Fig. 5.4). It is often used to treat germline cancer. In contrast to most anticancer drugs, bleomycin causes little myelosuppression: its most serious toxic effect is pulmonary fibrosis, which occurs in 10% of patients treated and is reported to be fatal in 1%. Allergic reactions can also occur. About half the patients manifest mucocutaneous reactions (the palms are frequently affected), and many develop hyperpyrexia.

Mitomycin

Following enzymic activation, **mitomycin** functions as a bifunctional alkylating agent, binding preferentially at O6 of the guanine nucleus. It cross-links DNA and may also degrade DNA through the generation of free radicals. It causes marked delayed myelosuppression and can also cause kidney damage and fibrosis of lung tissue.

> **Anticancer drugs: cytotoxic antibiotics**
>
> - **Doxorubicin** inhibits DNA and RNA synthesis; the DNA effect is mainly through interference with topoisomerase II action. Unwanted effects include nausea, vomiting, myelosuppression and hair loss. It is cardiotoxic in high doses.
> - **Bleomycin** causes fragmentation of DNA chains. It acts on non-dividing cells. Unwanted effects include fever, allergies, mucocutaneous reactions and pulmonary fibrosis. There is virtually no myelosuppression.
> - **Dactinomycin** intercalates in DNA, interfering with RNA polymerase and inhibiting transcription. It also interferes with the action of topoisomerase II. Unwanted effects include nausea, vomiting and myelosuppression.
> - **Mitomycin** is activated to give an alkylating metabolite.

PLANT DERIVATIVES

Several naturally occurring plant products exert potent cytotoxic effects and have a use as anticancer drugs.

Vinca alkaloids

The vinca alkaloids are derived from the Madagascar periwinkle (*Catharanthus roseus*). The principal members of the group are **vincristine**, **vinblastine** and **vindesine**. **Vinflumine**, a fluorinated vinca alkaloid, and **vinorelbine** are semisynthetic vinca alkaloids with similar properties. The drugs bind to tubulin and inhibit its polymerisation into microtubules, preventing spindle formation in dividing cells and causing arrest at metaphase. Their effects become manifest only during mitosis. They also inhibit other cellular activities that require functioning microtubules, such as leukocyte phagocytosis and chemotaxis, as well as axonal transport in neurons.

The adverse effects of vinca alkaloids differ from other anticancer drugs. Vincristine has very mild myelosuppressive activity but is neurotoxic and commonly causes *paraesthesias* (sensory changes), abdominal pain and weakness. Vinblastine is less neurotoxic but causes leukopenia, while vindesine has both moderate myelotoxicity and neurotoxicity. All members of the group can cause reversible hair loss.

Paclitaxel and related compounds

These *taxanes* are derived from a naturally occurring compound found in the bark of the Pacific yew tree (*Taxus* spp.). The group includes **paclitaxel** and the semisynthetic derivatives **docetaxel** and **cabazitaxel**. These agents act on microtubules, stabilising them (in effect 'freezing' them) in the polymerised state, achieving a similar effect to that of the vinca alkaloids. These drugs are usually given by intravenous infusion. They are generally used to treat breast and lung cancer and paclitaxel, given with carboplatin, is the treatment of choice for ovarian cancer.

Unwanted effects, which can be serious, include bone marrow suppression and cumulative neurotoxicity. Resistant fluid retention (particularly oedema of the legs) can occur with docetaxel. Hypersensitivity to these compounds is common and requires pretreatment with corticosteroids and antihistamines.

Camptothecins

The camptothecins **irinotecan** and **topotecan**, isolated from the stem of the tree *Camptotheca acuminata*, bind to and inhibit topoisomerase I, high levels of which are present throughout the cell cycle. Diarrhoea and reversible bone marrow depression occur but, in general, these alkaloids have fewer unwanted effects than most other anticancer agents.

Etoposide

Etoposide is derived from mandrake root (*Podophyllum peltatum*). Its mode of action is not clearly known, but it may act by inhibiting mitochondrial function and nucleoside transport, as well as having an effect on topoisomerase II similar to doxorubicin. *Unwanted effects* include nausea and vomiting, myelosuppression and hair loss.

▼ **Compounds from marine sponges. Eribulin** is a naturally occurring compound from marine sponges. Its main inhibitory action on cell division is through inhibition of microtubule function. **Trabectedin**, another compound derived from marine sponges, also disrupts DNA but utilizes a superoxide-related mechanism.

> ### Anticancer drugs: plant derivatives
>
> - **Vincristine** (and related alkaloids) inhibit mitosis at metaphase by binding to tubulin. It is relatively non-toxic but can cause unwanted neuromuscular effects.
> - **Etoposide** inhibits DNA synthesis by an action on topoisomerase II and also inhibits mitochondrial function. Common unwanted effects include vomiting, myelosuppression and alopecia.
> - **Paclitaxel** (and other taxanes) stabilise microtubules, inhibiting mitosis; it is relatively toxic and hypersensitivity reactions occur.
> - **Irinotecan** and **topotecan** inhibit topoisomerase I; They have relatively few toxic effects.

HORMONES

Tumours arising in hormone-sensitive tissues (e.g. breast, uterus, prostate gland) may be *hormone-dependent*, an effect related to the presence of hormone receptors in the malignant cells. Their growth can be inhibited by hormone agonists or antagonists, or by agents that inhibit the synthesis of the hormone.

Hormones or their analogues that have inhibitory actions on target tissues can be used in treatment of tumours of those tissues. Such procedures alone rarely effect a cure but do retard tumour growth and mitigate the symptoms of the cancer, and thus play an important part in the clinical management of sex hormone-dependent tumours.

Glucocorticoids

Glucocorticoids such as **prednisolone** have marked inhibitory effects on lymphocyte proliferation (see Chs 26 and 33) and are used in the treatment of leukaemias and lymphomas. The ability of **dexamethasone** to lower raised intracranial pressure is exploited in treating patients with brain tumours. Glucocorticoids mitigate some of the side effects of anticancer drugs, such as nausea and vomiting, making them useful as supportive therapy when treating other cancers, as well as in palliative care.

Oestrogens

Diethylstilbestrol and **ethinyloestradiol** are still occasionally used in the palliative treatment of androgen-dependent prostatic tumours. These tumours can also be treated with gonadotrophin-releasing hormone analogues (see Ch. 33).

Progestogens

Progestogens such as **megestrol**, **norehisterone** and **medroxyprogesterone** have a role in treatment of endometrial cancer.

Gonadotrophin-releasing hormone analogues

As explained in Chapter 35, analogues of the gonadotrophin-releasing hormones, such as **goserelin**, **buserelin**, **leuprorelin** and **triptorelin**, can, when administered chronically, inhibit gonadotrophin release. These agents are therefore used to treat advanced breast cancer in premenopausal women and prostate cancer. The effect of the transient surge of testosterone secretion that can occur in patients treated in this way for prostate cancer must be prevented by an antiandrogen such as **cyproterone**. **Degaralix** is a gonadotrophin-releasing hormone antagonist used for the treatment of prostate cancer.

Somatostatin analogues

Analogues of somatostatin such as **octreotide** and **lanreotide** (see Ch. 33) are used to relieve the symptoms of neuroendocrine tumours, including hormone-secreting tumours of the gastrointestinal tract such as VIPomas, glucagonomas, carcinoid tumours and gastrinomas. These tumours express somatostatin receptors, activation of which inhibits cell proliferation as well as hormone secretion.

HORMONE ANTAGONISTS

In addition to the hormones themselves, hormone antagonists can also be effective in the treatment of several types of hormone-sensitive tumours.

Antioestrogens

An antioestrogen, **tamoxifen**, is remarkably effective in some cases of hormone-dependent breast cancer and may have a role in preventing these cancers. In breast tissue, tamoxifen competes with endogenous oestrogens for the oestrogen receptors and therefore inhibits the transcription of oestrogen-responsive genes. Tamoxifen is also reported to have cardioprotective effects, partly by virtue of its ability to protect low-density lipoproteins against oxidative damage. Other oestrogen receptor antagonists include **toremifene** and **fulvestrant**.

Unwanted effects are similar to those experienced by women following the menopause. Potentially more serious are hyperplastic events in the endometrium, which may progress to malignant changes, and the risk of thromboembolism.

Aromatase inhibitors such as **anastrozole**, **letrozole** and **exemestane**, which suppress the synthesis of oestrogen from androgens in the adrenal cortex (but not in the ovary), are also effective in the treatment of breast cancer in postmenopausal (but not in premenopausal) women, in whom they are somewhat more effective than tamoxifen.

Antiandrogens

The androgen antagonists **flutamide**, **cyproterone** and **bicalutamide** may be used either alone or in combination with other agents to treat tumours of the prostate. They are also used to control the testosterone surge ('flare') that is seen when treating patients with gonadorelin analogues. Degarelix does not cause this flare.

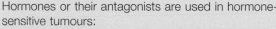

Anticancer agents: hormones

Hormones or their antagonists are used in hormone-sensitive tumours:

- **Glucocorticoids** for leukaemias and lymphomas.
- **Tamoxifen** for breast tumours.
- **Gonadotrophin-releasing hormone analogues** for prostate and breast tumours.
- **Antiandrogens** for prostate cancer.
- **Aromatase inhibitors** for postmenopausal breast cancer.

MONOCLONAL ANTIBODIES

Monoclonal antibodies (see Ch. 59) are relatively recent additions to the anticancer armamentarium. In some cases, binding of the antibody to its target activates the host's immune mechanisms and the cancer cell is killed by complement-mediated lysis or by killer T cells (see Ch. 6). Other monoclonal antibodies attach to and inactivate growth factors or their receptors on cancer cells, thus inhibiting the survival pathway and promoting apoptosis (Ch. 5, Fig. 5.5). Unlike most of the cytotoxic drugs described above, they offer the prospect of highly targeted therapy without many of the side effects of conventional chemotherapy. This advantage is offset in most instances as they are often given in combination with more traditional drugs. Several monoclonals are in current clinical use. Their high cost is a significant problem.

Rituximab

Rituximab is a monoclonal antibody that is used (in combination with other chemotherapeutic agents) for treatment of certain types of *lymphoma*. It lyses B lymphocytes by binding to the calcium-channel forming CD20 protein and activating complement. It also sensitises resistant cells to other chemotherapeutic drugs. It is effective in 40–50% of cases when combined with standard chemotherapy.

The drug is given by infusion, and its plasma half-life is approximately 3 days when first given, increasing with each administration to about 8 days by the fourth administration.

Unwanted effects include hypotension, chills and fever during the initial infusions and subsequent hypersensitivity reactions. A cytokine release reaction can occur and has been fatal. The drug may exacerbate cardiovascular disorders.

▼ **Alemtuzumab** is another monoclonal antibody that lyses B lymphocytes, and is used in the treatment of resistant chronic lymphocytic leukaemia. It may also cause a similar cytokine release reaction to that with rituximab. **Ofatumab** is similar. **Brentuximab** additionally targets T cells but in a different manner. It is a conjugate of a cytotoxic drug attached to an antibody that binds to CD30 on malignant cells. It is used to treat *Hodgkin's lymphoma*.

Trastuzumab

Trastuzumab (Herceptin) is a humanised murine monoclonal antibody that binds to an oncogenic protein termed *HER2* (the human epidermal growth factor receptor 2), a member of the wider family of receptors with integral tyrosine kinase activity (Fig. 56.1). There is some evidence that, in addition to inducing host immune responses, trastuzumab induces cell cycle inhibitors p21 and p27 (Ch. 5, Fig. 5.2). Tumour cells, in about 25% of breast cancer patients, overexpress this receptor and the cancer proliferates rapidly. Early results show that trastuzumab given with standard chemotherapy has resulted in a 79% 1-year survival rate in treatment-naive patients with this aggressive form of breast cancer. The drug is often given with a taxane such as docetaxel. Unwanted effects are similar to those with rituximab.

▼ Two mechanistically related compounds are **panitumumab** and **cetuximab**, which bind to epidermal growth factor (EGF) receptors (also overexpressed in a high proportion of tumours). They are used for the treatment of colorectal cancer usually in combination with other agents.

Bevacizumab

Bevacizumab is a humanised monoclonal antibody that is used for the treatment of colorectal cancer but would be expected to be useful for treating other cancers too. It neutralises *VEGF* (vascular endothelial growth factor), thereby preventing the angiogenesis that is crucial to tumour survival. It is administered by intravenous infusion and is generally combined with other agents. A closely related preparation is also given by direct injection into the eye to retard the progress of *acute macular degeneration* (AMD), a common cause of blindness associated with increased retinal vascularisation.

Catumaxomab

Catumaxomab attaches to an epithelial adhesion molecule, EpCAM, which is overexpressed in some malignant cells (e.g. malignant ascites in the peritoneal cavity). The antibody binds to this adhesion molecule and also to T lymphocytes and antigen-presenting cells, thus facilitating the action of the immune system in clearing the cancer.

PROTEIN KINASE INHIBITORS

Imatinib

Hailed as a conceptual breakthrough in targeted chemotherapy, **imatinib** (see Savage & Antman, 2002) is a small-molecule inhibitor of signalling pathway kinases. It inhibits an oncogenic cytoplasmic kinase (Bcr/Abl, see Fig. 56.1. and Fig. 56.8), considered to be a unique factor in the pathogenesis of chronic myeloid leukaemia (CML). It also inhibits platelet-derived growth factor (a receptor

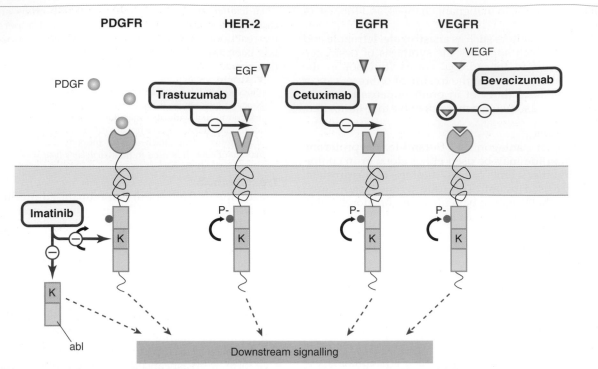

Fig. 56.8 The mechanism of action of anticancer monoclonal antibodies and protein kinase inhibitors. Many tumours overexpress growth factor receptors such as EGFR, the proto-oncogene HER2 or VEGFR. Therapeutic monoclonals can prevent this by interacting directly with the receptor itself (e.g. trastuzumab, cetuximab) or with the ligand (e.g. bevacizumab). An alternate way of reducing this drive on cell proliferation is by inhibiting the downstream signalling cascade. The receptor tyrosine kinases are good targets as are some oncongenic kinases such as bcr/abl. EGFR, epidermal growth factor receptor; HER, human epidermal growth factor; K, kinase domain in receptor; P-, phosphate group; PDGFR, platelet-derived growth factor receptor; VEGFR, vascular endothelial growth factor receptor.

tyrosine kinase; Fig. 56.1). It has greatly improved the (hitherto poor) prognosis of patients with CML, and is also used for the treatment of some gastrointestinal tumours not susceptible to surgery.

The drug is given orally. The half-life is about 18 h, and the main site of metabolism is in the liver, where approximately 75% of the drug is converted to a metabolite that is also biologically active. The bulk (81%) of the metabolised drug is excreted in the faeces.

Unwanted effects include gastrointestinal symptoms (pain, diarrhoea, nausea), fatigue, headaches and sometimes rashes. Resistance to imatinib, resulting from mutation of the kinase gene, is a growing problem. It results in little or no cross-resistance to other kinase inhibitors.

▼ Many similar tyrosine kinase inhibitors have recently been developed, including **axitinib**, **crizotinib**, **dastinib**, **erlotinib**, **gefitinib**, **imatinib**, **lapatinib**, **nilotinib**, **pazopanib**, **sunitinib** and **vandentanib**. Ruxolitinib inhibits the JAK1 and JAK2 kinases and **vemurafanib** inhibits BRAF kinase. **Sorafenib**, **everolimus** and **temsirolimus** are pan-kinase inhibitors with a similar utility.

MISCELLANEOUS AGENTS

Crisantaspase

▼ **Crisantaspase** is a preparation of the enzyme *asparaginase*, given by injection. It converts asparagine to aspartic acid and ammonia, and is active against tumour cells, such as those of acute lymphoblastic leukaemia, that have lost the capacity to synthesise asparagine and therefore require an exogenous source. As most normal cells are able to synthesise asparagine, the drug has a fairly selective action and has very little suppressive effect on the bone marrow, the mucosa of the gastrointestinal tract or hair follicles. It may cause

Anticancer drugs: monoclonal antibodies and protein kinase inhibitors

- Many tumours overexpress growth factor receptors that therefore stimulate cell proliferation and tumour growth. This can be inhibited by:
  - monoclonal antibodies, which bind to the extracellular domain of the EGF receptor (e.g. **panitumumab**), the oncogenic receptor HER2 receptor (e.g. **trastuzumab**), or which neutralise the growth factors themselves (e.g. VEGF; **bevacizumab**)
  - protein kinase inhibitors, which prevent downstream signalling triggered by growth factors by inhibiting specific oncogenic kinases (e.g. **imatinib**; bcr/abl) or by inhibiting specific receptor tyrosine kinases (e.g. EGF receptor; **erlotinib**) or several receptor-associated kinases (e.g. **sorefenib**).
- Some monoclonals act directly on lymphocyte cell surface proteins to cause lysis (e.g. **rituximab**), thereby preventing proliferation.

nausea and vomiting, central nervous system depression, anaphylactic reactions and liver damage.

Hydroxycarbamide

▼ **Hydroxycarbamide** (hydroxyurea) is a urea analogue that inhibits ribonucleotide reductase, thus interfering with the conversion of ribonucleotides to deoxyribonucleotides. It is mainly used to treat *polycythaemia rubra vera* (a myeloproliferative disorder of the red cell lineage) and (in the past) chronic myelogenous leukaemia. Its use (in somewhat lower dose) in sickle cell anaemia is described in Chapter 25. It has the familiar spectrum of unwanted effects, bone marrow depression being significant.

Bortezomib

▼ **Bortezomib** is a boron-containing tripeptide that inhibits cellular proteasome function. For some reason, rapidly dividing cells are more sensitive than normal cells to this drug, making it a useful anticancer agent. It is mainly used for the treatment of myeloma (a clonal malignancy of plasma cells).

Thalidomide

▼ Investigations of the notorious teratogenic effect of **thalidomide** showed that it has multiple effects on gene transcription, angiogenesis and proteasome function, leading to trials of its efficacy as an anticancer drug. In the event, it proved efficacious in myeloma, for which it is now widely used. The main adverse effect of thalidomide, apart from teratogenesis (irrelevant in myeloma treatment), is peripheral neuropathy, leading to irreversible weakness and sensory loss. It also increases the incidence of thrombosis and stroke.

A thalidomide derivative **lenalidomide** is thought to have fewer adverse effects, but unlike thalidomide, can cause bone marrow depression and neutropenia.

Biological response modifiers and others

▼ Agents that enhance the host's response are referred to as *biological response modifiers*. Some, for example **interferon-α** (and its pegylated derivative), are used in treating some solid tumours and lymphomas, and **aldesleukin** (recombinant interleukin-2) is used in some cases of renal tumours. **Tretinoin** (a form of vitamin A; see Ch. 27) is a powerful inducer of differentiation in leukaemic cells and is used as an adjunct to chemotherapy to induce remission. A related compound is **bexarotene**, a retinoid X receptor antagonist (see Ch. 3) that inhibits cell proliferation and differentiation.

Porfimer and **temoporfin** are haematoporphyrin photosensitizing agents. They accumulate in cells and kill them when excited by the appropriate wavelength light. They are usually used in cases where the light source can be selectively aimed at the tumour (e.g. in the case of obstructing oesophageal tumours).

RESISTANCE TO ANTICANCER DRUGS

The resistance that neoplastic cells manifest to cytotoxic drugs is said to be *primary* (present when the drug is first given) or *acquired* (developing during treatment with the drug). Acquired resistance may result from either *adaptation* of the tumour cells or *mutation*, with the emergence of cells that are less susceptible or resistant to the drug and consequently have a selective advantage over the sensitive cells. The following are examples of various mechanisms of resistance. See Mimeault et al. (2008) for a critical appraisal of this issue.

- *Decreased accumulation of cytotoxic drugs* in cells as a result of the increased expression of cell surface, energy-dependent drug transport proteins. These are responsible for multidrug resistance to many structurally dissimilar anticancer drugs (e.g. doxorubicin, vinblastine and dactinomycin; see Gottesman et al., 2002). An important member of this group is *P-glycoprotein* (P-gp/MDR1; see Ch. 8). P-glycoprotein protects cells against environmental toxins. It functions as a hydrophobic 'vacuum cleaner', picking up foreign chemicals, such as drugs, as they enter the cell membrane and expelling them. Non-cytotoxic agents that reverse

multidrug resistance are being investigated as potential adjuncts to treatment.

- *A decrease in the amount of drug taken up by the cell* (e.g. in the case of methotrexate).
- *Insufficient activation of the drug.* Some drugs require metabolic activation to manifest their antitumour activity. If this fails, they may no longer be effective. Examples include conversion of fluorouracil to FDUMP, phosphorylation of cytarabine and conversion of mercaptopurine to a fraudulent nucleotide.
- *Increase in inactivation* (e.g. cytarabine and mercaptopurine).
- *Increased concentration of target enzyme* (methotrexate).
- *Decreased requirement for substrate* (crisantaspase).
- *Increased utilisation of alternative metabolic pathways* (antimetabolites).
- *Rapid repair of drug-induced DNA damage* (alkylating agents).
- *Altered activity of target*, for example modified topoisomerase II (doxorubicin).
- *Mutations in various genes*, giving rise to resistant target molecules. For example, the *p53* gene and overexpression of the *Bcl-2* gene family (several cytotoxic drugs).

COMBINATION THERAPIES

Treatment with combinations of anticancer agents increases the cytotoxicity against cancer cells without necessarily increasing the general toxicity. For example, methotrexate, which mainly has myelosuppressive toxicity, may be used in a regimen with vincristine, which has mainly neurotoxicity. The few drugs we possess with low myelotoxicity, such as cisplatin and bleomycin, are good candidates for combination regimens. Treatment with combinations of drugs also decreases the possibility of the development of resistance to individual agents. Drugs are often given in large doses intermittently in several courses, with intervals of 2–3 weeks between courses, rather than in small doses continuously, because this permits the bone marrow to regenerate during the intervals. Furthermore, it has been shown that the same total dose of an agent is more effective when given in one or two large doses than in multiple small doses.

CONTROL OF EMESIS AND MYELOSUPPRESSION

EMESIS

The nausea and vomiting induced by many cancer chemotherapy agents are a serious deterrent to patient compliance (see also Ch. 30). It is a particular problem with cisplatin but also complicates therapy with many other compounds, such as the alkylating agents. 5-hydroxytryptamine $(HT)_3$-receptor antagonists such as **ondansetron** or **granisetron** (see Chs 15 and 30) are effective against cytotoxic drug-induced vomiting and have revolutionised cisplatin chemotherapy. Of the other antiemetic agents available, **metoclopramide**, given intravenously in high dose, has proved useful and is often combined with dexamethasone (Ch. 33) or **lorazepam** (Ch. 44), both of which further mitigate the unwanted effects of chemotherapy. As metoclopramide commonly causes extrapyramidal side effects in children and young adults, **diphenhydramine** (Ch. 26) can be used instead.

MYELOSUPPRESSION

Myelosuppression limits the use of many anticancer agents. Regimens contrived to surmount the problem have included removal of some of the patient's own bone marrow prior to treatment, purging it of cancer cells (using specific monoclonal antibodies) and replacing it after cytotoxic therapy is finished. A protocol in which aliquots of stem cells, harvested from the blood following administration of the growth factor **molgramostim**, which increases their abundance in blood, are expanded *in vitro* using further haemopoietic growth factors (Ch. 25) is now frequently used. The use of such growth factors after replacement of the marrow has been successful in some cases. A further possibility is the introduction, into the extracted bone marrow, of the mutated gene that confers multidrug resistance, so that when replaced, the marrow cells (but not the cancer cells) will be resistant to the cytotoxic action of the anticancer drugs. **Folinic acid** may be given as a supplement to prevent anaemia or as a 'rescue' after high-dose methotrexate.

FUTURE DEVELOPMENTS

As the reader will have judged by now, our current approach to cancer chemotherapy embraces an eclectic mixture of drugs – some very old and some very new – in an attempt to target selectively cancer cells. Real therapeutic progress has been achieved, although 'cancer' as a disease (actually many different diseases with a similar outcome) has not been comprehensively defeated and remains a massive challenge for future generations of researchers. In this therapeutic area, probably more than in any other, the debate about the risk–benefit of

treatment and the patient quality of life issues has taken centre stage and remains a major area of concern (see Duric & Stockler, 2001; Klastersky & Paesmans, 2001).

Of the recent advances in drug therapy, the tyrosine kinase inhibitors and the biologics have arguably been the most innovative advances. Further drugs of the kinase inhibitor type are under active investigation (see Vargas et al., 2013), as are anti-angiogenic drugs (similar to bevacizumab; see Ferrarotto & Hoff, 2013). Novel drugs targeting HER2-receptor in breast cancer have been reviewed by Abramson and Arteaga (2011). Warner and Gustafsson (2010) have highlighted the opportunities afforded by the discovery of a further isoform of the oestrogen receptor for the treatment of hormone-dependent breast and other cancers.

▼ For years, epidemiological and experimental evidence has been accumulating, which suggests that chronic use of cyclo-oxygenase (COX) inhibitors (see Ch. 26) protect against cancer of the gastrointestinal tract and possibly other sites as well. The COX-2 isoform is overexpressed in about 85% of cancers, and prostanoids originating from this source may activate signalling pathways that enable cells to escape from apoptotic death. The literature has been controversial but the balance of evidence now favours the notion that COX-2 may be a potentially important target for anticancer drug development (see Khan et al., 2011). COX-2 inhibitors could therefore be useful in the treatment of some cancers, either alone or in combination with conventional chemotherapeutic agents (Ghosh et al., 2010; Kraus et al., 2013). Ironically, some authors (Gurpinar et al., 2013) argue that the mechanism of action of these inhibitors in cancer models is unrelated to COX inhibition. No doubt these apparent paradoxes will be resolved with the passage of time.

Much work is going into genotyping of tumour tissue as a guide to selecting the best drug combination to use in treating an individual patient, based on the particular genetic abnormality present in the tumour cells (see Patel et al., 2013 for a short review). This approach, still in its early stages, is beginning to yield promising approaches to optimising treatment of melanoma and lung cancer, and is expected to develop rapidly.

REFERENCES AND FURTHER READING

General textbook

Airley, R., 2009. Anticancer Drugs. Wiley-Blackwell, Chichester. (*Recent textbook covering all aspects from basic pharmacology to clinical use*)

Mechanisms of carcinogenesis

Buys, C.H.C.M., 2000. Telomeres, telomerase and cancer. N. Engl. J. Med. 342, 1282–1283. (*Clear, concise coverage*)

Chambers, A.F., Groom, A.C., MacDonald, I.C., 2002. Dissemination and growth of cancer cells in metastatic sites. Nat. Rev. Cancer 2, 563–567. (*Review; stresses the importance of metastases in most cancer deaths, discusses the mechanisms involved in metastasis and raises the possibility of targeting these in anticancer drug development*)

Griffioen, A., Molema, G., 2000. Angiogenesis: potentials for pharmacologic intervention in the treatment of cancer, cardiovascular diseases and chronic inflammation. Pharmacol. Rev. 52, 237–268. (*Comprehensive review covering virtually all aspects of angiogenesis and the potential methods of modifying it to produce an antineoplastic effect*)

Mimeault, M., Hauke, R., Batra, S.K., 2008. Recent advances on the molecular mechanisms involved in the drug resistance of cancer cells and novel targeting therapies. Clin. Pharmacol. Ther. 83, 673–691. (*Comprehensive review covering all aspects of this field*)

Weinberg, R.A., 1996. How cancer arises. Sci. Am. Sept., 42–48. (*Simple, clear overview, listing main oncogenes, tumour suppressor genes and the cell cycle; excellent diagrams*)

Anticancer therapy

Gottesman, M.M., Fojo, T., Bates, S.E., 2002. Multidrug resistance in cancer: role of ATP-dependent transporters. Nat. Rev. Cancer 2,

48–56. (*Outlines cellular mechanisms of resistance; describes ATP-dependent transporters, emphasising those in human cancer; considers resistance reversal strategies*)

Krause, D.S., Van Etten, R., 2005. Tyrosine kinases as targets for cancer therapy. N. Engl. J. Med. 353, 172–187. (*Excellent review on tyrosine kinases as targets; good diagrams and tables as well as a highly readable style*)

Savage, D.G., Antman, K.H., 2002. Imatinib mesylate – a new oral targeted therapy. N. Engl. J. Med. 346, 683–693. (*Review with detailed coverage of this drug for chronic myelogenous leukaemia; very good diagrams*)

New directions and miscellaneous

Abramson, V., Arteaga, C.L., 2011. New strategies in HER2-overexpressing breast cancer: many combinations of targeted drugs available. Clin. Cancer Res. 17, 952–958. (*Deals mainly with ways in which the use of existing biologics can be optimized, but also discusses several new therapeutic directions*)

Duric, V., Stockler, M., 2001. Patients' preferences for adjuvant chemotherapy in early breast cancer. Lancet Oncol. 2, 691–697. (*The title is self-explanatory; deals with patients' assessment of quality of life issues*)

Ferrarotto, R., Hoff, P.M., 2013. Antiangiogenic drugs for colorectal cancer: exploring new possibilities. Clin. Colorect. Cancer 12, 1–7. (*Good review of this field, clinical in tone and content*)

Ghosh, N., Chaki, R., Mandal, V., Mandal, S.C., 2010. COX-2 as a target for cancer chemotherapy. Pharmacol. Rep. 62, 233–244. (*Excellent review of this, often controversial, area*)

Gurpinar, E., Grizzle, W.E., Piazza, G.A., 2013. COX-independent mechanisms of cancer chemoprevention by anti-inflammatory drugs. Frontiers Oncol. 3, 1–81. (*A contrarian viewpoint on the target of action of COX-2 inhibitors in cancer. Interesting reading*)

Keith, W.N., Bilsland, A., Hardie, M., Evans, T.R., 2004. Drug insight: cancer cell immortality – telomerase as a target for novel cancer gene therapies. Nat. Clin. Pract. Oncol. 1, 88–96.

Khan, Z., Khan, N., Tiwari, R.P., Sah, N.K., Prasad, G.B., Bisen, P.S., 2011. Biology of COX-2: an application in cancer therapeutics. Curr. Drug Targets 12, 1082–1093.

Klastersky, J., Paesmans, M., 2001. Response to chemotherapy, quality of life benefits and survival in advanced non-small lung cancer: review of literature results. Lung Cancer 34, S95–S101. (*Another paper that addresses quality of life issues surrounding chemotherapy*)

Kraus, S., Naumov, I., Arber, N., 2013. COX-2 active agents in the chemoprevention of colorectal cancer. Recent Results Cancer Res. 191, 95–103.

Patel, L., Parker, B., Yang, D., Zhang, W., 2013. Translational genomics in cancer research: converting profiles into personalized cancer medicine. Cancer Biol. Med. 10, 214–220. (*Discusses prospects for personalised cancer therapy based on genotyping*)

Tookman, L., Roylance, R., 2010. New drugs for breast cancer. Br. Med. Bull. 96, 111–129. (*Easy-to-read account of the use and actions of biologics in breast cancer and a review of some promising new leads in the field. Recommended*)

Vargas, L., Hamasy, A., Nore, B.F., Smith, C.I., 2013. Inhibitors of BTK and ITK: state of the new drugs for cancer, autoimmunity and inflammatory diseases. Scand. J. Immunol. 78, 130–139. (*An excellent account of this area together with a discussion of 'loss of function' mutations in these kinases that may predispose towards cancer. Good diagrams*)

Warner, M., Gustafsson, J.A., 2010. The role of estrogen receptor beta (ERbeta) in malignant diseases – a new potential target for antiproliferative drugs in prevention and treatment of cancer. Biochem. Biophys. Res. Commun. 396, 63–66. (*The title is self explanatory. A thought-provoking paper if you have an interest in oestrogen receptors and cancer*)

Useful Web resources

(*The US equivalent of the website below. The best sections for you are those marked* Health Information Seekers *and* Professionals)

<www.cancerresearchuk.org> (*The website of Cancer Research UK, the largest cancer charity in the UK. Contains valuable data on the epidemiology and treatment of cancer, including links to clinical trials. An excellent resource*)

57 Harmful effects of drugs

OVERVIEW

This chapter addresses harmful effects of drugs, both in the context of therapeutic use – so-called adverse drug reactions – and of deliberate or accidental overdose. We are concerned here with serious harm, sometimes life-threatening or irreversible, distinct from the minor side effects that virtually all drugs produce, as described throughout this book. The classification of adverse drug reactions is considered, followed by aspects of drug toxicity, namely toxicity testing in drug development, mechanisms of toxin-induced cell damage, mutagenesis and carcinogenicity, teratogenesis and allergic reactions.

INTRODUCTION

Paracelsus, a 16th-century alchemist, is credited with the aphorism that all drugs are poisons: '… the dosage makes it either a poison or a remedy'. Today, toxic effects of drugs remain clinically important in the context of overdose (self-poisoning accounts for approximately 10% of the workload of emergency medicine departments in the UK; by contrast, homicidal poisoning is extremely uncommon). Some susceptible individuals may experience dose-related toxicity even during therapeutic dosing; some of this susceptibility is genetically determined, and genomic testing as a means of avoiding such harms is beginning to make its way into the clinic (Ch. 11).

Rigorous toxicity testing in animals (see p. 693), including tests for carcinogenicity, teratogenicity and organ-specific toxicities, is carried out on potential new drugs during development (see Ch. 60), often leading to abandonment of the compound before it is tested in humans. These toxicity studies form part of the package of information routinely submitted to regulatory agencies by drug companies seeking approval to market a new drug. Nevertheless, harmful effects are often encountered after a drug is marketed for human use, due to the emergence of adverse effects not detected in animals. These harms are usually referred to as 'adverse drug reactions' (ADRs) and are of great concern to drug regulatory authorities, which are charged with establishing the safety as well as the efficacy of drugs. Unpredictable events are of particular concern. Some ADRs are predictable as a consequence of the main pharmacological effect of the drug and are relatively easily recognised, but some (e.g. immunological reactions), are unpredictable, sometimes serious, and likely to occur only in some patients.

Clinically important ADRs are common, costly and avoidable (see Pirmohamed et al., 2004).[1] Any organ can

be the principal target, and several organ systems can be involved simultaneously. The symptoms and signs sometimes closely shadow drug administration and discontinuation, but in other cases adverse effects only occur during prolonged use (*osteoporosis* during continued high-dose glucocorticoid therapy [Ch. 33], or *tardive dyskinesia* during continuous use of antipsychotic drugs [Ch. 46], for example). Some adverse effects occur on ending treatment, either within a few days (e.g. tachycardia on abrupt discontinuation of β-adrenoceptor blockade) or after a delay, first appearing months or years after treatment is discontinued, as in the case of some second malignancies following successful chemotherapy. Consequently, anticipating, avoiding, recognising and responding to adverse drug reactions are among the most challenging and important parts of clinical practice.

CLASSIFICATION OF ADVERSE DRUG REACTIONS

Harmful effects of drugs may or may not be related to the known mechanism of action of the drug In either case, individual variation (see Ch. 11) is a major factor in determining the response of a particular patient and their susceptibility to harm. Aronson & Ferner (2003) have suggested that ADRs be described according to the **do**se, **t**ime course and **s**usceptibility (DoTS).

ADVERSE EFFECTS RELATED TO THE KNOWN PHARMACOLOGICAL ACTION OF THE DRUG

Many adverse effects related to the known pharmacological actions of the drug are predictable, at least if these actions are well understood. They are sometimes referred to as type A ('augmented') adverse reactions (Rawlins & Thomson, 1985) and are related to dose and individual susceptibility. Many such reactions have been described in previous chapters. For example, postural hypotension occurs with α_1-adrenoceptor antagonists, bleeding with anticoagulants, sedation with anxiolytics and so on. In many instances, this type of unwanted effect is reversible, and the problem can often be dealt with by reducing the dose. Such effects are sometimes serious (e.g. intracerebral bleeding caused by anticoagulants, hypoglycaemic coma from insulin), and occasionally they are not easily reversible, for example drug dependence produced by opioid analgesics (see Ch. 49).

Some adverse effects related to the main action of a drug result in discrete events rather than graded symptoms, and can be difficult to detect. For example, drugs that block cyclo-oxygenase (COX)-2 (including 'coxibs', for example **rofecoxib**, **celecoxib**, **valdecoxib**, as well as some conventional non-steroidal anti-inflammatory drugs, NSAIDs) increase the risk of myocardial infarction in a dose-dependent manner (Ch. 26). This potential was predictable from the ability of these drugs to inhibit

---

[1] 6.5% of hospital admissions were due to ADRs at a projected annual cost of £466 million in the UK. Antiplatelet drugs, diuretics, non-steroidal anti-inflammatory drugs and anticoagulants between them accounted for 50% of the ADRs. 2.3% of the patients died. Most events were avoidable.

prostacyclin biosynthesis and increase arterial blood pressure, and early studies gave a hint of such problems. The effect was difficult to prove because of the high background incidence of coronary thrombosis, and it was only when placebo-controlled trials were performed for another indication (in the hope that COX-2 inhibitors could prevent bowel cancer) that this effect was confirmed unequivocally.

ADVERSE EFFECTS UNRELATED TO THE KNOWN PHARMACOLOGICAL ACTION OF THE DRUG

Adverse effects unrelated to the main pharmacological effect may be predictable when a drug is taken in excessive dose, for example **paracetamol** hepatotoxicity (see below) or **aspirin**-induced tinnitus; or when susceptibility is increased, for example during pregnancy or by a predisposing disorder such as glucose 6-phosphate dehydrogenase deficiency or a mutation in the mitochondrial DNA that predisposes to aminoglycoside ototoxicity (Ch. 11).

Unpredictable reactions unrelated to the main effect of the drug (sometimes termed *idiosyncratic reactions*, or type B for Bizarre in the Rawlins & Thomson (1985) classification) are often initiated by a chemically reactive metabolite rather than the parent drug. Examples of such ADRs, which are often immunological in nature, include drug-induced hepatic or renal necrosis, bone marrow suppression, carcinogenesis and disordered fetal development. Uncommon but severe unpredictable adverse effects that have been mentioned in earlier chapters include aplastic anaemia from **chloramphenicol** and anaphylaxis in response to **penicillin**. They are usually severe – otherwise they would go unrecognised – and their existence is important in establishing the safety of medicines.

DRUG TOXICITY

TOXICITY TESTING

Toxicity testing in animals is carried out on new drugs to identify potential hazards before administering them to humans. It involves the use of a wide range of tests in different species, with long-term administration of the drug, regular monitoring for physiological or biochemical abnormalities, and a detailed postmortem examination at the end of the trial to detect any gross or histological abnormalities. Toxicity testing is performed with doses well above the expected therapeutic range, and establishes which tissues or organs are likely 'targets' of toxic effects of the drug. Recovery studies are performed to assess whether toxic effects are reversible, and particular attention is paid to irreversible changes such as carcinogenesis or neurodegeneration. The basic premise is that toxic effects caused by a drug are similar in humans and other animals. There are, however, wide interspecies variations, especially in metabolising enzymes; consequently, a toxic metabolite formed in one species may not be formed in another, and so toxicity testing in animals is not always a reliable guide. **Pronethalol**, the first β-adrenoceptor antagonist synthesised, was not developed because it caused carcinogenicity in mice; it subsequently emerged that carcinogenicity occurred only in the one strain tested – but by then other β blockers were already in development.

Toxic effects can range from negligible to so severe as to preclude further development of the compound. Intermediate levels of toxicity are more acceptable in drugs intended for severe illnesses (e.g. AIDS or cancers), and decisions on whether or not to continue development are often difficult. If development does proceed, safety monitoring can be concentrated on the system 'flagged' as a potential target of toxicity by the animal studies.[2] *Safety* of a drug (as distinct from toxicity) can be established only during use in humans.

> **Types of drug toxicity**
>
> - Toxic effects of drugs can be:
>   - related to the principal pharmacological action (e.g. bleeding with anticoagulants)
>   - unrelated to the principal pharmacological action (e.g. liver damage with **paracetamol**).
> - Some adverse reactions that occur with ordinary therapeutic dosage are initially unpredictable, serious and uncommon (e.g. agranulocytosis with **carbimazole**). Such reactions (termed idiosyncratic) are almost inevitably detected only after widespread use of a new drug. It is sometimes possible to develop a test to exclude susceptible subjects from drug exposure (e.g. mitochondrial DNA variants/increased susceptibility to aminoglycoside ototoxicity).
> - Adverse effects unrelated to the main action of a drug are often caused by reactive metabolites and/or immunological reactions.

GENERAL MECHANISMS OF TOXIN-INDUCED CELL DAMAGE AND CELL DEATH

Toxic concentrations of drugs or drug metabolites can cause necrosis; however, programmed cell death (apoptosis; see Ch. 5) is increasingly recognised to be of equal or greater importance, especially in chronic toxicity.

Chemically reactive drug metabolites can form covalent bonds with target molecules, or can damage tissue by non-covalent mechanisms. The liver is of great importance in drug metabolism (Ch. 9), and hepatocytes are exposed to high concentrations of nascent metabolites. Drugs and their polar metabolites are concentrated in renal tubular fluid as water is reabsorbed, so renal tubules are exposed to higher concentrations than are other tissues. Several hepatotoxic drugs (e.g. paracetamol) are also nephrotoxic. Consequently, hepatic or renal damage are common reasons for abandoning development of drugs during toxicity testing and chemical pathology tests of hepatic damage (usually levels of transaminase

---

[2]The value of toxicity testing is illustrated by experience with **triparanol**, a cholesterol-lowering drug marketed in the USA in 1959. Three years later, a team from the Food and Drug Administration, acting on a tip-off, paid the manufacturer a surprise visit that revealed falsification of toxicology data demonstrating cataracts in rats and dogs. The drug was withdrawn, but some patients who had been taking it for a year or more did develop cataracts. Regulatory authorities now require that toxicity testing is performed under a tightly defined code of practice (Good Laboratory Practice), which incorporates many safeguards to minimise the risk of error or fraud.

enzymes measured in blood plasma or serum) and renal function (usually creatinine concentration) are routine.

NON-COVALENT INTERACTIONS

▼ Reactive metabolites of drugs are implicated in several potentially cytotoxic, non-covalent processes, including:

- lipid peroxidation
- generation of toxic reactive oxygen species
- depletion of reduced glutathione (GSH)
- modification of sulfhydryl groups.

Lipid peroxidation

▼ Peroxidation of unsaturated lipids can be initiated either by reactive metabolites or by reactive oxygen species (see Fig. 57.1). Lipid peroxyradicals (ROO$^{•}$) can produce lipid hydroperoxides (ROOH), which produce further lipid peroxyradicals. This chain reaction – a peroxidative cascade – may eventually affect much of the membrane lipid. Defence mechanisms, for example GSH peroxidase and vitamin E, protect against this. Cell damage results from alteration of membrane permeability or from reactions of the products of lipid peroxidation with proteins.

Reactive oxygen species

▼ Reduction of molecular oxygen to superoxide anion ($O_2^{-•}$) may be followed by enzymic conversion to hydrogen peroxide (H_2O_2), hydroperoxy (HOO$^{•}$) and hydroxyl (OH$^{•}$) radicals or singlet oxygen. These reactive oxygen species are cytotoxic, both directly and through lipid peroxidation, and are important in excitotoxicity and neurodegeneration (Ch. 40, Fig. 40.2).

Depletion of glutathione

▼ The GSH redox cycle protects cells from oxidative stress. GSH can be depleted by accumulation of normal oxidative products of cell metabolism, or by the action of toxic chemicals. GSH is normally maintained in a redox couple with its disulfide, GSSG. Oxidising species convert GSH to GSSG, GSH being regenerated by NADPH-dependent GSSG reductase. When cellular GSH falls to about 20–30% of normal, cellular defence against toxic compounds is impaired and cell death can result.

Modification of sulfhydryl groups

▼ Modification of sulfhydryl groups can be produced either by oxidising species that alter sulfhydryl groups reversibly or by covalent interaction. Free sulfhydryl groups have a critical role in the catalytic activity of many enzymes. Important targets for sulfhydryl modification by reactive metabolites include the cytoskeletal protein actin GSH reductase and Ca^{2+}-transporting ATPases in the plasma membrane and endoplasmic reticulum. These maintain cytoplasmic Ca^{2+} concentration at approximately 0.1 µmol/l in the face of an extracellular Ca^{2+} concentration of more than 1 mmol/l. A sustained rise in cell Ca^{2+} occurs with inactivation of these enzymes (or with increased membrane permeability; see above), and this compromises cell viability. Lethal processes leading to cell death after acute Ca^{2+} overload include activation of degradative enzymes (neutral proteases, phospholipases, endonucleases) and protein kinases, mitochondrial damage and cytoskeletal alterations (e.g. modification of association between actin and actin-binding proteins).

COVALENT INTERACTIONS

Targets for covalent interactions include DNA, proteins/peptides, lipids and carbohydrates. Covalent bonding to DNA is a basic mechanism of mutagenic chemicals; this is dealt with below. Several non-mutagenic chemicals also form covalent bonds with macromolecules, but the relationship between this and cell damage is incompletely understood. For example, the cholinesterase inhibitor paraoxon (the active metabolite of the insecticide parathion) binds acetylcholinesterase at the neuromuscular junction (Ch. 13) and causes necrosis of skeletal muscle.

One toxin from an exceptionally poisonous toadstool, *Amanita phalloides*, binds actin, and another binds RNA polymerase, interfering with actin depolymerisation and protein synthesis, respectively.

> ## General mechanisms of cell damage and cell death
>
> - Drug-induced cell damage/death is usually caused by reactive metabolites of the drug, involving non-covalent and/or covalent interactions with target molecules. Cell death often occurs by apoptosis.
> - Non-covalent interactions include:
>   - lipid peroxidation via a chain reaction
>   - generation of cytotoxic reactive oxygen species
>   - depletion of reduced glutathione
>   - modification of sulfhydryl groups on key enzymes (e.g. Ca^{2+}-ATPase) and structural proteins.
> - Covalent interactions, for example adduct formation between a metabolite of **paracetamol** (NAPBQI: *N*-acetyl-*p*-benzoquinone imine) and cellular macromolecules (Fig. 57.1). Covalent binding to protein can produce an immunogen; binding to DNA can cause carcinogenesis and teratogenesis.

HEPATOTOXICITY

Many therapeutic drugs cause liver damage, manifested clinically as hepatitis or (in less severe cases) only as laboratory abnormalities (e.g. increased activity of plasma aspartate transaminase, an enzyme released from damaged liver cells). Paracetamol and **halothane** cause hepatotoxicity by the mechanisms of cell damage outlined above. Genetic differences in drug metabolism (see Ch. 11) have been implicated in some instances (e.g. **isoniazid, phenytoin**). Mild drug-induced abnormalities of liver function are not uncommon, but the mechanism of liver injury is often uncertain (e.g. *statins*; Ch. 23). It is not always necessary to discontinue a drug when such mild laboratory abnormalities occur, but the occurrence of cirrhosis as a result of long-term low-dose **methotrexate** treatment for arthritis or psoriasis (see Chs 26 and 27) argues for caution. Hepatotoxicity of a different kind, namely reversible obstructive jaundice, occurs with **chlorpromazine** (Ch. 46) and androgens (Ch. 35).

Hepatotoxicity caused by **paracetamol** overdose remains a common cause of death following self-poisoning. An outline is given in Chapter 26. Paracetamol poisoning exemplifies many of the general mechanisms of cell damage outlined above. With toxic doses of paracetamol, the enzymes catalysing the normal conjugation reactions are saturated, and mixed-function oxidases instead convert the drug to the reactive metabolite *N*-acetyl-*p*-benzoquinone imine (NAPBQI). As explained in Chapter 9, paracetamol toxicity is increased in patients in whom P450 enzymes have been induced, for instance by chronic excessive consumption of alcohol. NAPBQI initiates several of the covalent and non-covalent interactions described above and illustrated in Figure 57.1. Oxidative stress from GSH depletion is important in leading

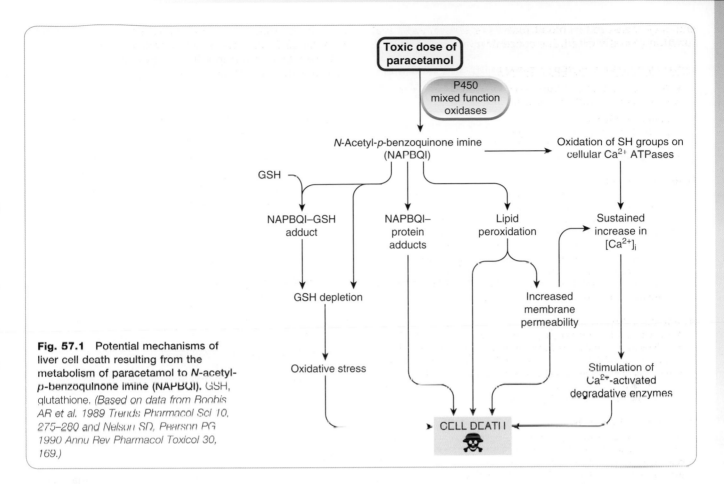

Fig. 57.1 Potential mechanisms of liver cell death resulting from the metabolism of paracetamol to *N*-acetyl-*p*-benzoquinone imine (NAPBQI). GSH, glutathione. (*Based on data from Boobis AR et al. 1989 Trends Pharmacol Sci 10, 275–280 and Nelson SD, Pearson PG 1990 Annu Rev Pharmacol Toxicol 30, 169.*)

to cell death. Regeneration of GSH from GSSG depends on the availability of cysteine, the intracellular availability of which can be limiting. *Acetylcysteine* or *methionine* can substitute for cysteine, increasing GSH availability; they are used to treat patients with paracetamol poisoning.

Liver damage can also be produced by immunological mechanisms (see p. 701), which have been particularly implicated in halothane hepatitis (see Ch. 41).

Hepatotoxicity

- Hepatocytes are exposed to reactive metabolites of drugs as these are formed by P450 enzymes.
- Liver damage is produced by several mechanisms of cell injury; **paracetamol** exemplifies many of these (see Fig. 57.1).
- Some drugs (e.g. **chlorpromazine**) can cause reversible cholestatic jaundice.
- Immunological mechanisms are sometimes implicated (e.g. **halothane**).

Table 57.1 Adverse effects of non-steroidal anti-inflammatory drugs on the kidney

Cause	Adverse effects
Principal pharmacological action (i.e. inhibition of prostaglandin biosynthesis)	Acute ischaemic renal failure Sodium retention (leading to or exacerbating hypertension and/or heart failure) Water retention Hyporeninaemic hypoaldosteronism (leading to hyperkalaemia)
Unrelated to principal pharmacological action (allergic-type interstitial nephritis)	Renal failure Proteinuria
Unknown whether or not related to principal pharmacological action (analgesic nephropathy)	Papillary necrosis Chronic renal failure

Adapted from Murray & Brater 1993.

NEPHROTOXICITY

Drug-induced nephrotoxicity is a common clinical problem: NSAIDs (Table 57.1) and angiotensin-converting enzyme (ACE) inhibitors are among the commonest precipitants of acute renal failure. This is usually caused by the principal pharmacological actions of these drugs, which, although well tolerated in healthy people, cause renal failure in patients with diseases that jeopardise glomerular filtration.

Nephrotoxicity

- Renal tubular cells are exposed to high concentrations of drugs and metabolites as urine is concentrated.
- Renal damage can cause papillary and/or tubular necrosis.
- Inhibition of prostaglandin synthesis by non-steroidal anti-inflammatory drugs causes vasoconstriction and lowers glomerular filtration rate.

MUTAGENESIS AND ASSESSMENT OF GENOTOXIC POTENTIAL

Drug-induced mutagenesis is one important cause of carcinogenesis and of teratogenesis. Registration of pharmaceuticals requires a comprehensive assessment of their genotoxic potential. Because no single test is adequate, the usual approach is to carry out a battery of *in vitro* and *in vivo* tests for genotoxicity, usually comprising tests for gene mutation in bacteria, *in vitro* and *in vivo* tests for chromosome damage, and *in vivo* tests for reproductive toxicity and carcinogenicity (see below).

BIOCHEMICAL MECHANISMS OF MUTAGENESIS

Chemical agents cause mutation by covalent modification of DNA. Certain mutations result in carcinogenesis, because the affected DNA sequence codes for a protein that regulates cell growth. It usually requires more than one mutation in a cell to initiate the changes that result in malignancy, mutations in proto-oncogenes (which regulate cell growth) and tumour suppressor genes (which code for products that inhibit the transcription of oncogenes) being particularly implicated (see Chs 5 and 56).

▼ Most chemical carcinogens act by modifying bases in DNA, particularly guanine, the O6 and N7 positions of which readily combine covalently with reactive metabolites of chemical carcinogens. Substitution at the O6 position is the more likely to produce a permanent mutagenic effect, because N7 substitutions are usually quickly repaired.

The accessibility of bases in DNA to chemical attack is greatest when DNA is in the process of replication (i.e. during cell division). The likelihood of genetic damage by many mutagens is therefore related to the frequency of cell division. The developing fetus is particularly susceptible, and mutagens are also potentially teratogenic for this reason (see p. 698). This is also important in relation to mutagenesis of germ cells, particularly in girls, because in humans the production of primary oocytes occurs by a rapid succession of mitotic divisions very early in embryogenesis. Each primary oocyte then undergoes only two further divisions much later in life, at the time of ovulation. It is consequently during early pregnancy that germ cells of the developing female embryo are most likely to undergo mutagenesis, the mutations being transmitted to progeny conceived many years later. In the male, germ cell divisions occur throughout life, and sensitivity of germ cells to mutagens is continuously present.

CARCINOGENESIS

Alteration of DNA is the first step in carcinogenesis (see Chs 5 and 56). Carcinogenic compounds can interact directly with DNA (genotoxic carcinogens) or act at a later stage to increase the likelihood that mutation will result in a tumour (epigenetic carcinogens; Fig. 57.2).

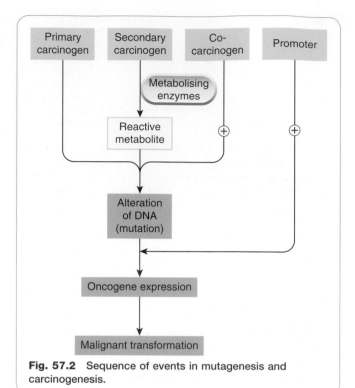

Fig. 57.2 Sequence of events in mutagenesis and carcinogenesis.

Mutagenesis and carcinogenicity

- Mutagenesis involves modification of DNA.
- Mutation of proto-oncogenes or tumour suppressor genes leads to carcinogenesis. More than one mutation is usually required.
- Drugs are relatively uncommon (but not unimportant) causes of birth defects and cancers.

MEASUREMENT OF MUTAGENICITY AND CARCINOGENICITY

Much effort has gone into developing assays to detect mutagenicity and carcinogenicity. *In vitro* tests for *mutagenicity* are used to screen large numbers of compounds but are unreliable as predictors of carcinogenicity. Whole-animal tests for carcinogenicity are expensive and time-consuming but are usually required by regulatory authorities before a new drug is licensed for use in humans. The main limitation of this kind of study is that there are important species differences, mainly to do with the metabolism of the foreign compound and the formation of reactive products.

The widely used *Ames test* for mutagenicity measures the effect of substances on the rate of back-mutation (i.e. reversion from mutant to wild-type form) in *Salmonella typhimurium*.

▼ The wild-type strain can grow in a medium containing no added amino acids, because it can synthesise all the amino acids it needs. A mutant form of the organism cannot make histidine in this way and therefore grows only on a medium containing this amino acid. The Ames test involves growing the mutant form on a medium containing a small amount of histidine, plus the drug to be tested. After several divisions, the histidine becomes depleted, and the only cells that continue dividing are those that have back-mutated to the wild type. A count of colonies following subculture on plates deficient in histidine gives a measure of the mutation rate.

Primary carcinogens cause mutation by a direct action on bacterial DNA, but most carcinogens have to be converted to an active metabolite (see Fig. 57.2). Therefore it is necessary to include, in the culture, enzymes that catalyse the necessary conversion. An extract of liver from a rat treated with **phenobarbital** to induce liver enzymes is usually employed. There are many variations based on the same principle.

Other short-term *in vitro* tests for genotoxic chemicals include measurements of mutagenesis in mouse lymphoma cells, and assays for chromosome aberrations and sister chromatid exchanges in Chinese hamster ovary cells. However, all the *in vitro* tests give some false-positive and some false-negative results.

In vivo tests for carcinogenicity entail detection of tumours in groups of test animals. Carcinogenicity tests are inevitably slow, because there is usually a latency of months or years before tumours develop. Furthermore, tumours can develop spontaneously in control animals, and the results often provide only equivocal evidence of carcinogenicity of the test drug, making it difficult for industry and regulatory authorities to decide on further development and possible licensing of a product. None of the tests so far described can reliably detect epigenetic carcinogens. To do this, tests that measure the effect of the substance on tumour formation in the presence of a threshold dose of a separate genotoxic agents are being evaluated.

Few therapeutic drugs in clinical use are known to increase the risk of cancer, the most important groups being drugs that act on DNA, i.e. cytotoxic and immunosuppressant drugs (Chs 56 and 26, respectively), and sex hormones (e.g. *oestrogens*, Ch. 35).

TERATOGENESIS AND DRUG-INDUCED FETAL DAMAGE

Teratogenesis signifies the production of gross structural malformations during fetal development, in distinction from other kinds of drug-induced fetal damage such as growth retardation, dysplasia (e.g. iodide-associated goitre) or the asymmetrical limb reduction resulting from vasoconstriction caused by **cocaine** (see Ch. 49) in an otherwise normally developing limb. Examples of drugs that affect fetal development adversely are given in Table 57.2.

The importance of X irradiation and rubella infection as causes of fetal malformation was recognised early in the 20th century, but it was not until 1960 that drugs were implicated as causative agents in teratogenesis: the shocking experience with **thalidomide** led to a widespread reappraisal of many other drugs in clinical use, and to the setting up of drug regulatory bodies in many countries. Most birth

Table 57.2 Some drugs reported to have adverse effects on human fetal development

Agent	Effect(s)	Teratogenicity[a]	See chapter
Thalidomide	Phocomelia, heart defects, gut atresia, etc.	K	This chapter
Penicillamine	Loose skin etc.	K	26
Warfarin	Saddle nose; retarded growth; defects of limbs, eyes, central nervous system	K	24
Corticosteroids	Cleft palate and congenital cataract – rare	–	33
Androgens	Masculinisation in female	–	35
Oestrogens	Testicular atrophy in male	–	35
Stilbestrol	Vaginal adenosis in female fetus, also vaginal or cervical cancer	20+ years later	35
Phenytoin	Cleft lip/palate, microcephaly, mental retardation	K	45
Valproate	Neural tube defects (e.g. spina bifida)	K	45
Carbamazepine	Retardation of fetal head growth	S	45
Cytotoxic drugs (especially folate antagonists)	Hydrocephalus, cleft palate, neural tube defects, etc.	K	56
Aminoglycosides	Deafness	–	51
Tetracycline	Staining of bones and teeth, thin tooth enamel, impaired bone growth	S	51
Ethanol	Fetal alcohol syndrome	K	49
Retinoids	Hydrocephalus etc.	K	27
Angiotensin-converting enzyme inhibitors	Oligohydramnios, renal failure	K	22

[a]K, known teratogen (in experimental animals and/or humans); S, suspected teratogen (in experimental animals and/or humans).

Adapted from Juchau MR 1989 Bioactivation in chemical teratogenesis. Ann Rev Pharmacol Toxicol 29, 165.

Carcinogens

- Carcinogens can be:
  - genotoxic, i.e. causing mutations directly (primary carcinogens) or after conversion to reactive metabolites (secondary carcinogens)
  - epigenetic, i.e. increasing the possibility that a mutagen will cause cancer, although not themselves mutagenic.
- New drugs are tested for mutagenicity and carcinogenicity.
- The Ames test for mutagenicity measures back-mutation, in histidine-free medium, of a mutant *Salmonella typhimurium* (which, unlike the wild-type, cannot grow without histidine) in the presence of:
  - the chemical to be tested
  - a liver microsomal enzyme preparation for generating reactive metabolites.
- Colony growth indicates that mutagenesis has occurred. The test is rapid and inexpensive, but some false-positives and false-negatives occur.
- Carcinogenicity testing:
  - involves chronic dosing of groups of animals
  - is expensive and time-consuming
  - does not readily detect epigenetic carcinogens.

defects (about 70%) occur with no recognisable causative factor. Drug or chemical exposure during pregnancy is estimated to account for only approximately 1% of all fetal malformations. Fetal malformations are common, so the absolute numbers of children affected are substantial.

MECHANISM OF TERATOGENESIS

The timing of the teratogenic insult in relation to fetal development is critical in determining the type and extent of damage. Mammalian fetal development passes through three phases (Table 57.3):

1. blastocyst formation
2. organogenesis
3. histogenesis and maturation of function.

Cell division is the main process occurring during blastocyst formation. During this phase, drugs can kill the embryo by inhibiting cell division, but provided the embryo survives, its subsequent development does not

generally seem to be compromised. Ethanol is an exception, affecting development even at this very early stage (Ch. 49).

Drugs can cause gross malformations if administered during organogenesis (days 17–60 in humans). The structural organisation of the embryo occurs in a well-defined sequence: eye and brain, skeleton and limbs, heart and major vessels, palate, genitourinary system. The type of malformation produced thus depends on the time of exposure to the teratogen.

The cellular mechanisms by which teratogenic substances produce their effects are not at all well understood. There is a considerable overlap between mutagenicity and teratogenicity. In one large survey, among 78 compounds, 34 were both teratogenic and mutagenic, 19 were negative in both tests and 25 (among them thalidomide) were positive in one but not the other. Damage to DNA is important but not the only factor. The control of morphogenesis is poorly understood; vitamin A derivatives (retinoids) are involved and are potent teratogens (see p. 699 and Ch. 27). Known teratogens also include several drugs (e.g. **methotrexate** and **phenytoin**) that do not react directly with DNA but which inhibit its synthesis by their effects on folate metabolism (see Ch. 25). Administration of **folate** during pregnancy reduces the frequency of both spontaneous and drug-induced malformations, especially neural tube defects.

The fetus depends on an adequate supply of nutrients during the final stage of histogenesis and functional maturation, and development is regulated by a variety of hormones. Gross structural malformations do not arise from exposure to mutagens at this stage, but drugs that interfere with the supply of nutrients or with the hormonal milieu may have deleterious effects on growth and development. Exposure of a female fetus to androgens at this stage can cause masculinisation. **Stilbestrol** (a synthetic estrogen, now seldom used, licensed to treat breast or prostate cancer) was commonly given to pregnant women with a history of recurrent miscarriage during the 1950s (for unsound reasons). Used in this way it caused dysplasia of the vagina of female infants and an increased incidence of carcinoma of the vagina, a rare malignancy with almost no background incidence, in such offspring in their teens and twenties. Angiotensin II plays an important part in the later stages of fetal development and in renal function in the fetus, and ACE inhibitors and angiotensin receptor antagonists (Ch. 22) cause oligohydramnios and renal failure if administered during later stages of pregnancy, and fetal malformations if given earlier.

Table 57.3 The nature of drug effects on fetal development

Stage	Gestation period in humans	Main cellular process(es)	Affected by
Blastocyst formation	0–16 days	Cell division	Cytotoxic drugs, ?alcohol
Organogenesis	17–60 days approximately	Division Migration Differentiation Death	Teratogens Teratogens Teratogens Teratogens
Histogenesis and functional maturation	60 days to term	As above	Miscellaneous drugs (e.g. alcohol, nicotine, antithyroid drugs, steroids)

TESTING FOR TERATOGENICITY

The thalidomide disaster dramatically brought home the need for teratogenicity studies on new therapeutic drugs. Detection of drug-induced teratogenesis in humans is a particularly difficult problem because the 'spontaneous' malformation rate is high (3–10% depending on the definition of a significant malformation) and highly variable between different regions, age groups and social classes. Large-scale long-term studies are required, and the results are often inconclusive.

▼ Studies using embryonic stem cells in assessing developmental toxicity are showing some promise. *In vitro* methods, based on the culture of cells, organs or whole embryos, have, however, not so far been developed to a level where they satisfactorily predict teratogenesis *in vivo*, and most regulatory authorities require teratogenicity testing in a rodent and a non-rodent species (e.g. rabbit). Pregnant females are dosed at various levels during the critical period of organogenesis, and the fetuses are examined for structural abnormalities. However, poor cross-species correlation means that tests of this kind are not reliably predictive in humans, and it is usually recommended that new drugs are not used in pregnancy unless it is essential.

SOME DEFINITE AND PROBABLE HUMAN TERATOGENS

Although many drugs have been found to be teratogenic in varying degrees in experimental animals, relatively few are known to be teratogenic in humans (see Table 57.2). Some of the more important are discussed below.

Thalidomide

Thalidomide is almost unique in producing, at therapeutic dosage, virtually 100% malformed infants when taken in the first 3–6 weeks of gestation. It was introduced in 1957 as a hypnotic and sedative with the special feature that it was much less hazardous in overdosage than barbiturates, and it was even recommended specifically for use in pregnancy (with the advertising slogan 'the safe hypnotic'). It had been subjected to toxicity testing only in mice, which are resistant to thalidomide teratogenicity. Thalidomide was marketed energetically and successfully, and the first suspicion of its teratogenicity arose early in 1961 with reports of a sudden increase in the incidence of phocomelia ('seal limbs', an absence of development of the long bones of the arms and legs) that had hitherto been virtually unknown. At this time, a million tablets were being sold daily in West Germany. Reports of phocomelia came simultaneously from Hamburg and Sydney, and the connection with thalidomide was made.[3] The drug was withdrawn late in 1961, by which time an estimated 10000 malformed babies had been born (Fig. 57.3 illustrates the use of data linkage in detecting delayed ADRs). Despite intensive study, its mechanism remains poorly understood, although epidemiological

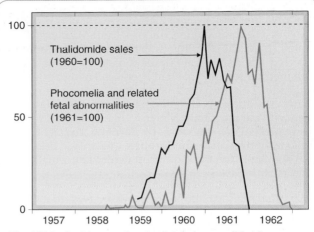

Fig. 57.3 Incidence of major fetal abnormalities in Western Europe following the introduction and withdrawal of thalidomide linked to sales data for thalidomide.

Table 57.4	Thalidomide teratogenesis
Day of gestation	**Type of deformity**
21–22	Malformation of ears Cranial nerve defects
24–27	Phocomelia of arms
28–29	Phocomelia of arms and legs
30–36	Malformation of hands Anorectal stenosis

investigation showed very clearly the correlation between the time of exposure and the type of malfunction produced (Table 57.4).

Cytotoxic drugs

Many alkylating agents (e.g. **chlorambucil** and **cyclophosphamide**) and antimetabolites (e.g. **azathioprine** and **mercaptopurine**) cause malformations when used in early pregnancy but more often lead to abortion (see Ch. 56). Folate antagonists (e.g. **methotrexate**) produce a much higher incidence of major malformations, evident in both live-born and stillborn fetuses.

Retinoids

Etretinate, a retinoid (i.e. vitamin A derivative) with marked effects on epidermal differentiation, is a known teratogen and causes a high proportion of serious abnormalities (notably skeletal deformities) in exposed fetuses. Dermatologists use retinoids to treat skin diseases, including several, such as acne and psoriasis, that are common in young women. Etretinate accumulates in subcutaneous fat and is eliminated extremely slowly, detectable amounts persisting for many months after chronic dosing is discontinued. Because of this, women should avoid pregnancy for at least 2 years after treatment. **Acitretin** is an active metabolite of etretinate. It is equally teratogenic, but tissue accumulation is less pronounced and elimination may be more rapid.

---

[3]A severe peripheral neuropathy, leading to irreversible paralysis and sensory loss, was reported within a year of the drug's introduction and subsequently confirmed in many reports. The drug company responsible was less than punctilious in acting on these reports (see Sjöström & Nilsson, 1972), which were soon eclipsed by the discovery of teratogenic effects, but the neurotoxic effect was severe enough in its own right to have necessitated restriction of the drug from general use. Today, use of thalidomide has had a resurgence related to several highly specialised applications. It is prescribed by specialists (in dermatology, oncology and in HIV infection, among others) under tightly controlled and restricted conditions.

Heavy metals

Lead, *cadmium* and *mercury* all cause fetal malformation in humans. The main evidence comes from *Minamata disease*, named after the locality in Japan where an epidemic occurred when the local population ate fish contaminated with methylmercury that had been used as an agricultural fungicide. This impaired brain development in exposed fetuses, resulting in cerebral palsy and mental retardation, often with microcephaly. Mercury, like other heavy metals, inactivates many enzymes by forming covalent bonds with sulfhydryl and other groups, and this is believed to be responsible for these developmental abnormalities.

Antiepileptic drugs (see Ch. 45)

Congenital malformations are increased two- to three-fold in babies of epileptic mothers, especially of mothers treated with two or more antiepileptic drugs during the first trimester, and in association with above-therapeutic plasma concentrations. Many antiepileptic drugs have been implicated, including **phenytoin** (particularly cleft lip/palate), **valproate** (neural tube defects) and **carbamazepine** (spina bifida and hypospadias, a malformation of the male urethra), as well as newer agents including **lamotrigine** and **topiramate** (Ch. 45). The relative risks attributable to different antiepileptic drugs are not well defined, but there is evidence that valproate is particularly harmful.

Warfarin

Administration of **warfarin** (Ch. 24) in the first trimester is associated with nasal hypoplasia and various central nervous system abnormalities, affecting roughly 25% of exposed babies. In the last trimester, it must not be used because of the risk of intracranial haemorrhage in the baby during delivery.

> ### Teratogenesis and drug-induced fetal damage
>
>
> - Teratogenesis means production of gross structural malformations of the fetus (e.g. the absence of limbs after **thalidomide**). Less comprehensive damage can be produced by several drugs (see Table 57.2). Less than 1% of congenital fetal defects are attributed to drugs given to the mother.
> - Gross malformations are produced only if teratogens act during organogenesis. This occurs during the first 3 months of pregnancy but after blastocyst formation. Drug-induced fetal damage is rare during blastocyst formation (exception: fetal alcohol syndrome) and after the first 3 months (exception: ACE inhibitors and sartans).
> - The mechanisms of action of teratogens are not clearly understood, although DNA damage is a factor.

IMMUNOLOGICAL REACTIONS TO DRUGS

Biological agents (Ch. 59) may provoke an immune response; anti-drug antibodies to insulin are common in diabetic patients, though they seldom cause problems (Ch. 31), but antidrug antibodies to erythropoietin and to thrombopoietin can have serious consequences for patients treated with these agents. (see Ch. 25). Measurement of antidrug antibodies is now routine during development of biological products. Seemingly trivial differences in manufacturing process (e.g. between different batches, or when a new manufacturer makes a copy of a biological product after it is no longer protected by patent – so-called 'biosimilar' products) can result in marked changes in immunogenicity.

Allergic reactions of various kinds are a common form of adverse drug reaction. Low-molecular-weight drugs are not immunogenic in themselves. A drug or its metabolites can, however, act as a *hapten* by interacting with protein to form a stable immunogenic conjugate (Ch. 6). The immunological basis of some allergic drug reactions has been well worked out, but often it is inferred from the clinical characteristics of the reaction, and direct evidence of an immunological mechanism is lacking. The existence of an allergic reaction is suggested by its delayed onset, or occurrence only after repeated exposure to the drug. Allergic reactions are generally unrelated to the main action of the drug, and conform to syndromes associated with types I, II, III and IV of the Gell and Coombs classification (see below and Ch. 6).

The overall incidence of allergic drug reactions is variously reported as being between 2% and 25%. Most are minor skin eruptions. Serious reactions (e.g. anaphylaxis, haemolysis and bone marrow depression) are rare. Penicillins, which are the commonest cause of drug-induced anaphylaxis, produce this response in an estimated 1 in 50 000 patients exposed. Rashes can be severe, and fatalities occur with Stevens–Johnson syndrome (provoked, for example, by sulfonamides), and toxic epidermal necrolysis (TEN, which can be caused for example by **allopurinol**). The association between **cabamazepine**-induced TEN and the gene for a particular human leukocyte antigen (HLA) allele *HLAB*1502* in people of Asian ancestry is mentioned in Chapter 11. Susceptibility to severe rashes in response to **abacavir** is closely linked to the variant *HLAB*5701* and this forms the basis of a clinically useful genomic test (Ch. 11).

IMMUNOLOGICAL MECHANISMS

The formation of an immunogenic conjugate between a small molecule and an endogenous protein requires covalent bonding. In most cases, reactive metabolites, rather than the drug itself, are responsible. Such reactive metabolites can be produced during drug oxidation or by photoactivation in the skin. They may also be produced by the action of toxic oxygen metabolites generated by activated leukocytes. Rarely (e.g. in drug-induced lupus erythematosus), the reactive moiety interacts to form an immunogen with nuclear components (DNA, histone) rather than proteins. Conjugation with a macromolecule is usually essential, although penicillin is an exception because it can form sufficiently large polymers in solution to elicit an anaphylactic reaction in a sensitised individual even without conjugation to protein, although penicillin-protein conjugates can also act as the immunogen.

CLINICAL TYPES OF ALLERGIC RESPONSE TO DRUGS

Hypersensitivity reactions of types I, II and III (Ch. 6) are antibody-mediated reactions while type IV is cell-mediated. Unwanted reactions to drugs involve both antibody- and cell-mediated reactions. The more important clinical manifestations of hypersensitivity include anaphylactic shock, haematological reactions, allergic liver damage and other hypersensitivity reactions.

ANAPHYLACTIC SHOCK

Anaphylactic shock – see also Chapters 6 and 28 – is a type I hypersensitivity response. It is a sudden and life-threatening reaction that results from the release of histamine, leukotrienes and other mediators. The main features include urticarial rash, swelling of soft tissues, bronchoconstriction and hypotension.

Penicillins account for about 75% of anaphylactic deaths, reflecting the frequency with which they are used in clinical practice. Other drugs that can cause anaphylaxis include enzymes, such as **asparaginase** (Ch. 56); therapeutic monoclonal antibodies (Ch. 59); hormones, for example **corticotropin** (Ch. 33); **heparin** (Ch. 24); dextrans; radiological contrast agents; vaccines; and other serological products. Anaphylaxis with local anaesthetics (Ch. 43), the antiseptic chlorhexidine and with many other drugs (sometimes as a consequence of contaminants such as latex used to seal reusable vials or of excipients and colouring agents rather than the drug itself) can occur. Treatment of anaphylaxis is mentioned in Chapter 28.

It is sometimes feasible to carry out a skin test for the presence of hypersensitivity, which involves injecting a minute dose intradermally. A patient who reports that she or he is allergic to a drug such as penicillin may actually be allergic to fungal contaminants, which were common in early preparations, rather than to penicillin itself. The use of penicilloylpolylysine as a skin test reagent for penicillin allergy is an improvement over the use of penicillin itself, because it bypasses the need for conjugation of the test substance, thereby reducing the likelihood of a false negative. Other specialised tests are available to detect the presence of specific immunoglobulin E in the plasma, or to measure histamine release from the patient's basophils, but these are not used routinely.

HAEMATOLOGICAL REACTIONS

Drug-induced haematological reactions can be produced by type II, III or IV hypersensitivity. Type II reactions can affect any or all of the formed elements of the blood, which may be destroyed by effects either on the circulating blood cells themselves or on their progenitors in the bone marrow. They involve antibody binding to a drug–macromolecule complex on the cell surface membrane. The antigen–antibody reaction activates complement, leading to lysis, or provokes attack by killer lymphocytes or phagocytic leukocytes (Ch. 6). *Haemolytic anaemia* has been most commonly reported with sulfonamides and related drugs (Ch. 51) and with an antihypertensive drug, **methyldopa** (Ch. 14), which is still widely used to treat hypertension during pregnancy. With methyldopa, significant haemolysis occurs in less than 1% of patients, but the appearance of antibodies directed against the surface of red cells is detectable in 15% by the Coombs test. The antibodies are directed against Rh antigens, but it is not known how methyldopa produces this effect.

Drug-induced *agranulocytosis* (complete absence of circulating neutrophils) is usually delayed 2–12 weeks after beginning drug treatment but may then be sudden in onset. It often presents with mouth ulcers, a severe sore throat or other infection. Serum from the patient lyses leukocytes from other individuals, and circulating anti-leukocyte antibodies can usually be detected immunologically. Drugs associated with agranulocytosis include NSAIDs, especially **phenylbutazone** (Ch. 26), **carbimazole** (Ch. 34) and **clozapine** (Ch. 46) (increased genetic susceptibility associated with *HLA-DQB1*0201* is mentioned in Ch. 11) and **sulfonamides** and related drugs (e.g. *thiazides* and *sulfonylureas*). Agranulocytosis is rare but life-threatening. Recovery when the offending drug is stopped is often slow or absent. Antibody-mediated leukocyte destruction must be distinguished from the direct effect of cytotoxic drugs (see Ch. 55), which cause granulocytopenia that is rapid in onset, predictably related to dose and reversible.

Thrombocytopenia (reduction in platelet numbers) can be caused by type II reactions to **quinine** (Ch. 54), **heparin** (Ch. 24) and thiazide diuretics (Ch. 29).

Some drugs (notably **chloramphenicol**) can suppress all three haemopoietic cell lineages, giving rise to *aplastic anaemia* (anaemia with associated agranulocytosis and thrombocytopenia).

The distinction between type III and type IV hypersensitivity reactions in the causation of haematological reactions is not clear-cut, and either or both mechanisms can be involved.

ALLERGIC LIVER DAMAGE

Most drug-induced liver damage results from the direct toxic effects of drugs or their metabolites, as described above. However, hypersensitivity reactions are sometimes involved, a particular example being **halothane**-induced hepatic necrosis (see Ch. 41). *Trifluoracetylchloride*, a reactive metabolite of halothane, couples to a macromolecule to form an immunogen. Most patients with halothane-induced liver damage have antibodies that react with halothane–carrier conjugates. Halothane–protein antigens can be expressed on the surface of hepatocytes. Destruction of the cells occurs by type II hypersensitivity reactions involving killer T cells, and type III reactions can also contribute.

OTHER HYPERSENSITIVITY REACTIONS

The clinical manifestations of type IV hypersensitivity reactions are diverse, ranging from minor skin rashes to generalised autoimmune disease. Fever may accompany these reactions. Rashes can be antibody mediated but are usually cell mediated. They range from mild eruptions to fatal exfoliation. Stevens–Johnson syndrome is a very severe generalised rash that extends into the alimentary tract and carries an appreciable mortality. In some cases, the lesions are photosensitive, probably because ultraviolet light converts the drug to reactive products.

▼ Some drugs (notably **hydralazine** and **procainamide**) can produce an autoimmune syndrome resembling systemic lupus erythematosus. This is a multisystem disorder in which there is immunological damage to many organs and tissues (including joints, skin, lung, central nervous system and kidney) caused particularly, but not exclusively, by type III hypersensitivity reactions. The prodigious array of antibodies directed against 'self' components has been termed an 'autoimmune thunderstorm'. The antibodies react with determinants shared by many molecules, for example the phosphodiester backbone of DNA, RNA and phospholipids. In drug-induced systemic lupus erythematosus, the immunogen may result from the reactive drug moiety interacting with nuclear material, and joint and pulmonary damage is common. The condition usually resolves when treatment with the offending drug is stopped.

Allergic reactions to drugs

- Drugs or their reactive metabolites can bind covalently to proteins to form immunogens. **Penicillin** (which can also form immunogenic polymers) is an important example.
- Drug-induced allergic (hypersensitivity) reactions may be antibody-mediated (types I, II, III) or cell-mediated (type IV). Important clinical manifestations include the following:
  - anaphylactic shock (type I): many drugs can cause this, and most deaths are caused by **penicillin**
  - haematological reactions (type II, III or IV): including haemolytic anaemia (e.g. **methyldopa**),

agranulocytosis (e.g. **carbimazole**), thrombocytopenia (e.g. **quinine**) and aplastic anaemia (e.g. **chloramphenicol**)
  - hepatitis (types II, III): for example, **halothane**, **phenytoin**
  - rashes (type I, IV): are usually mild but can be life-threatening (e.g. Stevens–Johnson syndrome)
  - drug-induced systemic lupus erythematosus (mainly type II): antibodies to nuclear material are formed (e.g. **hydralazine**).

REFERENCES AND FURTHER READING

Adverse drug reactions

Aronson, J.K., Ferner, R.E., 2003. Joining the DoTS: a new approach to classifying adverse drug reactions. Br. Med. J. 327, 1222–1225. (*Description of ADRs in terms of dose, time course and susceptibility*)

Pirmohamed, M., James, S., Meakin, S., et al., 2004. Adverse drug reactions as cause of admission to hospital: prospective analysis of 18 820 patients. Br. Med. J. 329, 15–19. (*A sobering analysis, emphasising the frequency and cost of adverse drug reactions, most of which were avoidable. Drugs most commonly implicated were aspirin and other NSAIDs, diuretics, warfarin; the most common reaction was gastrointestinal bleeding*)

Rawlins, M.D., Thomson, J.W., 1985. Mechanisms of adverse drug reactions. In: Davies, D.M. (Ed.), Textbook of Adverse Drug Reactions, third ed. Oxford University Press, Oxford, pp. 12–38. (*Type A/type B classification*)

Talbot, J., Aronson, J.K. (Eds.), 2012. Stephens' Detection and Evaluation of Adverse Drug Reactons, sixth ed. Wiley–Blackwell, Oxford. (*Invaluable reference book that is also readable*)

Drug toxicity: general and mechanistic aspects

Bhogal, N., Grindon, C., Combes, R., Balls, M., 2005. Toxicity testing: creating a revolution based on new technologies. Trends Biotechnol. 23, 299–307. (*Reviews current and likely future value of new technologies in relation to toxicological evaluation*)

Timbrell, J.A., 2009. Principles of Biochemical Toxicity. Informa Healthcare, New York.

Walker, D.K., 2004. The use of pharmacokinetic and pharmacodynamic data in the assessment of drug safety in early drug development. Br. J. Clin. Pharmacol. 58, 601–608. (*Pharmacokinetic profile is a factor in assessing safety during early drug development, especially in relation to safety parameters such as QT interval prolongation, where free plasma concentrations are predictive; procedures are available that allow this on the microdose scale – potential limitations are discussed*)

Wobus, A.M., Loser, P., 2011. Present state and future perspectives of using pluripotent stem cells in toxicology research. Arch. Toxicol. 85,

79–117. (*Describes methods for selection and differentiation of cardiac and hepatic cells from human pluripotent stem cells*)

Drug toxicity: carcinogenesis, teratogenesis

Briggs, G.G., Freeman, R.K., Yaffe, S.J., 2008. Drugs in Pregnancy and Lactation, eighth ed. Lippincott, Williams & Wilkins, Philadelphia. (*Invaluable reference guide to fetal and neonatal risk for clinicians caring for pregnant women*)

Collins, M.D., Mayo, G.E., 1999. Teratology of retinoids. Annu. Rev. Pharmacol. Toxicol. 39, 399–430. (*Overviews principles of teratology as they apply to the retinoids, describes signal transduction of retinoids and toxikinetics*)

Sjöström, H., Nilsson, R., 1972. Thalidomide and the Power of the Drug Companies. Penguin Books, London.

Drug toxicity: organ involvement

Murray, M.C., Brater, D.C., 1993. Renal toxicity of the nonsteroidal anti-inflammatory drugs. Annu. Rev. Pharmacol. Toxicol. 33, 435–465.

Park, B.K., Kitteringham, N.R., Maggs, J.L., et al., 2005. The role of metabolic activation in drug-induced hepatotoxicity. Annu. Rev. Pharmacol. Toxicol. 45, 177–202. (*Reviews evidence for reactive metabolite formation from hepatotoxic drugs such as paracetamol, tamoxifen, diclofenac and troglitazone, and the current hypotheses of how this leads to liver injury*)

Ritter, J.M., Harding, I., Warren, J.B., 2009. Precaution, cyclooxygenase inhibition, and cardiovascular risk. Trends Pharmacol. Sci. 30, 503–514.

Svensson, C.K., Cowen, E.W., Gaspari, A.A., 2001. Cutaneous drug reactions. Pharmacol. Rev. 53, 357–380. (*Covers epidemiology, clinical morphology and mechanisms. Assesses current knowledge of four types of cutaneous drug reaction: immediate-type immune mediated, delayed-type immune mediated, photosensitivity and autoimmune. Also reviews the role of viral infection as predisposing factor*)

Valentin, J.-P., 2010. Reducing QT liability and proarrhythmic risk in drug discovery and development. Br. J. Pharmacol. 159, 5–11. (*See also accompanying articles in this themed section on QT safety*)

Lifestyle drugs and drugs in sport

58

OVERVIEW

The term *lifestyle* is applied to drugs that are used for non-medical purposes. This is a diverse group that includes drugs of abuse, drugs used to enhance athletic or other performance, as well as those taken for cosmetic purposes or for purely social reasons. Many lifestyle drugs have dual uses and are also employed as conventional therapeutics and their pharmacological properties are described elsewhere in this book. In this chapter we present an overall summary of lifestyle drugs and discuss some of the social and medico-legal problems associated with their growing use.

Drugs that are used to enhance sporting performance, while being officially prohibited, represent a special category of lifestyle drugs. Once again, many types of substances are used for this purpose, including established medicines. Below, we discuss specific issues relating to their use in competitive sports.

WHAT ARE LIFESTYLE DRUGS?

This is a question that is sometimes difficult to answer. Here we define them as drugs or medicines that are taken by choice to give pleasure (e.g. cannabis, alcohol, cocaine), to improve performance (e.g. drugs in sport, cognition-enhancing drugs) or to improve appearance (e.g. **botox**, slimming aids for the non-obese), in other words to satisfy an aspiration or a non-health-related goal rather than to treat a clinical condition. Put simply, they are drugs taken by choice by people who are not ill. Examples include the use of the antihypertensive **minoxidil** for treating baldness. Oral contraceptives, which clearly lie in the domain of mainstream medicine, could also be considered lifestyle drugs. Also included in the lifestyle category are food supplements and other related preparations that are consumed because of some claimed benefit – even though there is often no good evidence that they are effective.

CLASSIFICATION OF LIFESTYLE DRUGS

The lifestyle category covers lifestyle *uses* of a wide variety of drugs and medicines and cuts across the pharmacological classification used throughout this book, so summarising it is difficult. The scheme in Table 58.1 is based largely on the work of Gilbert et al. (2000) and Young (2003). It embraces drugs that have been used for lifestyle choices based on historical precedent, such as oral contraceptives, as well as agents used to manage potentially debilitating lifestyle illnesses such as addiction to smoking (e.g. **bupropion**). It also includes drugs such as caffeine and alcohol that are consumed on a mass scale around the world, and drugs of abuse such as cocaine as well as nutritional supplements. Particularly topical is the controversial use of 'neuro-enhancers', such as **modafinil** and **methylphenidate** (Ch. 48), which are claimed to improve academic performance (see Sahakian & Morein-Zamir, 2007; Eickenhorst et al., 2012, for example), although much evidence is anecdotal.[1]

Over time, drugs can switch between 'lifestyle' and 'clinical' uses. For example, **cocaine** was used as a lifestyle drug by South American Indians. Early explorers commented that it 'satisfies the hungry, gives new strength to the weary and exhausted and makes the unhappy forget their sorrows'. Subsequently assimilated into European medicine as a local anaesthetic (Ch. 43), it is now largely returned to lifestyle drug status and, regrettably, is the basis of an illegal multimillion dollar international drugs industry. **Cannabis** is another good example of a drug that has been considered (in the West at least) as a purely recreational drug but which is now (as a plant extract containing **tetrahydrocannabinol** and **cannabidiol**) licensed for various clinical uses (see Chs 19, 42 and 49). There are many other examples (Flower, 2004).

Many widely used lifestyle 'drugs' or 'sports supplements' consist of natural products (e.g. *Ginkgo* extracts, melatonin, St John's wort, *Cinchona* extracts), whose manufacture and sale has not generally been controlled by regulatory bodies.[2] Their composition is therefore highly variable, and their efficacy and safety generally untested. Many contain active substances that, like synthetic drugs, can produce adverse as well as beneficial effects.

DRUGS IN SPORT

The American cyclist Lance Armstrong seemed to be an inspirational hero. Having overcome testicular cancer he went on to win the Tour de France on no less than seven occasions and the charity he founded raised millions of dollars for cancer relief. Persistent accusations of drug abuse surrounded the athlete but were strenuously denied, until January 2013 when Armstrong admitted, on a television chat show, that he had been using a cocktail of drugs to enhance his performance over the course of many years.[3] It prompted one commentator (Sparling, 2013) to despair of the 'charade of drug-free sport'.

The use of drugs to enhance sporting performance is evidently widespread, although officially prohibited.

---

[1]Drugs intended to give a competitive advantage in sport are, of course, considered unfair, banned and very actively policed. Will there come a time when taking drugs to improve examination performance will become illegal, with similar surveillance methods and sanctions? See Bostrom & Sandberg (2009) for a discussion of this ethical minefield.
[2]Things are changing. In the UK, the Medicines and Healthcare Products Regulatory Agency now has a Herbal Medicines Advisory Committee.
[3]Apparently including steroids, growth hormone and erythropoietin. He was later stripped of all his sporting honours.

Table 58.1 Lifestyle drugs and medicines, excluding drugs in sport

Category	Example(s)	Primary clinical use	'Lifestyle' use	Chapter
Medicines approved for specific indications but which also have other 'lifestyle' purposes	Sildenafil	Erectile dysfunction	Erectile enhancement	35
	Oral contraceptives	Preventing conception	Preventing conception	35
	Orlistat	Obesity	Weight loss	32
	Sibutramine	Anorectic agent (withdrawn in Europe)	Weight loss	32
Medicines approved for specific indications which can also be used to satisfy 'lifestyle choices' or to treat 'lifestyle diseases'	Minoxidil	Hypertension	Regrowth of hair	22
	Methylphenidate	Attention deficit/hyperactivity disorder (ADHD)	Improving academic performance	48
	Modafinil	Treatment of ADHD	Cognitive enhancement	48
	Opiates	Analgesia	'Recreational' usage	42, 49
Drugs that have only slight, or no, current clinical use but which fall into the lifestyle category	Alcohol	None as such	Widespread component of drinks	49
	Botulinum toxin	Relief of muscle spasm	Cosmetic alteration	13
	Caffeine	Migraine treatment	Widespread component of drinks	48
	Cannabis	Managing chronic pain, nausea and possibly muscle spasm	'Recreational' usage	19, 49
Drugs (generally illegal) that have no clinical utility but which are used to satisfy lifestyle requirements	Methylenedioxymethamphetamine (MDMA, 'ecstasy')	None	'Recreational' usage	48
	Tobacco (nicotine)	Nicotine preparations for tobacco addiction	'Recreational' usage	49
	Cocaine (some formulations)	Local anaesthesia (largely obsolete)	'Recreational' usage	42

In addition, there are countless herbal preparations and other natural products, largely unregulated, which are marketed as health-promoting, life-enhancing and beneficial for many disorders, despite lack of evidence of therapeutic efficacy. Many are claimed to 'boost the immune system'. Examples include numerous vitamin preparations, fish oils, melatonin, ginseng, *Echinacea*, *Ginkgo* and much besides.

From Flower 2004, after Gilbert et al., 2000 and Young, 2003.

Lifestyle drugs

- Comprise a group of drugs and medicines taken mainly for non-medical reasons. Should more accurately be called 'lifestyle uses'.
- Include prescription drugs such as **sildenafil** and **methylphenidate**, substances such as **alcohol** and **caffeine**, drugs of abuse and various nutritional preparations.
- Are linked to the concepts of 'self-diagnosis' and 'non-disease'.
- Are a growing sector of the pharmaceutical market.
- Are often brought to the consumer's attention through the Internet or direct marketing of drugs.

The World Anti-Doping Agency (www.wada-ama.org), which was established partly in response to some high-profile doping cases and drug-induced deaths among athletes, publishes an annually updated list of prohibited substances that may not be used by sportsmen or sportswomen either in, or out of, competition. Drug testing is based mainly on analysis of blood or urine samples according to strictly defined protocols. The chemical analyses, which rely mainly on gas chromatography/mass spectrometry or immunoassay techniques, must be carried out by approved laboratories.

Table 58.2 summarises the main classes of drugs that are prohibited for use in sports. Athletes are easily persuaded of the potential of a wide variety of drugs to increase their chances of winning, but it should be emphasised that in very few cases have controlled trials shown that the drugs actually improve sporting performance among trained athletes, and indeed many such trials have proved negative. However, marginal improvements in performance (often 1% or less), which are difficult to measure experimentally, may make the difference between winning and losing, and the competitive instincts of athletes and their trainers generally carry more weight than scientific evidence.

A brief account of some of the more important drugs in common use follows. For a broader and more complete coverage, see British Medical Association (2002) and

Table 58.2 Drugs used in sport

Drug class	Example(s)	Effects	Detection	Notes
Anabolic agents	Androgenic steroids (testosterone, nandrolone and many others; Ch. 35)	Increased muscle development, aggression and competitiveness Serious long-term side effects	Urine or blood samples	Many are endogenous hormones, so results significantly above normal range are required
	Clenbuterol (Ch. 14)	Combined anabolic and agonist action on β_2 adrenoceptors may increase muscle strength		Human chorionic gonadotrophin is sometimes used to increase androgen secretion
Hormones and related substances	Erythropoietin (Ch. 25)	Increased erythrocyte formation and oxygen transport. Increased blood viscosity causes hypertension and risk of strokes and coronary attacks Used mainly for endurance sports[a]	Plasma half-life is short, so detection is difficult	Use of other plasma markers indicating erythropoietin administration may be possible
	Human growth hormone (Ch. 33)	Increased lean body mass and reduced fat May accelerate recovery from tissue injury. Causes cardiac hypertrophy, acromegaly, liver damage and increased cancer risk	Blood testing	Distinguishing endogenous (highly variable) from exogenous human growth hormone can be difficult
	Insulin (Ch. 31)	Sometimes used (with glucose so as to avoid hypoglycaemia) to promote glucose uptake and energy production in muscle Probably ineffective in improving performance	Plasma samples	–
β_2-Adrenoceptor agonists	Salbutamol and others (Ch. 14)	Used by runners, cyclists, swimmers, etc. to increase oxygen uptake (by bronchodilatation) and increased cardiac function. Controlled studies show no improvement in performance	Urine samples	–
β-Adrenoceptor antagonists	Propranolol, etc. (Ch. 14)	Used to reduce tremor and anxiety in 'precision' sports (e.g. shooting, gymnastics, diving)	Urine samples	Not banned in most sports, where they actually impair performance
CNS 'stimulants'	Ephedrine and derivatives; amphetamines, cocaine, caffeine (Ch. 48)	Many trials show slight increase in muscle strength and performance in non-endurance events (sprint, swimming, field events, etc.)	Urine samples	The most widely used group, along with anabolic steroids
Diuretics	Thiazides, furosemide (Ch. 29)	Used mainly to achieve rapid weight loss before 'weighing in'. Also used to 'mask' the presence of other agents in urine by dilution	Urine samples	–
Narcotic analgesics	Codeine, morphine, etc. (Ch. 42)	Used to mask injury-associated pain	Urine samples	–

[a]'Blood doping' (removal of 1–2 l of blood well ahead of the competition, followed by re-transfusion immediately prior to the event) has a similar effect and is even more difficult to detect.

Mottram (2005). Gould (2013) has reviewed the potential use of gene therapy in promoting athletic performance. Another hurdle for the regulators!

ANABOLIC STEROIDS

Anabolic steroids (Ch. 35) include a large group of compounds with testosterone-like effects, including about 50 named compounds on the prohibited list. New chemical derivatives ('designer steroids'), such as **tetrahydrogestrinone** (THG), are regularly developed and offered illicitly to athletes, which represents a continuing problem to the authorities charged with detecting and identifying them. A further problem is that some of these drugs are endogenous compounds or their metabolites and their concentration can vary dramatically for physiological reasons. This makes it difficult to prove that the substance had been administered illegally. Isotope ratio techniques, based on the fact that endogenous and exogenous steroids have slightly different $^{12}C:^{13}C$ ratios, may enable the two to be distinguished analytically. Since anabolic steroids produce long-term effects and are normally used throughout training, rather than during the event itself, out-of-competition testing is essential.

When given in combination with training and high protein intake, anabolic steroids undoubtedly increase muscle mass and body weight, but there is little evidence that they increase muscle strength over and above the effect training could achieve alone, or that they improve sporting performance. On the other hand, they have serious long-term effects, including male infertility, female masculinisation, liver and kidney tumours, hypertension and increased cardiovascular risk, and (in adolescents) premature skeletal maturation causing irreversible cessation of growth. Anabolic steroids produce a feeling of physical well-being, increased competitiveness and aggressiveness, sometimes progressing to actual psychosis. Depression is common when the drugs are stopped, sometimes leading to long-term psychiatric problems.

Clenbuterol, is a β-adrenoceptor agonist (see Ch. 14). Through an unknown mechanism of action, it produces anabolic effects similar to those of androgenic steroids, with apparently fewer adverse effects. It can be detected in urine and its use in sport is banned.

HUMAN GROWTH HORMONE

The use of **human growth hormone** (hGH; see Ch. 33) by athletes followed the availability of the recombinant form of hGH, used to treat endocrine disorders. It is given by injection and its effects appear to be similar to those of anabolic steroids. hGH is also reported to produce a similar feeling of well-being, although without the accompanying aggression and changes in sexual development and behaviour. It increases lean body mass and reduces body fat, but its effects on muscle strength and athletic performance are unclear. It is claimed to increase the rate of recovery from tissue injury, allowing more intensive training routines. The main adverse effect of hGH is the development of acromegaly, causing overgrowth of the jaw and thickening of the fingers (Ch. 33), but it may also lead to cardiac hypertrophy and cardiomyopathy, and possibly also an increased cancer risk.

Detection of hGH administration is difficult because physiological secretion is pulsatile, so normal plasma concentrations vary widely. The plasma half-life is short (20–30 min), and only trace amounts are excreted in urine. However, secreted hGH consists of three isoforms varying in molecular weight, whereas recombinant hGH contains only one, so measuring the relative amounts of the isoforms can be used to detect the exogenous material. Growth hormone acts partly by releasing insulin-like growth factor from the liver, and this hormone itself is coming into use by athletes.

Another hormone, **erythropoietin**, which increases erythrocyte production (see Ch. 25), is given by injection for days or weeks to increase the erythrocyte count and hence boost the O_2-carrying capacity of blood. The development of recombinant erythropoietin has made it widely available, and detection of its use is difficult. It carries a risk of hypertension, neurologic disease and thrombosis.

STIMULANT DRUGS

The main drugs of this type used by athletes and officially prohibited are: **ephedrine** and **methylephedrine**; various amphetamines and similar drugs, such as **fenfluramine** and methylphenidate;[4] cocaine; and a variety of other CNS stimulants such as **nikethamide**, **amiphenazole** (no longer used clinically) and **strychnine** (see Ch. 48). **Caffeine** is also used: some commercially available 'energy drinks' contain taurine as well as caffeine. However, taurine is an agonist at glycine and extrasynaptic GABA$_A$ receptors (see Ch. 39). Its effects on the brain are therefore likely to be inhibitory rather than stimulatory. In this regard, taurine may be responsible for the post-energy-drink low that is experienced once the stimulatory effect of caffeine has worn off.

In contrast to steroids, some trials have shown stimulant drugs to improve performance in events such as sprinting and weightlifting, and under experimental conditions they increase muscle strength and reduce muscle fatigue significantly. The psychological effect of stimulants is probably more relevant than their physiological effects. Surprisingly, caffeine appears to be more consistently effective in improving muscle performance than other more powerful stimulants.

Several deaths have occurred among athletes taking amphetamines and ephedrine-like drugs in endurance events. The main causes are coronary insufficiency, associated with hypertension; hyperthermia, associated with cutaneous vasoconstriction; and dehydration.

From a pharmacological perspective, it is fair to say that the use of drugs to enhance sporting performance carries many risks and is of doubtful efficacy. Its growing prevalence reflects many of the same pressures as those driving the introduction of lifestyle drugs, namely the desire to enhance the performance of humans who are not impaired by disease, coupled with disregard for scientific evidence relating to efficacy and risk.

CONCLUSION

The lifestyle drug phenomenon is one aspect of a broader debate about what actually constitutes 'disease' and how far medical science should go to satisfy the needs and aspirations of otherwise healthy individuals or to alleviate human distress and dysfunction in the absence of pathology. Discussion of these issues is beyond the scope of this book but can be found in articles cited at the end of this chapter (see Flower 2004 and 2012).

There are several reasons why these drugs – no matter how we choose to define them – are of increasing concern. The increasing availability of drugs from 'e-pharmacies', coupled with the direct advertising by the pharmaceutical industry to the public that occurs in some countries, will ensure that demand is kept buoyant. Most sales are in the developed world and the pharmaceutical industry will undoubtedly develop more lifestyle agents to cater for this lucrative market. The lobbying power of patients advocating particular drugs, regardless of the potential costs or proven utility, causes major problems for drug regulators and those who set healthcare priorities for state-funded systems of social medicine.

---

[4]Also used to improve academic performance!

Drugs in sport

- Many drugs of different types are commonly used by sportsmen and sportswomen with the aim of improving performance in competition.
- The main types used are:
  - anabolic agents, mainly androgenic steroids and **clenbuterol**
  - hormones, particularly **erythropoietin** and **human growth hormone**
  - stimulants, mainly **amphetamine** and **ephedrine** derivatives and caffeine
  - β-adrenoceptor antagonists, to reduce anxiety and tremor in 'precision' sports.

- The use of drugs in sport is officially prohibited – in most cases, in or out of competition.
- Detection depends mainly on analysis of the drug or its metabolites in urine or blood samples. Detection of abuse is difficult in the case of endogenous hormones such as **erythropoietin**, **growth hormone** and **testosterone**.
- Controlled trials have mostly shown that drugs produce little improvement in sporting performance. Anabolic agents increase body weight and muscle volume without clearly increasing strength. The effect of stimulants is often psychological rather than physiological.

The use of drugs that improve short-term memory to treat patients with dementia (Ch. 40) is generally seen as desirable (even though current drugs are only marginally effective). Extending the use of existing and future drugs to give healthy children and students a competitive advantage in tests is much more controversial. Further off is the prospect of drugs that retard senescence and prolong life – another social and ethical minefield in an overpopulated world.

REFERENCES AND FURTHER READING

Lifestyle drugs and general reading

Bostrom, N., Sandberg, A., 2009. Cognitive enhancement: methods, ethics, regulatory challenges. Sci. Eng. Ethics 15, 343–349. (*Interesting discussion of a complex problem which will soon have to be faced*)

Eickenhorst, P., Vitzthum, K., Klapp, B.F., Groneberg, D., Mache, S., 2012. Neuroenhancement among German university students: motives, expectations, and relationship with psychoactive lifestyle drugs. J. Psychoactive Drugs 44, 418–427. (*The title is self explanatory. The efficacy of 'neuroenhancement' is not discussed*)

Flower, R.J., 2004. Lifestyle drugs: pharmacology and the social agenda. Trends Pharmacol. Sci. 25, 182–185. (*Accessible review that enlarges on some of the issues raised in this chapter*)

Flower, R., 2012. The Osler Lecture 2012: Pharmacology 2.0, medicines, drugs and human enhancement. QJM 105, 823–830. (*Discusses 'human enhancement' from a pharmacologist's viewpoint. Easy to read*)

Gilbert, D., Walley, T., New, B., 2000. Lifestyle medicines. BMJ 321, 1341–1344. (*Short but focused review dealing mainly with the clinical implications of the 'lifestyle medicine' phenomenon*)

Sahakian, B., Morein-Zamir, S., 2007. Professor's little helper. Nature 450, 1157–1159. (*Interesting 'commentary' of the use of neuroenhancers, especially by academics, and the ethical questions that this raises. Recommended*)

Walley, T., 2002. Lifestyle medicines and the elderly. Drugs Aging 19, 163–168. (*Excellent review of the whole area and its relevance to the treatment of the elderly*)

Young, S.N., 2003. Lifestyle drugs, mood, behaviour and cognition. J. Psychiatry Neurosci. 28, 87–89.

Drugs in sport

Avois, L., Robinson, N., Saudan, C., et al., 2006. Central nervous system stimulants and sport practice. Br. J. Sports Med. 40 (Suppl. 1), 16–20.

(*Deals mainly with the illegal use of stimulants such as ephedrine, amphetamine and cocaine in sport. Particularly highlights the dangers of misuse*)

British Medical Association, 2002. Drugs in Sport: The Pressure to Perform. BMJ Publications, London. (*Useful coverage of the whole topic*)

Catlin, D.H., Fitch, K.D., Ljungqvist, A., 2008. Medicine and science in the fight against doping in sport. J. Intern. Med. 264, 99–114. (*Very interesting review of the whole area and the establishment of antidoping agencies*)

Gould, D., 2013. Gene doping: gene delivery for Olympic victory. Br. J. Clin. Pharmacol. 76, 292–298. (*Discusses what must surely be the next challenge to the WADA: deliberately introducing into athletes genes that could boost performance*)

Mottram, D.R. (Ed.), 2005. Drugs in Sport, fourth ed. Routledge, London. (*Comprehensive description of pharmacological and regulatory aspects of drugs in sport, with balanced discussion of evidence relating to efficacy and risk*)

Munby, J., 2010. Drugs in sport. Scot. Med. J. 55, 29–30. (*Brief review of the use of drugs in sport – both professional and amateur – written from the point of view of a physician*)

Sparling, P.B., 2013. The Lance Armstrong saga: a wake-up call for drug reform in sports. Curr. Sports Med. Rep. 12, 53–54. (*Brief commentary on the Lance Armstrong affair*)

Spedding, M., Spedding, C., 2008. Drugs in sport: a scientist–athlete's perspective: from ambition to neurochemistry. Br. J. Pharmacol. 154, 496–501. (*Very accessible review written by two brothers, one of whom is an Olympic athlete and the other a pharmacologist. Unique insights. Highly recommended*)

59 Biopharmaceuticals and gene therapy

OVERVIEW

In this chapter, we review the impact of two therapeutic concepts based on our growing understanding and skill in manipulating genes. *Biopharmaceuticals* is an umbrella term applied to the use of 'engineered' proteins and antibodies or nucleic acids in medicine, while *gene therapy* refers specifically to attempts to use genes to reprogram cells to prevent, alleviate or cure disease. Engineered proteins, after some 30 years of (often frustrating) research and development, are well established in the clinic, while nucleic acid drugs and gene therapy are still in development.[1] In addition to introducing the central concepts in this chapter, we discuss the considerable problems associated with developing biopharmaceutical therapies, consider safety issues and review the progress made to date.

INTRODUCTION

The 'molecular biology revolution', which had its roots in the discovery of the structure of DNA in the 1950s, and the advances in cell biology that followed in its train, offered the prospect of manipulating the genetic material in ways that are useful in practical therapeutics. The seductive notion that a gene of interest can be expressed *in vitro* to generate useful proteins that could not be prepared synthetically or, more daringly, that a gene could be directly introduced *in vivo* and persuaded to synthesise some crucial cellular component, has driven this field at breakneck speed.

Biopharmaceuticals (often called *biologics*) are by now a well-recognised part of therapy, and we have already encountered them elsewhere in this book (see Tables 59.1 and 59.2). Widespread adoption of these drugs still faces many problems, not the least of which is the cost of manufacture, but the technology is now established and maturing fast. In a review of the area published in 2013, Wirth noted that some 211 biopharmaceuticals had been licensed around the world by 2011, earning some $113 billion revenue.[2] The veterinary use of these drugs is also increasing.

Gene therapy is the more considerable challenge. However, the idea commands such appeal that vast resources (both public and private) have been committed to its development. There are several reasons why it is so attractive. First, it is a (deceptively) simple approach to a radical cure of single-gene diseases such as *cystic fibrosis* and the *haemoglobinopathies*, which are collectively responsible for much misery throughout the world. Second, many other more common conditions, including malignant, neurodegenerative and infectious diseases, have a large genetic component. Conventional treatment of such disorders is (as readers of this book will have appreciated by now) far from ideal, so the promise of a completely new approach has enormous attraction. Finally, an ability to control gene expression (e.g. by antisense or siRNA oligonucleotides) could be used to treat many diseases that are not genetic in origin.

The gurus are emphatic that 'the conceptual part of the gene therapy revolution has indeed occurred ...' – so where are the therapies? The devil, of course, is in the detail: in this case, the details of:

- *pharmacokinetics*: delivery of the gene to the interior of appropriate target cells (especially in the central nervous system [CNS])
- *pharmacodynamics*: the controlled expression of the gene in question
- *safety*
- *clinical efficacy and long-term practicability.*

The first and most fundamental hurdle is the delivery problem; here, techniques borrowed from viruses, which are masters of the sort of molecular hijacking that is required to introduce functional genes into mammalian cells, have been used.

There is a broad consensus that the *Weismann barrier*[3] should not be breached and so a moratorium has been agreed on therapies intended to alter the DNA of germ cells (which could influence future generations) and gene therapy trials have focused on somatic cells.

BIOPHARMACEUTICALS

The use of proteins as therapeutic agents is not a novel idea; insulin, extracted from animal pancreas tissue (Ch. 31), and human growth hormone, extracted at one time from human cadaver pituitary glands (Ch. 33), were among the first therapeutic proteins to be used and, for many years, such purified extracts provided the only option for treating protein hormone deficiency disorders. However, there were problems. First, there were difficulties in extraction and often disappointing yields. Second, administration of animal hormones (e.g. pig insulin) to humans could evoke an immune response. Third, there was always a danger of the transmission of infectious agents across species, or between people. This was highlighted in the 1970s, when cases of *Creutzfeldt–Jakob disease* (see Ch. 40) occurred in patients treated with human growth hormone obtained from cadavers. This serious problem was later traced to contamination of the donor pituitary glands with infectious prions (Ch. 40). The advent of 'genetic engineering' techniques offered a new way to deal with these perennial problems.

---

[1]In Western countries anyway; a gene therapy product, **Gendicine**™, for treating cancer was licensed in China in 2003.
[2]Biopharmaceuticals currently comprise about 40% of new drugs approved.

[3]Named after August Weismann (1834–1914), who formulated the concept that inheritance utilises only germ, and not somatic, cells.

Table 59.1 Some examples of 'second-generation' biopharmaceuticals

Type of change	Protein	Indication	Reason for change
Altered amino acid sequence	Insulin	Diabetes	Faster-acting hormone
	Tissue plasminogen activator analogues	Thrombolysis	Longer circulating half-life
	Interferon analogue	Antiviral	Superior antiviral action
	Factor VIII analogue	Haemophilia	Smaller molecule, better activity
	Diphtheria toxin–interleukin-2 fusion protein	T-cell lymphoma	Targets toxin to appropriate cells
	Tumour necrosis factor receptor–human immunoglobulin G Fc fusion protein	Rheumatoid disease	Prolongs half-life
Altered carbohydrate residues	Glucocerebrosidase enzyme	Gaucher's disease	Promotes phagocyte uptake
	Erythropoietin analogue	Anaemia	Prolongs half-life
Covalent attachment to polyethylene glycol	Interferon	Hepatitis C	Prolongs half-life
	Human growth hormone	Acromegaly	Prolongs half-life

Modified from Walsh 2004.

Biopharmaceuticals and gene therapy: definition and potential uses

- *Biopharmaceuticals* include proteins, antibodies (and oligonucleotides) used as drugs:
  - *first-generation* biopharmaceuticals are mainly copies of endogenous proteins or antibodies, produced by recombinant DNA technology
  - *second-generation* biopharmaceuticals have been 'engineered' to improve the performance of the protein or antibody.
- Applications:
  - therapeutic monoclonal antibodies
  - recombinant hormones.
- *Gene therapy* is the genetic modification of cells to prevent, alleviate or cure disease.
- Potential applications:
  - radical cure of monogenic diseases (e.g. cystic fibrosis, haemoglobinopathies)
  - amelioration of diseases with or without a genetic component, including many malignant, neurodegenerative and infectious diseases.

PROTEINS AND POLYPEPTIDES

The biopharmaceuticals in use today are generally classified as first- or second-generation agents. *First-generation* biopharmaceuticals are usually straightforward copies of human hormones or other proteins prepared by transfecting the human gene into a suitable *expression system* (a cell line that produces the protein in good yield), harvesting and purifying the *recombinant protein* for use as a drug. The first agent to be produced in this way was human recombinant insulin in 1982.

Second-generation biopharmaceuticals are those that have been *engineered*: that is to say, either the gene has been deliberately altered prior to transfection such that

the structure of the expressed recombinant protein is changed, or some alteration is made to the purified end product. The reasons for making these changes are generally to improve some aspect of the protein's activity profile. Human recombinant insulins designed to act faster or last longer were among the first in this class to be marketed; Table 59.1 contains other examples.

Third-generation agents would be those in which macro molecules (including nucleic acid controllers of protein synthesis as well as proteins themselves) are designed from scratch to do a particular biological function. This technology is just beginning to bear fruit: **mipomersen**, the first antisense RNA product, was licensed in 2013.

Problems in manufacture

There are several problems associated with the manufacture of any type of recombinant protein, and one of the most pressing is the choice of expression system. Many recombinant proteins are expressed in bacterial systems (*Escherichia coli*, for example), which are useful because cultures grow quickly and are generally easy to manipulate. Disadvantages include the fact that the product may contain bacterial endotoxins, which must be meticulously removed before administration to patients, and that bacterial cells do not accomplish the same type of *post-translational processing* (e.g. glycosylation) as mammalian cells. This could pose problems if the protein's action is crucially dependent on this modification. To circumvent these problems, mammalian (e.g. Chinese hamster ovary, CHO) cells are also used as expression systems, although here the problem is often one of the final yields: such cells require more careful culture, grow more slowly and produce less product, all of which contributes to the cost of the final medicine.

There are, however, a number of emergent technologies that could transform the production process. The use of plants to produce recombinant proteins has attracted considerable interest (see Melnik & Stoger, 2013). Several species have shown promise, including the tobacco plant. Human genes of interest can readily be transfected into the plant by using tobacco mosaic virus as a vector; the crop grows rapidly (yields a high *biomass*) and offers a number of other advantages. Edible plants such as lettuce and bananas could be used to deliver some orally active proteins, such as vaccines, which could then be consumed directly without the need for prior purification. Several such proteins have already been produced in plants, and some are in clinical trial (Kwon et al., 2013).

Another technology that could dramatically increase the yield of human recombinant proteins is the use of transgenic cattle. A dairy cow can produce some 10 000 litres of milk per year, and recombinant proteins introduced into the genome, and under the control of promoters that regulate production of other milk proteins, can generate yields as high as 1 g/l (see Brink et al., 2000).

Engineered proteins

There are several ways in which proteins can be altered prior to expression. Alteration of the nucleotide sequence of the coding gene can be used to change single amino acids or, indeed, whole regions of the polypeptide chain. There are good reasons why it is an advantage to 'engineer' proteins prior to expression, including:

- modification of pharmacokinetic properties
- creation of novel *fusion* or other proteins
- reducing immunogenicity, e.g. by *humanising*.

It is frequently advantageous to modify the pharmacokinetic properties of recombinant proteins. Changes in the structure of human insulin, for example, provided diabetics with a form of the hormone that did not self-associate during storage and was thus faster-acting and easier to manage. The half-life of proteins in the blood can often be extended by *PEGylation* (see Ch. 10), the addition of polyethylene glycol to the molecule. This *post-translational engineering* approach has been applied to some human hormones, such as recombinant growth hormone, interferons and others. Prolonging half-life is not merely a convenience to patients; it also reduces the overall cost of the treatment, and economic factors are important in the adoption of this type of therapy.

Fusion proteins comprise two or more proteins engineered to be expressed as one single polypeptide chain, sometimes joined by a short linker. An example is **etanercept**, an anti-inflammatory drug used in the treatment of rheumatoid arthritis and other conditions (see Ch. 26). This consists of the ligand-binding domain taken from the tumour necrosis factor receptor, joined to the Fc domain of a human immunoglobulin G antibody. The receptor moiety sequesters tumour necrosis factor (TNF) in an inactive form, while the immunoglobulin increases its persistence in the blood. Reduction of immunogenicity through bioengineering is discussed below.

MONOCLONAL ANTIBODIES

Although antibodies are used to confer *passive immunity*, there are a number of disadvantages inherent in their production and use that limit their utility. Conventionally, antisera are produced from the blood of immunised humans or animals (e.g. to collect anti-tetanus serum). Antiserum containing high levels of specific antibodies is prepared from the plasma, which can then be used therapeutically to neutralise pathogens or other dangerous substances in the blood of the patient.

Such preparations contain *polyclonal antibodies* – that is, a *polyvalent* mixture of antibodies from all the plasma cell clones that reacted to that particular antigen. The actual composition and efficacy of these varies over time, and

obviously there is a limit to how much plasma can be collected on any one occasion. In 1975, Milstein and Köhler[4] discovered a method of producing from immunised mice an immortalised *hybridoma*, a fusion of one particular lymphocytic clone with an immortalised tumour cell. This furnished a method of producing *monoclonal antibodies* – a single species of monovalent antibody – at high abundance *in vitro*. The hybridoma cell line could be retained and expanded indefinitely while preserving the integrity of its product.

Monoclonal antibodies can be classified into first- or second-generation reagents along similar lines to other proteins discussed above. First-generation monoclonals were essentially murine monoclonals (or fragments thereof), but these suffered from several drawbacks. As mouse proteins, they provoked an immune response in 50–75% of all recipients. Other limiting factors were a short half-life in the circulation and the inability of the mouse antibodies to activate human complement.

Most of these problems have been surmounted by using either *chimeric* or *humanised* monoclonals. The two terms refer to the degree to which the monoclonals have been engineered. Figure 59.1 shows how this is done; the antibody molecule consists of a *constant* domain (Fc) and the antibody-binding domain (Fab), with *hypervariable* regions that recognise and bind to the antigen in question. The genes for chimeric monoclonals are engineered to contain the cDNA of the murine Fab domain coupled with the human Fc domain sequences. This greatly (around fivefold) extends the plasma half-life (most plasma proteins turn over quite rapidly; immunoglobulins are an exception, and it is easy to see how very long-lived antibodies provide selective advantage to the host). Incorporation of human Fc sequences also improves the functionality of the antibody in human medicine. A further development (and now the preferred approach) is to replace the entire Fc and Fab region with the human equivalent with the exception of the hypervariable regions, giving a molecule which, while essentially human in nature, contains the murine antibody-binding sites. The anticancer monoclonal **herceptin** (**trastuzumab**; see Ch. 56) is an example of such an antibody, and some others are given in Table 59.2.

THE PHARMACOLOGY OF BIOPHARMACEUTICALS

We are, by now, accustomed to the concept of using proteins and antibodies therapeutically, and many of the risks associated with (for example) anti-TNF therapy are well understood (see Ch. 26). For the most part, these medicines do not cause the range of toxic effects encountered with small molecules discussed in Chapter 57, but there are still very real dangers.

▼ In 2006, for example, a UK clinical trial of a new monoclonal antibody (TGN 1412) designed to activate T cells (see Ch. 6) and thus treat B-cell lymphocytic leukaemia went badly wrong. All six subjects became severely ill following a 'cytokine storm' and suffered lasting damage. The incident provoked wide media publicity[5] and, while the subsequent investigation blamed an 'unpredictable' biological reaction, it caused many to think hard about how such trials should be conducted in the future (see Muller & Brennan, 2009). Highly specific reagents such as monoclonals intended for human use, pose a particular problem as they may not cross-react with the corresponding proteins of other species, thus evading detection in the usual preclinical animal safety screens.

---

[4]They won the 1984 Nobel Prize for Physiology or Medicine for this work.
[5]One tabloid headline read: 'We saw human guinea pigs explode' (quoted by Stobbart et al., 2007).

Table 59.2 Some examples of 'second-generation' therapeutic monoclonal antibodies

Antibody	Type	Target	Use	See chapter
Infliximab	Chimeric Mab	Tumour necrosis factor	Crohn's disease, rheumatoid disease	26
Adalimumab	Humanised Mab	Tumour necrosis factor	Rheumatoid disease	26
Etanercept	Fusion protein	Tumour necrosis factor	Rheumatoid disease	26
Trastuzumab	Humanised Mab	HER2 epidermal growth factor receptor	Breast cancer	56
Palivizumab	Humanised Mab	Respiratory syncytial virus	Respiratory infections in young children	–
Omalizumab	Humanised Mab	Immunoglobulin E	Immunoglobulin E-mediated asthma	28
Abatacept	Fusion protein	B7 epitope on antigen presenting cells	Rheumatoid disease	26

Mab, monoclonal antibody. Therapeutic monoclonal antibody names all end in '-mab', prefixed by an indication of their species nature: -umab (human), -omab (mouse), -ximab (chimera), -zumab (humanised).
Source: Walsh 2004 and the British National Formulary.

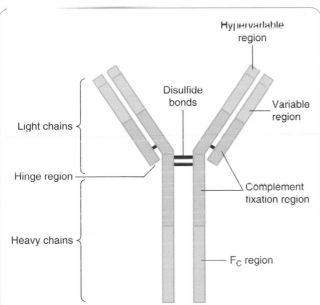

Fig. 59.1 Production of engineered 'chimeric' and 'humanised' monoclonal antibodies. The Y-shaped antibody molecule consists of two main domains: the Fc (constant) domain and the Fab (antibody-binding) domain. At the tip of the Fab regions (on the arms of the 'Y') are the hypervariable regions that actually bind the antigen. Chimeric antibodies are produced by replacing the murine Fc region with its human equivalent by altering and splicing the gene. For humanised antibodies, only the murine hypervariable regions are retained, the remainder of the molecule being human in origin. *(After Walsh, 2004.)*

The pharmacology of biopharmaceuticals is complicated because they may have multiple or even unknown modes of action, and partly because of their complex drug-receptor interactions many exhibit non-linear log dose-response curves. Erythropoietin, for example, has a bell-shaped dose response and, in the case of many monoclonal antibodies, there is a single optimal biological dose instead of the proportional effects that we are more accustomed to when dealing with small molecule drugs. Their pharmacokinetics are different too. We can no longer rely on the concepts such as Phase 1 and Phase 2 metabolism (see Ch. 9) to predict how they will be eliminated. Proteolytic degradation is more likely to be the important route for removal.

Whilst it is possible for generic manufacturers to copy conventional small molecule drugs when these come off patent, this cannot be done with biopharmaceuticals, which may depend upon the unique properties of a particular proprietary construct or clone. This means that *biosimilars*, as they are known in the argot of the industry, may not always have the same pharmacology as the original: obviously a big problem for regulators.

GENE THERAPY

Despite high hopes and intensive research efforts since the 1980s, realisation of the potential of gene therapy is still in its infancy. Here we focus first on the main problems and approaches being tried, with a final section on the limited success so far.

GENE DELIVERY

The transfer of recombinant nucleic acid into target cells – a special instance of the 'drug distribution' problem – is critical to the success of gene therapy. The constructs must pass from the extracellular space across the plasma and nuclear membranes, and be incorporated into the chromosomes. Because DNA is negatively charged and single genes have molecular weights around 10^4 times greater than conventional drugs, the problem is of a different order from the equivalent stage of routine drug development.

There are several important considerations in choosing a delivery system; these include:

- the *capacity* of the system (e.g. how much DNA it can carry)
- the *transfection efficiency* (its ability to enter and become utilised by cells)
- the *lifetime* of the transfected material (determined by the lifetime of the targeted cells)
- the *safety issue*, especially important in the case of viral delivery systems.

Table 59.3 Characteristics of some delivery systems for gene therapy

Vector	Advantages	Disadvantages	Utilisation of system*
Liposomes	Virus-free, cheap to produce	Low efficiency, sometimes cytotoxic	6%
DNA cassettes	Virus-free	Low efficiency, expression temporary	18%
Herpes simplex virus type I	Highly infective, persistent expression	No integration with host DNA, cytotoxic, difficult to handle	3%
Adenovirus	Highly infective in epithelia	Immunogenic and transient, requires repeated administration	23%
Adeno-associated virus	Stable	Low capacity	5%
Retrovirus	Efficient, permanent	Low capacity, unstable, must integrate into host DNA, requires dividing cells	22%

*The approximate percentage of trials employing this type of delivery system.
After Wolf & Jenkins 2002 and with data from Wirth et al. 2013.

Various approaches have been developed (see Table 59.3) in an attempt to produce the optimal system.

There are two main strategies for delivering genes into patients. Using the *in vivo strategy*, the vector containing the therapeutic gene is injected into the patient, either intravenously (in which case some form of organ or tissue targeting is required) or directly into the target tissue (e.g. the retina). The *ex vivo strategy* is to remove cells from the patient (e.g. stem cells from bone marrow or circulating blood, or myoblasts from a biopsy of striated muscle), treat them with the vector in the laboratory and inject the genetically altered cells back into the patient.

An ideal vector should be *safe*, highly *efficient* (i.e. insert the therapeutic gene into a high proportion of target cells) and *selective* in that it should lead to expression of the therapeutic protein in the target cells but *not* to the expression of other viral proteins. Provided that the cell into which it is inserted is itself long-lived, the vector should ideally cause persistent expression, avoiding the need for repeated treatment. The latter consideration can be a problem in some tissues. In the autosomal recessive disorder *cystic fibrosis*, for example, the airway epithelium malfunctions because it lacks a membrane Cl⁻ transporter known as the *cystic fibrosis transport regulator* (CFTR). Epithelial cells in the airways are continuously dying and being replaced, so even if the CFTR gene were stably transfected into the epithelium, there would still be a periodic need for further treatment unless the gene could be inserted into the progenitor (stem) cells. Similar problems are anticipated in other cells that turn over continuously, such as gastrointestinal epithelium and skin.

VIRAL VECTORS

▼ Many contemporary gene delivery strategies aim to capitalise on the capacity of viruses to subvert the transcriptional machinery of the cells they infect and their ability (in some cases) to fuse with the host genome. While seemingly simple, there remain substantial practical problems with the *viral vector* approach. As viruses have evolved the means to invade human cells, so humans have evolved immune responses and other protective counter-measures. Although irritating in some respects, this is not all bad news from the point of view of safety. As many of the viruses used for vectors are pathogenic, they are usually modified such that they are 'replication defective' to avoid toxicity.

Retroviruses

▼ If introduced into stem cells, retroviral vectors have the attraction that their effects are persistent because they are incorporated into, and replicate with, host DNA, and so the 'therapeutic' gene is passed down to each daughter cell during division. Against this, the *retroviral integrase* randomly inserts the construct into chromosomes, so it may cause damage. Also, retroviruses could infect germ or non-target cells and produce undesired effects if administered *in vivo*. For this reason, retroviruses have been used mainly for *ex vivo* gene therapy. The life cycle of naturally occurring retroviruses may be exploited to create useful vectors for gene therapy (see Fig. 59.2).

Many viruses are equipped to infect specific cell types, though not necessarily the target cell of interest. It is possible to alter the retroviral envelope to alter specificity, such that the vector could be administered systemically but would target only the desired cell population. An example of this approach with a *lentivirus* (a type of retrovirus) is the substitution of the envelope protein of a non-pathogenic vector (e.g. mouse leukaemia virus) with the envelope protein of human vesicular stomatitis virus, in order specifically to target human epithelial cells.

Most retrovirus vectors are unable to penetrate the nuclear envelope, and because the nuclear membrane dissolves during cell division, they only infect dividing cells rather than non-dividing cells (such as adult neurons).

Adenovirus

▼ Adenovirus vectors are popular because of the high transgene expression that can be achieved. They transfer genes to the nucleus of the host cell, but (unlike retroviruses) these are not inserted into the host genome and so do not produce effects that outlast the lifetime of the transfected cell. This property also obviates the risk of disturbing the function of other cellular genes and the theoretical risks of carcinogenicity and germ cell transfection. Because of these favourable properties, adenovirus vectors have been used for *in vivo* gene therapy. Engineered deletions in the viral genome, render it unable to replicate or to cause widespread infection in the host while at the same time creating space in the viral genome for the therapeutic transgene to be inserted.

One of the first adenoviral vectors lacked part of a growth-controlling region called E_1 while incorporating the desired transgene. This vector gave excellent results, demonstrating gene transfer to cell lines and animal models of disease, but it has been disappointing as a treatment for cystic fibrosis) in human trials. Low doses (administered by aerosol to patients with this disease) produced only a very low-efficiency transfer, whereas higher doses caused inflammation, a host immune response and short-lived gene expression. Furthermore, treatment could not be repeated because of neutralising antibodies. This has led to recent attempts to manipulate adenoviral vectors to mutate or remove the genes that are most strongly immunogenic.

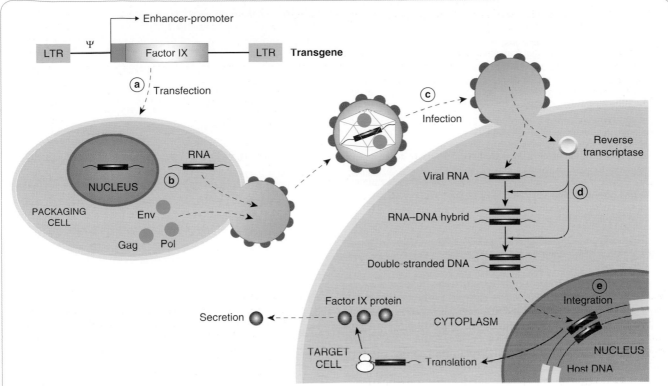

Fig. 59.2 Strategy for making retroviral vectors. The transgene (the example shows the gene for factor IX) in a vector backbone is introduced (a) into a packaging cell, where it is integrated into a chromosome in the nucleus, and (b) transcribed to make vector mRNA, which is packaged into the retroviral vector and shed from the packaging cell. It then infects the target cell (c). Virally encoded reverse transcriptase (d) converts vector RNA into an RNA–DNA hybrid, and then into double-stranded DNA, which is integrated (e) into the genome of the target cell. It can then be transcribed and translated to make factor IX protein. 'Env', 'Gag' and 'Pol' represent components of the retroviral vector. *(Redrawn from Verma, I.M., Somia, N., 1997. Gene therapy – promises, problems and prospects. Nature 389, 239–242.)*

Other viral vectors

▼ Other potential viral vectors under investigation include *adeno-associated virus*, *herpes virus* and disabled versions of *human immunodeficiency virus* (HIV). Adeno-associated virus associates with host DNA but is not activated unless the cell is infected with an adenovirus. It is less immunogenic than other vectors but is difficult to mass produce and cannot be used to carry large transgenes. Herpes virus does not associate with host DNA but is very long lived in nervous tissue (so could have a specific application in treating neurological disease). HIV, unlike most other retroviruses, can infect non-dividing cells such as neurons. It is possible to remove the genes from HIV that control replication and substitute other genes. Alternatively, it may prove possible to transfer to other non-pathogenic retroviruses those genes that permit HIV to penetrate the nuclear envelope.

NON-VIRAL VECTORS

Liposomes

▼ Non-viral vectors include a variant of liposomes (Ch. 8). Plasmids (diameter up to approximately 2 μm) are too big to package in regular liposomes (diameter 0.025–0.1 μm), but larger particles can be made from positively charged lipids ('lipoplexes'), which interact with both negatively charged cell membranes and DNA, improving delivery into the cell nucleus and incorporation into the host chromosome. Such particles have been used to deliver the genes for HLA-B7, interleukin-2 and CFTR. They are much less efficient than viruses, and attempts are currently under way to improve this by incorporating various viral signal proteins (membrane fusion proteins, for example) in their outer coat. Direct injection of these complexes into solid tumours (e.g. melanoma, breast, kidney and colon cancers) can, however, achieve high local concentrations within the tumour.

Microspheres

▼ Biodegradable microspheres made from polyanhydride co-polymers of fumaric and sebacic acids (see Ch. 8) can be loaded with plasmid DNA. A plasmid with bacterial β galactosidase activity formulated in this way and given by mouth to rats has resulted in systemic absorption and expression of the bacterial enzyme in the rat liver, raising the possibility of oral gene therapy.

Plasmid DNA

▼ Surprisingly, plasmid DNA itself ('naked DNA') enters the nucleus of some cells and is expressed, albeit much less efficiently than when it is packaged in a vector. Such DNA carries no risk of viral replication and is not usually immunogenic, but it cannot be targeted precisely. There is considerable interest in the possibility of using naked DNA for vaccines, because even very small amounts of foreign protein can stimulate an immune response. There are several theoretical advantages in this approach, numerous trials are taking place and several products have been licensed (Liu, 2011).

CONTROLLING GENE EXPRESSION

To realise the full potential of gene therapy, it is not enough to transfer the gene selectively to the desired target cells and maintain acceptable expression of its product – difficult though these goals are. It is also essential that the activity of the gene is controlled. Historically, it was the realisation of the magnitude of this task that diverted attention from the haemoglobinopathies (which were the first projected targets of gene therapy). Correction of these disorders demands an appropriate balance of normal α- and β-globin chain synthesis to be effective, and for this, and many other potential applications, precisely controlled gene expression will be essential.

▼ It has not yet proved possible to control transgenes precisely in human recipients, but there are techniques that may eventually enable us to achieve this goal. One hinges on the use of an inducible expression system. This is a fairly standard technique whereby the inserted gene also includes a **doxycycline**-inducible promoter such that expression of the gene can be switched on or off by treatment with, or withdrawal of, doxycycline.

The control of transfected genes is important in gene targeting as well. By splicing the gene of interest with a tissue-specific promoter, it should be possible to restrict expression of the gene to the target tissue. Such an approach has been used in the design of gene therapy constructs for use in ovarian cancer, the cells of which express several proteins at high abundance, including the proteinase inhibitor SLP1. In combination with the SLP1 promoter, plasmids carrying various genes were successfully and selectively expressed in ovarian cancer cell lines (Wolf & Jenkins, 2002).

SAFETY AND SOCIETAL ISSUES

Gene therapy tends to provoke deep unease in some sectors of society – witness the GM crop debate. Some of this reaction may be traced to ignorance or prejudice but it is nevertheless a problem that can hinder the introduction of new agents. Societal issues aside, the technique raises a number of specific concerns that generally relate to the use of viral vectors. These are usually selected because they are non-pathogenic, or modified to render them innocuous, but there is a concern that such agents might still acquire virulence during use. Retroviruses, which insert randomly into host DNA, could damage the genome and interfere with the protective mechanisms that normally regulate the cell cycle (see Ch. 5), and if they happen to disrupt essential cellular functions, this could increase the risk of malignancy.[6]

Another problem is that immunogenic viral proteins may be expressed that elicit an inflammatory response, and this could be harmful in some situations (e.g. in the airways of patients with cystic fibrosis). Initial clinical experience was reassuring, but the death of Jesse Gelsinger, an 18-year-old volunteer in a gene therapy trial for the non-fatal disease *ornithine decarboxylase deficiency* (which can be controlled by diet and drugs), led to the appreciation that safety concerns related to immune-mediated responses to vectors are very real (see Marshall, 1999).

THERAPEUTIC APPLICATIONS

Despite technical problems and safety concerns, there have been some encouraging successes. The European Medicines Agency granted its first license for a gene therapy product in 2012. **Glybera** is an adeno-associated virus construct that delivers a correct copy of lipoprotein lipase to patients lacking this enzyme (a very rare disorder, causing severe pancreatitis). Table 59.4 details some other examples and the area has been comprehensively reviewed by Wirth et al. (2013).

There are over 1800 gene therapy trials under way, recorded online at *Gene Therapy Review* (www.

genetherapyreview.com). Together with other resources (see Further Reading), this provides an enormous amount of relevant information. We conclude this section with a few comments on prominent applications of gene therapy.

GENE THERAPY FOR CANCER

Gene therapy for cancer and related diseases comprises almost 70% of all trials at the time of writing. Several therapeutic approaches (see Barar & Omidi, 2012) are under investigation, including:

Gene delivery and expression

- Gene delivery is one of the main hurdles to practical gene therapy.
- Recombinant genes are transferred using a vector, often a suitably modified virus.
- There are two main strategies for delivering genes into patients:
  - *in vivo* injection of the vector directly into the patient (e.g. into a malignant tumour)
  - *ex vivo* treatment of cells from the patient (e.g. stem cells from marrow or circulating blood), which are then returned to the patient.
- An ideal vector would be safe, efficient, selective and produce long-lasting expression of the therapeutic gene.
- Viral vectors include retroviruses, adenoviruses, adeno-associated virus, herpesvirus and disabled human immunodeficiency virus (HIV):
  - *retroviruses* infect many different types of dividing cells and become incorporated randomly into host DNA
  - *adenoviruses* are genetically modified to prevent replication and accommodate the therapeutic transgene. They transfer genes to the nucleus but not to the genome of the host cell. Problems include a strong host immune response, inflammation and short-lived expression. Treatment cannot be repeated because of neutralising antibodies
  - *adeno-associated virus* associates with host DNA and is non-immunogenic but is hard to mass-produce and has a small capacity
  - herpesvirus does not associate with host DNA but persists in nervous tissue and may be useful in treating neurological disease
  - disabled versions of HIV differ from most other retroviruses in that they infect non-dividing cells, including neurons.
- Non-viral vectors include:
  - a variant of liposomes, made using positively charged lipids and called 'lipoplexes'
  - biodegradable microspheres, which may offer orally active gene therapy
  - plasmid DNA ('naked DNA'), which can be used as a vaccine.
- A *tetracycline-inducible expression system* or similar technique can control the activity of the therapeutic gene.

---

[6]This risk is more than a theoretical possibility; several children treated for *severe combined immunodeficiency* (SCID) with a retrovirus vector developed a leukaemia-like illness (Woods et al., 2006). The retroviral vector was shown to have inserted itself into a gene called *LMO-2*, mutations of which are associated with childhood cancers.

Table 59.4 Some gene therapy successes

Disease target	Gene delivered	Vector	Technique	Reference
X-linked severe combined immunodeficiency	IL2 cytokine receptor subunit gamma chain	Murine leukaemia retrovirus	Transfusion of patient with bone marrow cells transfected *ex vivo*	Hacein-Bey-Abina et al., 2010
Leber's congenital amaurosis	Isomerohydrolase retinal pigment epithelium protein	Adeno-associated virus	Subretinal injection	Maguire et al., 2009
Heart failure	Ca^{2+}-ATPase	Adeno-associated virus	Intracoronary infusion	Jessup et al., 2011
β-thalassaemia	β-globin	Lentivirus	Transfusion of patient with bone marrow cells transfected *ex vivo*	Cavezzana-Calvo et al., 2010
Metachromatic leukodystrophy	Arylsulfatase	Lentivirus	*Ex vivo* transfection of haematopoietic stem cells and transfusion into patient	Biffi et al., 2013
Wiskott–Aldrich syndrome	WAS protein	Lentivirus	*Ex vivo* transfection of haematopoietic stem cells and transfusion into patient	Aiuti et al., 2013

Safety

- There are those safety concerns that are specific to any particular therapy (e.g. polycythaemia from overexpression of **erythropoietin**) and additional general concerns relating, for example, to the nature of vectors.
- Viral vectors:
  - might acquire virulence during use
  - contain viral proteins, which may be immunogenic
  - can elicit an inflammatory response
  - could damage the host genome and interfere with the cell cycle, provoking malignancy.
- The limited clinical experience to date has not so far provided evidence of insurmountable problems.

Gene therapy for cancer

- Promising approaches include:
  - restoring protective proteins such as p53
  - inactivating oncogenes
  - delivering a gene to malignant cells that renders them sensitive to drugs
  - delivering a gene to healthy host cells to protect them from chemotherapy
  - tagging cancer cells with genes that make them immunogenic.

- restoring 'protective' proteins, such as the tumour suppressor gene (see Ch. 5)
- inactivating oncogene expression (e.g. by using a retroviral vector bearing an antisense transcript RNA to the *k-ras* oncogene)
- delivering a gene to malignant cells that renders them sensitive to cytotoxic drugs (e.g. thymidylate kinase, which activates **ganciclovir**) – the so-called 'suicide gene' approach
- delivery of proteins to healthy host cells in order to protect them (e.g. addition of the multidrug resistance channel to bone marrow cells *ex vivo*, thereby rendering them resistant to drugs used in chemotherapy)
- tagging cancer cells with genes expressing proteins that render malignant cells more visible to the immune system (e.g. for antigens such as HLA-B7 or cytokines such as granulocyte-macrophage colony-stimulating factor and interleukin-2).

SINGLE-GENE DEFECTS

Single-gene (*monogenic*) disorders were the obvious starting point for gene therapy trials and haemoglobinopathies were the first projected targets, but early attempts (in the 1980s) were put 'on hold' because of the problem (mentioned above) posed by the need to control precisely the expression of the genes encoding the different polypeptide chains of the haemoglobin molecule. Patients with thalassaemia (the commonest monogenic disease) exhibit enormous phenotypic diversity and hence variable clinical symptoms because, even in monogenic disorders, other genes as well as environmental factors are also important. However, some successes have recently been reported following transfection of bone marrow cells with a correct copy of the β-globin gene (see Table 59.4).

Another early target was cystic fibrosis, but progress here has been slow (see Prickett & Jain, 2013 for details). There have been other successes though. For example, *X-linked chronic granulomatous disease* has been successfully treated using a retroviral technique to deliver a functional version of the mutated NADPH oxidase protein (Ott et al., 2006 and Fig. 59.3) and a form of inherited blindness, *Leber's congenital amaurosis*, associated with a mutation in a gene that produces retinal pigment, has been rectified

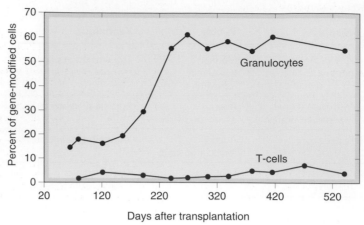

Fig. 59.3 Correcting an inherited defect using gene therapy. In this clinical trial, two patients with X-linked chronic granulomatous disease were transfused with GM–CSF-treated peripheral blood cells that had been genetically modified with a retroviral vector bearing the intact *gp91phox* gene ('*in vitro* protocol' – see text). The graph shows that the number of gene-modified peripheral blood leukocytes remained high for well over a year and this was accompanied by good levels of superoxide production in these cells – a clinical 'cure'. (*Data redrawn from Ott et al., 2006.*)

using an adeno-associated virus vector bearing a cDNA coding for the intact gene (Maguire et al., 2009).

GENE THERAPY AND INFECTIOUS DISEASE

In addition to DNA vaccines mentioned above, there is considerable interest in the potential of gene therapy for HIV infection. The aim is to render stem cells (which differentiate into immune cells) resistant to HIV before they mature. For an account of the strategies under investigation, see Chung et al. (2013).

GENE THERAPY AND CARDIOVASCULAR DISEASE

Gene therapy trials for treating cardiovascular diseases are reviewed by Bradshaw and Baker (2013). Vascular gene transfer is attractive not least because cardiologists and vascular surgeons routinely perform invasive studies that offer the opportunity to administer gene therapy vectors *ex vivo* (e.g. to a blood vessel that has been removed to use as an autograft) or locally *in vivo* (e.g. by injection through a catheter directly into a diseased coronary or femoral artery) (see Table 59.4). The nature of many vascular disorders, such as restenosis following angioplasty (stretching up a narrowed artery using a balloon that can be inflated via a catheter), is such that transient gene expression might be all that is needed therapeutically. Extension of vein graft patency by gene therapy approaches has been reviewed by Chandiwal et al. (2005). This is a promising area; for further details of angiogenic gene therapy see Hammond and McKirnan (2001) and of peripheral vascular disease, Ghosh et al. (2008).

OLIGONUCLEOTIDE APPROACHES

So far we have largely been considering the addition of entire genes, but there are other, related nucleic acid-based therapeutic strategies. Another approach is the use of *antisense oligonucleotides*. These are short (15–25 mer) oligonucleotides that are complementary to part of a gene

or gene product that it is desired to inhibit. These snippets of genetic material can be designed to suppress the expression of a harmful gene either by forming a triplex (three-stranded helix) with a regulatory component of chromosomal DNA, or by complexing a region of mRNA. Oligonucleotides can cross plasma and nuclear membranes by endocytosis as well as by direct diffusion, despite their molecular size and charge. However, there are abundant enzymes that cleave foreign DNA in plasma and in cell cytoplasm, so enzyme-resistant *methylphosphorate* and *phosphothiorate* analogues have been developed. The oligomer needs to be at least 15 bases long to confer specificity and tight binding

Following parenteral administration, such oligomers distribute widely (although not to the CNS) and work in part by interfering with the transcription of mRNA and in part by stimulating its breakdown by ribonuclease H, which cleaves the bound mRNA. Mipomersen, a phosphothiorate analogue that suppresses the expression of apolipoprotein B, to be used for the treatment of a rare form of hypercholesterolaemia, is the first licensed antisense therapeutic, registered in the USA in 2013. This approach is being used in clinical studies in patients with viral disease (including HIV infection) and malignancy (including the use of Bcl-2 antisense therapy administered subcutaneously in patients with non-Hodgkin's lymphoma).

A related approach (see Castanatto & Rossi, 2009), which provides more efficient gene silencing than antisense oligonucleotides, is the use of *short interfering RNA* (siRNA),[7] whereby short lengths of double-stranded RNA recruit an enzyme complex, known as RISC, which selectively degrades the corresponding mRNA produced by the cell, thereby blocking expression. Clinical trials of siRNA therapeutics are in progress.

---

[7]Discovered when it was found by plant scientists, to their surprise, that introducing RNA that encoded the colour-producing enzyme in petunias made the flowers less colourful, not more so. Subsequently siRNA has emerged as an important physiological mechanism for controlling gene expression, leading to the 2006 Nobel Prize award to Mello and Fire.

REFERENCES AND FURTHER READING

General reviews on biopharmaceuticals, gene therapy and utilities

Scientific American *published an issue devoted to gene therapy in June 1997, which is an excellent introduction, including articles by T. Friedmann ('Overcoming the obstacles to gene therapy'), P. L. Felgner (on non-viral strategies for gene therapy), R. M. Blaese (on gene therapy for cancer) and D. Y. Ho and R. M. Sapolsky (on gene therapy for the nervous system)*

Brink, M.F., Bishop, M.D., Pieper, F.R., 2000. Developing efficient strategies for the generation of transgenic cattle which produce biopharmaceuticals in milk. Theriogenology 53, 139–148. (*A bit specialised, as it focuses mainly on the husbandry of transgenic cattle, but interesting nonetheless*)

Castanatto, D., Rossi, J.J., 2009. The promises and pitfalls of RNA-interference-based therapeutics. Nature 457, 426–433. (*Useful review of the mechanism, current status and potential applications of RNAi as a means of controlling gene expression*)

Guttmacher, A.E., Collins, F.S., 2002. Genomic medicine: a primer. N. Engl. J. Med. 347, 1512–1520. (*First in a series on genomic medicine*)

Kwon, K.C., Verma, D., Singh, N.D., Herzog, R., Daniell, H., 2013. Oral delivery of human biopharmaceuticals, autoantigens and vaccine antigens bioencapsulated in plant cells. Adv. Drug Deliv. Rev. 65, 782–799. (*The title is self-explanatory*)

Liu, M.A., 2011. DNA vaccines: an historical perspective and view to the future. Immunol. Rev. 239, 62–84.

Melnik, S., Stoger, E., 2013. Green factories for biopharmaceuticals. Curr. Med. Chem. 20, 1038–1046. (*Another paper on the use of plants to produce biologics*)

Verma, I.M., Somia, N., 1997. Gene therapy – promises, problems and prospects. Nature 389, 239–242. (*The authors, from the Salk Institute, describe the principle of getting corrective genetic material into cells to alleviate disease, the practical obstacles to this and the hopes that better delivery systems will overcome them*)

Walsh, G., 2004. Second-generation biopharmaceuticals. Eur. J. Pharm. Biopharm. 58, 185–196. (*Excellent overview of therapeutic proteins and antibodies; some good tables and figures*)

Wirth, T., Parker, N., Yla-Herttuala, S., 2013. History of gene therapy. Gene 525, 162–169. (*An excellent review of the area from its very beginnings. Highly recommended*)

Problems

Check, E., 2002. A tragic setback. Nature 420, 116–118. (*News feature describing efforts to explain the mechanism underlying a leukaemia-like illness in a child previously cured of SCID by gene therapy*)

Marshall, E., 1999. Gene therapy death prompts review of adenovirus vector. Science 286, 2244–2245. (*Deals with the tragic 'Gelsinger affair'*)

Muller, P.Y., Brennan, F.R., 2009. Safety assessment and dose selection for first in-human clinical trials with immunomodulatory monoclonal antibodies. Clin. Pharmacol. Ther. 85, 247–258. (*A sober and, at times, very technical assessment of the safety procedures required for the 'first-in-man' testing of therapeutic monoclonals. Written in the wake of the TGN 1412 affair*)

Stobbart, L., Murtagh, M.J., Rapley, T., et al., 2007. We saw human guinea pigs explode. BMJ 334, 566–567. (*Analysis of the press coverage of the above clinical trial*)

Woods, N.B., Bottero, V., Schmidt, M., von Kalle, C., Verma, I.M., 2006. Gene therapy: therapeutic gene causing lymphoma. Nature 440, 1123.

Therapeutic uses

Aiuti, A., Biasco, L., Scaramuzza, S., et al., 2013. Lentiviral hematopoietic stem cell gene therapy in patients with Wiskott–Aldrich syndrome. Science 341 (6148), 1233151. PubMed PMID: 23845947. (*See Table 59.4*)

Barar, J., Omidi, Y., 2012. Translational approaches towards cancer gene therapy: hurdles and hopes. BioImpacts 2, 127–143.

Biffi, A., Montini, E., Lorioli, L., et al., 2013. Lentiviral hematopoietic stem cell gene therapy benefits metachromatic leukodystrophy. Science 341 (6148), 1233158. PubMed PMID: 23845948. (*See Table 59.4*)

Bradshaw, A.C., Baker, A.H., 2013. Gene therapy for cardiovascular disease: perspectives and potential. Vasc. Pharm. 58, 174–181.

Cavazzana-Calvo, M., Payen, E., Negre, O., et al., 2010. Transfusion independence and HMGA2 activation after gene therapy of human beta-thalassaemia. Nature 467, 318–322. (*See Table 59.4*)

Chandiwal, A., Balasubramanian, V., Baldwin, Z.K., Conte, M.S., Schwartz, L.B., 2005. Gene therapy for the extension of vein graft patency: a review. Vasc. Endovasc. Surg. 39, 1–14.

Chung, J., DiGiusto, D.L., Rossi, J.J., 2013. Combinatorial RNA-based gene therapy for the treatment of HIV/AIDS. Expert Opin. Biol. Ther. 13 (3), 437–445. (*Review on prophylactic gene therapy approaches for HIV*)

Ghosh, R., Walsh, S.R., Tang, T.Y., Noorani, A., Hayes, P.D., 2008. Gene therapy as a novel therapeutic option in the treatment of peripheral vascular disease: systematic review and meta-analysis. Int. J. Clin. Pract. 62, 1383–1390.

Hacein-Bey-Abina, S., Hauer, J., Lim, A., et al., 2010. Efficacy of gene therapy for X-linked severe combined immunodeficiency. N. Engl. J. Med. 363, 355–364. (*See Table 59.4*)

Hammond, H.K., McKirnan, M.D., 2001. Angiogenic gene therapy for heart disease: a review of animal studies and clinical trials. Cardiovasc. Res. 49, 561–567. (*Comprehensive review spanning animal and human trials of gene therapy for myocardial ischaemia*)

Jessup, M., Greenberg, B., Mancini, D., et al., 2011. Calcium upregulation by percutaneous administration of gene therapy in cardiac disease (CUPID): a phase 2 trial of intracoronary gene therapy of sarcoplasmic reticulum Ca²⁺-ATPase in patients with advanced heart failure. Circulation 124, 304–313. (*See Table 59.4*)

Maguire, A.M., High, K.A., Auricchio, A., et al., 2009. Age-dependent effects of RPE65 gene therapy for Leber's congenital amaurosis: a phase 1 dose-escalation trial. Lancet 374, 1597–1605. (*Clinical trial of gene therapy to correct a cause of congenital blindness. See Table 59.4*)

Nathwani, A.C., Davidoff, A.M., Linch, D.C., 2005. A review of gene therapy for haematological disorders. Br. J. Haematol. 128, 3–17. (*The title is self explanatory; easy to read and comprehensive in scope*)

Ott, M.G., Schmidt, M., Schwarzwaelder, K., et al., 2006. Correction of X-linked chronic granulomatous disease by gene therapy, augmented by insertional activation of MDS1-EVI1, PRDM16 or SETBP1. Nat. Med. 12, 401–409. (*Clinical trial of gene therapy to correct hereditary neutrophil dysfunction*)

Prickett, M., Jain, M., 2013. Gene therapy in cystic fibrosis. Transl. Res. 161, 255–264. (*Cystic fibrosis was one of the first monogenic disorders identified as a candidate for gene therapy. This review explains how and why things haven't quite worked out the way it was hoped*)

Wolf, J.K., Jenkins, A.D., 2002. Gene therapy for ovarian cancer (review). Int. J. Oncol. 21, 461–468. (*Excellent review and broad introduction to gene therapy in general*)

Useful Web resources

<www.genetherapynet.com> (*Gene Therapy Net – a fantastic resource for both patients and professionals. It is a veritable clearing house for information and up-to-date news on all aspects of gene therapy. It even advertises for volunteers and has a 'jobs' section, in case you are tempted! Has links to other related sites*)

60 Drug discovery and development

OVERVIEW

With the development of the pharmaceutical industry towards the end of the 19th century, drug discovery became a highly focused and managed process. Discovering new drugs moved from the domain of inventive doctors to that of scientists hired for the purpose. The bulk of modern therapeutics, and of modern pharmacology, is based on drugs that came from the laboratories of pharmaceutical companies, without which neither the practice of therapeutics nor the science of pharmacology would be more than a pale fragment of what they have become.

In this chapter we describe in outline the main stages of the process, namely (i) the discovery phase, i.e. the identification of a new chemical entity as a potential therapeutic agent; and (ii) the development phase, during which the compound is tested for safety and efficacy in one or more clinical indications, and suitable formulations and dosage forms devised. The aim is to achieve registration by one or more regulatory authorities, to allow the drug to be marketed legally as a medicine for human use.

Our account is necessarily brief and superficial, and more detail can be found elsewhere (Hill & Rang, 2013).

THE STAGES OF A PROJECT

Figure 60.1 shows in an idealised way the stages of a 'typical' project, aimed at producing a marketable drug that meets a particular medical need (e.g. to retard the progression of Parkinson's disease or cardiac failure, or to treat drug-resistant infections).

Broadly, the process can be divided into three main components:

1. *Drug discovery*, during which candidate molecules are chosen on the basis of their pharmacological properties.
2. *Preclinical development*, during which a wide range of non-human studies (e.g. toxicity testing, pharmacokinetic analysis and formulation) are performed.
3. *Clinical development*, during which the selected compound is tested for efficacy, side effects and potential dangers in volunteers and patients.

These phases do not necessarily follow in strict succession, as indicated in Figure 60.1, but generally overlap.

THE DRUG DISCOVERY PHASE

Given the task of planning a project to discover a new drug to treat – say, Parkinson's disease – where does one start? Assuming that we are looking for a novel drug rather than developing a slightly improved 'me-too' version of a drug already in use,[1] we first need to choose a new molecular target.

TARGET SELECTION

As discussed in Chapter 2, drug targets are currently, with few exceptions, functional proteins (e.g. receptors, enzymes, transport proteins). Although, in the past, drug discovery programmes were often based – successfully – on measuring a complex response *in vivo*, such as prevention of experimentally induced seizures, lowering of blood sugar or suppression of an inflammatory response, without the need for prior identification of a drug target, nowadays this is rare, and the first step is target identification. This most often comes from biological intelligence. It was known, for example, that inhibiting angiotensin-converting enzyme lowers blood pressure by suppressing angiotensin II formation, so it made sense to look for antagonists of the vascular angiotensin II receptor – hence the successful 'sartan' series of antihypertensive drugs (Ch. 22). Similarly, the knowledge that breast cancer is often oestrogen-sensitive led to the development of aromatase inhibitors such as **anastrozole**, which prevents oestrogen synthesis. Therapeutic drugs in use in 2005 addressed 266 distinct human targets (see Overington et al., 2006), but there are many proteins that are thought to play a role in disease for which we still have no cognate drug, and many of these represent potential starting points for drug discovery. Estimates range from a few hundred to several thousand potential drug targets that remain to be exploited therapeutically (see Betz, 2005). Selecting *valid* and '*druggable*' targets from this plethora is a major challenge.

Conventional biological wisdom, drawing on a rich fund of knowledge of disease mechanisms and chemical signalling pathways, coupled with genomic data, is the basis on which novel targets are most often chosen. Genomics is playing an increasing role by revealing new proteins involved in chemical signalling and new genes involved in disease. Space precludes discussion here of this burgeoning area; interested readers are referred to more detailed accounts (Lindsay, 2003; Kramer & Cohen, 2004; Semizarov & Blomme, 2008; Hill & Rang, 2013).

Overall, it is evident that in the foreseeable future there is ample biological scope in terms of novel drug targets for therapeutic innovation. What limits innovation is not the biology and primary pharmacology, but other factors, such as the emergence of unforeseen adverse effects during clinical testing, and the cost and complexity of drug discovery and development in relation to healthcare economics and increasing regulatory hurdles.

---

[1]Many commercially successful drugs have in the past emerged from exactly such 'me-too' projects, examples being the dozen or so β-adrenoceptor-blocking drugs developed in the wake of propranolol, and the many 'triptans' that followed the introduction of sumatriptan to treat migraine. Quite small improvements (e.g. in pharmacokinetics or side effects), coupled with aggressive marketing, have often proved enough, but the barriers to registration are getting higher, so the emphasis has shifted towards developing innovative (first in class) drugs aimed at novel molecular targets.

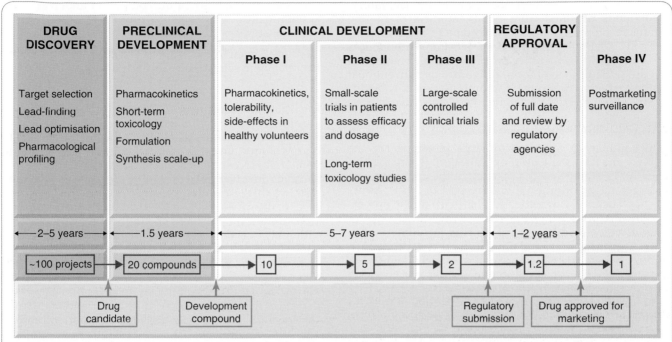

DRUG DISCOVERY	PRECLINICAL DEVELOPMENT	CLINICAL DEVELOPMENT			REGULATORY APPROVAL	
		Phase I	**Phase II**	**Phase III**		**Phase IV**
Target selection Lead-finding Lead optimisation Pharmacological profiling	Pharmacokinetics Short-term toxicology Formulation Synthesis scale-up	Pharmacokinetics, tolerability, side-effects in healthy volunteers	Small-scale trials in patients to assess efficacy and dosage Long-term toxicology studies	Large-scale controlled clinical trials	Submission of full date and review by regulatory agencies	Postmarketing surveillance

←—2–5 years—→ ←—1.5 years—→ ←———————5–7 years———————→ ←—1–2 years—→

~100 projects → 20 compounds → 10 → 5 → 2 → 1.2 → 1

| Drug candidate | Development compound | | | Regulatory submission | Drug approved for marketing |

Fig. 60.1 The stages of development of a 'typical' new drug, i.e. a synthetic compound being developed for systemic use. Only the main activities undertaken at each stage are shown, and the details vary greatly according to the kind of drug being developed.

LEAD FINDING

When the biochemical target has been decided and the feasibility of the project has been assessed, the next step is to find *lead compounds*. Commonly this involves cloning of the target protein – normally the human form, because the sequence variation among species is often associated with pharmacological differences, and it is essential to optimise for activity in humans. An assay system must then be developed, allowing the functional activity of the target protein to be measured. This could be a cell-free enzyme assay, a membrane-based binding assay or a cellular response assay. It must be engineered to run automatically, if possible with an optical read-out (e.g. fluorescence or optical absorbance), and in a miniaturised multiwell plate format for reasons of speed and economy. Robotically controlled assay facilities capable of testing tens of thousands of compounds per day in several parallel assays are now commonplace in the pharmaceutical industry, and have become the standard starting point for most drug discovery projects. For details on high-throughput screening, see Hüser (2006).

To keep such hungry monsters running requires very large compound libraries. Large companies will typically maintain a growing collection of a million or more synthetic compounds, which will be routinely screened whenever a new assay is set up. Whereas, in the past, compounds were generally synthesised and purified one by one, often taking a week or more for each, the use of combinatorial chemistry allows large families of related compounds to be made simultaneously. By coupling such high-speed chemistry to high-throughput assay systems, the time taken over the initial lead-finding stage of projects has been reduced to a few months in most cases, having previously often taken several years. Increasingly, use is being made of X-ray crystallography and other techniques to provide knowledge of the three-dimensional structure

of the target protein and computer-based molecular modelling to generate possible lead structures within the compound library, in order to reduce the number of compounds to be screened. Refined in this way, screening is often successful in identifying lead compounds that have the appropriate pharmacological activity and are amenable to further chemical modification.

'Hits' detected in the initial screen often turn out to be molecules that have features undesirable in a drug, such as too high a molecular weight, excessive polarity and possession of groups known to be associated with toxicity. Computational 'prescreening' of compound libraries is often used to eliminate such compounds.

The hits identified from the primary screen are used as the basis for preparing sets of homologues by combinatorial chemistry so as to establish the critical structural features necessary for binding selectively to the target. Several such iterative cycles of synthesis and screening are usually needed to identify one or more lead compounds for the next stage.

Natural products as lead compounds

Historically, natural products, derived mainly from fungal and plant sources, have proved to be a fruitful source of new therapeutic agents, particularly in the field of anti-infective, anticancer and immunosuppressant drugs. Familiar examples include **penicillin**, **streptomycin** and many other antibiotics; vinca alkaloids; **paclitaxel**; **ciclosporin**; and **sirolimus** (**rapamycin**). These substances presumably serve a specific protective function, having evolved to recognise with great precision vulnerable target molecules in an organism's enemies or competitors. The surface of this resource has barely been scratched, and many companies are actively engaged in generating and testing natural product libraries for lead-finding purposes. Fungi and other microorganisms are particularly suitable for this, because they are ubiquitous, highly diverse and easy to collect and grow in the laboratory. Compounds obtained from plants, animals or marine organisms are much more troublesome to produce commercially. The main disadvantage of natural products as lead compounds is that they are often complex molecules that are difficult to synthesise or modify by conventional synthetic chemistry, so that lead optimisation may be difficult and commercial production very expensive.

LEAD OPTIMISATION

Lead compounds found by random screening are the basis for the next stage, lead optimisation, where the aim (usually) is to increase the potency of the compound on its target and to optimise it with respect to other characteristics, such as selectivity and pharmacokinetic properties. In this phase, the tests applied include a broader range of assays on different test systems, including studies to measure the activity and time course of the compounds *in vivo* (where possible in animal models mimicking aspects of the clinical condition; see Ch. 7), and checking for unwanted effects in animals, evidence of genotoxicity and usually for oral absorption. The objective of the lead optimisation phase is to identify one or more *drug candidates* suitable for further development.

As shown in Figure 60.1, only about one project in five succeeds in generating a drug candidate, and it can take up to 5 years. The most common problem is that lead optimisation proves to be impossible; despite much ingenious and back-breaking chemistry, the lead compounds, like antisocial teenagers, refuse to give up their bad habits. In other cases, the compounds, although they produce the desired effects on the target molecule and have no other obvious defects, fail to produce the expected effects in animal models of the disease, implying that the target is probably not a good one. The virtuous minority proceed to the next phase, preclinical development.

PRECLINICAL DEVELOPMENT

The aim of preclinical development is to satisfy all the requirements that have to be met before a new compound is deemed ready to be tested for the first time in humans. The work falls into four main categories:

1. Pharmacological testing to check that the drug does not produce any obviously hazardous acute effects, such as bronchoconstriction, cardiac dysrhythmias, blood pressure changes and ataxia. This is termed *safety pharmacology*.
2. Preliminary toxicological testing to eliminate genotoxicity and to determine the maximum non-toxic dose of the drug (usually when given daily for 28 days, and tested in two species). As well as being checked regularly for weight loss and other gross changes, the animals so treated are examined minutely *post mortem* at the end of the experiment to look for histological and biochemical evidence of tissue damage (see also Ch. 57).
3. Pharmacokinetic testing, including studies on the absorption, metabolism, distribution and elimination (ADME studies) in the species of laboratory animals used for toxicology testing, so as to link the pharmacological and toxicological effects to plasma concentration and drug exposure.
4. Chemical and pharmaceutical development to assess the feasibility of large-scale synthesis and purification, to assess the stability of the compound under various conditions and to develop a formulation suitable for clinical studies.

Much of the work of preclinical development, especially that relating to safety issues, is done under a formal operating code, known as *Good Laboratory Practice* (GLP), which covers such aspects as record-keeping procedures, data analysis, instrument calibration and staff training. The aim of GLP is to eliminate human error as far as possible, and to ensure the reliability of the data submitted to the regulatory authority, and laboratories are regularly monitored for compliance to GLP standards. The strict discipline involved in working to this code is generally ill-suited to the creative research needed in the earlier stages of drug discovery, so GLP standards are not usually adopted until projects get beyond the discovery phase.

Roughly half the compounds identified as drug candidates fail during the preclinical development phase; for the rest, a detailed dossier (the 'investigator brochure') is prepared for submission alongside specific study protocols to the regulatory authority such as the European Medicines Evaluation Agency or the US Food and Drugs Administration, whose permission is required to proceed with studies in humans. This is not lightly given, and the regulatory authority may refuse permission or require further work to be done before giving approval.

Non-clinical development work continues throughout the clinical trials period, when much more data, particularly in relation to long-term and reproductive toxicity in animals, has to be generated. Failure of a compound at this stage is very costly, and considerable efforts are made to eliminate potentially toxic compounds much earlier in the drug discovery process by the use of *in vitro*, or even *in silico*, methods.

CLINICAL DEVELOPMENT

Clinical development proceeds through four distinct but overlapping phases of clinical trials (see Ch. 7). For detailed information, see Friedman et al. (2010).

- *Phase I studies* are performed on a small group (normally 20–80) of volunteers – often healthy young men but sometimes patients, and their aim is to check for signs of any potentially *dangerous effects*, for example on cardiovascular,[2] respiratory, hepatic or renal function; *tolerability* (does the drug produce any unpleasant symptoms, for example headache, nausea, drowsiness?); and *pharmacokinetic properties* (is the drug well absorbed? Is absorption affected by food? What is the time course of the plasma concentration? Is there evidence of cumulation or non-linear kinetics?). Phase I studies may also test for pharmacodynamic effects in volunteers, sometimes called 'proof-of-concept' studies (e.g. does a novel analgesic compound block experimentally induced pain in humans? How does the effect vary with dose?).
- *Phase II studies* are performed on groups of patients (normally 100–300) and are designed to determine pharmacodynamic effect in patients, and if this is confirmed, to establish the dose regimen to be used in the definitive phase III study. Often, such studies

---

[2]QT prolongation, a sign of potentially dangerous cardiac arrhythmias (see Ch. 21), is a common cause of failure in early development, and regulators demand extensive – and expensive – studies to test for this risk.

will cover several distinct clinical disorders (e.g. depression, anxiety states and phobias) to identify the possible therapeutic indications for the new compound and the dose required. When new drug targets are being studied, it is not until these phase II trials are completed that the team finds out whether or not its initial hypothesis was correct, and lack of the expected effect is a common reason for failure.

- *Phase III studies* are the definitive double-blind, randomised trials, commonly performed as multicentre trials on thousands of patients, aimed at comparing the new drug with commonly used alternatives. These are extremely costly, difficult to organise and often take years to complete, particularly if the treatment is designed to retard the progression of a chronic disease. It is not uncommon for a drug that seemed highly effective in the limited patient groups tested in phase II to look much less impressive under the more rigorous conditions of phase III trials.

▼ The conduct of trials has to comply with an elaborate code known as Good Clinical Practice, covering every detail of the patient group, data collection methods, recording of information, statistical analysis and documentation.[3]

Increasingly, phase III trials are being required to include a *pharmacoeconomic analysis* (see Ch. 1), such that not only clinical but also economic benefits of the new treatment are assessed.

At the end of phase III, the drug will be submitted to the relevant regulatory authority for licensing. The dossier required for this is a massive and detailed compilation of preclinical and clinical data. Evaluation by the regulatory authority normally takes a year or more, and further delays often arise when aspects of the submission have to be clarified or more data are required. Eventually, about two-thirds of submissions gain marketing approval. Overall, only 11.5% of compounds entering Phase I are eventually approved (see Munos, 2009). Increasing this proportion by better compound selection at the laboratory stage is one of the main challenges for the pharmaceutical industry.

- *Phase IV studies* comprise the obligatory postmarketing surveillance designed to detect any rare or long term adverse effects resulting from the use of the drug in a clinical setting in many thousands of patients. Such events may necessitate limiting the use of the drug to particular patient groups, or even withdrawal of the drug.[4]

BIOPHARMACEUTICALS

'Biopharmaceuticals', i.e. therapeutic agents produced by biotechnology rather than conventional synthetic chemistry, are discussed in Chapter 59. Such therapeutic agents comprise an increasing proportion – currently about 30% – of new products registered each year. The principles underlying the development and testing of biopharmaceuticals are basically the same as for synthetic drugs. In practice, biopharmaceuticals generally run into fewer toxicological problems than synthetic drugs,[5] but more

problems relating to production, quality control, immunogenicity and drug delivery. Walsh (2003) covers this specialised field in more detail.

COMMERCIAL ASPECTS

Figure 60.1 shows the approximate time taken for such a project and the attrition rate (at each stage and overall) based on recent data from several large pharmaceutical companies. The key messages are (i) that it is a high-risk business, with only about one drug discovery project in 50 reaching its goal of putting a new drug on the market, (ii) that it takes a long time – about 12 years on average and (iii) that it costs a lot of money to develop one drug (estimated at a mind-boggling $3.9 billion in 2008, see Munos, 2009).[6] For any one project, the costs escalate rapidly as development proceeds, phase III trials and long-term toxicology studies being particularly expensive. The time factor is crucial, because the new drug has to be patented, usually at the end of the discovery phase, and the period of exclusivity (20 years in most countries) during which the company is free from competition in the market starts on that date. After 20 years, the patent expires, and other companies, which have not supported the development costs, are free to make and sell the drug much more cheaply, so the revenues for the original company decrease rapidly thereafter. Many profitable drugs have come or are coming to the end of their patents between 2010 and 2015, adding to the industry's problems. Reducing the development time after patenting is a major concern for all companies, but so far it has remained stubbornly fixed at around 10 years, partly because the regulatory authorities are demanding more clinical data before they will grant a licence. In practice, only about one drug in three that goes on the market brings in enough revenue to cover its development costs. Success for the company relies on this one drug generating enough profit to pay for the rest.[7]

FUTURE PROSPECTS

Since about 1990, the drug discovery process has been in the throes of a substantial methodological revolution, following the rapid ascendancy of molecular biology, genomics and informatics, amid high expectations that this would bring remarkable dividends in terms of speed, cost and success rate. High-throughput screening has undoubtedly emerged as a powerful lead-finding technology, but overall the benefits are not yet clear: costs have risen steadily, the success rate has not improved (Fig. 60.2) and development times have not decreased.

Figure 60.2 illustrates the trend in the number of new drugs launched in the major markets worldwide, which has declined despite escalating costs and improved technology. There has been much speculation as to the causes, the optimistic view (see below) being that fewer but better

---

[3]Similar strict codes must be followed in laboratory tests to determine safety (Good Laboratory Practice; see text) and drug manufacture (Good Manufacturing Practice).
[4]Recent high-profile cases include the withdrawal of rofecoxib (a cyclo-oxygenase-2 inhibitor; see Ch. 26) when it was found (in a Phase III trial for a new indication) to increase the frequency of heart attacks, and of cerivastatin (Ch. 23), a cholesterol-lowering drug found to cause severe muscle damage in a few patients.

[5]The serious toxicity caused to human volunteers in the 2006 phase I trials of the monoclonal antibody TGN 1412 (see Ch. 59) showed that this could not be relied on, and has led to substantial tightening of standards (and slowdown of the development of biopharmaceuticals).
[6]These cost estimates have been strongly challenged by commentators (see Angell, 2004) who argue that the pharmaceutical companies overestimate their costs several-fold in order to justify high drug prices.
[7]Actually, companies spend about twice as much on marketing and administration as on research and development.

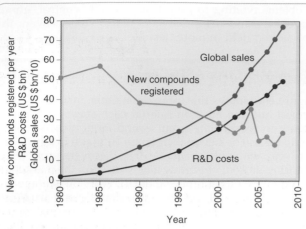

Fig. 60.2 Research and development (R&D) spend, sales and new drug registrations, 1980–2009. Registrations refer to new chemical entities (including biopharmaceuticals, excluding new formulations and combinations of existing registered compounds). The decline in registrations up to 2009 has since been halted (32 in 2012). *(Data from various sources, including the Centre for Medicines Research, Pharmaceutical Research and Manufacturers Association of America.)*

drugs are being introduced, and that the genomics revolution has yet to make its impact.

If the new drugs that are being developed improve the quality of medical care, there is room for optimism. In recent ('pre-revolutionary') years, synthetic drugs aimed at new targets (e.g. selective serotonin reuptake inhibitors, statins, kinase inhibitors and several monoclonal antibodies) have made major contributions to patient care. Even if the new technologies do not improve productivity, we can reasonably expect that their ability to make new targets available to the drug discovery machine will have a real effect on patient care. The decline in annual registrations between 1980 and 2000 (Fig. 60.2) has stabilised in the last decade, and even shows signs of an upturn more recently. Creativity remains high, despite the rising costs and declining profits that are a challenge to the pharmaceutical industry.

Trends to watch include the growing armoury of biopharmaceuticals, particularly monoclonal antibodies such as **trastuzumab** (an antibody directed against human epidermal growth factor receptor-2 – HER2 – which is used to treat breast cancers that overexpress this receptor) and **infliximab** (a tumour necrosis factor antibody used to treat inflammatory disorders; see Ch. 26); these are successful recent examples, and more are in the pipeline. Another likely change will be the use of genotyping to 'individualise' drug treatments, so as to reduce the likelihood of administering drugs to 'non-responders' (see Ch. 11, which summarises the current status of 'personalised medicine'). The implications for drug discovery will be profound, for the resulting therapeutic compartmentation of the patient population will mean that markets will decrease, bringing to an end the reliance on the 'blockbusters' referred to earlier. At the same time, clinical trials will become more complex (and expensive), as different genotypic groups will have to be included in the trial design. The hope is that therapeutic efficacy will be improved, not that it will be a route to developing drugs more cheaply and quickly. However, there is general agreement that the current modus operandi is commercially unsustainable (see Munos, 2009). Costs and regulatory requirements are continuing to rise, and the anticipated use of genomics to define subgroups of patients likely to respond to particular therapeutic agents (see Ch. 11) will mean fragmentation of the market, as we move away from the 'one-drug-suits-all' approach that encouraged companies to focus their efforts on blockbuster drugs. More niche products targeted at smaller patient groups will be needed, though each costs as much to develop as a blockbuster and carries a similar risk of failure.

A FINAL WORD

The pharmaceutical industry in recent years has attracted much adverse publicity, some of it well deserved, concerning drug pricing and profits, non-disclosure of adverse clinical trials data, reluctance to address major global heath problems such as tuberculosis and malaria, aggressive marketing practices and much else (see Angell, 2004; Goldacre, 2012). It needs to be remembered though that, despite its faults, the industry has been responsible for most of the therapeutic advances of the past half-century, without which medical care would effectively have stood still.

REFERENCES AND FURTHER READING

Angell, M., 2004. The Truth about the Drug Companies. Random House, New York. (*A powerful broadside directed against the commercial practices of pharmaceutical companies*)

Betz, U.A.K., 2005. How many genomics targets can a portfolio afford? Drug Discov. Today 10, 1057–1063. (*Interesting analysis – despite its odd title – of approaches to target identification in drug discovery programmes*)

Evans, W.E., Relling, M.V., 2004. Moving towards individualised medicine with pharmacogenomics. Nature 429, 464–468. (*Good review article discussing the likely influence of pharmacogenomics on therapeutics*)

Friedman, L.M., Furberg, C.D., DeMets, D.L., 2010. Fundamentals of Clinical Trials, fourth ed. Mosby, St Louis. (*Standard textbook*)

Goldacre, B., 2012. Bad Pharma, Fourth Estate, London. (*An outspoken polemic, flawed in places, that exposes malpractice in the industry*)

Hill, R.G., Rang, H.P. (Eds.), 2013. Drug Discovery and Development, second ed. Elsevier, Amsterdam. (*Short textbook describing the principles and practice of drug discovery and development in the modern era*)

Hüser, J. (Ed.), 2006. High Throughput Screening in Drug Discovery. Vol. 35 of Methods and Principles in Drug Discovery. Wiley–VCH, Weinheim. (*Comprehensive textbook covering all aspects of this technology*)

Kramer, R., Cohen, D., 2004. Functional genomics to new drug targets. Nat. Rev. Drug Discov. 3, 965–972. (*Describes the various approaches for finding new drug targets, starting from genomic data*)

Lindsay, M.A., 2003. Target discovery. Nat. Rev. Drug Discov. 2, 831–836. (*Well-balanced discussion of the application of genomics approaches to discovering new drug targets; more realistic in its stance than many*)

Munos, B., 2009. Lessons from 60 years of pharmaceutical innovation. Nat. Rev. Drug Discov. 8, 959–968. (*Informative summary of the current status of the drug discovery industry, making clear that the modus operandi that has been successful in the past is no longer sustainable*)

Overington, J.P., Al-Lazikani, B., Hopkins, A.L., 2006. How many drug targets are there? Nat. Rev. Drug Discov. 5, 993–996. (*Thoughtful analysis, concluding that we don't know the answer, but there are probably plenty of new targets on which to base future drug discovery*)

Semizarov, D., Blomme, E., 2008. Genomics in Drug Discovery and Development. Wiley, New York.

Walsh, G., 2003. Biopharmaceuticals, second ed. Wiley, Chichester. (*Comprehensive textbook covering all aspects of discovery, development and applications of biopharmaceuticals*)

Appendix
Some important pharmacological agents

Students may feel overwhelmed by the number of drugs described in pharmacology textbooks. We would emphasise that it is more important to understand general pharmacological principles, and to appreciate the pharmacology of the main classes of drug, than to attempt to memorise details of individual agents. Specific drugs are best learned about when they are encountered in the setting of particular topics (e.g. noradrenergic transmission), during practical classes or (for therapeutic drugs) near a patient's bedside. We provide a list (www.studentconsult.com) of examples of some of the most important pharmacological agents. It is not intended as a starting point to learning pharmacology, and we would caution against attempting to memorise lists of names and properties. The important agents we list here were selected subjectively; they include (but are not limited to) the 100 drugs most likely to be prescribed by newly qualified doctors in the UK (Baker et al., 2011) and are divided into agents of primary and secondary importance. For students of some subjects, and in different geographical areas, one or another class of drug will have more or less importance (e.g. anthelmintics are very important for veterinarians and for all clinicians in regions where helminthiasis is common), so these categories are meant only as a broad guide. The list includes not only drugs used therapeutically, but also endogenous mediators/transmitters (med/trnsm) and certain important drugs used mainly as experimental tools (exp.tool) – especially important for students studying basic or applied pharmacology as a science subject – and drugs used for recreational (recreat) rather than therapeutic purposes. Some endogenous mediators (e.g. adrenaline [epinephrine]) are also important therapeutic drugs.

The General Medical Council's 'Tomorrow's Doctors' (2009) specifies that students should be able to demonstrate knowledge of drug actions; therapeutics and pharmacokinetics; drug side effects and interactions, including for multiple treatments, long-term conditions and non-prescribed medication; and also including effects of drugs on the population, such as the spread of antibiotic resistance. A working knowledge of drugs in the 'primary importance' category should be built up gradually as they are encountered during training. For drugs in the second category, it is usually sufficient to be aware of the mechanism of action, supplemented by understanding how they differ from those in the primary category when relevant.

The choice of drugs in clinical use is somewhat arbitrary. Hospital formulary committees (on which pharmacists play a crucial role) grapple with choosing which individual drugs to stock in the pharmacy. There is a play-off between stocking several individual drugs of one category, for each of which there is good evidence of efficacy for distinct indications, and stocking a more restricted choice based on indirect evidence that efficacy is likely to be a common feature of different members of a class of drugs. Local variations will be encountered (e.g. as to which angiotensin-converting enzyme inhibitor or non-steroidal anti-inflammatory drugs are stocked in the hospital pharmacy). If the student or clinician (e.g. doctor, dentist, veterinarian or nurse) comes to these (e.g. when changing to a job in a new hospital) with a sound appreciation of the general principles of pharmacology and of the specifics of the various classes of agent involved, he or she will be able to look up and understand the details of agents favoured locally and use them sensibly. Drugs are grouped broadly as in the chapters of the text, and some appear more than once in the lists.

REFERENCES

Baker, E.H., Pryce Roberts, A., Wilde, K., et al., 2011. Development of a core drug list towards improving prescribing education and reducing errors in the UK. Br. J. Clin. Pharmacol. 71, 190–198.

GMC (General Medical Council), 2009. Tomorrow's Doctors: Outcomes and standards for undergraduate medical education. Online: <www.gmc-uk.org/education/undergraduate/tomorrows doctors_2009.asp> (accessed July 2014).

KEY

(Note: designation does not exclude a separate therapeutic role – for example, nicotine and cocaine are used therapeutically as well as recreationally, adrenaline is used therapeutically as well as being a mediator; conversely, some primarily therapeutic drugs such as morphine or other opioid analgesics are used recreationally by some individuals.)

med/trnsm = mediator/transmitter
exp.tool = experimental tool
recreat = drug used especially for recreational purposes
antag = antagonist

This appendix was originally adapted from that in Dale, M.M., Dickenson, A.H., Haylett, D.G. 1996. Companion to Pharmacology, second ed. Churchill Livingstone, Edinburgh, with permission.

Index

Page numbers followed by 'f' indicate figures, 't' indicate tables, and 'b' indicate boxes.

731

733